James Fawcett

PROGRESS IN BRAIN RESEARCH

VOLUME 137

SPINAL CORD TRAUMA: REGENERATION, NEURAL REPAIR AND FUNCTIONAL RECOVERY

PROGRESS IN BRAIN RESEARCH

VOLUME 137

SPINAL CORD TRAUMA: REGENERATION, NEURAL REPAIR AND FUNCTIONAL RECOVERY

EDITED BY

L. MCKERRACHER

Centre for Research in Neurological Sciences, Department of Pathology and Cellular Biology, Faculty of Medicine, Université de Montréal, 2900 Édouard-Montpetit, Montreal, QC H3T 1J8, Canada

G. DOUCET

Centre for Research in Neurological Sciences, Department of Pathology and Cellular Biology, Faculty of Medicine, Université de Montréal, 2900 Édouard-Montpetit, Montreal, QC H3T 1J8, Canada

S. ROSSIGNOL

Centre for Research in Neurological Sciences, Department of Physiology, Faculty of Medicine, Université de Montréal, 2900 Édouard-Montpetit, Montreal, QC H3T 1J8, Canada

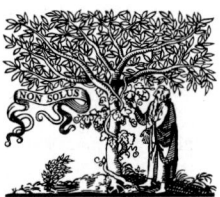

ELSEVIER
AMSTERDAM – BOSTON – LONDON – NEW YORK – OXFORD – PARIS – SAN DIEGO
SAN FRANCISCO – SINGAPORE – SYDNEY – TOKYO
2002

ELSEVIER SCIENCE B.V.
Sara Burgerhartstraat 25
P.O. Box 211, 1000 AE Amsterdam, The Netherlands

First edition 2002

Library of Congress Cataloging-in-Publication Data
Spinal cord trauma : neural repair and functional recovery / edited by L. McKerracher,
G. Doucet, S. Rossignol.
      p. cm. -- (Progress in brain research ; v. 137)
   Includes index.
   1. Spinal cord--Wounds and injuries--Congresses. 2. Spinal
cord--Regeneration--Congresses. I. McKerracher, L. (Lisa) II. Doucet, G. (Guy) III.
Rossignol, Serge, 1942- IV. Series.
   QP376 .P7 vol. 137
   [RD594.3]
   617.4'82044--dc21   2002070256

British Library Cataloguing in Publication Data
Spinal cord trauma : neural repair and functional recovery.
 - (Progress in brain research ; v. 137)
 1.Spinal cord - Wounds and injuries 2.Spinal cord - Wounds
and injuries - Treatment
 I.McKerracher, L. II.Doucet, G. III. Rossignol, Serge, 1942-
 617.4'82044

ISBN: 0-444-50817-1 (volume)
ISBN: 0-444-80104-9 (series)
ISSN: 0079-6123

⊗   The paper used in this publication meets the requirements of ANSI/NISO Z39.48-1992 (Permanence of Paper).
Printed in The Netherlands.

List of Contributors

Y. Adamchik, Toronto Western Research Institute, Room 12-413, 399 Bathurst Street, Toronto, ON M5T 2S8, Canada

M. Antri, Neurobiologie des Signaux Intercellulaires – CNRS UMR 7101, Institut de Biologie Intégrative (IFR 83), Université Pierre et Marie Curie, 7 Quai Saint Bernard – Boite 002, F-75252 Paris, France

R.A. Asher, Cambridge University Centre for Brain Repair, The E.D. Adrian Building, Forvie Site, Robinson Way, Cambridge CB2 2PY, UK

M. Avilés-Trigueros, Instituto de Bioingenieria, Universidad Miguel Hernández, 03550 San Juan (Alicante), Spain

H. Barbeau, Jewish Rehabilitation Hospital Research Center, 3205 Place Alton Goldbloom, Laval, Montreal, QC H7V 1R2, Canada

H. Barbeau, Centre de Recherche en Sciences Neurologiques, Faculté de Médecine, Université de Montréal, Pavillon Paul-G.-Desmarais, C.P. 6128, Succursale Centre-ville, Montreal, QC H3C 3J7, Canada

J.-Y. Barthe, Neurobiologie des Signaux Intercellulaires – CNRS UMR 7101, Institut de Biologie Intégrative (IFR 83), Université Pierre et Marie Curie, 7 Quai Saint Bernard – Boite 002, F-75252 Paris, France

D. Barthélemy, Centre de Recherche en Sciences Neurologiques, Faculté de Médecine, Université de Montréal, Pavillon Paul-G.-Desmarais, C.P. 6128, Succursale Centre-ville, Montreal, QC H3C 3J7, Canada

M.S. Beattie, Department of Neuroscience, Ohio State University Medical Center, 333 W. 10th Avenue, Columbus, OH 43210, USA

M. Bélanger, Dept. Kinanthropologie, Université du Québec à Montréal, C.P. 8888, Succursale Centre-ville, Montreal, QC H3C 3P8, Canada

G.J. Bell, Faculty of Physical Education, University of Alberta, 513 HMRC, Edmonton, AB T6G 2S2, Canada

L.I. Benowitz, Children's Hospital, Laboratories for Neuroscience Research in Neurosurgery and, Harvard Medical School, Department of Surgery, 300 Longwood Avenue, Boston, MA 02115, USA

A. Blesch, Department of Neurosciences-0626, University of California, San Diego, 9500 Gilman Drive, La Jolla, CA 92093-0626, USA

D.C. Bolser, Department of Physiological Sciences, University of Florida, College of Veterinary Medicine, P.O. Box 10144, Gainesville, FL 32610-0144, USA

L. Bouyer, Centre de Recherche en Sciences Neurologiques, Faculté de Médecine, Université de Montréal, Pavillon Paul-G.-Desmarais, C.P. 6128, Succursale Centre-ville, Montreal, QC H3C 3J7, Canada

B.S. Bregman, Georgetown University Medical Center, Department of Neuroscience, 3970 Reservoir Road NW, Washington, DC 20007, USA

J.C. Bresnahan, Department of Neuroscience, Ohio State University Medical Center, 333 W. 10th Avenue, Columbus, OH 43210, USA

E. Brustein, Centre de Recherche en Sciences Neurologiques, Faculté de Médecine, Université de Montréal, Pavillon Paul-G.-Desmarais, C.P. 6128, Succursale Centre-ville, Montreal, QC H3C 3J7, Canada

M.B. Bunge, The Miami Project to Cure Paralysis, University of Miami School of Medicine, The Lois Pope LIFE Center, P.O. Box 016960 (R-48), Miami, FL 33101, USA

D. Cai, Biology Department, Hunter College, City University of New York, 695 Park Avenue, New York, NY 10021, USA

P.L. Carlen, Toronto Western Research Institute, Room 12-413, 399 Bathurst Street, Toronto, ON M5T 2S8, Canada

C. Chau, Centre de Recherche en Sciences Neurologiques, Faculté de Médecine, Université de Montréal, Pavillon Paul-G.-Desmarais, C.P. 6128, Succursale Centre-ville, Montreal, QC H3C 3J7, Canada

S.-L. Chong, Centre for Neuroscience, University of Alberta, 513 HMRC, Edmonton, AB T6G 2S2, Canada

J.-V. Coumans, Georgetown University Medical Center, Department of Neuroscience, 3970 Reservoir Road NW, Washington, DC 20007, USA

H.-N. Dai, Georgetown University Medical Center, Department of Neuroscience, 3970 Reservoir Road NW, Washington, DC 20007, USA

S. David, Centre for Research in Neuroscience, Montreal General Hospital Research Institute, 1650 Cedar Avenue, Montreal, QC H3G 1A4, Canada

R.D. de Leon, Department of Physiological Sciences, University of California, Los Angeles, 1804 Life Sciences, 621 Charles E. Young Drive South, Los Angeles, CA 90095-1527, USA

G.A. Dekaban, BioTherapeutics Research Group, Robarts Research Institute, 100 Perth Drive, P.O. Box 5015, London, ON N6A 5K8, Canada

P. Dergham, Department of Pathology and Cell Biology, and Centre de Recherche en Sciences Neurologiques, Université de Montréal, Montreal, QC H3T 1J4, Canada

G. Doucet, Department of Pathology and Cell Biology, Université de Montréal, C.P. 6128, Succursale Centre-ville, Montreal, QC H3C 3J7, Canada

C. Dubreuil, Department of Pathology and Cell Biology, and Centre de Recherche en Sciences Neurologiques, Université de Montréal, Montreal, QC H3T 1J4, Canada

V.R. Edgerton, Department of Physiological Sciences, University of California, Los Angeles, 1804 Life Sciences, 621 Charles E. Young Drive South, Los Angeles, CA 90095-1527, USA

B. Ellezam, Department of Pathology and Cell Biology, and Centre de Recherche en Sciences Neurologiques, Université de Montréal, Montreal, QC H3T 1J4, Canada

J.W. Fawcett, Cambridge University Centre for Brain Repair, The E.D. Adrian Building, Forvie Site, Robinson Way, Cambridge, CB2 2PY, UK

M.G. Fehlings, Toronto Western Hospital Research Institute, McLaughlin Pavilion 2-417, 399 Bathurst Street, Toronto, ON M5T 2S8, Canada

D. Feraboli-Lohnherr, Neurobiologie des Signaux Intercellulaires – CNRS UMR 7101, Institut de Biologie Intégrative (IFR 83), Université Pierre et Marie Curie, 7 Quai Saint Bernard – Boite 002, F-75252 Paris, France

M.T. Filbin, Biology Department, Hunter College, City University of New York, 695 Park Avenue, New York, NY 10021, USA

A.E. Fournier, Department of Neurology and Section of Neurobiology, Yale University School of Medicine, P.O. Box 208018, New Haven, CT 06510, USA

M. Frantseva, Toronto Western Research Institute, Room 12-413, 399 Bathurst Street, Toronto, ON M5T 2X8, Canada

J. Fung, The Jewish Rehabilitation Hospital Research Center, 3205 Place Alton Goldbloom, Laval, Montreal, QC H7V 1R2, Canada

M. Gaviria, INSERM U 336, Université Montpellier II, B.P. 106, Place E. Bataillon, 34095 Montpellier, Cedex 05, France

M. Giménez y Ribotta, INSERM U 336, Université Montpellier II, B.P. 106, Place E. Bataillon, 34095 Montpellier, France

N. Giroux, Centre de Recherche en Sciences Neurologiques, Faculté de Médecine, Université de Montréal, Pavillon Paul-G.-Desmarais, C.P. 6128, Succursale Centre-ville, Montreal, QC H3C 3J7, Canada

D. Goldberg, Children's Hospital, Laboratories for Neuroscience Research in Neurosurgery, 300 Longwood Avenue, Boston, MA 02115, USA

F.J. Golder, Department of Physiological Sciences, University of Florida, College of Veterinary Medicine, P.O. Box 10144, Gainesville, FL 32610-0144, USA

G. Gould, Department of Neurology and Section of Neurobiology, Yale University School of Medicine, P.O. Box 208018, New Haven, CT 06510, USA

T. GrandPré, Department of Neurology and Section of Neurobiology, Yale University School of Medicine, P.O. Box 208018, New Haven, CT 06510, USA

S. Grillner, Nobel Institute for Neurophysiology, Department of Neuroscience, The Retzius Laboratory, Karolinska Institutet, SE-17177, Sweden

B. Grimpe, Case Western Reserve University, Dept of Neurosciences, 10900 Euclid Avenue, Cleveland, OH 44106, USA

D. Gris, BioTherapeutics Research Group, Robarts Research Institute, 100 Perth Drive, P.O. Box 5015, London, ON N6A 5K8, Canada

E. Hauben, Department of Neurobiology, The Weizmann Institute of Science, 76100 Rehovot, Israel

G.E. Hermann, Department of Neuroscience, Ohio State University Medical Center, 333 W. 10th Avenue, Columbus, OH 43210, USA

P.J. Horner, Department of Neurological Surgery, University of Washington, Harborview Medical Center, 325 Ninth Avenue, Box 359655, Seattle, WA 98104-2499, USA

M.J. Howard, Center for the Study of Nervous System Injury, Spinal Cord Injury Restorative Treatment and Research Program, and Department of Neurology, Washington University School of Medicine, Campus Box 8111, 660 S. Euclid Avenue, St. Louis MO 63110, USA

C.H. Hubscher, Department Anatomical Sciences and Neurobiology, University of Louisville, School of Medicine, Louisville, KY 40292, USA

N. Irwin, Children's Hospital, Laboratories for Neuroscience Research in Neurosurgery and, Harvard Medical School, Department of Surgery, 300 Longwood Avenue, Boston, MA 02115, USA

K.B. James, Centre for Neuroscience, University of Alberta, 513 HMRC, Edmonton, AB T6G 2S2, Canada

R.D. Johnson, Department of Physiological Sciences, University of Florida, College of Veterinary Medicine, P.O. Box 10144, Gainesville, FL 32610-0144, USA

L.M. Jordan, Department of Physiology, The University of Manitoba, Winnipeg, MB R3E 3J7, Canada

T.E. Kennedy, Centre for Neuronal Survival, Montreal Neurological Institute, McGill University, 3801 University Street, Montreal, QC H3A 2B4, Canada

A. Kido, Centre for Neuroscience, University of Alberta, 513 HMRC, Edmonton, AB T6G 2S2, Canada

P.L. Kuhn, Georgetown University Medical Center, Department of Neuroscience, 3970 Reservoir Road NW, Washington, DC 20007, USA

M. Ladouceur, Department of Physical Education, Brock University, 500 Glenridge Avenue, St. Catharine's, ON L2S 3A1, Canada

C. Langlet, Centre de Recherche en Sciences Neurologiques, Faculté de Médecine, Université de Montréal, Pavillon Paul-G.-Desmarais, C.P. 6128, Succursale Centre-ville, Montreal, QC H3C 3J7, Canada

H. Leblond, Centre de Recherche en Sciences Neurologiques, Faculté de Médecine, Université de Montréal, Pavillon Paul-G.-Desmarais, C.P. 6128, Succursale Centre-ville, Montreal, QC H3C 3J7, Canada

A. Leroux, Department of Physical Education, Concordia University, 1455 Boulevard de Maisonneuve O., Montreal, QC H4B 1R6, Canada

A.C. Lipson, Department of Neurological Surgery, University of Washington, Harborview Medical Center, 325 Ninth Avenue, Box 359655, Seattle, WA 98104-2499, USA

N.J. London, Department of Physiological Sciences, University of California, Los Angeles, 1804 Life Sciences, 621 Charles E. Young Drive South, Los Angeles, CA 90095-1527, USA

L. Loy, Department of Pathology and Cell Biology, and Centre de Recherche en Sciences Neurologiques, Université de Montréal, Montreal, QC H3T 1J4, Canada

R.D. Lund, Moran Eye Center, Health Science Center, University of Utah, 50 North Medical Drive, Salt Lake City, UT 84132, USA

J. Lynskey, Georgetown University Medical Center, Department of Neuroscience, 3970 Reservoir Road NW, Washington, DC 20007, USA

C. Manitt, Centre for Neuronal Survival, Montreal Neurological Institute, McGill University, 3801 University Street, Montreal, QC H3A 2B4, Canada

J. Marcoux, Centre de Recherche en Sciences Neurologiques, Faculté de Médecine, Université de Montréal, Pavillon Paul-G.-Desmarais, C.P. 6128, Succursale Centre-ville, Montreal, QC H3C 3J7, Canada

D.R. Marsh, BioTherapeutics Research Group, Robarts Research Institute, 100 Perth Drive, P.O. Box 5015, London, ON N6A 5K8, Canada

M. McAtee, Georgetown University Medical Center, Department of Neuroscience, 3970 Reservoir Road NW, Washington, DC 20007, USA

J.W. McDonald, Center for the Study of Nervous System Injury, Spinal Cord Injury Restorative Treatment and Research Program, and Department of Neurology, Washington University School of Medicine, Campus Box 8111, 660 S. Euclid Avenue, St. Louis MO 63110, USA

L. McKerracher, Department of Pathology and Cell Biology, and Centre de Recherche en Sciences Neurologiques, Université de Montréal, Montreal, QC H3T 1J4, Canada

S.O. Meakin, Cell Signalling Group, Robarts Research Institute, 100 Perth Drive, P.O. Box 5015, London, ON N6A 5K8, Canada

V. Menet, INSERM U 336, Université Montpellier II, B.P. 106, Place E. Bataillon, 34095 Montpellier, Cedex 05, France

D.A. Morgenstern, Cambridge University Centre for Brain Repair, The E.D. Adrian Building, Forvie Site, Robinson Way, Cambridge, CB2 2PY, UK

V. Mushahwar, Centre for Neuroscience, 507 HMRC, University of Alberta, Edmonton, AB T6G 2S2, Canada

D. Orsal, Neurobiologie des Signaux Intercellulaires – CNRS UMR 7101, Institut de Biologie Intégrative (IFR 83), Université Pierre et Marie Curie, 7 Quai Saint Bernard – Boite 002, F-75252 Paris, France

J.L. Perez Velazquez, Hospital for Sick Children, Department of Neurology, 555 University Avenue, Toronto, ON M5T 1X8, Canada

A. Petit, Department of Pathology and Cell Biology, Université de Montréal, C.P. 6128, Succursale Centre-ville, Montreal, QC H3C 3J7, Canada

A. Privat, INSERM U 336, Université Montpellier II, B.P. 106, Place E. Bataillon, 34095 Montpellier, Cedex 05, France

A. Prochazka, Centre for Neuroscience, 507 HMRC, University of Alberta, Edmonton, AB T6G 2S2, Canada

J. Provencher, Centre de Recherche en Sciences Neurologiques, Faculté de Médecine, Université de Montréal, Pavillon Paul-G.-Desmarais, C.P. 6128, Succursale Centre-ville, Montreal, QC H3C 3J7, Canada

J. Qiu, Biology Department, Hunter College, City University of New York, 695 Park Avenue, New York, NY 10021, USA

R.M. Quencer, Department of Radiology, University of Miami, School of Medicine, Miami, FL 33101, USA

T.A. Reader, Centre de Recherche en Sciences Neurologiques, Faculté de Médecine, Université de Montréal, Pavillon Paul-G.-Desmarais, C.P. 6128, Succursale Centre-ville, Montreal, QC H3C 3J7, Canada

P.J. Reier, McKnight Brain Institute of the University of Florida, Department of Neuro-science, Box 100244, Gainesville, FL 32610-0244, USA

D.J. Reinkensmeyer, Department of Mechanical and Aerospace Engineering, University of California, Irvine, CA 92697, USA

R.C. Rogers, Department of Neuroscience, Ohio State University Medical Center, 333 W. 10th Avenue, Columbus, OH 43210, USA

S. Rossignol, Centre de Recherche en Sciences Neurologiques, Faculté de Médecine, Université de Montréal, Pavillon Paul-G.-Desmarais, C.P. 6128, Succursale Centre-ville, Montreal, QC H3C 3J7, Canada

R.R. Roy, Brain Research Institute, University of California, Los Angeles, 621 Charles E. Young Drive South, Los Angeles, CA 90095-1527, USA

F. Sandhu, Georgetown University Medical Center, Department of Neuroscience, 3970 Reservoir Road NW, Washington, DC 20007, USA

Y. Sauvé, Moran Eye Center, Health Science Center, University of Utah, 50 North Medical Drive, Salt Lake City, UT 84132, USA

B.J. Schmidt, Department of Internal Medicine, The University of Manitoba, Winnipeg, MB R3E 3J7, Canada

G.W. Schrimsher, Department of Psychology, University of Houston, 4800 Calhoun, Houston, TX 77204, USA

M.E. Schwab, Department of Neuromorphology, Brain Research Institute, University of Zurich and Swiss Federal Institute of Technology, Winterthurerstr. 190, 8057 Zurich, Switzerland

G. Schwartz, Toronto Western Hospital Research Institute, McLaughlin Pavilion 2-417, 399 Bathurst Street, Toronto, ON MST 2S8, Canada

M. Schwartz, Department of Neurobiology, The Weizmann Institute of Science, 76100 Rehovot, Israel

I. Sellés-Navarro, Laboratorio de Oftalmologia Experimental, Facultad de Medicina, Universidad de Murcia, Murcia, H3T 1J4, Spain

S.J. Shefchyk, Department of Physiology, University of Manitoba, Winnipeg, MB R3E 3J7, Canada

J. Silver, Case Western University, School of Medicine, Department of Neurosciences, 10900 Euclid Avenue, Cleveland, OH 44106, USA

R.B. Stein, Centre for Neuroscience, 513 HMRC, University of Alberta, Edmonton, AB T6G 2S2, Canada

S.M. Strittmatter, Department of Neurology and Section of Neurobiology, Yale University School of Medicine, P.O. Box 208018, New Haven, CT 06510, USA

W.K. Timoszyk, Department of Mechanical and Aerospace Engineering, University of California, Irvine, Irvine, CA 92697, USA

A. Tonkikh, Toronto Western Research Institute, Room 12-413, 399 Bathurst Street, Toronto, ON M5T 2S8, Canada

L.A. Tubman, Faculty of Kinesiology, University of Calgary, Calgary, AB, Canada

M.H. Tuszynski, Department of Neuroscience-0626, University of California, San Diego, 9500 Gilman Drive, La Jolla, CA 92093-0626, USA

M.J. Velardo, McKnight Brain Institute of the University of Florida, Department of Neuroscience, Box 100244, Gainesville, FL 32610-0244, USA

M. Vidal-Sanz, Laboratorio de Oftalmologia Experimental, Universidad de Murcia, 30100 Murcia, Spain

X. Wang, Department of Neurology and Section of Neurobiology, Yale University School of Medicine, P.O. Box 208018, New Haven, CT 06510, USA

L.C. Weaver, BioTherapeutics Research Group, Robarts Research Institute, 100 Perth Drive, P.O. Box 5015, London, ON N6A 5K8, Canada

S.J.O. Whiteley, Department of Psychology, University of Sheffield, Sheffield, S10 2TP, UK

M. Winton, Department of Pathology and Cell Biology, and Centre de Recherche en Sciences Neurologiques, Université de Montréal, Montreal, QC H3T 1J4, Canada

S. Yakovenko, Centre for Neuroscience, 507 HMRC, University of Alberta, Edmonton, AB T6G 2S2, Canada

A. Yakovleff, Neurobiologie des Signaux Intercellulaires – CNRS UMR 7101, Institut de Biologie Intégrative (IFR 83), Université Pierre et Marie Curie, 7 Quai Saint Bernard – Boite 002, F-75252 Paris, France

W. Young, W.M. Keck Center for Collaborative Neuroscience, Rutgers, State University of New Jersey, 604 Allison Road, Piscataway, NJ 08854-8082, USA

Foreword by Christopher Reeve

Spinal cord research is a relatively new field of endeavor because of the age-old dogma that the spinal cord cannot be repaired after damage. But perceptions about the human spinal cord have undergone a revolutionary change in recent years as researchers have solved some of the riddles about preventing and reversing the damage that inevitably accompanies spinal cord injury. In the last twenty years scientists have proven that repair of the spinal cord is possible and the number of promising approaches to repair has grown exponentially. Because of these accomplishments, many no longer accept that they will be paralyzed for life.

Collaborative networks of international neuroscientists are pooling their wide-ranging expertise and working cooperatively to address the multifaceted challenges of spinal cord injury. These include learning how to use neurotrophins to the best advantage, understanding immune responses, promoting and directing nerve growth, bridging the gap and exploring ways to use stem cells to promote regeneration and repair of the cord as well as exploring ways to promote and maintain residual sensori-motor functions through bioengineering and physiotherapy approaches. Amazingly, it can be said that more research progress, including progress made through collaborative research, has been achieved in the past five years than in the previous fifty.

Research is truly the key to a cure for paralysis. With financial support, scientists can push toward cutting-edge discoveries and treatments to cure paralysis caused by spinal cord injury and other central nervous system disorders. Without sustained funding, scientists may fall short of their goals. Fostering public and private funding for spinal cord research will be the most instrumental component in the quest for the cure.

Preface

This book results from the XXIIIrd International Symposium of the Center for Research in Neurological Sciences of the Université de Montréal (held in Montréal, Québec, Canada from May 6 to 8, 2001). Our goal was to organize a symposium that would bridge different scientific approaches to the study of spinal cord injury, and to foster communication between scientists. We were particularly pleased that Mr. Christopher Reeve accepted to be Honorary Chair of the event, and that he addressed the scientific audience. Mr. Reeve emphasized the need to translate laboratory research to the clinical studies and this is also briefly stated in his foreword of this book. The symposium involved more than 300 registrants, 36 speakers and 75 posters. It was a special occasion to discuss the topic of spinal trauma at all scientific levels and share findings and progress with the international community of research scientists.

The chapters of this book summarize the platform presentations at the symposium, and present reviews of different studies, as well as new data. The aim was to cover, in a broad perspective, research on spinal cord injury, from its clinical aspects in humans to experimental studies in animals, as well as research on the molecular mechanisms of injury and regeneration. The scope of the book includes rehabilitation and functional repair in human patients and in animal models, strategies for neuroprotection and regeneration, cell transplantation into injured spinal cord, strategies to overcome growth inhibition, and axon guidance molecules in injury and regeneration. Accordingly, the chapters have been grouped in 4 sections: (1) Spinal Cord Injuries in Patients; (2) Animal Models of Spinal Cord Injuries; (3) Neuroprotection and Transplantation and (4) Molecular Targets to Promote Axon Regeneration in the CNS.

We wish to thank the authors for their contribution to the symposium and to this book. We also wish to express special thanks to Ms. Chantal Nault for organizing the logistics of the symposium. We also thank Mr. Daniel Cyr, Ms. Janyne Provencher and Ms. Suzanne Cabana for their precious help in the organization of this symposium. The generous help of many others, students and technicians, was greatly appreciated. We gratefully acknowledge the financial contribution of the André Senécal Foundation for Research on Spinal Cord that provided travel grants to enable students and postdoctoral trainees to travel to Montréal and attend the symposium. We also gratefully acknowledge the financial support of the following sponsors: Ministère de la Recherche, de la Science et de la Technologie du Québec, the Canadian Institutes of Health Research, the Université de Montréal, Quebecor Inc., AstraZeneca, the Kent Waldrep National Paralysis Foundation, the Rick Hansen Institute, Pharmacia, Merck Frosst Canada, the Fonds de la Recherche en Santé du Québec, the Fonds pour la Formation de Chercheurs et l'Aide à la Recherche, the Savoy Foundation for Epilepsy, the Société de l'Assurance Automobile du Québec, the Réseau Provincial de Recherche en Adaptation-Réadaptation, the Barbara Turnbull Foundation for Spinal Cord Research, the NeuroScience Canada Partnership, Yamaha, and Autobus Galland Ltée.

Lisa McKerracher
Guy Doucet
Serge Rossignol
(Editors)

Contents

xviii

Spinal cord injuries in patients

L. McKerracher, G. Doucet and S. Rossignol (Eds.)
Progress in Brain Research, Vol. 137

CHAPTER 1

Advances in imaging of spinal cord injury: implications for treatment and patient evaluation

Robert M. Quencer [*]

Department of Radiology, University of Miami School of Medicine, Miami, FL 33136, USA

Introduction

Detailed comparison of magnetic resonance (MR) images and histopathology of injured spinal cords has allowed a deeper understanding of the nature of such injuries in both the acute and chronic stages. In addition, abnormalities seen on MR explain many of the static and progressive neurologic symptoms experienced by spine injured patients. Future directions in treating patients with spinal cord injuries (SCI) will depend in large measure on the accurate interpretation of anatomic and physiologic information available on MR.

Acute spinal cord injury

In the acutely injured cord, hemorrhagic or non-hemorrhagic contusions result from the primary injury and are seen on MR as a hyperintense abnormal signal on T2 weighted images (non-hemorrhagic) as an area of low signal (hemorrhagic) on T2[*] gradient echo images, or a combination of these MR findings. Secondary effects resulting from the ongoing cascade of neural destruction, along with cord hypoperfusion (either local or systemic) result in abnormal signal, specifically hyperintensity on T2WIs,

below and above the epicenter of injury. It has long been noted that patients who have suffered a hemorrhagic contusive injury (Fig. 1) have a uniformly poor outcome with little or no return of neurologic function. It is possible that iron which diffuses out into the surrounding parenchyma from the hemorrhagic contusion potentiates lipid peroxidation of cell membranes and contributes significantly to the cascade of neural tissue destruction, thus explaining the worsened clinical outcome.

A forceful compression of the spinal cord may result in the displacement of gray matter superiorly and inferiorly from the epicenter of the injury (Becerra et al., 1995a). Thus displaced gray matter typically, but not exclusively, is found in the anterior portion of the dorsal columns. Because this gray matter loses its normal blood supply, a breakdown and necrosis of the tissue ensues, explaining in many instances, why eccentric cavities are seen in the chronically injured cord at a distance removed from the initial primary injury site (Fig. 2).

Acute compressive demyelination (Quencer et al., 1992) typically occurs in a low velocity hyperextension injury in a patient with a narrowed and/or spondolytic canal. Contrary to popular belief, the resulting neurological findings of severe upper extremity weakness out of proportion to the relatively less weak lower extremities is not due to a central cord hemorrhage (formerly but in most cases incorrectly described as an acute posttraumatic central cord syndrome). Rather the mechanism of injury is

---
[*] Correspondence to: R.M. Quencer, Department of Radiology, University of Miami School of Medicine, Miami, FL 33136, USA. Tel.: +1-305-243-4701; Fax: +1-305-247-7455; E-mail: rquencer@med.miami.edu

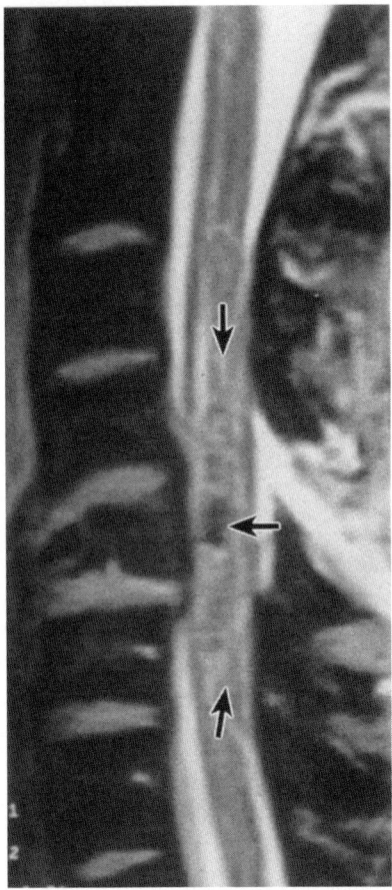

Fig. 1. Hemorrhagic cord contusion. Sagittal gradient echo image (T2* weighted) shows a hypointense signal (arrow) representing hemorrhage within a cord which shows signal changes above and below the epicenter of injury. These secondary effects of injury are manifested by increased signal (arrowheads). See text. A retropulsed, fractured C5 vertebral body caused continued cord compression, despite external distraction/reduction efforts. A non-reversible and poor clinical outcome is a result of this type hemorrhagic injury.

secondary to a squeezing mechanism of the cord often in a canal narrowed by bony spurs, disc protrusion and a hypertrophied ligamentum flava. The lateral cortical spinal tracts bear the brunt of this injury (Fig. 3) and a loss of the myelin-axon units predominately in the lateral columns results.

Subacute spinal cord injury

In weeks following a spinal cord injury, abnormal signal is noted in the dorsal columns (ascending

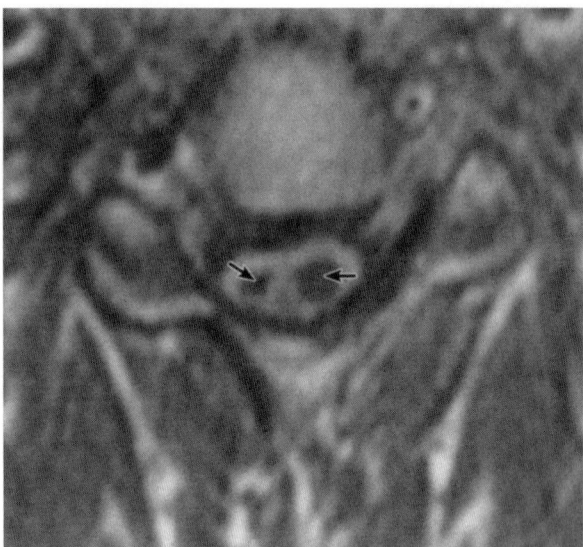

Fig. 2. Eccentric cysts in a chronically injured cord. At a level (C4) above the primary injury site, two eccentric cysts within the cord are noted (arrows) on this T1WI. As explained in the text, this may result from the breakdown of displaced, and subsequently devitalized gray matter. Such cysts may gradually expand over time and affect previously normal spinal cord tissue.

tracts) above the level of injury and in the lateral corticospinal tracts (descending tracts) below the level of injury. Such Wallerian degeneration (Becerra et al., 1995b) can be seen on routine T2 spin echo (either conventional or fast spin echo) or gradient echo imaging approximately 1.5–2 months following injury (Fig. 4). It is probable that with improvements in diffusion weighted imaging (DWI) and calculated apparent diffusion coefficient maps (ADC maps), earlier acute changes along the white matter tracts which reflect restricted water diffusion in the myelin sheaths will be noted (bright signal on DWIs and hypointensity on ADC maps). In Wallerian degeneration, detailed high resolution post mortem MR imaging and histopathology comparison show precise anatomic correlation with these MR findings. Tract involvement and tract sparing can, by inference, predict the level of primary injury.

Chronic spinal cord injury: delayed sequela of SCI

After a period of relatively stable neurological dysfunction following a spinal cord injury, approxi-

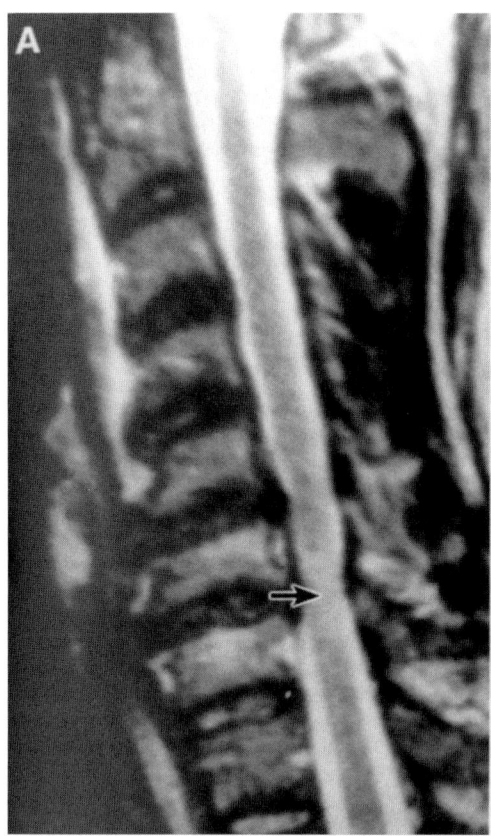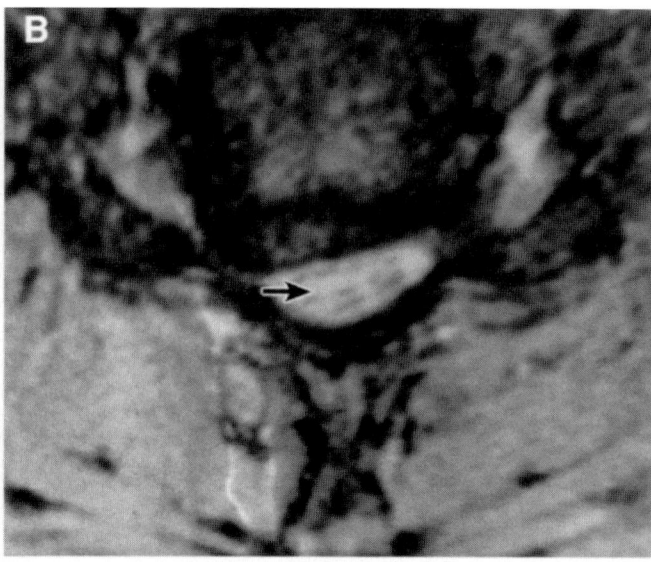

Fig. 3. Acute compression of the lateral columns of the cord. In this low velocity hyperextension injury, the sagittal (A) and axial (B) T2 weighted MR images show a spondylitic, narrow canal with abnormal high signal (arrowheads) at the C6–C7 level in the cord. The axial image shows the signal abnormality predominately in the lateral portion of the cord (right greater than left). Note the lack of hemorrhage in the cord. Refer to text for explanation of the injury mechanism.

mately 5–10% of patients may suffer clinical deterioration manifested by worsening motor or sensory function, increasing pain, and/or dysautonomia. A number of progressive and often insidious findings can underlie these symptoms including: enlarging intramedullary or subarachnoid cysts; progressive myelomalacia; ascending cord atrophy; cord scarring with distortion and tethering of the cord to the dura; progressive instability of the spinal column; or any combination of these abnormalities.

Progressive posttraumatic myelomalacia (PPTM) (Falcone et al., 1994) superficially shares MR findings often associated with cystic changes within the cord, however in PPTM, the spin density image shows that the abnormality does not match the intensity of CSF. Routine MR imaging of the spine usually does not include spin density images, so that the

appearance of PPTM is quite similar to an expanding cord cyst. The cord appears enlarged because the pial/arachnoid layer is tethered often circumferentially to the dura, so that in essence the cord is pulled out to the edges of the canal. CSF flow studies may assist in differential diagnosis so because PPTM will not show the typical flow flows associated with cord cysts. Treatment, if undertaken, consist of release of the scarring and establishing free flow of CSF in the subarachnoid space via a wide expansile duraplasty (Lee et al., 1997). With intraoperative ultrasound, a dramatic change in the apparent size of the cord can be seen once the tethering adhesions are released.

CSF equivalent lesions within the injured spinal cord may either represent non-expanding flaccid cavities or expanding tense cysts (Quencer et al., 1986); histopathologically the former have no discrete pe-

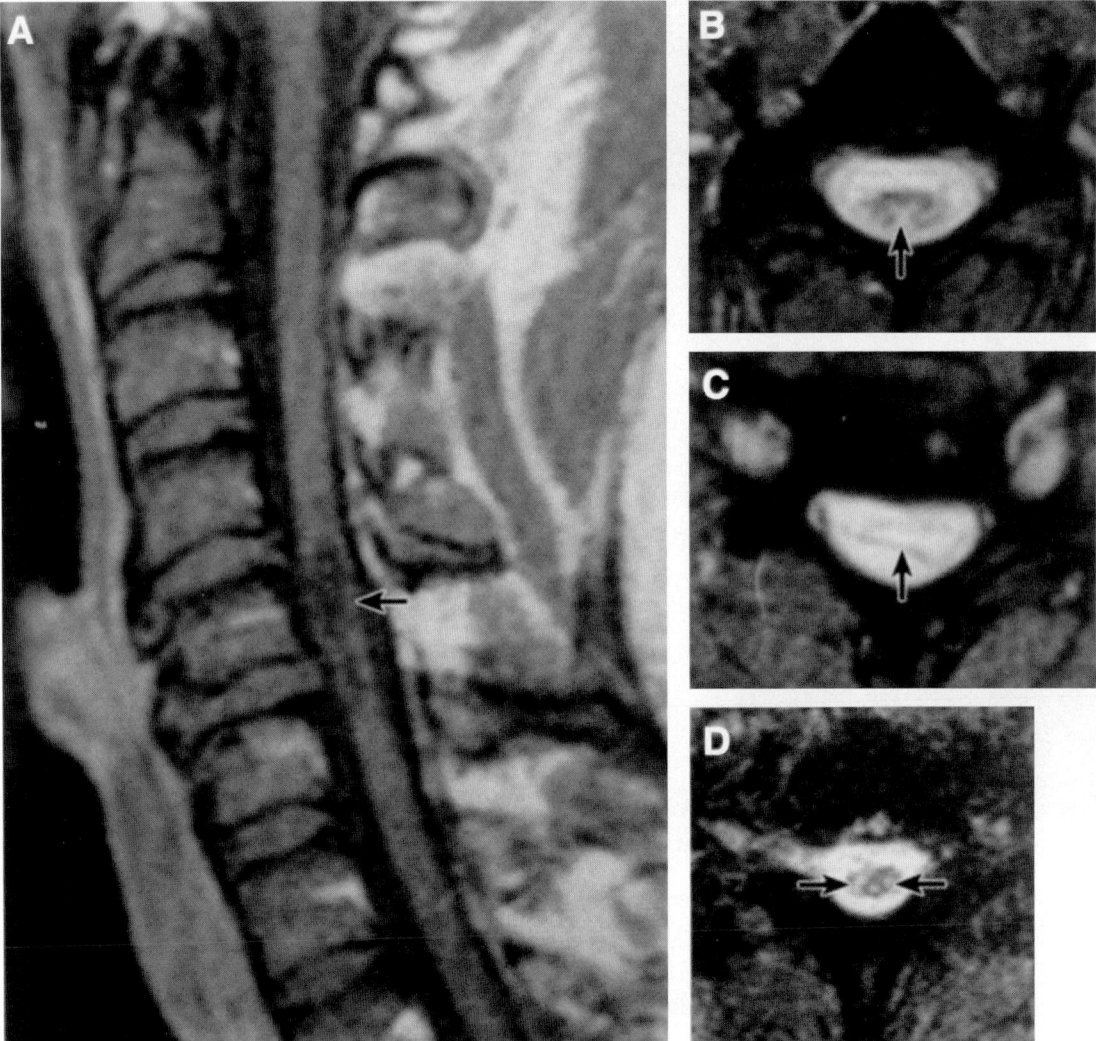

Fig. 4. Wallerian degeneration above and below the epicenter of a cord injury (7 weeks postinjury). At C5, the T1WI (A) and the axial T2 weighted image (C) show the result of direct injury of the cord (arrows in A and C). Note above the injury level at C3 (B) and below the injury level at C7 (D) the bright signal in the dorsal columns and the lateral columns (arrowheads in B and D).

ripheral border zones whereas the latter may demonstrate well-defined astrocytic borders (Quencer and Bunge, 1996). Expanding cysts often have associated with the zones of abnormal signal or MR, above and below the cyst itself (Fig. 5). Whether this represents pericystic fluid (analogous to periventricular edema in obstructive hydrocephalus) or represents ongoing myelomalacic/metabolic/vascular changes is unclear, however such a finding does suggest the possibility of cord parenchymal changes in re-

sponse to an enlarging cyst. Restoration of a patent subarachnoid space to permit normal flow of CSF around the injury site is a method to surgically treat both PPCM and an enlarging spinal cord cyst (Schwartz et al., 1999a). In both instances, opening the dura, reducing the cord tethering, resection of the thickened and scarred dura, and performing a wide duroplasty may be performed. Resultant collapse of extensive cysts can be verified on follow-up MR imaging.

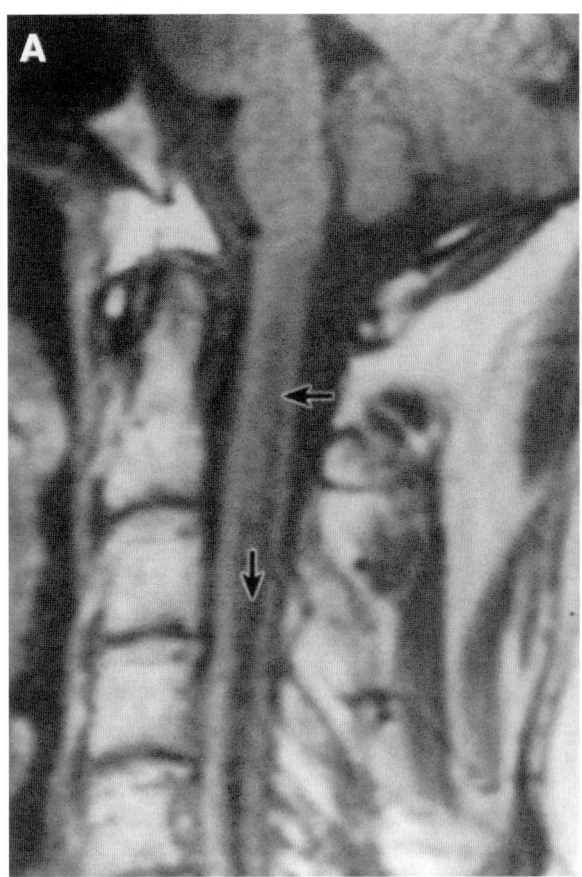 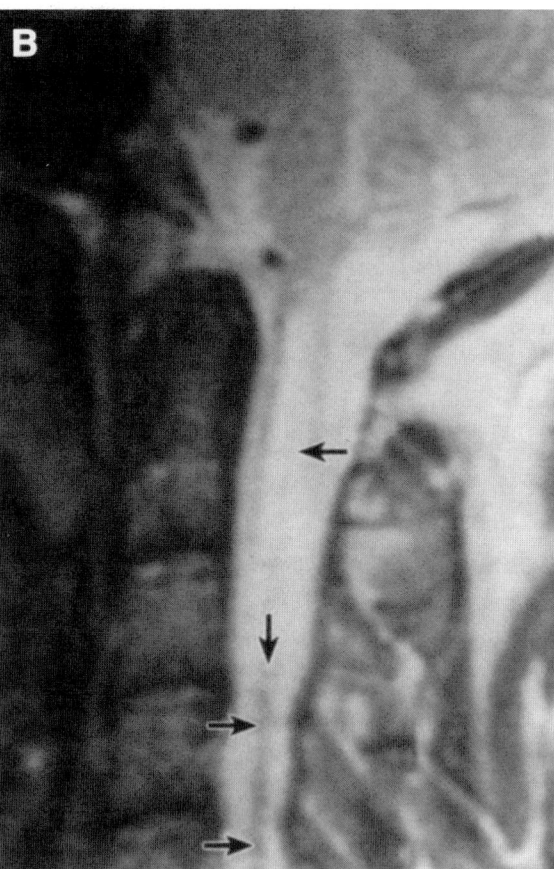

Fig. 5. Signal changes above an expanding posttraumatic syrinx. Both the T1WI (A) and the T2WI (B) show the upper end of a posttraumatic syrinx (arrows). On the T2WI (5B), there is loss of signal within the cyst (arrowheads) because of brisk flow within the cyst cavity. Signal changes above the upper end of the syrinx ascend to the C1 level (curved arrows). Pericystic fluid and/or ongoing metabolic alterations in the cord explains this finding and is frequently seen in patients with expanding cysts who are worsening clinically.

Cord tethering and scarring is a frequent sequela of severe SCI and the scarring can be progressive over time, resulting in more and more cord distortion (Fig. 6). Deciding whether such abnormalities are responsible for on-going and/or new neurological symptoms is a difficult clinical problem. Release of the tethering bands may reduce symptoms if a clear cut and unequivocal association between the clinical picture and the MR can be established.

Summary

Close inspection of MR images in all stages of SCI can reveal alterations which are important for our understanding of the changes which occur in SCI and may be crucial for planning surgical intervention. Importantly also, these observations may assist in the evaluation of novel therapies in SCI, such as cellular transplantation. It is hopeful that MR strategies which are currently in routine use in the brain, such as diffusion weighted imaging, perfusion studies, spectroscopy, and magnetization transfer can be adopted for use in the spine (Schwartz et al., 1999b). Because of the small size of the cord, the magnetic suspectability problems caused by surrounding air and bone, and nearby vascular and CSF flow/pulsations, these techniques are currently very difficult to employ in the cord. They will, however, evolve over time and give us greater insights into the in vivo status of the injured cord.

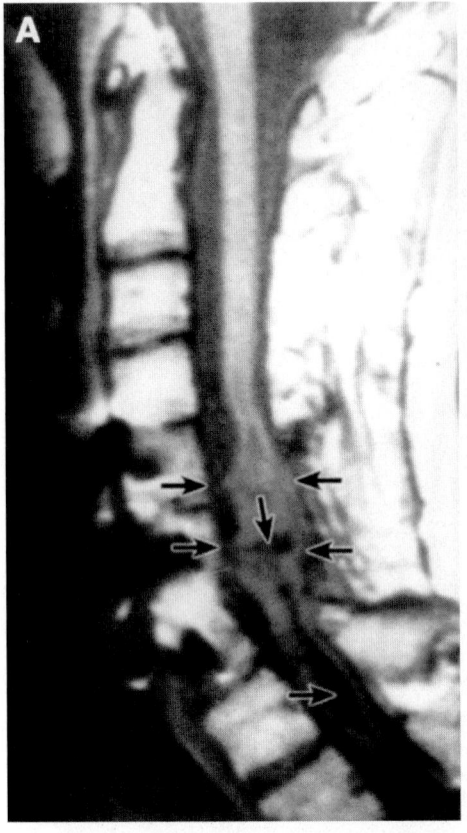 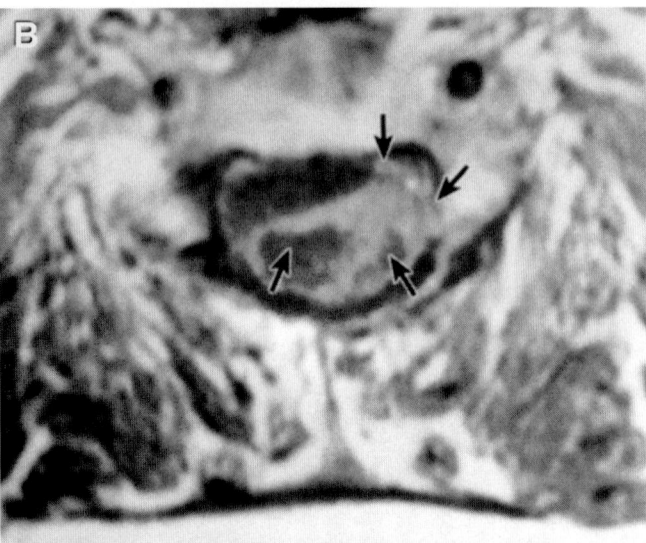

Fig. 6. Tethering and severe cord distortion. In a patient with progressive neurological symptoms and increasing pain in the left arm, the MR shows cord scarring, distortion and tethering (arrowheads), both posteriorly and to the anteriolateral aspect of the spinal canal. Note also the prior anterior cervical decompression and fusion with plate and screws from C4 to C7, the focal cavities with the cord (arrows), an expanding central cyst (curved white arrow) extending inferiorly from the injury site, and cord atrophy at the C4–C5 level. This case shows the multiple and complex abnormalities seen in the previously injured spinal cord. Which of these abnormalities is responsible for new and/or progressive symptoms is often difficult to answer.

References

Becerra, J.L., Puckett, W.R., Marcillo, A.E. and Quencer, R.M. et al. (1995a) Human spinal cord injury: MRI and histopathology. *Neuroradiol. Suppl.*, 37: 307–309.

Becerra, J.L., Puckett, W.R., Hiester, E.D., Quencer, R.M., Marcillo, A.E., Post, M.J.D. and Bunge, R.P. (1995b) MR/pathological comparisons of Wallerian degeneration in spinal cord injury. *Am. J. Neuroradiol.*, 16: 125–133.

Falcone, S., Quencer, R.M., Green, B.A., Patchen, S. and Post, M.J.D. (1994) Progressive posttraumatic myelomalacic myelopathy: imaging and clinical features. *Am. J. Neuroradiol.*, 15: 747–754.

Lee, T.T., Arias, J.M., Andrus, H.L., Quencer, R.M., Falcone, S.F. and Green, B.A. (1997) Progressive posttraumatic myelomalacic myelopathy: treatment with untethering and expansive duraplasty. *J. Neurosurg.*, 86: 624–628.

Quencer, R.M. and Bunge, R. (1996) The injured spinal cord: imaging, histopathological, clinical correlates and basic science approaches to enhancing neural function after spinal cord injury. *Spine*, 21: 2064–2066.

Quencer, R.M., Sheldon, J.J. and Post, M.J.D. et al. (1986) MRI in the chronically injured cervical spinal cord. *Am. J. Neuroradiol.*, 7: 457–464.

Quencer, R.M., Bunge, R., Egnor, M., Puckett, W., Naidich, T.P., Green, B.A. and Post, M.J.D. (1992) MR/pathological correlations in the acute post-traumatic central cervical spinal cord syndrome. *Neuroradiology*, 34: 85–94.

Schwartz, E.D., Falcone, S., Quencer, R.M. and Green, B.A. (1999a) Posttraumatic syringomyelia: pathogenesis, imaging and treatment: pictorial essay. *Am. J. Roentgenol.*, 173: 487–492.

Schwartz, E.D., Yezierski, R.P., Pattany, P.M., Quencer, R.M. and Weaver, R.G. (1999b) MR and diffusion weighted imaging in a rat model of syringomyelia following excitotoxic spinal cord injury. *Am. J. Neuroradiol.*, 20: 1422–1428.

L. McKerracher, G. Doucet and S. Rossignol (Eds.)
Progress in Brain Research, Vol. 137

CHAPTER 2

A review of the adaptability and recovery of locomotion after spinal cord injury

H. Barbeau [1,2,*], J. Fung [1,2], A. Leroux [1,2,3] and M. Ladouceur [1,2,4]

[1] *School of Physical and Occupational Therapy, McGill University, 3645 Drummond Street, Montreal, QC H39 1Y5, Canada*
[2] *Jewish Rehabilitation Hospital Research Center, 3205 Place Alton Goldbloom, Haval, QC H7V 1R2, Canada*

Abstract: Spinal cord injury (SCI) is associated with multiple motor problems leading to the alteration and limited adaptation in the walking and postural behavior. This review addresses recent findings on locomotor and postural adaptations after spinal cord injury. The adaptation of the locomotor behavior to behavioral goals and external constraints constitute important functional prerequisites in the recovery of locomotion after spinal cord injury. Functional prerequisites in locomotion include coping with changes in speed, slope obstacle, weight support, interaction with walking aids, energy consumption and attentional demands. Various treatment approaches such as locomotor training using body weight support (BWS) and functional electrical stimulation (FES) will be discussed, in the context of functional prerequisites necessary in the recovery of locomotion. Understanding locomotor and postural adaptations will lead to a better appreciation of the normal and dysfunctional mechanisms, and culminate eventually in the development of appropriate rehabilitation assessment and treatment strategies.

Introduction

The human locomotor pattern can be easily and rapidly adapted to changes in the environment and external demands, such as speed (Murray et al., 1966; Brandell, 1977; Nilsson et al., 1985), slope (Brandell, 1977; Wall et al., 1981; Simonsen et al., 1995; Lange et al., 1996) and obstacles (Chen et al., 1991; McFadyen and Winter, 1991; Patla et al., 1991; McFadyen et al., 1993; Patla and Rietdyk, 1993; Patla and Prentice, 1995; Chou et al., 1997; Chou and Draganich, 1997, 1998; McFadyen

---

* Correspondence to: H. Barbeau, Jewish Rehabilitation Hospital Research Center, 3205 Place Alton Goldbloom, Laval, QC, H7V 1R2 Canada.
E-mail: hugues.barbeau@mcgill.ca
[3] Present address: Department of Physical Education, Concordia University, Montreal, QC Canada
[4] Present address: Department of Physical Education, Brock University, St. Catharine's, ON, Canada

and Carnahan, 1997). The adaptation is normally achieved by changing the movement patterns of the trunk, pelvis and lower limb segments (Murray et al., 1966; Wall et al., 1981; Nilsson et al., 1985; Lange et al., 1996) and by changing the motor recruitment of the relevant flexor and extensor muscles (Brandell, 1977; Nilsson et al., 1985; Simonsen et al., 1995; Lange et al., 1996).

Following a spinal cord injury, descending pathways are usually damaged, affecting the adaptability of the locomotor pattern. Animal studies have shown that cats with complete spinal cord transection can recover locomotion on the treadmill when trained and can adapt to limited changes in speed (Rossignol, 2000 for a comprehensive review). However, the spinal cat has great difficulty in adapting its walking pattern to changes in incline. In contrast to the adaptability of the EMG and movement patterns in the intact cat, only minor changes in the electromyographic (EMG) activity were observed during uphill (15°) and downhill (20°) walking in the spinal animal (Bélanger, 1990). Moreover, without manually supporting the spinal cat, the animal could only adapt to a few degrees' changes in roll-plane incline, as compared to least 20° observed in the intact cat (Bélanger, 1990).

In humans, uphill walking is a demanding task that requires specific modifications in lower-limb movements (Wall et al., 1981; Lange et al., 1996) and muscle activation (Brandell, 1977; Simonsen et al., 1995; Lange et al., 1996). As the walking grade increases, more propulsion has to be generated from the lower limbs (Brandell, 1977), and postural adjustments must be performed to maintain equilibrium. Following spinal cord injury (SCI), the basic locomotor pattern is altered (Barbeau et al., 1998a), and the ability to adapt to changes in the environment could be affected. However, it remains relatively unknown to which extent persons with SCI can adapt to external demands. This review will assess the adaptability of the walking pattern in the context of behavioral goals and external constraints following SCI.

Adaptation to changes in walking speed

A first striking difference of gait observed in most SCI subjects and in most cases of spastic paresis resulting from different neurological disorders is the reduced walking speed as compared to normal subjects (Fig. 1). In a retrospective review, the speed data were pooled from 162 subjects across 20 studies (Barbeau et al., 1998b). The SCI subjects showed a wide spectrum of walking speed abilities, ranging from total incapacity to near normal speed.

More than 20% of the SCI population that we have evaluated thus far (in ASIA C category) were unable to walk overground following spinal cord injury. They needed to be supported by a walking harness to partially unload their weight (Fig. 1, black histogram). The body weight support (BWS) system developed in the eighties in Montreal allowed this subgroup of SCI subjects to be evaluated and to eventually participate in new locomotor training approaches (Barbeau et al., 1987; Norman et al., 1995).

Fig. 2A shows the curvilinear relationship between the cycle duration and the walking speed in both healthy and SCI subjects. This relationship has been shown before for healthy subjects walking at

speeds above 0.4 m/s (Nilsson et al., 1985). Indeed, in healthy normal subjects walking at low speed, the cycle, stance, and swing durations were increased, and the stride length decreased as compared to the values obtained at comfortable gait speed.

A prolonged cycle duration that results from an increase in both stance and swing duration is usually observed in most SCI subjects walking at their own preferred gait speed. To characterize the walking patterns of SCI subjects, it is important to make comparisons with normal subjects walking at matched speeds. Some of the characteristics of normal and SCI subjects walking patterns are presented in Fig. 2C.

When compared at the same speed (0.3 m/s), the cycle duration measured from most SCI subjects was greater than that of normal subjects (Fig. 2A). Angular displacement of lower limb joints in the sagittal plane in SCI subjects revealed that the total hip joint angular excursion was much greater than that expressed by the normal subjects. The SCI subjects made foot contact with the knee in a flexed position (see arrow, Fig. 2C, knee), and for some, the knee remained flexed throughout stance. Some SCI subjects tended to walk with a more dorsiflexed ankle at the beginning of stance (see arrow), and the ankle remained more dorsiflexed than normal even at push-off or at the end of stance. This is mainly a passive consequence of the walking with a flexed knee during stance. During swing, the ankle joint could remain dorsiflexed, or in contrast, it could be plantarflexed because of a foot-drop weakness (see asterisk). Several other groups have made similar observations with SCI subjects (Dietz et al., 1981; Conrad et al., 1985).

The electromyographic (EMG) activity of lower limb muscles during walking reveals alterations in both timing and amplitude in SCI subjects as compared to normal subjects. Coactivation of muscle activity at proximal and distal joints is often reported in SCI subjects (Fung et al., 1990). Further, abnormal activation of the soleus muscle, including clonus, is commonly seen in early stance, especially when the walking speed is increased (Fig. 2B).

Joint stiffness, including the relative contribution of the stretch reflex and the intrinsic properties of the ankle extensors in normal and spastic subjects has been studied (Dietz et al., 1981; Dietz and Berger,

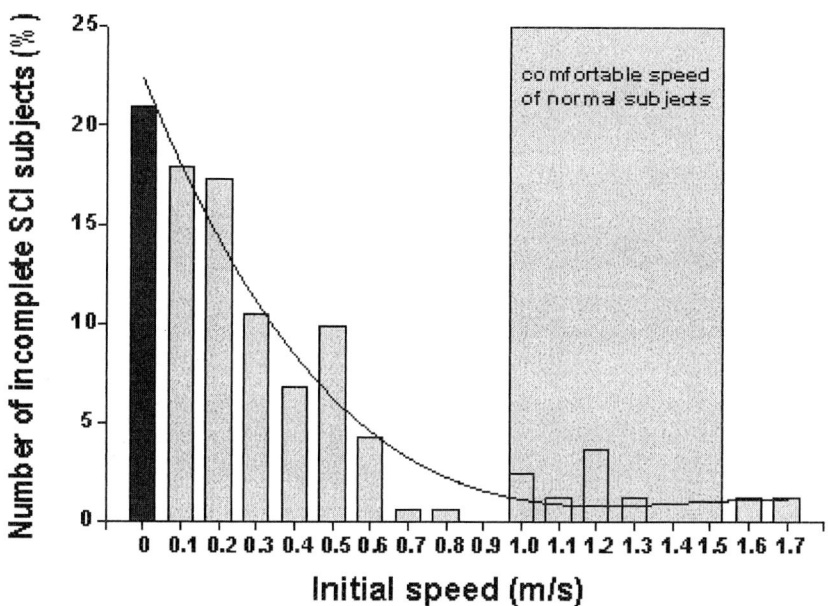

Fig. 1. Representation of the spectrum of walking speeds achieved by the SCI subjects (Asia C and D) before initiating rehabilitation. The black histogram represents the number of SCI subjects who were unable to walk overground following the injury; thus, necessitating a body weight support system to achieve very limited walking speed. For each level of walking speed, the number of SCI subjects is expressed as a percentage of the whole group ($n = 162$).

1983; Thilmann et al., 1991; Sinkjaer and Magnussen, 1994; Mirbagheri et al., 1998a,b). An increase of the reflex gain and a decrease of inhibition during the swing phase have been reported in SCI subjects (Yang et al., 1991; Sinkjaer et al., 1996). These findings suggest that increases in both the reflex gain and the non-reflex torque could contribute to the increased stiffness of the ankle joint seen in SCI subjects during walking. Hence, both alterations in central mechanisms and changes in intrinsic properties of the muscle fibers could be responsible for the increased stiffness. (Mirbagheri et al., 2001).

Adaptation to assistive devices

There have been few studies examining the contribution of an ambulatory assistive device to gait in incomplete spinal cord injured individuals. Many individuals who have sustained incomplete SCI are able to ambulate but rely heavily on walking aids. Without the assistive walking devices, incomplete spinal cord injured individuals are often limited to wheelchair usage for mobility. Although wheelchair usage is generally a more practical mode of locomo-

tion, assisted weight-bearing ambulation has many benefits to the user including increased blood flow, decreased risk of osteoporosis, and increased physical fitness and well being (Go et al., 1995).

The interaction between gait of incomplete spinal cord injured individuals and their usage of walking aids has been relatively under-investigated. Recent studies that have attempted to examine these interactions in the incomplete spinal cord injured population have shown interesting relationships between gait and walking aid usage. Melis et al. (1999), proposed two possible connections both relevant to the type of walking aid used: walker, crutches or canes (Fig. 3A,B). Their data showed that individuals who used walkers tended to walk slower than crutch users who tended to walk slower than cane users. The opposite relationship existed for the maximal amount of force exerted on an instrumented walking aid during gait, where walker users tended to place the most amount of force on their aid, and cane users, the least. These results suggest that walking speed might be related to maximal axial force, or that the limiting factor in the speed of an individual's gait might be, in fact, the type of walking aid itself.

12

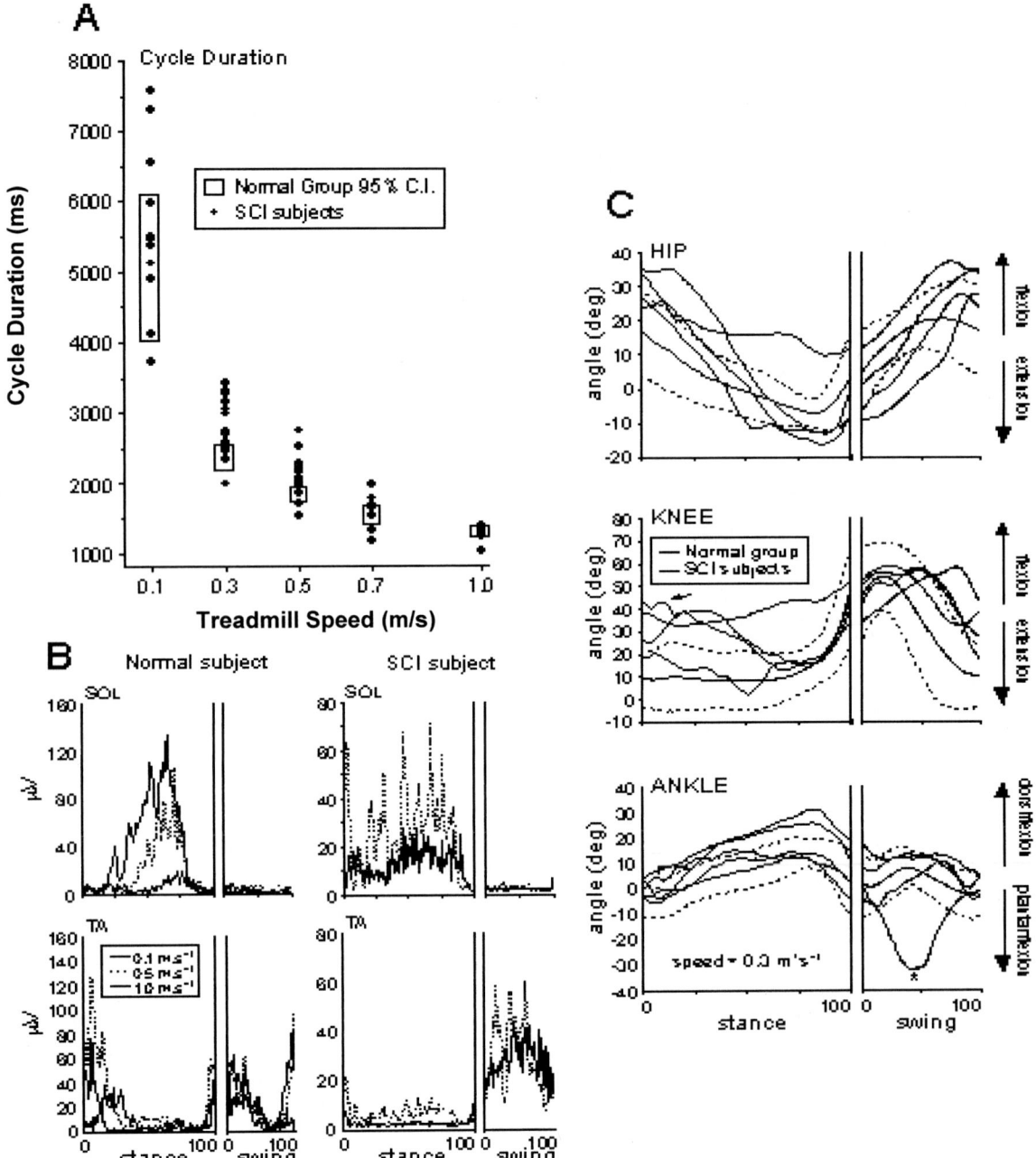

Fig. 2. (A) Cycle duration as a function of treadmill speed in 11 SCI subjects, as compared to the 95% confidence interval of the mean of seven normal subjects (rectangle). (B) Soleus and tibialis anterior EMG activity at different walking speeds for one normal (0.1, 0.5 and 1.0 m/s) and one SCI subject (0.1 and 0.5 m/s). (C) Comparison of the joint angular excursions at the hip, knee, and ankle of seven SCI subjects compared with the average of a normal group at 0.3 m/s. Arrows indicate the presence of knee flexion during stance. The dotted lines represent the 95% confidence interval for the normal group.

13

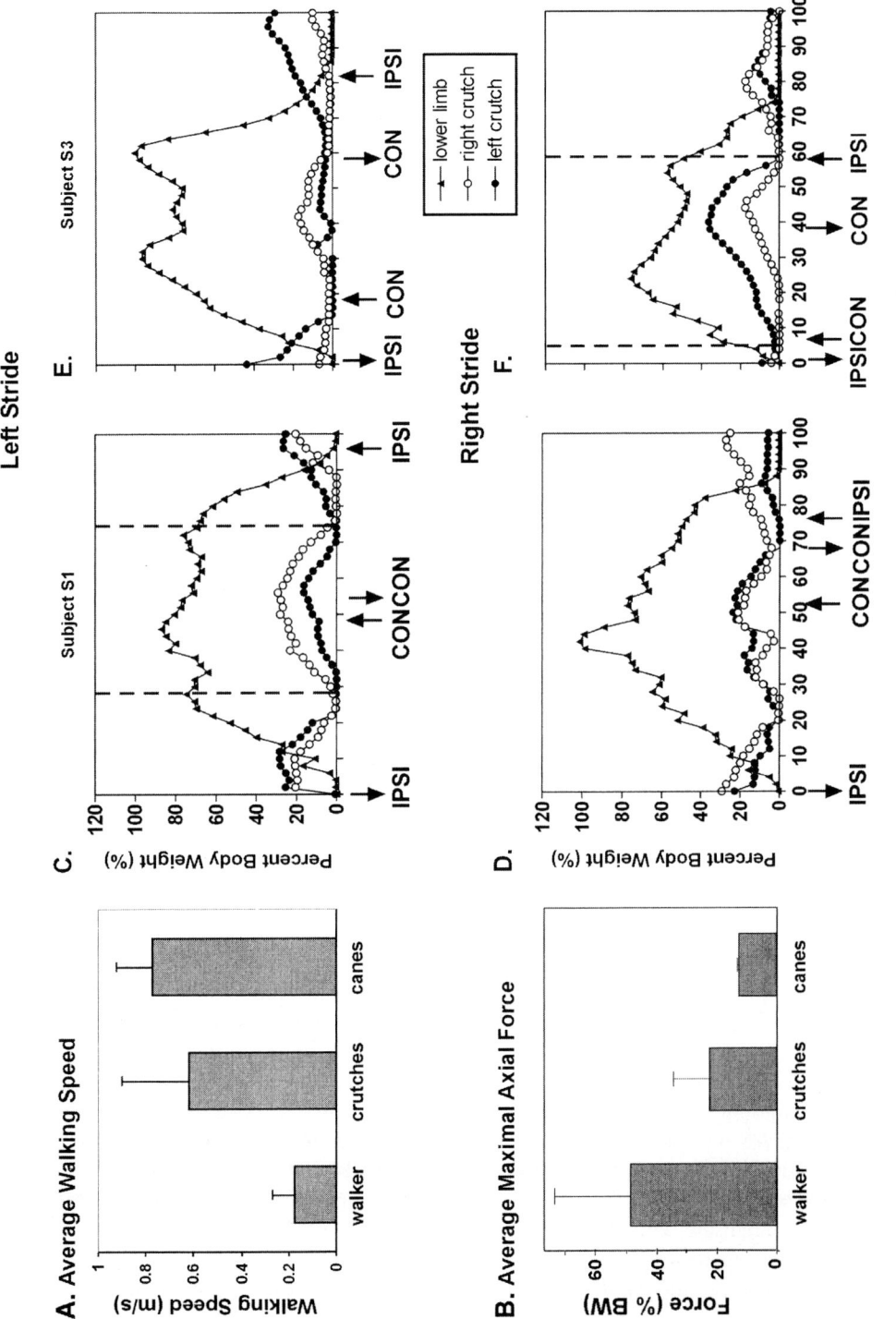

Fig. 3. (A) Average walking speed in relation to walking aids (walker, crutches and canes). (B) Average maximal axial force in relation to walking aids. (C–F) Force exerted on the lower limb and axial loading on left and right crutches in two subjects, S1 (C and D) and subject S3 (E and F). C and E indicated the left stride while D and F indicated the right stride.

Chung et al. (2001) investigated similar gait characteristics in a group of incomplete SCI individuals using the elbow crutches. A notable difference in crutch usage was observed between subjects who walked at lower gait speeds (0.08 m/s (Fig. 3C,D) and 0.38 m/s (Fig. 3E,F)) than those who walked at higher speeds. Between the subjects with the highest speed and the subjects with the lowest gait speed, the magnitude of force exerted on the subject's crutches was observed to be related to the force exerted on the lower limb contralateral to the crutch (Chung et al., 2001). However, SCI subjects (Fig. 3E,F) whose right leg exerted less force than the left on the ground platform also exerted more force on the left (contralateral) crutch than the right one. This suggests that loading of crutches in the axial direction may be affected more by lower limb loading than by gait speed, though gait speed may be an important contributing factor.

It is often assumed that the SCI subjects are highly variable from one person to another. It becomes apparent that there may be some common factors that can be used to develop quantitative, objective measures to quantify and to develop criteria for progressing walking aids to other assisted gait in incomplete spinal cord injured individuals, but this needs further investigation.

In chronic SCI subjects who walked with an asymmetrical walking pattern, BWS also appeared to have positive effects on the gait parameters. This is illustrated in Fig. 4, which compares the effects of 40% BWS on an SCI subject walking with or without parallel bars. As the SCI subject walked on the treadmill holding onto parallel bars with no BWS, the SCI subject compensated by pushing with his upper extremities and the less affected lower limb. The resulting lower limb kinematics showed an increase in ankle plantarflexion in the left limb (less affected limb, not illustrated) at the end of stance, while swinging the right leg (more affected, illustrated in Fig. 4) with a minimal amount of hip, knee and ankle flexion. When 40% BWS was provided, while the SCI subject walked with parallel bars, minimal changes were noted in the walking pattern (Fig. 4) as the subject continued to compensate with the upper extremities and the less affected lower limb. However, when the SCI subject released the parallel bars while walking at 40% BWS, a more normal gait

pattern emerged. This was characterized by an appropriate swing phase with flexion at the hip, knee and ankle (Fig. 4), as well as a burst of activity in the tibialis anterior muscle (not illustrated) (Visintin and Barbeau, 1994). These results suggest that BWS induced a 'forced-use' regime of the paretic limb such that the patients could not compensate by using the non-paretic upper and lower limbs.

Energy cost in SCI subjects

An example of the energy cost recorded by a heart rate monitor is illustrated in Fig. 5. The heart rate increased for an SCI subject from about 110 beats/min when he was sitting, to about 160 beats/min when he was walking at 0.13 m/s and then decreased progressively to approximately the same baseline level when he was sitting again.

Fig. 5 also illustrates the relationship of the physiological cost index (PCI = (active-resting heart rate)/(gait speed), measured in heart beats/m) as a function of the walking speed in both normal and SCI subjects. It can be noted that the physiological cost index was 2–5 times more than that of normal subjects walking at very low speed. As for the SCI subjects who have higher speed (from 0.8 m/s to above) the PCI is closely related to that of normal subjects. An important observation is that the SCI subjects at low gait speeds are usually ambulating with walkers whereas the SCI subjects at higher speeds often need a single cane or no assisted walking aids (see previous section).

Attentional requirement during walking in SCI subjects

Cognitive central processing plays an important role in sensory integration as well as movement planning and execution while performing walking and standing. In order to reach a functional status for the maintenance of posture and gait, the quantity of cognitive resources available (not used by the standing or walking tasks) need to be efficient. These resources are used by other regulatory systems to adapt to the environmental constraints or to the subjects' own goals. Fig. 6A summarizes the results of a study on cognitive requirement in normal subjects and SCI subjects (Lajoie and Barbeau, 1999). Au-

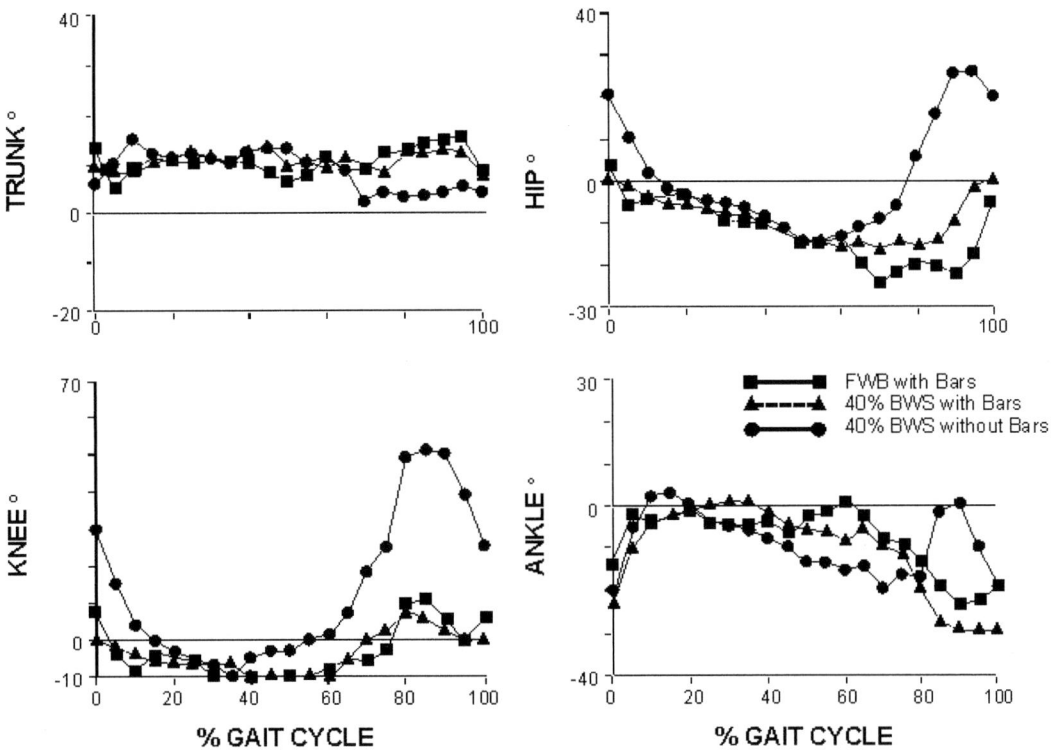

Fig. 4. The right lower limb kinematics of a SCI subject walking on the treadmill, at a speed of 0.08 ms^{-1}, at 0% BWS with parallel bars. 40% BWS with parallel bars, and 40% BWS without parallel bars. The sagittal angular displacement patterns of a representative cycle for the trunk, hip, knee and ankle are illustrated. Note the presence of hip and knee flexion and ankle dorsiflexion at 40% BWS without parallel bars.

ditory stimuli were presented at the onset of single-support or double-support phase of locomotion and reaction times (RTs) for both groups of subjects were evaluated during sitting, standing and walking. Normal subjects walked at preferred and lower speeds (0.5 m/s) to match those of SCI subjects, such that attentional demands could be compared between the two groups of subjects for a similar walking speed. SCI subjects performed very well in both static tasks (better than in normal subjects) but were significantly slower than normal at preferred speed when walking, especially during the single-support phase of walking ($P < 0.01$). The differences, however, became minimal when SCI subjects were compared to normal subjects walking at matched speeds.

Even though SCI subjects compared well in their RTs with normal subjects walking at matched speeds, it is possible that they still need more attention than normal subjects do during walking. For this

reason, the difference between sitting and walking RTs was computed as a new variable, to remove individual differences and to illustrate the real attentional cost of walking (Fig. 6B). This transformed RT was significantly higher in SCI subjects as compared to normal subjects ($P < 0.05$).

In general, results of RTs reveal that SCI subjects need to allocate significantly more of their attentional resources to walking than normal subjects. Several arguments may explain this difference. SCI subjects experienced impaired postural stability, lack of equilibrium, muscle weakness, sensory loss and spasticity. To counterbalance those problems, they must closely monitor their movements and evaluate the impact of those during walking. This evaluation requires more attentional resources given to sensory integration (visual, vestibular and proprioceptive). The implication is that production of walking in SCI subjects is very demanding. Any change in environ-

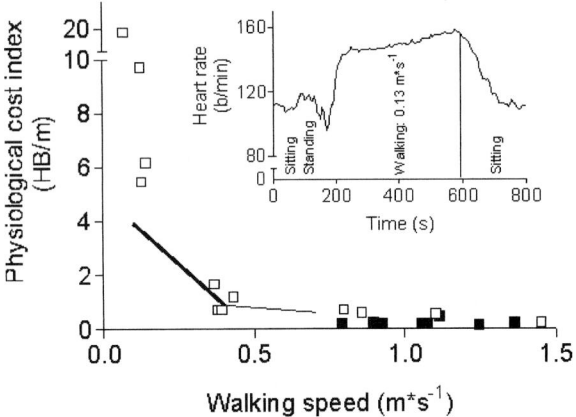

Fig. 5. Physiological cost index (PCI) of walking in normal (■) and SCI (□) subjects, expressed in heart beats per meter walked. The right top panel shows an example of the raw data used to calculate the PCI in sitting, standing, during walking and then back to sitting. The bottom panel illustrates the PCI in relation of the walking speed in both normal and SCI subjects. The bold line represents the upper 95% confidence interval of the PCI of able-bodied participants at the 0.7, 0.4 and 0.1 m/s conditions.

ment or external demands, such as crossing a traffic intersection or obstacles, would pose increased risk on the walking behavior.

Adaptation to inclined walking

Fig. 7 shows the kinematics and muscle patterns of normal and SCI subjects during inclined walking. Increasing the treadmill slope from 0 to 15° induced a gradual increase in hip and knee flexion and in ankle dorsiflexion from late swing through the stance phase in all normal subjects. The vertical displacement of the greater trochanter, as shown on top of Fig. 7, was quite stable across the different grades. In the group of seven SCI subjects, however, lower limb motions did not show consistent patterns of adaptation. Rather, a spectrum of adaptation was found and ranged from a near normal adaptation to an adaptation involving mainly the hip joint. SCI subjects who were unable to achieve the steepest slope (15%), showed only an increased hip flexion in early stance combined with an elevation of the greater trochanter (hip hiking) during the swing phase in all walking conditions (see example in Fig. 7). This hip hiking was used to compensate for the absence of TA activity during the swing phase (Leroux et al., 1999).

Increasing the treadmill slope from 0 to 15 induced a gradual increase in the amplitude of EMG activity of all muscles in normal subjects (Fig. 7). The most marked changes occurred in the medial gastrocnemius (MG). When the treadmill slope was raised to 15, the peak amplitude of MG activity increased 3.5 times the control value (level walking) during push-off. In most of the SCI subjects, the amplitude of EMG activity of thigh muscles (VL and MH) also increased during uphill walking, although to a lesser extent than in normal subjects (an example of one SCI subject is shown on Fig. 7). For the leg muscles, soleus and MG, a prolongation of the EMG activity and an absence of peak activity during the push-off phase were found in all SCI subjects. Further, an increase in slope was not associated with an increase in the amplitude of EMG activity in SCI subjects. For the TA, the modulation ranged from near normal (in four subjects) to a complete absence of activity (see Fig. 7) during inclined walking. The absence of increase in the level of activation of MG likely results in a weak push off and compensatory mechanisms from proximal segments might be used to adapt to uphill walking (Leroux et al., 1999).

A recent study has been conducted to investigate the contribution of the trunk and pelvis during inclined walking in normal and SCI subjects (Leroux et al., 2001). Briefly, results showed the importance of trunk and pelvic segments in the postural adaptation to inclined walking. Trunk and pelvic movements do not seem to participate directly in the generation or absorption of energy required for walking up-and-down slope. It was shown that total angular excursions were consistent across walking grades in sagittal and transverse planes and varied to a small degree in the frontal plane (not illustrated). However, modifications in trunk and pelvic vertical alignment would allow lower limbs to perform the most efficient patterns of movements during uphill and downhill walking. It is proposed that trunk and pelvic postural modifications are mainly performed to assist lower limbs when adapting to inclined walking.

Adaptation to speed and obstacles

Fig. 8 shows the average angular displacement profiles as a function of the walking speed in the normal

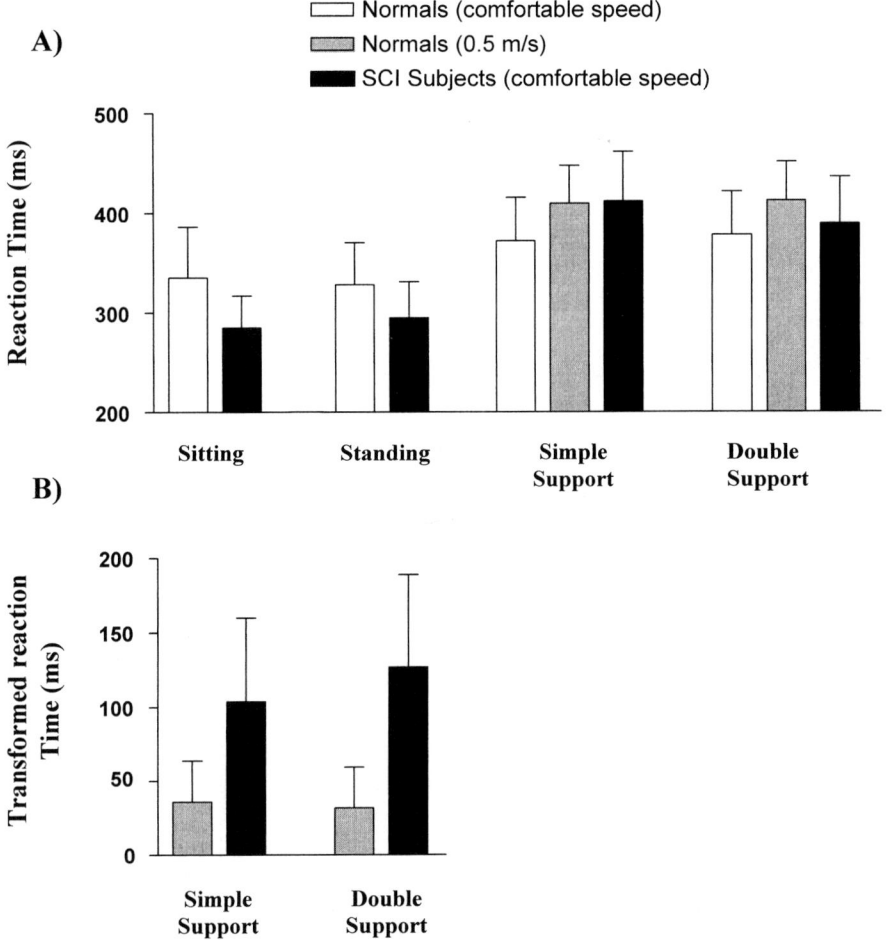

Fig. 6. (A) Reaction time for the different conditions; sitting, standing and walking when stimuli were presented in single-support (SS) and double-support (DS) phases of locomotion at preferred speed and at 0.5 m/s. (B) Average transformed reaction time (individual walking reaction time minus individual setting reaction time) during walking when stimuli was presented in SS or in DS at 0.5 m/s.

group (Fig. 8A) and in one SCI subject (Fig. 8B). The SCI subject could walk at a maximal speed of 1.0 m/s on the treadmill, and was graded as a D according to the ASIA impairment scale (Ditunno et al., 1994; Maynard et al., 1997). Functionally, he could walk overground without a walking aid although he normally used one forearm crutch.

For normal subjects (Fig. 8A), the mean angular displacement profiles are shown for speeds of 0.1, 0.3, 0.5 and 1.0 m/s along with the 95% confidence interval for the 1.0 m/s condition. Some striking changes as a function of the speed can be observed for all three joints. For the lower speed conditions, the amount of hip extension at the end of stance

and the amount of hip flexion during swing and early stance are substantially reduced as compared to values obtained at 1.0 m/s. These results are directly linked to the reduced stride length. Similarly, at the knee joint, the brief flexion associated with weight acceptance normally occurring in early stance, is greatly reduced or absent at speeds of 0.5 m/s or less, and the amount of knee flexion during the swing phase is reduced as the walking speed decreases. In contrast, the amount of knee flexion at foot-contact for the 0.1 m/s condition is increased by about 8° as compared to the 1.0 m/s condition. At the ankle joint, there is a small decrease in the passive dorsiflexion during stance when speed decreases. In

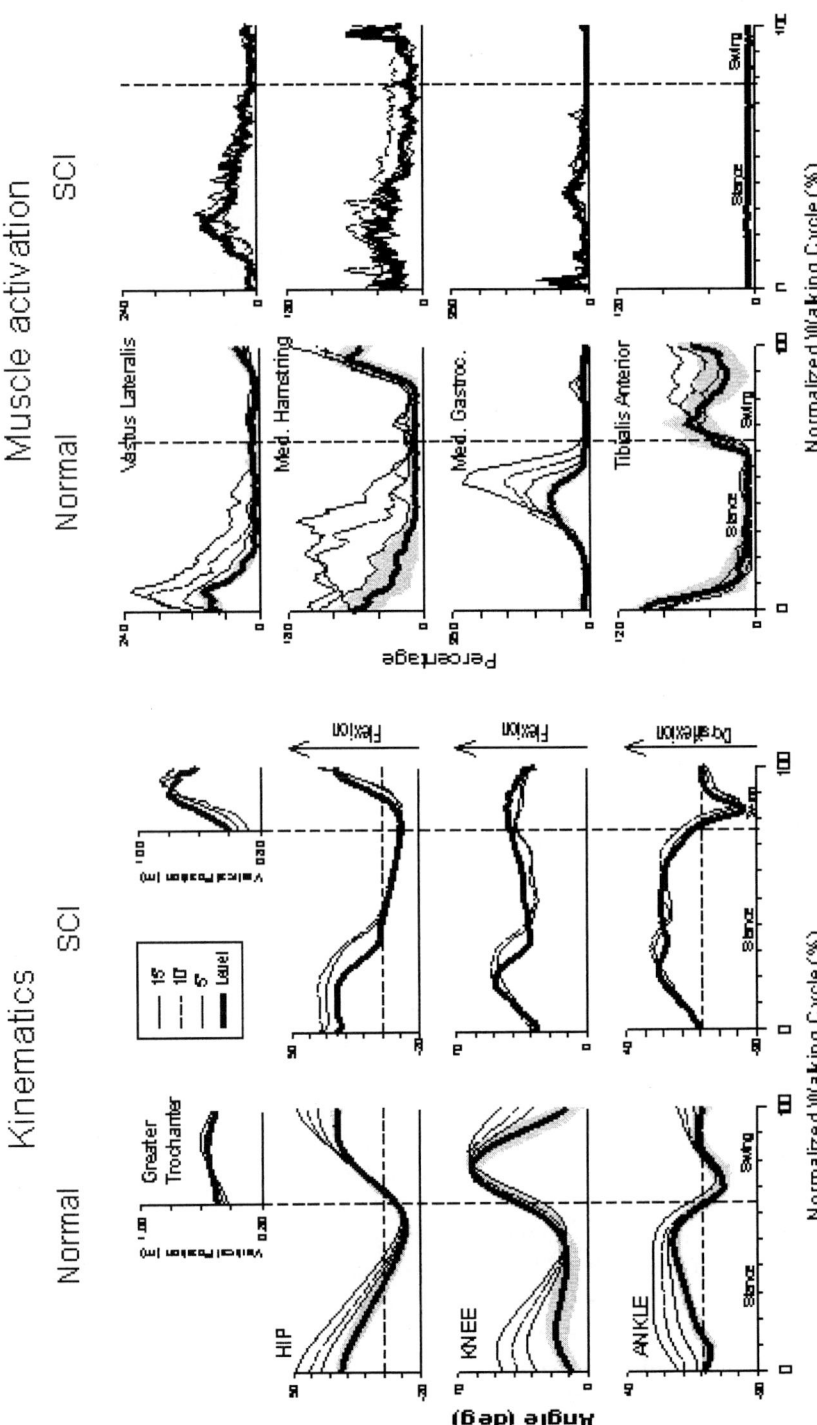

Fig. 7. Angular excursions of hip, knee and ankle joints, as well as EMG ensemble averages of lower limb muscles during uphill walking normalized to the gait cycle (from one foot contact −0% to the next 100%). The trajectory of the greater trochanter is shown on top. This figure shows the average of the seven normal subjects and one SCI subject (each line represents the average of 5 cycles). The gray area represents the 95% confidence interval for the normal group. Amplitude of EMG activity was normalized and expressed as a percentage of the level condition. Note that locomotor adaptation is very limited in this SCI subject.

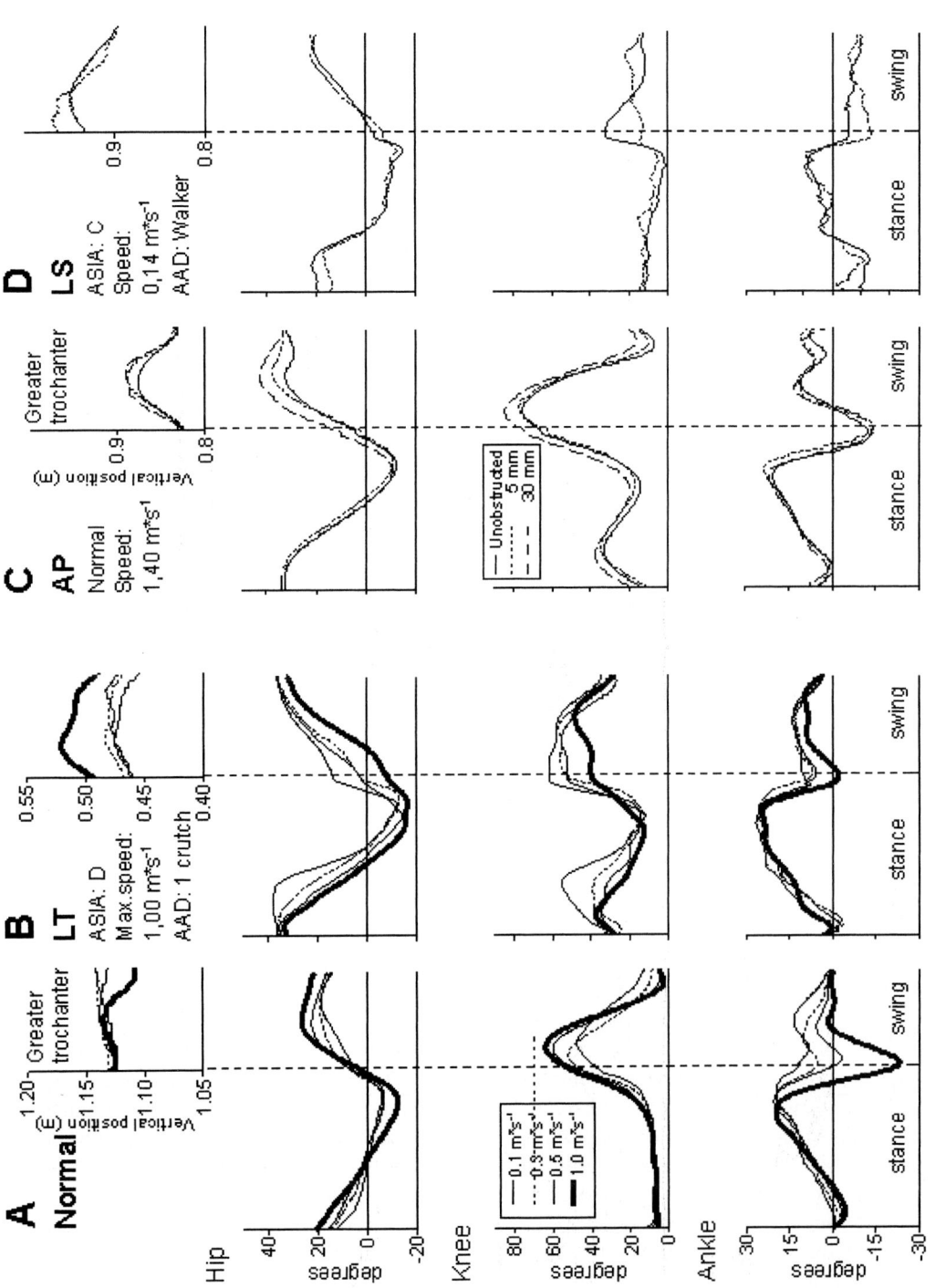

Fig. 8. Angular excursions of hip, knee and ankle during different speeds (A and B) and different obstacles (C and D) in normal (A and C) and SCI subjects (B and D).

contrast, at push-off, the ankle joint remains in a dorsiflexed position during push-off at 0.1 and 0.3 m/s and the amount of dorsiflexion increased at lower speeds during swing.

When the angular displacements of the lower limb joints of SCI subjects (Fig. 8B) are compared to those of the normal group (Fig. 8A), striking differences can be observed both in terms of amplitude and profiles. First, there was a greater amount of flexion at the hip and knee joints at foot-contact for all speeds (0.1–1.0 m/s). This finding was also observed in the average angular displacement patterns of a group of SCI subjects (Fig. 2C). A striking finding is the high variability in the displacement profiles among the SCI subjects (not illustrated). For all SCI subjects, the profiles of the hip, knee and ankle angular displacements fell outside of the normal 95% confidence interval, either in part or for the whole profile (not illustrated). For example, the hip joint remained in extension longer than that of the normal group, and showed increased flexion during the swing period as function of the speed. At the knee joint, as presented above, it is clear that most of the subjects made foot-contact with the knee in a flexed position and some of them maintained knee flexion throughout stance (Fig. 2C and Fig. 8B). During the swing phase, the knee decreased in maximum flexion later than compared to the normal group. At the ankle joint, SCI subjects show more dorsiflexion throughout stance as compared the normal group at the same speed. During swing, the individual profiles are very variable going from extreme plantarflexion to dorsiflexion (Fig. 2C) and plantarflexion was generally decreased as a function of speed.

Examples of normal and SCI anticipatory locomotor adjustments are also shown in Fig. 8C and D. The extreme of the adaptation spectrum is represented in Fig. 8D. The upper part of panels, Fig. 8A and B, show the relative vertical displacements of GT relative to its position in quiet standing. The normal subject increases both the flexion of hip and during the early swing with 5 and 30 mm obstacles. At the opposite end of the spectrum of adaptations, the SCI subject was capable of clearing only the 5-mm obstacle. He did not adapt the trajectory of the fifth metatarsal during the obstructed condition (30 mm) showing that the unobstructed foot trajectory was sufficient to clear such a low height obstacle.

However, there were changes in the locomotor pattern with an elevation of the greater trochanter and a decrease in knee flexion at the initiation of the swing phase (Fig. 8D). Therefore, different strategies can be adopted by the SCI subjects, such as elevating the greater trochanter to adapt to increased speed, or increasing knee flexion to clear obstacles as used by normal subjects.

Effect of treatment approaches on functional prerequisites in the recovery of locomotion

The combination of a simple functional electrical stimulation (FES) system with locomotor training shows the usefulness of such devices to improve walking (Wieler et al., 1999). Fig. 9A illustrates the increase of maximal walking speed of an SCI subject using a single-channel FES system over a period of more than 3 years. For the group of chronic SCI subjects, a gradual improvement of the maximal walking speed was observed within the first year, with the mean magnitude increase of 0.50 m/s. However, more remarkably, walking speed of the SCI subjects was increased even when the stimulator was temporarily turned off. This retained increase of walking speed without FES has been termed the therapeutic effect and is of the same magnitude as reported earlier (Ladouceur and Barbeau, 2000a,b). This therapeutic effect on walking has been reported anecdotally for hemiplegic patients (Liberson et al., 1961) and in SCI subjects (Granat et al., 1993; Ladouceur and Barbeau, 1997). Changes in their assistive ambulatory devices (Fig. 9A from crutches to canes), as well decreases in their energy cost (Fig. 9B) of the walking behavior were also observed. From these results, it was concluded that increases in maximal walking speed during training with the FES orthosis is mostly due to a therapeutic effect, which implies that mechanisms of plasticity occurred during the training paradigm. The locomotor recovery observed with this training paradigm appears to result from the interaction between these plastic changes in combination with the proper activation of peripheral afferents (including cutaneous and proprioceptive) (Ladouceur and Barbeau, 2000a,b).

The effect of FES assisted walking on the physiological cost index and walking speed during the 5-min walk was examined in 12 participants that

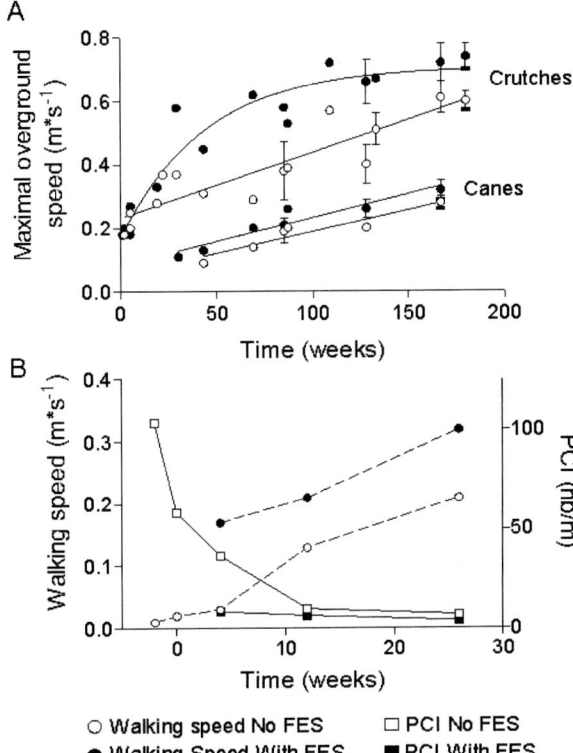

Fig. 9. (A) One SCI subject showing the longitudinal changes of the maximal overground walking speed occurring with locomotor training using FES-assisted walking. This panel is an example of a quantitative change between the combined (open squares) and therapeutic (filled squares) conditions, as well as example of the similar longitudinal changes occurring when the person uses different ambulatory assistive devices. Squares represent the condition with forearm crutches; circles represent the condition with two canes. (B) The same SCI subject showing the overground speed (left axes) and the energy cost (right axis).

had been using FES assisted walking for at least 3 months (Ladouceur and Barbeau, 2000b). Because initial measurement of the physiological cost index was not acquired at the onset of FES assisted walking, not all participants were followed in time. An example of the data recorded by the heart rate monitor can be found in Fig. 5. To evaluate the effect of training with FES assisted walking on the physiological cost of walking we studied SCI participants longitudinally from onset of FES assisted walking. When combined with time, the results showed a positive effect diminished the physiological cost of walking by a factor of two for all SCI subjects that

were evaluated for a duration of more than 3 months (Ladouceur and Barbeau, 2000b).

Functional implication

In summary, the results from this review demonstrated that SCI subjects can adapt to a certain limit of the functional prerequisite of posture and walking, such as speed, slope, obstacles, walking aids, energy, and attentional demand. Understanding the strategy that SCI subjects used can lead us to develop concepts and principles that can be included in rehabilitation. Fig. 10 illustrated a comprehensive schematic of several important factors necessary to achieve functional recovery. Several new approaches have been developed in the last 20 years, such as locomotor training using BWS or FES; pharmacological approaches and their combination to enhanced recovery in the neurological population particularly SCI subjects. These approaches have shown great potential and are in the process of validation in the rehabilitation setting. Recent reviews summarize those findings (Barbeau et al., 1998a,b; Rossignol, 2000).

Fig. 10 also illustrates several important prerequisites necessary to achieve functional recovery and how treatment approaches affect such prerequisites, as reviewed in the present paper. From the present review, several important principles for rehabilitation have emerged.

Specificity of the task

Locomotor training is task specific. For example, if the spinal animal is trained to stand and not to walk, they will perform very well during standing but not as well during walking, as for the group of spinal cats that have been trained to walk could walk very well at higher speed (Lovely et al., 1986). In humans with stroke or spinal cord injury, it has been demonstrated that locomotor training in different forms could be more powerful than conventional treatment using more traditional concepts, such as standing and exercising while aligned on the ground (Barbeau et al., 1992; Werning and Müller, 1992; Hesse et al., 1995; Werning et al., 1995; Visintin et al., 1998).

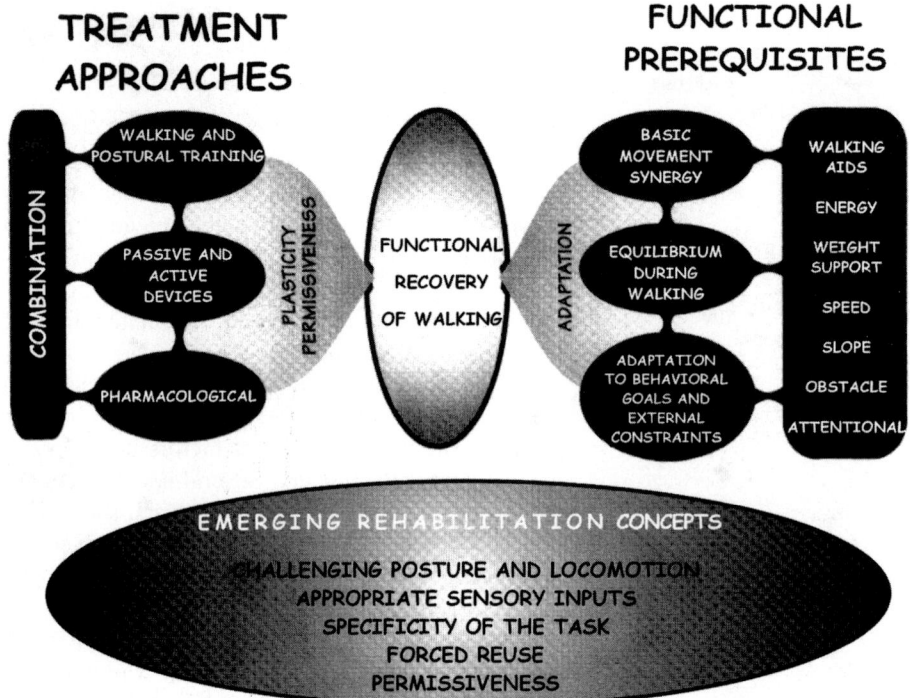

Fig. 10. A model of recovery of walking following spinal cord injury. In the left panel, treatment approaches, such as pharmacological, locomotor training, and their combination can enhance the functional recovery of walking, suggesting that plastic changes occur several years after spinal cord injury. In the right panel, several important prerequisites to achieve adaptation, walking posture and navigation are illustrated. In the bottom panel, proposed emerging rehabilitation concepts, both from animal and human studies, are illustrated.

Appropriate sensory inputs

It appears from animal and human studies that the locomotor training does not consist of only putting the spinal animal or the SCI subjects on the treadmill. Appropriate inputs, such as giving just enough weight that the animal is able to cope with are essential to maximize the functional recovery. The same strategy should by applied in SCI and stroke subjects (Visintin and Barbeau, 1989 and Visintin et al., 1998).

The important role of sensory inputs has been shown in animal studies. First, Grillner and Rossignol provided evidence indicating that afferent from the hip joint are very important in resetting and entraining the locomotor rhythm (see Rossignol, 1996 for comprehensive review). Secondly, the modulation of reflexes has been shown to be task and phase specific in intact and spinalized cats as well as in human subjects. For example, mechanical or electrical stimulation to the paw or to the sural nerve during the flexor activity enhanced the ipsilateral flexor activity as well the contralateral extensor activity but when the stimulus was delivered during the ipsilateral extensor activity it increased the extensor activity (see Rossignol, 1996). Thirdly, appropriate loading has been considered as a very important input from animal studies (Rossignol, 1996; Dietz, 2000).

In fact, there is increased evidence that Ib afferent from ankle extensors during locomotion leads to autogenic excitation rather than inhibition (Dietz, 2000). The mechanism of the effect was still unclear but recent animal studies strongly support the role of modulation of the extensor load receptors probably arising from Golgi tendon organs (Dietz and Duysens, 2000). This represents a newly discovered function of these receptors in the regulation of stance and walking. In spinal cord population, appropriate loading during the support phase can enhance the extensor activity as well as increased the vertical force during support phase and also trigger swing phase in the contralateral limb (Barbeau et al., 1992; Werning et al., 1995) and can be incorporated in the locomotor training strategy. The benefit of locomotor training using BWS may depend partly on the degree of body unloading during walking but this needs further investigation.

Challenging posture and walking adaptation

Incorporating posture and speed demands with a locomotor intervention are essential to increase the maximal walking speed, decrease energy cost and to change walking aids (Ladouceur and Barbeau, 2000a,b). Training and staying at a comfortable speed level will not challenge the patient. Thus, to improve locomotor and postural adaptation, it is important, first, to understand the limiting control mechanisms and second, to identify important determinant variables that could be used to evaluate proper locomotion and posture and incorporate them into a locomotor and posture training strategy.

Forced reuse

The use of assistive walking devices, such as parallel bars while necessary for the expression of the locomotor behavior, can also lead to over compensation and limited adaptive capacity. It is important to identify different means of achieving locomotion at the early stages of training, such as the use of BWS, and progressively decrease the weight support over the training period. In addition, BWS induced a pattern of forced-reuse of the paretic limb such that the patients could not compensate by using the non-paretic upper and/or lower limbs.

Plasticity and permissiveness

Results from animal and human studies revealed that several important factors could allow permissive walking in SCI subjects and other neurological population. For example, in the behaving spinal cat preparations, some drugs such as noradrenergic agents combined with locomotor training can accelerate the recovery of walking (Chau et al., 1998). When recovery occurred, the locomotor pattern could be maintained even if the noradrenergic drugs have been removed. In SCI subjects, cloni-

dine could also express a limited walking behavior (Rémy-Neris et al., 1999) but when combined with locomotor training using body weight support, the recovery of walking was greatly enhanced (Fung et al., 1990).

Other permissive situations, such as using a passive (body weight support) or/and active device (functional electrical stimulation) could enhance the recovery of walking when combined with locomotor training (Visintin and Barbeau, 1989; Visintin et al., 1998; Ladouceur and Barbeau, 2000a,b).

Conclusion

In conclusion, this review summarizes very important aspects of locomotor adaptations that are relevant to neurorehabilitation. First, understanding the basic mechanism of adaptation of locomotion and posture leads to the identification of control variables that are important to properly evaluate and treat neurological patient populations. Secondly, understanding the effect of new treatment approaches such as BWS or/and FES, pharmacological interventions and their combinations on locomotor adaptation will lead to a more comprehensive and integrative approach in the development of rehabilitation strategies. Finally, emerging rehabilitation principles based on both from animals and human findings should recognized as important concepts in neuroplasticity that can impact on motor learning and rehabilitation.

References

Barbeau, H., Danakas, M.B. and Arsenault (1992) The effects of locomotor training in spinal cord injured subjects: a preliminary study. *Restor. Neurol. Neurosci.*, 5: 81–84.

Barbeau, H., Pépin, A., Norman, K.E., Ladouceur, M. and Leroux, A. (1998a) Walking after spinal cord injury: control and recovery. *Neuroscientist*, 4: 14–24.

Barbeau, H., Norman, K., Fung, J., Visintin, M. and Ladouceur, M. (1998b) Does neurorehabilitation play a role in the recovery of walking in neurological populations? In: O. Kiehn, R.M. Harris-Warrick, L.M. Jordan, H. Hultborn and N. Kudo (Eds.), Neuronal mechanisms for generating locomotor activity. *Ann. N.Y. Acad. Sci.*, 860: 377–392.

Barbeau, H., Wainberg, M. and Finch, L. (1987) Description and application of a system for locomotor rehabilitation. *Med. Diol. Eng. Comput.*, 25: 341–344.

Bélanger, M. (1990) A quantitative comparison of the locomotor patterns and the capacity for adaptation before and after spinalisation of the cat. Ph.D. Thesis, University of Montreal.

Brandell, B.R. (1977) Functional roles of the calf and vastus muscles in locomotion. *Am. J. Phys. Med.*, 56: 59–74.

Chau, C., Barbeau, H. and Rossignol, S. (1998) Early locomotor training with clonidine in spinal cats. *J. Neurophysiol.*, 79(1): 392–409.

Chen, H.C., Ashton-Miller, J.A., Alexander, N.B. and Schults, A.B. (1991) Stepping over obstacles: gait patterns of healthy young and old adults. *J. Gerontol.*, 46: 196–203.

Chou, L.S. and Draganich, L.F. (1997) Stepping over an obstacle increases the motions and moments of the joints of the trailing limb in young adults. *J. Biomech.*, 30: 331–337.

Chou, L.S., Draganich, L.F. and Song, S.M. (1997) Minimum energy trajectories of the swing ankle when stepping over obstacles of different heights. *J. Biomech.*, 30: 115–120.

Chou, L.S. and Draganich, L.F. (1998) Increasing obstacle height and decreasing toe–obstacle distance affect the joint moments of the stance limb differently when stepping over an obstacle. *Gait Posture*, 8: 186–204.

Chung, B., Barbeau, H., Torres-Moreno, R. and Gravel, D. (2001) Biomechanical analysis of crutch assisted walking in persons with incomplete spinal cord injury. *Spinal Cord*, in press.

Conrad, B., Benecke, R. and Meinck, H.M. (1985) Gait disturbances in paraspastic patients. In: P.J. Delwaide and R.R. Young (Eds.), *Clinical Neurophysiology in Spasticity*. Elsevier Science Publishers, Amsterdam, pp. 155–174.

Dietz, V. and Berger, W. (1983) Normal and impaired regulation of muscle stiffness in gait: a new hypothesis about muscle hypertonia. *Exp. Neurol.*, 79: 680–687.

Dietz, V. and Duysens, J. (2000) Significance of load receptor input during locomotion: a review. *Gait Posture*, 11(2): 102–110.

Dietz, V.S.J.D. (2000) Significance of load receptor input during locomotion: a review. *Gait Posture*, 11(2): 102–110.

Dietz, V., Quintern, J. and Berger, W. (1981) Electrophysiological studies of gait in spasticity and rigidity. Evidence that altered mechanical properties of muscle contribute to hypertonia. *Brain*, 104: 431–449.

Ditunno Jr., J.F., Young, W., Donovan, W.H. and Creasey, G. (1994) The international standards booklet for neurological and functional classification of spinal cord injury. *Am. Spinal Injury Assoc. Paraplegia*, 32: 70–80.

Fung, J. and Barbeau, H. (1990) A dynamic EMG profile index to quantify muscular activation disorder in spastic paretic gait. *Electroencephalogr. Clin. Neurophysiol.*, 73: 491–495.

Fung, J., Stewart, J.E. and Barbeau, H. (1990) The combined effects of clonidine and cyproheptadine with interactive training on the modulation of locomotion in spinal cord injured subjects. *J. Neurol. Sci.*, 100(1–2): 85–93.

Go, B.K., DeVivo, M.J. and Richards, J.S. (1995) The epidemiology of spinal cord injury. In: S.L. Stover, J.A. DeLisa and G.G. Whiteneck (Eds.), *Spinal Cord Injury: Clinical Outcomes from the Model Systems*. Aspen, Gaithersberg, MD, 21–55.

Granat, M.H., Ferguson, A.C.B., Andrews, B.J. and Delargy, M. (1993) The role of functional electrical stimulation in the rehabilitation of patients with incomplete spinal cord injury: observed benefits during gait studies. *Paraplegia*, 31: 207–215.

Hesse, S., Bertelt, C., Jahnke, M.T., Schaffrin, A., Baake, P., Malezic, M. and Mauritz, K.H. (1995) Treadmill training with partial body weight support compared with physiotherapy in nonambulatory hemiparetic patients. *Stroke*, 26: 976–981.

Ladouceur, M. and Barbeau, H. (1997) Effects of walking training with a functional electrical stimulation assisted orthosis for spinal cord injured persons: a longitudinal study. In: D. Propovic (Ed.), *Proceedings of the Second Annual Conference of the International Functional Electrical Stimulation Society and Fifth Triennial Conference Neural Protheses: Motor Systems 5*, pp. 193–194.

Ladouceur, M. and Barbeau, H. (2000a) Functional electrical stimulation-assisted walking for persons with incomplete spinal injuries: changes in the kinematics and physiological cost of overground walking. *Scand. J. Rehabil. Med.*, 32(2): 72–79.

Ladouceur, M. and Barbeau, H. (2000b) Functional electrical stimulation-assisted walking for persons with incomplete spinal cord injury: longitudinal changes in maxial overground walking speed. *Scand. J. Rehabil. Med.*, 32(1): 28–36.

Lajoie, Y. and Barbeau, H. (1999) Attentional requirements of walking in spinal cord injured subjects compared to normal subjects. *Spinal Cord*, 37: 245–250.

Lange, G.W., Hintermeister, R.A., Schlegel, T., Dillman, C.J. and Steadman, J.R. (1996) Electromyographic and kinematic analysis of graded treadmill walking and the implications for knee rehabilitation. *J. Orthop. Sports Phys. Ther.*, 23: 294–301.

Leroux, A., Fung, J. and Barbeau, H. (1999) Adaptation of the walking pattern to uphill walking in normal and spinal-cord injured subjects. *Exp. Brain Res.*, 126: 359–368.

Leroux, A., Fung, J. and Barbeau, H. (2001) Postural adaptation to inclined walking. I. Normal Strategies. *Gait Posture*, in press.

Liberson, W.T., Holmquest, H.J., Scott, D. and Dow, A. (1961) Functional electrotherapy: stimulation of the peroneal nerve synchronized with the swing phase of the gait in hemiplegic patients. *Arch. Phys. Med. Rehabil.*, 42: 101–105.

Lovely, R.G., Gregor, R.J., Roy, R.R. and Edgerton, V.R. (1986) Effects of training on the recovery of full-weight-bearing stepping in the adult spinal cat. *Exp. Neurol.*, 92: 421–435.

Maynard Jr., F.M., Bracken, M.B., Creasey, G., Ditunno Jr., J.F., Donovan, W.H., Ducker, T.B., Garber, S.L., Marino, R.J., Stover, S.L., Tator, C.H., Waters, R.L., Wilberger, J.E. and Young, W. (1997) International standards for neurological and functional classification of spinal cord injury. *Spinal Cord*, 35: 266–274.

McFadyen, B.J. and Carnahan, H. (1997) Anticipatory locomotor adjustments for accommodating versus avoiding level changes in humans. *Exp. Brain Res.*, 114: 500–506.

McFadyen, B.J. and Winter, D.A. (1991) Anticipatory locomotor adjustments during obstructed human walking. *Neurosci. Res. Commun.*, 9: 37–44.

McFadyen, B.J., Magan, G.A. and Boucher, J.P. (1993) Anticipatory locomotor adjustments for avoiding visible, fixed obstacles of varying proximity. *Hum. Mov. Sci.*, 12: 259–272.

Melis, E., Torres-Moreno, R., Barbeau, H., Chilco, L. and Lemaire, E.D. (1999) Analysis of assisted-gait characteristics in persons with incomplete spinal cord injury. *Spinal Cord*, 37: 430–435.

Mirbagheri, M.M., Kearney, R.E. and Barbeau, H. (1998a) Stretch reflex behavior of spastic ankle under passive and active conditions. *Annu. Int. Conf. IEEE Eng. Med. Biol. Soc.*, 20: 2325–2327.

Mirbagheri, M.M., Kearney, R.E. and Barbeau, H. (1998b) Abnormal passive and intrinsic stiffness in the spastic ankle. *Annu. Int. Conf. IEEE Eng. Med. Biol. Soc.*, 20: 2338–2340.

Mirbagheri, M.M., Kearney, R.E., Ladouceur, M. and Barbeau, H. (2001) Abnormal stretch reflex mechanics in spastic spinal cord injured subjects. *Brain Res.*, in press.

Murray, M.P., Kory, R.C., Clarkson, B.H. and Sepic, S.B. (1966) Comparison of free and fast speed walking patterns of normal men. *Am. J. Phys. Med.*, 45: 8–24.

Nilsson, J., Thorstensson, A. and Halbertsma, J. (1985) Changes in leg movements and muscle activity with speed of locomotion and mode of progression in humans. *Acta Physiol. Scand.*, 123: 457–475.

Norman, K.E., Pépin, A., Ladouceur, M. and Barbeau, H. (1995) A treadmill apparatus and harness support for evaluation and rehabilitation of gait. *Arch. Phys. Med. Rehabil.*, 76: 772–778.

Patla, A.E. and Prentice, S.D. (1995) The role of active forces and intersegmental dynamics in the control of limb trajectory over obstacles during locomotion in humans. *Exp. Brain Res.*, 106: 499–504.

Patla, A.E. and Rietdyk, S. (1993) Visual control of limb trajectory over obstacles during locomotion: effect of obstacle height and width. *Gait Posture*, 1: 45–60.

Patla, A.E., Prentice, S.D., Robinson, C. and Neufeld, J. (1991) Visual control of locomotion: strategies for changing direction and for going over obstacles. *J. Exp. Psychol. Hum. Percept. Perform.*, 17: 603–634.

Rémy-Neris, O., Barbeau, H., Daniel, O., Boiteau, F., Cambeau, M. and Bussel, B. (1999) The effects of intrathecalclonidine on spinal reflexes and on locomotion in incomplete paraplegic subjects. *Exp. Brain Res*, 129(3): 433–440.

Rossignol, S. (1996) Neural control of stereotypic limb movements. In: L.B. Rowell and J.T. Shepherd (Eds.), *Handbook of Physiology, Section 12. Exercise: Regulation and Integration of Multiple Systems.* American Physiological Society, Bethesda, MD, pp. 173–216.

Rossignol, S. (2000) Locomotion and its recovery after spinal injury. *Curr. Opin. Neurobiol.*, 10(6): 708–716.

Rossignol, S., Drew, T., Brustein, E. and Jiang, W. (1999) Locomotor performance and adaptation after partial or complete spinal cord lesions in the cat. *Prog. Brain Res.*, 123: 349–365.

Simonsen, E.B., Dyhre-Poulsen, P. and Voigt, M. (1995) Excitability of the soleus H-reflex during graded walking in humans. *Acta Physiol. Scand.*, 153: 21–32.

Sinkjaer, T. and Magnussen, I. (1994) Passive, intrinsic, and reflex-mediated stiffness in the ankle extensors of hemiparetic patients. *Brain*, 117: 355–363.

Sinkjaer, T., Andersen, J.B. and Nielsen, J.F. (1996) Impaired stretch reflex and joint torque modulation during spastic gait. *J. Neurophysiol.*, 76: 1112–1120.

Thilmann, A.F., Fellows, S.J. and Garms, E. (1991) The mechanism of spastic muscle hypertonus. Variation in reflex gain over the time course of spasticity. *Brain*, 114: 233–244.

Visintin, M. and Barbeau, H. (1989) The effects of body weight support with locomotor pattern of spastic paretic patients. *Can. J. Neurol. Sci.*, 16(3): 315–325.

Visintin, M. and Barbeau, H. (1994) The effect of parallel bars, body weight support and speed on the modulation of the locomotor pattern of spastic paretic gait. *Paraplegia*, 32: 540–553.

Visintin, M., Barbeau, H., Korner-Bitensky, N. and Mayo, N.E. (1998) A new approach to retrain gait in stroke patients through body weight support and treadmill stimulation. *Stroke*, 29(6): 1122–1128.

Wall, J.C., Nottrodt, J.W. and Charteris, J. (1981) The effects of uphill and downhill walking on pelvic oscillations in transverse plane. *Ergonomics*, 24: 807–816.

Werning, A. and Müller, S. (1992) Laufband locomotion with body weight support improved walking in persons with severe spinal cord injuries. *Paraplegia*, 30: 229–238.

Werning, A., Nanassy, S.M., Nanassy, A. and Cagol, E. (1995) Short Communication: Laufband therapy based on 'rules of spinal locomotion' is effective in spinal cord injured persons. *Eur. J. Neurosci.*, 7: 823–829.

Wieler, M., Stein, R.B., Ladouceur, M., Whittaker, M., Smith, A.W., Nieman, S., Barbeau, H., Bugaresti, J., Aimone, E. and Biemann, I. (1999) Multi-center evaluation of electrical stimulation systems for walking. *Arch. Phys. Med. Rehabil.*, 80(5): 495–500.

Yang, J.F., Fung, J., Edamura, M., Blunt, R., Stein, R.B. and Barbeau, H. (1991) H-reflex modulation during walking in spastic paretic subjects. *Can. J. Neurol. Sci.*, 18: 443–452.

L. McKerracher, G. Doucet and S. Rossignol (Eds.)
Progress in Brain Research, Vol. 137

CHAPTER 3

Electrical stimulation for therapy and mobility after spinal cord injury

Richard B. Stein [1,*], Su Ling Chong [1], Kelvin B. James [1], Aiko Kido [1], Gordon J. Bell [2], L. Aaron Tubman [3] and Marc Bélanger [4]

[1] *Centre for Neuroscience, University of Alberta, Edmonton, AB T6G 2S2, Canada*
[2] *Faculty of Physical Education, University of Alberta, Edmonton, AB T6G 2S2, Canada*
[3] *Faculty of Kinesiology, University of Calgary, AB, Canada*
[4] *Department Kinanthropologie, Université du Québec à Montréal, Montreal, QC, Canada*

Abstract: This article reviews the use of therapeutic and functional electrical stimulation in subjects after a spinal cord injury (SCI). Muscles become much weaker and more fatigable, while bone density decreases dramatically after SCI. Therapeutic stimulation of paralyzed muscles for about 1 h/day can reverse the atrophic changes and markedly increase muscle strength and endurance as well as bone density. Functional electrical stimulation can also improve the speed and efficiency of walking in people with an incomplete SCI. Finally, a modified wheelchair is described in which electrical stimulation or residual voluntary activation of leg muscles can produce movements of a footrest that is coupled to the wheels. The wheelchair can provide greater mobility and fitness to persons who are not functional walkers and currently use their arms to propel a wheelchair.

Introduction

The emphasis in this symposium is justifiably on neural repair following a spinal cord injury (SCI). Although this remains the ultimate goal, much can currently be done to improve function for people with complete and incomplete lesions using electrical stimulation. To the extent that improved function by means of regeneration becomes possible in the coming years, the methods described here may still be helpful to supplement the recovery that occurs naturally or through external means. Electrical stimulation is commonly applied for therapy (therapeutic

electrical stimulation or TES) or for specific functions (functional electrical stimulation or FES). FES has been applied to restore leg function, arm function, breathing, bowel, bladder and sexual function (Peckham and Creasey, 1992; Rushton, 1997). In this short review I will limit my scope to TES and FES for leg function (e.g., walking).

Following spinal cord injury a number of dramatic changes take place. Fig. 1 shows the effects on muscle fiber types after complete SCI. Biopsy samples were taken from the vastus lateralis muscle of human subjects at various times after a complete spinal cord injury (Burnham et al., 1997). In control subjects about 2/3 of the fibers are slow and 1/3 are fast fibers, when stained using antibodies to the fast and slow isoforms of the myosin heavy chains. After SCI the percentage of slow fibers decreases over time almost to zero with a time constant of about 17 months and this is the most complete change in

* Correspondence to: R.B. Stein, Centre for Neuroscience, 513 HMRC, University of Alberta, Edmonton, AB T6G 2S2, Canada. Tel.: +1-780-492-1618; Fax: +1-780-492-1617; E-mail: richard.stein@ualberta.ca

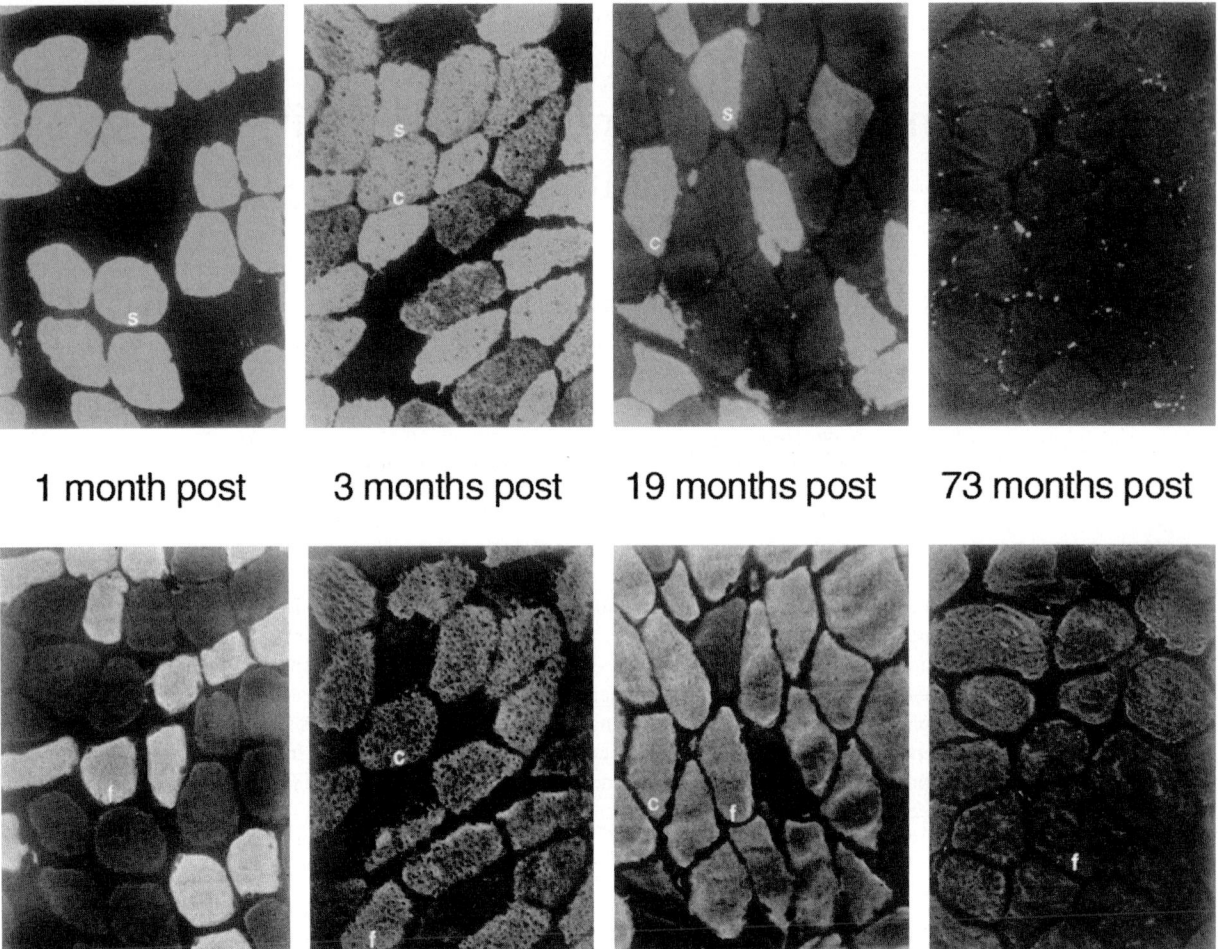

1 month post   3 months post   19 months post   73 months post

Fig. 1. Immunofluorescence labeling of *vastus lateralis* muscle of human subjects studied at different times after spinal cord injury. Muscles were labeled with antibodies to slow (top four panels) and fast (bottom four panels) myosin heavy chain isoforms. Note that the numbers of slow (s) fibers decrease over time and are converted to fast (f) fibers. At intermediate times some fibers coexpress (c) both fast and slow myosin heavy chains. Modified from Burnham et al. (1997).

muscle fiber types that has been described (Andersen et al., 2000). Interestingly, at shorter times after SCI, many of the fibers express both fast and slow myosin isoforms, presumably because the gene for fast myosin has been turned on, but slow myosin molecules remain in many of the fibers.

There is an equally dramatic change in bone density as shown in Fig. 2 (Bélanger et al., 2000). After only 1 year from the lesion the bone density around the knee joint (i.e., distal femur and proximal tibia) has decreased to about 50% of control subjects. Over the next 10–15 years the bone density in that region has fallen to between 20 and 30% of control values.

This severe osteoporosis results in a very high rate of fractures in the distal femur and proximal tibia of long-term SCI subjects, accounting for 34% of all fractures in long-term SCI subjects (Freehafer, 1995).

Therapeutic electrical stimulation

Associated with the change in fiber type is a change in fatigue resistance. Fig. 3 shows the effect of daily stimulation of between 15 min and 8 h on the endurance of tibialis anterior muscles in subjects with a complete SCI (Stein et al., 1992). The muscles were stimulated at 20 Hz and an intensity sufficient to pro-

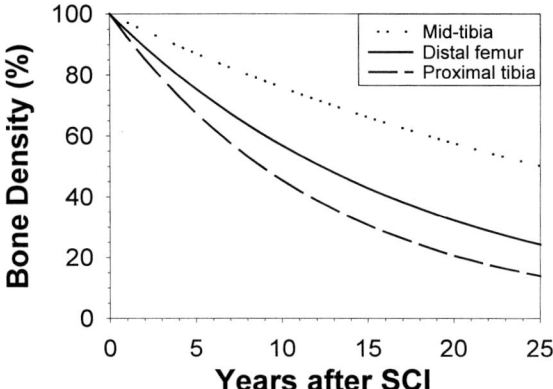

Fig. 2. Bone density falls dramatically after spinal cord injury. Only the fitted curves are shown for 12 subjects who were studied up to 25 years after spinal cord injury. Values are expressed as a percent of the values for control subjects. Density was measured by dual energy X-ray absorptiometry at three places along the leg (Bélanger et al., 2000).

duce a maximal contraction, using a cycle of 5 s on and 5 s off for the periods indicated in Fig. 3. At the start of training the muscles fatigued to about 40% of the initial value within 3–4 min. This is indicated as an endurance index of 0.4, compared to a value of nearly 0.8 in control subjects. This did not change significantly during a 6 week period of stimulation at 15 min/day, but did increase progressively when the stimulation was increased in 6-week blocks to 45

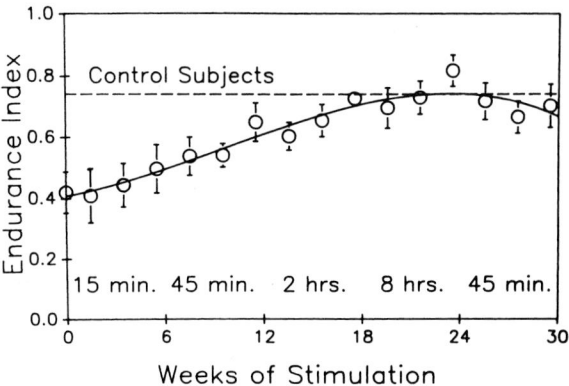

Fig. 3. After SCI, the tibialis anterior muscle becomes much more fatigable. Electrical stimulation can increase the endurance (decrease fatigue) to control values or even above with sufficiently long periods of daily stimulation. Stimulation duration was 15 min/day for 6 weeks, increasing in 6-week blocks to 45 min, 2 h, 8 h and finally a repeat of 45 min. Mean values (± S.E.) are shown (Stein et al., 1992).

min and 2 h. With 8 h/day the endurance reached or even exceeded that of control subjects. Thus, the stimulation was effective in reversing the increased fatigability associated with the change in fiber type after spinal cord injury. However, regular stimulation is required to maintain the endurance, since after a further 6 weeks of stimulation at 45 min/day, the endurance had decreased to the value found earlier in the trial after 6 weeks of stimulation at 45 min/day. This suggests that the value of endurance reached in 6 weeks for a given level of stimulation was due to that level of stimulation, rather than the cumulative history of stimulation.

Thus, the changes in fatigue are not a direct consequence of the SCI itself, but of the disuse of muscles after the SCI. In the 30 weeks of the study some fibers changed from fast to slow (Martin et al., 1992), but longer periods may be required for complete restoration of the changes that had occurred over years (see Fig. 1). Presumably, many fibers had converted from a fast fatigable (FF) to a fast, fatigue-resistant (FR) fiber type. Thus, the maxim, 'Use it or lose it', applies to TES after SCI, as it does to training of muscles under voluntary control. Interestingly, there were no significant changes in muscle strength in these subjects, but a marked increase was seen with a similar program for stimulating the quadriceps muscles of SCI subjects (Bélanger et al., 2000). However, the quadriceps muscles did not show the endurance changes observed for the tibialis anterior muscles. The reasons for these differences are not known, but clearly different muscles can respond differently to similar training protocols.

The amount of torque generated also depended on whether the stimulated muscle moved against a resistance or not (Fig. 4). The SCI subjects were seated, so stimulating the quadriceps will extend the knee and straighten the limb. One leg was free to move with only the resistance of gravity, whereas the other leg moved against a resistance provided by an isokinetic device (Hydragym or a Cybex). The resistance was increased progressively as the muscles became stronger. The fitted torque is shown with the 95% confidence intervals for the two legs and increased nearly 75% in the unresisted muscles and nearly 150% in the resisted muscles.

The changes in bone density from the TES are shown in Fig. 5. There was a 10–11% change in

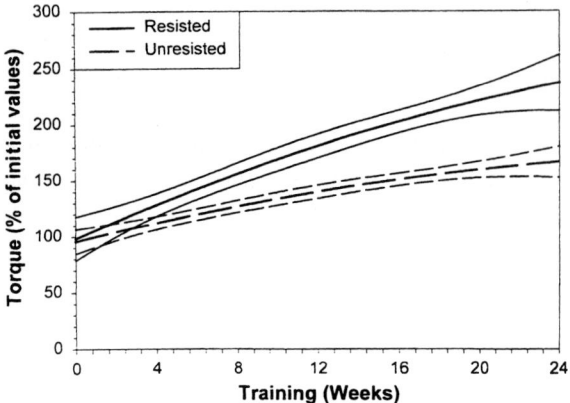

Fig. 4. The strength of quadriceps muscles increases dramatically after stimulation for a number of weeks. One leg of each subject worked against resistance and showed a greater increase (solid line). The other leg only contracted against the force of gravity (dashed lines). The best-fitting parabola and the 95% confidence intervals are shown for the 14 subjects studied (Bélanger et al., 2000).

the distal femur and the proximal tibia, but almost no change in the mid-tibia. The mid-tibia showed no change since the stimulation of the quadriceps muscle primarily stressed the structures around the knee joint and not this part of the leg. Thus, no systemic effects were observed, but only ones that were related to stress on the bone. The increases in

the distal femur and the proximal tibia represent 28% of the bone density lost in these subjects after SCI, compared to control subjects and may substantially reduce fractures in this population. No difference was observed between the resisted and unresisted legs, suggesting that even the resistance of gravity during stimulation was sufficient to generate enough stress on the bone to regenerate at least part of the lost bone mineral density. In conclusion to this section, about 1 h/day of TES is able to reverse many of the atrophic changes that result after SCI in muscles and bones as a result of disuse.

Functional electrical stimulation

The previous section dealt with persons having a complete SCI. By using patterned stimulation of flexor and extensor muscles, even persons with a complete SCI can walk limited distances, but the speed is low and the energy cost is high (Marsolais and Kobetic, 1987; Kralj and Bajd, 1989; Graupe and Kohn, 1994). Use of bracing can reduce the energy cost to some extent, but speed and effort are still high enough that relatively few subjects use FES as their major means of transport in place of a wheelchair (Hirokawa et al., 1990; Nene and Patrick, 1990). We have concentrated in the last few years instead on people with incomplete SCI in the hope that they

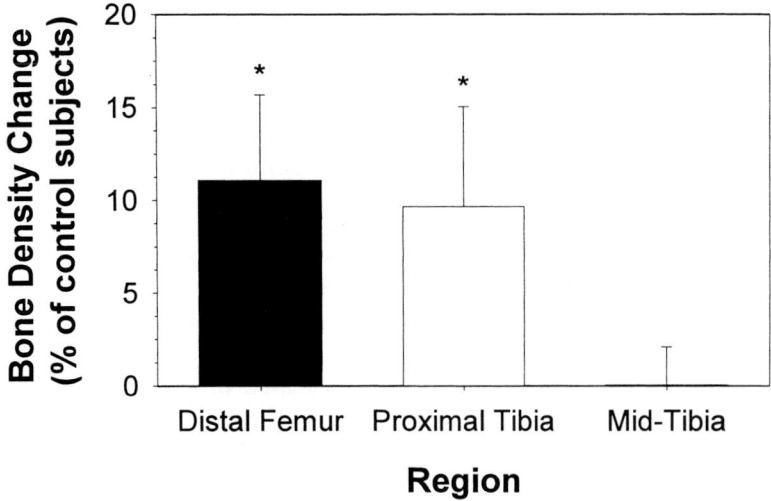

Fig. 5. Bone density increases after electrical stimulation of the quadriceps muscles in the distal femur and the proximal tibia, but not in the mid-tibia. Mean values (+ S.E.) are expressed as a percentage of the bone density for control subjects. The increases represent 28% of the bone density lost after SCI and were statistically significant (*) at $P < 0.05$ (Bélanger et al., 2000).

could use walking with FES as their major means of locomotion. We have also tried to use FES with a modified wheelchair to provide improved mobility and fitness for complete SCI subjects. These two topics are presented here.

Fig. 6 shows the effect of using FES systems with 40 subjects (31 had SCI) in a multi-center trial across Canada (Montreal, Toronto, Edmonton and Vancouver) (Wieler et al., 1999). The FES systems consisted of one to four channels of surface stimulation and were used by subjects on average for a period of 1 year. Since the subjects had a wide range of walking speeds, all values were normalized to the mean for each subject over the period of the trial. At each recording session speed was measured with and without stimulation. The mean values are shown in Fig. 6 for subjects at the beginning and end of the trials. Subjects with SCI (gray bars) showed more improvement than did subjects with damage to the brain (white bars), but the increase was significant for both groups. The use of FES produced an increase in walking speed at both time points, but an increase in walking speed is also seen between the initial and final times without FES. All subjects started more than a year after their injury, so the increase is unlikely to be due to spontaneous recovery. Rather, the increase without FES is probably a training effect, since the subjects were walking more and faster with FES and hence built up their muscles and coordination. The overall increase from initial values

without FES to the final values with FES represents a 55% increase in speed for the SCI subjects, so even relatively simple, non-invasive systems can improve walking abilities substantially.

In the last couple of years we have concentrated on stimulators for foot drop. If the foot drops and drags on the ground during the swing phase of the gait cycle, even a single channel of stimulation to the common peroneal nerve can correct the foot drop. We developed a foot drop stimulator using the tilt of the leg with respect to gravity as a means of turning the stimulus on and off during the step cycle (Dai et al., 1996) and the stimulator is currently being tested in several centers.

In addition to speed, we also measure the effort required, using changes in heart rate. Fig. 7 shows results for one person with an incomplete SCI. The resting heart rate was measured over a period of 2 min. Then, the subject walked for 4 min and rested for another 4 min while his heart rate returned to resting values. Fig. 7B shows that he walked over 20 m/min with FES (×), but only 17 m/min without FES (o). The change in heart rate was virtually identical. Also shown is the physiological cost index or PCI (MacGregor, 1981). The PCI is calculated by dividing the speed (m/min) by the change in heart rate in beats/min. This gives a value for the number of extra heartbeats required to walk 1 m. The value was decreased from 1.88 to 1.55 for this subject using FES. Although only about a 20% decrease, the

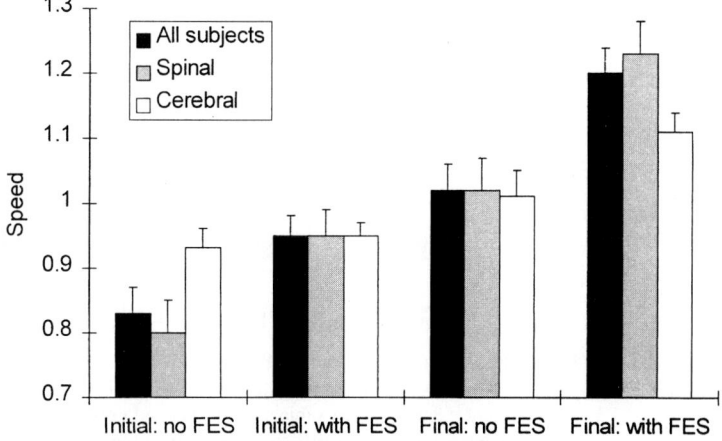

Fig. 6. Changes in walking speed relative to each subject's mean value over an average period of a year. Data are plotted for all subjects and separately for those with spinal or cerebral injury (stroke or traumatic brain injury). Mean values (+ S.E.) are shown for the initial and final speeds with and without FES (Wieler et al., 1999).

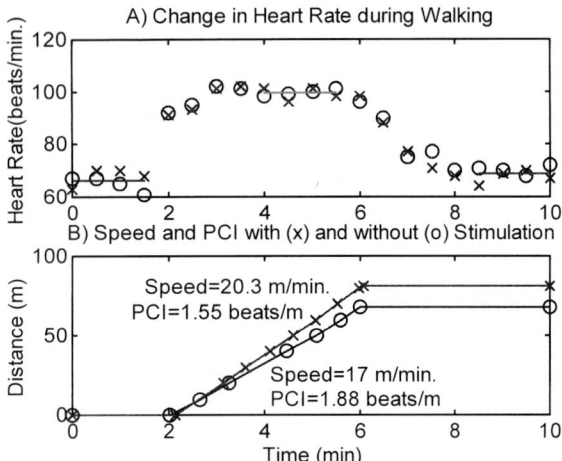

Fig. 7. Heart rate (A) and distance covered (B) for one SCI subject walking with and without an FES stimulator to prevent foot drop. The speed increases and the physiological cost index (PCI = velocity/change in heart rate) decreases with FES.

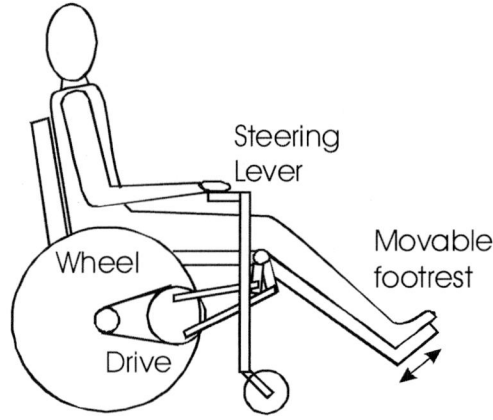

Fig. 8. Schematic diagram of the modified wheelchair. A modified footrest allows rotation about a virtual knee center. The rotation is coupled to movement of the wheels by a drive mechanism a chain and a one-way clutch that converts bidirectional to unidirectional movement for forward propulsion of the wheelchair. A lever connected to the front wheel enables the wheelchair to be steered.

energy required is often a good indicator of whether a subject will become a community walker or not (Cerny et al., 1980).

As mentioned above, FES for people with a complete SCI is not a viable alternative to a wheelchair for most subjects. Furthermore, the energy cost of a wheelchair is similar or even lower than normal locomotion, which is why people in a wheelchair can often post faster times for endurance races than can able-bodied runners. Fig. 8 shows a schematic diagram of a modified wheelchair in which the legs and footrests can move and the movements are coupled via a chain and two, one-way clutches to the wheel. We studied the effort needed to use the modified wheelchair for three groups of subjects: (1) control subjects ($n = 13$); (2) subjects with complete SCI who moved their legs with FES ($n = 9$); and (3) other disabled subjects who retained enough voluntary activity to move the foot rests ($n = 13$). This last group included four people with incomplete SCI.

Fig. 9 shows the results of measuring the PCI in these three groups (Stein et al., 2001). The test was repeated for three conditions: walking, propelling the chair with the arms and propelling the chair with the legs. Leg propulsion was the most efficient for the control subjects, taking less than half the effort of arm propulsion and 30% less effort than walking. The improved efficiency results from the fact that

in normal walking energy must be expended to lift the body up against gravity during each step, as well as propelling the body forward. With a wheelchair energy is only expended to propel the chair forward, although this may require more effort because of the added weight of the chair. Subjects with a complete SCI could not walk, so the comparison is only between propelling the wheelchair with the arms and

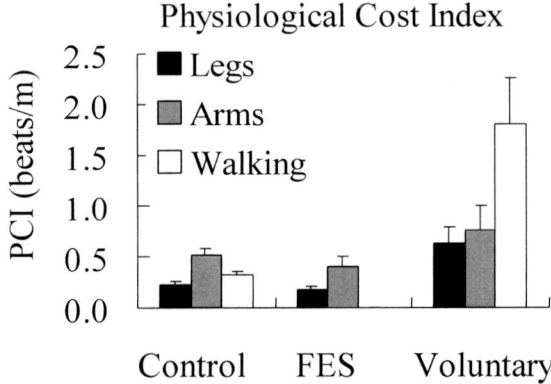

Fig. 9. Physiological cost index (PCI) for three groups: control subjects, subjects with a complete SCI who used FES to propel the wheelchair and disabled subjects who retained enough voluntary control to walk and propel the wheelchair voluntarily. Note that the effort, as measured by the PCI, was smaller in all three groups for leg propulsion than arm propulsion or walking. Mean values + S.E. are shown.

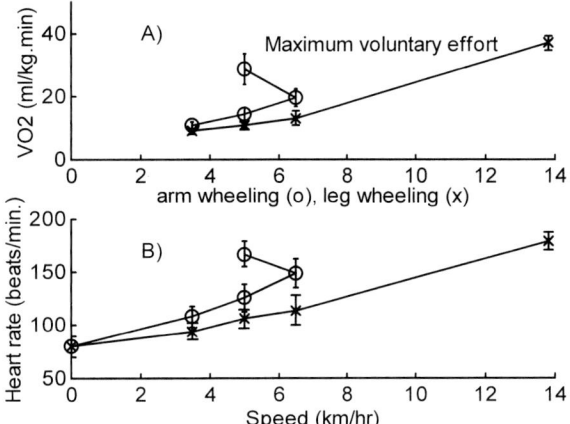

Fig. 10. (A) Oxygen consumption (VO$_2$) and (B) heart rate were always higher for submaximal speeds (3.5, 5 and 6.5 km/h) using the arms to propel the wheelchair, compared to the legs (i.e., using the legs is more efficient). However, for arm propulsion even 6.5 km/h could not be maintained with maximum effort because of fatigue. In contrast, with maximal effort using leg propulsion subjects could go nearly 14 km/h and get a better aerobic workout (higher VO$_2$). Note also the parallel changes in VO$_2$ and heart rate under the various conditions.

the legs. Again, propulsion with the legs required less than half the effort compared to arm propulsion. The third group was quite mixed so the differences were not significant. However, by analyzing individual subjects it became clear that subjects with little or no spasticity performed similarly to the other two groups. For subjects with substantial spasticity in their legs, the effort required to move the wheelchair with their legs could be greater than for the arms. Therefore, subjects with substantial spasticity would not be suitable candidates for the new wheelchair.

Finally, we studied both submaximal and maximal exercise with the wheelchair mounted over a treadmill, so that oxygen consumption (VO$_2$) as well as heart rate could be measured. Nine able-bodied, female, university subjects participated. Weights were added to the wheelchair so that a total weight of 77 kg (subject + added weights) was used for all subjects. Leg propulsion and arm propulsion were studied on separate days. For each condition subjects worked for 2 min each at three submaximal speeds (3.5, 5 and 6.5 km/h). In Fig. 10, the VO$_2$ (Fig. 10A) and the heart rate (Fig. 10B) were lower for all three speeds with leg propulsion than with arm propulsion (greater efficiency). When asked to

produce a maximum voluntary effort, subjects were unable to increase or even maintain the speed for another 2 min with arm propulsion. The speed actually declined as a result of fatigue, although the VO$_2$ and heart rate increased with maximum voluntary effort. In contrast, with leg propulsion, subjects were able to increase speed by 1.5 km/h each minute, even with added loads of 4.5 kg/min until they reached nearly 14 km/h on average. Thus, leg propulsion was more efficient than arm propulsion at all submaximal speeds (better efficiency), but could produce much higher speeds and reached a higher aerobic level. The higher speeds presumably result from the use of the large muscles of the leg, rather than the smaller arm muscles, and the direct linkage of leg movements to moving the wheels. The larger leg muscles will also consume more oxygen and give a better aerobic workout. Thus, there is a potential in SCI subjects of improving cardio-respiratory fitness as well as reversing the atrophy of muscles and bones in the leg. This may be important since heart disease is now the major killer of people with SCI and the rate is considerably higher for this group than for the general population (Geisler et al., 1983). Finally, many people who are long-term users of a wheelchair develop pain and overuse injuries in their arms (Nichols et al., 1979; Subbarao et al., 1995) which may be alleviated by using leg muscles. Thus, this new wheelchair provides a potentially exciting combination of increased mobility and fitness while reducing some injuries and pain. We are currently testing these effects in longer-term trials with subjects who have a SCI or other disabilities. In conclusion, methods are available today, both for preventing atrophy of bones and muscles after SCI, and improving mobility and fitness using voluntary and stimulated activity of the nervous system below the level of the injury.

References

Andersen, J.L., Schjerling, P. and Saltin, B. (2000) Muscles, genes and athletic performance. *Sci. Am.*, 283(3): 48–55.

Bélanger, M., Stein, R.B., Wheeler, G.D., Gordon, T. and Leduc, B. (2000) Electrical stimulation increases muscle strength and reverses osteopenia in spinal cord injured individuals. *Arch. Phys. Med. Rehab.*, 81: 1090–1098.

Burnham, R., Martin, T., Stein, R., Bell, G., MacLean, I. and Steadward, R. (1997) Skeletal muscle fibre type transformation

34

following spinal cord injury. *Spinal Cord*, 35: 86–91.

Cerny, K., Waters, R., Hislop, H. and Perry, J. (1980) Walking and wheelchair energetics in persons with paraplegia. *Phys. Ther.*, 60: 1133–1139.

Dai, R.C., Stein, R.B., Andrews, B.J., James, K.B. and Wieler, M. (1996) Application of tilt sensors in functional electrical stimulation. *I.E.E.E. Trans. Rehab. Eng.*, 4: 63–72.

Freehafer, A.A. (1995) Limb fractures in patients with spinal cord injury. *Arch. Phys. Med. Rehabil.*, 76: 823–827.

Geisler, W.O., Jousse, A.T., Wynne-Jones, M. and Breithaupt, D. (1983) Survival in traumatic spinal cord injury. *Paraplegia*, 21: 364–373.

Graupe, D. and Kohn, K.H. (1994) *Functional Electrical Stimulation for Ambulation by Paraplegics: twelve years of clinical observations and system studies*. Krieger, Malabar, FL.

Hirokawa, S., Grimm, M., Le, T., Solomonow, M., Baratta, R.V., Shoji, H. and D'Ambrosia, R.D. (1990) Energy consumption in paraplegic ambulation using the reciprocating gait orthosis and electrical stimulation of the thigh muscles. *Arch. Phys. Med. Rehab.*, 71: 687–694.

Kralj, A. and Bajd, T. (1989) *Functional Electrical Stimulation, Standing and Walking after Spinal Cord Injury*. Boca Raton, FL, CRC Press.

MacGregor, J. (1981) The evaluation of patient performance using long-term ambulatory monitoring technique in the domiciliary environment. *Physiotherapy*, 67: 30–33.

Marsolais, E.B. and Kobetic, R. (1987) Functional electrical stimulation for walking in paraplegia. *J. Bone Joint Surg.*, 69A: 728–733.

Martin, T.P., Stein, R.B., Hoeppner, P.H. and Reid, D.R. (1992) Influence of electrical stimulation on the morphological and metabolic properties of paralyzed muscle. *J. Appl. Physiol.*, 72: 1401–1406.

Nene, A.V. and Patrick, J.H. (1990) Energy cost of paraplegic locomotion using the ParaWalker — electrical stimulation 'hybrid' orthosis. *Arch. Phys. Med. Rehab.*, 71: 116–120.

Nichols, P.J.R., Norman, P.A. and Ennis, J.R. (1979) Wheelchair user's shoulder? Shoulder pain in patients with spinal cord lesions. *Scand. J. Rehab. Med.*, 11: 29–32.

Peckham, P.H. and Creasey, G.H. (1992) Neural prostheses: clinical applications of functional electrical stimulation in spinal cord injury. *Paraplegia*, 30: 96–101.

Rushton, D.N. (1997) *Neuroprostheses, Neuromodulators and Rehabilitation*. British Society of Rehabilation Medicine, London.

Stein, R.B., Gordon, T., Jefferson, J., Sharfenberger, A., Yang, J., Totosy de Zepetnek, J. and Bélanger, M. (1992) Optimal stimulation of paralysed muscle in spinal cord injured patients. *J. Appl. Physiol.*, 72: 1393–1400.

Stein, R.B., Chong, S.L., James, K.B. and Bell, G.J. (2001) Improved efficiency with a wheelchair propelled by the legs using voluntary activity or electrical stimulation. *Arch. Phys. Med. Rehab.*, in press.

Subbarao, J.V., Klopstein, J. and Turpin, R. (1995) Prevalence and impact of wrist and shoulder pain in patients with spinal cord injury. *J. Spinal Cord Med.*, 18: 9–13.

Wieler, M., Stein, R.B., Ladouceur, M., Whittaker, M., Smith, A.W., Naaman, S., Barbeau, H., Bugaresti, J. and Aimone, E. (1999) Multi-center evaluation of electrical stimulation systems for walking. *Arch. Phys. Med. Rehab.*, 80: 495–500.

Spinal cord injuries in animal models

L. McKerracher, G. Doucet and S. Rossignol (Eds.)
Progress in Brain Research, Vol. 137
© 2002 Elsevier Science B.V. All rights reserved

CHAPTER 4

Cell death in models of spinal cord injury

Michael S. Beattie *, Gerlinda E. Hermann, Richard C. Rogers and
Jacqueline C. Bresnahan

Department of Neuroscience, The Ohio State University Medical Center, 333 W. 10th Avenue, Columbus, OH 43210, USA

Abstract: Current treatments for acute spinal cord injury are based on animal models of human spinal cord injury (SCI). These models have shown that the initial traumatic injury to cord tissue is followed by a long period of secondary injury that includes a number of cellular and biochemical cascades. These secondary injury processes are potential targets for therapies. Continued refinement of rat and mouse models of SCI, along with more detailed analyses of the biology of the lesion in these models, points to both necrotic and apoptotic mechanisms of cell death after SCI. In this chapter, we review recent evidence for long-term apoptotic death of oligodendrocytes in long tracts undergoing Wallerian degeneration following SCI. This process appears to be related closely to activation of microglial cells. It is has been thought that microglial cells might be the source of cytotoxic cytokines, such as tumor necrosis factor-α (TNF-α), that kill oligodendrocytes. However, more recent evidence in vivo suggests that TNF-α by itself may not induce necrosis or apoptosis in oligodendrocytes. We review data that suggests other possible pathways for apoptosis, such as the neurotrophin receptor p75 which is expressed in both neurons and oligodendrocytes after SCI in rats and mice. In addition, it appears that microglial activation and TNF-α may be important in acute SCI. Ninety minutes after a moderate contusion lesion, microglia are activated and surround dying neurons. In an 'atraumatic' model of SCI, we have now shown that TNF-α appears to greatly potentiate cell death mediated by glutamate receptors. These studies emphasize that multiple mechanisms and interactions contribute to secondary injury after SCI. Continued study of both contusion models and other new approaches to studying these mechanisms will be needed to maximize strategies for acute and chronic therapies, and for neural repair.

Introduction

Human spinal cord injury (SCI) is now treated acutely by the administration of methylprednisolone (MP), a steroid with several proposed mechanisms of action. These include anti-oxidant and anti-lipid peroxidation properties (Hall, 1992, 1996) as well as anti-inflammatory effects mediated through glucocorticoid receptors (Hall, 1992, 1996; Xu et al., 1998). Clinical trials of MP were initiated after a

series of preclinical animal studies, some of which showed efficacy, and some which did not. The first clinical trial (Bracken et al., 1984) showed no benefit, with adverse effects. A second trial was initiated on the basis of animal studies that showed that the first trial may have used an inadequate dosing schedule. This trial showed a modest but significant effect on recovery of function (Bracken et al., 1990). A third major, NIH-funded trial has since been completed that also included the use of the 17-amino-steroid tirilizad methylate that lacks glucocorticoid receptor activity, but retains anti-lipid peroxidation properties (Bracken et al., 1997). This trial was also interpreted to support the efficacy of MP (and tirilizad), especially when MP was given within 4 h of injury. Thus, there is one widely (but not universally)

---

* Correspondence to: M.S. Beattie, Department of Neuroscience, Ohio State University Medical Center, 333 W. 10th Ave., Columbus, OH 43210, USA. Tel.: +1-614-292-6639; Fax: +1-614-688-8742; E-mail: beattie.2@osu.edu

accepted treatment for acute spinal cord injury, and that treatment must be given within hours of trauma. The animal models that were used to study MP and other potential therapeutic agents showed early on that the outcome of SCI depended not only on the initial tissue injury at the time of trauma, but also on secondary injury processes that could extend for hours or even days. Indeed, these models formed the basis for the rationale for using MP and other agents that could block secondary biochemical and cellular cascades initiated by tissue damage. The models have now been studied in more detail, and it is clear that there are multiple cascades involved in the production of cell death and secondary degeneration after SCI. For example, in addition to the 'necrotic' cell death produced by frank damage, excitotoxic amino acids and lipid peroxidation, it is now clear that cells that have received less severe injuries can undergo cell death mediated by active processes, i.e. apoptosis. This chapter will explore some of the newer findings from our laboratory and others that have identified new possible therapeutic targets for acute and sub-acute intervention based on animal models of SCI. It is also noted that the cell death described here is accompanied by endogenous repair mechanisms that provide for cellular proliferation and differentiation during the same time periods as cell death is occurring. Thus, strategies aimed at reducing cell death need to be coordinated with strategies that direct effective repair.

Contusion models of SCI

Contusion or compression models of SCI attempt to mimic the mechanical events that produce pathophysiology in human SCI. Some models use devices that induce rapid mechanical deformation of the spinal cord by dropping an impactor rod (e.g. the 'MASCIS' device, Gruner, 1992; Constantini and Young, 1994; Basso et al., 1996) a weight (Noble and Wrathall, 1985; Kuhn and Wrathall, 1998) or using a computer controlled impounder (e.g. the 'Ohio State or OSU' device: Bresnahan et al., 1987; Behrmann et al., 1992; Stokes et al., 1992; Jakeman et al., 2000). Other laboratories use compression injuries by applying weights to the cord (Li et al., 1996, 1999; Farooque, 2000) or an aneurysm clip (Tator and Fehlings, 1991; Fehlings and Tator, 1995).

There are many common features of these models: a laminectomy is performed, and the injury is applied to the dorsal surface of the cord with the dura intact. And, while there are differences in the injury and recovery depending upon the method used, there are more commonalities to the resulting progression of events than there are differences. Cord injuries that actually open the dura and cut the cord substance, like transections or hemisections, have more different features, and will not be discussed here.

Many authors have described the progression of events in these models, and there have been corroborating or validating studies of human pathology specimens (e.g. Bunge et al., 1993; Metz et al., 2000). Depending upon its severity, the initial impact or compression results in remarkably little gross damage to the cord substance. Typically there will be gray matter hemorrhage, but the white matter looks remarkably intact. There have only been a few studies of the truly acute pathology of the cord after contusion lesions (Balentine, 1978a,b; Noble and Wrathall, 1985; Rosenberg and Wrathall, 1997; Grossman et al., 2001; Hermann et al., 2001, discussed below). However, it is clear that cellular disruption at the center of the lesion initiates a cascade of centripetal and rostro-caudal tissue destruction (Fig. 1) that includes membrane damage by lipid peroxidation (Hall, 1996), massive Ca^{2+} influx into the intracellular compartment (Young and Flamm, 1982; Stokes et al., 1983; Young, 1985), and necrotic cell death. There is strong evidence that excitatory amino acids are released and involved in these early death events (Faden and Simon, 1988; Panter et al., 1990). There is also an early invasion of neutrophils from the blood, and cytokine levels can rise rapidly (e.g. tumor necrosis factor-α (TNF-α): Wang et al., 1997; Xu et al., 1998; Bethea et al., 1999). By 24 h post injury, macrophages have invaded the lesion, and a cavity begins to form. Axons, damaged by the initial injury, continue to die back over a long period of time (Fig. 1A–N; Hill et al., 2001). The distal ends of these injured axons undergo Wallerian degeneration, contributing to further loss of tissue and changes in circuitry in regions remote from the lesion (see Beattie and Bresnahan, 2000, for a review). In addition to invading macrophages, the resident microglia seem to play an important role in post-injury lesion progression. These cells are activated immediately

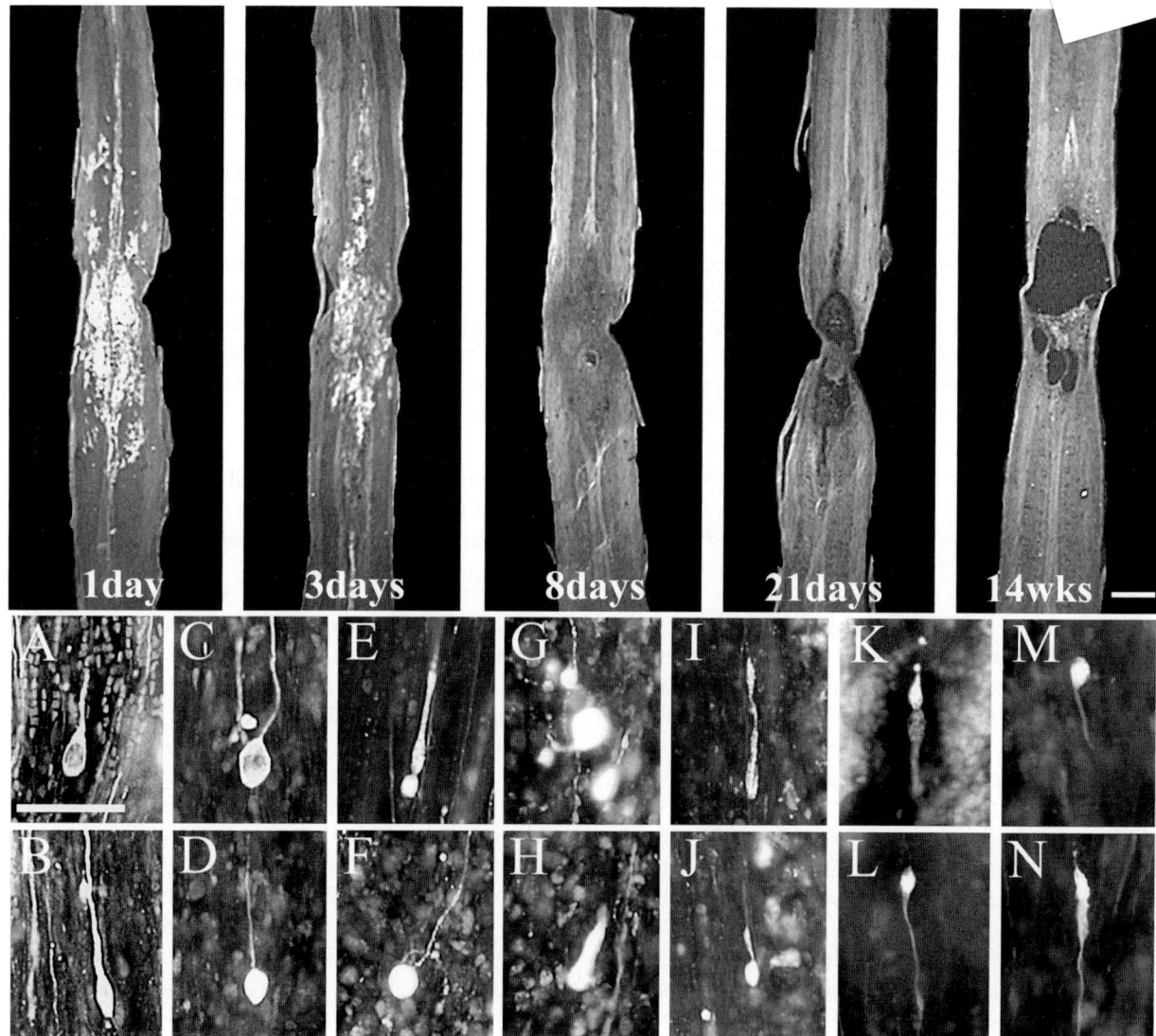

Fig. 1. Top: the progression of the injury from 1 day to 3.5 months is shown. Horizontal sections through the rat spinal cord at the level of the central canal after a moderate contusion injury (12.5 mm MASCIS device injury), were taken from a series of cases surviving from 24 h to 14 weeks. At 1 and 3 days the hemorrhagic regions are evident as bright areas due to the autofluorescence of red blood cells in the fluorescent light. At 8 days, the lesion region contains large numbers of macrophages and cellular debris. At 21 days, cavitation is clearly evident. At 14 weeks, the lesion has open cystic regions and areas of tissue ingrowth which contain astrocytes, Schwann cells, axons, fibroblasts, and macrophages Scale bar: 1 mm. Bottom: after contusion lesions, dying back axons have retraction bulbs of various sizes and morphologies. Rostral to the injury, endbulbs of corticospinal tract (CST) axons (labeled with fluororuby) are shown after 1 day (A,B), 3 days (C,D), 8 days (E,F), 21 days (G,H), and 14 weeks (I,J). The distal ends of severed CST axons (labeled before injury) also show swellings due to continued retrograde transport; some were visible for up to 21 days after injury although they become progressively fragmented as they undergo Wallerian degeneration. Scale bar: 50 μm. Adapted from Hill et al. (2001).

following injury at the lesion site (e.g. Hermann et al., 2001), and activated microglia are present within long tract undergoing Wallerian degeneration (Popovich et al., 1997; Shuman et al., 1997).

Necrosis followed by apoptosis

Recently, renewed attention has been given to the distinction between necrotic or 'passive' cell death, and active forms of cell death that produce 'apopto-tis' (Ankarcrona et al., 1995; Majno and Joris, 1995; Portera-Cailliau et al., 1997). Apoptosis is important in the elimination of unwanted cells during develop-ment, and in the regulation of the immune system, and all cells seem to have the equipment needed to produce death by, ultimately, the controlled destruc-tion of their DNA (see Nagata, 1997 for a review). It is now well established that both forms, and no doubt intermediary forms, of cell death occur after CNS trauma (Zipfel et al., 2000), including SCI (see Beattie et al., 2000a for a review).

In addition to the shearing of membranes that cause immediate necrotic death of some cells after contusion SCI, intact and partially damaged cells are vulnerable to death by biochemical attack by free radicals (Hall, 1996) and excitatory amino acids that can be released by dying neurons and other cells. In addition, loss of blood flow makes the cord en-vironment hypoxic. Cell death caused by hypoxia and excitotoxicity have been studied extensively in vitro (Choi, 1994; Mattson, 1998; Toborek et al., 1999), and it is now known that these stimuli can cause death by both necrosis and apoptosis, and that the interactions between intracellular Ca^{2+}, free rad-icals, and cell protective mechanisms are extremely complex (Azbill et al., 1997). However, it is clear that a massive amount of glutamate can kill cells by activating AMPA and subsequently NMDA receptors which allow so much Ca^{2+} influx that cells swell and burst, typical necrotic cell death. On the other hand, cells that receive a lower challenge can recover, al-though some then go on to die not by necrosis, but by apoptosis (Choi, 1996). In addition, hypoxia makes cells more sensitive to glutamate challenge (Choi, 1996). Glutamate levels rise dramatically in the cord following injury (Panter et al., 1990), in a hypoxic environment. Thus, it is likely that excitatory amino acids like glutamate play a very important role in mediating the progression of secondary injury that is seen following SCI. This idea is strengthened by findings that show that pharmacologic blockade of glutamate receptors, specifically AMPA/kainate re-ceptors, reduce gray and white matter damage after contusion SCI (Wrathall et al., 1994, 1996, 1997). AMPA receptors are present not only on neurons, but on oligodendrocytes as well, and AMPA-receptor mediated death of oligodendrocytes has been demon-strated in vitro (McDonald et al., 1998). However, it has been difficult to parcel out the role that different aspects of the secondary injury play in the com-plicated and rapidly changing post-contusion spinal cord. For example, cytokines including TNF-α and IL1-β rise rapidly after SCI. Do they play a role in necrotic or apoptotic cell death after SCI, as some recent evidence would suggest (e.g. Bethea et al., 1999)? In an attempt to examine early post-injury mediators of cell death in vivo, we have developed an 'atraumatic' model of SCI in the rat. Our first use of that model has been to examine the question of the role of cytokines and excitatory amino acids in secondary injury.

TNF and glutamate interactions in the brainstem suggest a possible mechanism for potentiation of cell death in the spinal cord after injury

Recent studies in the Rogers and Hermann labora-tory have shown that TNF-α is a potent inhibitor of gastric motility. Lipopolysaccharide (LPS)-induced increases in circulating TNF inhibit gastric motil-ity by direct activation of neurons in the nucleus of the solitary tract (NTS). These second order vis-ceral sensory neurons in turn inhibit vagal efferent neurons in the vagal motor nucleus (n. X) (Her-mann and Rogers, 1995). Indeed, TNF appears to also potentiate the effects of vagal afferent inputs from the stomach. When femtomolar quantities of TNF are microinjected onto NTS neurons, the subse-quent effects of gastric distention are much enhanced (Emch et al., 2000). The vagal afferents that convey the information on gastric distention are, of course, glutamatergic (Talman et al., 1980; McCann and Rogers, 1994). These results, and the considerations of the acute rise in both TNF and glutamate af-ter cord injury led us to design a simple means of testing whether TNF and glutamate interact in SCI.

Under some conditions, TNF in high concentra-tions can be cytotoxic; it can kill oligodendrocytes by apoptosis in vitro (Louis et al., 1993; D'Sousa et al., 1995), and can kill tumor cells as well (Granger et al., 1969; Carswell et al., 1975). However, even relatively high concentrations injected into the spinal cord, result in only minimal damage (Schnell et al., 1999; Hall et al., 2000). We used a fine micropipette to pressure-inject small quantities of TNF and kainic acid (KA), a glutamate agonist into the spinal gray matter after a laminectomy at T9. As controls, we injected albumin (MW similar to active, trimeric TNF). The doses of TNF were based on those that could excite neurons in the NTS (from 10^{-7} to 10^{-9} M, in volumes of 30–35 nl, for total doses of 0.04–35 fmol, or 0.06–60.0 pg of TNF protein). We chose a dose of KA known to excite neurons but not cause frank damage (5 mM, same volume, 150 pmol). In order to determine whether TNF (and KA) injections were having excitatory effects on neurons like those seen in the NTS, we used immunocytochemistry to detect the nuclear immediate early gene, c-fos (Rinaman et al., 1993). To study the acute effects of these compounds, we sacrificed rats 90 min after injection (Hermann et al., 2001).

Control injections (albumin) produced no lesions and no c-fos activation. TNF injections alone produced no lesions, and a small area containing cells with c-fos staining surrounding the injection site. The injections of KA produced a very small area of damaged neurons surrounded by a small region of c-fos-stained cells. However, when KA was paired with TNF at the 60-pg dose, a dramatic loss of neurons over a large area of gray matter was seen; c-fos activation was found in many cells surrounding the area of neuronal loss, and activated microglia were seen in the middle of the lesion site in areas devoid of neurons (Fig. 2A), and engulfing neurons at the margins of the dead zone (Fig. 2B). TNF at very low doses (one and two orders of magnitude less) did not potentiate KA-induced neuronal loss. When CNQX (6-cyano-7-nitroquinoxaline 2,3-(1H,4H)-dione), an AMPA/kainate receptor antagonist was co-injected with the lethal TNF-KA combination, the damage was completely blocked, although some c-fos induction was still observed.

Together, these results suggest that TNF can activate neurons in both the brainstem and the spinal cord, and that this activation is associated with a potentiation of the effects of local glutamate release. When that release is under physiological conditions, e.g. release from vagal afferents, TNF tends to potentiate activation of second order neurons. However, when some threshold of glutamate concentration is reached, even low levels of TNF can push neurons into excitotoxic cell death. Further, this potentiation is associated with AMPA/kainate type receptors.

The glutamate trigger requirement for the initiation of cell death secondary to injury makes sense in light of current knowledge of immune–neural interactions. It is highly disadvantageous for cytokines alone to have the power to induce wide-spread CNS cell death. It is now well accepted that the CNS is not an immune-privileged organ when the peripheral immune system is activated. Cytokines, TNF especially, can gain easy access to the CNS by regulating the blood–brain barrier permeability (Pan et al., 1999). If TNF were the sole determinant of CNS cell death, then influenza could set off a wave of neural apoptosis.

The relationship between microglial activation, glutamate release, and neuronal death is likely to be a feed-forward cascade that once started may spread to adjacent areas. Indeed, preliminary studies of 2- and 8-day post-injection spinal cords show wider areas of damage (Beattie et al., 2000c). In addition, the margins of the lesions at later time points contained evidence for apoptotic cells, suggesting that the spread of the lesion involves initiation of secondary damage by necrosis caused by excitotoxic cell death, followed by apoptosis (and see below).

We had not examined contusion injury sites as early as 90 min prior to this study. What we saw 90 min following a mild contusion to the T9 spinal cord using the MASCIS model (6.25 mm injury) was virtually indistinguishable from the TNF+KA lesion: a central core devoid of neurons, with no evidence of apoptosis, and activated microglia, as well as fos-positive neurons and microglia at the margins of the lesion. This nanoinjection model may thus be a useful tool for predicting which neuroprotective strategies and agents might be effective in stopping the initiation of the cascade.

Long-term events: neuronal and oligodendrocyte apoptosis

The initial findings that apoptosis occurs in oligodendrocytes in long tracts, days and weeks following SCI (Crowe et al., 1995, 1997; Li et al., 1996, 1997), have been repeated and expanded by many laboratories (Yong et al., 1998; Abe et al., 1999; Arnold et al., 2000; Warden et al., 2001; see review in Beattie et al., 2000a). It is also known that this apoptosis involves the activation of intracellu-

42

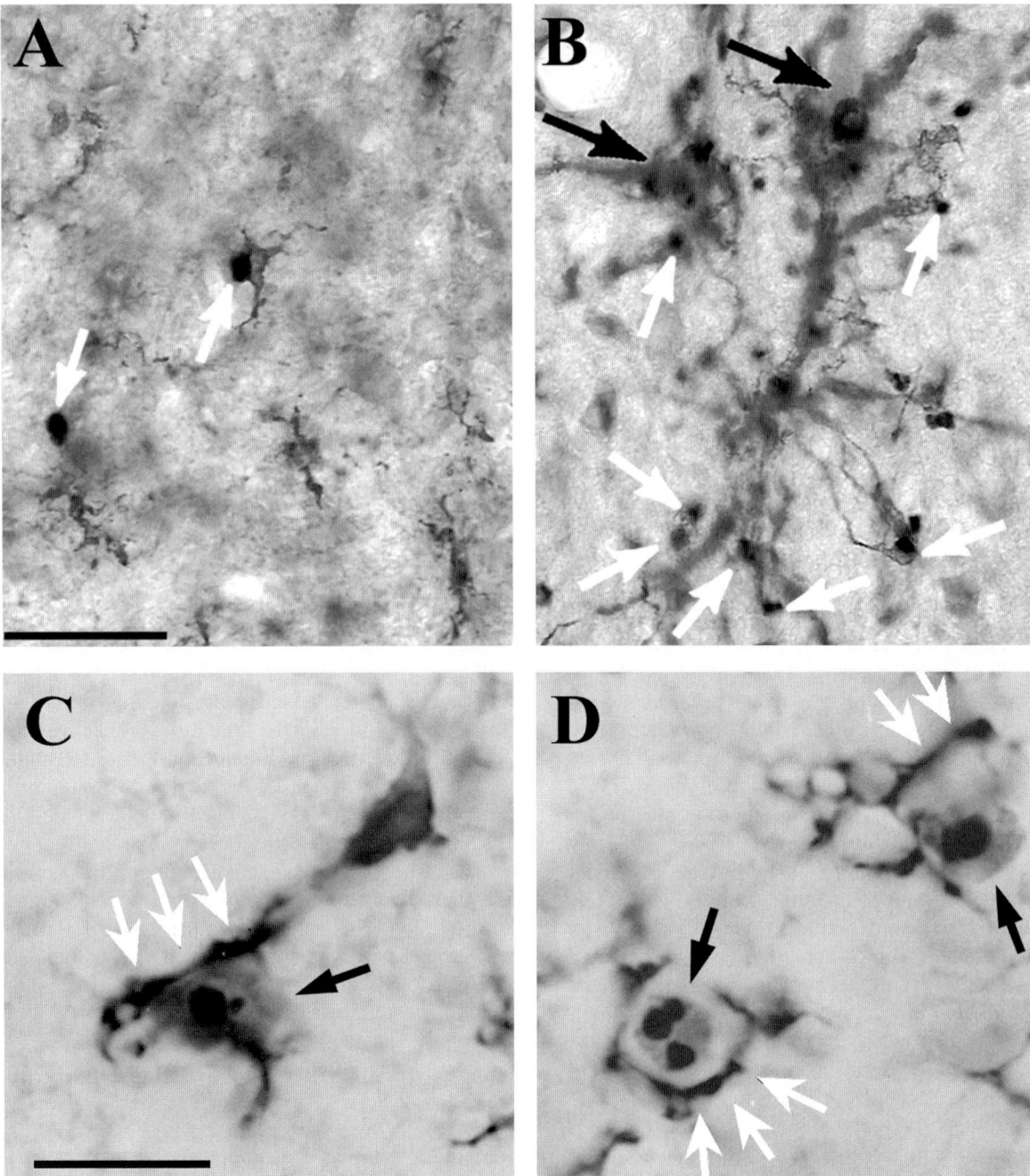

Fig. 2. (A,B) Activated microglia (white arrows) are evident within 90 min at TNF-α plus kainate injection sites. At the center of the injection (A), microglia are the only cells remaining whereas at the periphery, many neurons (black arrows) remain, have c-*fos* positive nuclei, but are encrusted by activated microglial cell processes. Activated microglia are OX-42 immunopositive (gray) and have c-*fos* positive (black) nuclei (white arrows). (C,D) Activated microglia (white arrows) are also present in regions remote from a spinal cord injury lesion site in fiber tracts (dorsal columns rostral to an injury, in this case) undergoing Wallerian degeneration. The microglial processes (OX-42 immunopositive, reaction product appears black) are engulfing oligodendrocytes (CC-1 immunopositive, reaction product appears gray) which are undergoing apoptosis as evidenced by nuclear condensation (apoptotic bodies). Scale bar in A: 30 μm (also applies to B). Scale bar in C: 20 μm (also applies to D). A and B were adapted from Hermann et al. (2001); C and D were adapted from Shuman et al. (1997).

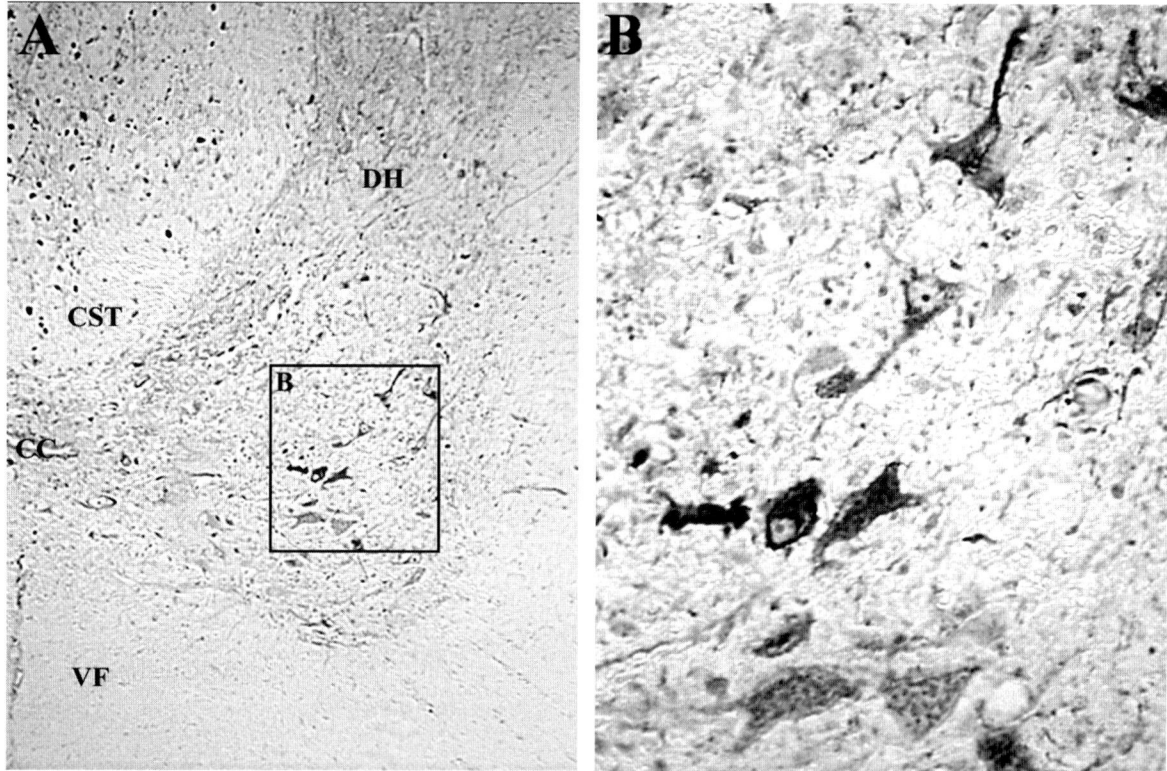

Fig. 3. p75 Neurotrophin receptor expression in spinal cord cells 24 h after a moderately severe contusion injury (25 mm MASCIS injury). The cross section shown was taken 2.5 mm rostral to the lesion center and shows immunostaining (black reaction product) in both the gray and white matter. Immunopositive glial cells in the dorsal columns (presumably oligodendrocytes) are evident especially above the corticospinal tract (CST), and neurons in the intermediate gray and ventral horn are immunostained (B). Note the two large cells at the bottom, center of B which have reaction product in a clumped pattern similar to Nissl staining of rough endoplasmic reticulum. CC, central canal; CST, corticospinal tract; DH, dorsal horn; VF, ventral funiculus.

lar cysteine–aspartate proteases known as 'caspases' (see Springer et al., 1999). Oligodendrocytes very far away from the injury site undergo apoptosis in areas where axons are dying, and it is thought that this may contribute to demyelination that adds to the functional deficit (Shuman et al., 1997; Beattie et al., 2000a). However, the signals (or lack thereof) that induce this death are not known. Microglial cells are seen in direct apposition to dying oligodendrocytes in white matter tracts (Fig. 2C,D; Shuman et al., 1997). These microglia may be acting as mediators of cell death, or they may be cleaning up the debris after oligodendrocytes have died. The microglial apposition to oligodendrocytes remote to the lesion in time and distance looks similar, however, to the activated microglia seen at the injury site 90 min after a contusion lesion or injection of TNF and kainic

acid (Fig. 2). Since activated microglia can release TNF-α and IL1-β, it might be that these or other factors released by microglia (or astrocytes) are involved. However, as noted above, the direct injection of TNF-α into the spinal white matter does not produce a large amount of either necrotic or apoptotic cell death. Parallel to the story in acute injury, it has been shown that oligodendrocytes are susceptible to excitotoxic cell death mediated by AMPA receptors (McDonald et al., 1998). Perhaps there is an interaction between TNF and glutamate receptors in long-term apoptotic cell death as well. In addition, there is evidence that the p75 neurotrophin receptor may participate in oligodendrocyte cell death in vitro, and that p75 is expressed in oligodendrocytes in the white matter after spinal cord injury (Beattie et al., 1999; Casha et al., 2001). SCI also induces p75 in spinal neurons shortly after injury (Fig. 3), suggesting that p75 may be expressed in response to cellular stress, and may in some cases be an apoptosis receptor rather than being neuroprotective, as it seems to be in concert with the NGF receptor trk A (Casaccia-Bonnefil et al., 1998; Chao et al., 1998; Yoon et al., 1998).

An alternative hypothesis must be considered: oligodendrocytes seem to require axons for survival during development (Barres et al., 1992, 1993; Raff et al., 1993). The loss of axons after SCI might deprive oligodendrocytes of a needed trophic factor, and induce apoptosis. In this case, the prominent microglial response would be in response to oligodendroglial rather than axonal degeneration. Of course, it may be in response to both stimuli.

Implications for therapies

The cascade of secondary injury after SCI is complex, and no doubt involves the interactions of a wide variety of events, beginning with frank membrane disruption, leading to receptor-mediated necrosis, and later to apoptosis of cells far from the original lesion site. Here we have discussed only a few of the possible players, i.e. glutamate, cytokines, and perhaps trophic factors. We also know that injury to the CNS initiates repair responses that include the elaboration of growth and trophic factors (Dougherty et al., 2000; Hayashi et al., 2000), cellular proliferation (Beattie et al., 1997; Horner et al., 2000), and abortive attempts at regeneration and sprouting at the lesion site (e.g. Hill et al., 2001). There may indeed be attempts at remyelination by means of proliferation of oligodendrocyte precursors, or glial progenitors (McTigue et al., 1998). In circuits remote from the lesion where deafferentation has occurred, there is often evidence of collateral sprouting and reorganization (Beattie et al., 2000b; Pikov and Wrathall, 2001). This sprouting may be beneficial, or it may contribute to adverse effects, such as spasticity (Liu and Chambers, 1958). Therapeutics aimed at reducing the secondary injury may also affect some or all of these other aspects of the long-term resolution of SCI. For example, reduction of excitotoxic cell death early after injury will likely spare more axons, resulting in a decrease of the later glial cell death. Together, these events should spare more

patent connections, and result in a better long-term outcome. The effects of blocking secondary injury on the reparative responses are unknown. However, it might be that some effective blockers of injury also might block parts of the repair response, such as growth factor production, or even sprouting.

Such complexity only reiterates the importance of understanding the multiple biological responses of the CNS to injury, and designing therapeutics with multiple targets. Pre-clinical in vivo testing will play a critical role in the implementation of therapies based on new biological findings, since the complexity of both the response to injury and the response to drugs makes predicting outcomes difficult. This will be especially true when combination therapies are employed.

Acknowledgements

Thanks are extended to John Komon for preparing the illustrations. This work was supported by NIH Grants NS38079 and DK52142.

References

Abe, Y., Yamamoto, T., Sugiyama, Y., Watanabe, T., Saito, N., Kayama, H. and Kumagai, T. (1999) Apoptotic cells associated with Wallerian degeneration after experimental spinal cord injury: a possible mechanism of oligodendroglial death. *J. Neurotrauma*, 16: 946–952.

Ankarcrona, M., Dypbukt, J.M., Bonfoco, E., Zhivotovsky, B., Orrenius, S., Lipton, S.A. and Nicotera, P. (1995) Glutamate-induced neuronal death: a succession of necrosis or apoptosis depending on mitochondrial function. *Neuron*, 15: 961–973.

Arnold, P.M., Citron, B.A., Ameenudin, S., Malladi, S., Wang, X. and Festoff, B.W. (2000) Caspase-3 inhibition is neuroprotective after spinal cord injury. *J. Neurochem.*, 74: S73.

Azbill, R.D., Mu, X., Bruce-Keller, A.J., Mattson, M.P. and Springer, J.E. (1997) Impaired mitochondrial function, oxidative stress and altered antioxidant enzyme activities following traumatic spinal cord injury. *Brain Res.*, 765: 283–290.

Balentine, J.D. (1978a) Pathology of experimental spinal cord trauma. I. The necrotic lesion as a function of vascular injury. *Lab. Invest.*, 39: 236–253.

Balentine, J.D. (1978b) Pathology of experimental spinal cord trauma. II. Ultrastructure of axons and myelin. *Lab. Invest.*, 39: 254–266.

Barres, B.A., Hart, I.K., Coles, H.S., Burne, J.F., Voyvodic, J.T., Richardson, W.D. and Raff, M.C. (1992) Cell death in the oligodendrocyte lineage. *J. Neurobiol.*, 23: 1221–1230.

Barres, B.A., Jacobson, M.D., Schmid, R., Sendtner, M. and

Raff, M.C. (1993) Does oligodendrocyte survival depend on axons? *Curr. Biol.*, 3: 489–497.

Basso, D.M., Beattie, M.S. and Bresnahan, J.C. (1996) Histological and locomotor studies of graded spinal cord contusion using the NYU weight-drop device versus transection. *Exp. Neurol.*, 139: 224–256.

Beattie, M.S. and Bresnahan, J.C. (2000) Cell death, repair, and recovery of function after spinal cord contusion injuries in rats. In: R.G. Kalb and W.J. Strittmatter (Eds.), *Neurobiology of Spinal Cord Injury*. Humana Press, Totowa, NJ, pp. 1–22.

Beattie, M.S., Bresnahan, J.C., Koman, J., Tovar, C.A. and Anderson, D.K. et al. (1997) Endogenous repair after spinal cord contusion injuries in the rat. *Exp. Neurol.*, 148: 453–463.

Beattie, M.S., Boyce, S.L., Yoon, S.O., Longo, F.M., Yeo, T.T. and Bresnahan, J.C. (1999) Expression of p75 NTFR in neurons and oligodendrocytes after spinal cord injury in rats: neurotrophin-induced apoptosis in vivo? *Soc. Neurosci. Abstr.*, 25: 762.

Beattie, M.S., Farooqui, A.A. and Bresnahan, J.C. (2000a) A review of current evidence for apoptosis after spinal cord injury. *J. Neurotrauma*, 17: 915–925.

Beattie, M.S., Li, Q. and Bresnahan, J.C. (2000b) Cell death and plasticity after experimental spinal cord injury. In: F. Seil (Ed.), *Progress in Brain Research*, Vol. 128. Elsevier Science, Amsterdam, pp. 9–21.

Beattie, M.S., Rogers, R.C., Hermann, G.E. and Bresnahan, J.C. (2000c) TNF, glutamate and neurodegeneration in the rat spinal cord. *Soc. Neurosci. Abstr.*, 26: 2279.

Behrmann, D.L., Bresnahan, J.C. and Beattie, M.S. (1992) Spinal cord injury produced by consistent mechanical displacement of the cord in rats: behavioral and histologic analysis. *J. Neurotrauma*, 9: 197–217.

Bethea, J.R., Nagashima, H., Acosta, M.C., Briceno, C., Gomez, F., Marcillo, A.E., Loor, K., Green, J. and Dietrich, W.D. (1999) Systemically administered interleukin-10 reduces tumor necrosis factor-alpha production and significantly improves functional recovery following traumatic spinal cord injury in rats. *J. Neurotrauma*, 16: 851–863.

Bracken, M.B., Collins, W.F., Freeman, D.F., Shepard, M.J., Wagner, F.W., Silten, R.M., Hellenbrand, K.G., Ransohoff, J., Hunt, W.E., Perot, P.L., Grossman, R.G., Green, B.A., Eisenberg, H.M., Rifkinson, N., Goodman, J.H., Meagher, J.N., Fischer, B., Clifton, G.L., Flamm, E.S. and Rawe, S.E. (1984) Efficacy of methylprednisolone in acute spinal-cord injury. *J. Am. Med. Assoc.*, 251: 45–52.

Bracken, M.B., Shepard, M.J., Collins, W.F., Holford, T.R., Young, W., Baskin, D.S., Eisenberg, H.M., Flamm, E., Leo-Summers, L. and Maroon, J. et al. (1990) A randomized controlled trial of methylprednisolone or naloxone in the treatment of acute spinal-cord injury. *New Engl. J. Med.*, 322: 1405–1461.

Bracken, M.B., Shepard, M.J., Holford, T.R., Leo-Summers, L., Aldrich, E.F., Fazl, M., Fehlings, M., Herr, D.L., Hitchon, P.W. and Marshall, L.F. et al. (1997) Administration of methylprednisolone for 24 or 48 hours or tirilazad mesylate for 48 hours in the treatment of acute spinal cord injury — results of the Third National Acute Spinal Cord Injury Randomized Controlled Trial. *J. Am. Med. Assoc.*, 277: 1597–1604.

Bresnahan, J.C., Todd, F., Beattie, M.S. and Noyes, D.H. (1987) A behavioral and morphological analysis of spinal cord injuries produced by a feedback controlled impact device. *Exp. Neurol.*, 95: 548–570.

Bunge, R.P., Puckett, W.R., Becerra, J.L., Marcillo, A. and Quencer, R.M. (1993) Observations of the pathology of human spinal cord injury. A review and classification of 22 new cases with details from a case of cord compression with extensive focal demyelination. *Adv. Neurol.*, 59: 75–89.

Carswell, E.A., Old, L.J., Kassel, R.L., Green, S., Fiore, N. and Williamson, B. (1975) An endotoxin-induced serum factor that causes necrosis of tumors. *Proc. Natl. Acad. Sci. USA*, 72: 3666–3670.

Casaccia-Bonnefil, P., Kong, H. and Chao, M.V. (1998) Neurotrophins: the biological paradox of survival factors eliciting apoptosis. *Cell Death Differ.*, 5: 354–367.

Casha, S., Yu, W.R. and Fehlings, M.G. (2001) Oligodendroglial apoptosis occurs along degenerating axons and is associated with Fas and p75 expression following spinal cord injury in the rat. *Neuroscience*, 103: 203–218.

Chao, M., Casaccia-Bonnefil, P. and Carter, B. et al. (1998) Neurotrophin receptors: mediators of life and death. *Brain Res. Rev.*, 26: 295–301.

Choi, D.W. (1994) Glutamate receptors and the induction of excitotoxic neuronal death. In: *Neuroscience: From the Molecular to the Cognitive. Progress in Brain Research*, Vol. 100, Elsevier Science, Amsterdam, pp. 47–51.

Choi, D.W. (1996) Ischemia-induced neuronal apoptosis. *Curr. Opin. Neurobiol.*, 6: 667–672.

Constantini, S. and Young, W. (1994) The effects of methylprednisolone and the ganglioside GM1 on acute spinal cord injury in rats. *J. Neurosurg.*, 80: 97–111.

Crowe, M.J., Shuman, S.L., Masters, J.N., Bresnahan, J.C. and Beattie, M.S. (1995) Morphological evidence suggesting apoptotic nuclei in spinal cord injury. *Soc. Neurosci. Abstr.*, 21: 232.

Crowe, M.J., Bresnahan, J.C., Shuman, S.L., Masters, J.N. and Beattie, M.S. (1997) Apoptosis and delayed degeneration after spinal injury in rats and monkeys. *Nat. Med.*, 3: 73–76.

D'Sousa, S., Alinauskas, K., McCrea, E., Goodyear, C. and Antel, J.P. (1995) Differential susceptibility of human CNS-derived cell populations to TNF-dependent and independent immune-mediated injury. *J. Neurosci.*, 15: 7293–7300.

Dougherty, K.D., Dreyfus, C.F. and Black, I.B. (2000) Brain-derived neurotrophic factor in astrocytes, oligodendrocytes, and microglia/macrophages after spinal cord injury. *Neurobiol. Dis.*, 7: 574–585.

Emch, G., Hermann, G.E. and Rogers, R.C. (2000) TNF activates solitary nucleus neurons responsive to gastric distention. *Am. J. Physiol.*, 279: G582–G586.

Faden, A.I. and Simon, R.P. (1988) A potential role for excitotoxins in the pathophysiology of spinal cord injury. *Ann. Neurol.*, 23: 623–626.

Farooque, M. (2000) Spinal cord compression injury in the

46

mouse: Presentation of a model including assessment of motor dysfunction. *Acta Neuropathol.*, 100: 13–22.

Fehlings, M.G. and Tator, C.H. (1995) The relationships among the severity of spinal cord injury, residual neurological function, axon counts, and counts of retrogradely labeled neurons after experimental spinal cord injury. *Exp. Neurol.*, 132: 220–228.

Granger, G.A., Shacks, S.J., Williams, T.W. and Kolb, W.P. (1969) Lymphocyte in vitro cytotoxicity: specific release of lymphotoxin-like materials from tuberculin-sensitive lymphoid cells. *Nature*, 221: 1155–1157.

Grossman, S.D., Rosenberg, L.J. and Wrathall, J.R. (2001) Relationship of altered glutamate receptor subunit mRNA expression to acute cell loss after spinal cord contusion. *Exp. Neurol.*, 168: 273.

Gruner, J. (1992) A monitored contusion model of spinal cord injury in the rat. *J. Neurotrauma*, 9: 123–128.

Hall, E.D. (1992) The neuroprotective pharmacology of methylprednisolone. *J. Neurosurg.*, 76: 13–22.

Hall, E.D. (1996) Free radicals and lipid peroxidation. In: R.K. Narayan, J.E. Wilberger Jr. and J.T. Povlishock (Eds.), *Neurotrauma*. McGraw Hill, New York, pp. 1405–1419.

Hall, S.M., Redford, E.J. and Smith, K.J. (2000) Tumor necrosis factor-alpha has morphological effects within the dorsal columns of the spinal cord in contrast to its effect in the peripheral nervous system. *J. Neuroimmunol.*, 106: 130–136.

Hayashi, M., Ueyama, T. and Nemoto, K. et al. (2000) Sequential mRNA expression for immediate early genes, cytokines, and neurotrophins in spinal cord injury. *J. Neurotrauma*, 17: 203–218.

Hermann, G.E. and Rogers, R.C. (1995) TNF in the dorsal vagal complex suppresses gastric motility. *Neuroimmunomodulation*, 2: 74–81.

Hermann, G.E., Rogers, R.C., Bresnahan, J.C. and Beattie, M.S. (2001) Tumor necrosis factor induces cFOS and strongly potentiates glutamate-mediated cell death in rat spinal cord. *Neurobiol. Dis.*, 8: 590–599.

Hill, C.E., Beattie, M.S. and Bresnahan, J.C. (2001) Degeneration and sprouting of identified descending supraspinal axons after contusive spinal cord injury in the rat. *Exp. Neurol.*, 171: 153–169.

Horner, P.J., Power, A.E., Kenpermann, G., Kuhn, H.G., Palmer, T.D., Winkler, J., Thal, L.J. and Gage, F.H. (2000) Proliferation and differentiation of progenitor cells throughout the intact adult rat spinal cord. *J. Neurosci.*, 20(6): 2218–2228.

Jakeman, L.B., Guan, Z., Wei, P., Ponnappan, R., Dzwonczyk, R., Popovich, P. and Stokes, B.T. (2000) Traumatic spinal cord injury produced by controlled contusion in mouse. *J. Neurotrauma*, 17: 299–319.

Kuhn, P. and Wrathall, J. (1998) A mouse model of graded contusive spinal cord injury. *J. Neurotrauma*, 15: 125–140.

Li, G., Brodin, G., Farooque, M., Funa, K., Holtz, A., Wang, W. and Olsson, Y. (1996) Apoptosis and expression of bcl-2 after compression trauma to rat spinal cord. *J. Exp. Neuropathol. Exp. Neurol.*, 55: 280–289.

Li, G.L., Farooque, M., Holtz, A. and Olsson, Y. (1999) Apoptosis of oligodendrocytes occurs for long distances away from

the primary injury after compression trauma to rat spinal cord. *Acta Neuropathol.*, 98: 473–480.

Liu, C.N. and Chambers, W.W. (1958) Intraspinal sprouting of dorsal root axons. *Arch. Neurol. Psychiatry*, 79: 46–61.

Liu, X.Z., Xu, X.M., Hu, R., Zhang, S.X., Mcdonald, J.W., Dong, H.X., Wu, Y.J., Fan, G.S., Jacquin, M.F., Hsu, C.Y. and Choi, D.W. (1997) Neuronal and glial apoptosis after traumatic spinal cord injury. *J. Neurosci.*, 17: 5395–5406.

Louis, J.-C., Magal, E., Takayama, S. and Varon, S. (1993) CNTF protection of oligodendrocytes against natural and tumor necrosis factor-induced cell death. *Science*, 259: 689–692.

Majno, G. and Joris, I. (1995) Apoptosis, oncosis, and necrosis: an overview of cell death. *Am. J. Pathol.*, 146: 3–15.

Mattson, M.P. (1998) Modification of ion homeostasis by lipid peroxidation: roles in neuronal degeneration and adaptive plasticity. *Trends Neurosci.*, 21: 721.

McCann, M.J. and Rogers, R.C. (1994) Functional and chemical anatomy of a gastric vago-vagal reflex. In: D.L. Wingate and T.F. Burks (Eds.), *Innervation of the Gut: Pathophysiological Implications*. CRC Press, Boca Raton, FL, pp. 81-92.

McDonald, J.W., Althomsons, S.P., Hyrc, K.L., Choi, D.W. and Goldberg, M.P. (1998) Oligodendrocytes from forebrain are highly vulnerable to AMPA/kainate receptor-mediated excitotoxicity. *Nat. Med.*, 4: 291–297.

McTigue, D.M., Horner, P.J., Stokes, B.T. and Gage, F.H. (1998) Neurotrophin-3 and brain-derived neurotrophic factor induce oligodendrocyte proliferation and myelination of regenerating axons in the contused adult rat spinal cord. *J. Neurosci.*, 18: 5354–5365.

Metz, G.A., Curt, A., Van de Meent, H., Klusman, I., Schwab, M. and Dietz, V. (2000) Validation of the weight drop contusion model in rats: a comparative study of human spinal cord injury. *J. Neurotrauma*, 17: 1–17.

Nagata, S. (1997) Apoptosis by death factor. *Cell*, 88: 355–365.

Noble, L. and Wrathall, J. (1985) Spinal cord contusion in the rat: morphometric analyses of alterations in the spinal cord. *Exp. Neurol.*, 88: 135–149.

Pan, W.H., Kastin, A.J., Bell, R.L. and Olson, R.D. (1999) Upregulation of tumor necrosis factor alpha transport across the blood–brain barrier after acute compressive spinal cord injury. *J. Neurosci.*, 19: 3649–3655.

Panter, S.S., Yum, S.W. and Faden, A.I. (1990) Alteration in extracellular amino acids after traumatic spinal cord injury. *Ann. Neurol.*, 27: 96–99.

Pikov, V. and Wrathall, J.R. (2001) Coordination of the bladder detrusor and the external urethral sphincter in a rat model of spinal cord injury: effect of injury severity. *J. Neurosci.*, 21: 559–569.

Popovich, P.G., Wei, P. and Stokes, B.T. (1997) Cellular inflammatory response after spinal cord injury in Sprague–Dawley and Lewis rats. *J. Comp. Neurol.*, 377: 443–464.

Portera-Cailliau, C., Price, D.L. and Martin, L.J. (1997) Excitotoxic neuronal death in the immature brain is an apoptosis–necrosis morphological continuum. *J. Comp. Neurol.*, 378: 70–87.

Raff, M.C., Barres, B.A., Burne, J.F., Coles, H.S., Ishizaki, Y.

and Jacobsen, M.D. (1993) Programmed cell death and the control of cell survival: lessons from the nervous system. *Science*, 262: 695–700.

Rinaman, L., Verbalis, J.G., Striker, E.M. and Hoffman, G.E. (1993) Distribution and neurochemical phenotypes of caudal medullary neurons activated to express cFOS following peripheral administration of cholecystokinin. *J. Comp. Neurol.*, 338: 475–490.

Rosenberg, L.J. and Wrathall, J.R. (1997) Quantitative analysis of acute axonal pathology in experimental spinal cord contusion. *J. Neurotrauma*, 14: 823–838.

Rosenberg, L.J., Teng, Y.D. and Wrathall, J.R. (2000) 2,3-Dihydroxy-6-nitro-7-sulfamoyl-benzo(f)quinoxaline reduces glial loss and acute white matter pathology after experimental spinal cord contusion. *J. Neurosci.*, 19: 464–475.

Schnell, L., Fearn, S., Schwab, M.E., Perry, V.H. and Anthony, D.C. (1999) Cytokine-induced acute inflammation in brain and spinal cord. *J. Neuropathol. Exp. Neurol.*, 58: 245–254.

Shuman, S.L., Bresnahan, J.C. and Beattie, M.S. (1997) Apoptosis of microglia and oligodendrocytes after spinal cord contusion in rats. *J. Neurosci. Res.*, 50: 798–808.

Springer, J.E., Azbill, R.D. and Knapp, P.E. (1999) Activation of the caspase-3 apoptotic cascade in traumatic spinal cord injury. *Nat. Med.*, 5: 943–946.

Stokes, B.T., Fox, P. and Hollinder, G. (1983) Extracellular calcium activity in the injured spinal cord. *Exp. Neurol.*, 80: 561–572.

Stokes, B.T., Behrmann, D.L. and Noyes, D.H. (1992) An electromechanical spinal injury device with dynamic sensitivity. *J. Neurotrauma*, 9: 187–195.

Talman, W., Peronne, M. and Reis, D.J. (1980) Evidence for L-glutamate as the neurotransmitter of baroreceptor afferent nerve fibers. *Science*, 209: 813–815.

Tator, C.H. and Fehlings, M.G. (1991) Review of the secondary injury theory of acute spinal cord trauma with emphasis on vascular mechanisms. *J. Neurosurg.*, 75: 15–26.

Toborek, M., Malecki, A., Garrido, R., Mattson, M.P., Hennig, B. and Young, B. (1999) Arachidonic acid-induced oxidative injury to cultured spinal cord neurons. *J. Neurochem.*, 73: 684–692.

Wang, C.X., Olschowka, J.A. and Wrathall, J.R. (1997) Increase of interleukin-1 beta mRNA and protein in the spinal cord following experimental traumatic injury in the rat. *Brain Res.*, 759: 190–196.

Warden, P., Bamber, N.I., Li, G., Esposito, A., Ahmad, K.A., Hsu, C.Y. and Xu, X.-M. (2001) Delayed glial cell death following Wallerian degeneration in white matter tracts after spinal cord dorsal column cordotomy in adult rats. *Exp. Neurol.*, 168: 213–224.

Wrathall, J.R., Choiniere, D. and Teng, Y.D. (1994) Dose-dependent reduction of tissue loss and functional impairment after spinal cord trauma with the AMPA-kainate antagonist NBQX. *J. Neurosci.*, 14: 6598–6607.

Wrathall, J.R., Teng, Y.D. and Choiniere, D. (1996) Amelioration of functional deficits from spinal cord trauma with systemically administered NBQX, an antagonist of non-N-methyl-D-aspartate receptors. *Exp. Neurol.*, 137: 119–126.

Wrathall, J.R., Teng, Y.D. and Marriott, R. (1997) Delayed antagonism of AMPA/kainate receptors reduces long-term functional deficits resulting from spinal cord trauma. *Exp. Neurol.*, 145: 565–573.

Xu, J., Fan, G., Chen, S., Wu, Y., Xu, X.M. and Hsu, C. (1998) Methylprednisolone inhibition of TNF-α expression and NF-κB activation after spinal cord injury in rats. *Mol. Brain Res.*, 59: 135–142.

Yong, C., Arnold, P.M., Zoubine, M.N., Citron, B.A., Watanabe, I., Berman, N.E. and Festoff, B.W. (1998) Apoptosis in cellular compartment of rat spinal cord after severe contusion injury. *J. Neurotrauma*, 15: 459–472.

Yoon, S.O., Casaccia-Bonnefil, P., Carter, B. and Chao, M. (1998) Competitive signaling between TrkA and p75 nerve growth factor receptors determines cell survival. *J. Neurosci.*, 18: 3273–3281.

Young, W. (1985) The role of calcium in spinal cord injury. *CNS Trauma*, 2: 109–115.

Young, W. and Flamm, E. (1982) Effects of high dose corticosteroid therapy on blood flow, evoked potentials and extracellular calcium in experimental spinal cord injury. *J. Neurosurg.*, 57: 667–673.

Zipfel, G.J., Babcock, D.J., Lee, J.-M. and Choi, D.W. (2000) Neuronal apoptosis after CNS injury: the roles of glutamate and calcium. *J. Neurotrauma*, 17: 857–869.

L. McKerracher, G. Doucet and S. Rossignol (Eds.)
Progress in Brain Research, Vol. 137
© 2002 Elsevier Science B.V. All rights reserved

CHAPTER 5

Gray matter repair in the cervical spinal cord

Paul J. Reier [1,*], Francis J. Golder [1,2], Donald C. Bolser [1,2], Charles Hubscher [2,**],
Richard Johnson [2], Gregory W. Schrimsher [3] and Margaret J. Velardo [1]

[1] *Department of Neuroscience, McKnight Brain Institute of the University of Florida, Box 100244, Gainesville, FL 32610-0244, USA*
[2] *Department of Physiological Sciences, University of Florida College of Veterinary Medicine, Box 10144,*
Gainesville, FL 32610-0144, USA
[3] *Department of Psychology, University of Houston, 4800 Calhoun, Houston, TX 77204, USA*

Introduction

The advent of fetal CNS tissue transplantation research over two decades ago has led to many new insights about neuronal replacement and functional synaptic network reconstruction. More recently, the prospects of stem cell research (Gage, 2000; Ourednik et al., 2000; Whittemore and Onifer, 2000) have raised the level of optimism to yet another level. Nonetheless, gray matter repair remains elusive in a variety of neurological disorders. This certainly holds true for spinal cord injury (SCI) (Onifer et al., 2000), where regeneration of long tracts alone may be insufficient for optimum recovery, especially with injuries at cervical or lumbar levels. Therefore, while cellular interventions for SCI show promise, very little is known about how to specifically rebuild segmental circuits, many of which are still poorly understood. As shown elsewhere in this volume (Bregman et al., 2002), grafts of naïve neurons also may promote locomotor improvements by forming functional bridges (Jakeman and Reier, 1991; Reier et al., 1992, 1993) in conjunction with other therapeutic approaches. This is theoretically compelling, and it will be important to elucidate how such relays are synaptically integrated with segmental circuits — particularly those that may be undergoing extensive neuroplastic modifications.

With emphasis on gray matter repair in the injured spinal cord, this chapter reviews two separate, but complementary, areas of ongoing investigation in this laboratory. The first set of experiments concentrates on the phrenic motoneuron (PhMN) system as an experimental model for testing transplantation safety and efficacy, as well as for exploring possibilities for beneficially interfacing neuronal grafts with ongoing neuroplasticity. We thus wanted to gain a more comprehensive view of functional neuroplasticity in the PhMN system and a perspective of how, at the segmental spinal level, the presence of novel neuronal populations, derived from primary fetal spinal cord tissue, affects spontaneous repair processes. The second part of this review focuses on the issue of defining alternative sources of donor tissue for gray matter repair. We describe our early findings involving grafts of the neuronal precursor-rich Ntera2 human cell line in chronic contusion lesions of the midcervical spinal cord. As will be discussed, both fetal tissue and the Ntera2 cell line

---

* Correspondence to: P.J. Reier, Department of Neuroscience, McKnight Brain Institute of the University of Florida, Box 100244, Gainesville, FL 32610-0244, USA. Tel.: +1-352-392-5644; Fax: +1-352-392-0431; E-mail: reier@mbi.ufl.edu

** Present address: Department Anatomical Sciences and Neurobiology, University of Louisville School of Medicine, Louisville, KY 40292, USA.

provide important templates for the future experimental and clinical application of other neural and non-neural stem cell lines for neuronal replacement in the injured spinal cord, as well as other regions of the CNS. A brief discussion of the rationale for the concept of gray matter repair and SCI is presented as a prelude to the summary of experimental findings that have been obtained to date.

Gray matter repair

SCI has been commonly regarded as primarily a 'white matter problem'. Some literature suggests that even very extensive gray matter loss in humans may be of little consequence to motor function (Goldstein et al., 1998). This agrees with earlier experiments in which hindlimb function was permanently abolished (Stelzner and Cullen, 1991) following staggered lateral hemisections which left a continuous gray matter, propriospinal circuit between the lesions. Therefore, most efforts to establish therapeutic strategies for improving functional outcomes — including several represented by other chapters in this volume — have concentrated on neuroprotection to enhance fiber sparing shortly after injury or on combined treatments to promote axonal regeneration (Bregman, 1998; Horner and Gage, 2001; Murray, 2001).

This emphasis on long-tract preservation and regeneration, however, is largely predicated by the predominant use of thoracic SCI models and the prevailing focus on motor function. In that region of the spinal cord, gray matter loss appears to be of little consequence as far as hindlimb locomotion is concerned (Magnuson et al., 1999). The case for gray matter repair is far more compelling in the instance of lesions occurring at cervical or lumbar levels (Hadi et al., 2000). For example, restricted gray matter deletion at the L_1–L_2 level of the adult rat spinal cord, without compromise of surrounding white matter, has been elegantly shown to result in locomotor deficits equivalent to those produced by severe thoracic spinal contusion injuries (Magnuson et al., 1999). This is explained by the fact that a significant part of the hindlimb central pattern generator appears to reside at that level of the rat spinal cord (Cowley and Schmidt, 1997; Magnuson and Trinder, 1997). Similarly, cervical cord injuries can lead to deficits in forelimb (Schrimsher and Reier, 1992, 1993; Onifer et al., 1997; McKenna and Whishaw, 1999) and respiratory (el-Bohy et al., 1998) function that relate to both white and gray matter damage.

It has to be stressed, however, that the importance of gray matter repair may not be so regionally restricted for other modalities. Central gray matter destruction alone at thoracic or lumbar levels can profoundly alter neuronal excitability (Yezierski, 1996) and dramatically modify behaviors related to sensation and the expression of central pain (Yezierski et al., 1998). The relatively modest emphasis on gray matter and SCI also is difficult to reconcile when considering short distance, propriospinal cells that can have significant input onto motoneurons at neighboring segmental levels. For example, C_3–C_4 propriospinal neurons in the cat project monosynaptically onto motoneurons, Ia inhibitory interneurons, and spinoreticular and -cerebellar neurons at the forelimb segments of C_6–T_1 (Alstermark et al., 1987, 1990). These cells receive converging cortico-, rubro-, tecto-, and reticulospinal projections and mediate the command for visually guided target-reaching movements and conjoint control of axial muscles to stabilize the trunk during target reaching (Tantisira et al., 1996).

Together, these and other findings, which are beyond the scope of this review, suggest that the issue of gray matter repair after SCI may be more significant than the general SCI literature would suggest (Magnuson et al., 1999; Reier et al., 2000). Furthermore, it is likely that interruption of a cascade of intersegmental, propriospinal coupling, such as in lower vertebrates (e.g. lampreys: Mellen et al., 1995; McClellan and Hagevik, 1999), could contribute to the manifestation of some functional consequences of SCI that are masked by the more obvious motor deficits caused by white matter damage. Therefore, restoration of the continuity of spinal gray matter may prove more vital to the overall recovery process than recognized thus far.

We have recently started to investigate some of these issues of gray matter repair and functional bridging with the intent of superimposing neurotransplantation strategies onto spontaneous repair processes in the injured cervical spinal cord. The PhMN system of the adult rat C_3–C_6 spinal cord is the primary model we have been using because of this system's demonstrated neuroplasticity (O'Hara

Jr. and Goshgarian, 1991) and recovery properties (Nantwi et al., 2000). The PhMN system also has inherent value in relation to preclinical research, since any consideration of future clinical trials, involving subjects with cervical SCI must circumvent the possibility of compromising diaphragm function. However, aside from the obvious question of safety, it is equally important to learn if the introduction of neuronal populations into this or other regions of the spinal cord could adversely affect the expression of intrinsic repair processes. Alternatively, the PhMN system could provide a model for testing if treatments can be used to marshal endogenous self-repair mechanisms and thereby promote even greater degrees of functional improvement. The PhMN system also offers a unique opportunity to explore whether its patterned neural activity can influence the functional integration of neural tissue transplants. This may entail a form of native, neurophysiological 'training' or entrainment of donor neurons through supraspinal respiratory pattern generators that rhythmically drive phrenic motoneurons. Lastly, the functional neuroanatomy of this system provides an ideal setting in which to investigate modes of functional bridging by novel relay circuits and other related considerations.

Neuroplasticity in the phrenic motor system

Organization of the phrenic motor system and its inherent neuroplasticity

Brainstem projections to the phrenic motoneuron pool arise primarily, though not exclusively, from the brainstem ventral respiratory group (VRG). These premotor neurons in the rat provide direct descending inspiratory drive to phrenic motoneurons via monosynaptic projections. In addition, many VRG neurons have bilateral phrenic projections in the adult rat (Fig. 1a) (Lipski et al., 1994), and this may partially account for the fact that these cells are among the least susceptible to axotomy-induced retrograde degeneration (Houlé et al., 1998). Interestingly, VRG neurons retain the longest post-axotomy potential for regeneration compared to other supraspinal neuronal populations (Ye and Houlé, 1997). Previous studies have demonstrated that these neurons can be coaxed to regenerate cut axons into

peripheral nerve grafts where they exhibit spontaneous, phasic bursting activity even in the absence of a target (Decherchi et al., 1996). Experiments described below are based on the neuroanatomical and regenerative features of this system.

One also can appreciate from Fig. 1a that a unilateral lesion of the spinal cord above the phrenic motoneuron pool (i.e., at C_2) will lead to a hemiparalysis of the ipsilateral diaphragm. This provides the setting for one of the more definitive demonstrations of spinal neuroplasticity — namely, the crossed phrenic phenomenon (CPP), which Goshgarian and colleagues (Goshgarian, 1981; O'Hara Jr. and Goshgarian, 1991; Yu and Goshgarian, 1993) have systematically documented over the last two decades. These studies have shown that under rigorously controlled terminal electrophysiological recording conditions, a previously paralyzed hemidiaphragm can suddenly recover function when a contralateral phrenicotomy is made sometime after the original C_2 hemisection. Several lines of evidence suggest that the asphyxic condition caused by an immediate or delayed phrenic nerve lesion activates a previously latent, crossed pathway (Fig. 1b).

More recently, it has been found that the CPP is not limited to terminal, electrophysiological conditions. In one collaborative (Nantwi et al., 2000) and one independently conducted set of experiments (Golder et al., 2001), it has been found that some phrenic functional activity is spontaneously restored on the side of a previous C_2 hemilesion over the course of 1–2 months post-injury (Fig. 2). No evidence of any possible regeneration of descending VRG axons on the side of injury was noted. While the magnitude of this recovery is well below normal, the consistent appearance of this recovery raises questions related to the development of therapeutic approaches for the cervical spinal cord that could enhance this intrinsic repair process. Alternatively, as addressed below, the issue of therapeutic safety emerges in whether or not a particular treatment would interfere with such functional neuroplasticity.

Contralateral plasticity following high cervical hemisection

In theory, axotomy by way of a hemilesion could have retrograde effects on VRG neurons in terms

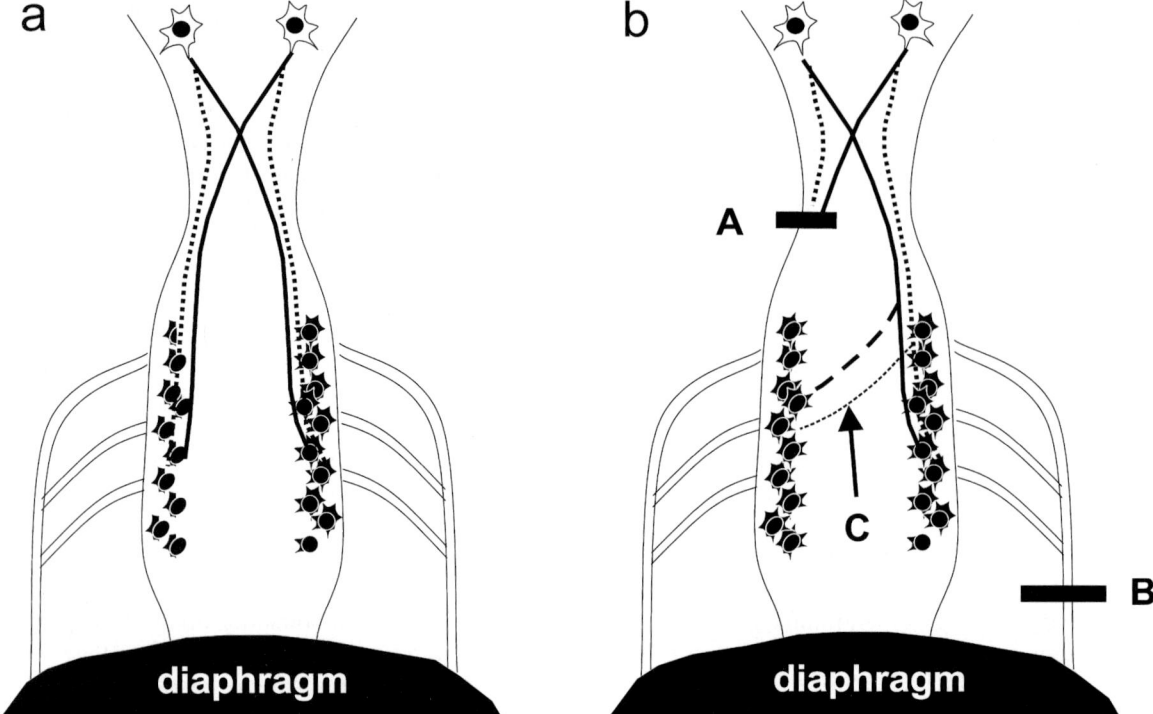

Fig. 1. Diagrams showing the basic neuroanatomy of the phrenic motoneuron (PhMN) system (a) and the proposed plasticity associated with the crossed phrenic phenomenon (CPP) which may also be the basis for spontaneous recovery seen in C_2 hemisected rats and some human conditions as described in the text. As seen in a, premotor neurons form monosynaptic projections on phrenic motoneurons at C_3–C_6 of the spinal cord. Some of these cells have bilateral ipsi- and contralateral projections. A hemilesion could thus axotomize premotor cells bilaterally and affect the physiology of the contralateral PhMN pool. Under terminal electrophysiological conditions in which brainstem drive to the PhMN pool is essentially isolated, the CPP was shown in experiments where a C_2 hemisection (lesion A) was first made followed by a contralateral phrenicotomy (lesion B) (b). The combination of the two lesions should cause complete paralysis of the diaphragm; however, some recovery of function is seen on the side ipsilateral to the hemicord lesion. This is thought to be due to activation of a latent crossed pathway (C) involving collaterals from the contralateral descending premotor fibers.

of their supraspinal activity, as well as their influences on the contralateral phrenic motoneurons via intact, descending collaterals (Fig. 1a). To characterize further the effects of cervical SCI on respiratory function/physiology in the mature rat, we thus became interested in exploring whether a unilateral cord injury would alter activity in the contralateral phrenic motoneuron pool. The recently published findings of that study demonstrated that at 2 months after a C_2 hemisection, supraspinal and contralateral phrenic motoneurons in operated animals vs. unoperated controls showed certain differential alterations in phrenic and hypoglossal motoneuron activity when subjected to set durations of either hypercapnia or hypoxia (Golder et al., 2001). Such altered responses to chemical challenges were not seen, however, at 1 month post-injury (Fig. 3), thereby suggesting that progressive neuroplastic changes may be associated with these electrophysiological responses. As shown in Fig. 3a, before either hypercapnic or hypoxic challenges, the starting respiratory rate (RR) was significantly less in the C_2 hemisected rats than their controls. The peak RR during hypercapnia, however, was similar in both animal groups (Fig. 3b). In contrast, the lesioned rats showed a significantly elevated peak RR during hypoxia (Fig. 4a). Examination of contralateral phrenic neurogram amplitudes showed that during hypercapnia, the hemilesioned rats showed a marked attenuation in the increase of output amplitude (Fig. 3c), whereas no differences were seen during hypoxic challenge (Fig. 4b).

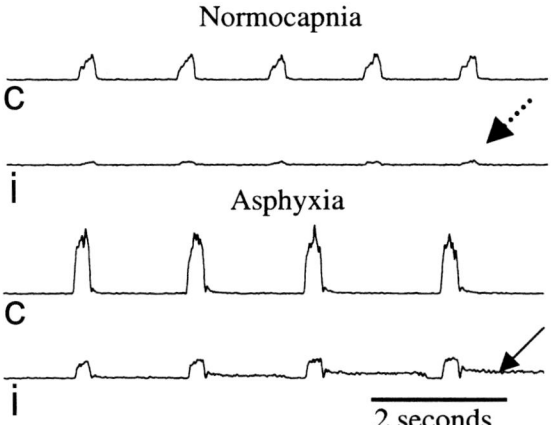

Normocapnia

c

i

Asphyxia

c

i

2 seconds

Fig. 2. Spontaneous recovery of PhMN activity ipsilateral to a hemicord lesion. Integrated neurograms from the contralateral (c) and ipsilateral (i) phrenic nerves in a rat with a complete C_2 hemisection were obtained 2 months post-injury during normocapnia and asphyxic challenge. (Vertical scales (in mV) are the same for all traces.) Synchronous phasic inspiratory activity is seen in the ipsilateral nerve (dotted arrow) under normocapnic conditions. During asphyxia, increased tonic activity is seen during the expiratory phase in the ipsilateral, but not contralateral, neurogram (solid arrow). (Adapted from Golder et al., 2001, Fig. 5.)

A thoracic contusive injury in rats also results in an elevated RR during hypercapnia (Teng et al., 1999). In humans, cervical SCI alters hypercapnic and hypoxic ventilatory responses by increasing minute ventilation thus involving a higher RR and lower tidal volume than normal (Pokorski et al., 1989; Gorini et al., 2000). Although the altered phrenic output in response to chemical challenges could result from segmental changes alone via synaptic/glial plasticity within the phrenic motoneuron pool (Hadley et al., 1999), the changes in respiratory rate which we observed after C_2 injury suggests a possible supraspinal involvement. Those RR data are of exceptional interest as they imply a retrograde axotomy effect leading to alterations in the medullary respiratory pattern generator.

To explore further whether C_2 hemisection had induced supraspinal changes in respiratory motor drive, we recorded ipsilateral and contralateral hypoglossal neurograms during hypercapnia. The rationale for this approach is based on the fact that some VRG bulbospinal premotor neurons with bilateral projections to the phrenic nuclei also project towards the ipsilateral hypoglossal nucleus (Lipski et al., 1994). A C_2

hemisection could thus potentially alter respiratory motor output from both hypoglossal nuclei (Golder et al., 2001). Interestingly, recordings of the hypoglossal neurogram response to a pulsed hypercapnic interval showed significant bilateral reductions in hypoglossal neurogram amplitudes at 2 months, but not 1 month, after the spinal injury (Fig. 3d).

These findings suggest that common segmental and supraspinal mechanisms are involved or that cellular-functional reorganization within or extrinsic to the premotor neurons (Tseng et al., 1996; Bernstein-Goral et al., 1997; Chen and Tseng, 1997; Hubscher and Johnson, 1999a; Jain ct al., 2000; Wang et al., 2000) is occurring between 1 and 2 months after high cervical hemisection. While an axotomy-related change is the favored interpretation of the findings to date, the mechanisms underlying the phenomena observed require further analysis (for additional discussion, see Golder et al., 2001). Accordingly, we cannot discount the effect of interrupted ascending spinobulbar projections as illustrated by other functional model systems that involve neighboring regions of the brainstem (Hubscher and Johnson, 1999a,b).

Contralateral and ipsilateral phrenic plasticity overlap

Both the contralateral and supraspinal effects of C_2 hemisection temporally coincided with the onset of a limited recovery of ipsilateral phrenic motoneuron function. The incidence of spontaneous recovery increased from 25% to 73% between 1 and 2 months, which is consistent with other findings (Nantwi et al., 2000). A similar onset of functional plasticity in the ipsilateral and contralateral PhMN pools suggests these events share a common mechanism or that one is very intimately dependent on the other. Functional recovery in the ipsilateral hemidiaphragm could result, for example, in decreased motor output in the contralateral phrenic nerve via renewed inhibitory phrenic afferent feedback and respiratory plasticity.

Transplantation in the phrenic motor system

The results outlined above have shown for the first time a contralateral effect of a high cervical spinal cord hemisection on phrenic neurogram amplitude,

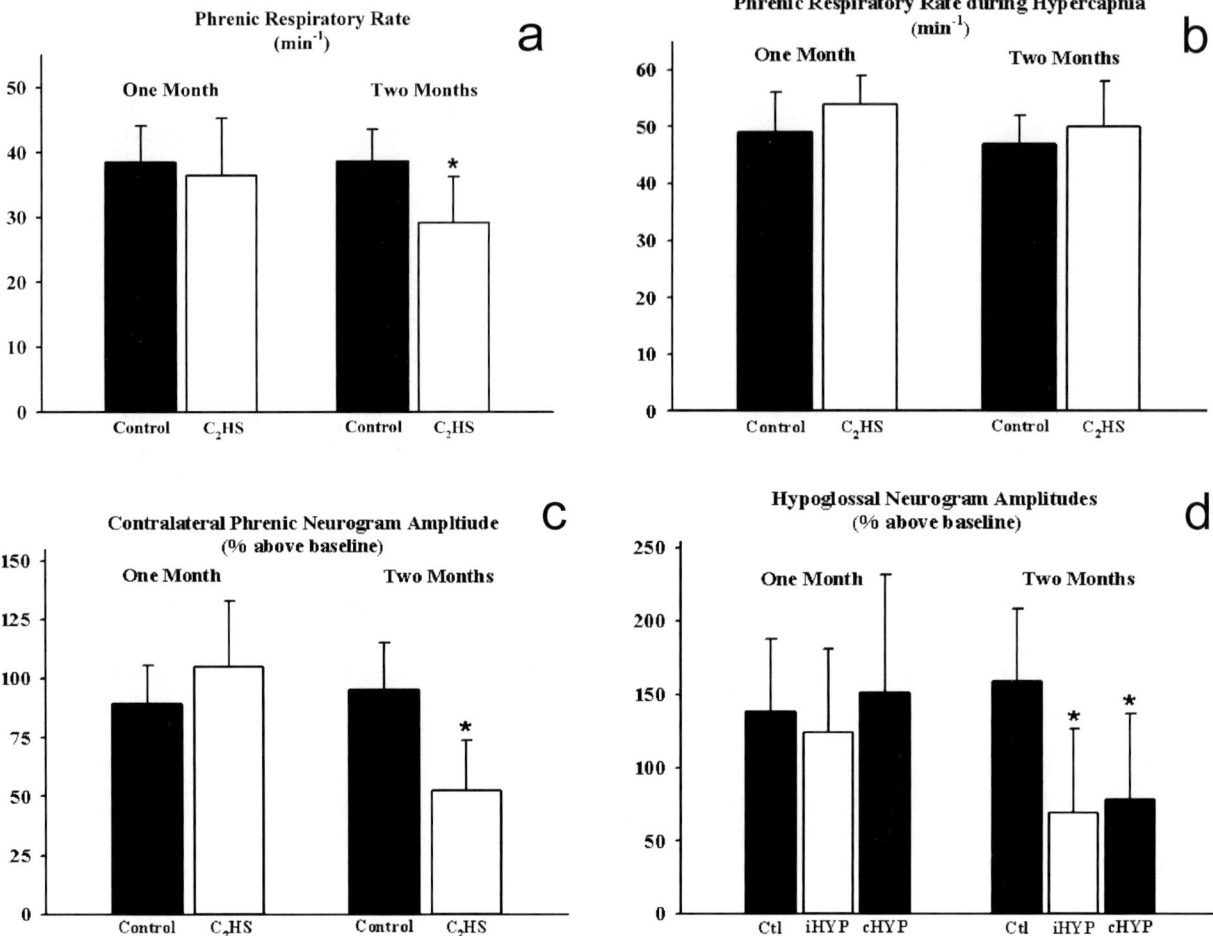

Fig. 3. Summary of changes in phrenic motor (a–c) and hypoglossal (d) activity during normocapnic (a) and hypercapnic (b–d) conditions as a function of time post-C_2 hemisection. Details are explained in the text. C_2HS, C_2 hemisection. (Adapted from Figs. 2 and 4 in Golder et al., 2001.)

as well as a bilateral supraspinal effect on the control of breathing. These responses were not present until 2 months after injury — a time when a modest spontaneous recovery of ipsilateral phrenic motoneuron function also became evident. Whether the ipsi- and contralateral changes are functionally linked is currently under investigation. This study has thus extended our understanding of the range of plasticity that can be expressed in the PhMN system. In addition to revealing more about the basic functional plasticity of this system, these results provide additional endpoints for investigating both the positive and negative effects of various therapeutic interventions addressing high cervical injury.

Fetal cell transplantation and ipsi- and contralateral phrenic plasticity

As shown in Fig. 2, a C_2 hemisection lesion results in an immediate hemiparalysis of the ipsilateral diaphragm; however, within 2 months, a significant number of animals showed a detectable level of spontaneous recovery. In view of this, we were interested in testing whether E14 fetal spinal cord (FSC) grafts into an acute C_2 hemilesion would either interfere or enhance this intrinsic neuroplastic process. Consistent with our previous studies noted above, spontaneous diaphragm function was restored ipsilateral to the spinal lesion by 2 months in lesion-only

55

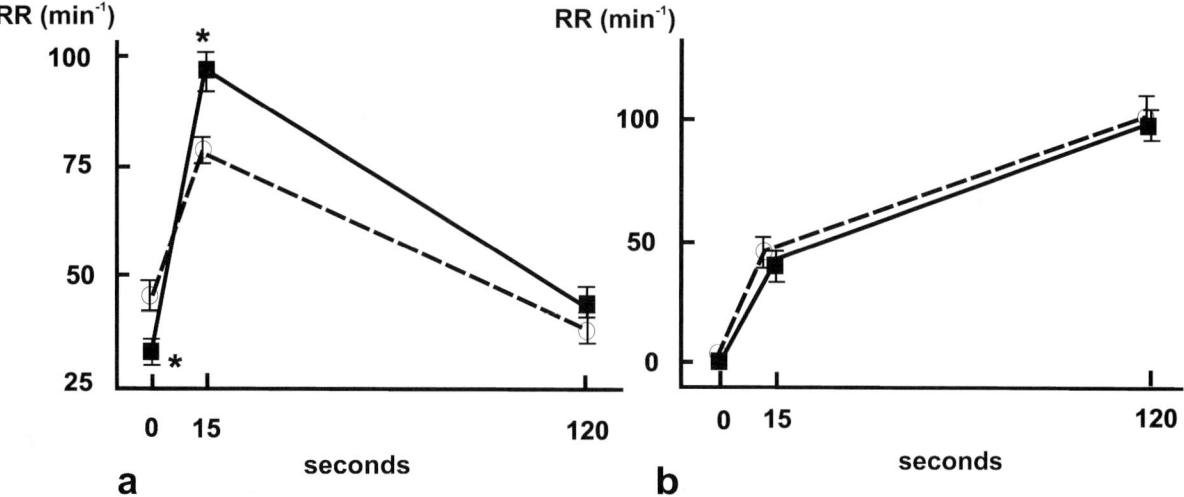

Fig. 4. Respiratory rate (a) and contralateral phrenic output amplitude (b) changes as seen in phrenic neurograms in response to a 2-min hypoxic challenge. Dashed lines and ○ represent unoperated controls; solid lines and ■ represent C_2 hemisected rats. The data reflect means ± S.E.; asterisks denote statistically significant ($P < 0.05$) differences between control and lesioned animals.

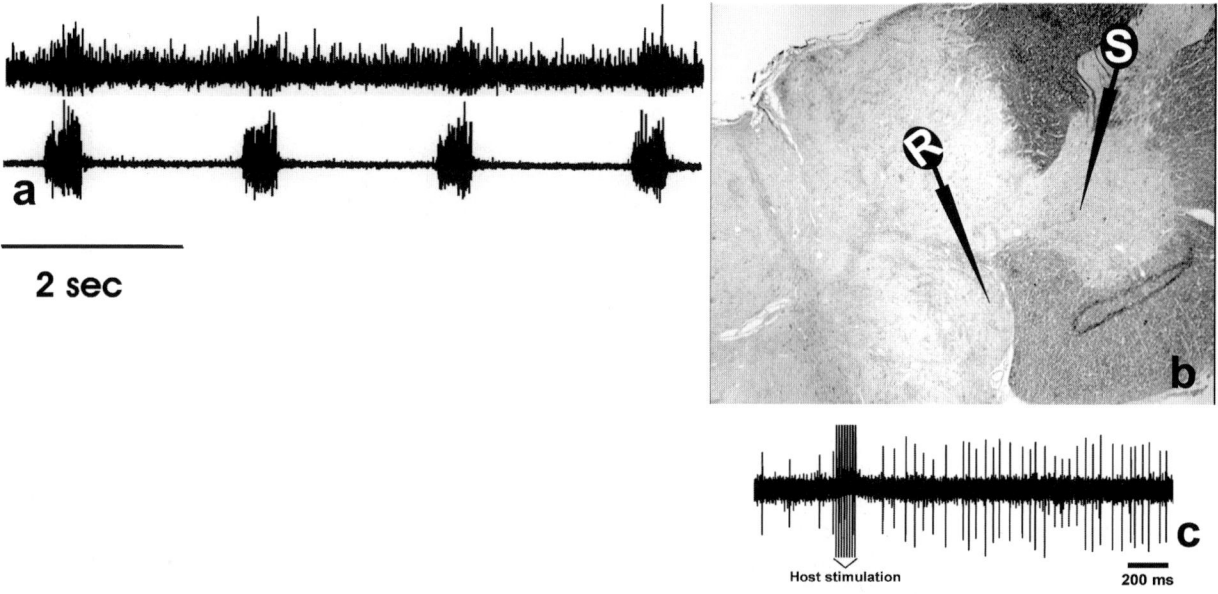

Fig. 5. (a) Raw neurograms obtained from the ipsi- (top trace) and contralateral (lower) trace phrenic nerves of a rat that had a C_2 hemisection followed immediately with a transplant of fetal spinal cord tissue. Note the spontaneous activity in the ipsilateral nerve which was detected 2 months after surgery. (b) Histological example of a fetal spinal cord graft as seen 2 months after transplantation into an acute C_4–C_5 hemisection lesion. This figure also provides some orientation for the positioning of stimulating (S, host) and recording (R, graft) electrodes that were used to demonstrate physiological connectivity between the host and transplant. (c) Shown is one trace demonstrating evoked activation of donor cells near the graft periphery following stimulation of the host contralateral spinal cord.

control rats (Fig. 2). Transplant recipients also exhibited a similar functional return (Fig. 5a), and the degree of spontaneous ipsilateral diaphragm recov-

ery that had resulted seemed comparable to that in the controls. There also appeared to be no deleterious transplant effects on contralateral phrenic function.

Hypercapnic Ventilatory Response

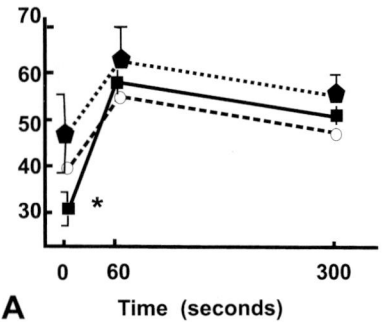

A Time (seconds)

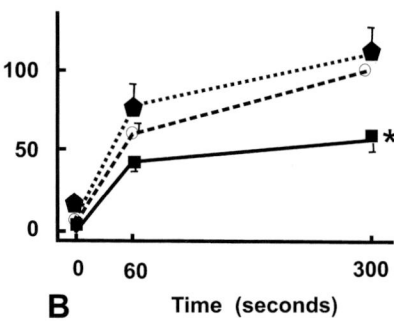

B Time (seconds)

Hypoxic Ventilatory Response

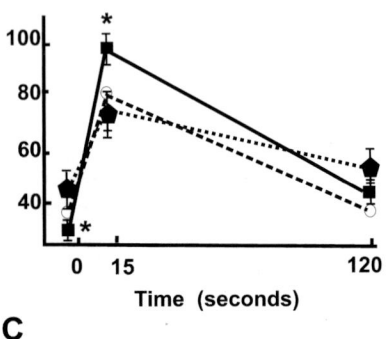

C Time (seconds)

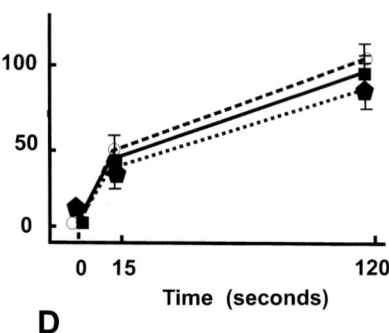

D Time (seconds)

Fig. 6. Transplant modulation of post-C_2 respiratory rate (RR) (A,C) phrenic motoneuron amplitude (B,D) responses to hypercapnic and hypoxic challenges. Dashed lines and ○ represent unoperated controls; solid lines and ■ represent C_2 hemisected rats; ●, solid polygons represent graft recipients. The data reflect means ± S.E.; asterisks denote statistically significant ($P < 0.05$) differences between control and lesioned animals and between graft and lesion-only animals. These initial data suggest that the presence of embryonic spinal cord tissue appeared to normalize normocapnic RR (A,C). Phrenic peak amplitude during hypercapnia also was modulated by the transplants (B). Under hypoxic conditions, lesioned animals showed an increase in RR, but this did not occur in either the unoperated controls or graft recipients (C). The presence of a graft did not appear to alter phrenic amplitudes during hypoxic challenge consistent with what was seen with lesion-only animals (D).

In the same group of transplant recipients, we examined whether the presence of FSC grafts altered contralateral phrenic responses to hypercapnic or hypoxic challenges under comparable physiological conditions relative to arterial blood gases, heart rate, and blood pressure (Golder et al., 2001). Baseline phrenic RR, as noted earlier, was significantly reduced in control rats 2 months post-injury, whereas in transplant recipients, this value was not statistically different from that of unoperated controls (Fig. 6A). Following 5 min of hypercapnic challenge, the lesion only and unoperated controls both showed a rise in phrenic RR. The transplant recipients likewise showed a similar response pattern, and

the graft effect was thus restricted to baseline phrenic RR. Whether these transplants affected hypoglossal output as seen in our previous study (Golder et al., 2001) has not yet been determined. Therefore, it is unknown whether the FSC grafts modulated phrenic RR at the brainstem or indirectly at the segmental level. C_2 hemisection also reduces the rise in phrenic amplitude, which ensues hypercapnic challenge in normal animals (Fig. 6B). Meanwhile, transplant recipients showed no attenuation in phrenic amplitude but instead showed a response to hypercapnia similar to that seen in the intact controls (Fig. 6B).

At 2 months post-C_2 hemisection, a 2-min hypoxic challenge caused an elevated peak phrenic

RR in normal rats. The same occurs in lesioned-only animals, although the RR values were significantly higher (Fig. 6C). Transplant recipients showed changes in RR after hypoxic challenge comparable to that seen in normal controls, although the RR never returned to the prechallenge baseline level as it did in the other animal groups (Fig. 6C). No significant differences were seen between the three groups of rats in relation to phrenic amplitude changes following hypoxic challenge (Fig. 6D).

Neuroanatomical features of host–graft neuronal interaction: grafts as functional bridges

The above data thus showed both safety and efficacy of fetal spinal cord grafts into acute C_2 hemisection lesions by not compromising spontaneous ipsilateral diaphragm functional recovery or preserved contralateral phrenic function. At the same time, these grafts did not appear to be entirely passive because their presence was associated with a modulation of the contralateral neuroplastic phrenic responses to chemical challenges that follow a C_2 hemisection. The fact that the recovery of ipsilateral diaphragm function was not amplified suggests that the transplants might not be serving as a functional relay coupling descending inspiratory drive via projections from the VRG. On the other hand, the apparent graft-associated modulation of post-hemisection changes in contralateral phrenic function could reflect graft–host neuronal interactions at the segmental level. Correlative neuroanatomical and neurophysiological approaches were thus employed in order to define the extent to which a relay setting may be established between VRG axons, the transplants, and the host phrenic motoneuron pool, as well as to gain some insights on potential short-range inter-/intrasegmental host–graft connectivity.

Pseudorabies virus (PRV) transsynaptic tracing (Yates et al., 1999; Billig et al., 2000) was first employed to determine the pattern of potential synaptic connectivity of phrenic motoneurons with fetal spinal cord grafts. Following microinjection of the phrenic nerve ipsilateral to a transplant, robust PRV labeling of the phrenic motoneuron pool was obtained, along with labeling of other neuronal populations both ipsi- and contralateral to the PRV-injected phrenic nerve. Inspection of the transplants also re-

vealed variable numbers of PRV labeled donor neurons. In the more conservative cases (Fig. 7a), very modest donor neuron labeling was observed (i.e., as little as five cells per section), and the majority of those cells were located at the caudal host–graft interface (i.e., just rostral to the labeled phrenic motoneuron pool). This observation is consistent with our earlier retrograde tracing results (Jakeman and Reier, 1991) in which injection of the host spinal cord with Fluorogold resulted in labeled graft neurons close to the corresponding host–graft interface relative to the site of tracer injection. In other cases, a far more robust labeling of graft neurons was seen throughout the transplants (Fig. 7b), and this increased transsynaptic labeling could have been due to virus taken up by phrenic afferents since concomitant infection of dorsal root ganglion cells was indicated in such robustly PRV-labeled specimens. In separate experiments, we performed ipsilateral dorsal rhizotomies at the time of PRV injection. In the three rats studied thus far, all had extremely dense graft infection. Two of the rats had more extensive host label than had been noted previously, while one had immunoreactivity limited to the phrenic motoneuron pool and graft.

The presence of some transsynaptically labeled donor neurons following phrenic nerve injection with PRV and subsequent infection of phrenic motoneurons and other host neuronal populations indicates that these fetal grafts can form short-range synaptic relationships with the host spinal cord and that an efferent limb of a graft-mediated relay can be established in the phrenic motor system. To determine the presence of a VRG afferent component, the anterograde tracer, *Phaseolus vulgaris* leucoagglutinin (PHAL), was iontophoretically injected bilaterally into the region of brainstem based on anatomical coordinates and physiological recordings of VRG multiunit activity that was phase-locked to inspiratory activity. PHAL-labeled axons, detected by immunohistochemistry, were seen approximating the rostral host–graft interface, and in some cases, a few fibers could be seen extending deeper into the grafts but not traversing them. Anatomically, these findings thus demonstrated the potential for a graft-mediated relay that may functionally reconstruct interactions between VRG and phrenic neurons that were previously linked monosynaptically (Ellenberger et al., 1990).

58

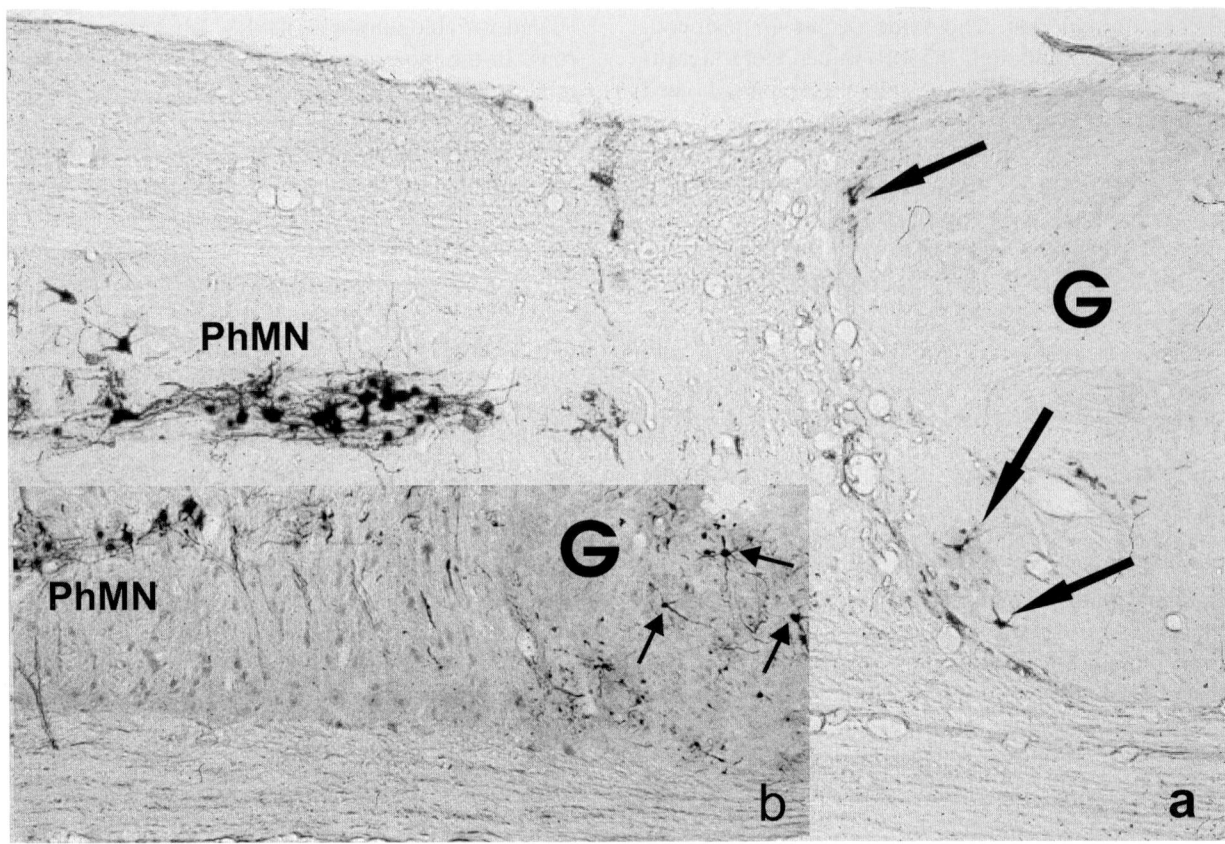

Fig. 7. Pseudorabies virus transsynaptic immunolabeling in two animals with high-to-midcervical hemilesions and grafts of fetal spinal cord tissue (sagittal sections). In both illustrations, robust labeling of the phrenic motoneuron (PhMN) pool is seen. In a, some PRV-immunoreactive neurons (arrows) are seen which are predominantly at the periphery of the graft (G). In b, a greater number of PRV-immunoreactive cells (arrows) is seen, and most of these cells are localized toward the caudal pole of the transplant.

Neurophysiological analyses of host–graft interactions in the cervical spinal cord

Under these transplantation conditions, however, it is obvious that a polysynaptic circuit would have to be involved and previous findings (Jakeman and Reier, 1991) had shown that neuronal populations within these grafts were highly interconnected. Thus, even with restricted ingrowth of VRG axons, it is conceivable that activation of donor cells at the rostral graft pole could ultimately lead to activation of graft neurons at the other pole — some of which are likely to be synaptically linked with the phrenic motoneuron pool based on the PRV results above. To determine whether VRG axons approximating matured fetal spinal cord transplants could make any functional connections, experiments were carried out

in which bilateral microstimulation of the VRG were performed and extracellular recordings were then made from selected donor neurons with identified spontaneous firing properties (see below). Unfortunately, no evoked activity has been detected using this approach (Johnson et al., 2000).

However, relative to our findings regarding the modulation of contralateral phrenic plasticity by grafts into acute C_2 hemisections, we did find that stimulation of the host spinal cord contralateral to a transplant could lead to activation of donor neurons (Johnson et al., 2000) (Fig. 5a,b). Consistent with the PRV labeling results, all of the graft neurons showing evoked activity appeared to be close to the host–graft interface. Many of these cells also showed characteristic spontaneous 'on/off', 'intermittent' or 'slow down/speed up' activity. To determine whether this was a natural feature of these grafts or a type of activity associated with the surrounding environment, E14 FSC tissue also was transplanted into the choroidal fissure region of the brain (Reier et al., 1983). The site of engraftment appeared to influence the frequency at which neurons with these spontaneous firing characteristics were seen. Both spontaneous 'on/off' and 'slow down/speed up' cells were found almost exclusively within grafts placed at C_4–C_5, whereas neurons exhibiting 'intermittent' firing characteristics were common to these grafts in both transplant sites (Johnson et al., unpublished). While there are several possible explanations for these results, the neuroanatomical findings coupled with the evoked activity results just noted, lean towards a synaptically based neuronal conditioning by surrounding host neurons.

Sources of donor tissue for experimental gray matter repair

Many possible sources of stem or precursor cells have been identified for the purposes of 'gray matter repair' — or more specifically 'neuronal replacement' — including neural stem cells from the adult CNS (Kukekov et al., 1999; Laywell et al., 1999, 2000; Palmer et al., 2001) and transdifferentiated non-neural cell types (Pittenger et al., 1999; Brazelton et al., 2000; Mezey et al., 2000; Woodbury et al., 2000). Studies are thus also ongoing in this laboratory, in tandem with the PhMN experiments just described, to explore the safety, feasibility, and efficacy of various sources of donor tissue, and we describe below our initial experience with one neuronally restricted precursor cell line. At the same time, a retrospective analysis of primary fetal CNS tissue grafts has revealed that as an experimental template for gray matter repair, at the very least, these cells may have more in common with neural stem cell related therapies of the future than fully recognized thus far.

Fetal CNS transplants

As in the experiments just described, this laboratory continues to use primary fetal tissue as a template for cellular functional repair in the injured spinal cord. This is based on two considerations. First is that little is known about what will be required in terms of neuronal cell numbers, phenotypes, connectivity and related issues for circuit reconstruction in the injured spinal cord. In that regard, our understanding of neural stem cell biology has yet to reach the level at which high yields of different neuronal phenotypes are available for systematic development of gray matter reconstruction protocols for SCI. Primary fetal cells thus offer a considerable experimental advantage by providing the degree and diversity of neuronal replacement that is required for this purpose (Jakeman et al., 1989).

The second consideration is that matured fetal grafts appear to emerge de novo as the product of the development of lineage-restricted precursors and residual stem cells rather than more differentiated elements already present at the time of donor tissue harvesting and transplantation. This view derives from a previous study in which we examined the early post-graft history of fetal spinal cord tissue as part of an investigation of allograft rejection in the injured spinal cord (Theele et al., 1996). In contrast to the more selective donor cell loss that others have described with fetal CNS grafts (e.g., mesencephalic tyrosine-positive neurons: Boonman and Isacson, 1999; Sortwell et al., 2000), we subsequently found that in the case of rat fetal spinal cord tissue, there is nearly a complete loss of donor tissue by 4 days post-transplantation (Theele et al., 1996). Instead of the cavities being completely filled by graft tissue, as seen at more advanced post-transplantation intervals, all that is present soon after transplantation are small islands of germinal neuroepithelial cells (for illustration, see Reier et al., 2000). From such vestiges of fetal spinal cord tissue, there is a rapid cellular rebound over the course of the next 7–10 days such that by 1 month, the lesion cavities are usually filled by matured donor neural tissue. In more recent experiments (Velardo et al., 1999), we found that grafts of regionally microdissected E14 spinal cord tissue exhibited very distinct cytological and cytoarchitectural features depending upon the derivation of graft tissue from either the extreme ventral or alar aspect of the embryonic spinal cord. These results are consistent with reported differences in the developmental fates of floor plate derivatives (Noll and Miller, 1993), as well as differential expression of positional transcription factors and other neurogenic genes in different regions of the embryonic spinal cord (Tanabe and Jessell, 1996; Lee and Jessell, 1999). It thus appears that fetal spinal cord grafts actually represent transplants of lineage-restricted precursors, as well as residual populations of stem cells (Chow et al., 2000) and thus are a closer prototype to stem cell grafts than previously considered. Fetal CNS transplants thus can still serve as a benchmark against which one can compare outcomes with other alternative sources of donor tissue, particularly neural precursor cell populations.

A neuronally restricted cell line

From this discussion, it is apparent that cell lines yielding high percentages of differentiated neurons after transplantation offer other sources of donor tissue that could have interesting properties with regard to gray matter repair (Whittemore and Onifer, 2000). Intriguing experimental opportunities in that regard are presented by the hNT cell line derived from human embryonal carcinoma-derived cells (NT2/D1, Ntera2). In our experience, the hNT line has provided intraspinal grafts having three-dimensional integrity and neuronal composition approximating primary fetal CNS grafts more closely than what has been obtained with grafts from other stem or stem-like sources (Liu et al., 1999; McDonald et al., 1999; Chow et al., 2000).

Ntera2 cells can be induced with retinoic acid and mitotic inhibitors to differentiate into post-mitotic, neuronal-like cells (Pleasure and Lee, 1993). The hNT neurons then retain a stable neuronal phenotype after RetA withdrawal (Gao et al., 1998; Guillemain et al., 2000). In tissue culture, hNT cells exhibit many bona fide features of CNS neurons and form functional connections with each other (Hartley et al., 1999a). Survival, growth, and differentiation of hNT neurons occurs following transplantation into the developing (Zigova et al., 2000) and injured CNS (Trojanowski et al., 1993). In the case of CNS damage, different degrees of engraftment and cellular differentiation have been described (Pleasure and Lee, 1993).

The most extensive description of the intraspinal engraftment of these neurons has emerged from a recent study in which hNT cells were implanted into the normal spinal cords of neonatal, adolescent, and adult nude mice (Hartley et al., 1999b). The hNT cells remained at the implantation site where they survived throughout the 15-month study period and extended processes into the surrounding host neural parenchyma. The transplanted cells expressed a variety of markers characteristic of mature neurons, such as synaptophysin, hNCAM, hNFM, adult tau, GAD, and TH. Synaptophysin immunoreactivity was localized near the hNT axons, implying the formation of synaptic connections. In contrast to other stem cells (McKay, 1997; Flax et al., 1998; Fricker et al., 1999; Armstrong and Svendsen, 2000), these grafts did not exhibit site-specific differentiation. They did show, however, differential patterns of neuritic outgrowth in the host such that short projections were formed in gray matter and long-distance elongation (>2 cm) occurred in white matter.

Transplants of a neuronally enriched cell line

We have carried out a comprehensive series of studies in which we have tested various preparations of these cells in acute and chronic contusion injuries. A more detailed description of the post-transplantation development of these cells and their integration with the host CNS is in progress (Velardo and Reier, in preparation). For the purposes of this review, we will present some of the cytological features of these hNT xenografts and their neuritic interaction with the surrounding host CNS. The results to be described primarily derive from experiments in which hNT cells were placed into chronic (i.e., 1–6-month-old) contusion injuries of the adult rat C_4–C_5 spinal cord. The animals were then allowed to survive as long as 14 months after transplantation with daily administration of cyclosporine A (10 mg/kg, s.c.). These experimental conditions provided an optimal setting in which to address some issues of safety that immediately are raised by cells having a neoplastic history. This challenging and clinically relevant lesion condition allows exploration of basic questions of graft survival and maturation, host–graft integration, host cell infiltration of the grafts, and host immune responses to these xenotransplants.

Intraspinal grafts of hNT neurons into chronic mid-cervical contusion injuries

Similar to what has been observed with human fetal CNS transplants into the rodent (Giovanini et al., 1997; Akesson et al., 2001), the hNT grafts differentiated very slowly. Thus, at post-graft intervals of <120 days, the cells are typically very immature in appearance. It should be noted that in other experiments (Marsala et al., unpublished observations), the hNT cells differentiated at a faster rate in the presence of FK506, rather than cyclosporine A immunosuppression.

As with fetal tissue, these grafts formed a cohesive mass of cells that often filled the lesion, but did not overgrow. The fact that some cysts were incompletely filled even after several month survival times speaks to this issue and argues against the notion that the hNT cells might revert to their tumorigenic lineage and thus resume proliferative activity. In these experiments, we also used nuclear magnetic resonance (NMR) microimaging of fixed tissue specimens to facilitate our reconstruction of these transplants and to survey whether any hNT cells had migrated and seeded themselves in other regions of the neuraxis. All grafts, even those at the longest survival intervals, were completely confined to the lesion site. In light of these observations, it appears that once rendered postmitotic, hNT cells remain stable under the conditions of spinal cord engraftment. While further analysis is still necessary, it seems that these cells do not migrate. Specific functional studies have not been carried out at this time, however, there was no initial neurophysiological or overall behavioral indications of respiratory compromise despite these cells having been placed into injuries at the level of the phrenic motoneuron pool. The potential of life-threatening respiratory compromise by transplant overgrowth was previously shown in experiments in which fetal neocortical tissue, with a very high proliferative potential, was introduced into upper thoracic spinal lesions (Reier et al., 1992). Under those conditions, the fetal neocortical tissues grew beyond the lesion rostrally to the brainstem, and animals became progressively quadriplegic and exhibited increasing respiratory distress. This has never been observed with the hNT grafts we have studied to date.

As observed with primary fetal grafts in acute and chronic spinal lesions (Houlé and Reier, 1988; Anderson et al., 1989; Reier et al., 1994), the hNT cells showed a high degree of host–graft integration, although some glial demarcation between donor and host tissue was present. In fact, the level of integration with white matter (Fig. 8) rivaled the best seen with fetal grafts into the neonatal rat spinal cord (Reier et al., 1985). At later post-graft intervals, an interesting feature of these grafts was the increasing presence of astrocytes and central myelin profiles (Hartley et al., 1999b). Because hNT cells apparently do not give rise to glia in vivo, the latter observation suggests that these grafts may be recruiting host astrocytes and oligodendrocytes by activation of intrinsic glial precursors.

By 120 days post-transplantation, matured neuronal profiles were observed at the host–graft interface, and thereafter more widespread cell differentiation was apparent throughout the grafts. Immunostaining revealed mature neuronal profiles expressing a variety of neurotransmitters or neurotransmitter receptor phenotypes. GABAergic and tyrosine hydroxylase (Fig. 9a) positive profiles, however, were among the most prominent neuronal populations in these grafts. In several grafts, GAD$^+$ cells near the periphery of the grafts also expressed GluR1 immunoreactivity (data not shown). GluR1 is the structural subunit of the AMPA subtype of glutamate receptors. It is characteristic of spinal interneurons to be GAD$^+$ while expressing glutamatergic receptors. These data are thus suggestive that the majority of the hNT cells may be acquiring a spinal inhibitory interneuronal-like phenotype. While strongly staining ChAT neuronal profiles were not seen in these grafts, faint ChAT-like neuronal IR was observed in some grafts suggesting that hNT cells may have potential to acquire a cholinergic phenotype.

Connectivity and long-distance axonal outgrowth from hNT neuron grafts

Immunocytochemistry demonstrating serotonergic, CGRP, tyrosine hydroxylase, and human neurofilament-specific axons have provided indications of the establishment of both afferent and efferent host–graft neuritic projections. For example, intraspinal grafts of hNT cells appeared to attract

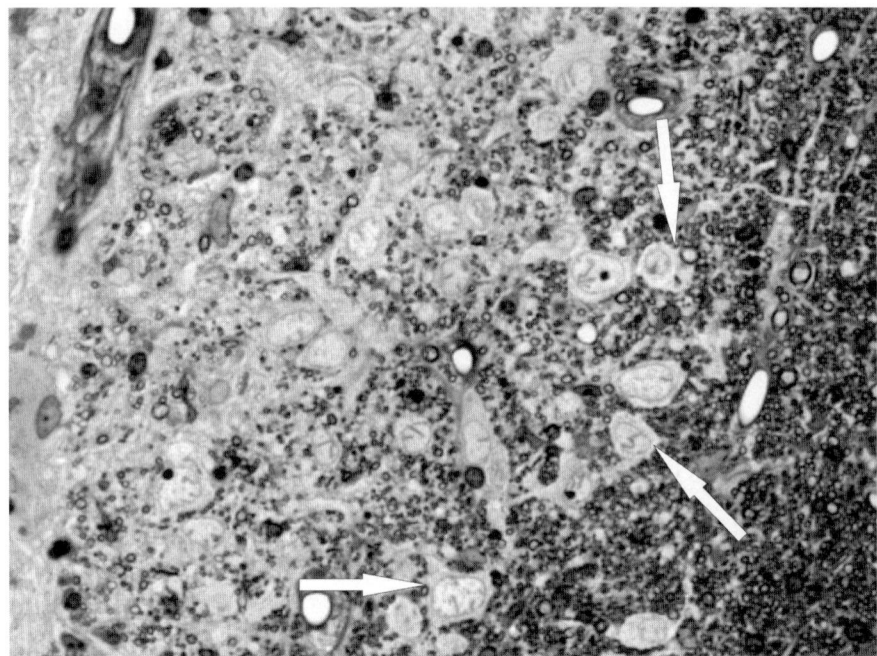

Fig. 8. Ntera 2 neurons (arrows) are seen engrafted in dorsal column white matter of a rat that had sustained a chronic C_4–C_5 cervical contusion injury. These human neurons are highly integrated within rat white matter with no overt evidence of surrounding gliosis or inflammation. These donor cells are easily distinguished from rodent neurons by virtue of their large, and irregular appearing nuclei showing numerous incisure-like infoldings. Two-micron plastic section stained with Toluidine blue.

host 5-HT fibers at sites of graft approximation with regions of host gray matter that are normal targets for 5-HT innervation. This included the ingrowth of 5-HT axons from adjacent motoneuron pools into either the primary mass of transplant tissue or small, ectopic islands of graft cells. Serotonergic axons from Lamina X (around the central canal) also extended across the midline into the hNT grafts. In some cases, the 5-HT fibers were seen deep within the interior of hNT transplants. The pattern of 5-HT innervation of hNT grafts was very striking and appeared to be more robust than that previously observed in fetal spinal cord grafts. Host CGRP-positive fibers also were observed in these grafts. Collectively, these early TH, ChAT, 5-HT, and CGRP fiber immunostaining results suggest that the hNT graft microenvironment is conducive to axonal growth and that these grafts may even have neuritic growth-promoting/neurotrophic properties.

The most striking feature of the hNT grafts was the extensive axonal outgrowth in the host spinal cord, which they exhibited even in the chronic contusion lesion setting. Human neurofilament-specific

(HO14) immunostaining showed prolific process outgrowth within the grafts, which extended into surrounding regions of white matter (Fig. 9b). From the graft site, these hNT cell-derived axons then extended for over long distances (i.e., several spinal cord segments) in both white and gray matter (Fig. 10a,b). Particularly notable was the fact that these axons appeared to favor white matter more than gray and were especially prone to grow in regions of white matter degeneration. Such long-range growth in CNS white matter is considered to be under potent inhibitory influences of myelin-associated inhibitors (Huang et al., 1999; Chen et al., 2000; GrandPre et al., 2000; Huber and Schwab, 2000). However, the elaborate growth of hNT axons could be due to the absence of appropriate receptors for Nogo. Whether this principle applies to other molecules as well, such as inhibitory extracellular matrix proteins (Davies et al., 1997; Fitch and Silver, 1999; Lemons et al., 1999; Moon et al., 2001), remains to be evaluated more directly.

The long distance outgrowth of hNT fibers is very consistent with previous descriptions of axonal

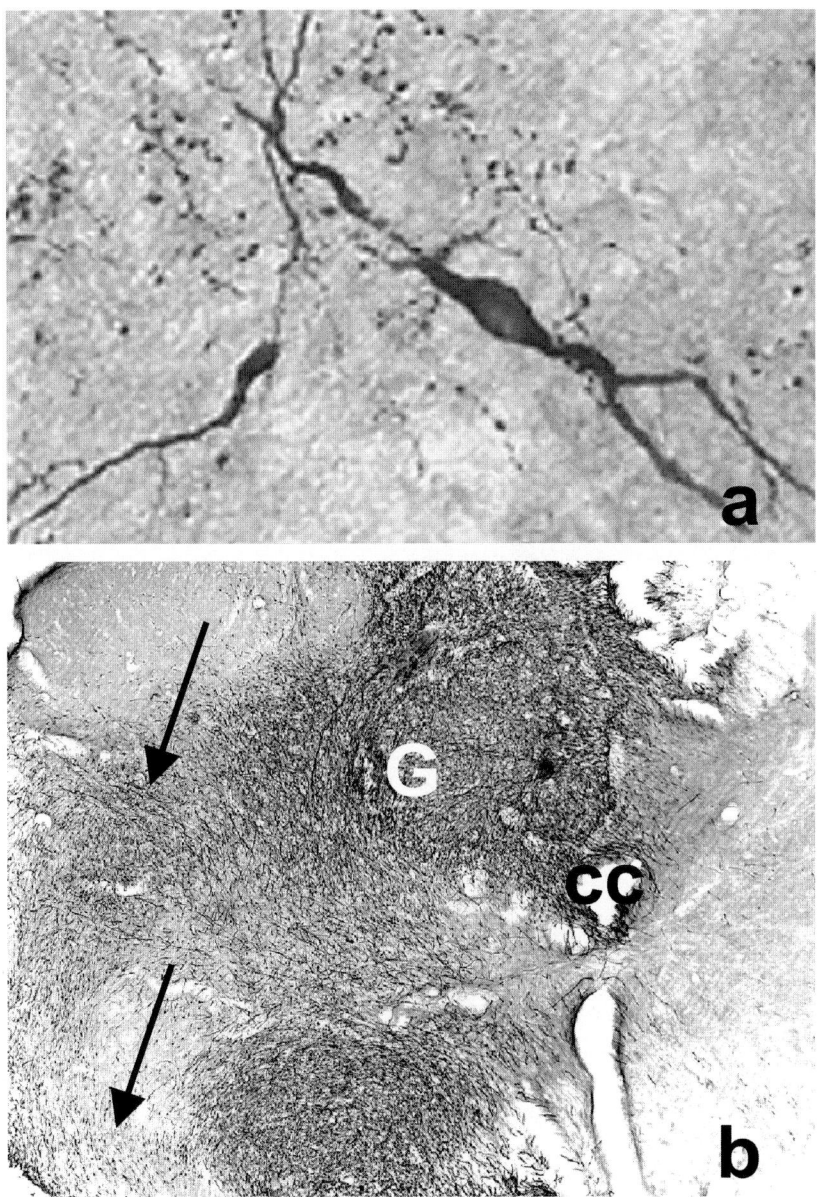

Fig. 9. (a) TH immunoreactivity of Ntera2 neurons over 1 year after transplantation into a chronic midcervical contusion injury of the rat spinal cord. Note bouton-like profiles in the surrounding neuropil of the graft. (b) A large Ntera2 graft (G) is seen in a hemicontusion cavity of the rat cervical spinal cord at 1 year posttransplantation. cc, host spinal central canal. The section was stained with the human neurofilament antibody, HO14. Arrows denote robust neuritic outgrowth from the hNT transplant into surrounding host white matter.

outgrowth from primary human fetal CNS tissue in the adult rat CNS (Wictorin et al., 1990; Wictorin and Bjorklund, 1992). However, while some human fetal CNS neurons in the rat CNS have been reported to establish terminal arbors in certain target sites (Wictorin et al., 1992), the hNT fibers appeared to be more preferentially attracted to white matter. Even when axons were seen coursing through gray matter, there was no indication of terminal arborizations. Instead, in regions such as the dorsal horn, the hNT axons appeared to favor primary afferent fiber tracking. The presence of terminal arbors

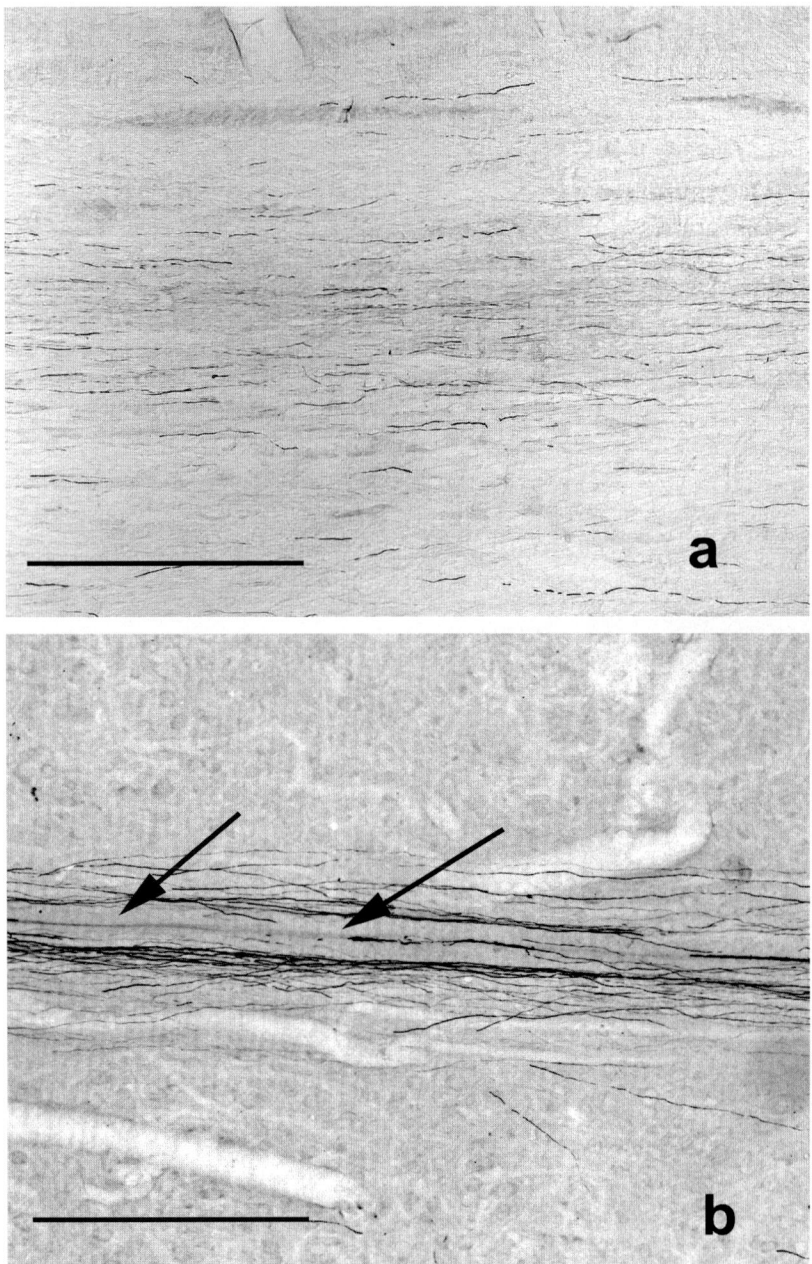

Fig. 10. Longitudinal sections of HO14 stained sections of the rat spinal cord several segments rostral (a) or caudal (b) from the hNT graft illustrated in Fig. 9. Numerous axons are seen in lateral white matter (a), as well as in gray matter coursing adjacent to the host central canal (arrows) in lamina X (b). Scale bars in a and b: 40 μm.

within hNT grafts (Fig. 9a), combined with preliminary results with anti-synaptophysin staining, have suggested, however, that the grafted hNT cells can form synapses with each other as they do in vitro (Hartley et al., 1999a). These initial findings thus leave the impression that any functional outcomes obtained with hNT xenografts in the rat (e.g., Borlongan et al., 1998; Hurlbert et al., 1999) would most likely be attributed to non-synaptic mechanisms. Since this would have profound significance in terms of preclinical investigations and potential mechanisms being invoked, further studies of this important issue are warranted.

Concluding remarks

Many experimental strategies have emerged that now underscore the potential for promoting neuronal survival, axonal regeneration, and functional improvement following SCI. Given the complexity of the problem, however, a proverbial 'magic bullet' cure is doubtful. Future treatments will instead involve a synthesis of complementary approaches (Bregman, 1998; Bregman et al., 2002, this volume; Murray, 2001), and it is likely that many such treatments will require common modalities. Neurotransplantation and interactive (i.e., rehabilitative) training could easily represent two universal therapeutic components.

While the regeneration of long-tract systems is certainly a vital issue, it should not be overlooked that in many cases of human SCI these axons may not be completely compromised. For that reason, the repair process is obviously a far more complex and challenging problem. Furthermore, the necessity of gray matter repair cannot be dismissed especially with regard to lesions at cervical and lumbar levels. In that context, there are now many novel options for donor tissue and neuronal replacement available, including sources of cells that circumvent many of the political and ethical issues that are associated with the use of primary fetal tissue and ES cells. While these alternatives offer great promise, much remains to be learned about how to effectively reconstruct a damaged nervous system before the value of any cell source for this purpose can be fully recognized. From that perspective, transplantation of fetal CNS tissue continues to be an effective experimental tool and a benchmark for many evolving cellular technologies. In addition, the nature of primary fetal grafts appears to represent more of a neural stem cell/lineage-restricted progenitor transplant format than has been acknowledged. Thus, in several respects, primary fetal tissue could arguably represent a template for the ideal stem/precursor cell graft. Furthermore, the cellular diversity of fetal CNS grafts offers many

opportunities for defining what neuronal populations are critical to the recovery of certain functions via segmental circuit reconstruction.

The ultimate success of functional spinal cord repair will largely entail a normalized modulation of motoneuron excitability (Ribotta et al., 2000). In the experiments described in this overview, we have addressed this issue in the phrenic motor system, and the initial data suggest that FSC tissue into acute C_2 hemisections is able to modulate some aspects of the neuroplastic responses of phrenic motoneurons contralateral to the injury. Previous studies in this laboratory have explored gray matter reconstruction relative to hind limb reflexes in the rat (Thompson et al., 1993) and tail reflexes in the adult cat (Friedman et al., 2000) and demonstrated a capacity of fetal spinal cord tissue grafts to modulate motoneuron hyperexcitability. It remains to be determined whether the effect in the PhMN system or elsewhere is unique to the embryonic spinal cord. Anatomical evidence derived from the use of a transsynaptic tracing approach also indicated the possibility of these grafts being synaptically related with surrounding segmental host neurons. This was further underscored by some initial neurophysiological findings showing evoked responses by donor neurons following microstimulation of the contralateral spinal cord and spontaneous firing properties that were unique to intraspinal vs. intracerebral grafts. While many issues remain to be pursued, the trend of results thus far suggest that at least FSC tissue is able to restructure gray matter in such a way as to influence local segmental circuits and thus motoneuron excitability.

The phrenic motor system also provides an excellent opportunity in which to assess the highly relevant issue of procedural/biological safety. Neither primary fetal tissue nor hNT grafts — both of which showed robust growth — had any life threatening or other obviously deleterious effects on phrenic function. The vigorous neuroplasticity of the phrenic motor system also presented an opportunity to look at a subtle, yet relevant, issue of safety — namely, the possibility of intraspinal grafts interfering with self-repair. It was thus important to find that the spontaneous recovery of ipsilateral diaphragm function after a C_2 hemisection was not suppressed by the presence of graft tissue. Under these conditions, however, the transplants did not augment that repair process at least by any mechanism associated with a crossed phrenic phenomenon.

Theoretically, the possibility existed for the grafts to have amplified the recovery process by providing a bridge for regeneration of VRG axons across the lesion. This did not occur in these experiments, however, where grafting alone was performed. Whether the addition of neurotrophic factors could have promoted the regrowth of those axons, as others have reported with PNS or CNS grafts (Bregman and McAtee, 1995; Ye and Houlé, 1997) is a consideration for future investigation.

Likewise, these transplants could have improved spontaneous diaphragm functional recovery by serving as a neuronal relay. PRV transsynaptic tracing and PHAL anterograde labeling showed that both the efferent and afferent limb, respectively, of such a relay to be in place, at least in principle. Again, the combined used of neurotrophic factors may be required to enhance the extent of host–graft interaction. On the other hand, such a novel circuit may not work in this VRG-to-phrenic motoneuron pathway simply because of neurophysiological considerations associated with the conversion of a monosynaptic system to a polysynaptic one. In addition, there is the issue of pharmacological coupling between VRG axons whose inspiratory drive involves NMDA and non-NMDA receptor mechanisms (Greer et al., 1991; Connelly et al., 1992). It may thus require a 'designer' approach to establish a pharmacologically suitable graft construct that FSC tissue in the form presently used falls short of doing without more extensive pre-graft manipulations.

As these considerations illustrate, many questions remain to be explored that apply not only to experimental fetal CNS tissue transplantation, but also to a host of new cell sources that are rapidly becoming available. At the same time, it is important to concurrently explore the merits and shortcomings of alternative cell types for CNS repair. In addition to a variety of other stem cell preparations we and others are currently investigating, the hNT cell line is attractive for several reasons outlined above. Since the use of these cells in a clinical trial has attracted some criticism (Bjorklund and Lindvall, 2000), it seemed important to obtain a better appreciation for their inherent biology under a defined set of neu-

ropathological conditions in the laboratory. As our initial results show, these human cells have many attributes that more closely resemble primary fetal grafts than any other cell line described in the literature thus far especially in terms of their capacity to replace large expanses of tissue destruction with three-dimensionally integrated transplants and their high neuronal yields. Transplants of postmitotic hNT cells provide a remarkably cohesive and safe degree of tissue reconstruction for over 1 year after grafting into contusions of the adult rat cervical spinal cord. The virtually exclusive neuronal composition of these transplants, with subsequent population by macroglial and vascular elements, unequivocally surpassed the extent of tissue repair that has been reported to date with other sources of neural precursors. These observations establish an essential framework for multidisciplinary investigations of the in vivo neurobiology and functional benefits of a human cell line that does not originate from embryos or fetuses but which exhibits primary fetal- and neural stem cell-like features in a clinically relevant model of SCI.

Acknowledgements

These studies were supported by research awards from the National Institutes of Health (1 PO1 NS35702, 1 R443NS38828), the State of Florida Brain and Spinal Cord Injury Trust Fund, and the Mark F. Overstreet Chair for Spinal Cord Regeneration Research. The hNT cells used in the studies reviewed were kindly provided by Dr. Michael McGrogan (Layton Biosciences, Inc.).

References

Akesson, E., Holmberg, L., Jonhagen, M.E., Kjaeldgaard, A., Falci, S., Sundstrom, E. and Seiger, A. (2001) Solid human embryonic spinal cord xenografts in acute and chronic spinal cord cavities: a morphological and functional study. *Exp. Neurol.*, 170: 305–316.

Alstermark, B., Kummel, B.H., Pinter, M.J. and Tantisira, B. (1987) Branching and termination of C3–C4 propriospinal neurones in the cervical spinal cord of the cat. *Neurosci. Lett.*, 74: 291–296.

Alstermark, B., Isa, T. and Tantisira, B. (1990) Projection from excitatory C3–C4 propriospinal neurones to spinocerebellar and spinoreticular neurones in the C6–Th1 segments of the cat. *Neurosci. Res.*, 8: 124–130.

Anderson, D.K., Reier, P.J., Theele, D.P., Munson, J.B., Ritz, L.A., Brown, S.A. and Zeller, B.E. (1989) Development of fetal cat neural grafts in acute and chronic lesions of the adult cat spinal cord. *Soc. Neurosci. Abstr.*, 15: 1242–1242.

Armstrong, R.J. and Svendsen, C.N. (2000) Neural stem cells: from cell biology to cell replacement. *Cell Transplant.*, 9: 139–152.

Bernstein-Goral, H., Diener, P.S. and Bregman, B.S. (1997) Regenerating and sprouting axons differ in their requirements for growth after injury. *Exp. Neurol.*, 148: 51–72.

Billig, I., Foris, J.M., Enquist, L.W., Card, J.P. and Yates, B.J. (2000) Definition of neuronal circuitry controlling the activity of phrenic and abdominal motoneurons in the ferret using recombinant strains of pseudorabies virus. *J. Neurosci.*, 20: 7446–7454.

Bjorklund, A. and Lindvall, O. (2000) Cell replacement therapies for central nervous system disorders. *Nat. Neurosci.*, 3: 537–544.

Boonman, Z. and Isacson, O. (1999) Apoptosis in neuronal development and transplantation: role of caspases and trophic factors. *Exp. Neurol.*, 156: 1–15.

Borlongan, C.V., Saporta, S., Poulos, S.G., Othberg, A. and Sanberg, P.R. (1998) Viability and survival of hNT neurons determine degree of functional recovery in grafted ischemic rats. *NeuroReport*, 9: 2837–2842.

Brazelton, T.R., Rossi, F.M., Keshet, G.I. and Blau, H.M. (2000) From marrow to brain: expression of neuronal phenotypes in adult mice. *Science*, 290: 1775–1779.

Bregman, B.S. (1998) Regeneration in the spinal cord. *Curr. Opin. Neurobiol.*, 8: 800–807.

Bregman, B.S. and McAtee, M. (1995) Neurotrophic factors increase axonal growth after spinal cord lesions and transplants in adult rats. *Soc. Neurosci. Abstr.*, 21: 1056.

Bregman, B.S., Coumans, J.-V., Dai, H.N., Kuhn, P.L., Lynskey, J., McAtee, M. and Sandhu, F. (2002) Transplants and neurotrophic factors increase regeneration and recovery of function after spinal cord injury. In: L. McKerracher, G. Douchet and S. Rossignol (Eds.), *Spinal Cord Trauma: Neural Repair and Functional Recovery. Progress in Brain Research*, Vol. 137. Elsevier Science, Amsterdam, pp. 257–273.

Chen, J.R. and Tseng, G.F. (1997) Membrane properties and inhibitory connections of normal and upper cervically axotomized rubrospinal neurons in the rat. *Neuroscience*, 79: 449–462.

Chen, M.S., Huber, A.B., van der Haar, M.E., Frank, M., Schnell, L., Spillmann, A.A., Christ, F. and Schwab, M.E. (2000) Nogo-A is a myelin-associated neurite outgrowth inhibitor and an antigen for monoclonal antibody IN-1. *Nature*, 403: 434–439.

Chow, S.Y., Moul, J., Tobias, C.A., Himes, B.T., Liu, Y., Obrocka, M., Hodge, L., Tessler, A. and Fischer, I. (2000) Characterization and intraspinal grafting of EGF/bFGF-dependent neurospheres derived from embryonic rat spinal cord. *Brain Res.*, 874: 87–106.

Connelly, C.A., Otto Smith, M.R. and Feldman, J.L. (1992) Blockade of NMDA receptor-channels by MK-801 alters breathing in adult rats. *Brain Res.*, 596: 99–110.

Cowley, K.C. and Schmidt, B.J. (1997) Regional distribution of the locomotor pattern-generating network in the neonatal rat spinal cord. *J. Neurophysiol.*, 77: 247–259.

Davies, S.J., Fitch, M.T., Memberg, S.P., Hall, A.K., Raisman, G. and Silver, J. (1997) Regeneration of adult axons in white matter tracts of the central nervous system. *Nature*, 390: 680–683.

Decherchi, P., Lammari-Barreault, N. and Gauthier, P. (1996) Regeneration of respiratory pathways within spinal peripheral nerve grafts. *Exp. Neurol.*, 137: 1–14.

el-Bohy, A.A., Schrimsher, G.W., Reier, P.J. and Goshgarian, H.G. (1998) Quantitative assessment of respiratory function following contusion injury of the cervical spinal cord. *Exp. Neurol.*, 150: 143–152.

Ellenberger, H.H., Feldman, J.L. and Goshgarian, H.G. (1990) Ventral respiratory group projections to phrenic motoneurons — electron microscopic evidence for monosynaptic connections. *J. Comp. Neurol.*, 302: 707–714.

Fitch, M.T. and Silver, J. (1999) Beyond the glial scar. In: M.H. Tuszynski and J.H. Kordower (Eds.), *CNS Regeneration: Basic Science and Clinical Advances*. Academic Press, New York, pp. 55–88.

Flax, J.D., Aurora, S., Yang, C., Simonin, C., Wills, A.M., Billinghurst, L.L., Jendoubi, M., Sidman, R.L., Wolfe, J.H., Kim, S.U. and Snyder, E.Y. (1998) Engraftable human neural stem cells respond to developmental cues, replace neurons, and express foreign genes. *Nat. Biotechnol.*, 16: 1033–1039.

Fricker, R.A., Carpenter, M.K., Winkler, C., Greco, C., Gates, M.A. and Bjorklund, A. (1999) Site-specific migration and neuronal differentiation of human neural progenitor cells after transplantation in the adult rat brain. *J. Neurosci.*, 19: 5990–6005.

Friedman, R.M., Ritz, L.A., Reier, P.J. and Vierck Jr., C.J. (2000) Effects of sacrocaudal spinal cord transection and transplantation of fetal spinal tissue on withdrawal reflexes of the tail. *Neurorehabil. Neural Repair*, 14: 331–343.

Gage, F.H. (2000) Mammalian neural stem cells. *Science*, 287: 1433–1438.

Gao, Z.Y., Xu, G., Stwora, W.M., Matschinsky, F.M., Lee, V.M. and Wolf, B.A. (1998) Retinoic acid induction of calcium channel expression in human NT2N neurons. *Biochem. Biophys. Res. Commun.*, 247: 407–413.

Giovanini, M.A., Reier, P.J., Eskin, T.A. and Anderson, D.K. (1997) MAP2 expression in the developing human fetal spinal cord and following xenotransplantation. *Cell Transplant.*, 6: 339–346.

Golder, F.J., Reier, P.J. and Bolser, D.C. (2001) Altered respiratory motor drive after spinal cord injury: supraspinal and bilateral effects of a unilateral lesion. *J. Neurosci.*, 21: 8680–8689.

Goldstein, B., Hammond, M.C., Stiens, S.A. and Little, J.W. (1998) Posttraumatic syringomyelia: profound neuronal loss, yet preserved function. *Arch. Phys. Med. Rehabil.*, 79: 107–112.

Gorini, M., Corrado, A., Aito, S., Ginanni, R., Villella, G., Lucchesi, G. and De Paola, E. (2000) Ventilatory and respiratory muscle responses to hypercapnia in patients with paraplegia. *Am. J. Respir. Crit Care Med.*, 162: 203–208.

Goshgarian, H.G. (1981) The role of cervical afferent nerve fiber inhibition of the crossed phrenic phenomenon. *Exp. Neurol.*, 72: 211–225.

GrandPre, T., Nakamura, F., Vartanian, T. and Strittmatter, S.M. (2000) Identification of the Nogo inhibitor of axon regeneration as a reticulon protein. *Nature*, 403: 439–444.

Greer, J.J., Smith, J.C. and Feldman, J.L. (1991) Role of excitatory amino acids in the generation and transmission of respiratory drive in neonatal rat. *J. Physiol. Lond.*, 437: 727–749.

Guillemain, I., Alonso, G., Patey, G., Privat, A. and Chaudieu, I. (2000) Human NT2 neurons express a large variety of neurotransmission phenotypes in vitro. *J. Comp. Neurol.*, 422: 380–395.

Hadi, B., Zhang, Y.P., Burke, D.A., Shields, C.B. and Magnuson, D.S. (2000) Lasting paraplegia caused by loss of lumbar spinal cord interneurons in rats: no direct correlation with motor neuron loss. *J. Neurosurg.*, 93: 266–275.

Hadley, S.D., Walker, P.D. and Goshgarian, H.G. (1999) Effects of serotonin inhibition on neuronal and astrocyte plasticity in the phrenic nucleus 4 h following C2 spinal cord hemisection. *Exp. Neurol.*, 160: 433–445.

Hartley, R.S., Margulis, M., Fishman, P.S., Lee, V.M. and Tang, C.M. (1999a) Functional synapses are formed between human NTera2 (NT2N, hNT) neurons grown on astrocytes. *J. Comp. Neurol.*, 407: 1–10.

Hartley, R.S., Trojanowski, J.Q. and Lee, V.M. (1999b) Differential effects of spinal cord gray and white matter on process outgrowth from grafted human NTERA2 neurons (NT2N, hNT). *J. Comp. Neurol.*, 415: 404–418.

Horner, P.J. and Gage, F.H. (2001) Regenerating the damaged central nervous system. *Nature*, 407: 963–970.

Houlé, J.D. and Reier, P.J. (1988) Transplantation of fetal spinal cord tissue into the chronically injured adult rat spinal cord. *J. Comp. Neurol.*, 269: 535–547.

Houlé, J.D., Schramm, P. and Herdegen, T. (1998) Trophic factor modulation of c-Jun expression in supraspinal neurons after chronic spinal cord injury. *Exp. Neurol.*, 154: 602–611.

Huang, D.W., McKerracher, L., Braun, P. and David, S. (1999) A therapeutic vaccine approach to stimulate axon regeneration in the adult mammalian spinal cord. *Neuron*, 24: 639–647.

Huber, A.B. and Schwab, M.E. (2000) Nogo-A, a potent inhibitor of neurite outgrowth and regeneration. *Biol. Chem.*, 381: 407–419.

Hubscher, C.H. and Johnson, R.D. (1999a) Changes in neuronal receptive field characteristics in caudal brain stem following chronic spinal cord injury. *J. Neurotrauma*, 16: 533–541.

Hubscher, C.H. and Johnson, R.D. (1999b) Effects of acute and chronic midthoracic spinal cord injury on neural circuits for male sexual function. I. Ascending pathways. *J. Neurophysiol.*, 82: 1381–1389.

Hurlbert, M.S., Gianani, R.I., Hutt, C., Freed, C.R. and Kaddis, F.G. (1999) Neural transplantation of hNT neurons for Huntington's disease. *Cell Transplant.*, 8: 143–151.

Jain, N., Florence, S.L., Qi, H.X. and Kaas, J.H. (2000) Growth of new brainstem connections in adult monkeys with massive sensory loss. *Proc. Natl. Acad. Sci. USA*, 97: 5546–5550.

Jakeman, L.B. and Reier, P.J. (1991) Axonal projections between fetal spinal cord transplants and the adult rat spinal cord: a neuroanatomical tracing study of local interactions. *J. Comp. Neurol.*, 307: 311–334.

Jakeman, L.B., Reier, P.J., Bregman, B.S., Wade, E.B., Kastner, R.J. and Dailey, M. (1989) Differentiation of substantia gelatinosa-like regions in intraspinal and intracerebral transplants of embryonic spinal cord tissue in the rat. *Exp. Neurol.*, 103: 17–33.

Johnson, R.D., Hubscher, C., Schrimsher, G., O'Steen, B. and Reier, P. (2000) Graft neuron firing patterns recorded in vivo following long-term recovery in cervical hemisection cavities of adult rats. *Soc. Neurosci. Abstr.*, 26: 1102.

Kukekov, V.G., Laywell, E.D., Suslov, O., Davies, K., Scheffler, B., Thomas, L.B., O'Brien, T.F., Kusakabe, M. and Steindler, D.A. (1999) Multipotent stem/progenitor cells with similar properties arise from two neurogenic regions of adult human brain. *Exp. Neurol.*, 156: 333–344.

Laywell, E.D., Kukekov, V.G. and Steindler, D.A. (1999) Multipotent neurospheres can be derived from forebrain subependymal zone and spinal cord of adult mice after protracted postmortem intervals. *Exp. Neurol.*, 156: 430–433.

Laywell, E.D., Rakic, P., Kukekov, V.G., Holland, E.C. and Steindler, D.A. (2000) Identification of a multipotent astrocytic stem cell in the immature and adult mouse brain. *Proc. Natl. Acad. Sci. USA*, 97: 13883–13888.

Lee, K.J. and Jessell, T.M. (1999) The specification of dorsal cell fates in the vertebrate central nervous system. *Annu. Rev. Neurosci.*, 22: 261–294.

Lemons, M.L., Howland, D.R. and Anderson, D.K. (1999) Chondroitin sulfate proteoglycan immunoreactivity increases following spinal cord injury and transplantation [In process citation]. *Exp. Neurol.*, 160: 51–65.

Lipski, J., Zhang, X., Kruszewska, B. and Kanjhan, R. (1994) Morphological study of long axonal projections of ventral medullary inspiratory neurons in the rat. *Brain Res.*, 640: 171–184.

Liu, Y., Himes, B.T., Solowska, J., Moul, J., Chow, S.Y., Park, K.I., Tessler, A., Murray, M., Snyder, E.Y. and Fischer, I. (1999) Intraspinal delivery of neurotrophin-3 using neural stem cells genetically modified by recombinant retrovirus. *Exp. Neurol.*, 158: 9–26.

Magnuson, D.S. and Trinder, T.C. (1997) Locomotor rhythm evoked by ventrolateral funiculus stimulation in the neonatal rat spinal cord in vitro. *J. Neurophysiol.*, 77: 200–206.

Magnuson, D.S.K., Trinder, T.C., Zhang, Y.P., Burke, D., Morassutti, D.J. and Shields, C.B. (1999) Comparing deficits following excitotoxic and contusion injuries in the thoracic and lumbar spinal cord of the adult rat. *Exp. Neurol.*, 156: 191–204.

McClellan, A.D. and Hagevik, A. (1999) Coordination of spinal locomotor activity in the lamprey: long-distance coupling of spinal oscillators. *Exp. Brain Res.*, 126: 93–108.

McDonald, J.W., Liu, X.Z., Qu, Y., Liu, S., Mickey, S.K., Turetsky, D., Gottlieb, D.I. and Choi, D.W. (1999) Transplanted embryonic stem cells survive, differentiate and promote recovery in injured rat spinal cord. *Nat. Med.*, 5: 1410–1412.

McKay, R. (1997) Stem cells in the central nervous system. *Science*, 276: 66–71.

McKenna, J.E. and Whishaw, I.Q. (1999) Complete compensation in skilled reaching success with associated impairments in limb synergies, after dorsal column lesion in the rat. *J. Neurosci.*, 19: 1885–1894.

Mellen, N., Kiemel, T. and Cohen, A.H. (1995) Correlational analysis of fictive swimming in the lamprey reveals strong functional intersegmental coupling. *J. Neurophysiol.*, 73: 1020–1030.

Mezey, E., Chandross, K.J., Harta, G., Maki, R.A. and McKercher, S.R. (2000) Turning blood into brain: cells bearing neuronal antigens generated in vivo from bone marrow. *Science*, 290: 1779–1782.

Moon, L.D., Asher, R.A., Rhodes, K.E. and Fawcett, J.W. (2001) Regeneration of CNS axons back to their target following treatment of adult rat brain with chondroitinase ABC. *Nat. Neurosci.*, 4: 465–466.

Murray, M. (2001) Therapies to promote CNS repair. In: M. Murray and N.A. Ingoglia (Eds.), *Regeneration in the Central Nervous System*. Marcel Dekker, New York, pp. 649–673.

Nantwi, K.D., El-Bohy, A., Schrimscher, G.W., Reier, P.J. and Goshgarian, H.G. (2000) Spontaneous functional recovery in a paralyzed hemidiaphragm following upper cervical spinal cord injury in adult rats. *Neurorehab. Neural Repair*, 13: 225–234.

Noll, E. and Miller, R.H. (1993) Oligodendrocyte precursors originate at the ventral ventricular zone dorsal to the ventral midline region in the embryonic rat spinal cord. *Development*, 118: 563–573.

O'Hara Jr., T.E. and Goshgarian, H.G. (1991) Quantitative assessment of phrenic nerve functional recovery mediated by the crossed phrenic reflex at various time intervals after spinal cord injury. *Exp. Neurol.*, 111: 244–250.

Onifer, S.M., Rodriguez, J.F., Santiago, D.I., Beneitez, J.C., Kim, D.T., Brunschwig, J.P.R., Pacheco, J.T., Perrone, J.V., Llorente, O., Hesse, D.H. and Martinez-Arizalla, A. (1997) Cervical spinal cord injury in the adult rat: assessment of forelimb dysfunction. *Restor. Neurol. Neurosci.*, 11: 211–223.

Onifer, S.M., Magnuson, D.S.K., Shields, C.B. and Whittemore, S.B. (2000) Grafting into the injured spinal cord to restore locomotion: two decades of promise yet to be filled. *NeuroSci. News*, 3: 50–55.

Ourednik, V., Ourednik, J., Park, K.I., Teng, Y.D., Aboody, K.A., Auguste, K.I., Taylor, R.M., Tate, B.A. and Snyder, E.Y. (2000) Neural stem cells are uniquely suited for cell replacement and gene therapy in the CNS. *Novartis. Found. Symp.*, 231: 242–262.

Palmer, T.D., Schwartz, P.H., Taupin, P., Kaspar, B., Stein, S.A. and Gage, F.H. (2001) Cell culture. Progenitor cells from human brain after death. *Nature*, 411: 42–43.

Pittenger, M.F., Mackay, A.M., Beck, S.C., Jaiswal, R.K., Douglas, R., Mosca, J.D., Moorman, M.A., Simonetti, D.W., Craig, S. and Marshak, D.R. (1999) Multilineage potential of adult human mesenchymal stem cells. *Science*, 284: 143–147.

Pleasure, S.J. and Lee, V.M.Y. (1993) Ntera 2 cells: a human cell line which displays characteristics expected of a human committed neuronal progenitor cell. *J. Neurosci. Res.*, 35: 585–602.

Pokorski, M., Morikawa, T., Takaishi, S., Masuda, A., Ahn, B. and Honda, Y. (1989) Paralysis of respiratory muscles and hypoxic ventilatory chemoreflex. *Biomed. Biochim. Acta*, 48: S573–S577.

Reier, P.J., Bregman, B.S. and Wujek, J.R. (1985) Intraspinal transplants of embryonic spinal cord tissue in adult and neonatal rats: evidence for topographical differentiation and axonal interactions with the host CNS. In: A. Bjorklund and U. Stenevi (Eds.), *Neural Grafting in the Mammalian CNS*. Elsevier, Amsterdam, pp. 257–263.

Reier, P.J., Anderson, D.K. and Stokes, B.T. (1992) Neural tissue transplantation and CNS trauma: anatomical and functional repair of the injured spinal cord. In: J.A. Jane, D.K. Anderson, J.C. Torner and W. Young (Eds.), *Central Nervous System Status Report. J. Neurotrauma*, 9 (Suppl. 1): pp. S223–S248.

Reier, P.J., Perlow, M.J. and Guth, L. (1983) Development of embryonic spinal cord transplants in the rat. *Dev. Brain Res.*, 10: 201–219.

Reier, P.J., Anderson, D.K., Schrimsher, G.W., Bao, J., Friedman, R.M., Ritz, L.A. and Stokes, B.T. (1993) Neural cell grafting: anatomical and functional repair of the spinal cord. In: S.K. Salzman and A.I. Faden (Eds.), *The Neurobiology of Central Nervous System Trauma*. Oxford University Press, New York, pp. 288–311.

Reier, P.J., Anderson, D.K., Schrimsher, G.W., Bao, J., Friedman, R.M., Ritz, L.A. and Stokes, B. (1994) Neural cell grafting: anatomical and functional repair of the spinal cord. In: S.K. Salzman and A.I. Faden (Eds.), *The Neurobiology of Central Nervous System Trauma*. Oxford University Press, New York, pp. 288–311.

Reier, P.J., Thompson, F.J., Fessler, R.G., Anderson, D.K. and Wirth III, E.D. (2000) Spinal cord injury and fetal cns tissue transplantation: an initial 'bench-to-bedside' translational research experience. In: N.A. Ingoglia and M. Murray (Eds.), *Regeneration in the Central Nervous System*. Marcel Dekker, New York, pp. 603–647.

Ribotta, M.G., Provencher, J., Feraboli-Lohnherr, D., Rossignol, S., Privat, A. and Orsal, D. (2000) Activation of locomotion in adult chronic spinal rats is achieved by transplantation of embryonic raphe cells reinnervating a precise lumbar level. *J. Neurosci.*, 20: 5144–5152.

Schrimsher, G.W. and Reier, P.J. (1992) Forelimb motor performance following cervical spinal cord contusion injury in the rat. *Exp. Neurol.*, 117: 287–298.

Schrimsher, G.W. and Reier, P.J. (1993) Forelimb motor performance following dorsal column, dorsolateral funiculi, or ventrolateral funiculi lesions of the cervical spinal cord in the rat. *Exp. Neurol.*, 120: 264–276.

Sortwell, C.E., Pitzer, M.R. and Collier, T.J. (2000) Time course of apoptotic cell death within mesencephalic cell suspension grafts: implications for improving grafted dopamine neuron survival. *Exp. Neurol.*, 165: 268–277.

Stelzner, D.J. and Cullen, J.M. (1991) Do propriospinal projections contribute to hindlimb recovery when all long tracts are cut in neonatal or weanling rats? *Exp. Neurol.*, 114: 193–205.

Tanabe, Y. and Jessell, T.M. (1996) Diversity and pattern in the developing spinal cord [published erratum appears in Science 1997 Apr 4; 276(5309): 21]. *Science*, 274: 1115–1123.

Tantisira, B., Alstermark, B., Isa, T., Kummel, H. and Pinter, M. (1996) Motoneuronal projection pattern of single C3–C4 propriospinal neurones. *Can. J. Physiol. Pharmacol.*, 74: 518–530.

Teng, Y.D., Mocchetti, I., Taveira-DaSilva, A.M., Gillis, R.A. and Wrathall, J.R. (1999) Basic fibroblast growth factor increases long-term survival of spinal motor neurons and improves respiratory function after experimental spinal cord injury. *J. Neurosci.*, 19: 7037–7047.

Theele, D.P., Schrimsher, G.W. and Reier, P.J. (1996) Comparison of the growth and fate of fetal spinal iso- and allografts in the adult rat injured spinal cord. *Exp. Neurol.*, 142: 128–143.

Thompson, F.J., Reier, P.J., Parmer, R. and Lucas, C.C. (1993) Inhibitory control of reflex excitability following contusion injury and neural tissue transplantation. In: F.J. Seil (Eds.), *Advances in Neurology*, Vol. 59. Raven Press, New York, pp. 175–184.

Trojanowski, J.Q., Mantione, J.R., Lee, J.H., Seid, D.P., You, T., Inge, L.J. and Lee, V.M. (1993) Neurons derived from a human teratocarcinoma cell line establish molecular and structural polarity following transplantation into the rodent brain. *Exp. Neurol.*, 122: 283–294.

Tseng, G.F., Wang, Y.J. and Lai, Q.C. (1996) Rubral astrocytic reactions to proximal and distal axotomy of rubrospinal neurons in the rat. *Brain Res.*, 742: 115–128.

Velardo, M.J., O'Steen, B.E. and Reier, P.J. (1999) Regional differentiation of dorsal and ventral fetal spinal cord (FSC) transplants into adult rat spinal cord. *Soc. Neurosci. Abstr.*, 24: 524.

Wang, Y.J., Ho, H.W. and Tseng, G.F. (2000) Fate of the supraspinal collaterals of cord-projection neurons following upper spinal axonal injury. *J. Neurotrauma*, 17: 231–241.

Whittemore, S.R. and Onifer, S.M. (2000) Immortalized neural cell lines for CNS transplantation. *Prog. Brain Res.*, 127: 49–65.

Wictorin, K. and Bjorklund, A. (1992) Axon outgrowth from grafts of human embryonic spinal cord in the lesioned adult rat spinal cord. *NeuroReport*, 3: 1045–1048.

Wictorin, K., Brundin, P., Gustavii, B., Lindvall, O. and Björklund, A. (1990) Reformation of long axon pathways in adult rat central nervous system by human forebrain neuroblasts. *Nature*, 347: 556–558.

Wictorin, K., Brundin, P., Sauer, H., Lindvall, O. and Bjorklund, A. (1992) Long distance directed axonal growth from human dopaminergic mesencephalic neuroblasts implanted along the nigrostriatal pathway in 6-hydroxydopamine lesioned adult rats. *J. Comp. Neurol.*, 323: 475–494.

Woodbury, D., Schwarz, E.J., Prockop, D.J. and Black, I.B. (2000) Adult rat and human bone marrow stromal cells differentiate into neurons. *J. Neurosci. Res.*, 61: 364–370.

Yates, B.J., Smail, J.A., Stocker, S.D. and Card, J.P. (1999) Transneuronal tracing of neural pathways controlling activity of diaphragm motoneurons in the ferret. *Neuroscience*, 90: 1501–1513.

Ye, J.H. and Houlé, J.D. (1997) Treatment of the chronically injured spinal cord with neurotrophic factors can promote axonal regeneration from supraspinal neurons. *Exp. Neurol.*, 143: 70–81.

Yezierski, R.P. (1996) Pain following spinal cord injury: the clinical problem and experimental studies [see comments]. *Pain*, 68: 185–194.

Yezierski, R.P., Liu, S., Ruenes, G.L., Kajander, K.J. and Brewer, K.L. (1998) Excitotoxic spinal cord injury: behavioral and morphological characteristics of a central pain model. *Pain*, 75: 141–155.

Yu, X.-J. and Goshgarian, H.G. (1993) Aging enhances synaptic efficacy in a latent motor pathway following spinal cord hemisection in adult rats. *Exp. Neurol.*, 121: 231–238.

Zigova, T., Pencea, V., Sanberg, P.R. and Luskin, M.B. (2000) The properties of hNT cells following transplantation into the subventricular zone of the neonatal forebrain. *Exp. Neurol.*, 163: 31–38.

L. McKerracher, G. Doucet and S. Rossignol (Eds.)
Progress in Brain Research, Vol. 137

CHAPTER 6

Spinal cord neural organization controlling the urinary bladder and striated sphincter

Susan J. Shefchyk [*]

Department of Physiology, University of Manitoba, Winnipeg, MB R3E 3J7, Canada

Abstract: The storage and elimination of urine requires the coordination of activity between the autonomic nervous system (thoracolumbar sympathetic and sacral parasympathetic divisions) controlling the urinary bladder and urethra and the lumbosacral somatic motoneurons innervating the striated sphincter and pelvic floor muscles. These three efferent systems involved in the control of lower urinary tract function receive segmental sensory information from various visceral organs and the perineum, as well as inputs from supraspinal regions. Ascending and descending connections between the various spinal segments levels and supraspinal regions provide the reflex substrates participating in normal bladder continence and micturition reflexes. Many of the actions of descending and segmental reflexes are mediated by excitatory and inhibitory sacral spinal interneurons located within the region of the parasympathetic preganglionic autonomic neurons and the sphincter ventral horn motoneurons. This review will: (1) discuss the basic organization and spinal elements of the reflex pathways subserving continence and micturition; (2) describe features of the identified sacral interneuronal circuitry contributing to the control of the bladder and sphincter function; and (3) discuss how changes in the control of these reflex pathways and neurons may contribute to abnormal patterns of bladder and sphincter function commonly observed following spinal cord injury.

Introduction

Bladder continence and micturition reflexes are mediated by spinal and spinobulbospinal reflexes involving the coordination of the sympathetic and parasympathetic autonomic control of the lower urinary tract smooth muscle and the somatic motoneurons innervating the striated sphincter and pelvic floor muscles. This review will highlight the organization of spinal cord neurons and pathways controlling the bladder and striated urethral sphincter and discuss some of the changes that may contribute to altered lower urinary tract function following suprasacral spinal cord injury.

---

[*] Correspondence to: S.J. Shefchyk, Department of Physiology, University of Manitoba, Winnipeg, MB R3E 3J7, Canada. Tel.: +1-204-789-3736; Fax: +1-204-789-3930; E-mail: sjs@scrc.umanitoba.ca

Several levels of the spinal cord are involved in sensory and motor integration controlling the lower urinary tract, including both the thoracolumbar and sacral spinal segments. The sympathetic autonomic outflow to the bladder and urethra originates in the lower thoracic and upper lumbar spinal segments and travels via the hypogastric nerves and sympathetic chain to the lower urinary tract. Disruption of the sympathetic outflow to the bladder, while not producing life-threatening complications, does result in a decrease in bladder storage volumes and competency of the bladder neck and proximal urethra. In addition to the sympathetic efferents, there are both nociceptive and non-nociceptive afferents from the lower urinary tract travelling in the hypogastric nerve to the thoracolumbar spinal cord segments. Normally, this sensory input does not play a major role in distension-evoked micturition reflexes but may relay vague sensations of distension in patients with lower lumbar or sacral spinal cord damage.

It is in the sacral spinal segments that one finds the excitatory bladder parasympathetic efferents and afferents associated with the lower urinary tract. The bladder efferents and afferents (distension, pain, temperature) travel in the pelvic nerves and are the basis for the micturition reflex (de Groat, 1975, 1986; Elbadawi, 1996; de Groat et al., 1999). In addition, within the caudal lumbar and rostral sacral segments one finds the ventral horn motoneurons innervating the striated muscles of the external urethral sphincter, which innervate the striated muscle largely via the motor branch of the pudendal nerve (Onuf, 1899; McKenna and Nadelhaft, 1986; Thor et al., 1989; Dubrovsky and Filipini, 1990; Vanderhorst and Holstege, 1997). The sensory branch of the pudendal nerve carries sensory information from the glans of the penis, clitoris and perineal skin (Thor et al., 1989) as well as afferent information from the urethra (Buss and Shefchyk, 1999) to the sacral spinal cord. The basic components of these afferent and efferent pathways are illustrated in Fig. 1. Unlike the situation with the sympathetic innervation of the lower urinary tract, damage to the sacral spinal cord or pelvic nerves results in major disruptions of lower urinary tract function.

Continence

Since the bladder is in a storage mode most of the time, the mechanisms underlying continence are tonically active and only periodically interrupted during micturition. Closure of the bladder neck and proximal urethra is achieved through a combination of mechanical and physical arrangements as well as the neurally mediated contraction of the smooth muscle (reviewed in Vaughan and Satchell, 1995; de Groat et al., 1999). Between voids, the sympathetic system is active and facilitates bladder filling via a β-adrenergic receptor-mediated relaxation of the bladder smooth muscle and an α-adrenergic receptor-mediated contraction of the smooth muscle of the bladder neck and urethra (reviewed in de Groat et al., 1999; Andersson, 2000). de Groat and Saum (1972) found that in the cat, the sympathetic efferents may suppress transmission between parasympathetic preganglionic and postganglionic neurons within the

pelvic ganglia. They proposed that this resulted in decreased cholinergic parasympathetic excitation of the bladder smooth muscle and may contribute to continence. However, there is some debate about the contribution of this mechanism to continence in the cat (Vaughan and Satchell, 1995) and it has yet to be confirmed in humans.

Another major component contributing to continence is the striated muscle of the external urethral sphincter and pelvic floor. The external urethral sphincter (EUS) muscle, which is tonically active during bladder filling, is innervated by somatic motoneurons located in the ventral horn in caudal lumbar or sacral segments. Neuroanatomical and electrophysiological examinations of cat sphincter motoneurons have revealed a number of features that differ from either ventral horn motoneurons innervating hindlimb muscles or spinal autonomic preganglionic neurons. Hochman et al. (1991) and Sasaki (1991) described high membrane input resistance values, short duration afterhyperpolarizations and low rheobase values in sacral sphincter motoneurons — features indicating these are highly excitable cells capable of firing rapid trains of action potentials. Furthermore, Paroschy and Shefchyk (2000) demonstrated the presence of non-linear membrane properties, or plateau potentials, in sphincter motoneurons. Such membrane properties can act to amplify and prolong motoneuron firing initiated by a phasic segmental and descending excitatory input to the motoneuron and thus could contribute to tonic sphincter activity. There is no evidence of recurrent inhibition (Jankowska et al., 1978; Mackel, 1979) of these motoneurons. Furthermore, the presence of axon collaterals which appear to project back to the region of the sphincter motoneuron somatas (Sasaki, 1994) suggests a positive feedback loop capable of sustaining firing. Although lacking a significant segmental monosynaptic excitatory input, a variety of pelvic visceral and cutaneous perineal afferents have powerful excitatory actions on sphincter motoneurons (Garry et al., 1959; McMahon et al., 1982; Fedirchuk et al., 1992). In addition to the tonic activity, phasic bursts of sphincter activity can be evoked during challenges to continence such as sneezing, coughing or postural changes. Presumably, these phasic responses are mediated by pelvic visceral afferents which excite sacral spinal reflex

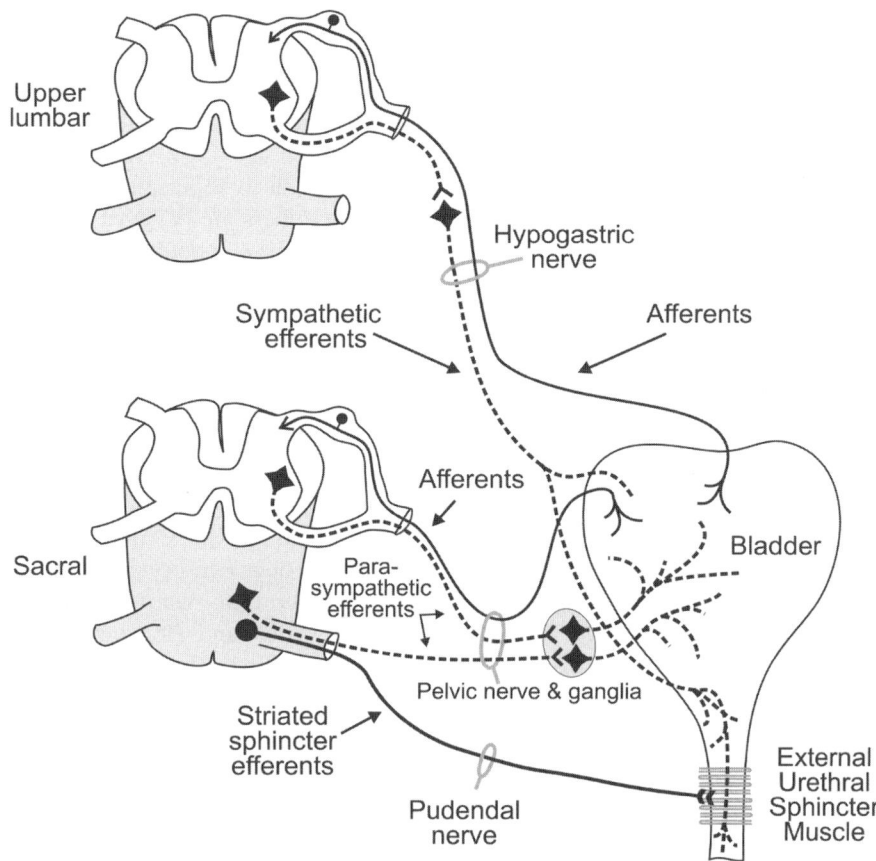

Fig. 1. Schematic of the upper lumbar and sacral spinal cord segments and the innervation of the lower urinary tract. Star-shaped cells in the spinal gray matter represent autonomic neurons (sympathetic preganglionic neurons in the upper lumbar segments; parasympathetic preganglionic neurons in the mid-sacral segments); the dashed lines are the autonomic efferent fibers including both preganglionic and postganglionic fibers. Sphincter ventral horn motoneurons are represented by solid filled circles in the sacral gray matter. Afferents are shown entering the dorsal horn and terminating with an arrow since details about the terminations are omitted for simplicity of presentation.

excitation of the sphincter motoneurons. Descending pathways from the brainstem and cortex to the sphincter and/or pelvic floor motoneurons have also been described (Mackel, 1979; Nakagawa, 1980; Dubrovsky and Filipini, 1990). While voluntary interruption of urine flow by sphincter and pelvic floor contraction presumably is mediated by one or more of these descending pathways, the roles of these various pathways in continence and micturition have yet to be elaborated (Blok et al., 1997b,c).

In summary, both the anatomical arrangement of the lower urinary tract within the pelvis along with neural mechanisms, including lumbar sympathetic efferents and sacral somatic efferents innervating the pelvic floor and sphincter muscles, all contribute to

continence. This multiplicity of mechanisms for continence including both physical anatomical arrangements and neurally controlled factors creates a situation in which damage to descending pathways, such as might occur with suprasacral spinal cord injury, do not necessarily result in complete or even significant incontinence. If the damage leaves the thoracolumbar sympathetic efferent outflow to the bladder intact, sympathetic system-mediated continence mechanisms may be overactive (Krane and Olsson, 1973; Awad and Downie, 1977) as may be the sacral spinal circuitry controlling the efferent output to the striated muscles of the sphincter and pelvic floor (Sethi et al., 1989; Walter et al., 1994). In fact, the inability to control these continence mechanisms can lead to inappropriate continence reflexes during micturition and thus difficulty in emptying the bladder during micturition (Blaivas et al., 1981; Rudy et al., 1988).

Micturition

As mentioned earlier, both the spinal cord and the brainstem are thought to participate in the coordination of autonomic and somatic motor systems during micturition (see Fig. 2). The micturition reflex is initiated by activity in pelvic nerve Aδ-fibers that relay information about the degree of bladder distension to the sacral spinal cord. Pain and temperature information from the bladder is carried by C-fibers (for reviews see de Groat, 1986; de Groat et al., 1997), which in the absence of bladder irritation or spinal cord injury, do not appear to play a major role in micturition reflexes, at least in the cat model examined (Häbler et al., 1990, 1993; Häbler and Janig, 1993). In addition to the role of glutamate, a variety of neuropeptides associated with pelvic afferents have been described (reviewed in de Groat, 1986). Much of the focus has been on substance C and vasoactive intestinal polypeptide, the latter which appears may be concentrated selectively in pelvic visceral afferents (Basbaum and Glazer, 1983).

Once reaching the spinal cord, sensory information from the lower urinary tract has both segmental and supraspinal actions (reviewed in Barrington, 1921, 1925, 1931, 1933). A number of laboratories have described spinal and spinobulbospinal bladder and striated sphincter reflexes evoked by various types of stimulation of the bladder itself, urethra, colon and perineal skin (for examples see Garry et al., 1959; de Groat and Ryall, 1969; de Groat, 1971; McMahon and Morrison, 1982a,c; Mallory et al., 1989; Fall et al., 1990; Mazieres et al., 1997). In the spinal intact anesthetized or decerebrated animal, prior to initiating the micturition reflex bladder and urethral afferents can evoke activity in the striated sphincter and facilitate bladder relaxation (Barrington, 1931; reviewed in Fall et al., 1977; Shefchyk and Buss, 1998; Thor and Muhlhauser, 1999). Stimulation of the pudendal afferents innervating the clitoris, vaginal, anus, glans and perineal skin inhibits bladder contractility (Fall et al., 1977) as well as activates the sphincter efferents (Fedirchuk et al., 1992), actions that oppose emptying the bladder.

Ascending fibers in the dorsal columns, dorsolateral and lateral funiculi (Nathan and Smith, 1951; Nathan, 1952, 1956; McMahon and Morrison, 1982b; Fedirchuk and Shefchyk, 1991; Al-Chaer et al., 1996, 1997; Espey et al., 1998) carry pelvic visceral sensory information to supraspinal regions. Some of these ascending fibers are believed to comprise the ascending arm of the spinobulbospinal micturition reflex present in the mature adult nervous system. Transmission in these ascending pathways is sensitive to serotonin (Espey et al., 1998) as well as excitatory and inhibitory amino acids (reviewed in Downie, 1999).

In the rostral pons is a region, first described in detail by Barrington (1925), now commonly referred to as the pontine micturition center (PMC) (Satoh et al., 1978; Holstege et al., 1986; Griffiths et al., 1990). The ascending bladder sensory information appears to be relayed to the PMC via the periaqueductal gray (Liu, 1983; Blok and Holstege, 1994; Blok et al., 1995; Ding et al., 1997, 1998; Marson, 1997; Matsuura et al., 1998, 2000). The PMC is also subject to both excitation and inhibition from other brainstem, subcortical and cortical regions (several models are presented in a review by Kinder et al., 1995). It has been proposed that the PMC functions as a switch for continence and micturition (reviewed in de Groat, 1995; de Groat et al., 1997) with the descending pathways from the PMC comprising the bulbospinal arm of the spinobulbospinal micturition reflex loop. However, the PMC may have be more complex role to play with more recent evidence that it is involved in the integration for other visceral sensory information and autonomic functions (McMahon and Morrison, 1982a,c; Pavcovich et al., 1998; Valentino et al., 1999; Cano et al., 2000).

When the level of bladder afferent activity reaches a particular magnitude (micturition threshold), continence is turned off and micturition initiated. A variety of descending actions have been described (McMahon and Spillane, 1982). Descending pathways from the PMC may have both direct connections to the sacral parasympathetic preganglionic neurons (Blok and Holstege, 1997) as well as actions mediated by sacral spinal interneurons (reviewed in de Groat et al., 1996; Blok and Holstege, 1999; Shefchyk, 2001). Efforts have been made to identify the descending pathways involved in micturition in both

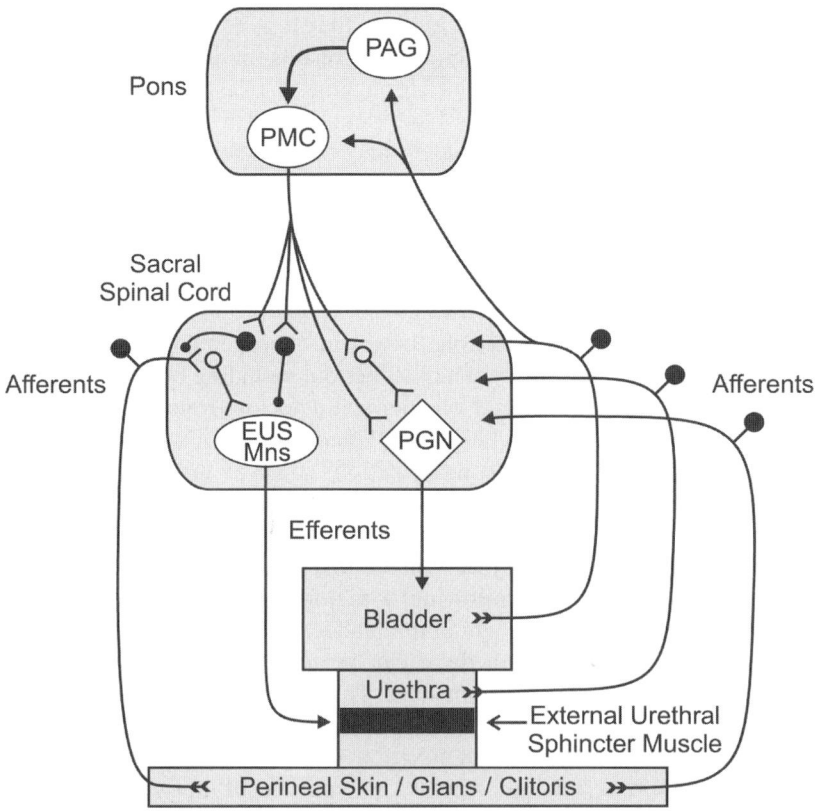

Fig. 2. Schematic of the basic components of the brainstem and sacral spinal neural control of the lower urinary tract during micturition in the adult cat model. The afferents from the bladder, urethra and perineal skin evoke both ascending and segmental reflex actions. The small cells within the sacral spinal box represent several of the major interneuron populations thought to have excitatory (open circle somatas) and inhibitory (filled circle somatas) actions during micturition. Arrows are used to present polysynaptic pathways whose connections are not fully defined. EUS, external urethral sphincter; PAG, periaqueductal gray; PGN, parasympathetic preganglionic neurons; PMC, pontine micturition center; Mns, ventral horn motoneurons.

animals (McMahon and Morrison, 1982b) and humans (Nathan and Smith, 1958) and the general consensus appears to be that the descending fibers travel in the lateral columns of the spinal white matter. Unfortunately, our ability to distinguish damage to ascending versus descending fibers related to micturition is often limited and so it is often not possible to draw conclusions as to whether disruption of lower urinary tract function is due to damage of the ascending or descending arms of the spinobulbospinal micturition reflex loop. Although identification of the descending pathways have sometimes eluded investigators, this has not prevented identification of transmitter systems linked with the pathways that are able to alter excitability of the sacral spinal neurons (reviewed in Downie, 1999). In addition to

evidence that glutamate is involved in the descending micturition pathways (Matsumoto et al., 1995), noradrenaline (Ishizuka et al., 1996), serotonin (Thor et al., 1990) and corticotrophin-releasing factor (CRF, Valentino et al., 1999) have also been implicated.

When micturition occurs, the sympathetic efferent output to the bladder and urethra is depressed while sacral bladder parasympathetic preganglionic neurons are recruited (reviewed in de Groat et al., 1999; however also see McMahon and Morrison, 1982a,c). In order for the bladder to contract and expel fluid through the urethra, not only must their be adequate parasympathetic efferent output to the bladder smooth muscle, but the striated muscles of the sphincter and pelvic floor must relax during the bladder contraction. Evidence in the cat model suggests that the ventral horn motoneurons innervating the sphincter muscles are hyperpolarized by a chloride-sensitive conductance (Fedirchuk and Shefchyk, 1993). Shefchyk et al. (1998) reported that the decrease in sphincter activity that accompanies micturition bladder contractions was sensitive to the glycine-antagonist strychnine and that the sphincter motoneurons appeared to have glycine receptors. Recently, Sie et al. (2001) provided evidence for a direct projection from the PMC to a group of glycine-containing interneurons in the sacral cord, a group which are located within the region that Blok et al. (1998) stimulated to decrease urethral pressure. A percentage of these interneurons also contained GABA (also see Blok et al., 1997a). The presence of GABA-ergic terminals on the motoneurons (Ramirez-Leon and Ulfhake, 1993) suggests that GABA may also contribute to the direct inhibition of the motoneurons. Depression of the sphincter efferent activity appears to be achieved not only by a postsynaptic inhibition of the sphincter motoneurons as just described but may also involve depression of synaptic transmission from perineal sacral afferents which evoked strong excitatory responses in the sphincter efferents (Angel et al., 1994; Shefchyk, 1998; Buss and Shefchyk, 1999). This form of presynaptic inhibition or primary afferent depolarization may be mediated by activation of segmental sacral interneurons (Jankowska et al., 2000) that are recruited during micturition.

The sacral spinal cord houses not only the output cells (preganglionic neurons and sphincter motoneurons) that are targets of the descending micturition pathway, but also contains a rich supply of segmental interneurons involved in the control of sacral efferent outflow (de Groat et al., 1996; Shefchyk, 2001). These various interneuron populations appear to contribute to the excitation of the autonomic parasympathetic efferents, mediate the postsynaptic inhibition of urethral sphincter motoneurons and the modulation of transmission (i.e. presynaptic inhibition) from particular sacral segmental afferents during micturition.

Impact of spinal cord injury to micturition

Since the early work of Barrington at the turn of the century (Barrington, 1921, 1925, 1931, 1933),

it has been evident that loss of descending signals from the brainstem results in lower urinary tract dysfunction. Throughout the last 25 years, numerous studies have documented a variety of changes in the bladder smooth muscle itself, as well as the neural control over the bladder and sphincter in both animal models (de Groat, 1995) and human clinical populations (Fowler, 1999). Attempts to manipulate or reverse some of these changes have been made in efforts to restore more efficient bladder function, however, management of the lower urinary tract dysfunction, including bladder hyperactivity and bladder-sphincter dyssynergia, remains a major clinical challenge.

In the next section, some of the changes in the neural and smooth muscle components of the lower urinary tract described following suprasacral spinal cord injury will be discussed. The period immediately following a major spinal cord injury is one during which the bladder is non-responsive (flaccid) although there can be tonic activity in the striated sphincter muscles. This initial post-injury period will not be discussed further in this review. Rather, the changes in function occurring weeks to years following a suprasacral spinal cord injury will be highlighted.

Bladder smooth muscle

Within days to weeks of the spinal cord injury above the sacral segments, the bladder smooth muscle weight increases and muscle hypertrophy is evident. The changes in the smooth muscle itself, and perhaps also the resulting changes in afferent sensory feedback from the hypertrophies organ, are thought to contribute to the decreased compliance and hyperactivity of the bladder smooth muscle. Bladder hyperactivity manifests itself as frequent small amplitude bladder contractions evoked at low intravesical volumes. The factors responsible for these smooth muscle changes are not well understood. It may be that the overactivity in the sphincter muscle seen after suprasacral spinal cord injury functionally obstructs the urethral and this evoked the bladder smooth muscle changes (Brading, 1997). The important point is that the changes observed in the bladder smooth muscle following spinal cord injury or urethral obstruction appear to be long lasting and not easily reversed. Thus, the presence of these changes in the bladder may seriously confound the effectiveness of successful restoration of normal central nervous system output to the lower urinary tract.

Afferents

As mentioned earlier, normally Aδ-afferents that relay information about bladder distension initiate micturition. A variety of changes in the bladder afferents have been reported following spinal cord injury (reviewed in Yoshimura, 1999). From animal model work, it appears that following suprasacral spinal cord lesions the normally Aδ-fiber-evoked spinobulbospinal bladder reflex is replaced by C-fiber-activated reflex actions in the sacral spinal cord (de Groat, 1995). Sprouting of bladder afferent terminals, presumably mainly C-fibers containing vasoactive intestinal polypeptide (VIP) and substance P, is seen in the sacral spinal cord following transection of the cord at a more rostral level (reviewed in Thor et al., 1986; de Groat et al., 1990). It has been proposed that the expansion of the afferent terminal fields contributes to the bladder hyper-reflexia and decreased micturition threshold. The proposed increased C-fiber contribution to bladder reflexes seen with bladder irritation and spinal cord injury has been the target for manipulation with C-fiber-specific neurotoxins such as capsaicin and resiniferatoxin. Intravesical administration of these neurotoxins presumably desensitizes C-fiber afferents in the bladder and decreases the bladder hyperactivity (Chancellor and de Groat, 1999; Fowler, 2000). Side effects such as bladder pain and irritation associated with the administration of capsaicin have been a problem clinically, however, resiniferatoxin does not produce these side effects and may be a more viable approach for treatment of the hyperexcitable bladder conditions in humans.

Along with the C-fibers afferents from the bladder, a different role for perineal cutaneous afferents appears to emerge following supraspinal cord injury. While perineal stimulation inhibits bladder contractility and evokes sphincter activity in the adult spinal intact animal, this stimulation appears to facilitate bladder emptying in chronic spinal animals, perhaps via activation of spinal neonatal micturition pathways (see Thor et al., 1986; de Groat et al., 1990,

1997). Unfortunately, perineal stimulation also tends to evoke sphincter activity in lesioned animals leading to inefficient voiding.

Parasympathetic efferent changes (preganglionic and postganglionic neurons)

Beattie et al. (1993) described changes in the synaptic contacts on sacral preganglionic autonomic neurons and sphincter motoneurons in acute and chronic spinal cats. They documented a decrease in synaptic contact on the preganglionic neuron somata and proximal dendrites in chronically spinalized animals suggesting the loss of the descending inputs did not initiate the same type of synaptic replacement and reorganization as was seen in sphincter motoneurons. Changes in excitatory amino acid receptor expression on sympathetic preganglionic neurons may contribute to the altered sympathetic efferent responses following spinal cord injury (Llewellyn-Smith et al., 1997). However, no evidence for similar changes in the sacral parasympathetic preganglionic neurons has been reported at this time. Because there is evidence that descending projections activate interneurons that in turn can influence the preganglionic neurons, one might predict that perhaps some of the reorganization could occur at the interneuronal level. This possibility remains to be examined. In addition to the classic spinobulbospinal synaptic reflex connections, it remains to be determined whether or not some of these descending fibers may be the source of neuromodulatory substances that are released less specifically within the sacral segments where they function to modify the responsiveness or firing properties of interneurons and preganglionic neurons.

Bladder-sphincter dyssynergia

Following disruption of the descending pathways to the sacral spinal cord, the normally occurring decrease in striated sphincter activity during voiding may be disrupted producing a condition referred to as bladder-sphincter dyssynergia (Blaivas et al., 1981; Siroky and Krane, 1982; Galeano et al., 1986; Rudy et al., 1988; Sethi et al., 1989; Kruse and de Groat, 1990; Walter et al., 1994; Pikov and Wrathall, 2001). This dyssynergia leads to incomplete bladder emptying and high intravesical pressures which in turn are linked to the deterioration of the upper urinary tract. While normally there is a decrease or absence of sphincter muscle activity during the void, when bladder-sphincter dyssynergia is present, the bladder contraction coincides with tonic or even increased activity in the sphincter muscle (Rudy et al., 1988; Chancellor et al., 1990) resulting in obstruction of the urethra and decreased flow from the bladder. Intramuscular injections of botulinum toxin have been used to eliminate or decrease hyperactive external urethral sphincter muscles in clinical populations (Dykstra and Sidi, 1990; Petit et al., 1998).

It has been proposed that descending signals from the pontine micturition center not only activate the preganglionic neurons (Blok and Holstege, 1997) but are also directly responsible for activation of interneurons that contribute to decreased sphincter activity (Blok et al., 1997a, 1998; Sie et al., 2001). Thus, the loss of the descending excitatory pathway of these inhibitory interneurons would result in weakened inhibition of the motoneurons during voiding. The lack of any significant segmentally evoked inhibition of the sphincter motoneurons, paired with the release of segmental excitatory reflexes to the motoneurons, further contributes to the overactivity of the muscle. These inhibitory interneurons, some of which have been described by Holstege and coworkers (Blok et al., 1997a; Sie et al., 2001) could either mediate a postsynaptic inhibition of the sphincter motoneurons (Fedirchuk and Shefchyk, 1993) or presynaptic inhibition of transmission from sacral primary afferents (Angel et al., 1994; Buss and Shefchyk, 1999; Jankowska et al., 2000). Thus, appropriately timed recruitment of these inhibitory populations could be disrupted or prevented with loss of descending projections and thus contribute to sphincter dyssynergia. In an effort to enhance spinal inhibition and depress the hyperactive sphincter reflexes evoked by segmental afferents, oral and intrathecal Baclofen, a GABA agonist have been used clinically (Hachen and Krucker, 1977; Nanninga et al., 1989; Steers et al., 1992). The depression of afferent transmission seen in the sacral spinal cord with this approach however, also tended to depress bladder and sexual reflex function, thus limited the applicability to sub-populations of carefully screened patients.

Functional electrical stimulation in the control of bladder and sphincter function

Strategies employing electrical stimulation of sacral spinal roots or peripheral nerves to promote bladder emptying following spinal cord injury have been proposed for several decades. Many of these approaches quickly encountered the problem of evoking undesired sphincter activity during stimulation of spinal roots that carry both parasympathetic and sphincter efferents (or afferents capable of reflexively activating the sphincter). The introduction of a variety of manipulations ranging from dorsal root rhizotomies to customized stimulation parameters/methods have been introduced to deal with this challenge (for instance, see Tanago and Schmidt, 1988; Walter et al., 1989; Brindley and Rushton, 1990; Haleem et al., 1993; Sawan et al., 1996). More recently, with a better understanding of the spinal cord circuitry subserving micturition and advances in biomedical technology, the approach of focal intraspinal stimulation (Woodford et al., 1996; Grill et al., 1998; Prochzska et al., 2001) may provide a means of overcoming many of the difficulties encountered with functional electrical stimulation for bladder function.

Conclusions

In summary, over the last 20 years, a picture of the elegance of the sacral network organization responsible for the coordination of bladder parasympathetic neurons and sphincter motoneurons has developed (reviewed in de Groat et al., 1996; Shefchyk, 2001). The contributions of plastic changes in the afferents controlling bladder reflexes, while long recognized, must now be put in a more refined context of the normal or abnormal activation of this sacral neural circuitry. The challenge remains to identify: (1) the various populations of sacral spinal interneurons key to the activation and coordination of the bladder parasympathetics and sphincter somatic efferent activity; (2) the segmental and descending pathways and transmitters controlling these interneurons; and (3) the transmitters used by these various interneurons to control the efferent outputs from the sacral spinal cord. With this information, it may be possible to develop new approaches to re-balancing the system and restoring efficient bladder filling and emptying following brain or spinal cord injury.

Acknowledgements

This work was supported by a grant from the Canadian Institutes for Health Research. I would like to thank Shannon Deschamps and Maria Setterbom for their secretarial/graphics assistance in preparing this review and Dr. John Downie for his helpful comments.

References

Al-Chaer, E.D., Lawand, N.B., Westlund, K.N. and Willis, W.D. (1996) Pelvic visceral input into the nucleus gracilis is largely mediated by the postsynaptic dorsal column pathway. *J. Neurophysiol.*, 76: 2675–2690.

Al-Chaer, E.D., Westlund, K.N. and Willis, W.D. (1997) Nucleus gracilis: an integrator for visceral and somatic information. *J. Neurophysiol.*, 78: 521–527.

Andersson, K.-E. (2000) Treatment of overactive bladder: other drug mechanisms. *Urology*, 55(Suppl. 5A): 51–57.

Angel, M.J., Fyda, D., McCrea, D.A. and Shefchyk, S.J. (1994) Primary afferent depolarization of cat pudendal afferents during micturition and segmental afferent stimulation. *J. Physiol.*, 479: 451–461.

Awad, S.A. and Downie, J.W. (1977) Sympathetic dyssynergia in the region of the external sphincter: a possible source of lower urinary tract obstruction. *J. Urol.*, 118: 636–640.

Barrington, F.J.F. (1921) The relation of the hind-brain to micturition. *Brain*, 4: 23–53.

Barrington, F.J.F. (1925) The effect of lesions of the hind- and mid-brain on micturition in the cat. *Q. J. Exp. Physiol.*, 15: 81–102.

Barrington, F.J.F. (1931) The component reflexes of micturition in the cat. Parts I and II. *Brain*, 54: 177–188.

Barrington, F.J.F. (1933) The localization of the paths subserving micturition in the spinal cord of the cat. *Brain*, 56: 126–148.

Basbaum, A.I. and Glazer, E.J. (1983) Immunoreactive vasoactive intestinal polypeptide is concentrated in the sacral spinal cord: a possible marker for pelvic visceral afferent fibers. *Somatosensory Res.*, 1: 69–82.

Beattie, M.S., Leedy, M.G. and Bresnahan, J.C. (1993) Evidence for alterations of synaptic inputs to sacral spinal reflex circuits after spinal cord transection in the cat. *Exp. Neurol.*, 123: 35–50.

Blaivas, J.G., Sinha, H.P., Zayed, A.A.H. and Labib, K.B. (1981) Detrusor-external sphincter dyssynergia: a detailed electromyographic study. *J. Urol.*, 125: 545–548.

Blok, B.F.M. and Holstege, G. (1994) Direct projections from the periaqueductal gray to the pontine micturition center (M-region). An anterograde and retrograde tracing study in the cat. *Neurosci. Lett.*, 166: 93–96.

Blok, B.F.M. and Holstege, G. (1997) Ultrastructural evidence for a direct pathway from the pontine micturition center to the parasympathetic preganglionic motoneurons of the bladder of the cat. *Neurosci. Lett.*, 222: 195–198.

Blok, B.F.M. and Holstege, G. (1999) The central control of micturition and continence: implications for urology. *B.J.U. Int.*, 83(Suppl. 2): 1–6.

Blok, B.F.M., De Weerd, H. and Holstege, G. (1995) Ultrastructural evidence for a paucity of projections from the lumbosacral cord to the pontine micturition center or M-region in the cat: a new concept for the organization of the micturition reflex with the periaqueductal gray as central relay. *J. Comp. Neurol.*, 359: 300–309.

Blok, B.F.M., DeWeerd, H. and Holstege, G. (1997a) The pontine micturition center projects to sacral cord GABA immunoreactive neurons in the cat. *Neurosci. Lett.*, 233: 109–112.

Blok, B.F.M., Sturms, L.M. and Holstege, G. (1997b) A PET study on cortical and subcortical control of pelvic floor musculature in women. *J. Comp. Neurol.*, 389: 535–544.

Blok, B.F.M., Willemsen, A.T.M. and Holstege, G. (1997c) A PET study on brain control of micturition in humans. *Brain*, 120: 111–121.

Blok, B.F.M., Van Maarseveen, J.T.P.W. and Holstege, G. (1998) Electrical stimulation of the sacral dorsal gray commissure evokes relaxation of the external urethral sphincter in the cat. *Neurosci. Lett.*, 249: 68–70.

Brading, A. (1997) Alterations in the physiological properties of urinary bladder smooth muscle caused by bladder emptying against an obstruction. *Scand. J. Urol. Nephrol.*, Suppl. 184: 51–58.

Brindley, G.S. and Rushton, D.N. (1990) Long-term follow-up of patients with sacral anterior root stimulator implants. *Paraplegia*, 28: 469–475.

Buss, R.R. and Shefchyk, S.J. (1999) Excitability changes in sacral afferents innervating the urethra, perineum and hindlimb skin of the cat during micturition. *J. Physiol.*, 514(2): 593–607.

Cano, G., Card, J.P., Rinaman, L. and Sved, A.F. (2000) Connections of Barrington's nucleus to the sympathetic nervous system in rats. *J. Auton. Nerv. Syst.*, 79: 117–128.

Chancellor, M.B. and de Groat, W.C. (1999) Intravesical capsaicin and resiniferatoxin therapy: spicing up the ways to treat the overactive bladder. *J. Urol.*, 162: 3–11.

Chancellor, M.B., Kaplan, S.A. and Blaivas, J.G. (1990) Detrusor-external sphincter dyssynergia. *Ciba Found. Symp.*, 151: 207–213.

de Groat, W.C. (1971) Inhibition and excitation of sacral parasympathetic neurons by visceral and cutaneous stimuli in the cat. *Brain Res.*, 33: 499–503.

de Groat, W.C. (1975) Nervous control of the urinary bladder of the cat. *Brain Res.*, 87: 201–211.

de Groat, W.C. (1986) Spinal cord projections and neuropeptides in visceral afferent neurons. *Prog. Brain Res.*, 67: 165–187.

de Groat, W.C. (1995) Mechanisms underlying the recovery of lower urinary tract function following spinal cord injury. *Paraplegia*, 33: 493–505.

de Groat, W.C. and Ryall, R.W. (1969) Reflexes to sacral parasympathetic neurones concerned with micturition in the cat. *J. Physiol.*, 200: 87–108.

de Groat, W.C. and Saum, W.R. (1972) Sympathetic inhibition of the urinary bladder and of pelvic ganglionic transmission in the cat. *J. Physiol.*, 220: 297–314.

de Groat, W.C., Kawatani, M., Hisamitsu, T., Cheng, C.-L., Ma, C.-P., Thor, K., Steers, W. and Roppolo, J.R. (1990) Mechanisms underlying the recovery of urinary bladder function following spinal cord injury. *J. Auton. Nerv. Syst.*, 30: S71–S78.

de Groat, W.C., Vizzard, M.A., Araki, I. and Roppolo, J. (1996) Spinal interneurons and preganglionic neurons in sacral autonomic reflex pathways. *Prog. Brain Res.*, 107: 97–111.

de Groat, W.C., Kruse, M.N., Vizzard, M.A., Cheng, C.-L., Araki, I. and Yoshimura, N. (1997) Modification of urinary bladder function after spinal cord injury. *Adv. Neurol.*, 72: 347–364.

de Groat, W.C., Downie, J.W., Levin, R.M., Long Lin, A.T., Morrison, J.F.B., Nishizawa, O., Steers, W.D. and Thor, K.B. (1999) Basic neurophysiology and neuropharmacology. In: P. Abrams, S. Khoury, A. Wein (Eds)., *Incontinence*. Plymbridge Distributors Ltd, Plymouth, pp. 107–154.

Ding, Y.-Q., Zeng, H.-X., Gong, L.-W., Lu, Y., Zhao, H. and Qin, B.-Z. (1997) Direct projections from the lumbosacral spinal cord to Barrington's nucleus in the rat: a special reference to micturition circuitry. *J. Comp. Neurol.*, 387: 149–160.

Ding, Y.-Q., Wang, D., Nie, H., Guan, Z.-L., Lu, B.-Z. and Li, J.-S. (1998) Direct projections from the periaqueductal gray to pontine micturition center neurons projecting to the lumbosacral cord segments: an electron microscopic study in the rat. *Neurosci. Lett.*, 242: 97–100.

Downie, J.W. (1999) Pharmacological manipulation of central micturition circuitry. *Curr. Opin. CPNS Invest. Drugs*, 1(2): 231–239.

Dubrovsky, B. and Filipini, D. (1990) Neurobiological aspects of the pelvic floor muscles involved in defecation. *Neurosci. Biobehav. Rev.*, 14: 157–168.

Dykstra, D.D. and Sidi, A.A. (1990) Treatment of detrusor-sphincter dyssynergia with botulinum A toxin: a double-blind study. *Arch. Phys. Med. Rehabil.*, 71: 24–26.

Elbadawi, A. (1996) Functional anatomy of the organs of micturition. *Urol. Clin. N. Am.*, 23: 177–210.

Espey, M.J., Du, H.-J. and Downie, J.W. (1998) Serotonergic modulation of spinal ascending activity and sacral reflex activity evoked by pelvic nerve stimulation in cats. *Brain Res.*, 798: 101–108.

Fall,M., Erlandson, B.E., Carlsson, C.A. and Lindstrom, S. (1977) The effect of intravaginal electrical stimulation on the feline urethra and urinary bladder. Neuronal mechanisms. *Scand. J. Urol. Nephrol.*, Suppl. 44: 19–30.

Fall, M., Lindstrom, S. and Mazieres, L. (1990) A bladder-to-bladder cooling reflex in the cat. *J. Physiol.*, 427: 281–300.

Fedirchuk, B. and Shefchyk, S.J. (1991) Effects of electrical stimulation of the thoracic spinal cord on bladder and external urethral sphincter activity in the decerebrate cat. *Exp. Brain Res.*, 84: 635–642.

Fedirchuk, B. and Shefchyk, S.J. (1993) Membrane potential changes in sphincter motoneurons during micturition in the decerebrate cat. *J. Neurosci.*, 13: 3090–3094.

Fedirchuk, B., Hochman, S. and Shefchyk, S.J. (1992) An intracellular study of perineal and hindlimb afferent inputs onto sphincter motoneurons in the decerebrate cat. *Exp. Brain Res.*, 89: 511–516.

Fowler, C.J. (1999) Neurological disorders of micturition and their treatment. *Brain*, 122: 1213–1231.

Fowler, C.J. (2000) Intravesical treatment of overactive bladder. *Urology*, 55: 60–64; discussion 66.

Galeano, C., Jubelin, B., Germain, L. and Guenette, L. (1986) Micturitional reflexes in chronic spinalized cats: the underactive detrusor and detrusor-sphincter dyssynergia. *Neurourol. Urodyn.*, 5: 45–63.

Garry, R.C., Roberts, T.D.M. and Todd, J.K. (1959) Reflexes involving the external urethral sphincter in the cat. *J. Physiol.*, 149: 653–665.

Griffiths, D., Holstege, G., Dalm, E. and de Wall, H. (1990) Control and coordination of bladder and urethral function in the brainstem of the cat. *Neurourol. Urodyn.*, 9: 63–82.

Grill, W.M., Wang, B., Hadziefendic, S. and Haxhiu, M.A. (1998) Identification of the spinal neural network involved in coordination of micturition in the male cat. *Brain Res.*, 796: 150–160.

Häbler, H.J. and Janig, W.K.M. (1993) Myelinated primary afferents of the sacral spinal cord responding to slow filling and distension of the cat urinary bladder. *J. Physiol.*, 463: 449–460.

Häbler, H.-J., Janig, W. and Koltzenburg, M. (1990) Activation of unmyelinated afferent fibers by mechanical stimuli and inflammation of the urinary bladder in the cat. *J. Physiol.*, 425: 545–562.

Häbler, H.-J., Janig, W. and Koltzenburg, M. (1993) Receptive properties of myelinated primary afferents innervating the inflamed urinary bladder of the cat. *J. Neurophysiol.*, 69: 395–405.

Hachen, H.J. and Krucker, V. (1977) Clinical and laboratory assessment of the efficacy of Baclofen (Lioresal®) on urethral sphincter spasticity in patients with traumatic paraplegia. *Eur. Urol.*, 3: 237–240.

Haleem, A.S., Boehm, F., Legatt, A.D., Kantrowitz, A., Stone, B. and Melman, A. (1993) Sacral root stimulation for controlled micturition: prevention of detrusor-external sphincter dyssynergia by intraoperative identification and selective section of sacral nerve branches. *J. Urol.*, 149: 1607–1612.

Hochman, S., Fedirchuk, B. and Shefchyk, S.J. (1991) Membrane electrical properties of external urethral and external anal sphincter somatic motoneurons in the decerebrate cat. *Neurosci. Lett.*, 127: 87–90.

Holstege, G., Griffiths, D., de Wall, H. and Dalm, E. (1986) Anatomical and physiological observations on supraspinal control of bladder and urethral sphincter muscles in the cat. *J. Comp. Neurol.*, 250: 449–461.

Ishizuka, O., Mattiasson, A. and Andersson, K.-E. (1996) Role of spinal and peripheral alpha2 adrenoceptors in micturition in normal conscious rats. *J. Urol.*, 156: 1853–1857.

Jankowska, E., Padel, Y. and Zarzecki, P. (1978) Crossed disynaptic inhibition of sacral motoneurones. *J. Physiol.*, 285: 425–444.

Jankowska, E., Bichler, E. and Hammer, I. (2000) Areas of operation of interneurons mediating presynaptic inhibition in sacral spinal segments. *Exp. Brain Res.*, 133(3): 402–406.

Kinder, M.V., Bastiaanssen, E.H.C., Janknegt, R.A. and Marani, E. (1995) Neuronal circuitry of the lower urinary tract; central and peripheral neuronal control of the micturition circuitry. *Anat. Embryol.*, 192: 195–209.

Krane, R.J. and Olsson, C.A. (1973) Phenoxybenzamine in neurogenic bladder dysfunction. I. A theory of micturition. *J. Urol.*, 110(6): 650–652.

Kruse, M.N. and de Groat, W.C. (1990) Micturition reflexes in decerebrate and spinalized neonatal rats. *Am. J. Physiol.*, 258: R1508–R1511.

Liu, R.P.C. (1983) Laminar origins of spinal projection neurons to the periaqueductal gray of the rat. *Brain Res.*, 264: 118–122.

Llewellyn-Smith, I.J., Cassam, A.K., Krenz, N.R., Krassioukov, A.V. and Weaver, L.C. (1997) Glutamate- and GABA-immunoreactive synapses on sympathetic preganglionic neurons caudal to a spinal cord transection in rats. *Neuroscience*, 80: 1225–1235.

Mackel, R. (1979) Segmental and descending control of the external urethral and anal sphincters in the cat. *J. Physiol.*, 294: 105–122.

Mallory, B., Steers, W.D. and de Groat, W.C. (1989) Electrophysiological study of micturition reflexes in rats. *Am. J. Physiol.*, 257: R410–R421.

Marson, L. (1997) Identification of central nervous system neurons that innervate the bladder body, bladder base, or external urethral sphincter of female rats: a transneuronal tracing study using pseudorabies virus. *J. Comp. Neurol.*, 389: 584–602.

Matsumoto, G., Hisamitsu, T. and de Groat, W.C. (1995) Role of glutamate and NMDA receptors in the descending limb of the spinobulbospinal micturition reflex pathway of the rat. *Neurosci. Lett.*, 183: 58–61.

Matsuura, S., Allen, G.V. and Downie, J.W. (1998) Volume-evoked micturition reflex is mediated by the ventrolateral periaqueductal gray in anesthetized rats. *Am. J. Physiol.*, 275: R2049–R2055.

Matsuura, S., Downie, J.W. and Allen, G.V. (2000) Micturition evoked by glutamate microinjection in the ventrolateral periaqueductal gray is mediated through Barrington's nucleus in the rat. *Neuroscience*, 101(4): 1053–1061.

Mazieres, L., Jiang, C. and Lindstrom, S. (1997) Bladder parasympathetic response to electrical stimulation of urethral afferents in the cat. *Neurourol. Urodyn.*, 16: 471–472.

McKenna, K.E. and Nadelhaft, I. (1986) The organization of the pudendal nerve in the male and female rat. *J. Comp. Neurol.*, 248: 532–549.

McMahon, S.B. and Morrison, J.F. (1982a) Factors that determine the excitability of parasympathetic reflexes to the cat bladder. *J. Physiol.*, 322: 35–43.

McMahon, S.B. and Morrison, J.F.B. (1982b) Spinal neurones with long projections activated from the abdominal viscera of the cat. *J. Physiol.*, 322: 1–20.

McMahon, S.B. and Morrison, J.F. (1982c) Two group of spinal interneurones that respond to stimulation of the abdominal viscera of the cat. *J. Physiol.*, 322: 21–34.

McMahon, S.B. and Spillane, K. (1982) Brain stem influences on the parasympathetic supply to the urinary bladder of the cat. *Brain Res.*, 234(2): 237–249.

McMahon, S.B., Morrison, J.F. and Spillane, K. (1982) An electrophysiological study of somatic and visceral convergence in the reflex control of the external sphincters. *J. Physiol.*, 328: 379–387.

Nakagawa, S. (1980) Onuf's nucleus of the sacral cord in a South American monkey (Saimiri): Its location and bilateral cortical input from area 4. *Brain Res.*, 191: 337–344.

Nanninga, J.B., Frost, F. and Penn, R. (1989) Effect of intrathecal Baclofen on bladder and sphincter function. *J. Urol.*, 142: 101–105.

Nathan, P.W. (1952) Thermal sensation in the bladder. *J. Neurol. Neurosurg. Psychiatry*, 15: 150–151.

Nathan, P.W. (1956) Sensations associated with micturition. *Br. J. Urol.*, 28: 126–131.

Nathan, P.W. and Smith, M.C. (1951) The centripetal pathway from the bladder and urethra within the spinal cord. *J. Neurol. Neurosurg. Psychiatry*, 14: 262–280.

Nathan, P.W. and Smith, M.C. (1958) The centrifugal pathway for micturition within the spinal cord. *J. Neurol. Neurosurg. Psychiatry*, 21: 177–189.

Onuf, B. (1899) Notes on the arrangement and function of the cell groups in the sacral region of the spinal cord. *J. Nerv. Ment. Dis.*, 26: 498–504.

Paroschy, K.L. and Shefchyk, S.J. (2000) Non-linear membrane properties of sacral sphincter motoneurones in the cat. *J. Physiol.*, 523(3): 741–753.

Pavcovich, L.A., Yang, M., Miselis, R.R. and Valentino, R.J. (1998) Novel role for the pontine micturition center, Barrington's nucleus: evidence for coordination of colonic and forebrain activity. *Brain Res.*, 784: 355–361.

Petit, H., Wiart, L., Gaujard, E., Le Breton, F., Ferriere, J.M., Lagueny, A., Joseph, P.A. and Barat, M. (1998) Botulinum A toxin treatment for detrusor-sphincter dyssynergia in spinal cord disease. *Spinal Cord*, 36: 91–94.

Pikov, V. and Wrathall, J.R. (2001) Coordination of the bladder detrusor and the external urethral sphincter in a rat model of spinal cord injury: effect of injury severity. *J. Neurosci.*, 21: 559–569.

Prochzska, A., Mushahwar, V.M. and McCreery, D.B. (2001) Neural Prothesis. *J. Physiol.* 533(1): 99–109.

Ramirez-Leon, V. and Ulfhake, B. (1993) GABA-like immunoreactive innervation and dendro-dendritic contacts in the ventrolateral dendritic bundle in the cat S1 spinal cord segment: an electron microscopic study. *Exp. Brain Res.*, 97: 1–12.

Rudy, D.C., Awad, S.A. and Downie, J.W. (1988) External sphincter dyssynergia: an abnormal continence reflex. *J. Urol.*, 140: 105–110.

Sasaki, M. (1991) Membrane properties of external urethral and external anal sphincter motoneurones in the cat. *J. Physiol.*, 440: 345–366.

Sasaki, M. (1994) Morphological analysis of external urethral and external anal sphincter motoneurones of cat. *J. Comp. Neurol.*, 349: 269–287.

Satoh, K., Shimizu, N., Tohyama, M. and Maeda, T. (1978) Localization of the micturition reflex center at dorsolateral pontine tegmentum of the rat. *Neurosci. Lett.*, 8: 27–33.

Sawan, M., Hassouna, M.M., Li, J., Duval, F. and Elhilali, M.M. (1996) Stimulator design and subsequent stimulation parameter optimization for controlling micturition and reducing urethral resistance. *IEEE Trans. Rehabil. Eng.*, 4: 39–46.

Sethi, R.K., Bauer, S.B., Dyro, F.M. and Krarup, C. (1989) Modulation of the bulbocavernosus reflex during voiding: loss of inhibition in upper motor neuron lesions. *Muscle Nerve*, 12: 892–897.

Shefchyk, S.J. (1998) Modulation of excitatory perineal reflexes and sacral striated sphincter motoneurons during micturition in the cat. In: P. Rudomin, R. Romo and L.M. Mendell (Eds.), *Presynaptic Inhibition and Neural Control*. Oxford University Press, New York, pp. 398–406.

Shefchyk, S.J. (2001) Sacral spinal interneurones and the control of urinary bladder and urethral striated sphincter muscle function. *J. Physiol.*, 533: 57–63.

Shefchyk, S.J. and Buss, R.R. (1998) Urethral pudendal afferent-evoked bladder and sphincter reflexes in decerebrate and acute spinal cats. *Neurosci. Lett.*, 244: 137–140.

Shefchyk, S.J., Espey, M.J., Carr, P., Nance, D., Sawchuk, M. and Buss, R. (1998) Evidence for a strychnine-sensitive mechanism and glycine receptors involved in the control of urethral sphincter activity during micturition in the cat. *Exp. Brain Res.*, 119: 297–306.

Sie, J.A., Blok, B.F., de Weerd, H. and Holstege, G. (2001) Ultrastructural evidence for direct projections from the pontine micturition center to glycine-immunoreactive neurons in the sacral dorsal gray commissure in the cat. *J. Comp. Neurol.*, 429: 631–637.

Siroky, M.B. and Krane, R.J. (1982) Neurologic aspects of detrusor-sphincter dyssynergia, with reference to the guarding reflex. *J. Urol.*, 127: 953–957.

Steers, W.D., Meythaler, J.M., Haworth, C., Herrell, D. and Park, T.S. (1992) Effects of acute bolus and chronic continuous intrathecal baclofen on genitourinary dysfunction due to spinal cord pathology. *J. Urol.*, 148: 1849–1855.

Tanago, E.A. and Schmidt, R.A. (1988) Electrical stimulation in the clinical management of the neurogenic bladder. *J. Urol.*, 140: 1331–1339.

Thor, K.B. and Muhlhauser, M.A. (1999) Vesicoanal, urethroanal and urethrovesical reflexes initiated by lower urinary tract irritation in the rat. *Am. J. Physiol.*, 277: R1002–R1012.

Thor, K., Kawatani, M. and de Groat, W.C. (1986) Plasticity in the reflex pathways to the lower urinary tract of the cat during postnatal development and following spinal cord injury. In: Goldberger, M.E., Gorio, A. and Murray, M.(Eds.), *Development and Plasticity of the Mammalian Spinal Cord*. Vol. III, Section II. Fidia Research Series, pp. 65–80.

Thor, K.B., Morgan, C., Nadelhaft, I., Houston, M. and de Groat, W.C. (1989) Organization of afferent and efferent pathways in the pudendal nerve of the female cat. *J. Comp. Neurol.*, 288: 263–279.

Thor, K.B., Hisamitsu, T. and de Groat, W.C. (1990) Unmasking of a neonatal somatovesical reflex in adult cats by the serotonin autoreceptor agonist 5-methoxy-*N,N*-dimethyltryptamine. *Brain Res. Dev. Brain Res.*, 54: 35–42.

Valentino, R.J., Miselis, R.R. and Pavcovich, L.A. (1999) Pontine regulation of pelvic viscera: pharmacological target for pelvic visceral dysfunctions. *Trends Pharmacol. Sci.*, 20: 253–260.

Vanderhorst, V.G.J.M. and Holstege, G. (1997) Organization of lumbosacral motoneuronal cell groups innervating hindlimb, pelvic floor and axial muscles in the cat. *J. Comp. Neurol.*, 382: 46–76.

Vaughan, C.W. and Satchell, P.M. (1995) Urine storage mechanisms. *Prog. Neurobiol.*, 46: 215–237.

Walter, J.S., Wheeler, J.S., Robinson, C.J., Khan, T. and Wurster, R.D. (1989) Urethral responses to sacral stimulation in chronic spinal dog. *Am. J. Physiol.*, 257: R284–R291.

Walter, J.S., Wheeler, J.S. and Dunn, R.B. (1994) Dynamic bulbocavernosus reflex: dyssynergia evaluation following SCI. *J. Am. Paraplegia Soc.*, 17: 140–145.

Woodford, B.J., Carter, R.R., McCreery, D., Bullara, L.A. and Agnrew, W.F. (1996) Histopathological and physiologic effects of chronic implantation of microelectrodes in sacral spinal cord of the cat. *J. Neuropathol. Exp. Neurol.*, 55(9): 982–991.

Yoshimura, N. (1999) Bladder afferent pathway and spinal cord injury: possible mechanisms inducing hyperreflexia of the urinary bladder. *Prog. Neurobiol.*, 57: 583–606.

L. McKerracher, G. Doucet and S. Rossignol (Eds.)
Progress in Brain Research, Vol. 137

CHAPTER 7

Central mechanisms for autonomic dysreflexia after spinal cord injury

Lynne C. Weaver [*], Daniel R. Marsh, Denis Gris, Susan O. Meakin and Gregory A. Dekaban

Spinal Cord Injury Laboratory, BioTherapeutics Research Group, The John P. Robarts Research Institute, 100 Perth Drive, P.O. Box 5015, London ON N6A 5K8, Canada

Characteristics of autonomic dysreflexia after spinal cord injury

After spinal cord injury, life-threatening increases in arterial pressure can develop in response to sensory input entering the spinal cord below the level of the lesion (Lee et al., 1994; Maiorov et al., 1998; Mathias and Frankel, 1999). This hypertension, part of a condition termed autonomic dysreflexia, occurs in 50–90% of people with tetraplegia or high paraplegia and correlates with the severity and location of injury (Corbett et al., 1975; Erickson, 1980; Lindan et al., 1980; Lee et al., 1994; Giannantoni et al., 1998; Karlsson, 1999; Mathias and Frankel, 1999). The hypertension can result in debilitating headaches, seizures, strokes and even death. SCI seriously disturbs blood pressure control that normally depends upon supraspinal regulation of sympathetic preganglionic neurons (SPNs) (Calaresu and Yardley, 1988). After such injury, CNS regulation of arterial pressure is dominated by spinal reflex control of the SPNs. The unchecked activity of spinal reflexes leads to autonomic dysreflexia. This condition is most prevalent after severe cord injury, when supraspinal inhibitory influences on spinal circuits are lost (Dembowsky et al., 1978). Furthermore, dysreflexia occurs after injury at or rostral to the 6th thoracic spinal segment, because injury at this level leaves the sympathetic control of the extensive abdominal circulation amenable to unrestrained spinal reflexes (Mathias and Frankel, 1999). These exaggerated reflexes begin within weeks of the cord injury and can be caused by stimulation of the skin, pressure sores, distension or inflammation of the urinary bladder or gastrointestinal tract and also by muscle spasms that often develop after spinal cord injury (Guttman and Whitteridge, 1947; Corbett et al., 1975; Mathias and Frankel, 1999). They can be initiated by routine daily procedures such as bladder catheterization and bowel evacuation. Dysreflexia is not always severe and may be characterized only by sweating, flushed skin, piloerection and small increases in arterial pressure. However, even in rehabilitated tetraplegics and paraplegics, this condition can become uncontrolled, leading to life-threatening hypertension (Shea et al., 1973; Naftchi, 1990; Lee et al., 1994; Mathias and Frankel, 1999; Giannantoni et al., 1998).

Mechanisms for autonomic dysreflexia

Mechanisms for autonomic dysreflexia that have been considered include upregulation of vascular catecholamine receptors, increased neural release of

---

* Correspondence to: G.A. Dekaban, Spinal Cord Injury Laboratory, BioTherapeutics Research Group, The John P. Robarts Research Institute, 100 Perth Drive, P.O. Box 5015, London ON N6A 5K8, Canada. Tel.: +1-519-663-3776; Fax: +1-519-663-3789; E-mail: lcweaver@rri.on.ca

catecholamines, loss of the baroreceptor reflex and loss of tonic bulbospinal inhibitory input to spinal neurons (Naftchi, 1990; Lee et al., 1994; Arnold et al., 1995; Karlsson et al., 1998; Karlsson, 1999; Mathias and Frankel, 1999; Teasell et al., 2000; Collins and DiCarlo, 2002). Indeed, the modulation of spinal reflex excitation of SPNs by baroreceptors and other supraspinal inhibitory systems is either lost or reduced. This lack of inhibition likely has a role in determining the magnitude and duration of the hypertensive episodes. The loss of inhibition, however, develops almost instantaneously after the injury, whereas autonomic dysreflexia in humans or experimental animals takes weeks or months to develop (Mathias and Frankel, 1992; Krassioukov and Weaver, 1995; Maiorov et al., 1997a). The time-dependent, progressive development of autonomic dysreflexia suggests that gradual reactions of the spinal cord or cardiovascular system (Mathias and Frankel, 1992; Karlsson, 1999; Teasell et al., 2000) to the injury are major causes of the condition (Lee et al., 1994).

Peripheral mechanisms

The increased vascular response to the activation of a spinal reflex after injury has been documented in human studies, and evidence has been obtained for altered α-receptor expression or responsiveness and for marked noradrenaline spillover in beds below the level of the injury (Arnold et al., 1995; Karlsson, 1999; Teasell et al., 2000). The potential contribution of depressed catecholamine uptake by nerve terminals at these sites has not been assessed. A recent study in rats, months after spinal cord injury, has confirmed role of vascular hyper-responsiveness in autonomic dysreflexia and assessed its contribution to the induced hypertension (Collins and DiCarlo, 2002). These investigators found that upper body exercise was sufficient to normalize constrictor responses to close arterial injections of the α-receptor agonist phenylephrine, rendering the responses of spinal rats identical to those of uninjured rats. At this time, the dysreflexic, hypertensive responses to colon stimulation were decreased by 50% in the cord-injured rats, revealing that enhanced vascular responsiveness was responsible for about half of the autonomic dysreflexia. A vascular mechanism has

been credited a large responsibility for the induction of autonomic dysreflexia, in part because evidence for central mechanisms in tetraplegic or paraplegic human patients is not easily obtained. Electrophysiological studies in tetraplegic patients have been limited to recordings from lower leg vasoconstrictor nerves that likely are not engaged greatly in the reflexes that cause the hypertension (Wallin and Stjernberg, 1984; Stjernberg et al., 1986). Instead constriction of the abdominal visceral beds is more important and discharge of vasomotor sympathetic nerves innervating these beds is a better indicator of the contribution of changes in the spinal sympathetic reflex after cord injury. However the large increase in noradrenaline spillover during dysreflexia suggests intense sympathetic firing (Karlsson et al., 1998). Indeed, renal sympathetic firing recorded in conscious, chronic cord-injured rats increases massively during episodes of autonomic dysreflexia (Maiorov et al., 1997b). This chapter will address experimental evidence, obtained in animals, for plastic changes within the injured spinal cord that lead to autonomic dysreflexia. Such changes act in concert with enhanced catecholaminergic vasoconstriction to cause the large increases in arterial pressure characteristic of this condition.

Central mechanisms

Rats and mice readily develop autonomic dysreflexia after spinal cord injury (Osborn et al., 1990; Krassioukov and Weaver, 1995; Maiorov et al., 1997a,b). After spinal cord transection in the rat at the 4th (T$_4$) thoracic segment, exaggerated spinal reflexes below the site of injury lead to major excitation of visceral sympathetic vasomotor nerves and underlie the episodic hypertension (Fig. 1) (Krassioukov and Weaver, 1995; Maiorov et al., 1997a,b). Reorganization of the spinal pathways controlling SPNs after the loss of supraspinal input is the likely cause of the exaggerated sympathetic reflexes (Krassioukov and Weaver, 1996; Cassam et al., 1997, 1999; Weaver et al., 1997). Enhanced transmission through the spinal reflex circuits could be mediated by changes in the afferent, interneuronal or preganglionic neuronal components of the arc. Earlier studies lead to the hypothesis that synaptic input to preganglionic neurons undergoes plastic reorganization after cord injury,

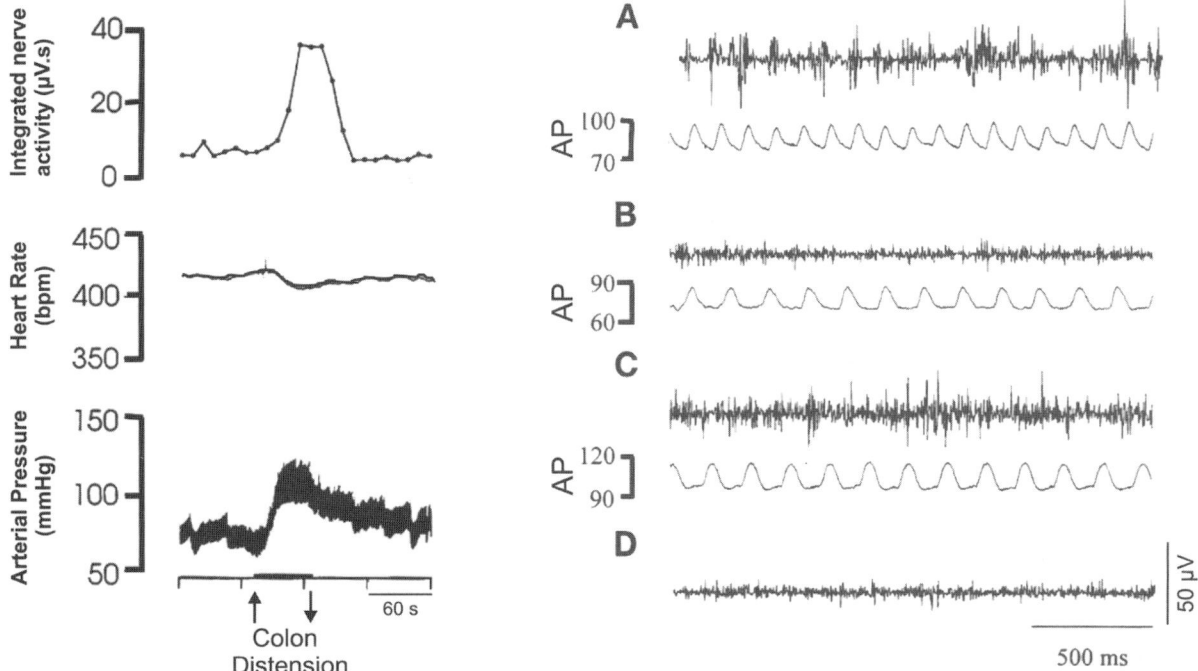

Fig. 1. Autonomic dysreflexia and renal sympathetic nerve activity in rats after spinal cord transection (SCT). Left panel: Colon distension in an anesthetized rat 24 h after SCT markedly increases integrated renal nerve activity and arterial pressure, while decreasing heart rate. Right panel: (A) Renal sympathetic nerve activity and arterial pressure (AP, mmHg) before SCT. (B) Control recordings 24 h after SCT. (C) Increased sympathetic nerve firing at peak autonomic dysreflexia response of arterial pressure during colon distension. (D) Residual neural signal after hexamethonium blockade. Reproduced with permission from Maiorov et al., 1997b.

resulting in replacement of inputs from bulbospinal neurons with those from interneurons (Krassioukov and Weaver, 1996; Weaver et al., 1997). Although this was an appealing model for the generation of exaggerated spinal reflexes, a recent electron microscopic study has demonstrated that the loss of bulbospinal synaptic input to SPNs reduces synaptic input to these neurons by 50–70% and this loss does not appear to be replaced by intraspinal inputs (Llewellyn-Smith and Weaver, 2001). The innervation of SPN from spinal interneurons after cord injury clearly can mediate the spinal reflexes but the number of synapses from the interneurons after cord injury does not appear to increase. Accordingly, such a change does not mediate the time-dependent increases in the spinal sympathetic reflexes. The interneurons may still play a role if they are more excited by an afferent input to the spinal cord and provide increased excitation of SPNs through temporal summation. A recent electrophysiological study of responses of spinal interneurons in sympathetic

reflex circuits suggests that this may be the case (Krassioukov et al., 2000). If the interneurons respond excessively to afferent input, one interpretation is that the input is greater after cord injury. Much experimental evidence demonstrates that this is true. The arbors in the dorsal horn of small-diameter primary afferent neurons enlarge greatly in rats and mice after SCI (Krenz et al., 1999; Wong et al., 2000; Weaver et al., 2001) and could readily lead to increased reflex excitation of SPNs. These calcitonin gene-related peptide-immunoreactive (CGRP-Ir) afferent neurons and the interneurons in laminae III–VII make up the pathway mediating spinal reflex excitation of SPNs (Sato and Schmidt, 1973; Cabot et al., 1994; Joshi et al., 1995; Clarke et al., 1998). In experimental animals, the 2-week time course for the increased arbor size correlates with the period of time required for development of autonomic dysreflexia; the size of the increase correlates with the magnitude of dysreflexia (Krenz et al., 1999). This afferent arbor remains enlarged at 1 month after cord injury, a time when autonomic dysreflexia is well developed in rats (Krassioukov and Weaver, 1995).

A clinically relevant model of autonomic dysreflexia

Autonomic dysreflexia is readily apparent in rats when spinal cord injury is caused by a method that reproduces the typical clinical injury. This method entails brief (60 s) extradural compression of the cord with a calibrated, modified aneurysm clip. The clip-model mimics the key pathophysiological features of human spinal cord injury. This model produces mechanical injury (primary injury) and secondary damage by a variety of well characterized mechanisms including microvasculature disruption, hemorrhage, ischemia, increases in intracellular calcium, calpain activation, progressive axonal injury and glutamate toxicity (Wallace and Tator, 1986; Wallace et al., 1986; Fehlings et al., 1989; Koyanagi et al., 1993a,b; Agrawal and Fehlings, 1996, 1997a,b; Agrawal et al., 1998; Schumacher et al., 1999). Marked autonomic dysreflexia is readily evoked after severe (50 g) clip-spinal cord injury at T_4 (Maiorov et al., 1998; Weaver et al., 2001). Distension of the colon with a small balloon-tipped catheter or cutaneous stimulation in conscious rats at 2 weeks after injury causes large increases in arterial pressure (mean change $= 42 \pm 3$ mmHg) (see Fig. 3A below). Enlargement of the CGRP-Ir primary afferent arbor is also characteristic of this injury model (Fig. 2). Similar to the human condition, injury to the cord must be severe for enlargement of the primary afferent arbor and autonomic dysreflexia to occur. At two weeks after moderate/mild (20 g) clip-spinal cord injury at T_4, rats have no autonomic dysreflexia in response to colon distension and no change in the small-diameter CGRP-Ir afferent arbor.

Association between nerve growth factor and autonomic dysreflexia

Enlargement of the afferent arbor depends upon actions of nerve growth factor (NGF) in the injured rat spinal cord. Intrathecal delivery of a highly selective neutralizing antibody to NGF for 2 weeks after cord injury at T_4 completely blocked the sprouting of the small-diameter afferent fibers in the dorsal horn (Krenz et al., 1999). Delivery of the antibody subcutaneously to peripheral targets of the sensory neurons had no effect, demonstrating that the afferent sprouting was not caused by a target-derived source of NGF. Blockade of the sprouting response was due to neutralizing the effects of the anti-NGF antibody on the trkA-expressing central arbors of these sensory neurons. Autonomic dysreflexia was measured in the same rats and the increases in arterial pressure caused by visceral stimulation were reduced by 43% in the (intrathecal) antibody-treated rats. This reduced the dysreflexia to the magnitude of the spinal reflex that is present in the conscious rat within 48 h of cord transection, before enlargement of the afferent arbor could occur (Maiorov et al., 1997a). These data led to two major conclusions. First, afferent sprouting in the spinal cord dorsal horn is clearly associated with the time-dependent increase in hypertensive responses to sensory stimulation, characteristic of autonomic dysreflexia. Second, the sprouting is caused by an intraspinal action of NGF, presumably at the central arbors of the sensory neurons.

Other methods of blocking NGF in the injured spinal cord also prevent the development of secondary disorders such as autonomic dysreflexia. For example, a soluble trkA receptor protein that sequesters NGF is highly effective. This protein includes the extracellular portion of trkA fused to the Fc portion of human IgG and is expressed using a baculovirus system. This trkA-IgG fusion protein bound NGF specifically with a $K_d = 4.26 \times 10^{-11} M$ and blocked NGF-dependent neuritogenesis in cultured neuron-like cells. Intrathecal infusions (4 μg/day) of trkA-IgG for 14 days after severe, high thoracic (T_4) clip-spinal cord injury in rats markedly reduced autonomic dysreflexia (Fig. 3B). The increases in mean arterial pressure in rats treated with trkA-IgG were approximately 50% as large as those in rats treated control IgG infusions. These results indicate that treatment with trkA-IgG to block NGF, like the polyclonal antibody used earlier (Krenz et al., 1999), blocks the component of the spinal reflex attributable to secondary plastic changes and suppresses autonomic dysreflexia.

These studies suggest that NGF is a culprit in the development of autonomic dysreflexia. Normally the spinal cord contains very little NGF but NGF

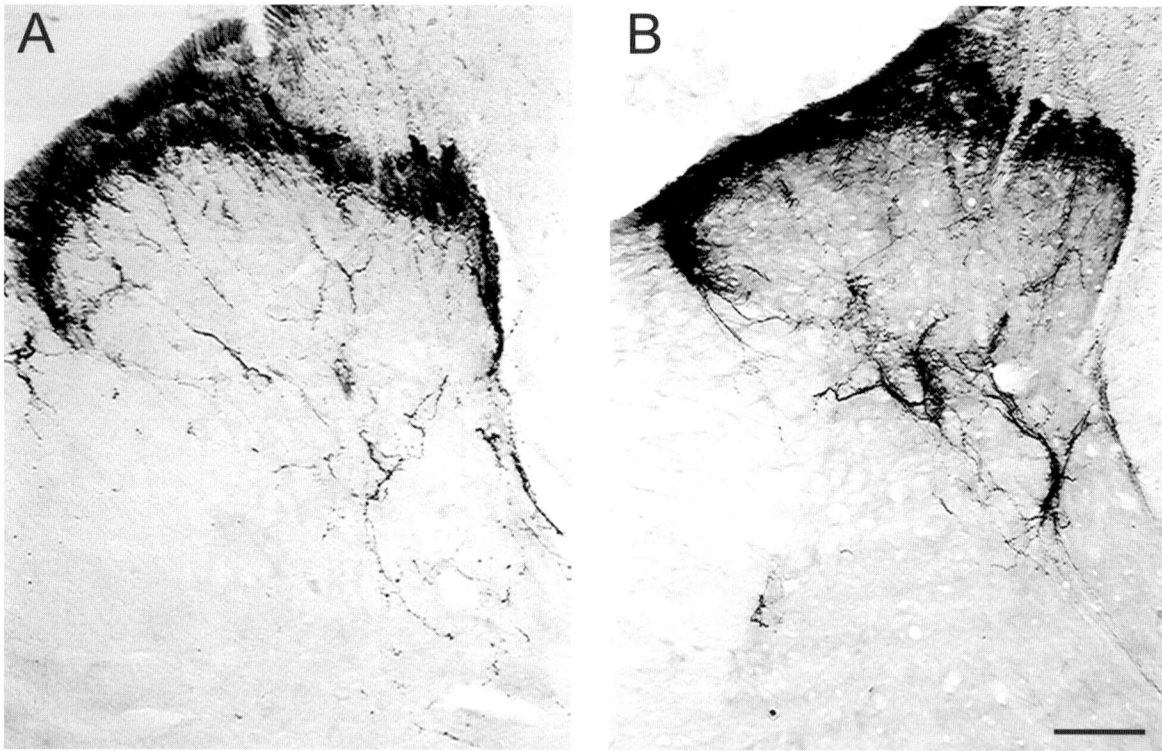

Fig. 2. Photomicrographs of CGRP-Ir fibers in the dorsal horn of thoracic cord segment T_{10} in a sham-injured rat (A) and 2 weeks after 50 g clip compression injury (B). The CGRP-Ir in laminae V–VII is greater in the 50 g clip-injured rat. Scale bar is 100 μm and applies to A and B.

levels within a few segments of a cord injury site have been reported to increase to a peak at 1 week post-injury, remaining increased for 4 weeks (Bakhit et al., 1991). Using a two-site enzyme-linked immunosorbant assay (ELISA) we have confirmed that NGF levels in the injured rat spinal cord are significantly greater close to the injury than rostral to the injury or in the lumbar cord. NGF at the injury site was ~2-fold greater than the content in this region in un-injured rats (1.5 ± 0.8 pg/mg). Immunocytochemistry on spinal cord sections, revealed increased NGF-immunoreactivity in cells and fibers in the dorsal root entry zone, and in astrocytes, microglia and leptomeningeal cells of cord-injured rats (Fig. 4) (Krenz and Weaver, 2000). These were prevalent in segments T_3–T_8. The stimulus for the increased intraspinal NGF is now in question. The inflammatory response to traumatic injury of the spinal cord is likely to promote the production of NGF. This NGF may be generated within the injured cord or it may enter the cord after production by surrounding damaged muscle, skin or dorsal root ganglia.

Inflammation, spinal cord injury and autonomic dysreflexia

The inflammatory response to SCI begin within minutes and evolve for days, spreading throughout the damaged cord and into adjacent, non-injured, regions (Blight, 1985; Tator and Fehlings, 1991; Young, 1993; Popovich et al., 1997; Taoka and Okajima, 1998). First pro-inflammatory chemokines and cytokines are released into the injured area by astrocytes, microglia and endothelial cells (Prewitt et al., 1997). Next, activation and proliferation of glia (gliosis), and influx of neutrophils and monocyte/macrophages from the circulation leads to phagocytosis of debris and release of cytokines important to wound healing. The inflammatory response also has pathological outcomes (Blight, 1992; Barone et al., 1997; Hanisch et al., 1997; Streit et al., 1998) including the release of reactive oxy-

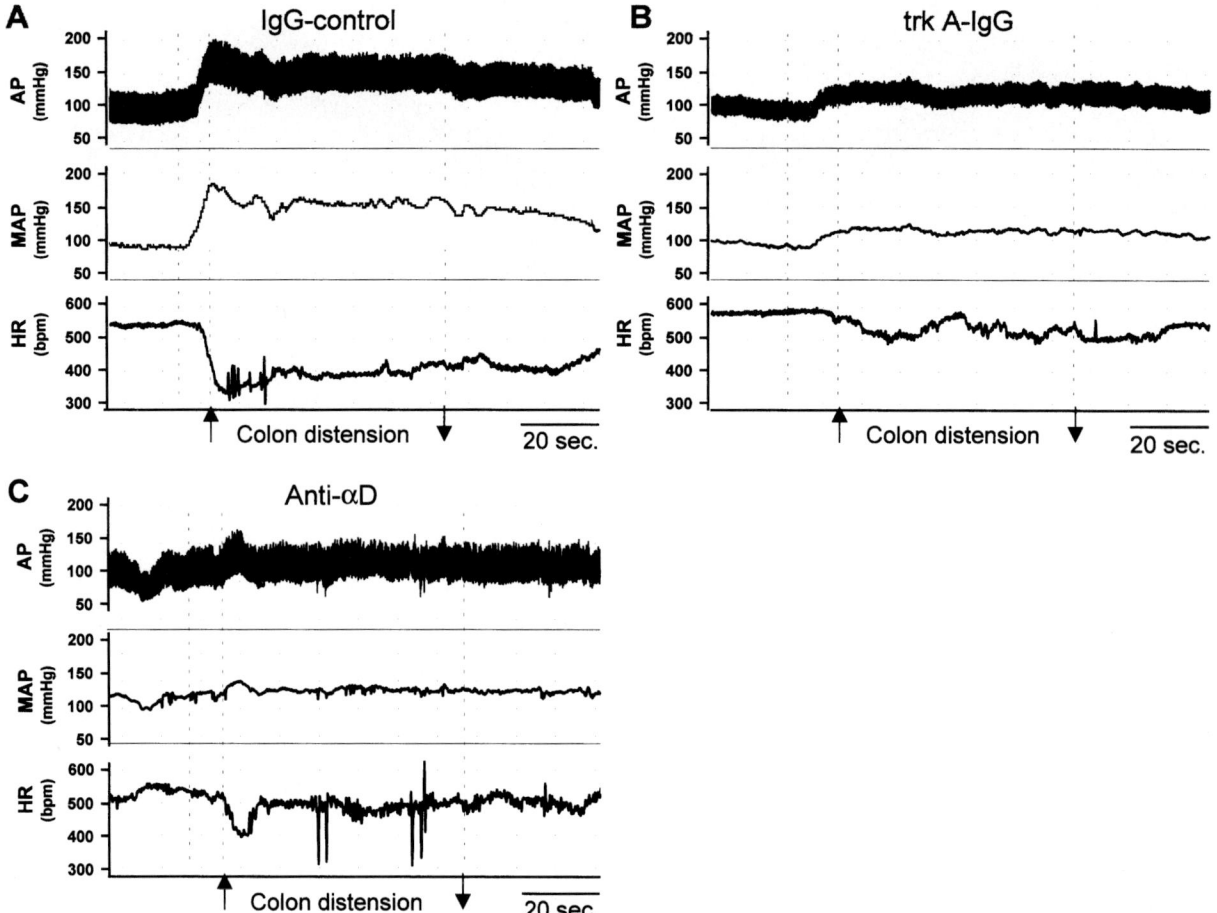

Fig. 3. Mean and pulsatile arterial pressure and heart rate responses to colon distension in rats 2 weeks after 50 g clip compression spinal cord injury. In a rat treated with the control IgG protein (A), colon distension caused large increases in arterial pressure and decreases in heart rate, typical of this severe spinal cord injury. In contrast, the autonomic dysreflexia caused by colon distension was markedly reduced in a rat treated with trkA-IgG (B). Likewise, anti-αD treatment suppressed the development of autonomic dysreflexia after spinal cord injury. Consequently, little cardiovascular responses were elicited by colon distension (C).

gen species that causes further tissue damage (Balentine and Paris, 1978; Kwo et al., 1989; Zeidman et al., 1996; Azbill et al., 1997; Klusman and Schwab, 1997; Streit et al., 1998). Leukocytes are major players after SCI and contribute to the release of cytokines and chemokines, the induction of reactive microglia and endothelial damage (Taoka and Okajima, 1998; Taoka et al., 1998). Infiltrating macrophages and neutrophils and glial cells express cytokines such as interleukin-1β (IL-1β), IL-6, tumor necrosis factor-α (TNF-α), and transforming growth factor-β (TGF-β) (Barone et al., 1997; Hanisch et al., 1997; Streit et al., 1998).

Inflammation and nerve growth factor

Inflammation and NGF expression and/or signaling are clearly related. IL-6 and IL-1β, two cytokines found in the injured cord (Streit et al., 1998; Hayashi et al., 2000) have well-documented actions to increase the expression of NGF in the CNS (Bandtlow et al., 1990; Spranger et al., 1990; Saporito et al., 1993) and in Schwann cells of peripheral nerves (Heumann et al., 1987a,b; Lindholm et al., 1987). In response to cord injury, microglial NGF mRNA transcription and NGF protein release (Heese et al., 1998a,b) are stimulated synergistically by IL-1 and

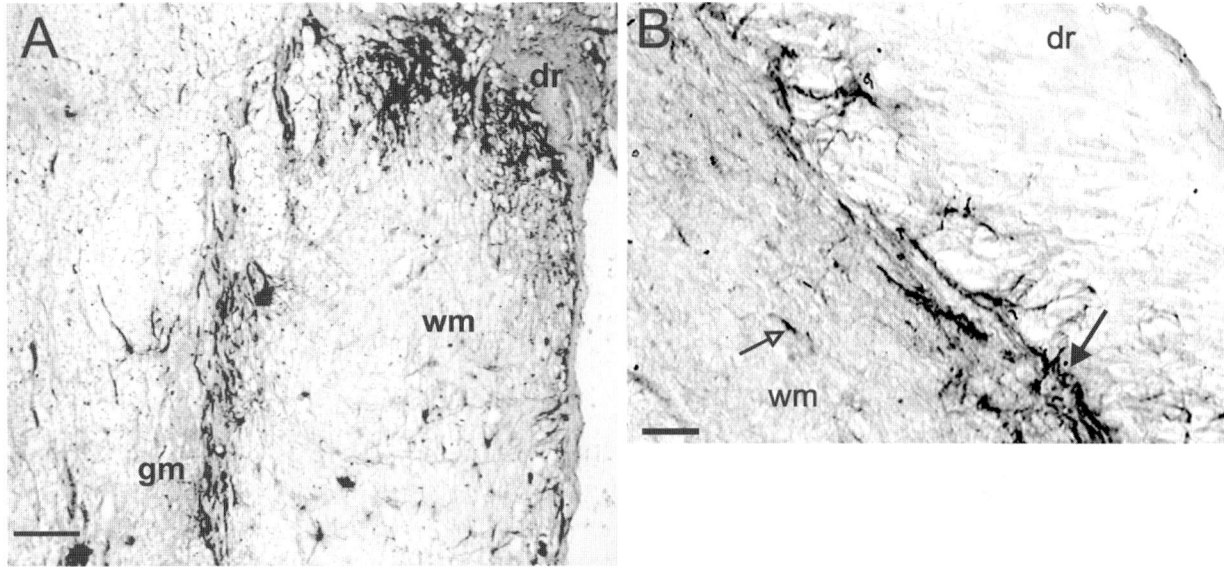

Fig. 4. Photomicrographs of horizontal sections of spinal cord 7 days after spinal cord transection. (A) Immunoreactivity to NGF in cells and fibers in the white (wm) and gray (gm) matter near the lesion site (thoracic cord T_4). (B) Cells immunoreactive for NGF in the subpial white matter near the dorsal root (dr) entry zone caudal to the lesion site at T_6 are indicated with arrows. Scale bars: A, 100 μm; B, 25 μm. From Krenz and Weaver, 2000. Reproduced with permission of Blackwell Science Ltd.

TNF-α. IL-1 and its receptors are expressed at low levels in the brain, putatively by oligodendrocytes, and this expression increases rapidly after brain injury (Yan et al., 1992). IL-6 is found in the cerebrospinal fluid after traumatic brain injury and peak increases in IL-6 occur in parallel with peak increases in NGF in the cerebrospinal fluid (Kossmann et al., 1996). The central processes of sensory neurons have IL-6 receptors that would be exposed to IL-6 in the injured cord, leading to stimulation of NGF expression. NGF also has pro-inflammatory actions (see LaSala et al., 2000). The high affinity trkA receptor is expressed on monocytes, B-lymphocytes and T-lymphocytes. Although the signaling caused by NGF on these receptors is not fully understood, NGF promotes expression of Bcl-2 in monocytes and mast cells, conferring resistance to cell death (Bullock and Johnson, 1996; LaSala et al., 2000; Saragovi and Gehring, 2000). NGF also can facilitate inflammation by promoting differentiation of myeloid progenitor cells, inducing proliferation and maturation of B-lymphocytes and stimulating the release of inflammatory cytokines (IL-3, IL-4, IL-10, TNF-α) from basophils and mast cells. Binding of NGF to mast cells causes degranulation, contributing

to peripheral inflammation (Shu and Mendell, 1999). In summary, inflammation can promote NGF expression and NGF can promote the process of inflammation. Clearly the relationship between inflammation and NGF could contribute to the NGF-dependent increases in primary afferent arbors in the spinal cord and the development of autonomic dysreflexia.

Leukocyte adhesion and spinal cord inflammation

The essential role of leukocyte adhesion in immune-mediated inflammatory responses is a possible target for therapeutic anti-inflammatory intervention (Archelos et al., 1993; Cannella et al., 1993; Yenari et al., 1998). Antibodies to adhesion molecules on leukocytes inhibit adhesion-dependent processes including leukocyte transendothelial migration (Smith et al., 1989), leukocyte–leukocyte adhesion and leukocyte–extracellular matrix adhesion (Haskard et al., 1986; Bevilacqua et al., 1987). In animal models of cord injury, the concentration of adhesion molecules is increased on the surface of endothelial cells at the SCI site. This leads to the extravasation and activation of inflammatory cells into the spinal cord (Carlson et al., 1998). Monoclonal antibodies (mAb) to adhesion molecules reduce the inflammatory infiltrate at the SCI site (Hamada et al., 1996; Taoka and Okajima, 1998). The integrins are a family of α/β heterodimeric membrane-bound glycoproteins that mediate cell–cell adhesion (Larson and Springer, 1990). Adhesion and extravasation of leukocytes are mediated by α4β1 and the β2 subfamily of integrins on the surface of leukocytes that bind immunoglobulin-like adhesion molecules on endothelia (Bevilacqua, 1993). β2 integrins play an essential role in leukocyte trafficking and activation and arbitrate cell–cell interactions during inflammation (van Kooyk and Figdor, 1993). The novel β2 integrin family member, αD, is highly expressed on the surface of monocyte/macrophages and to a lesser extent on neutrophils and other leukocytes (Grayson et al., 1997). αD plays an important role in cell–cell interactions during an immune response. The concentration of cell adhesion molecules, such as the intracellular and vascular adhesion molecules-1 (ICAM-1 and VCAM-1), is increased at sites of CNS inflammation, contributing to the extravasation of leukocytes across the blood–brain barrier (Barten and Ruddle, 1994; Cannella and Raine, 1995). The concentrations of proinflammatory cytokines TNF-α, IL-1β, and interferon-γ (IFN-γ) are increased in response to injury and these cytokines induce expression of ICAM-1 and VCAM-1 (Van der Vieren et al., 1999) on endothelial cells, monocytes and astrocytes (Frohman et al., 1989; Hurwitz et al., 1992; Rosenman et al., 1993; Bevilacqua et al., 1994; Henninger et al., 1997). The ligand for αD in the rat appears to be VCAM-1. Both cell surface and soluble forms of recombinant αD bind to VCAM-1, interactions that can be blocked with mAb to αD and VCAM-1 (Rice and Bevilacqua, 1989). αD expression also contributes to the homing/retention of cells at VCAM-1 expressing sites.

A novel anti-inflammatory strategy after spinal cord injury

We have shown a significant anti-inflammatory effect of an intravenous anti-αD mAb treatment (ICOS Corporation, Seattle, WA) that reduced the infiltration of macrophages into the injured spinal cord (Mabon et al., 2000). Delivery of anti-αD mAb at 2, 24 and 48 h after severe clip-SCI at T_4 diminishes

(by 60%) the macrophage infiltrates in the injured cord at 72 h post-injury and improves autonomic and locomotor outcome at 2–4 weeks after injury (Dekaban et al., 2000). At 3 weeks after this injury, these rats scored significantly higher (6.6 ± 1) on a 21 point open field locomotor rating scale (Basso et al., 1995) compared to the typical scores of untreated rats (~3.1 points). When assessed for autonomic dysreflexia, they had increases in arterial pressure in response to colon distension that were 50% of those typically observed in untreated rats 2 weeks after this injury (Weaver et al., 2001). In some rats dysreflexia was completely blocked (Fig. 3C). These experiments reveal a powerful effect of this anti-inflammatory treatment on autonomic dysreflexia. Secondary damage to the cord after this severe clip-SCI was assessed quantitatively by evaluating the white matter sparing at the lesion site and within 2 cm rostral and caudal to the epicenter of the lesion. Treatment with the anti-αD mAb led to significant white matter sparing (Fig. 5). This neuroprotective action could underlie the improved locomotor performance and would contribute to suppression of autonomic dysreflexia through sparing of descending inhibitory pathways. The relationship between this treatment effect and NGF-dependent primary afferent sprouting remains to be determined.

Conclusion

In conclusion, spinal cord injury leads to a host of changes within the injured cord that promote pathological secondary outcomes such as autonomic dysreflexia. Although neurotrophic factors are useful and probably necessary for the process of regeneration of injured tracts and neurons, NGF does not appear to be a good candidate for this task as it clearly contributes to secondary disorders. Likewise, inflammation is a necessary part of healing but, in the CNS, inflammation can cause great damage that is not readily reversed. Therefore, the inflammatory response to cord injury also is an ideal target for manipulation to maintain its useful functions while limiting its capacity to cause destructive or maladaptive responses. Autonomic dysreflexia is one of many secondary consequences of cord injury such as bladder and sexual dysfunction, chronic pain, muscle spasticity. Understanding the mechanisms of auto-

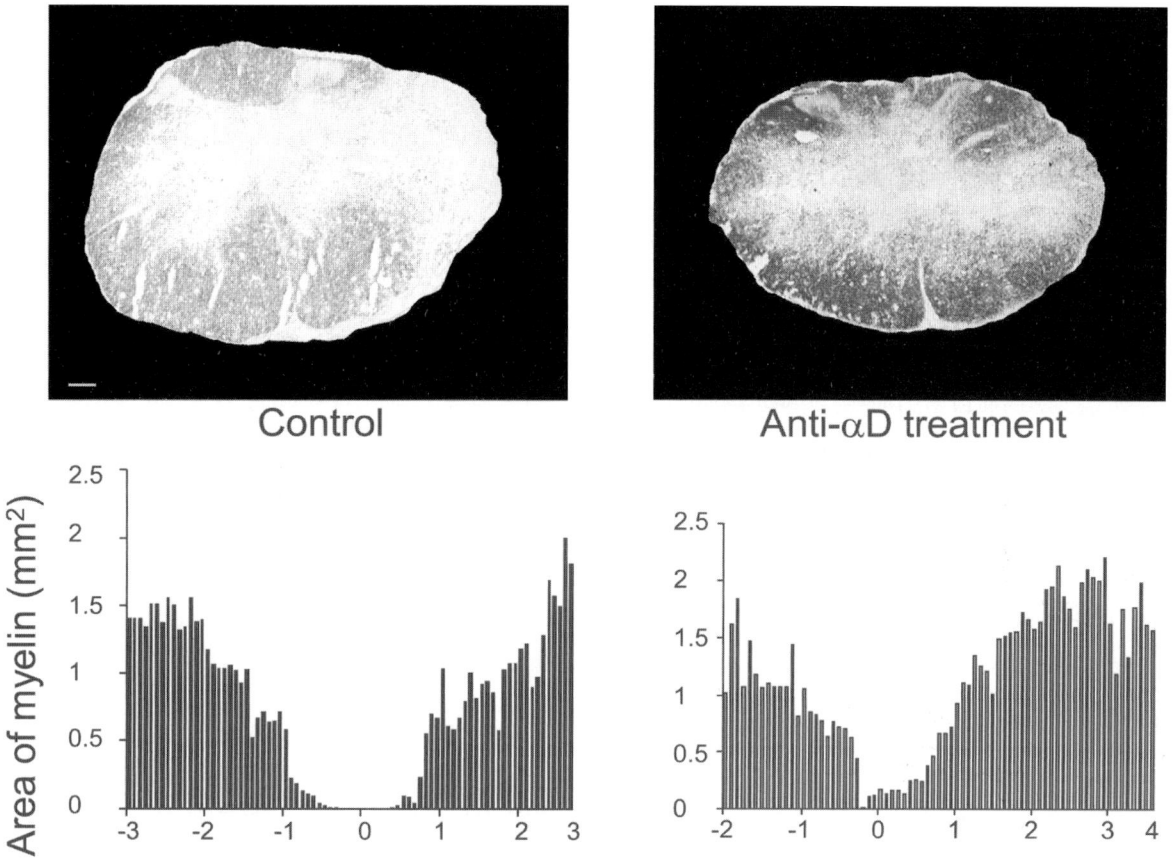

Fig. 5. Area of lesion in a control and an anti-αD mAb-treated rat after 50 g clip compression spinal cord injury at T₄. Anti-αD mAb was injected at 2, 24 and 48 h after cord injury. Top panels: Luxol fast blue-stained sections of thoracic spinal cord 1.0 mm caudal to the epicenter of the lesion. Note the darker, more extensive staining after treatment indicating white matter sparing. Scale bar: 200 μm. Lower panels: areas of myelin staining were measured in each of the two rats in serial 25-μm sections rostral (negative values) and caudal (positive values) to the injury site. The lesion size was markedly reduced after treatment with anti-αD mAb.

nomic dysreflexia and development of treatments to prevent its development may impact on many of these disabling secondary disorders.

References

Agrawal, S.K. and Fehlings, M.G. (1996) Mechanisms of secondary injury to spinal cord axons in vitro role Na⁺, Na⁺–K⁺-ATPase, the Na⁺–H⁺ exchanger, and the Na⁺–Ca⁺ exchanger. *J. Neurosci.*, 16(2): 545–552.

Agrawal, S.K. and Fehlings, M.G. (1997a) Role of NMDA and non-NMDA ionotropic glutamate receptors in traumatic spinal cord axonal injury. *J. Neurosci.*, 17(3): 1055–1063.

Agrawal, S.K. and Fehlings, M.G. (1997b) The effect of the sodium channel blocker QX-314 on recovery after acute spinal cord injury. *J. Neurotrauma*, 14: 81–88.

Agrawal, S.K., Theriault, E. and Fehlings, M.G. (1998) Role of group I metabotropic glutamate receptors in traumatic spinal cord white matter injury. *J. Neurotrauma*, 15: 929–941.

Archelos, J.J., Jung, S. and Maurer, M. (1993) Inhibition of experimental autoimmune encephalomyelitis by an antibody to the intercellular adhesion molecule ICAM-1. *Ann. Neurol.*, 34: 145–154.

Arnold, J.M.O., Feng, Q.P., Delaney, G.A. and Teasell, R.W. (1995) Autonomic dysreflexia in tetraplegic patients: evidence for α-adrenoceptor hyper-responsiveness. *Clin. Auton. Res.*, 5: 267–270.

Azbill, R.D., Mu, X., Bruce-Keller, A.J., Mattson, M.P. and Springer, J.E. (1997) Impaired mitochondrial function, oxidative stress and altered antioxidant enzyme activities following traumatic spinal cord injury. *Brain Res.*, 765: 283–290.

Bakhit, C., Armanini, M., Wong, W.L.T., Bennett, G.L. and Wrathall, J.R. (1991) Increase in nerve growth factor-like immunoreactivity and decrease in choline acetyltransferase following contusive spinal cord injury. *Brain Res.*, 554: 264–271.

Balentine, J.D. and Paris, D. (1978) Pathology of experimental spinal cord trauma. I. The necrotic lesion as a function of vascular injury. *Lab. Invest.*, 39: 236–253.

Bandtlow, C.E., Meyer, M., Lindholm, D., Spranger, M., Heumann, R. and Thoenen, H. (1990) Regional and cellular codistribution of interleukin 1 beta and nerve growth factor mRNA in the adult rat brain: possible relationship to the regulation of nerve growth factor synthesis. *J. Cell Biol.*, 111: 1701–1711.

Barone, F.C., Arvin, B., White, R.F., Miller, A., Webb, C.L., Willette, R.N., Lysko, P.G. and Feuerstein, G.Z. (1997) Tumour necrosis factor-alpha. A mediator of focal ischemic brain injury. *Stroke*, 28: 1233–1244.

Barten, D.M. and Ruddle, N.H. (1994) Vascular cell adhesion molecule-1 modulation by tumour necrosis factor in experimental allergic encephalomyelitis. *J. Neuroimmunol.*, 51(2): 123–133.

Basso, D.M., Beattie, M.S. and Bresnahan, J.C. (1995) A sensitive and reliable locomotor rating scale for open field testing in rats. *J. Neurotrauma*, 12: 1–21.

Bevilacqua, M.P. (1993) Endothelial–leukocyte adhesion molecules. *Annu. Rev. Immunol.*, 11: 767–804.

Bevilacqua, M.P., Pober, J.S., Mendrick, D.L., Cotran, R.S. and Gimbrone Jr., M.A. (1987) Identification of an inducible endothelial–leukocyte adhesion molecule. *Proc. Natl. Acad. Sci. USA*, 84(24): 9238–9242.

Bevilacqua, M.P., Nelson, R.M., Mannori, G. and Cecconi, O. (1994) Endothelial–leukocyte adhesion molecules in human disease. *Annu. Rev. Med.*, 45: 361–387.

Blight, A.R. (1985) Delayed demyelination and macrophage invasion: a candidate for 'secondary' cell damage in spinal cord injury. *Cent. Nerv. Syst. Trauma*, 2: 299–315.

Blight, A.R. (1992) Macrophages and inflammatory damage in spinal cord injury. *J. Neurotrauma*, 9(Suppl. 1): S83–S91.

Bullock, E.D. and Johnson, E.M. (1996) Nerve growth factor induces the expression of certain cytokine genes and bcl-2 in mast cells. Potential role in survival promotion. *J. Biol. Chem.*, 271: 27500–27508.

Cabot, J., Alessi, V., Carroll, J. and Ligorio, M. (1994) Spinal cord lamina V and lamina VII interneuronal projections to sympathetic preganglionic neurons. *J. Comp. Neurol.*, 347: 515–530.

Calaresu, F.R. and Yardley, C.P. (1988) Medullary basal sympathetic tone. *Annu. Rev. Physiol.*, 50: 511–524.

Cannella, B. and Raine, C.S. (1995) The adhesion molecule and cytokine profile of multiple sclerosis lesions. *Ann. Neurol.*, 37(4): 424–435.

Cannella, B., Cross, A.H. and Raine, C.S. (1993) Anti-adhesion molecule therapy in experimental autoimmune encephalomyelitis. *J. Neuroimmunol.*, 46: 1–2.

Carlson, S.L., Parrish, M.E., Springer, J.E., Doty, K. and Dossett, L. (1998) Acute inflammatory response in spinal cord following impact injury. *Exp. Neurol.*, 151: 77–81.

Cassam, A.K., Llewellyn-Smith, I.J. and Weaver, L.C. (1997) Catecholamine enzymes and neuropeptides are expressed in fibres and somata in the intermediate grey matter in chronic spinal rats. *Neuroscience*, 78: 829–841.

Cassam, A.K., Rogers, K.A. and Weaver, L.C. (1999) Co-localization of substance P and dopamine β-hydroxylase with growth associated protein-43 is lost caudal to a spinal cord transection. *Neuroscience*, 88: 1275–1288.

Clarke, H.A., Dekaban, G.A. and Weaver, L.C. (1998) Identification of lamina V and VII interneurons presynaptic to adrenal sympathetic preganglionic neurons in rats using a recombinant herpes simplex virus type 1. *Neuroscience*, 85: 863–872.

Collins, H.L. and DiCarlo, S.E. (2002) Acute exercise reduces the response to colon distension in T5 spinal rats. *Am. J. Physiol. Heart Circ. Physiol.*, 282: H1566–H1570.

Corbett, J.L., Debarge, O., Frankel, H.L. and Mathias, C. (1975) Cardiovascular responses in tetraplegic man to muscle spasm, bladder percussion and head-up tilt. *Clin. Exp. Pharmacol. Physiol.*, Suppl. 2: 189–193.

Dekaban, G., Semidrea, C., Peters, A. and Weaver, L.C. (2000) Inhibition of ED-1+ macrophage migration to the site of spinal cord injury by a monoclonal antibody to the integrin alpha D. *Neurosci. Abstr.*, 26: 512 (abstract).

Dembowsky, K., Czachurski, J., Amendt, K. and Seller, H. (1978) Tonic, supraspinal, monoaminergic inhibition on spinal somato-sympathetic reflexes. *Pflugers Arch.*, 373: R76.

Erickson, R.P. (1980) Autonomic hyperreflexia: pathophysiology and medical management. *Arch. Phys. Med. Rehabil.*, 61: 431–440.

Fehlings, M.G., Tator, C.H. and Linden, R.D. (1989) The effect of nimodipine and dextran on axonal function and blood flow following experimental spinal cord injury. *J. Neurosurg.*, 71: 403–416.

Frohman, E.M., Frohman, T.C., Dustin, M.L., Vayuvegula, B., Choi, B., Gupta, A., van den Noort, S. and Gupta, S. (1989) The induction of intercellular adhesion molecule 1 (ICAM-1) expression on human fetal astrocytes by interferon-gamma, tumour necrosis factor alpha, lymphotoxin, and interleukin-1: relevance to intracerebral antigen presentation. *J. Neuroimmunol.*, 23: 117–124.

Giannantoni, A., Di, S.S., Scivoletto, G., Mollo, A., Silecchia, A., Fuoco, U. and Vespasiani, G. (1998) Autonomic dysreflexia during urodynamics. *Spinal Cord*, 36: 756–760.

Grayson, M.H., Van der Vieren, M., Gallatin, W.M., Hoffman, P.A. and Bochner, B.S. (1997) Expression of a novel β2 integrin (αdβ2) on human leukocytes and mast cells. *J. Allergy Clin. Immunol.*, 99: 5386 (abstract).

Guttman, F.L. and Whitteridge, D. (1947) Effects of bladder distention on autonomic mechanisms after spinal cord injuries. *Brain*, 70: 361–404.

Hamada, Y., Ikata, T., Katoh, S., Kauchi, K., Wa, M., Wai, Y. and Kuzawa, K. (1996) Involvement of an intercellular adhesion molecule 1-dependent pathway in the pathogenesis of secondary changes after spinal cord injury in rats. *J. Neurochem.*, 66: 1525–1531.

Hanisch, U.K., Neuhaus, J., Rowe, W., Van Rossum, D., Moller, T., Kettenmann, H. and Quirion, R. (1997) Neurotoxic consequences of central long-term administration of interleukin-2 in rats. *Neuroscience*, 79(3): 799–818.

Haskard, D., Cavender, D., Beatty, P., Springer, T. and Ziff, M. (1986) T lymphocyte adhesion to endothelial cells: mechanisms demonstrated by anti-LFA-1 monoclonal antibodies. *J. Immunol.*, 137(9): 2901–2906.

Hayashi, M., Ueyama, T., Nemoto, K., Tamaki, T. and Senba, E. (2000) Sequential MRNA expression for immediate early genes, cytokines, and neurotrophins in spinal cord injury. *J. Neurotrauma*, 17: 203–218.

Heese, K., Fiebich, B.L., Bauer, J. and Otten, U. (1998a) NF-kappaB modulates lipopolysaccharide-induced microglial nerve growth factor expression. *Glia*, 22: 401–407.

Heese, K., Hock, C. and Otten, U. (1998b) Inflammatory signals induce neurotrophin expression in human microglial cells. *J. Neurochem.*, 70: 699–707.

Henninger, D.D., Panes, J., Eppihimer, M., Russel, J., Gerritsen, M., Anderson, D.C. and Granger, D.N. (1997) Cytokine-induced VCAM-1 and ICAM-1 expression in different organs of the mouse. *J. Immunol.*, 158(4): 1825–1832.

Heumann, R., Korsching, S., Bandtlow, C. and Thoenen, H. (1987a) Changes of nerve growth factor synthesis in nonneuronal cells in response to sciatic nerve transection. *J. Cell Biol.*, 104: 1623–1631.

Heumann, R., Lindholm, D., Bandtlow, C., Meyer, M., Radeke, M.J., Misko, T.P., Shooter, E. and Thoenen, H. (1987b) Differential regulation of MRNA encoding nerve growth factor and its receptor in rat sciatic nerve during development, degeneration, and regeneration: role of macrophages. *Proc. Natl. Acad. Sci. USA*, 84: 8735–8739.

Hurwitz, A.A., Lyman, W.D., Guida, M.P., Calderon, T.M. and Berman, J.W. (1992) Tumour necrosis factor alpha induces adhesion molecule expression on human fetal astrocytes. *J. Exp. Med.*, 176(6): 1631–1636.

Joshi, S., LeVatte, M.A., Dekaban, G.A. and Weaver, L.C. (1995) Identification of spinal interneurons antecedent to adrenal sympathetic preganglionic neurons using trans-synaptic transport of herpes simplex virus type 1. *Neuroscience*, 65: 893–903.

Karlsson, A.-K. (1999) Autonomic dysreflexia. *Spinal Cord*, 37: 383–391.

Karlsson, A.-K., Friden, P.M., Lonnroth, P., Sullivan, L. and Elam, M. (1998) Regional sympathetic function in high spinal cord injury during mental stress and autonomic dysreflexia. *Brain*, 121: 1711–1719.

Klusman, I. and Schwab, M.E. (1997) Effects of pro-inflammatory cytokines in experimental spinal cord injury. *Brain Res.*, 762: 173–184.

Kossmann, T., Hans, V., Imhof, H.G., Trentz, O. and Morganti-Kossmann, M.C. (1996) Interleukin-6 released in human cerebrospinal fluid following traumatic brain injury may trigger nerve growth factor production in astrocytes. *Brain Res.*, 713: 143–152.

Koyanagi, I., Tator, C.H. and Lea, P.J. (1993a) Three-dimensional analysis of the vascular system in the rat spinal cord with scanning electron microscopy of vascular corrosion casts. Part 2: Acute spinal cord injury. *Neurosurgery*, 33: 285–291.

Koyanagi, I., Tator, C.H. and Theriault, E. (1993b) Silicone rubber microangiography of acute spinal cord injury in the rat. *Neurosurgery*, 32: 260–268.

Krassioukov, A.V. and Weaver, L.C. (1995) Episodic hypertension due to autonomic dysreflexia in acute and chronic spinal cord-injured rats. *Am. J. Physiol.*, 268: H2077–H2083.

Krassioukov, A.V. and Weaver, L.C. (1996) Morphological changes in sympathetic preganglionic neurons after spinal cord injury in rats. *Neuroscience*, 70: 211–226.

Krassioukov, A.V., Jonson, D.G. and Schramm, L.P. (2000) Spinal interneurons are hyperresponsive to somatic and visceral stimuli after chronic spinal cord transection in rat. *Neurosci. Abstr.*, 26: 1191 (abstract).

Krenz, N.R. and Weaver, L.C. (2000) Nerve growth factor in glia and inflammatory cells of the injured rat spinal cord. *J. Neurochem.*, 74: 730–739.

Krenz, N.R., Meakin, S.O., Krassioukov, A.V. and Weaver, L.C. (1999) Neutralizing intraspinal nerve growth factor blocks autonomic dysreflexia caused by spinal cord injury. *J. Neurosci.*, 19(17): 7405–7414.

Kwo, S., Young, W. and DeCrescito, V. (1989) Spinal cord sodium, potassium, calcium and water concentration changes in rats after graded contusion injury. *J. Neurotrauma*, 6: 4–24 (abstract).

Larson, R.S. and Springer, T.A. (1990) Structure and function of leukocyte integrins. *Immunol. Rev.*, 114: 181–217.

LaSala, A., Corinti, S., Federici, M., Saragovi, H.U. and Girolomoni, G. (2000) Ligand activation of nerve growth factor receptor TrkA protects monocytes from apoptosis. *J. Leukocyte Biol.*, 68: 104–110.

Lee, B.Y., Karmakar, M.G., Herz, B.L. and Sturgill, R.A. (1994) Autonomic dysreflexia revisited. *J. Spinal Cord Med.*, 18: 75–87.

Lindan, R., Joiner, E., Freehafer, A.A. and Hazel, C. (1980) Incidence and clinical features of autonomic dysreflexia in patients with spinal cord injury. *Paraplegia*, 18: 285–292.

Lindholm, D., Heumann, R., Meyer, M. and Thoenen, H. (1987) Interleukin-1 regulates synthesis of nerve growth factor in non-neuronal cells of rat sciatic nerve. *Nature*, 330: 658–659.

Llewellyn-Smith, I.J. and Weaver, L.C. (2001) Changes in synaptic inputs to sympathetic preganglionic neurons after spinal cord injury. *J. Comp. Neurol.*, 435: 226–240.

Mabon, P.J., Weaver, L.C. and Dekaban, G.A. (2000) Inhibition of monocyte/macrophage migration to a spinal cord injury site by an antibody to the integrin alphaD: a potential new anti-inflammatory treatment. *Exp. Neurol.*, 166: 52–64.

Maiorov, D.N., Fehlings, M.G. and Krassioukov, A.V. (1998) Relationship between severity of spinal cord injury and abnormalities in neurogenic cardiovascular control in conscious rats. *J. Neurotrauma*, 15(5): 365–374.

Maiorov, D.N., Krenz, N.R., Krassioukov, A.V. and Weaver, L.C. (1997a) Role of spinal NMDA and AMPA receptors in episodic hypertension in conscious spinal rats. *Am. J. Physiol.*, 273: H1266–H1274.

Maiorov, D.N., Weaver, L.C. and Krassioukov, A.V. (1997b) Relationship between sympathetic activity and arterial pressure in conscious spinal rats. *Am. J. Physiol.*, 272: H625–H631.

Mathias, C.J. and Frankel, H.L. (1992) The cardiovascular system in tetraplegia and paraplegia. In: H.L. Frankel (Ed.), *Handbook of Clinical Neurology*, 17th edn. Elsevier Science, Amsterdam, pp. 435–456.

Mathias, C.J. and Frankel, H.L. (1999) Autonomic disturbances in spinal cord lesions. In: C.J. Mathias and R. Bannister (Eds.), *Autonomic Failure. A Textbook of Clinical Disorders of the Autonomic Nervous System*, 4th edn. Oxford University Press, Oxford, pp. 494–513.

Naftchi, N.E. (1990) Mechanism of autonomic dysreflexia; contributions of cathecholamine and peptide neurotransmitters. *Ann. New York Acad. Sci.*, 579: 133–148.

Osborn, J.W., Taylor, R.F. and Schramm, L.P. (1990) Chronic cervical spinal cord injury and autonomic hyperreflexia in rats. *Am. J. Physiol.*, 258: R169–R174.

Popovich, P.G., Wei, P. and Stokes, B.T. (1997) Cellular inflammatory response after spinal cord injury in Sprague–Dawley and Lewis rats. *J. Comp. Neurol.*, 377: 443–464.

Prewitt, C.M.F., Niesman, I.R., Kane, C.J.M. and Houle, J.D. (1997) Activated macrophage/microglial cells can promote the regeneration of sensory axons into the injured spinal cord. *Exp. Neurol.*, 148: 433–443.

Rice, G.E. and Bevilacqua, M.P. (1989) An inducible endothelial cell surface glycoprotein mediates melanoma adhesion. *Science*, 246(4935): 1303–1306.

Rosenman, S.J., Ganji, A.A., Tedder, T.F. and Gallatin, W.M. (1993) Syn-capping of human T lymphocyte adhesion/activation molecules and their redistribution during interaction with endothelial cells. *J. Leukocyte Biol.*, 53(1): 1–10.

Saporito, M.S., Wilcox, H.M., Hartpence, K.C., Lewis, M.E., Vaught, J.L. and Carswell, S. (1993) Pharmacological induction of nerve growth factor MRNA in adult rat brain. *Exp. Neurol.*, 123: 295–302.

Saragovi, H.U. and Gehring, K. (2000) Development of pharmacological agents for targeting neurotrophins and their receptors. *Trends Pharmacol. Sci.*, 21: 93–98.

Sato, A. and Schmidt, R.F. (1973) Somatosympathetic reflexes: afferent fibers, central pathways, discharge characteristics. *Physiol. Rev.*, 53(4): 916–947.

Schumacher, P.A., Eubanks, J.H. and Fehlings, M.G. (1999) Increased calpain I-mediated proteolysis, and preferential loss of dephosphorylated NF200, following traumatic spinal cord injury. *Neuroscience*, 91: 733–744.

Shea, J.D., Gioffre, R., Carrion, H. and Small, M.P. (1973) Autonomic hyperreflexia in spinal cord injury. *South. Med. J.*, 66(8): 869–872.

Shu, X.-Q. and Mendell, L.M. (1999) Neurotrophins and hyperalgesia. *Proc. Natl. Acad. Sci. USA*, 96: 7693–7696.

Smith, C.W., Marlin, S.D., Rothlein, R., Toman, C. and Anderson, D.C. (1989) Cooperative interactions of LFA-1 and Mac-1 with intercellular adhesion molecule-1 in facilitating adher-
ence and transendothelial migration of human neutrophils in vitro. *J. Clin. Invest.*, 83(6): 2008–2017.

Spranger, M., Lindholm, D., Bandtlow, C., Heumann, R., Gnahn, H., Naher-Noe, M. and Thoenen, H. (1990) Regulation of nerve growth factor (NGF) synthesis in the rat central nervous system: comparison between the effects of interleukin-1 and various growth factors in astrocyte cultures and in vivo. *Eur. J. Neurosci.*, 2: 69–76.

Stjernberg, L., Blumberg, H. and Wallin, B.G. (1986) Sympathetic activity in man after spinal cord injury. Outflow to muscle below the lesion. *Brain*, 109: 695–715.

Streit, W.J., Semple-Rowland, S.L., Hurley, S.D., Miller, R.C., Popovich, P.G. and Stokes, B.T. (1998) Cytokine MRNA profiles in contused spinal cord and axotomized facial nucleus suggest a beneficial role for inflammation and gliosis. *Exp. Neurol.*, 152: 74–87.

Taoka, Y. and Okajima, K. (1998) Spinal cord injury in the rat. *Prog. Neurobiol.*, 56: 341–358.

Taoka, Y., Okajima, K., Uchiba, M., Murakami, K., Harada, N., Johno, M. and Naruo, M. (1998) Activated protein C reduces the severity of compression-induced spinal cord injury in rats by inhibiting activation of leukocytes. *J. Neurosci.*, 18(4): 1393–1398.

Tator, C.H. and Fehlings, M.G. (1991) Review of the secondary injury theory of acute spinal cord trauma with emphasis on vascular mechanisms. *J. Neurosurg.*, 75: 15–26.

Teasell, R.W., Arnold, J.M.O., Krassioukov, A.V. and Delaney, G.A. (2000) Cardiovascular consequences of loss of supraspinal control of the sympathetic nervous system after spinal cord injury. *Arch. Phys. Med. Rehabil.*, 81: 506–516.

Van der Vieren, M., Crowe, D.T., Hoekstra, D., Vazeux, R., Hoffman, P.A., Grayson, M.H., Bochner, B.S., Gallatin, W.M. and Staunton, D.E. (1999) The leukocyte integrin $\alpha D\beta 2$ binds VCAM-1: evidence for a binding interface between I domain and VCAM-1. *J. Immunol.*, 163: 1984–1990.

van Kooyk, Y. and Figdor, C.G. (1993) Lymphocyte adhesion mediated by integrins. *Res. Immunol.*, 144: 709–722.

Wallace, M.C. and Tator, C.H. (1986) Spinal cord blood flow measured with microspheres following spinal cord injury in the rat. *Can. J. Neurol. Sci.*, 13: 91–96.

Wallace, M.C., Tator, C.H. and Frazee, P. (1986) Relationship between posttraumatic ischemia and hemorrhage in the injured rat spinal cord as shown by colloidal carbon angiography. *Neurosurgery*, 18: 433–439.

Wallin, B.G. and Stjernberg, L. (1984) Sympathetic activity in man after spinal cord injury. *Brain*, 107: 183–198.

Weaver, L.C., Cassam, A.K., Krassioukov, A.V. and Llewellyn-Smith, I.J. (1997) Changes in immunoreactivity for growth associated protein-43 suggest reorganization of synapses on spinal sympathetic neurons after cord transection. *Neuroscience*, 81: 535–551.

Weaver, L.C., Verghese, P., Bruce, J.C., Fehlings, M.G., Krenz, N.R. and Marsh, D.R. (2001) Autonomic dysreflexia and primary afferent sprouting after clip-compression injury of the rat spinal cord. *J. Neurotrauma*, 18: 1107–1119.

Wong, S.T., Atkinson, B.A. and Weaver, L.C. (2000) Confocal microscopic analysis of sprouting small-diameter primary afferent fibres after spinal cord injury. *Neurosci. Lett.*, 296: 65–68.

Yan, H.Q., Banos, M.A., Herregodts, P., Hooghe, R. and Hooghe-Peters, E.L. (1992) Expression of interleukin (IL)-1 beta, IL-6 and their respective receptors in the normal rat brain and after injury. *Eur. J. Immunol.*, 22: 2963–2971.

Yenari, Q., Kunis, D., Sun, G.H., Onley, D., Watson, L., Turner, S., Whitaker, S. and Steinberg, G.K. (1998) Hu23F2G, an anti-body recognizing the leukocyte CD11/CD18 integrin, reduces injury in a rabbit model of transient focal cerebral ischemia. *Exp. Neurol.*, 153: 223–233.

Young, W. (1993) Secondary injury mechanisms in acute spinal cord injury. *J. Emerg. Med.*, 11: 13–22.

Zeidman, S.M., Ling, G.S., Ducker, T.B. and Ellenbogen, R.G. (1996) Clinical applications of pharmacologic therapies for spinal cord injury. *J. Spinal Disord.*, 9: 367–380.

L. McKerracher, G. Doucet and S. Rossignol (Eds.)
Progress in Brain Research, Vol. 137

CHAPTER 8

The spinal locomotor CPG: a target after spinal cord injury

Sten Grillner[*]

Nobel institute for Neurophysiology, Department of Neuroscience, The Retzius laboratory, Karolinska Institutet, SE-17177 Stockholm, Sweden

Introduction

In all vertebrate classes from mammals to fish and cyclostomes, the spinal cord has proven to contain the necessary information to coordinate the propulsive aspect of locomotor movement (Grillner, 1985). In some species, like the dogfish and the eel, the spinal cord generates locomotor movements directly after a spinal transection and continues to do so for days and weeks. After a transection of the spinal cord at lower thoracic level, young mammals like kittens can also generate alternating hind limb movements, thus under the control of the lumbosacral spinal cord isolated from the rest of the central nervous system. If regularly trained they are able to support themselves for shorter periods while performing locomotor movements with the hind limbs. The pattern of muscle activation in each step cycle is similar to that of the intact walking cat (Forssberg et al., 1980a,b).

After a similar transection in the adult spinal cat, the situation is different, no locomotor activity is observed initially. If, however, the cat is trained on a treadmill regularly, alternating limb movements will develop that improve in quality progressively, to finally present appropriate locomotor coordination

*Correspondence to: S. Grillner, Nobel Institute for Neurophysiology, Department of Neuroscience, The Retzius Laboratory, Karolinska Institutet, SE-17177 Stockholm, Sweden. Tel.: +46-8-7286900; Fax: +46-8-349544; E-mail: sten.grillner@neuro.ki.se

with weight support after several weeks (Smith et al., 1982; Rossignol, 1996; Edgerton et al., 2001; de Leon et al., 2002). If no training takes place, some sort of alternating limb movements may still occur but not with a locomotor-like coordination. If training only involves standing, but not walking, only positive effects on the former will result (de Leon et al., 1999). Thus training can affect the motor pattern in a striking and specific way, which testifies to a spinal plasticity at some level.

If noradrenergic agonists are injected after an acute transection, however, locomotor movements develop within some minutes (Forssberg and Grillner, 1973). These movements adapt to the treadmill speed within a certain range of velocities. Thus, locomotor circuits are available also in the adult spinal cord, provided that they receive an appropriate activation. In rats the situation is similar, locomotor movements can be produced in the chronic spinal state, but be much improved by 5-HT agonists, or by transplantation of monoamine neurons, in particular in the rostral lumbar spinal cord (Rossignol, 1996; Ribotta et al., 2000; Giménez y Ribotta et al., 2002; Orsal et al., 2002). Also in spinal primates locomotor-like movements can be produced. In all classes of vertebrates it has, in addition, been possible to develop isolated spinal cord preparations that via different experimental interventions have been able to produce fictive locomotor activity. These preparations are important for the analysis of the intrinsic function of the spinal locomotor networks, and the neuropharmacology of these neuronal systems. The latter aspect may also be important and contribute to the design of pharmacological means of regulating the level of excitability in the spinal cord networks.

These spinal locomotor circuits depend on a central network often referred to as the central pattern generator network (CPG), but there is also a powerful sensory component from afferents activated during the locomotor movement (Fig. 1). This sensory input influences the duration of for instance the support phase, and also, at least at slower speeds, the degree of muscle activation. In spinal animals the sensory component is clearly of critical importance, and accounts for the fact that spinal animals can adapt to the treadmill speed within a certain range (see Grillner, 1981, 1985, 1996; Pearson, 2000).

From these and similar data, we can extrapolate that the spinal cord of all vertebrates including humans contain the necessary circuitry to provide the basic locomotor coordination. In some species, the activity is displayed spontaneously, in other cases training is required. In most cases monoaminergic agents or transplantation of monoaminergic neurons can promote the expression of locomotor activity. The problem is, however, that this activity cannot be controlled from the brainstem, which normally initiates the locomotor activity. Essentially, these different spinal preparations acquire a moderately high excitability in their spinal CPGs at rest. They do not, as a rule, perform spontaneous locomotor movements, but respond with well-coordinated locomotor movements when placed on a moving treadmill belt. The spinal locomotor circuit is thus independent from any control from the brain. One goal of this symposium is to explore how this control can be regained.

What types of supraspinal control are used in the normal control of locomotion?

Slow and fast descending control of the spinal CPGs

The spinal CPGs are controlled by reasonably fast conducting reticulospinal pathways (Figs. 1 and 2) that in turn become activated from the mesencephalic (MLR) and diencephalic (DLR) locomotor regions (Noga et al., 1988, 1991; see Grillner et al., 1997; Orlovsky et al., 1999). They control the level of activity in the CPGs, and can induce rapid changes

in the level of locomotor activity. In addition, slow monoaminergic pathways (5-HT, NA, Fig. 2) affect the level of responsiveness in the spinal circuits (Grillner and Shik, 1973; Jordan and Steeves, 1976; Noga et al., 1999). These two control systems appear to function in a very different way. The monoamine system sets the level of background tone, whereas the fast reticulospinal system is in the command role (on–off and level of activity).

Accurate positioning of the foot during each step

In addition to the slow and the fast descending control of the locomotor CPGs other types of control are also needed for a behaviorally successful locomotor activity. In most mammals, visuomotor coordination plays an important role to adapt each step to avoid obstacles, and place each foot in an optimal spot in each step. This type of control is of little importance, if we walk on a flat open surface like a large floor, but very much needed as soon as we enter a more complex terrain. The corticospinal system, in particular, is involved in this type of control, which helps to position the foot accurately in each step (Liddell and Phillips, 1944; Georgopoulos and Grillner, 1989; Drew, 1993; Widajewicz et al., 1994; see Orlovsky et al., 1999), but indirect effects via reticulospinal pathways also contribute (Prentice and Drew, 2001). In this case the basic locomotor drive is still produced by the spinal locomotor CPGs, but the corticospinal system provides superimposed signals, which will add targeted excitation (or inhibition) on certain spinal inter- and motoneurons. This will result in a modification of the foot trajectory and an accurate positioning of the foot. A similar type of control is also involved in the control of turning or changing direction of the locomotor movements.

Control of body equilibrium during locomotion

A third control system of equal importance is that controlling body equilibrium during walking (orientation of the body in general). In each step there are lateral movements of the trunk to move the projection of the center of gravity close to that of the supporting limb (Thorstensson et al., 1984). These postural commands are programmed into the locomotor control system, but as we walk along there

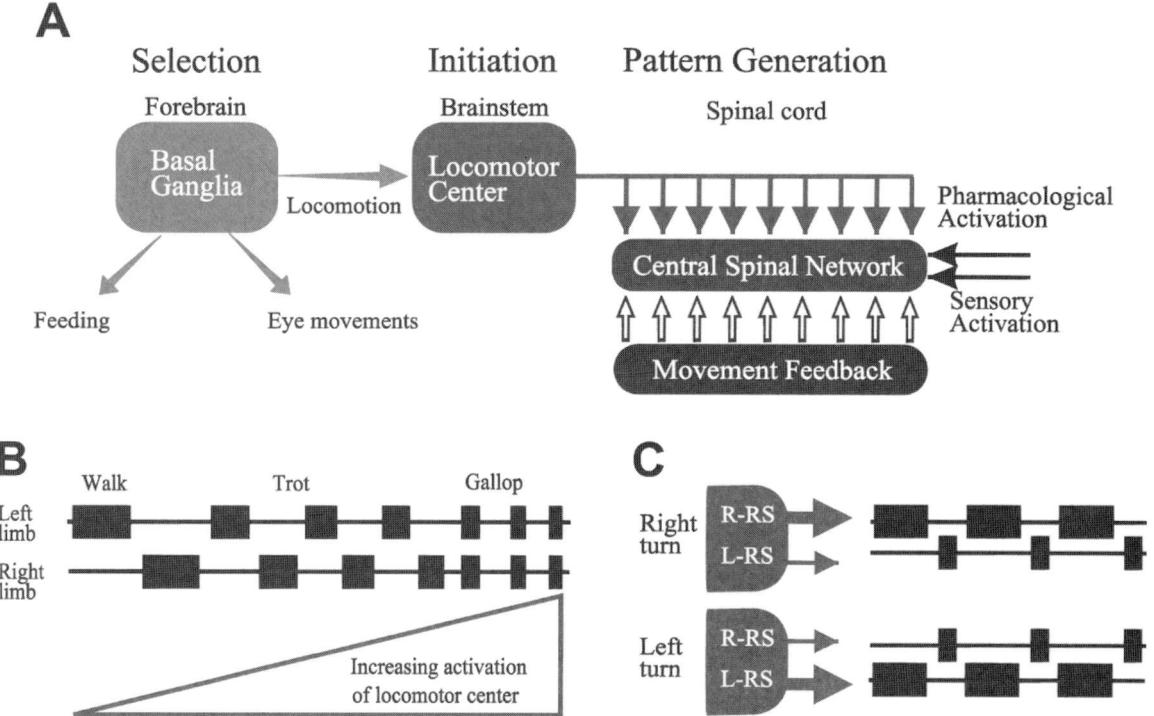

Fig. 1. General control strategy for vertebrate locomotion (A). Locomotion is initiated by an increased activity in reticulospinal neurons of the brainstem locomotor center, which in turn produces the locomotor pattern in close interaction with sensory feedback. With increased activation of the locomotor center, the speed of locomotion will also increase (B). In quadrupeds this also leads to a shift in interlimb coordination, from walk to trot and then to gallop. The basal ganglia exert a tonic inhibitory influence on different motor centers. Once a pattern of motor behavior is selected, the inhibition is released, in this case allowing the locomotor center in the brainstem to be activated. Experimentally, locomotion can also be elicited pharmacologically by administration of excitatory amino acid agonists and by sensory input. (C) Shows that an asymmetric activation of reticulospinal (RS) neurons gives rise to an asymmetric output in the left (L) and right (R) sides. This will result in a turning movement to one side or the other.

may also be smaller or larger unexpected perturbations, which need to be counteracted instantly. These perturbations are detected by a variety of receptors in both the vestibular organ, and in muscles, joints and skin particularly under the feet. These correcting signals include cerebellum (see Orlovsky et al., 1999) and are mediated preferentially via vestibulo- and reticulospinal pathways to a variety of motoneurons/muscles that collectively compensate for the particular perturbation that has occurred.

In which pathways would it be most important to recover function, after a spinal cord injury?

Consider a patient with a complete spinal cord lesion at lower thoracic level. If he/she is to be partially restored in locomotor function so that he/she will be

able to walk over an even floor, supraspinal access to the spinal cord CPGs will be required. On the other hand, an accurate foot placement is not critical (corticospinal control), and the equilibrium control can be aided by an extrinsic 'walking aid'. Such a partial restitution could allow the patient to take a limited number of steps in the home environment and perhaps to a waiting taxi. Clearly, bladder and bowel function also have a very high priority. For a complete restitution the different descending and ascending sensory systems will, however, most likely be required.

From this follows that it would be important that the primary focus, in the different animal models that seek to establish functional regeneration across a spinal cord lesion, should be on the descending reticulospinal pathways that control the locomotor

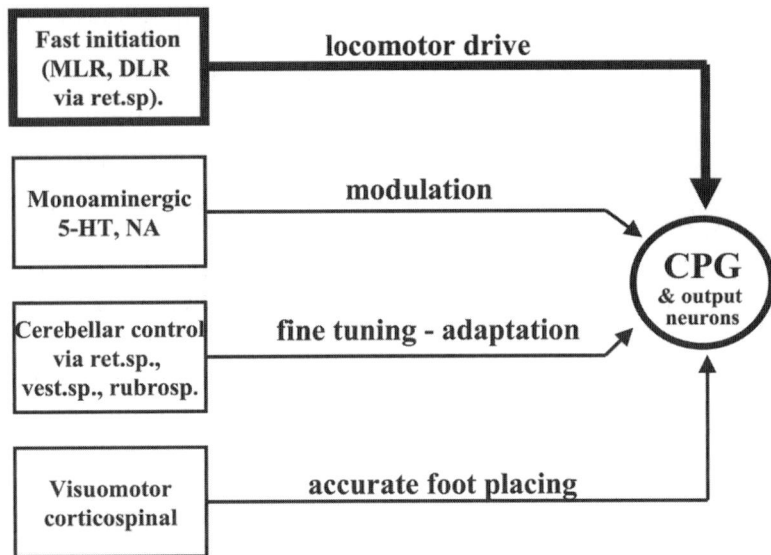

Fig. 2. Four descending systems control different aspects of the locomotor behavior. The uppermost system regulates the initiation of locomotion from the mesencephalic (MLR) and diencephalic (DLR) locomotor regions. The monoaminergic systems are able to modulate the responsiveness of the CPG and the quality of the motor pattern. Postural adaptations involve cerebellar control via vestibulo-, reticulo-, and rubrospinal pathways. Visuomotor coordination to achieve, for instance, an accurate foot placement in a complex terrain is mediated via the corticospinal pathways.

CPGs, at least in models of paraplegia (Fig. 2). A secondary requirement is to restore the function to some degree of the equilibrium control systems, and only as a third priority the precise foot placing systems (corticospinal projections). It is thus very surprising to see that the different research groups that address regeneration of descending pathways in the context of spinal cord injury, use preferentially the corticospinal tract, as the pathway of choice for establishing regeneration. One methodological reason may be the morphological approach used, and the circumscribed location of the corticospinal tract in rat. A lack of communication between research areas appears to account for this unfortunate fact.

Recovery of function in patients with partial lesions of the spinal cord

Recent studies have shown that certain patients with partial lesions that have been paraplegic (incomplete lesions) and bound to a wheel chair, even for years can regain locomotor movements with the legs to some degree (Dobkin et al., 1995; Wernig et al., 1995, 1999, 2000; Barbeau et al., 1999, 2002; de Leon et al., 2002). The requirement has been a very

active training on a treadmill, initially with support of most of the body through a harness, and a physical therapist for each leg, moving the two legs back and forth on the treadmill, with locomotor-like movements. After some time the legs of the patients will start to contribute actively, and the weight support of the patient will progressively increase. After some months, some of these patients are able to walk across the floor, in the best case with the support of a cane, in other cases with a walker. What has happened? Presumably, the locomotor-like sensory input from the two limbs will entrain the locomotor CPGs, and there may be a use-dependent facilitation of synapses within the spinal locomotor system. This may be a similar mechanism to that operating in the spinal cats referred to above — they perform well-coordinated movements, if they are trained regularly on the treadmill. If not, the motor pattern degenerates but can be regained by training. The previously paraplegic patients that became able to walk after the training program obviously cannot have had a complete spinal cord lesion. The result of the training is presumably to make the spinal cord locomotor circuitry operational again. The remaining axons at the lesion site are thus able to regain access to the spinal cord circuitry to a sufficient degree to initiate locomotor activity. Once the patients have started to walk, they will themselves take care of the daily retraining required.

This process can most likely be facilitated by a variety of drugs that affect for instance monoaminergic receptors in the spinal cord (Barbeau et al., 1999). Ideally, pumps with intrathecal catheters should be used to administer the drugs locally over the lumbar spinal cord rather than systemically. Other therapeutical possibilities would be to transplant; e.g. monoaminergic neurons in the lumbar cord as done on spinal animals (Kim et al., 1999; Ribotta et al., 2000; Orsal et al., 2002). Such manipulations can lower the threshold for activation of the spinal locomotor CPG, and facilitate for a supraspinal control via the few remaining axons. The results indicate that a proportion of incomplete paraplegic patients can regain walking and a certain degree of independence with appropriate training. In this case we are not dealing with regeneration, but with mechanisms to facilitate the control of the spinal locomotor CPGs for the benefit of the patients.

One may also ask, if there are pharmacological tools that would allow a patient to recover faster directly after the lesion, among other things to reduce the period referred to as spinal shock. A variety of drugs, for instance monoaminergic drugs, have been considered in this context (Barbeau et al., 1999; Rossignol et al., 2002). This may be another important avenue to take for patients with partial lesions, if combined with the type of treadmill training referred to above. In general, it will also be important to investigate which parts of the spinal cord white matter are most likely to convey the necessary signals to the spinal cord.

Evaluation of recovery of function in experimental models

It is obviously very important to have stringent criteria for evaluation of recovery of function. The scoring systems that have been developed are therefore useful, although not without problems, particularly with regard to effects presumed to be signs of regeneration (see Young, 2002). The fact that the isolated spinal cord in itself under certain conditions is able to generate a coordination and impressive motor repertoire, complicates the scientific evaluation of a given score level (Bregman et al., 2002).

If a control and experimental group with spinal cord lesion is compared, and the latter gains a somewhat higher score, this could be due to either an actual regeneration, but alternatively to an effect on the intrinsic spinal circuitry caused by the manipulation (e.g. pharmacological effects, growth factors, etc.). From the above, it is clear that the spinal cord below the lesion has a 'dormant' capacity to coordinate movements. The interpretation of data of this type requires great caution, and a detailed knowledge of the experimental history of the two groups compared.

If regenerating fibers cross the lesion area and affect the caudal spinal cord, the effects can be of very different nature. Slow unmyelinated fiber systems, like the monoaminergic, may cause a change in excitability in the spinal cord, and thereby the responsiveness to a variety of stimuli (Fig. 2). This can be important, but will not suffice to permit a 'voluntary' control of the locomotion. It is noteworthy that monoaminergic unmyelinated fibers appear to regenerate comparatively well within the gray rather than the white matter, in which they are normally located (Björklund et al., 1986).

To achieve a dynamic interaction between the brainstem locomotor centers and the spinal cord CPGs, most likely a regeneration of part of the fast reticulospinal glutamatergic axons will be required. It is possible that only a comparatively unspecific connectivity to the spinal cord interneuronal circuitry will be necessary in order to turn on and conversely switch off the spinal CPGs. One reason for suggesting this possibility is that in the isolated spinal cord of mammals as well as lower vertebrates, the CPGs can be turned on by bath applied glutamate agonists (see below), which indeed is a very unspecific mode of activation. This is probably due to the fact that the spinal locomotor circuitry has priority and a dominating role at the spinal level.

Furthermore, it would seem useful to compare experimental groups that in addition to the experimental manipulation also are trained on the treadmill. If the spinal cord circuitry is kept at its best, it is probably easier for the presumed regenerating descending fibers to acquire control of the spinal CPG circuits, rather than to start with having to re-activate a 'dormant' structure.

The intrinsic function of the spinal CPGs: the mammalian CPGs

In mammals, the spinal CPGs are known to be organized such that there is a CPG for each limb and also for the trunk and tail muscles. The different CPGs can be recombined to achieve the different gaits. In trot and walk fore- and hind-limbs, respectively, strictly alternate, whereas they are coordinated in a more or less synchronous way during the different types of gallop. In man, walking and running are both coordinated with an alternation of the two legs. The difference between walking and running lies in the leg movements and the foot placements. In walking there is a clear heel strike, whereas in running the forefoot or the whole foot is placed in each step. It is possible that the CPGs can be further subdivided into unit pattern generators that control groups of close synergistic muscles (Grillner, 1981).

Whereas there is no question that CPGs exist (combined with sensory movement-related feedback), few hard facts are available on the intrinsic function of the mammalian CPGs. The inhibitory premotor interneuron subtype, referred to as the 1a interneuron, is activated during locomotion and provides inhibition of motoneurons antagonistic to muscles active at a given instant of the step cycle (Edgerton et al., 1976; Pratt and Jordan, 1987). In addition, the inhibition at each girdle is known to be glycinergic (responsible for the alternation). However, the interaction between CPG interneurons is not yet understood. The development of the rat/mouse neonatal isolated spinal cord models most likely will help to remedy this lack of information on the functional organization of the mammalian CPGs (Kudo and Yamada, 1987; Kiehn and Kjaerulff, 1998; Huang et al., 2000; Kjaerulff and Kiehn, 2001). With regard to transmitters involved, glutamatergic excitatory interneurons activate both NMDA and AMPA receptors, and glycinergic inhibition is responsible for the reciprocal inhibition between antagonist muscles and limbs (for review see Rossignol, 1996; Orlovsky et al., 1999). In addition, these circuits are modulated by a variety of monoaminergic, peptidergic, and other metabotropic (GABAergic, glutamatergic) receptors that can modify the motor pattern in a variety of ways. It is also important to consider the evolution of the expression of different receptors after spinalization and during training (Giroux et al., 1999).

To facilitate the motor coordination of the spinal CPGs in paraplegic patients it will be important to define with great accuracy the different modulator systems (receptors) and their target ion channels, which can influence different aspects of the detailed motor burst generation, both with regard to timing and degree of activation. Only with such knowledge there is the possibility to develop a rational drug therapy, rather than the more common trial and error strategy.

Lower vertebrate models

In contrast to mammals the CPGs underlying locomotion are well described in lamprey (see Grillner et al., 2000) and the frog tadpole (see Dale and Kuenzi, 1997; Sillar et al., 1997; Roberts, 2000). The circuitry is described in some detail as well as the transmitters/receptors involved and the ion channels of importance for the pattern generation. This is all information that is required for an understanding of the intrinsic function of the CPGs, and also for defining appropriate drug targets. I will very briefly review the lamprey system.

The lamprey brainstem–spinal cord can be maintained in vitro over several days (Fig. 3). Moreover, the motor coordination underlying locomotion can be elicited by stimulation of the brainstem locomotor centers in the isolated nervous system, while the efferent motor pattern is recorded from the cut ventral roots. Only with an active nervous system it is possible to elucidate the underlying network function. By simultaneous paired recordings from pre- and postsynaptic interneurons, it has been possible to identify network interneurons in the spinal cord (Fig. 4). The excitatory spinal premotor interneurons (E in Fig. 4) are glutamatergic and activate other E interneurons via mutual excitation and inhibitory glycinergic interneurons and motoneurons. The excitory drives from E interneurons and from descending reticulospinal neurons activate both AMPA and NMDA receptors. The interaction between E interneurons are sufficient to produce rhythmic bursting unilaterally (Cangiano et al., 2000; and unpublished) without any concomitant glycinergic contribution. The primary role of the crossed glycinergic interneuron

103

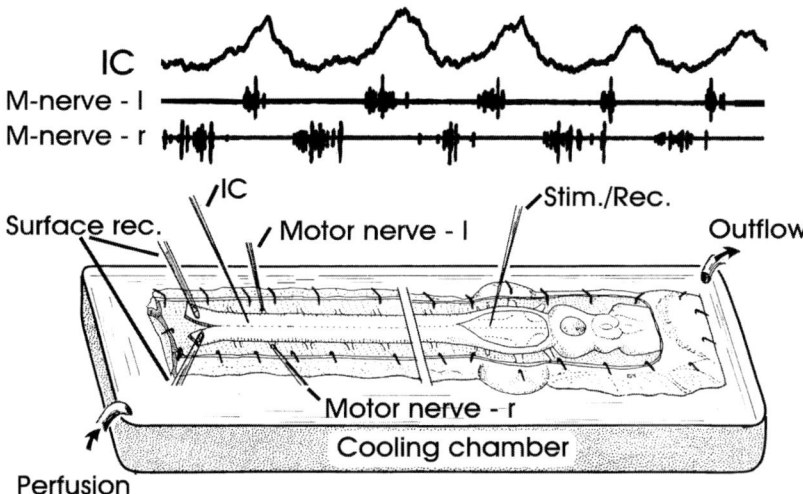

Fig. 3. In vitro preparation of the lamprey CNS. The brainstem–spinal cord of the lamprey can be maintained alive for several days in isolation, and the motor pattern underlying locomotion can be produced by stimulating the brainstem locomotor centers. The motor activity can be recorded in the ventral roots (motor nerves) that normally activate the musculature on the left (l) and right (r) sides. The activity in single or pairs of cells can be recorded intracellularly with microelectrodes (IC). An intracellular record (IC) of a network neuron with subthreshold membrane potential oscillations is shown above together with the alternating motor activity in the ventral roots on the left and right sides. The experimental chamber is kept cold (4–7°C) and it is continuously perfused with physiological solution.

is to generate the alternating activity between the left and the right side.

Essentially, the supraspinal drive from RS neurons will elevate the excitability in the spinal interneurons, such that the interneurons will tend to fire action potential when not actively inhibited from contralateral inhibitory interneurons. Thus, there are mechanisms on each side that will help terminating the burst on that side. When this happens the contralateral side will automatically start, due to the background excitatory drive from the supraspinal RS drive. The control of the burst termination is thus one critical factor. Membrane properties contribute importantly. Fig. 5 illustrates the membrane oscillation throughout a locomotor cycle. After the schematically illustrated neuron comes out of the crossed inhibition, the background excitation will depolarize the cell, leading to an activation of voltage-dependent NMDA and low-voltage-activated (LVA) Ca^{2+} channels, which will further depolarize the cell. During the depolarizing plateau, there will be a Ca^{2+} entry through NMDA channels and Ca^{2+} channels activated by each action potential and through LVA Ca^{2+} channels (Bacskai et al., 1995). This in turn will lead to an activation of Ca^{2+}-dependent K^+ channels (K_{Ca}) that will progressively hyperpolarize the membrane to a level when the voltage-dependent NMDA channels start to close again, leading to a rapid hyperpolarization and a cessation of the burst. Since there is a spike frequency adaptation in the E-IN interneurons due to a summation of the post-spike after-hyperpolarization (due to K_{Ca}), this will lead to a decreased mutual excitation between E-INs, which will lead to a reduction of the excitatory drive.

In the isolated nervous system there is obviously no sensory movement-related feed back. During actual locomotion, however, stretch receptors will be activated that sense the locomotor movements (Grillner et al., 1984; Viana di Prisco et al., 1990). When the segmental muscles on one side contract, the contralateral stretch receptor (SR-I in Fig. 4) will become activated. There are two types of stretch receptors, an inhibitory one with crossed glycinergic axons (SR-I) that provides inhibition to contralateral network neurons, and thus contributes to burst termination (see also Fig. 5); stretch receptors with ipsilateral axons are excitatory (SR-E), and provide excitation to the side that is to become active. The sensory feedback is a very important part of the control circuit and will act to correct perturbations of the locomotor movements.

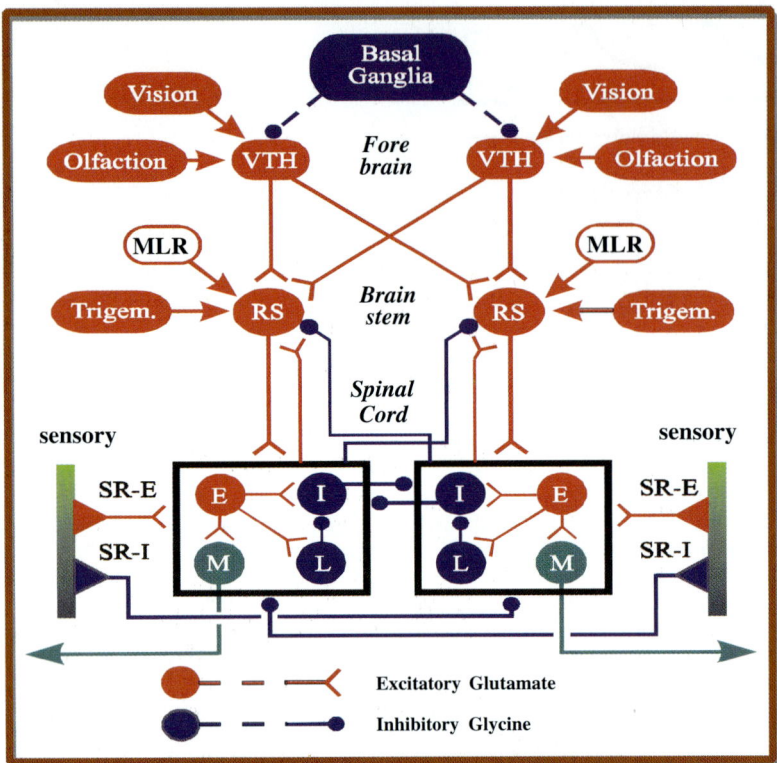

Fig. 4. Lamprey locomotor network. A schematic representation of the forebrain, brainstem and spinal components of the neural network that generate locomotor burst activity. All neuron symbols denote populations of neurons rather than single cells. The reticulospinal (RS) glutamatergic neurons excite all classes of spinal interneurons. The excitatory interneurons (E) excite all types of spinal neurons, that is, the inhibitory glycinergic interneurons (I) that cross the midline and inhibits all classes of neurons on the contralateral side, the lateral interneurons (L), which inhibits I interneurons and motoneurons (M). The stretch receptor neurons are of an excitatory type (SR-E) that excites neurons on the ipsilateral side and an inhibitory type (SR-I) that inhibits all neurons on the contralateral side. RS neurons receive excitatory synaptic inputs from cutaneous afferents (Trigem.) the mesencephalic locomotor region (MLR) and from the ventral thalamus (VTH), which in turn receives inputs from the basal ganglia and olfactory bulb and optic nerve. Olfactory and visual stimuli are very effective in evolving locomotion and can act via VTH. VTH seems as the diencephalic locomotor region.

Although we have extensive knowledge of the properties of the interneurons and their synaptic interaction, it is nevertheless difficult to comprehend the complex and interactive process that goes on within each network interneuron (different types of ion channels), as well as between population of cells. Therefore, we have made extensive use of detailed mathematical modelling to test whether the circuit that is presented here operates. This work is published in some detail (Hellgren et al., 1992, 1999; Yang et al., 2000), but will not be reviewed further here.

The fast network interaction between interneurons and with motoneurons is due to ionotropic glutamate and glycine receptors. In addition, a number of G-protein-mediated receptors have marked effects on the locomotor network. These include different types of 5-HT, DA, GABA$_B$, metabotropic glutamate receptors (mGluR I–III) and peptides (see Table I). We know their target ion channels at the soma-dendritic or presynaptic level, and thereby also their effects on the properties of the different cell types. Since we have a good knowledge of the network we can also predict the effect of a given modulation on the network level, and thus also on the motor behavior. We can thus essentially bridge from ion channels to cell, synapse, network and behavior within this vertebrate system.

In conclusion, the lamprey locomotor network can be regarded as a model system for that of higher

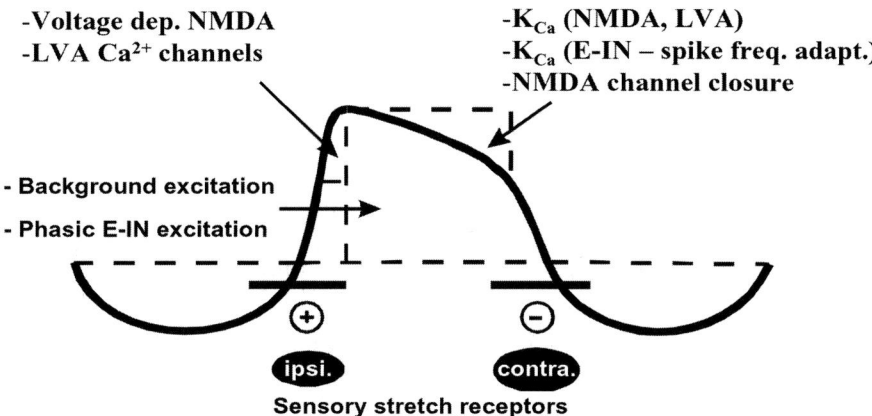

Fig. 5. Factors controlling burst onset and termination. Several different factors contribute to the initiation of the depolarizing phase, its maintenance, and its termination. In addition to conventional synaptic, voltage-dependent NMDA receptors and low-voltage-activated Ca^{2+} channels (LVA-CA) are activated. Ca^{2+} will enter the cell through these channels, cause activation of K_{Ca}, and thereby a progressive hyperpolarization leading to closure of the NMDA channels. The initiation of the depolarizing phase is facilitated by activation of ipsilateral excitatory stretch receptor neurons (SR-E), while the termination of the depolarized phase is partially a result of activation of contralateral inhibitory stretch receptor neurons (SR-I). Abbreviation: E = excitatory interneuron.

TABLE I

Metabotropic animo acid, aminergic and peptidergic G-protein-mediated modulation of ion channel, synaptic, cellular and network activity in the lamprey spinal cord

Spinal modulation: G-protein-coupled receptors

	Presyn	HVA_{Ca}	LVA_{Ca}	K_{Ca}	K^+	NMDA	Network
$GABA_B$	I	↘	↘				↘
$mGluR_I$	0	0	0			↗	↗
$mGluR_{II}$	I	0	0				↘
$mGluR_{III}$	I	0	0				↘
$5\text{-}HT_{1A}$	0			↘			↘
$5\text{-}HT_x$	I	↘					
D_2	I	↘	↘				↘
TK	F			↘	↗		↗
NPY	I						0
Som.		0	0	0	↗		↘
NT		0	0	0			↗

The table summarizes the results of a number of studies (see text as well). The effects of different transmitters and receptors on different targets are listed in the columns on the right. The presynaptic actions can be targeted to sensory afferents, excitatory or inhibitory interneurons and descending reticulospinal axons (Alford et al., 1991; Alford and Grillner, 1991; El Manira et al., 1997; Parker, 2000). Different transmitters have selective actions on different cellular targets (I, indicates presynaptic inhibition; F, indicates facilitation). The locomotor network modulated phasically, in each cycle, the synaptic transmission from sensory afferents and interneurons. The modulation of HVA_{Ca}, LVA_{Ca}, K_{Ca} and K^+ and NMDA channels is indicated with a downward arrow for depression and an upward arrow for facilitation (cf. Hellgren et al., 1992; Matsushima et al., 1993; Schotland et al., 1995; Krieger et al., 1998; Parker et al., 1998). Again, the effects may be specific to particular cell types. Finally, the effects on the network level have been studied on the background of locomotor activity (arrows relate to locomotion burst frequency), and in related modelling experiments (Tegnér et al., 1993, 1997, 1998; Schotland et al., 1995). 5-HT = 5-hydroxytryptamine (serotonin) receptor; D_2 = type-2 dopamine receptor; HVA = high-voltage-activated; mGluR = metabotropic glutamate receptor; NPY = neuropeptide Y; NT = neurotensin; TK = tachykinin.

vertebrates. Although, the network remains to be identified in mammals, the pharmacological analysis of the different vertebrate locomotor systems from lamprey to primate appear similar in design. This may not be too surprising, since during phylogeny the different species have emerged out of another in an evolutionary chain. This, however, suggests that information on, for instance, the different modulator systems in the lamprey may give rise to insight on the pharmacological optimization of the mammalian locomotor systems of the spinal cord injury.

Acknowledgements

The support from the Science Council of Sweden (project 03026-32A) and the Marianne and Marcus Wallenberg Foundation is gratefully acknowledged, as is the valuable help of Mrs I. Sylvander.

References

Alford, S. and Grillner, S. (1991) The involvement of GABA$_B$ receptors and coupled G-proteins in spinal GABAergic presynaptic inhibition. *J. Neurosci.*, 11: 3718–3726.

Alford, S., Christenson, J. and Grillner, S. (1991) Presynaptic GABA$_A$ and GABA$_B$ receptor-mediated phasic modulation in axons of spinal motor interneurons. *Eur. J. Neurosci.*, 3: 107–117.

Bacskai, B.J., Wallén, P., Lev-Ram, V., Grillner, S. and Tsien, R.Y. (1995) Activity-related calcium dynamics in lamprey motoneurons as revealed by video-rate confocal microscopy. *Neuron*, 14: 19–28.

Barbeau, H., McCrea, D.A., O'Donovan, M.J., Rossignol, S., Grill, W.M. and Lemay, M.A. (1999) Tapping into spinal circuits to restore motor function. *Brain Res. Rev.*, 30: 27–51.

Barbeau, H., Fung, J., Leroux, A. and Ladouceur, M. (2002) A review of the adaptability and recovery of locomotion after spinal cord injury. In: L. McKerracher, G. Doucet and S. Rossignol (Eds.), *Spinal Cord Trauma: Neural Repair and Functional Recovery*. Progress in Brain Research, Vol. 137, Elsevier, Amsterdam, pp. 9–25.

Bregman, B.S., Coumans, J.-V., Dai, H.N., Kuhn, P.L., Lynskey, J., McAtee, M. and Sandhu, F. (2002) Transplants and neurotrophic factors increase regeneration and recovery of function after spinal cord injury. In: L. McKerracher, G. Doucet and S. Rossignol (Eds.), *Spinal Cord Trauma: Neural Repair and Functional Recovery*. Progress in Brain Research, Vol. 137, Elsevier, Amsterdam, pp. 257–273.

Björklund, A., Nornes, H. and Gage, F.H. (1986) Cell suspension grafts of noradrenergic locus coeruleus neurons in rat hippocampus and spinal cord: reinnervation and transmitter turnover. *Neuroscience*, 18: 685–698.

Cangiano, L., Woolley, J.D., Wallén, P. and Grillner, S. (2000) The isolated lamprey hemicord is capable of generating coordinated rhythmic motor activity. *Soc. Neurosci.*, 26: 1997.

Dale, N. and Kuenzi, F. (1997) Ionic currents, transmitters and models of motor pattern generators (review). *Curr. Opin. Neurobiol.*, 7: 790–796.

De Leon, R.D., Tamaki, H., Hodgson, J.A., Roy, R.R. and Edgerton, V.R. (1999) Hindlimb locomotor and postural train-ing modulates glycinergic inhibition in the spinal cord of the adult spinal cat. *J. Neurophysiol.*, 82: 359–369.

De Leon, R.D., Reinkensmeyer, D.J., Timoszyk, W.K., London, N.J., Roy, R.R. and Edgerton, V.R. (2002) Use of robotics in assessing the adaptive capacity of the rat lumbar spinal cord. In: L. McKerracher, G. Doucet and S. Rossignol (Eds.), *Spinal Cord Trauma: Neural Repair and Functional Recovery*. Progress in Brain Research, Vol. 137, Elsevier, Amsterdam, pp. 141–149.

Dobkin, B.H., Harkema, S., Requejo, P. and Edgerton, V.R. (1995) Modulation of locomotor-like EMG activity in subjects with complete and incomplete spinal cord injury. *J. Neurol. Rehabil.*, 9: 183–190.

Drew, T. (1993) Motor cortical activity during voluntary gait modifications in the cat, I. Cells related to the forelimbs. *J. Neurosci.*, 70: 179–199.

Edgerton, V.R., Grillner, S., Sjöström, A. and Zangger, P. (1976) Central generation of locomotion in vertebrates. In: R. Herman, S. Grillner, P. Stein and D. Stuart (Eds.), *Neural Control of Locomotion*. Plenum Press, New York, pp. 181–201.

Edgerton, V.R., de Leon, R.R., Harkema, S.J., Hodgson, J.A., London, N., Reinkensmeyer, D.J., Roy, R.R., Talmadge, R.J., Tillakaratne, N.J., Timoszyk, W. and Tobin, A. (2001) Retraining the injured spinal cord. *J. Physiol.*, 533: 15–22.

El Manira, A., Tegnér, J. and Grillner, S. (1997) Locomotor-related presynaptic modulation of primary afferents in the lamprey. *Eur. J Neurosci.*, 9: 696–705.

Forssberg, H. and Grillner, S. (1973) The locomotor of the acute spinal cat injected with clinidine i.v. *Brain Res.*, 50: 184–186.

Forssberg, H., Grillner, S. and Halbertsma, J. (1980a) The locomotion of the low spinal cat, I. Coordination within a hindlimb. *Acta Physiol. Scand.*, 108: 269–281.

Forssberg, H., Grillner, S., Halbertsma, J. and Rossignol, S. (1980b) The locomotion of the low spinal cat, II. Interlimb coordination. *Acta Physiol. Scand.*, 108: 283–295.

Georgopoulos, A.P. and Grillner, S. (1989) Visuomotor coordination in reaching and locomotion. *Science*, 345: 1209–1210.

Giménez y Ribotta, M., Gaviria, M., Menet, V. and Privat, A. (2002) Strategies for regeneration and repair in spinal cord traumatic injury. In: L. McKerracher, G. Doucet and S. Rossignol (Eds.), *Spinal Cord Trauma: Neural Repair and Functional Recovery*. Progress in Brain Research, Vol. 137, Elsevier, Amsterdam, pp. 191–212.

Giroux, N., Rossignol, S. and Reader, T.A. (1999) Autoradiographic study of α1, α2-noradrenergic and Serotonin 1A receptors in the spinal cord of normal and chronically transected cats. *J. Comp. Neurol.*, 406: 402–414.

Grillner, S. (1981) Control of locomotion in bipeds, tetrapods and fish (1981). In: V.B. Brooks (Ed.), *Handbook of Physiology, Sect. 1. The Nervous System II. Motor Control*. Am. Physiol. Soc., Waverly Press, MD, pp. 1179–1236.

Grillner, S. (1985) Neurobiological bases of rhythmic motor acts in vertebrates. *Science*, 228: 143–149.

Grillner, S. (1996) Neural networks for vertebrate locomotion. *Sci. Am.*, 274: 64–69.

Grillner, S. and Shik, M.L. (1973) On the descending control of the lumbosacral spinal cord from the mesencephalic locomotor region. *Acta Physiol. Scand.*, 87: 320–333.

Grillner, S., Williams, T. and Lagerback, P. (1984) The edge cell, a possible intraspinal mechanoreceptor. *Science*, 223: 500–503.

Grillner, S., Georgopoulos, A. and Jordan, L. (1997) Selection and initiation of motor behavior. In: P. Stein, S. Grillner, A.I. Selverston and D.G. Stuart (Eds.), *Neurons, Networks and Motor Behavior*. MIT Press, Cambridge, MA, pp. 3–19.

Grillner, S., Cangiano, L., Hu, G.-Y., Thompson, R., Hill, R. and Wallén, P. (2000) The intrinsic function of a motor system: from ion channels to networks and behavior. *Brain Res.*, 886: 224–236.

Hellgren, J., Grillner, S. and Lansner, A. (1992) Computer simulation of the segmental neural network generating locomotion in lamprey by using populations of network interneurons. *Biol. Cybern.*, 68: 1–13.

Hellgren Kotaleski, J., Lansner, A. and Grillner, S. (1999) Neural mechanisms potentially contributing to the intersegmental phase lag in lamprey, II. Hemisegmental oscillations produced by mutually coupled excitatory neurons. *Biol. Cybern.*, 81: 299–315.

Huang, A., Noga, B.R., Carr, P.A., Fedirchuk, B. and Jordan, L.M. (2000) Spinal cholinergic neurons activated during locomotion: localization and electrophysiological characterization. *J. Neurophysiol.*, 83: 3537–3547.

Jordan, L.M. and Steeves, J.D. (1976) Chemical lesioning of the spinal noradrenaline pathway: Effects on locomotion in the cat. In: R.M. Herman, S. Grillner, P.S.G. Stein and D.G. Stuart (Eds.), *Neural Control of Locomotion*. Advances in Behavioral Biology, Vol. 18, Plenum Press, New York, pp. 769–773.

Kiehn, O. and Kjaerulff, O. (1998) Distribution of central pattern generators for rhythmic motor outputs in spinal cord of limbed vertebrates. *Ann. N.Y. Acad. Sci.*, 860: 110–129.

Kim, D., Adipudi, V., Shibayama, M., Giszter, S., Tessler, A., Murray, M. and Simansky, K.J. (1999) Direct agonists for serotonin receptors enhance locomotor function in rats that received neural transplants after neonatal spinal transection. *J. Neurosci.*, 19: 6213–6224.

Kjaerulff, O. and Kiehn, O. (2001) 5-HT modulation of multiple inward rectifiers in motoneurons in intact preparations of the neonatal rat spinal cord. *J. Neurophysiol.*, 85: 580–593.

Krieger, P., Grillner, S. and El Manira, A. (1998) Endogenous activation of metabotropic glutamate receptors contributes to burst frequency regulation in the lamprey locomotor network. *Eur. J. Neurosci.*, 10: 3333–3342.

Kudo, N. and Yamada, T. (1987) N-Methyl-D, L-aspartate-induced locomotor activity in a spinal cord–hindlimb muscles preparation of the newborn rat studied in vitro. *Neurosci. Lett.*, 75: 43–48.

Liddell, E.G.T. and Phillips, C.G. (1944) Pyramidal section in the cat. *Brain*, 67: 1–9.

Matsushima, T., Tegnér, J., Hill, R. and Grillner, S. (1993) GABA_B receptor activation causes a depression of low- and high-voltage-activated (Ca^{2+}) currents, postinhibitory rebound, and postspike afterhyperpolarization in lamprey neurons. *J. Neurophysiol.*, 70: 2606–2619.

Noga, B.R., Kettler, J. and Jordan, L.M. (1988) Locomotion produced in mesencephalic cats by injections of putative transmitter substances and antagonists into the medial reticular formation and the pontomedullary locomotor strip. *J. Neurosci.*, 8: 2074–2086.

Noga, B.R., Kriellaars, D.J. and Jordan, L.M. (1991) The effect of selective brainstem or spinal cord lesions on treadmill locomotion evoked by stimulation of the mesencephalic or pontomedullary locomotor regions. *J. Neurosci.*, 11: 1691–1700.

Noga, B.R., Mesigil, R., Hentall, L.D. and Hesse, D. (1999) Real-time measurement of monamine release in the cat lumbar spinal cord during brainstem-evoked fictive locomotion. *Soc. Neurosci.*, 25: 1152.

Orlovsky, G.N., Deliagina, T.G. and Grillner, S. (1999) *Neuronal Control of Locomotion. From Mollusc to Man*. Oxford Press, New York, 322 pp.

Orsal, D., Barthe, J.-Y., Antri, M., Feraboli-Lohnherr, D., Yakovleff, A., Giménez y ribotta, M., Privat, A., Provencher, J. and Rossignol, S. (2002) Locomotor recovery in chronic spinal rat; long-term pharmacological treatment or transplantation of embryonic neurons. In: L. McKerracher, G. Doucet and S. Rossignol (Eds.), *Spinal Cord Trauma: Neural Repair and Functional Recovery*. Progress in Brain Research, Vol. 137, Elsevier, Amsterdam, pp. 213–230.

Parker, D. (2000) Presynaptic and interactive peptidergic modulation of reticulospinal synaptic inputs in the lamprey. *J. Neurophysiol.*, 83: 2497–2507.

Parker, D., Zhang, W. and Grillner, S. (1998) Substance P modulated NMDA responses and causes long-term protein synthesis-dependent modulation of the lamprey locomotor network. *J. Neurosci.*, 18: 4800–4813.

Pearson, K.G. (2000) Neuronal adaptation in the generation of rhythmic behavior. *Annu. Rev. Physiol.*, 62: 723–753.

Pratt, C.A. and Jordan, L.M. (1987) Ia inhibitory interneurons and Renshaw cells as contributors to the spinal mechanisms of fictive locomotion. *J. Neurophysiol.*, 57: 56–71.

Prentice, S.D. and Drew, T. (2001) Contributions of the reticulospinal system to the postural adjustments occurring during voluntary gait modifications. *J. Neurophysiol.*, 85: 679–698.

Ribotta, M.G., Provencher, J., Feraboli-Lohnherr, D., Rossignol, S., Privat, A. and Orsal, D. (2000) Activation of locomotion in adult chronic spinal rats is achieved by transplantation of embryonic raphe cells reinnervating a precise lumbar level. *J. Neurosci.*, 20: 5144–5152.

Roberts, A. (2000) Early functional organization of spinal neurons in developing lower vertebrates. *Brain Res. Bull.*, 13: 617–627.

Rossignol, S. (1996) Neural control of stereotypic limb movements. In: L.B. Rowell and J.T. Shepherd (Eds.), *Handbook of Physiology*. Oxford University Press, New York, pp. 173–216.

Rossignol, S., Chau, C., Giroux, N., Brustein, E., Bouyer, L., Marcoux, J., Lanlet, C., Barthelémy, D., Provencher, J., Leblond, H., Drew, T., Barbeu, H. and Reader, T. (2002) The cat model of spinal cat. In: L. McKerracher, G. Doucet and S. Rossignol (Eds.), *Spinal Cord Trauma: Neural Repair and*

Functional Recovery. Progress in Brain Research, Vol. 137, Elsevier, Amsterdam, pp. 151–168.

Schotland, J., Schupliakov, O., Wikström, M., Brodin, L., Srinivasan, M., You, Z., Herrera-Marschitz, M., Zhang, W., Hökfelt, T. and Grillner, S. (1995) Control of lamprey locomotor neurons by co-localized monoamine transmitters. *Nature*, 374: 266–268.

Sillar, K., Kiehn, O. and Kudo, N. (1997) Chemical modulation of vertebrate motor circuits. In: P. Sten, D. Stuart, A. Selverson, S. Grillner (Eds.), *Neurons, Networks, and Motor Behaviour*. MIT Press, Cambridge, MA, Ch. 17, pp. 183–193.

Smith, J.L., Smith, L.A., Zernicke, R.F. and Hoy, M. (1982) Locomotion in exercised and non-exercised cats cordotomized at two or twelve weeks of age. *Exp. Neurol.*, 76: 393–413.

Tegnér, J., Matsushima, T., El Manira, A. and Grillner, S. (1993) The spinal GABA system modulated burst frequency and intersegmental coordination in the lamprey: differential effects of $GABA_A$ and $GABA_B$ receptors. *J. Neuropphysiol.*, 69: 647–657.

Tegnér, J., Hellgren-Kotaleski, J., Lansner, A. and Grillner, S. (1997) Low voltage activated calcium channels in the lamprey locomotor network-simulation and experiment. *J. Neurophysiol.*, 77: 1795–1812.

Tegnér, J., Lansner, A. and Grillner, S. (1998) Modulation of burst frequency by calcium-dependent potassium channels in the lamprey locomotor system. Dependence of the activity level. *J. Comput. Neurosci.*, 5: 121–140.

Thorstensson, A., Nilsson, J., Carlson, H. and Zomlefer, M.R. (1984) Trunk movements in human locomotion. *Acta Physiol. Scand.*, 121: 9–22.

Viana di Prisco, G., Pearlstein, E., Robitaille, R. and Dubuc, R. (1990) Role of sensory-evoked NMDA plateau potentials in the initiation of locomotion. *Science*, 278: 1122–1125.

Wernig, A., Muller, S., Nanassy, A. and Cagol, E. (1995) Laufband therapy based on 'rules of spinal locomotion' is effective in spinal cord injured persons. *Eur. J. Neurosci.*, 7: 823–829.

Wernig, A., Nanassy, A. and Muller, S. (1999) Laufband (LB) therapy in incomplete paraplegia and tetraplegia. *J. Neurotrauma*, 16: 719–726.

Wernig, A., Nanassy, A. and Muller, S. (2000) Laufband (LB) therapy in spinal cord lesioned persons. *Prog. Brain Res.*, 128: 89–97.

Widajewicz, W., Kably, B. and Drew, T. (1994) Motor cortical activity during voluntary gait modifications within cat, II. Cells related to the hindlimbs. *J. Neurophysiol.*, 72: 2070–2089.

Yang, K.H., Hellgren-Kotaleski, J. and Blackwell, K.T. (2000) The role of PKC in temporal specificity of classical conditioning of purkinje cells. *Soc. Neurosci.*, 26: 718.

Young, W. (2002) Spinal cord contusion models. In: L. McKerracher, G. Doucet and S. Rossignol (Eds.), *Spinal Cord Trauma: Neural Repair and Functional Recovery*. Progress in Brain Research, Vol. 137, Elsevier, Amsterdam, pp. 231–255.

L. McKerracher, G. Doucet and S. Rossignol (Eds.)
Progress in Brain Research, Vol. 137

CHAPTER 9

Activation and coordination of spinal motoneuron pools after spinal cord injury

Arthur Prochazka *, Vivian Mushahwar and Sergiy Yakovenko

Centre for Neuroscience, University of Alberta, 507 HMRC, Edmonton, AB T6G 252, Canada

Abstract: Goal-directed movements of the limbs involve the coordinated activation of dozens of muscles. The neural signals activating these muscles are organized at spinal and supraspinal levels, the end result being trains of action potentials delivered to muscles by ensembles of spinal motoneurons (MNs). A new modelling approach has allowed us to visualize the activity of MNs controlling cat hindlimb locomotion. This reveals a rostrocaudal oscillation of MN activity distributed over about 30 mm of the lumbosacral spinal cord. The coordination and topographical distribution of MN pools thus revealed put an interesting perspective on the restoration of motor function with regeneration and neuroprosthetic techniques. Recent progress in the area of intraspinal microstimulation (ISMS) is reviewed, including the synthesis of locomotor movements with a small number of implanted microwires, eliciting movements after a spinal transection and facilitating weak voluntary movements with subliminal ISMS. We suggest that neuroprostheses may be useful in maximizing the benefits of neural regeneration in the future.

Introduction

Bridging the gap in the spinal cord

In the last few years much progress has been made in the field of spinal cord regeneration (Schwab, 1996; Hulsebosch et al., 2000; McKerracher, 2001). Many approaches to 'bridging the gap' in the transected or injured spinal cord are being pursued, several of which are reviewed in this volume. Some reports have now been published detailing significant improvements in motor function of the limbs in spinal-cord-injured rats in which these bridging procedures have been used (Diener and Bregman, 1998; Blits et al., 2000; Ramon-Cueto et al., 2000). At the Montreal meeting there was clearly an air of

excitement and expectancy that these advances could soon translate into significant clinical advances in the restoration of functions in humans with spinal cord injury (SCI). In this chapter, we will first comment on the distribution of the neural circuitry and mechanisms required for the recovery of locomotion. Second, we will discuss the potential role of ISMS as an adjunct to regeneration in maximizing the recovery of these functions in people with SCI.

Bridging the gap in our understanding

One of the neurophysiological puzzles of recent neural regeneration research is that the functional improvements in locomotion reported in experiments in rats with complete thoracic spinal cord transections and grafts of different types are hard to explain in relation to the extent of axonal growth and reconnection that have been documented. Unlike cats, rats with complete thoracic transections do not recover hindlimb locomotion without intensive treadmill training (Edgerton et al., 2001). It is therefore

---

* Correspondence to: A. Prochazka, Centre for Neuroscience, 507 HMRC, University of Alberta, Edmonton, AB T6G 2S2, Canada. Tel.: +1-780-492-3783; Fax: +1-780-492-1617; E-mail: arthur.prochazka@ualberta.ca

very significant when coordinated, weight-bearing hindlimb locomotion is restored in untrained rats with complete spinal cord transections either as a result of bridging grafts (Ramon-Cueto et al., 2000) or cell transplants caudal to the transection (Gimenez y Ribotta et al., 1998, 2000).

Depending on the bridge or graft used, when regenerating axons were traced caudal to the spinal cord transections they were usually relatively few in number and generally extended only a few millimeters caudal to the lesion (Zompa et al., 1993; Xu et al., 1999; Bamber et al., 2001), though more extensive regeneration has been claimed (Ramon-Cueto et al., 2000). For the mid-thoracic sites of lesions studied, the regenerating axons would barely reach the T_{12}, T_{13}, L_1 and L_2 segments thought to be the 'lead areas' of the hindlimb locomotor pattern generator (Cazalets et al., 1995; Cowley and Schmidt, 1997; Marcoux and Rossignol, 2000). How is the functional recovery then to be explained in these cases? Perhaps the regenerating axons make functional contacts with propriospinal interneurons that project caudally and activate neurons of the locomotor pattern generator directly. Perhaps these interneurons activate MNs of the trunk musculature, contractions of which might then elicit sensory input to the spinal cord caudal to the transection that entrains the hindlimb locomotor pattern generator (Giszter et al., 1998). Or perhaps they release neuromodulators that non-specifically increase lumbosacral spinal cord activity, facilitating locomotor reflexes evoked by sensory activity from the abdomen and hindlimbs generated as the forelimbs drag the body forward.

Fig. 1 puts some of these issues into perspective. The data refer to the cat rather than the rat, but the organizational features of MN pools are similar in the two species (Nicolopoulos-Stournaras and Iles, 1983). The figure shows the distributions of flexor and extensor MN pools of muscles acting about the hip, knee and ankle, and is derived from the data of VanderHorst and Holstege (1997). The MN pools responsible for contractions of the hip muscles are not only very widely distributed along the rostro-caudal axis, but their flexor and extensor divisions are nearly completely separated. The MN pools controlling the ankle muscles are more localized and the flexor and extensor divisions overlap. It is clear that a proper coordination of all these pools dur-

ing the step cycle would require neuronal circuitry that could appropriately sequence the activation of these MN pools from their most rostral to their most caudal ends. The rhythmical rostrocaudal oscillation of lumbosacral MN activity underlying cat locomotion has recently been modeled by activating MNs of hindlimb muscles in a three-dimensional model according to the EMG patterns of these muscles in the step cycle (Yakovenko et al., 2000). Calcium-sensitive dyes have since been used to visualize rhythmical rostrocaudal migrations of MN activity in the isolated in vitro neonatal mouse spinal cord (Bonnot-Vrillaud et al., 2001).

If the alternation between swing and stance in the step cycle is largely due to a centrally generated pattern, the main requirement for restoring locomotion would be to activate the central pattern generator (CPG). If the hindlimb CPG is localized within a 'leading area' just rostral to the hindlimb MN pools as has been suggested (Cazalets et al., 1995; Marcoux and Rossignol, 2000), this would provide a relatively close and circumscribed target for propriospinal axons descending from the mid-thoracic region. However, if the pattern generator includes hindlimb MN pools (Perrins and Roberts, 1995) and if these also require innervation, the target is clearly far more distributed and distant.

Well-coordinated locomotion depends heavily on sensory inputs signaling limb kinematics and loading (Pearson, 1995; Rossignol, 1996; Duysens et al., 2000). In fact one could view the CPG as a 'default' oscillator that is deeply modulated or even overridden by these sensory inputs (Prochazka, 1996). It is therefore also quite relevant to know how descending propriospinal systems might enhance transmission in the sensorimotor pathways responsible for modulating weight-support and phase-switching (Shik, 1997). Sensory axons bifurcate close to where they enter the spinal cord and their ascending and descending branches innervate MNs and premotoneurons in several segments rostrally and caudally. Thus afferents from ankle extensors project to hip MN regions and vice versa. The central neuronal systems controlling a limb are thereby extensively coupled by sensory pathways and their associated interneurons. It is usually assumed that the sensory inputs that cause phase-switching act directly on the locomotor CPG and modulate its cycle frequency, but it is also possible

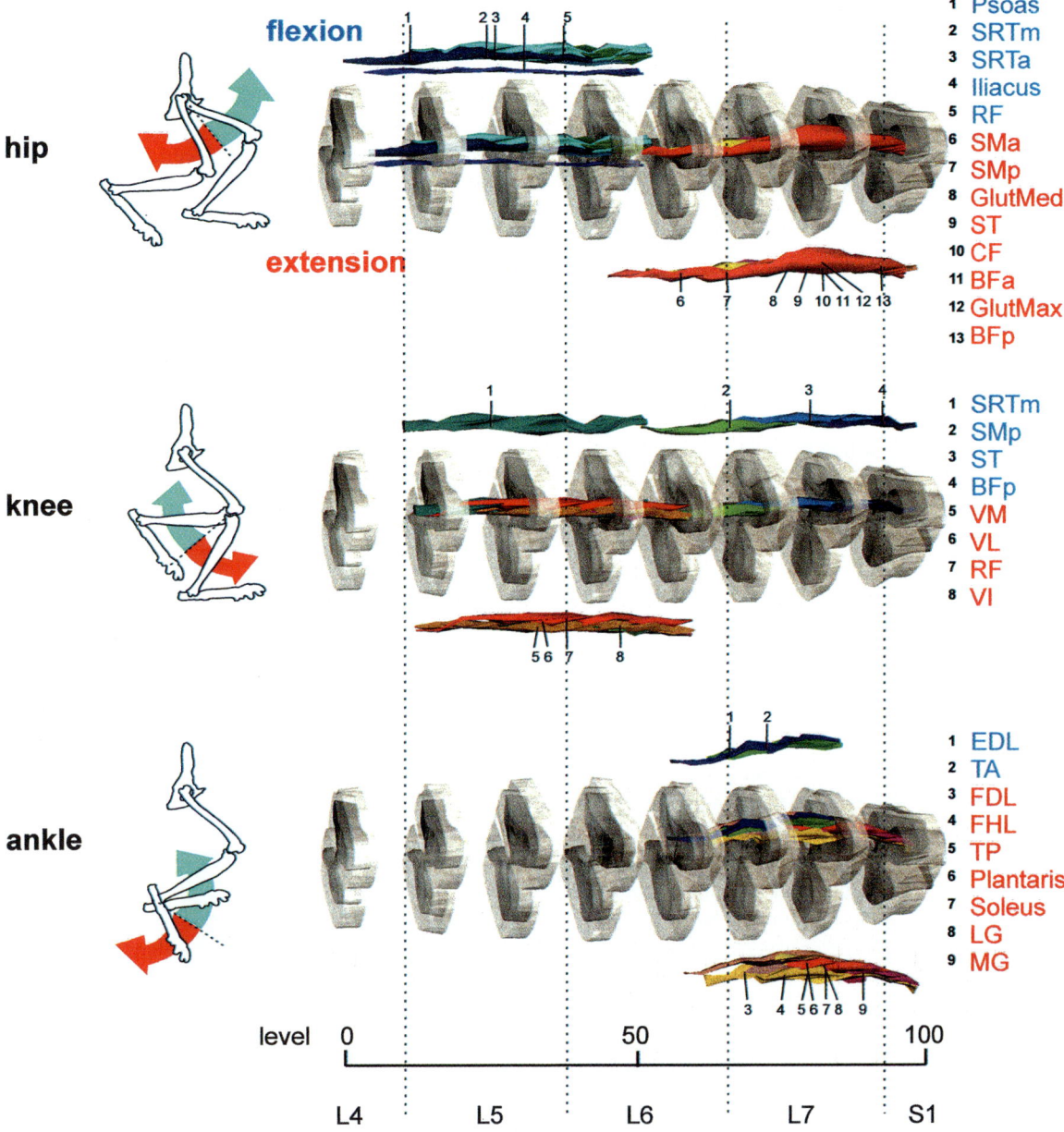

Fig. 1. Hip, knee and ankle motoneuron (MN) pools of the cat lumbosacral spinal cord and their activation during flexion and extension around hip, knee and ankle. Notice the long, thin distributions, particularly of the hip MN pools. Hip flexors and extensors hardly overlap whereas knee and ankle flexors and extensors overlap considerably. If MNs are integral to the central pattern generator (CPG) for locomotion, descending inputs controlling them would have to be widely distributed along the rostrocaudal axis.

that sensory integration is performed by separate neuronal circuits (e.g. the interneurons of Clarke's column (Bosco and Poppele, 2001)) that provide inputs for supraspinal mechanisms as well as the CPG.

Neuroprostheses, ISMS

In a recent article, we reviewed the many different types of neuroprostheses currently available or under development (Prochazka et al., 2001). Neuroprostheses have been developed that use electrical stimulation of peripheral nerves and muscles to improve respiration, micturition and motor function (Kralj and Bajd, 1989; Stein et al., 1992). Though some of these approaches have been very successful, e.g. cardiac pacemakers, phrenic nerve stimulators (Baer et al., 1990) and bladder control stimulators (Brindley, 1977; Brindley et al., 1986), the restoration of limb movements remains a challenge because implanted wires are vulnerable and surgery is required to tunnel wires subcutaneously from an implanted pacemaker-like stimulator to the numerous muscles of a limb (Peckham et al., 1980; Peckham and Keith, 1992; Prochazka and Davis, 1992).

In the last few years it has become apparent that ISMS may provide an effective alternative approach to some of the shortcomings of peripheral nerve neuroprostheses (Mushahwar and Horch, 1997, 1998; Tai et al., 1999). We recently showed that ISMS through microwires chronically implanted in the spinal cords of normal cats can be used to elicit synergistic, coordinated movements of the hindlimbs (Mushahwar et al., 2000a). Furthermore, we were able to produce graded, controlled contractions of paralyzed tail muscles up to 2 weeks after a complete spinal transection in rats (Prochazka and Mushahwar, 2001). The lumbar enlargement of the adult human spinal cord is about 5 cm long. Electrodes implanted in this relatively small, mechanically stable region, might therefore suffice to activate the main leg muscles to produce standing and locomotor movements. Electrodes implanted in the *cervical* enlargement could in principle be used to elicit movements of the upper extremity too (Saxena et al., 1995). Finally, electrodes implanted in the sacral spinal cord could help improve the control over bladder and bowel function (Agnew et al., 1998; Grill et al., 1999; Tai et al., 1999; Prochazka et al., 2001).

In what follows we will focus on two potential applications of ISMS: synthesis of standing and locomotion, and facilitation of weak voluntary contractions.

Synthesis of standing and locomotion

ISMS was first used as a neurophysiological tool to explore the organization of synergistic movements in the frog spinal cord (Giszter et al., 1993). This led to the concept of 'movement primitives', i.e. elementary muscle synergies evoked from circumscribed regions in the intermediate parts of the grey matter. The idea of using ISMS as a neuroprosthetic application was first explored by Mushahwar and Horch (1997), who found that focal stimulation through microelectrodes placed within MN pools in anesthetized cats could produce isolated contractions of individual muscles. Systematic studies produced detailed maps of spinal MN pools that corresponded reasonably well with the familiar anatomical data of Romanes (1951), recently extended by VanderHorst and Holstege (1997).

The next step was to test the neuroprosthetic application of ISMS with implanted electrode arrays. The main hurdle was to develop a technique of fixation that would ensure stable and reproducible ISMS for long periods after implantation. This was achieved by modifying a technique originally developed for recording from single sensory afferent cell bodies in the dorsal root ganglia of freely moving cats (Prochazka et al., 1976). The implantation technique is briefly summarized as follows. In a sterile surgical procedure under pentobarbital or fluothane anesthesia, a laminectomy is performed at L_6–S_1. Up to 20 microwires are inserted into the lumbosacral spinal cord bilaterally, 1.7–2.1 mm from the midline (Fig. 2A) through minute puncture holes made in the dura mater with a sharp needle. Electrode placement is based on functional and anatomical maps (VanderHorst and Holstege, 1997; Mushahwar and Horch, 2000). The microwires are pre-cut and bent so that after insertion in the spinal cord to depths of 3.0–4.5 mm, their epidural portions can be sutured and spot-glued to the dura mater with cyanoacrylate, fixed to the L_6 spinous process with bone pins and dental acrylic and led subcutaneously to a headpiece connector. Stimulation is used to guide placement. Plastic thin film glued to the dura mater over the microwires serves as a barrier to the growth of connective tissue around the electrodes. EMG electrodes are implanted in flexor and extensor muscles acting about the knee and ankle of each hindlimb (BF, VL, TA, LG). Animals are tested for up to 6 months. They are then deeply anesthetized and perfused with a 3.7% formaldehyde solution. The lumbosacral portion of the spinal cord is re-

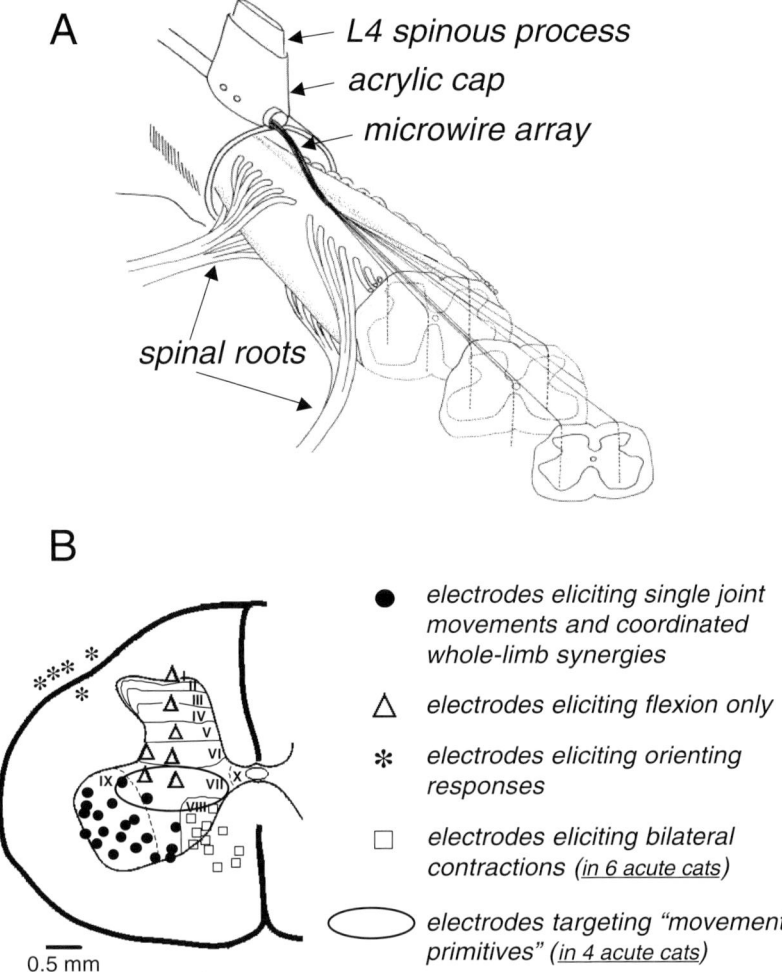

Fig. 2. (A) Schematic showing layout of implanted intraspinal microstimulation (ISMS) microwires and means of fixation to the L$_4$ spinous process (Mushahwar et al., 2000a). (B) Schematic summarizing histologically determined locations of stimulating tips of microwires in 12 chronically implanted cats and 10 cats in which acute experiments were performed during anaesthesia. The sensory and motor functions evoked by ISMS are specified by the different symbols.

moved with the microwires in place. The cord is sectioned and the locations of the microwire tips are determined. Histology of spinal cords implanted with microwires for up to 6 months has revealed minor glial reactions restricted to the microwire tracks, but an absence of secondary inflammatory processes (Woodford et al., 1996; Prochazka et al., 2001).

Fig. 2B provides an overview of the types of sensory and motor reactions we have observed in our study of ISMS in 12 chronically implanted cats and in 10 acute experiments on anesthetized cats. Elec-trodes in or near the ventral horn elicited discrete movements or synergies, the more medial group producing movements bilaterally. Dorsally located electrodes elicited flexion movements only, and it is possible that at least some of these resulted from sensory perception of the stimuli, though frank orienting responses were only observed in electrodes in or close to dorsal roots (asterisks in Fig. 2C). In some experiments we specifically targeted the intermediate region hypothesized to contain neuronal ensembles responsible for generating movement primitives (Giszter et al., 1993).

One of the first things we noticed when we stimulated through microwires implanted in chronically implanted cats was that although single muscles were often activated at low stimulus strengths (typically 10–60 µA pulses, 300 µs in duration), other muscles became activated as stimulus strength was increased. About half the time the muscles activated were synergists. Consequently, some microwires produced synergistic contractions of muscles that fully extended the hip, knee and ankle joints with enough force for weight-bearing. Note that threshold currents for microwires are higher than for microelectrodes (Mushahwar and Horch, 1998), presumably because of the larger tip areas and thus lower current densities.

The muscles activated did not always correspond in a simple way to the MN pools closest to the electrode tips. Thus microstimulation in the rostral part of the lumbosacral enlargement could elicit hip and ankle flexion, though ankle flexor MNs were not in the immediate vicinity (Fig. 1). It is possible that groups of interneurons in nearby intermediate laminae are activated, and these in turn activate widely distributed synergistic MN pools. Similarly, antidromically activated sensory afferents may reflexly excite synergistic MN pools through propriospinal mechanisms. Whether the synergies we elicited corresponded to 'movement primitives' or whether they were simply classical extensor or flexor reflexes (Sherrington, 1910) is the topic of a paper in preparation (Mushahwar, Stein, Aoyagi and Prochazka). Suffice it to say that the movements elicited from one and the same microwire could switch from flexion to extension as stimulus strength increased, which is not consistent with the idea that stimulation at one site activates a specific movement primitive regardless of intensity. It is possible that extensor MN pools and even ventral roots underlying the microwire tips may become activated as the stimuli spread beyond the confines of the grey matter (Giszter et al., 2000). Because extensor motoneurons greatly outnumber flexor motoneurons in much of the lumbosacral enlargement (VanderHorst and Holstege, 1997), these would tend to dominate as more and more ventral rootlets were activated.

Regardless of the mechanisms, our chronic implants showed that useful movements can be elicited from within the spinal cord of normal animals with ISMS. We then explored whether flexion and extension synergies could be coordinated in two limbs to produce locomotor like movements. Experiments in three anesthetized cats were performed, in which we delivered amplitude-modulated pulse trains through microwires implanted in the ventral horn of the spinal cord in the lumbosacral enlargement. As anticipated from the elementary movements observed in the chronic cats, it was indeed possible to generate weight-bearing stepping movements. In all three cases just 4 microwires selected from 10 implanted on each side of the spinal cord sufficed to elicit weight-bearing locomotor-like movements of the two hindlimbs (Mushahwar et al., 2000b).

It remained to be verified that functional movements could be elicited and controlled with ISMS after a complete chronic spinal cord transection. As a first approach to this question, we performed complete spinal cord transections at S_2–S_3 level in four rats and implanted four to six microwires caudal to the transections. In this low-spinal preparation the tail musculature is paralyzed, but locomotion as well as bladder and bowel function are all spared (Bennett et al., 1999). Stimulus trains applied through the implanted microwires produced tail movements whose force could be graded by modulating the amplitude of the stimulus pulses in the range of 2–250 µA. This demonstrates that in principle, muscle contractions could be graded to produce controlled movements with ISMS after chronic spinal cord injury, though of course this needs to be confirmed and characterized over longer periods of time in cats and perhaps primates before human implants should be contemplated. The question of whether ISMS can elicit graded, synergistic contractions of limb muscles to produce locomotion after chronic spinal injury must also be confirmed in experiments with more rostral lesions.

Facilitation of weak voluntary contractions

Fortunately about 80% of people with SCI have incomplete injuries and can weakly contract some of their paretic muscles. If these weak muscle contractions could be augmented, voluntary control would be significantly improved. In what follows we will describe the interaction between natural muscle activation and that produced by ISMS in normal cats implanted with microwires. The main finding was that in many cases the responses to steady, low-level ISMS were facilitated during weak 'voluntary' contractions, which had the effect of increasing the total mean level of EMG.

Twelve cats were implanted with between 6 and 20 microwires using the technique summarized above. Facilitation of weak voluntary contractions by ISMS was noted in all cats, but it was only quantified in three. Starting 4 to 7 days after surgery and twice a week thereafter, stimulation was applied through individual spinal cord microwires during testing sessions lasting up to 3 h. Stimulus pulses (2 s^{-1}, 300 μs, 10–240 μA) were delivered through each electrode individually and visual inspection, palpation and intramuscular EMG recordings were used to determine threshold and range over which individual muscles were activated (Mushahwar and Horch, 1998, 2000).

EMG signals were amplified, bandpass filtered (30–3,000 Hz), recorded on magnetic tape and subsequently digitized (11 kHz). Custom software was used to analyze the EMG signals in a variety of ways. Fig. 3 shows an example of VL EMG responses in a cat to three short bursts of five ISMS pulses of constant duration, current and rate (300 μs, 50 μA, 50 s^{-1}) for three levels of background EMG elicited by lowering the animal onto a supporting surface. The top trace shows the timing of the stimulus pulses, to which all three segments of recording were aligned. VL EMG responses to each stimulus pulse occurred at a latency of about 3 ms. The responses were superimposed on a background of unsynchronized EMG activity. The amplitude of the background activity could be estimated by blocking off an interval after each stimulus pulse in which there was no synchronized response (shaded in Fig. 3). In Fig. 3A, the background EMG level happened to be low (the animal was not bearing weight) and the responses to the stimulus pulses were close to threshold. As background EMG increased (Fig. 3B,C), so did the responses to ISMS of constant amplitude (i.e. the responses were facilitated during increased background EMG). From a physiological point of view, this raises the question of whether the responses were due to direct stimulation of motoneurons, or whether they were mediated by premotoneuronal pathways. Clearly the *total* EMG activity including the stimulus responses in Fig. 3 was larger than the background activity without the responses. From a

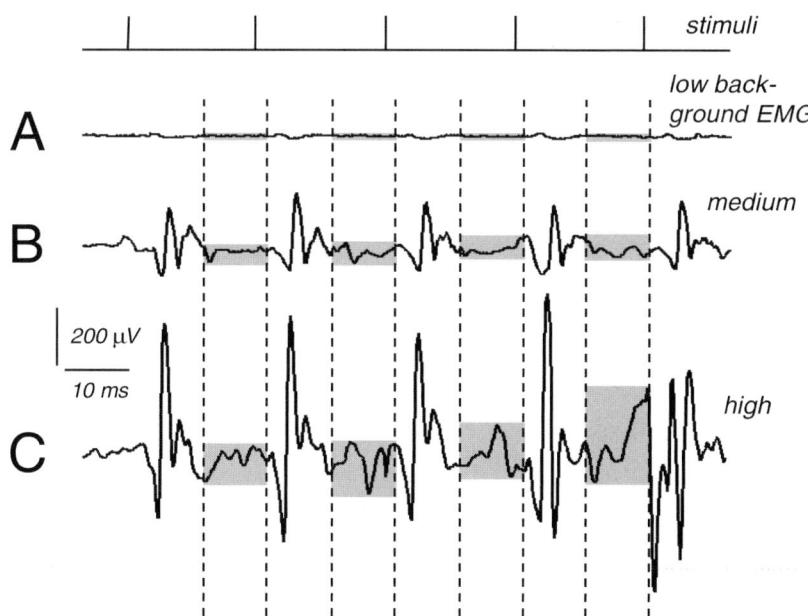

Fig. 3. Quadriceps EMG responses to trains of identical ISMS pulses for three levels of background EMG in the normal cat (A, B, C). Top: timing of stimulus pulses. (A–C) Increasing levels of background EMG. Background EMG is identified by the shaded rectangles between responses to the stimuli.

116

neuroprosthetic point of view, the interesting conclusion is that tonic, low-level ISMS might have the effect of amplifying weak voluntary contractions.

The facilitation of VL EMG responses to bursts of constant-amplitude ISMS pulses as background EMG increases is shown in Fig. 4. In the upper panel the rectified background EMG signal was very low during the first stimulus train (pulses at 50 s^{-1}) and then increased spontaneously at the arrow. The stimuli in the first train were evidently close to threshold, as evidenced by response dropouts. Responses to the second train followed the stimuli 1 : 1 and were much larger. The lower panel is a plot of mean total EMG versus mean background EMG just before the stimulus train in the intervals defined in the upper panel. The plot represents 1952 stimuli and each ordinate represents the mean total EMG associated with a 100-μV range of background EMG. When mean background EMG was zero, the stimuli were sub-threshold for evoking responses. As mean background EMG increased, individual ISMS responses also increased and this led to increases in mean total EMG. The three diagonal reference lines in the plot have slopes of 1 (total EMG = background EMG, no facilitation), 2 (total EMG = 2 × background EMG) and 3 (total EMG = 3 × background EMG), respectively. The data points in the plot are above the third line, i.e. in the presence of ISMS the mean total EMG was more than three times the mean background EMG.

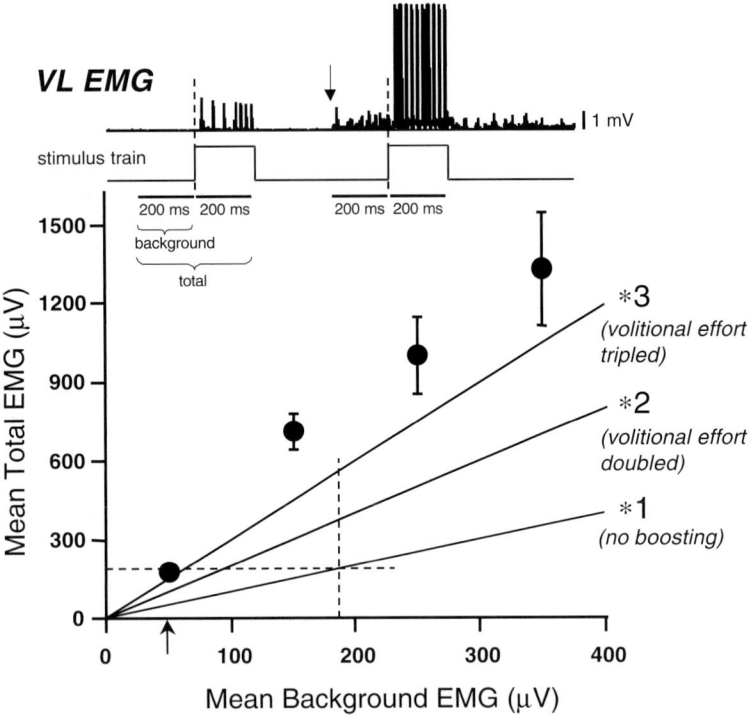

Fig. 4. Facilitation of VL EMG responses to ISMS pulses when background EMG increased as the cat's foot was lowered onto a support surface. Top: background EMG was nearly zero during first stimulus train (10 pulses at 50 s^{-1}) and the responses were small and in some cases missing. Background EMG increased at the arrow, subsequent responses to another train of 10 stimuli were much larger. Plot shows mean total EMG in the presence of intraspinal stimulation (computed over the 400-ms interval shown) versus mean background EMG in the 200 ms before the stimulus train. As mean background EMG increased, individual ISMS responses also increased and this led to increases in mean total EMG. The three diagonal reference lines in the plot have slopes of 1 (total EMG = background EMG, no facilitation), 2 (total EMG = 2 × background EMG) and 3 (total EMG = 3 × background EMG), respectively. The data points in the plot are above the third line, i.e. in the presence of ISMS the mean total EMG was more than three times the mean background EMG. Dashed reference lines show mean EMG level during stance phases of gait, measured separately (187 μV). Data point on far left shows that during ISMS the cat only needed to generate 50 μV of background EMG to achieve the 187-μV mean total EMG level required for gait.

If we assume an approximately linear relationship between mean EMG and isometric muscle force in weak to moderate-strength contractions (Bigland and Lippold, 1954; Basmajian and De Luca, 1985), the isometric force associated with the background EMG would in this case have been more than tripled in the presence of ISMS. The dashed reference lines show the mean level of EMG bursts in the stance phases of step cycles measured during medium-speed gait in separate trials (187 μV). The data point on the far left confirms that during ISMS this level of *total* EMG (i.e. background plus responses to ISMS) was achieved at about 50 μV background EMG.

To avoid carry-over effects from one response to the next during the 50-s^{-1} trains, in most cases we studied responses to stimuli of $1\ \text{s}^{-1}$. Fig. 5 shows an example of superimposed TA EMG responses to 230 such stimuli aligned to the stimulus trigger pulses (for clarity every sixth response is displayed in Fig. 5A, and the mean of all responses is superimposed as a thick line. To compute mean background and mean total EMG, first the stimulus artifact (∼1 ms in duration) was replaced by the mean EMG level immediately preceding the trigger (Fig. 5B). Next, the standard deviation (SD) of mean background EMG in the 10 ms prior to each stimulus was calculated from all the single sweeps. Mean onset latency was then taken as the time after the trigger at which the mean EMG signal first deviated from mean background level by 3 SD ($p < 0.001$). Mean background EMG and mean total EMG were then computed in each of the single sweeps over the intervals specified in Fig. 5C (note that in single sweeps the 1 ms segments of EMG in which stimulus artifacts might have been present were replaced by the EMG levels just prior to the stimulus triggers, as described above). The reason for estimating mean total and background EMG from the EMG in the 20-ms straddling response onset was to provide a measure of increase or decrease in EMG that would occur at a stimulus rate of $50\ \text{s}^{-1}$, as might be used in a neuroprosthetic application.

Fig. 6 shows the results of this analysis performed on the responses of four muscles to ISMS pulses at a rate of $1\ \text{s}^{-1}$ in cat #2 (the location of the microwire tip is indicated by the number 18 in the right portions of the spinal cord sections in Fig. 8). For

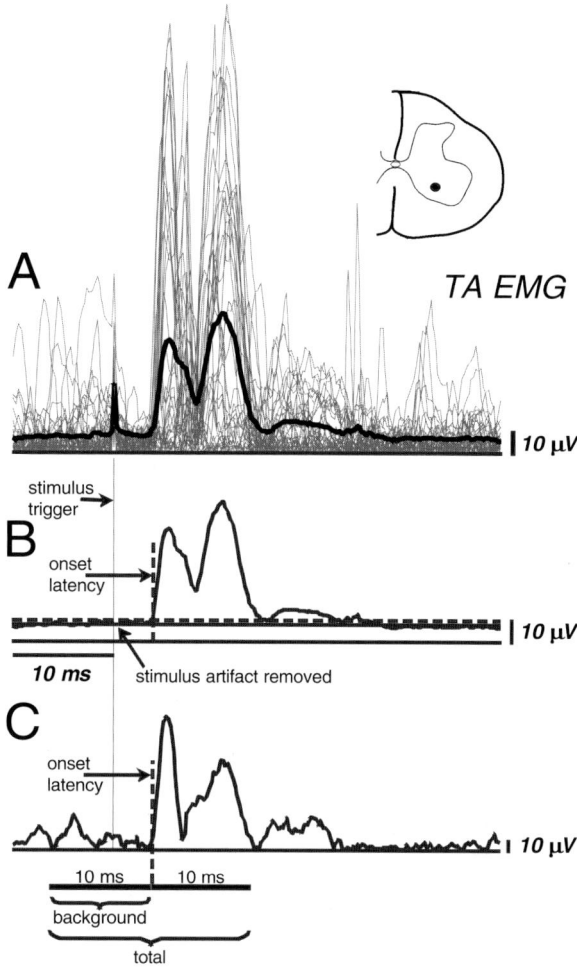

Fig. 5. Method of computing modulation ratio (mean total EMG/mean background EMG) of responses to ISMS delivered at $1\ \text{s}^{-1}$. (A) Superimposed TA EMG responses to 230 stimuli aligned to the stimulus trigger pulses (every sixth response is displayed, mean of all responses superimposed as thick line). (B) Mean onset latency was computed as the time after the trigger at which the mean EMG deviated from mean background level by 3 standard deviations. (C) Mean background EMG and mean total EMG were then computed in each of the single sweeps over the intervals specified.

each muscle a pair of plots is shown in Fig. 6, the upper being the averaged EMG response to ISMS and the lower being a plot of the mean total EMG versus mean background EMG. In VL and TA there were short-latency (2–4 ms) increases in EMG in response to ISMS (Fig. 6A,D) and in BF (Fig. 6B)

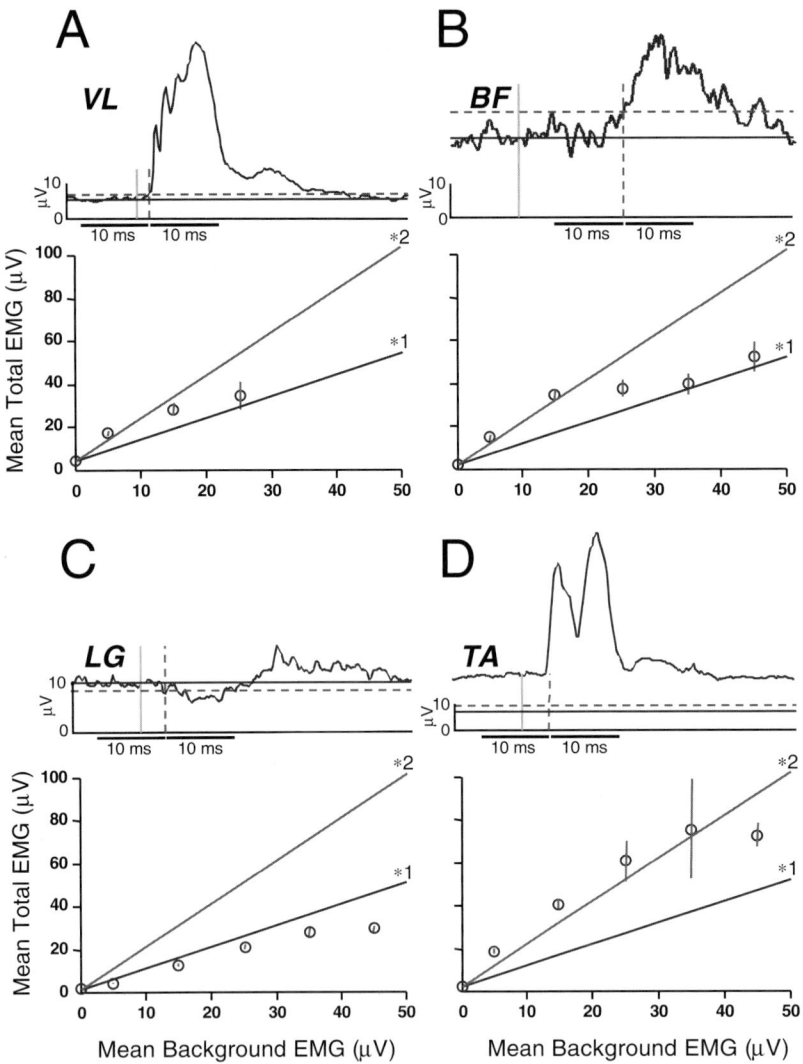

Fig. 6. Four examples of mean EMG responses and corresponding plots of total versus background EMG. (A,D) VL and TA had short-latency (2–4 ms) excitatory EMG responses to ISMS. (B) BF had a long-latency excitatory response (~15 ms). (C) LG: small short-latency *reduction* in EMG followed by a longer-latency increase. The differences in the averaged responses were reflected in the corresponding plots of total EMG versus background EMG (see text).

there was a long-latency increase (~15 ms). In LG on the other hand there was a small short-latency *reduction* in EMG followed by a longer-latency increase (Fig. 6C). The differences in the averaged responses were reflected in the corresponding plots of total EMG versus background EMG. Thus in Fig. 6A,B,D, over the first half of the range shown, the mean total EMG rose more rapidly than the mean background EMG. This occurred because the EMG

responses to ISMS were progressively facilitated with increases in background EMG. In contrast, for LG (Fig. 6C), the mean total EMG rose more slowly than the mean background EMG, because the short-latency responses to ISMS consisted of *reductions* in EMG. These reductions were also augmented with increasing background EMG, as evidenced by the increasing divergence of mean total EMG from the unity slope line (i.e. inhibition increased with increasing background EMG in this case). Note that in the trials represented in Fig. 6, in some cases ISMS was just supra-threshold when background EMG was zero. This produced small positive offsets of total EMG. These offsets were subtracted from all ordinates in the calculations of facilitation/inhibition ratios (see below), as they represented a constant level of stimulus-evoked response that did not scale with background EMG.

The modulation of EMG response to ISMS is attributable to local premotoneuronal and motoneuronal actions rather than to any generalized reflex arousal. This was shown by gradually increasing the rate of stimulation from 10 s^{-1} to 50 s^{-1}. Regardless of the rate, the EMG signal just prior to stimulus onset remained constant (i.e. there was no generalized increase or decrease of background EMG).

To evaluate facilitation or inhibition in all 34 electrodes in which interactions between ISMS and background EMG were quantified, we computed a modulation ratio: (mean total EMG)/(mean background EMG) over two ranges of background EMG (0–50, 150–200 μV) for each individual electrode in all the muscles studied. Modulation ratios above 1.15 were statistically larger than unity ($p < 0.05$) and thus represented clear facilitation. Modulation ratios under 0.85 were statistically smaller than unity ($p < 0.05$) and thus represented clear inhibition. Fig. 7 shows the complete distributions of modulation ratios over the two ranges of mean background EMG in the four muscles tested. Facilitation predominated in VL and TA, particularly in the range of 0–50 μV (ratios > 1.15), whereas inhibition predominated in BF and in LG in the range of 150–250 μV (ratios < 0.85). In all, there were 63 statistically significant facilitatory interactions, 40 statistically significant inhibitory interactions and 23 cases in which there was no significant interaction. Note that

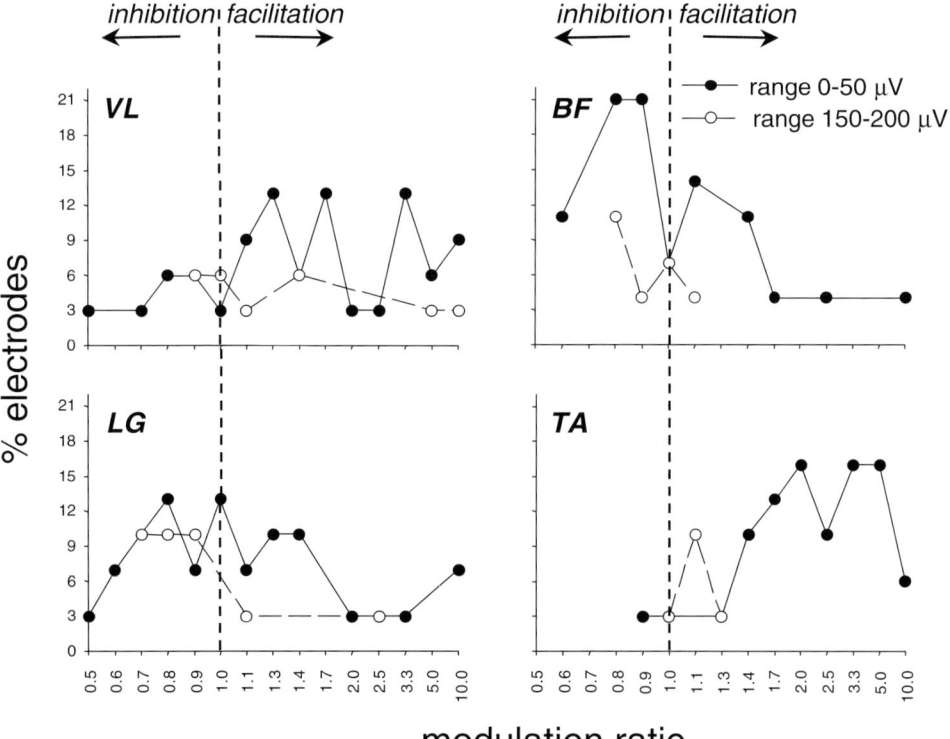

Fig. 7. Distributions of modulation ratios for all 34 microwires and 4 muscles tested. Distributions were computed for two ranges of mean background EMG: 0–50 μV (dots), 150–250 μV (circles). Modulation ratios > 1.15 and < 0.85 were significantly different than unity ($p < 0.05$) and thus represented facilitation and inhibition, respectively. Across the whole sample, facilitation predominated in VL and TA, particularly in the range 0–50 μV (ratios > 1.15). Inhibition predominated in BF and in LG in the range 150–250 μV.

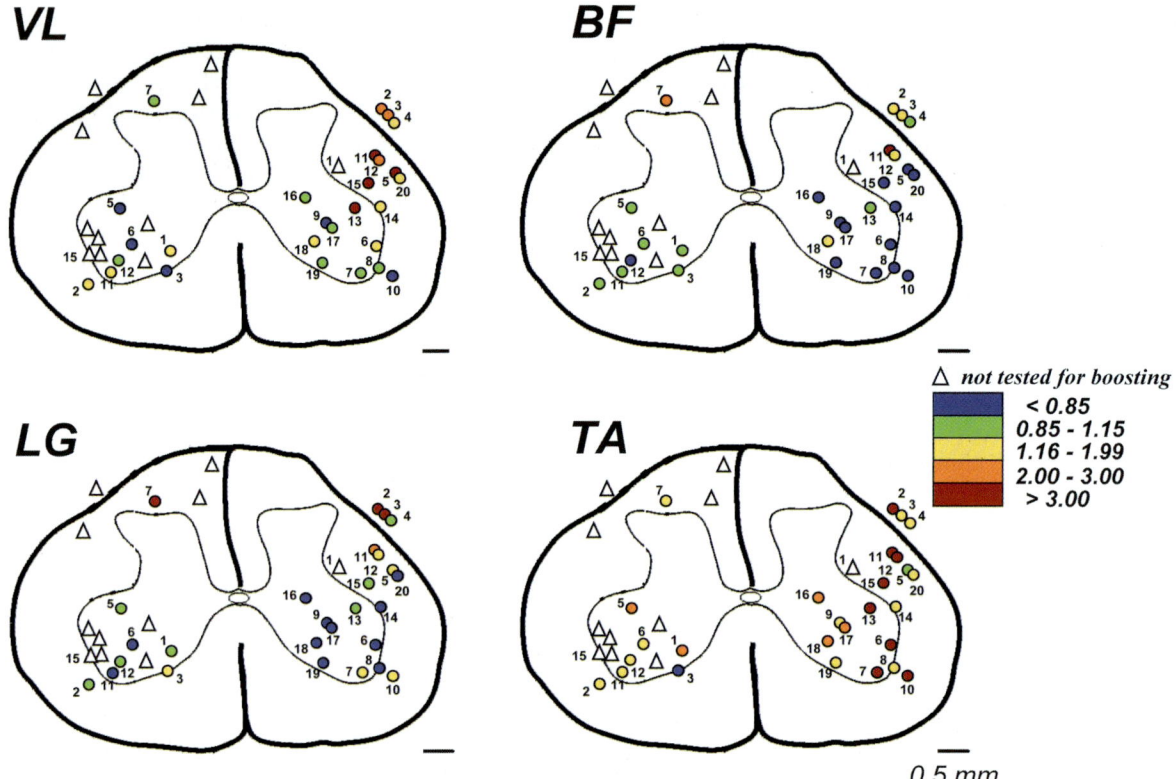

Fig. 8. Schematic of microwire tip locations in two cats and their corresponding modulation ratios in the four muscles tested. Numbers identify electrodes in cat #2 (right side of each section) and cat #3 (left side of each section). Color-coded circular symbols indicate both the position of an electrode tip and its corresponding modulation ratio for a given muscle (color bar). Triangles indicate positions of electrodes in which interactions between background EMG and ISMS were not tested. The four tips outside the perimeter of each schematic represent microwire tips located in dorsal roots.

although inhibition was common in LG and BF, there were enough facilitatory interactions to suggest that weak contractions in these muscles could be augmented in a neuroprosthetic application by the appropriate choice of electrode. It is also worth noting that each of the 34 electrodes in which the effect was quantified produced facilitatory effects in at least one muscle.

Fig. 8 shows the locations of the tips of the electrodes referred to above, with respect to a schematic cross-section of the spinal cord representative of the lower lumbar region. The numbers identify specific electrodes in cat #3 (left side of each section) and cat #2 (right side of each section). Though the majority of electrode tips were located in the grey matter of the ventral horn, a few were located in dorsal white matter or even in dorsal roots. The color-coded

circular symbols indicate both the position of an electrode tip and the modulation ratio with which it was associated for a given muscle. Dorsolateral stimulation sites were more likely to be facilitatory, but otherwise there was no obvious correlation between electrode tip position and the type or amplitude of interaction.

On the assumption that some of the normal EMG background activity depended on drive descending from cortical areas, we wondered whether an interaction between cortex-evoked EMG responses and ISMS could be verified directly. We tested this in one cat by stimulating electrically between two of the screws that anchored the headpiece. One of these screws was located over motor cortex (Nieoullon and Rispal-Padel, 1976; Armstrong and Drew, 1984). This produced small twitches of the contralateral

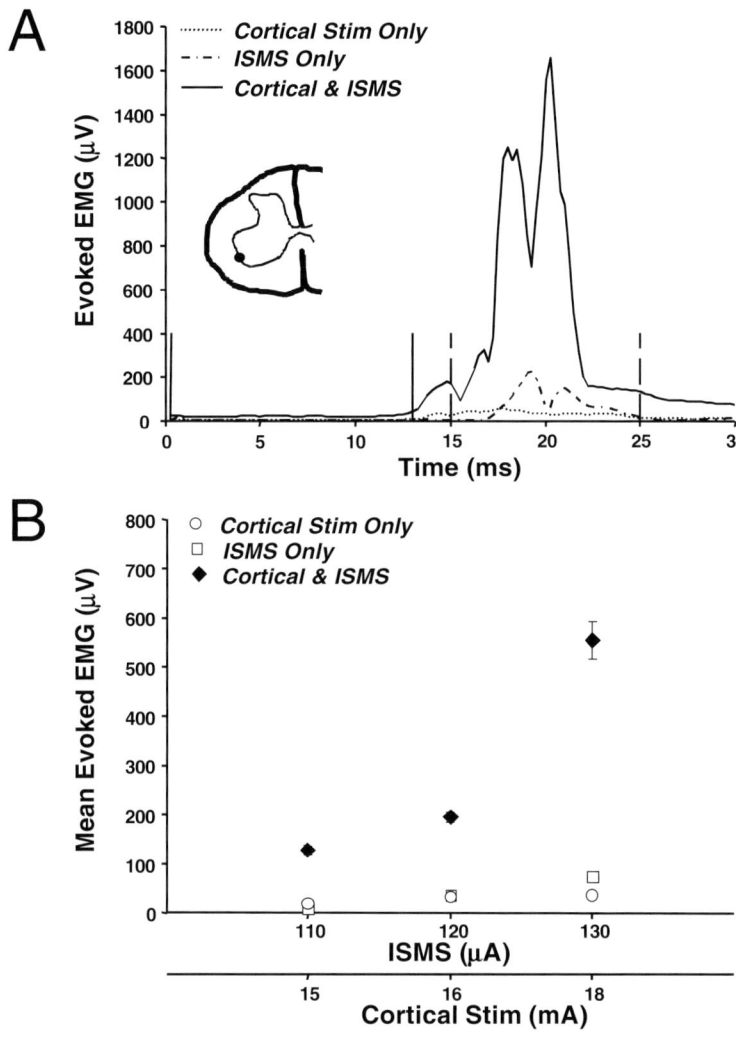

Fig. 9. (A) TA EMG responses to cortical stimuli, ISMS pulses and paired cortical and ISMS pulses delivered 13 ms apart so that their respective EMG responses coincided. (B) Mean EMG over the interval between the dashed lines in A. Responses to paired stimuli were larger than the sum of individual responses. This indicates that background EMG generated by descending commands would be boosted by SCμstim.

limbs to which the animal paid little if any attention. Fig. 9A shows TA EMG responses to cortical stimuli, ISMS pulses (2 s^{-1}, 300 μs, 14–18 mA), and paired cortical and ISMS pulses delivered 13 ms apart so that their respective EMG responses coincided. The responses to paired stimuli were clearly larger than the sum of the individual responses. EMG was averaged over the interval 2–12 ms after the second (intraspinal) pulse (Fig. 9B). Paired stimuli produced mean EMG responses far in excess of the responses

produced from cortical and intraspinal electrodes individually. This is consistent with the doubling or tripling of background EMG described earlier, suggesting that similar mechanisms might have been involved.

Neuroprostheses, summary

To summarize, our basic finding was that the EMG responses evoked in limb muscles by ISMS were

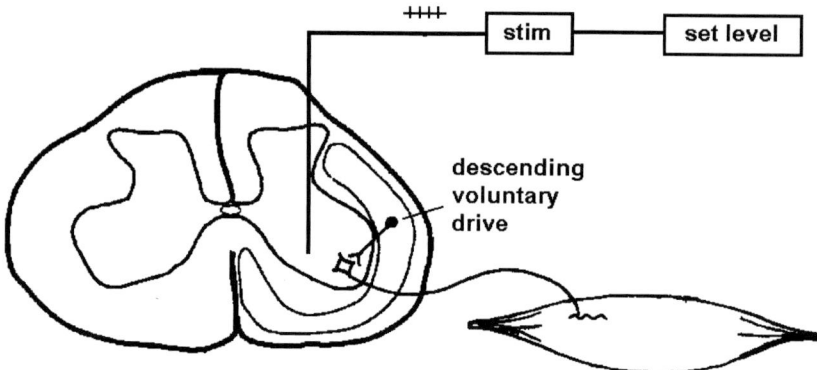

Fig. 10. Schematic showing how steady ISMS at a level close to threshold for eliciting muscle contraction at rest, could boost descending commands to that muscle in a person with incomplete SCI.

either facilitated or inhibited during naturally evoked increases in background EMG activity of the muscles. Facilitation was more common at the lower levels of background EMG, and inhibition became progressively more apparent as EMG levels rose. Accordingly, when trains of stimuli were delivered, the total EMG, comprising the sum of the naturally occurring background EMG and the responses to the stimulus trains, tended to be significantly facilitated at the lower background levels, but less so at the higher levels. The practical implication of this result is that in people with incomplete SCI who have weak voluntary control over some muscles, ISMS through microwires implanted caudal to the lesion could provide useful facilitation of these muscle contractions that might be enough to improve overall motor function significantly (Fig. 10). It is also possible that sub-threshold ISMS could be used to boost patterns of activation produced by the spinal cord such as the locomotor rhythm. Finally, though the use of ISMS to restore bladder, bowel and sexual function was not the focus of this chapter, these are extremely important potential applications of ISMS (Agnew et al., 1998; Grill et al., 1999; Tai et al., 1999; Prochazka et al., 2001). Because key excitatory and inhibitory areas for bladder and bowel control are localized within a relatively small region of the sacral spinal cord, and because the control task is essentially switch-like (Shefchyk, 2001), these may in fact be the first applications of ISMS to reach clinical application.

Concluding remarks

In this chapter we first used some recent anatomical modelling data to help clarify the location and migration of activity in spinal MN pools underlying locomotion. We identified the interesting gap in knowledge that is important to fill in with regard to the restoration of locomotor function after incomplete spinal cord regeneration. Then we concentrated on the restoration of movement with ISMS. Controlled movements of the legs can be achieved with ISMS but the challenging task of producing coordinated locomotion with ISMS alone remains to be tested in both animals and humans with SCI. Clearly the boosting of weak voluntary contractions has important potential but it needs to be verified and characterized more thoroughly in both normal animals and those with partial spinal cord lesions before it can be tested in humans with SCI. At this point it constitutes an interesting approach to the augmentation of residual voluntary movement and could eventually be a very useful adjunct in maximizing the benefits of regeneration therapies as these become more widespread in the future.

Acknowledgements

This work was supported by the Canadian Institutes of Health Research (CIHR) and the Alberta Heritage Foundation for Medical Research.

References

Agnew, W.F., McCreery, D.B., Lossinsky, A. and Bullara, L. (1998) *Microstimulation of the Lumbosacral Spinal Cord.* Huntington Medical Research Institutes, Pasadena.

Armstrong, D.M. and Drew, T. (1984) Discharges of pyramidal tract and other motor cortical neurones during locomotion in the cat. *J. Physiol.*, 346: 471–495.

Baer, G.A., Talonen, P.P., Hakkinen, V., Exner, G. and Yrjola, H. (1990) Phrenic nerve stimulation in tetraplegia. *Scand. J. Rehabil. Med.*, 22: 107–111.

Bamber, N.I., Li, H., Lu, X., Oudega, M., Aebischer, P. and Xu, X.M. (2001) Neurotrophins BDNF and NT-3 promote axonal re-entry into the distal host spinal cord through Schwann cell-seeded mini-channels. *Eur. J. Neurosci.*, 13: 257–268.

Basmajian, J.V. and De Luca, C.J. (1985) EMG signal amplitude and force. In: *Muscles Alive. Their Functions Revealed by Electromyography* 5th edn. Williams and Wilkins, Baltimore, pp. 187–222.

Bennett, D.J., Gorassini, M., Fouad, K., Sanelli, L., Han, Y. and Cheng, J. (1999) Spasticity in rats with sacral spinal cord injury. *J. Neurotrauma*, 16: 69–84.

Bigland, B. and Lippold, O. (1954) The relation between force, velocity and integrated electrical activity motor unit activity in the voluntary contraction of human muscle. *J. Physiol.*, 125: 322–335.

Blits, B., Dijkhuizen, P.A., Boer, G.J. and Verhaagen, J. (2000) Intercostal nerve implants transduced with an adenoviral vector encoding neurotrophin-3 promote regrowth of injured rat corticospinal tract fibers and improve hindlimb function. *Exp. Neurol.*, 164: 25–37.

Bonnot-Vrillaud, A., Whelan, P., Mentis, G. and O'Donovan, M. (2001) Calcium imaging of network activity in the neonatal mouse spinal cord during electrically-induced alternating rhythmic activity in vitro. *XXIII Int. Symp. CRSN: Spinal Cord Trauma: Neural Repair and Functional Recovery, Montreal.*

Bosco, G. and Poppele, R.E. (2001) Proprioception from a spinocerebellar perspective. *Physiol. Rev.*, 81: 539–568.

Brindley, G.S. (1977) An implant to empty the bladder or close the urethra. *J. Neurol., Neurosurg. Psychiatry*, 40: 358–369.

Brindley, G.S., Polkey, C.E., Rushton, D.N. and Cardozo, L. (1986) Sacral anterior root stimulators for bladder control in paraplegia: the first 50 cases. *J. Neurol., Neurosurg. Psychiatry*, 49: 1104–1114.

Cazalets, J.R., Borde, M. and Clarac, F. (1995) Localization and organization of the central pattern generator for hindlimb locomotion in newborn rat. *J. Neurosci.*, 15: 4943–4951.

Cowley, K.C. and Schmidt, B.J. (1997) Regional distribution of the locomotor pattern-generating network in the neonatal rat spinal cord. *J. Neurophysiol.*, 77: 247–259.

Diener, P.S. and Bregman, B.S. (1998) Fetal spinal cord transplants support the development of target reaching and coordinated postural adjustments after neonatal cervical spinal cord injury. *J. Neurosci.*, 18: 763–778.

Duysens, J., Clarac, F. and Cruse, H. (2000) Load-regulating mechanisms in gait and posture: comparative aspects. *Physiol. Rev.*, 80: 83–133.

Edgerton, V.R., De Leon, R.D., Harkema, S.J., Hodgson, J.A., London, N., Reinkensmeyer, D.J., Roy, R.R., Talmadge, R.J., Tillakaratne, N.J., Timoszyk, W. and Tobin, A. (2001) Retraining the injured spinal cord. *J. Physiol.*, 533: 15–22.

Gimenez y Ribotta, M., Orsal, D., Feraboli-Lohnherr, D. and Privat, A. (1998) Recovery of locomotion following transplantation of monoaminergic neurons in the spinal cord of paraplegic rats. *Ann. N.Y. Acad. Sci.*, 860: 393–411.

Gimenez y Ribotta, M., Provencher, J., Feraboli-Lohnherr, D., Rossignol, S., Privat, A. and Orsal, D. (2000) Activation of locomotion in adult chronic spinal rats is achieved by transplantation of embryonic raphe cells reinnervating a precise lumbar level. *J. Neurosci.*, 20: 5144–5152.

Giszter, S.F., Mussa-Ivaldi, F.A. and Bizzi, E. (1993) Convergent force fields organized in the frog's spinal cord. *J. Neurosci.*, 13: 467–491.

Giszter, S., Graziani, V., Kargo, W., Hockensmith, G., Davies, M.R., Smeraski, C.S. and Murray, M. (1998) Pattern generators and cortical maps in locomotion of spinal injured rats. *Ann. N.Y. Acad. Sci.*, 860: 554–555.

Giszter, S.F., Grill, W.M., Lemay, M.A., Mushahwar, V.K. and Prochazka, A. (2000) Intraspinal microstimulation: techniques, perspectives and prospects for FES. In: J.K. Chapin and K.A. Moxon (Eds.), *Neural Prostheses for Restoration of Sensory and Motor Function.* CRC Press, London.

Grill, W.M., Bhadra, N. and Wang, B. (1999) Bladder and urethral pressures evoked by microstimulation of the sacral spinal cord in cats. *Brain Res.*, 836: 19–30.

Hulsebosch, C.E., Hains, B.C., Waldrep, K. and Young, W. (2000) Bridging the gap: from discovery to clinical trials in spinal cord injury. *J. Neurotrauma*, 17: 1117–1128.

Kralj, A.R. and Bajd, T. (1989) *Functional Electrical Stimulation: Standing and Walking after Spinal Cord Injury.* CRC Press, Boca Raton, FL.

Marcoux, J. and Rossignol, S. (2000) Initiating or blocking locomotion in spinal cats by applying noradrenergic drugs to restricted lumbar spinal segments. *J. Neurosci.*, 20: 8577–8585.

McKerracher, L. (2001) Spinal cord repair: strategies to promote axon regeneration. *Neurobiol. Dis.*, 8: 11–18.

Mushahwar, V.K. and Horch, K.W. (1997) Proposed specifications for a lumbar spinal cord electrode array for control of lower extremities in paraplegia. *IEEE Trans. Rehabil. Eng.*, 5: 237–243.

Mushahwar, V.K. and Horch, K.W. (1998) Selective activation and graded recruitment of functional muscle groups through spinal cord stimulation. *Ann. N.Y. Acad. Sci.*, 860: 531–535.

Mushahwar, V.K. and Horch, K.W. (2000) Selective activation of muscle groups in the feline hindlimb through electrical microstimulation of the ventral lumbo-sacral spinal cord. *IEEE Trans. Rehabil. Eng.*, 8: 11–21.

Mushahwar, V.K., Collins, D.F. and Prochazka, A. (2000a) Spinal cord microstimulation generates functional limb movements in chronically implanted cats. *Exp. Neurol.*, 163: 422–429.

Mushahwar, V.K., Gillard, D.N., Gauthier, M.J.A. and Prochazka, A. (2000b). Spinal cord microstimulation generates locomotor and target-directed movements. *Soc. Neurosci. Abstr.*

Nicolopoulos-Stournaras, S. and Iles, J.F. (1983) Motor neuron columns in the lumbar spinal cord of the rat. *J. Comp. Neurol.*, 217: 75–85.

Nieoullon, A. and Rispal-Padel, L. (1976) Somatotopic localization in cat motor cortex. *Brain Res.*, 105: 405–422.

Pearson, K.G. (1995) Proprioceptive regulation of locomotion. *Curr. Opin. Neurobiol.*, 5: 786–791.

Peckham, P.H. and Keith, M.W. (1992) Motor prostheses for restoration of upper extremity function. In: R.B. Stein, P.H. Peckham and D.B. Popovic (Eds.), *Neural Prostheses: Replacing Motor Function After Disease or Disability*. Oxford University Press, New York, NY.

Peckham, P.H., Marsolais, E.B. and Mortimer, J.T. (1980) Restoration of key grip and release in the C6 tetraplegic patient through functional electrical stimulation. *J. Hand Surg.*, 5: 462–469.

Perrins, R. and Roberts, A. (1995) Cholinergic contribution to excitation in a spinal locomotor central pattern generator in *Xenopus* embryos. *J. Neurophysiol.*, 73: 1013–1019.

Prochazka, A. (1996) Proprioceptive feedback and movement regulation. In: L. Rowell and J.T. Sheperd (Eds.), *Handbook of Physiology, Section 12. Exercise: Regulation and Integration of Multiple Systems*. American Physiological Society, New York, NY.

Prochazka, A. and Davis, L.A. (1992) Clinical experience with reinforced, anchored intramuscular electrodes for functional neuromuscular stimulation. *J. Neurosci. Methods*, 42: 175–184.

Prochazka, A. and Mushahwar, V.K. (2001) Activation of paralyzed muscles with intraspinal microstimulation after chronic spinal cord transection. *Soc. Neurosci. Abstr.*, 27 (in press).

Prochazka, A., Westerman, R.A. and Ziccone, S.P. (1976) Discharges of single hindlimb afferents in the freely moving cat. *J. Neurophysiol.*, 39: 1090–1104.

Prochazka, A., Mushahwar, V.K. and McCreery, D.B.N.P. (2001) Neural prostheses. *J. Physiol.*, 533: 99–109.

Ramon-Cueto, A., Cordero, M.I., Santos-Benito, F.F. and Avila, J. (2000) Functional recovery of paraplegic rats and motor axon regeneration in their spinal cords by olfactory ensheathing glia. *Neuron*, 25: 425–435.

Romanes, G.J. (1951) The motor cell columns of the lumbosacral spinal cord of the cat. *J. Comp. Neurol.*, 94: 313–358.

Rossignol, S. (1996) Neural control of stereotypic limb movements. In: L. Rowell and J.T. Sheperd (Eds.), *Handbook of Physiology, Section 12. Exercise: Regulation and Integration of Multiple Systems*. American Physiological Society, New York, NY.

Saxena, S., Nikolic, S. and Popovic, D. (1995) An EMG-controlled grasping system for tetraplegics. *J. Rehabil. Res. Dev.*, 32: 17–24.

Schwab, M.E. (1996) Bridging the gap in spinal cord regeneration. *Nat. Med.*, 2: 976–977.

Shefchyk, S.J. (2001) Sacral spinal interneurons and the control of urinary bladder and urethral striated sphincter muscle function. *J. Physiol.*, 533: 57–63.

Sherrington, C.S. (1910) Flexion-reflex of the limb, crossed extension-reflex, and reflex stepping and standing. *J. Physiol.*, 40: 28–121.

Shik, M.L. (1997) Recognizing propriospinal and reticulospinal systems of initiation of stepping. *Motor Control*, 1: 310–313.

Stein, R.B., Peckham, P.H. and Popovic, D.B. (Eds.) (1992) *Neural Prostheses. Replacing Motor Function After Disease or Disability*. Oxford Univ. Press, New York.

Tai, C., Booth, A.M., Robinson, C.J., de Groat, W.C. and Roppolo, J.R. (1999) Isometric torque about the knee joint generated by microstimulation of the cat L6 spinal cord. *IEEE Trans. Rehabil. Eng.*, 7: 46–55.

VanderHorst, V.G.J.M. and Holstege, G. (1997) Organization of lumbosacral motoneuronal cell groups innervating hindlimb, pelvic floor, and axial muscles in the cat. *J. Comp. Neurol.*, 382: 46–76.

Woodford, B.J., Carter, R.R., McCreery, D., Bullara, L.A. and Agnew, W.F. (1996) Histopathologic and physiologic effects of chronic implantation of microelectrodes in sacral spinal cord of the cat. *J. Neuropathol. Exp. Neurol.*, 55: 982–991.

Xu, X.M., Zhang, S.X., Li, H., Aebischer, P. and Bunge, M.B. (1999) Regrowth of axons into the distal spinal cord through a Schwann-cell-seeded mini-channel implanted into hemisected adult rat spinal cord. *Eur. J. Neurosci.*, 11: 1723–1740.

Yakovenko, S., Mushahwar, V.K., Vanderhorst, V., Holstege, G. and Prochazka, A. (2000) Locus of activation of spinal motoneuron pools in the cat step cycle. *J. Physiol.*, 525P: 42P.

Zompa, E.A., Pizzo, D.P. and Hulsebosch, C.E. (1993) Migration and differentiation of PC12 cells transplanted into the rat spinal cord. *Int. J. Dev. Neurosci.*, 11: 535–544.

L. McKerracher, G. Doucet and S. Rossignol (Eds.)
Progress in Brain Research, Vol. 137
© 2002 Elsevier Science B.V. All rights reserved

CHAPTER 10

Propriospinal neurons involved in the control of locomotion: potential targets for repair strategies?

Larry M. Jordan * and Brian J. Schmidt

Departments of Physiology and Internal Medicine, The University of Manitoba, Winnipeg, MB R3E 3J7, Canada

Propriospinal systems and their importance in the control of locomotion

Numerous studies have attempted to determine which spinal cord pathways mediate descending activation of the mammalian central pattern generator (CPG) for locomotion. In the acute decerebrate cat, the pontomedullary medial reticular formation is the origin of long fast-conducting descending projections that travel in the ventrolateral funiculus; this pathway must remain intact in order to elicit hindlimb locomotor activity in response to brainstem electrical stimulation (Steeves and Jordan, 1980; Noga et al., 1991). Similarly, the ventrolateral white matter appears to be critical for the preservation of locomotor responses in the rat (Iwahara et al., 1991; Stelzner and Cullen, 1991; Magnuson et al., 1995).

However, locomotor capacity changes as a function of time and training. Therefore any effort to define descending pathways that are essential or sufficient for the activation of locomotion must also consider observations obtained from the study of animals with chronic lesions. In their review of the locomotor capabilities of cats and primates after various

chronic spinal cord lesions, Rossignol and colleagues concluded that there is "no indication that any particular descending pathway is unique or essential for triggering locomotion" (Rossignol et al., 1996).

In addition to direct bulbospinal projections, there is evidence that a propriospinal system exists in the dorsolateral region of the cat spinal cord, which may be continuous with the pontomedullary locomotor region (e.g. Kazennikov et al., 1983; Shik, 1983; Yamaguchi, 1986; Kazennikov and Shik, 1988). Although not essential for the production of stepping while electrically stimulating the mesencephalic locomotor region (MLR) (Noga et al., 1991), stimulation of the dorsolateral propriospinal system, either directly or via segmental afferents, does produce locomotor activity in all four limbs and may be sufficient for the activation of forelimb stepping in response to MLR stimulation (Yamaguchi, 1986). Descending propriospinal systems are also thought to be involved in other rhythmic behaviors such as turtle scratching (Berkowitz and Stein, 1994). Despite this evidence, important issues raised by Shik, on the role of a locomotor-related propriospinal system in the mammalian spinal cord, remain largely unanswered. He stated, "unfortunately the properties of this system are scarcely known, and further analytic research is necessary to decide if this system provides the role that is ascribed here. . . probably its neurons take part in propagation of activity along the spinal cord as well as in generation of stepping." (Shik, 1983).

* Correspondence to: L.M. Jordan, Department of Physiology, The University of Manitoba, Winnipeg, MB R3E 3J7, Canada. Tel.: +1-204-789-3694/3761; Fax: +1-204-789-3930; E-mail: larry@scrc.umanitoba.ca

In contrast to the concept of a distributed CPG is the proposal that the rat CPG is anatomically localized to the L_1/L_2 segments (Cazalets et al., 1995, 1996). However, we showed that the network is distributed throughout the spinal cord, including supralumbar regions (Cowley and Schmidt, 1997), a finding consistent with the 'unit burst generator' hypothesis proposed by Grillner (Grillner, 1981), in which discrete areas of the spinal cord responsible for rhythmic activity around one joint are expected to possess rhythmogenic properties. Cells with specific receptors for neuroactive substances capable of eliciting locomotion may be restricted to specific sites in the spinal cord (Giménez y Ribotta et al., 2000; Marcoux and Rossignol, 2000; Fyda et al., 2002), but CPG elements elsewhere may be activated by other means (Cowley and Schmidt, 1997), so that restricted sites of action for certain drugs does not invalidate the notion of a distributed CPG. Other studies of the rat spinal cord (lumbar region) also suggest that the CPG is distributed (Kjaerulff and Kiehn, 1996; Kremer and Lev-Tov, 1997). Furthermore, the idea of a distributed CPG is consistent with studies of locomotion and scratching in other preparations (e.g. Grillner, 1974; Cohen and Wallen, 1980; Roberts and Khan, 1982; Deliagina et al., 1983; Mortin and Stein, 1989; Ho and O'Donovan, 1993). Such a distributed system suggests that propriospinal links within the network may mediate rostrocaudal activation by supraspinal input.

Studies of spinal cord regeneration stimulate further interest in the functional role of descending propriospinal pathways. Although some models have demonstrated that the spinal cord contains the capacity for long-distance axonal regeneration (e.g. Hasan et al., 1993; Cheng et al., 1996), generally this has been more difficult to achieve, especially in adult mammalian preparations, compared with short-distance regrowth of axons (Bregman et al., 1997). For instance, after spinal cord transection, the axons of several types of neurons, including brainstem cells, enter into Schwann cell grafts at the lesion site; however, only propriospinal and sensory axons also have the capacity to exit the graft and re-enter the spinal cord distal to the transection/graft site (Guest et al., 1997).

From a functional perspective, it is possible that propriospinal relay pathways contribute to descend-ing CPG activation, yet this system may not be essential under normal (pre-lesion) conditions, as suggested by transection studies in the cat (see above) and lamprey (McClellan, 1994). However, after cord transection, regrowth of short propriospinal connections across the transection may become critically important. Such links could compensate for the loss of direct bulbospinal projections to more caudal regions of the cord, as demonstrated in the lamprey spinal cord (McClellan, 1994; Rouse and McClellan, 1997). Thus, "the possibility that regeneration of intrinsic [propriospinal] spinal cord neurons may augment behavioral recovery, possibly by linking supraspinal inputs to the locomotor pattern generators, should be further explored" (Guest et al., 1997). If propriospinal connections are able to mediate supraspinal activation of the mammalian CPG, then attempts to restore spinal cord function using strategies aimed at regeneration or replacement of propriospinal cells involved in the control of locomotion may be a realistic goal. Clearly, more information about the identification, properties, and roles of mammalian CPG-related propriospinal pathways is needed if such strategies are to be successful.

In order to test the notion that propriospinal cells can relay a locomotor message descending from the brain, we (Cowley and Schmidt, 2000) suppressed synaptic transmission in the thoracic region of the isolated neonatal rat spinal cord and showed that coupling of motor rhythms between the cervical and lumbar regions can be disrupted. This implicates propriospinal cells in the relay of locomotor information between the cervical and lumbar enlargements. We have also recently observed that locomotor-like activity in the lumbar region, evoked by neurochemical stimulation of the brainstem (using an isolated brainstem–spinal cord preparation), was abolished during suppression of synaptic transmission in the thoracic cord (Zaporozhets and Schmidt, 2001); this suggests that propriospinal cells make a powerful contribution to the transmission of the descending message that activates the locomotor network.

5-HT responsive cells involved in the spinal networks for locomotion

There is strong evidence that 5-HT responsive propriospinal cells are involved in the spinal control of locomotion, and might be suitable targets for repair strategies (reviewed in Schmidt and Jordan, 2000). We have attempted to identify cells which could be involved in this propriospinal system and capable of relaying a locomotor message. In the isolated neonatal rat spinal cord, various agents, including N-methyl-D-aspartate (NMDA), DA, 5-HT, NE and acetylcholine (ACh), are capable of inducing locomotor-like activity (Kudo and Yamada, 1987; Smith et al., 1988; Atsuta et al., 1991; Cazalets et al., 1992; Cowley and Schmidt, 1994, 1997; Kiehn and Kjaerulff, 1996; Kiehn et al., 1999). We showed that, of these various agents, 5-HT was the most reliable in eliciting a locomotor-like pattern of hindlimb nerve activity (Cowley and Schmidt, 1994). In addition, we demonstrated that pharmacological blockade of 5-HT impaired the ability of 5-HT and other neurochemicals to elicit locomotor-like activity (MacLean et al., 1998), suggesting that 5-HT receptor activation may be critical for the production of rhythmic motor behavior in the neonatal rat spinal cord. Brownstone and colleagues (Jiang et al., 1999) demonstrated that 5-HT can contribute to the production of fictive locomotion in the functionally mature isolated mouse spinal cord. 5-HT also contributes to locomotion in younger mice (Nishimaru et al., 2000; Whelan et al., 2000). Jacobs and co-workers (Fornal et al., 1985; Jacobs and Azmitia, 1992; Veasey et al., 1995) suggested that 5-HT cells projecting to the spinal cord have a role in locomotion, on the basis of their activity in freely moving cats. 5-HT agonists enhanced the locomotor output, but did not result in the initiation of locomotion in chronic spinal cats (Barbeau and Rossignol, 1990, 1991; Rossignol et al., 1998). In spinal rabbits (Viala and Buser, 1969) and rats (Feraboli-Lohnherr et al., 1999), however, 5-HT agonists are effective for the initiation of locomotion, and 5-HT enhanced locomotor activity in marmoset monkeys (Fedirchuk et al., 1998). As discussed in a previous review (Schmidt and Jordan, 2000), successful serotonergic activation of locomotor rhythms in mammals has involved preparations that preserve at least a few thoracic segments.

The role of 5-HT in the production of locomotion has been exploited successfully in experiments designed to restore locomotor function after injury. 5-HT has recently been shown to activate the locomotor network in adult spinal rats (Feraboli-Lohnherr et al., 1999), and 5-HT agonists increased weight-supported stepping in spinal rats with neural transplants (Kim et al., 1999). Transplantation of monoaminergic neurons in adult spinal rats restores locomotor capability (for review see Giménez y Ribotta et al., 1998, 2000; Orsal et al., 2002).

Gerin et al. (1995) showed that 5-HT, DA and their respective metabolites are released in the ventral funiculus of the lumbar cord during exercise in the adult rat. However, samples taken from the ventral horn gray matter revealed no increase in 5-HT or 5-HIAA release during exercise, with a small increase in DA release (Gerin and Privat, 1998). We have shown regional differences in responsiveness of the neonatal rat locomotor network to 5-HT. First, using bath partitions at T_{13}/L_1 we demonstrated that activation of 5-HT-sensitive neurons in the supralumbar portions of the cord was required to induce rhythmic locomotor discharge in the lumbar cord (Cowley and Schmidt, 1997). 5-HT application to the lumbar cord was also required in these experiments; however, when applied to the lumbar cord alone, 5-HT promoted only tonic discharge. We then tested for possible regional differences in the distributions of monoamine release that might suggest differences in their sites of action in the spinal cord. Using an isolated neonatal rat brainstem–spinal cord preparation (Fyda et al., 2002), locomotor-like activity was elicited by electrical stimulation of the brainstem (Fig. 1). 5-HT and other amines, as well as their respective metabolites, were released during locomotor-like activity, and there were regional differences in the sites of release along the rostrocaudal extent of the spinal cord. The site of maximal release of 5-HT was within the lower thoracic spinal cord, with a second peak in the lumbar region.

In the same study (Fyda et al., 2002), application of monoamine antagonists, restricted to rostral or caudal sites of release, suggested that activation of cells possessing 5-HT7 receptors is essential for brainstem-evoked locomotion, and that the neurons with these receptors are located in the thoracic and upper lumbar segments (Fig. 2A). Furthermore, antagonism of 5-HT2A receptors with ketanserin blocked locomotion, and this effect was predominantly on neurons located in the L_3–L_4 region (Fig. 2A). Our findings confirm the suggestion by

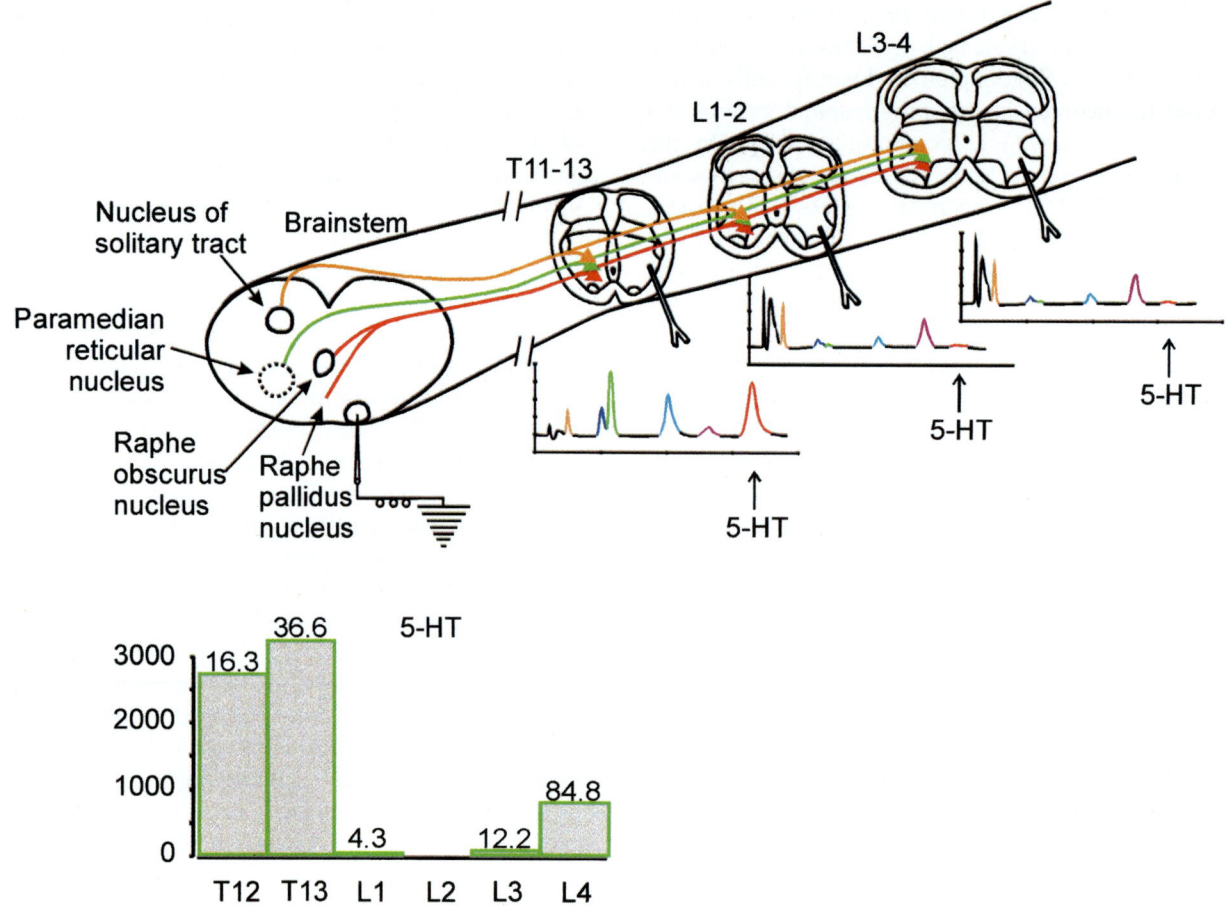

Fig. 1. 5-HT release from the isolated neonatal rat spinal cord monitored using microdialysis probes inserted into the ventral horn and HPLC analysis. (Top) Schematic drawing of the brainstem–spinal cord preparation used for determining the release of 5-HT during brainstem-evoked fictive locomotion. 5-HT peaks are indicated (arrows) in examples of HPLC records at three different levels of the spinal cord. (Bottom) The rostrocaudal distribution of 5-HT release is illustrated (mean $\pm$ SEM, pg/20 μl, $n = 9$ per segment). Modified from Fyda et al. (2002).

Hochman (Cina and Hochman, 1998) that 5-HT7 receptors in particular may be required for the initiation of locomotion in the neonatal rat spinal cord, and demonstrate a regional differentiation between the effects of 5-HT7 and 5-HT2A receptors. This rostrocaudal differential distribution of 5-HT7 versus 5-HT2A receptors may also underlie our initial observations of the differential effect of 5-HT application on supralumbar versus lumbar regions (Cowley and Schmidt, 1997). We found that 5-HT was required at both sites, but that its rhythmogenic effects were restricted to the supralumbar region. These results pertain specifically to interneurons possessing 5-HT receptors, and should not be confused with the

effects of co-application of 5-HT and NMDA on a wide range of segments throughout the supralumbar, as well as upper, mid, and lower lumbar spinal cord (Kjaerulff and Kiehn, 1996; Cowley and Schmidt, 1997; Kremer and Lev-Tov, 1997).

Further evidence for an action of 5-HT on elements of the CPG at the supralumbar level emerges when the time course of the action of clozapine is examined (Fig. 2B). When applied to the supralumbar cord, the locomotor rhythm slowly declines in frequency, consistent with an action on rhythmogenic elements. We hypothesize that some elements of the CPG for locomotion must be excited by 5-HT, and that the cells involved are located at supralumbar

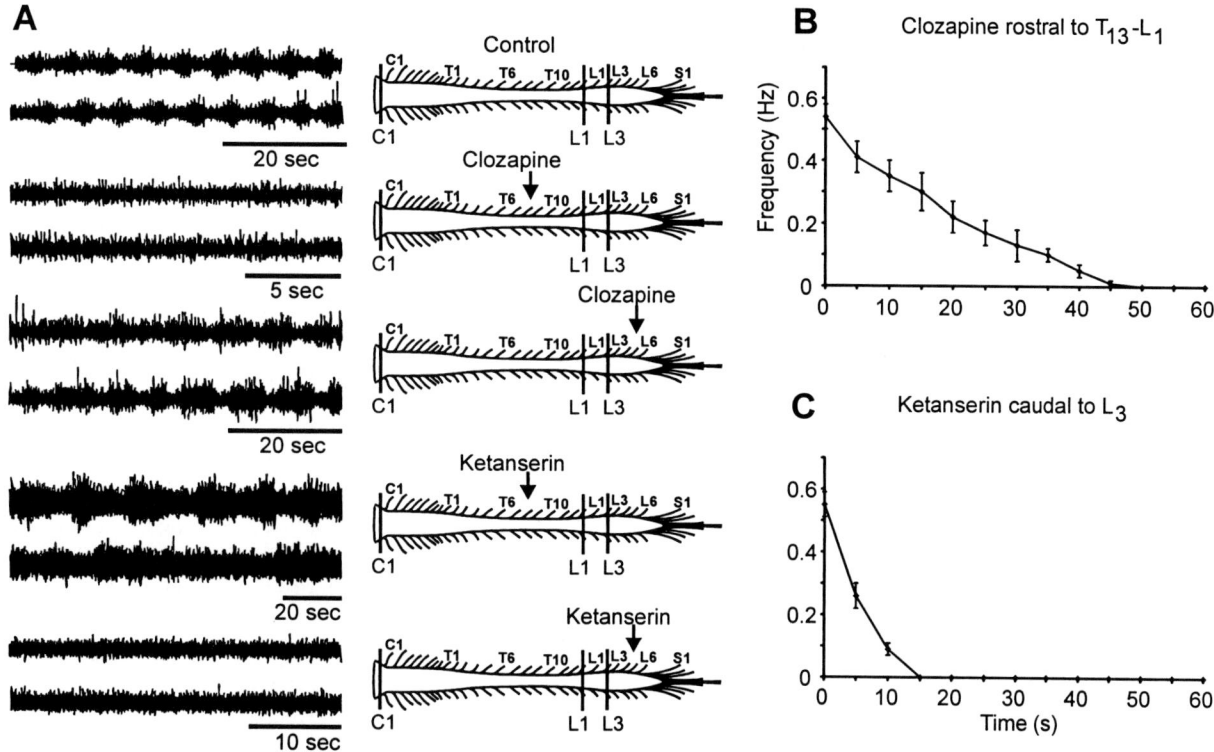

Fig. 2. Effects of the 5-HT7 antagonist clozapine and the 5-HT2A antagonist ketanserin on brainstem-evoked fictive locomotion in vitro. (A) Electroneurographic recordings from the right and left L_2 (for rostral drug applications) or L_5 (for caudal drug applications) ventral roots during clozapine (0.25 μM) or ketanserin (20 μM) application to the bath. Clozapine applied rostral to a barrier at L_1 blocked locomotion, but was without effect when applied caudal to a barrier at L_3. Ketanserin was without effect when applied rostral to L_1, but blocked locomotion when applied caudal to L_3. (B) Mean $\pm$ SEM of the frequency (Hz) of ventral root electroneurographic recordings as a function of time following application of clozapine, showing the gradual decline in locomotor frequency, consistent with an action of 5-HT on elements of the CPG in the rostral portion of the spinal cord. (C) Mean $\pm$ SEM of the frequency (Hz) of ventral root electroneurographic recordings as a function of time following application of ketanserin, showing a relatively abrupt decrease in locomotor frequency, consistent with an action of 5-HT on motoneurons or other output elements of the locomotor network in caudal parts of the lumbar enlargement. Modified from Fyda et al. (2002).

levels in the neonatal rat spinal cord. It is interesting to note that 5-HT excites isolated spinal cord cells with 'pacemaker' properties (Legendre et al., 1989). Furthermore, transplantation of serotonergic neurons into the lower thoracic region resulted in activation of the locomotor central pattern generator in spinal rats (Giménez y Ribotta et al., 2000).

The effects of the 5-HT2A antagonist ketanserin on the locomotor rhythm are not only restricted to the lumbar level of the cord, but the time course of action of ketanserine is much more abrupt than that of clozapine (Fig. 2B), consistent with an action directly upon motoneurons rather than on rhythmogenic elements of the CPG. It has been demonstrated

that 5-HT2A receptors are abundant on spinal motoneurons (Cornea-Hébert et al., 1999).

5-HT has a well-documented excitatory action on spinal motoneurons (White and Neuman, 1980; Connell and Wallis, 1989; White and Fung, 1989; Takahashi and Berger, 1990; Ziskind-Conhaim et al., 1993). It also promotes plateau potentials (Hounsgaard and Kiehn, 1989) and is essential for NMDA receptor-induced voltage oscillatory activity in amphibian (Sillar and Simmers, 1994) and mammalian (MacLean et al., 1998) motoneurons. Stimulation of raphespinal pathways can induce plateau properties in motoneurons in anesthetized cats (Brownstone and Hultborn, 1992; R.M. Brownstone, T. Toth and

H. Hultborn, unpublished). We also showed that 5-HT modulates NMDA receptor-mediated nonlinear membrane behavior in neonatal rat motoneurons (MacLean and Schmidt, 2001).

We recently embarked upon a series of experiments aimed at revealing the locations of neurons in the adult rat spinal cord that are active during locomotion and which possess 5-HT7 receptors. Cells activated in response to a treadmill locomotor task were detected using c-*fos* immunochemistry, and the same sections were double-labeled with an antibody to the 5-HT7 receptor (Jordan et al., 2000). In the lower thoracic cord, double-labeled cells were numerous (Fig. 3), and over 80% of the c-fos-positive cells were also labeled with the 5-HT7 antibody. This indicates that cells active during locomotion in these rats possess 5-HT7 receptors, consistent with the observations that clozapine blocks brainstem-evoked locomotion when applied into the lower thoracic and upper lumbar cord (Fig. 2), and that the release of 5-HT in this preparation is maximal in the lower thoracic cord (Fig. 1).

There is thus a firm basis for a thorough characterization of the properties and connections of the spinal cord propriospinal cells which are activated by 5-HT. It is clear that 5-HT can elicit or enhance locomotor activity after spinal cord injury. 5-HT and other amines are released in the spinal cord during brainstem-evoked locomotion, and the sites of maximal 5-HT release correspond to the thoracic and lumbar sites of action of 5-HT (Fig. 4). It appears that there are at least two important sites of action of 5-HT with potent effects on the control of locomotion: one in the lower thoracic–upper lumbar region, where 5-HT induces locomotor activity, possibly by activating 5-HT7 receptors; and one in the lower lumbar cord involving 5-HT2A receptors on output elements of the CPG, including, if not confined to, motoneurons. Future studies examining the upper thoracic and cervical cord segments, which also contain elements of a distributed locomotor network (Cowley and Schmidt, 1997), may clarify a role for neurons with 5-HT receptors in these more rostral regions also. We hypothesize that an important component of the propriospinal cell population forming part of the CPG for locomotion can be characterized by the presence of 5-HT7 receptors, and that these propriospinal cells are suitable targets for attempts to restore locomotion using regeneration or transplantation approaches.

Cholinergic propriospinal and commissural interneurons involved in the control of locomotion

There is also compelling evidence that cholinergic propriospinal cells, as well as cells with acetylcholine (ACh) receptors, are involved in the control of locomotion, and it is possible that these cells could be exploited to relay a locomotor message after injury. Recovery of hindlimb stepping has been related to sprouting of cholinergic fibers after spinal cord injury (Jakeman et al., 1998). A role for ACh in the initiation and control of locomotion in vertebrates is suggested on the basis of several lines of evidence. In the *Xenopus* embryo, Roberts and his colleagues (Panchin et al., 1991) observed that bath application of ACh evoked a burst of activity, followed by an increased frequency of spontaneous swimming episodes. The muscarinic antagonist atropine reversibly blocked the effects of ACh. Atropine also considerably shortened both spontaneous and evoked bursts of fictive swimming, while nicotinic antagonists appeared to have little effect. A portion of the drive to motoneurons during swimming in these animals is derived from a cholinergic input (Perrins and Roberts, 1995a,b, 1995c).

In the newborn rat, rhythmic motor activity can be elicited by bath application of ACh and edrophonium, an anticholinesterase, to the spinal cord of an in vitro brainstem–spinal cord preparation (Smith and Feldman, 1987; Smith et al., 1988; Cowley and Schmidt, 1994). The effects appear to be mediated through the activation of muscarinic receptors at the spinal level since the muscarinic receptor antagonist atropine can completely suppress ACh-induced rhythmic activity in this preparation (Smith et al., 1988). Neurons containing cholinergic receptors may be involved in interlimb coordination, because the motor rhythm induced by ACh in the neonatal rat cord is characterized by ipsilateral synchronous flexor and extensor bursts which regularly alternate between the two hindlimbs (Cowley and Schmidt, 1994). Thus it appears that a system of commissural and propriospinal cells which are sensitive to ACh plays a prominent role in the generation

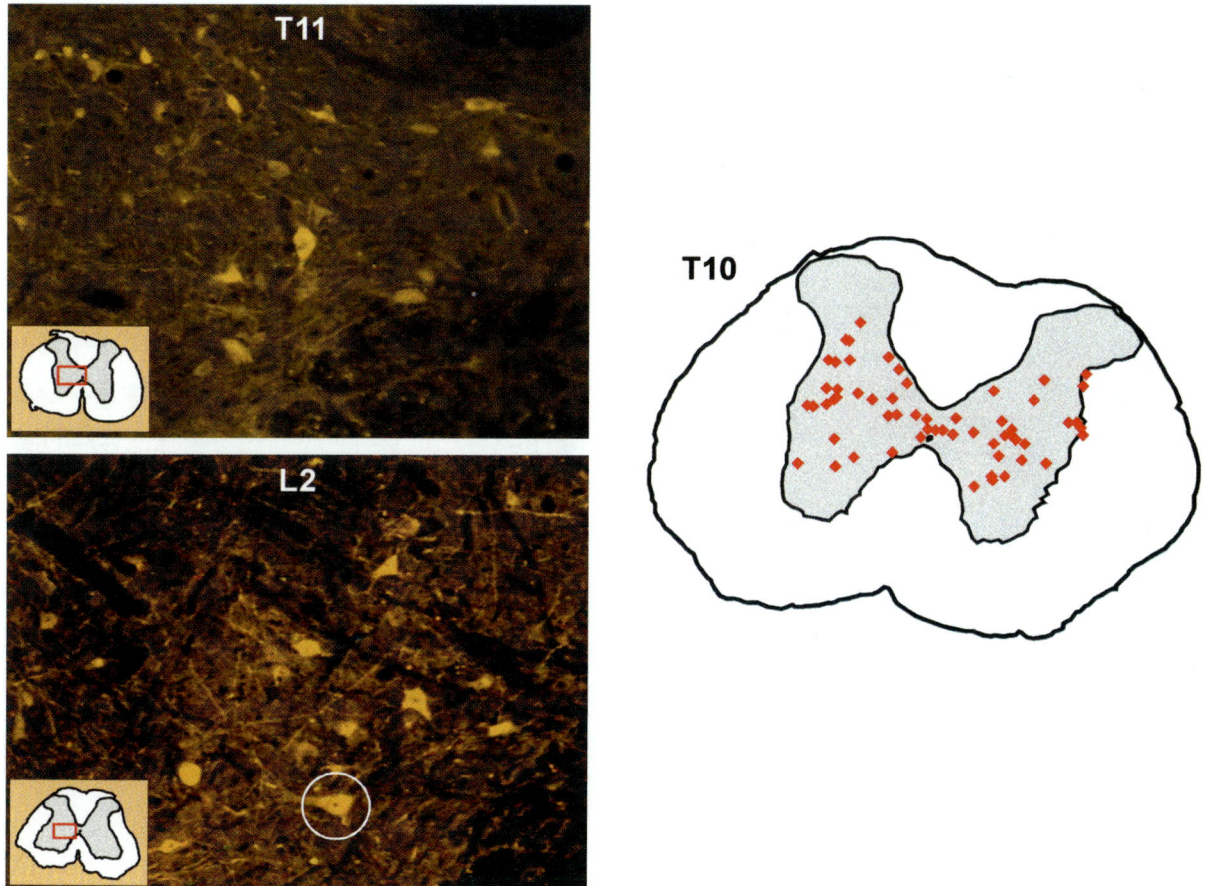

Fig. 3. Immunohistochemical detection of locomotor neurons of the spinal cord with 5-HT7 receptors. Locomotor neurons were detected in the spinal cords of adult rats subjected to a treadmill locomotor task using an antibody to c-*fos* (nuclear labeling, see circled cell for example). Cytoplasmic labeling represents 5-HT7 receptor. The drawing is a representative section showing the distribution of double-labeled cells at the T_{10} level.

of rhythmic activity in the spinal cord, and that pharmacological methods can be used to isolate key elements of the CPG for locomotion. We have preliminary evidence that some propriospinal cells that are excited by ACh are also strongly excited by 5-HT, so that these two populations may overlap (K.P. Carlin and L.M. Jordan, unpublished observation). The fact that acetylcholine-sensitive propriospinal cells are capable of relaying a locomotor message along the length of the spinal cord is illustrated by experiments in which the coupling of rhythmic activity between the cervical and lumbar enlargements was disrupted by application of atropine restricted to the mid-thoracic region of the cord (Cowley and Schmidt, 2000).

Commissural propriospinal cells are an important component of the spinal locomotor network. They appear to be involved in the first rhythmic activity which appears during development of the fetal rat (Kudo et al., 1991). In the adult cat, crossed excitatory effects on movement can be very powerful (Prochazka and Mushahwar, 1999). Commissural connections have also been shown to be remarkably powerful in the neonatal rat spinal cord, because left–right coordination persists when only a small portion of the commissural white matter remains intact (Cowley and Schmidt, 1997). Commissural and propriospinal neurons appear to form a coupled system with excitatory interconnections involved in rhythmogenesis in the lamprey (Hagevik and Mc-

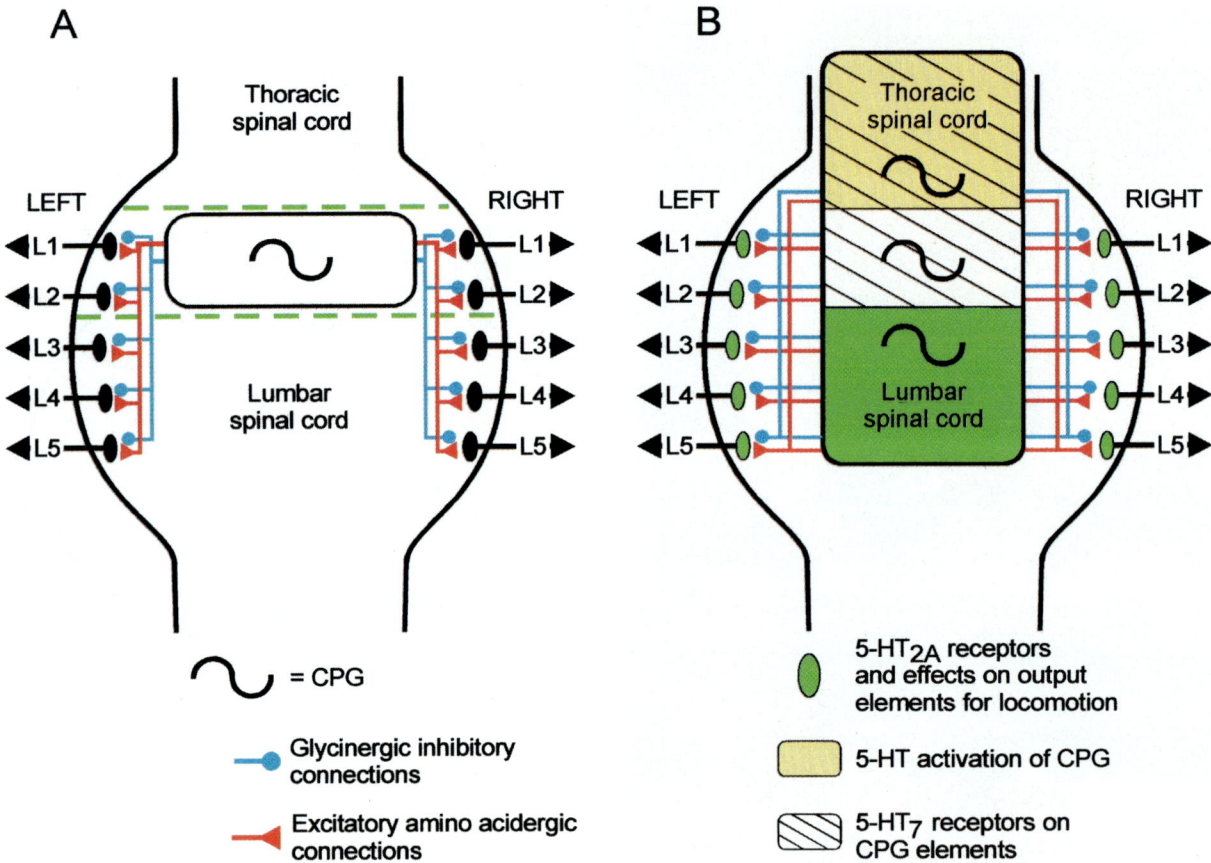

Fig. 4. Comparison of the CPG localization proposed by Cazalets et al. (A) and the probable sites of action of 5-HT revealed in the studies reviewed here (B). In contrast to the proposal by Cazalets et al. (1996), we believe that the rhythmogenic mechanism is more widely distributed, and the action of 5-HT to induce the locomotor rhythm is exerted primarily on the thoracic region of the neonatal rat cord, while the actions of 5-HT in the lumbar cord are likely to be on motoneurons and possibly premotor interneurons. 5-HT 7 receptor distribution on locomotor neurons is also shown, based on double-labeling experiments using antibodies to 5-HT7 receptors and c-fos in adult rats subjected to a treadmill locomotor task (Fig. 3).

Clellan, 1994), neonatal rat (Cowley and Schmidt, 1995, 1997; Kjaerulff and Kiehn, 1997; Kremer and Lev-Tov, 1997) and adult cat (Noga et al., 1993). Commissural cells crossing in the upper lumbar cord appear to be essential for VLF stimulation-evoked locomotor-like activity in the neonatal rat cord (Magnuson and Trinder, 1997); excitotoxic lesions of cells in this region impair locomotion in adult rats (Magnuson et al., 1999).

We have attempted to identify ACh-releasing spinal interneurons involved in the production of locomotor activity in the cat, using intracellular dye injection into physiologically identified neurons coupled with immunohistochemical markers (Carr et

al., 1994, 1995). These experiments showed that a population of interneurons active during fictive locomotion (produced by stimulation of the (MLR)) contained choline acetyltransferase (ChAT) and thus may be cholinergic (Fig. 5). We have combined c-fos with ChAT immunohistochemistry to map the segmental and laminar distributions of spinal cholinergic interneurons activated during locomotion, and we have used intracellular labeling combined with immunohistochemistry for ChAT to determine the activity pattern during locomotion and axonal trajectory of a specific population of cholinergic partition cells (Fig. 6) (Huang et al., 2000). The results suggest that a new population of spinal locomotor

ChAT

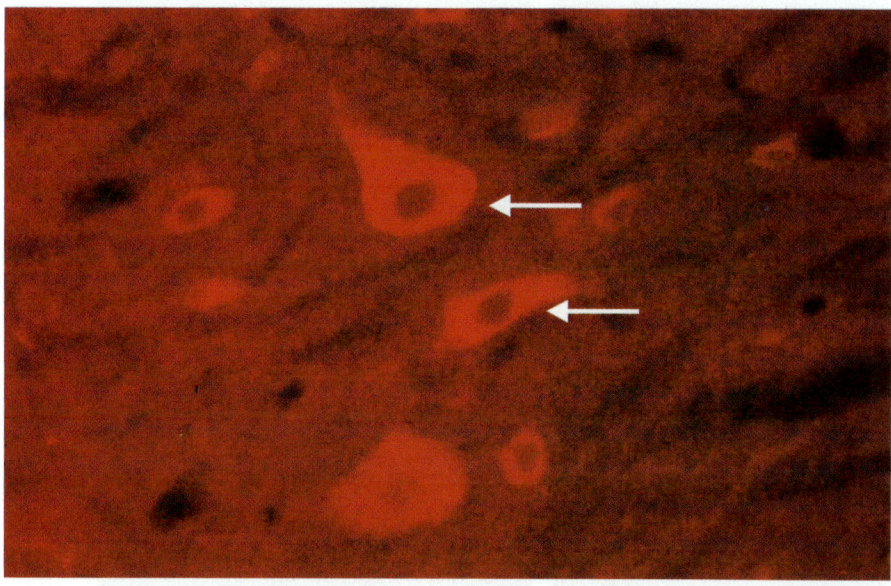

c-fos

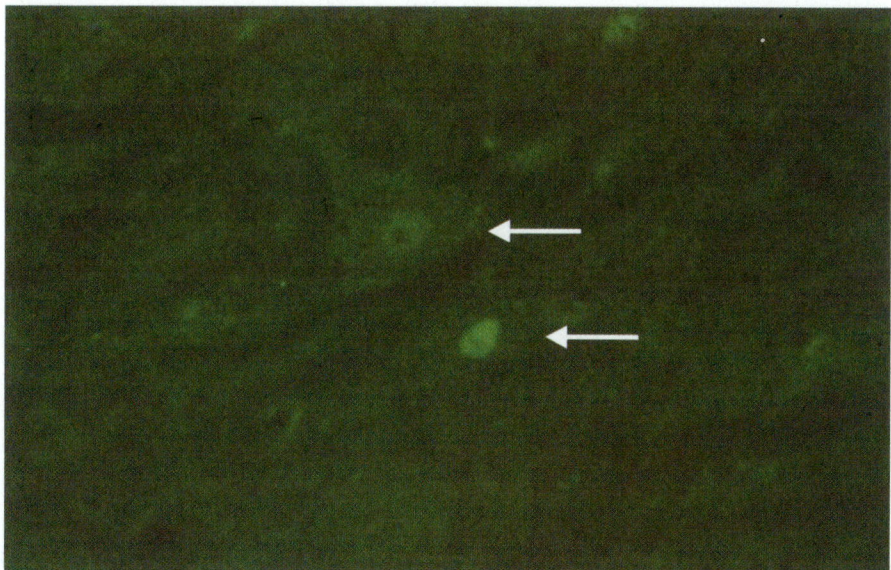

Fig. 5. Double labeling with antibodies to choline acetyltransferase (ChAT) and c-fos in the cat spinal cord in which c-fos expression was induced in locomotor neurons during fictive locomotion. Details of the methods are given in Carr et al. (1995) and Huang et al. (2000).

network-related neurons can be defined. These are cholinergic cells with contralateral projections, that are active during the extension phase of locomotion. The pattern of activity and high firing rates of these cells indicate that they should make a significant contribution to the control of locomotion. Their ac-

134

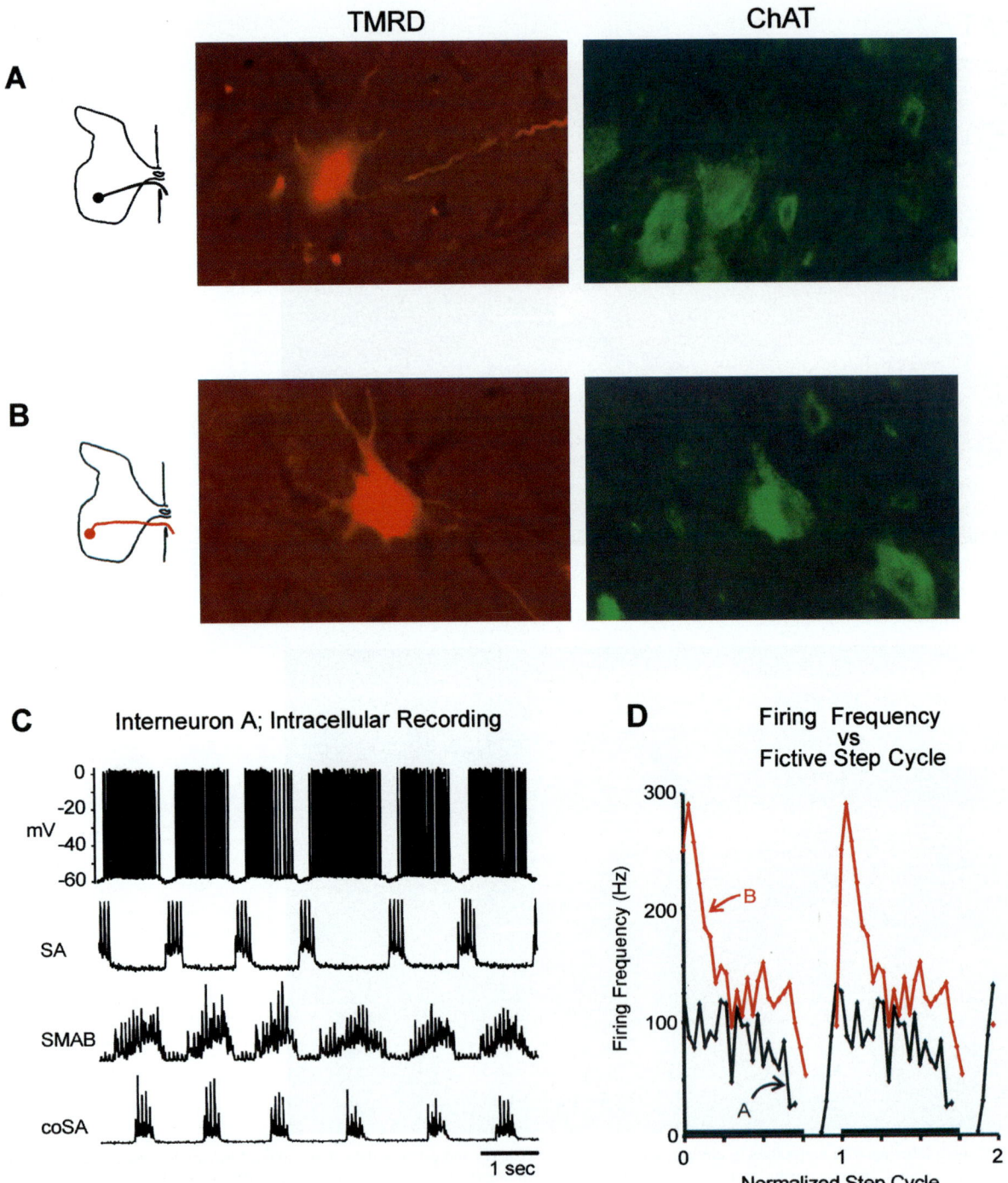

Fig. 6. Intracellular labeling with tetramethyl rhodamine (TMRD) of ChAT-positive interneurons (A and B, ×155) and intracellular recording during locomotion from the same neurons (C and D). Reprinted with permission from Huang et al. (2000).

tivity spanned the entire ipsilateral extensor phase of the locomotor cycle, and the peak firing rate was over 100 Hz.

Attempts to show that interneurons which release and/or respond to ACh contribute to the control of locomotion and might be suitable targets for locomotor repair strategies include the recent demonstration by Cowley and Schmidt (2000) that blockage of cholinergic transmission in the thoracic region of the isolated neonatal rat spinal cord reduces the coupling of rhythmic activity between the cervical and lumbar regions. Further studies to evaluate any contribution of such propriospinal cells to the recovery of locomotion after spinal injury are warranted. There is evidence that the sprouting of cholinergic fibers is associated with recovery of hindlimb stepping after spinal cord injury (Jakeman et al., 1998). BDNF was reported to enhance sprouting of cholinergic fibers into the lesion site, and to acutely activate the spinal locomotor network when applied intrathecally onto the thoracic cord (Ankeny et al., 2001). BDNF has also been shown to enhance propriospinal axonal regeneration (Xu et al., 1995). It is obviously important to determine the identity of cells with BDNF receptors in the spinal cord and test the hypothesis that these cells may be involved in locomotion and may contribute to locomotor recovery after spinal cord injury.

The spinal cord of vertebrates contains several types of cholinergic neurons, including motoneurons, preganglionic autonomic neurons, partition cells (lamina VII), central canal cluster cells (lamina X) and small dorsal horn cells scattered in lamina III–V (Houser et al., 1983; Barber et al., 1984; Phelps et al., 1984; Borges and Iversen, 1986; Sherriff and Henderson, 1994). There is consensus that the cholinergic cells in lamina VII and around the central canal form an extensive propriospinal system of interconnected neurons (Sherriff and Henderson, 1994), and may therefore play a role in activities requiring coordination among several spinal segments.

ChAT-positive commissural and propriospinal cells are present throughout the length of the spinal cord (Barber et al., 1984; Phelps et al., 1984). If they are capable of relaying a locomotor message from one segment of the spinal cord to another, they would be obvious targets for attempts to bridge the lesions site to restore walking after injury. Cholinergic 'partition cells' are intensely stained with ChAT on postnatal day 1, and they represent some of the largest cells in the spinal cord. Retrograde transport of fluorescent microspheres injected into selected motor nuclei has revealed that the commissural cells which project to motoneurons overlap with the location of partition cells and cluster cells (Hoover and Durkovic, 1992). Partition cells have been shown to send axons into the motoneuron pools (Phelps et al., 1984). It is likely, therefore, that some of the cholinergic propriospinal cells involved in locomotion have actions directly on spinal motoneurons.

Spinal motoneurons receive prominent cholinergic terminals (Nagy et al., 1993; Li et al., 1995; Arvidsson et al., 1997; Heisler and Tecott, 2000), and large cholinergic terminals on motoneurons, termed C terminals (Nagy et al., 1993; Li et al., 1995) have been implicated in spinal cord plasticity (Pullen and Sears, 1983; Feng-Chen and Wolpaw, 1996). Muscarinic cholinergic inputs to motoneurons have been shown to produce plateau potentials and rhythmicity in turtle motoneurons (Hounsgaard and Svirskis, 1998; Guertin and Hounsgaard, 1999). In adult mammalian motoneurons, cholinergic agents produce plateau-like responses (Zieglgansberger and Reiter, 1974), consistent with the cholinergic effects in the turtle spinal cord slice. Cholinergic plateau potentials have been described elsewhere in the CNS (Fraser and MacVicar, 1996). Spinal motoneurons have recently been shown to possess M2 receptors (Heisler and Tecott, 2000). Identification of the cholinergic propriospinal cells that project to motoneurons has not yet been accomplished, and their role in the control of locomotion needs to be determined.

We hypothesize that cholinergic propriospinal cells can contribute to the restoration of locomotion after spinal cord injury, and that they are suitable targets for regeneration or transplantation strategies to restore locomotion. We have preliminary evidence from recordings of commissural cells in spinal cord slices that these neurons can be strongly activated by both 5-HT and acetylcholine. This suggests that there may be overlap between the neurons possessing 5-HT receptors and the commissural cells that are active during locomotion. The ability of acetylcholine to depolarize these cells is consistent with their participation in a system of coupled propriospinal neurons that can relay a locomotor message. Further experiments are warranted to test these suggestions.

References

Ankeny, D.P., McTigue, D.M., Guan, Z., Yan, Q., Kinstler, O. and Stokes, B.T. (2001) Pegylated brain-derived neurotrophic factor shows improved distribution into the spinal cord and stimulates locomotor activity and morphological changes after injury. *Exp. Neurol.*, 170: 85–100.

Arvidsson, U., Riedl, M., Elde, R. and Meister, B. (1997) Vesicular acetylcholine transporter (VAChT) protein: A novel and unique marker for cholinergic neurons in the central and peripheral nervous systems. *J. Comp. Neurol.*, 378: 454–467.

Atsuta, Y., Abraham, P., Iwahara, T., Garcia-Rill, E. and Skinner, R.D. (1991) Control of locomotion in vitro, II. Chemical stimulation. *Somatosens. Mot. Res.*, 8: 55–63.

Barbeau, H. and Rossignol, S. (1990) The effects of serotonergic drugs on the locomotor pattern and on cutaneous reflexes of the adult chronic spinal cat. *Brain Res.*, 514: 55–67.

Barbeau, H. and Rossignol, S. (1991) Initiation and modulation of the locomotor pattern in the adult chronic spinal cat by noradrenergic, serotonergic and dopaminergic drugs. *Brain Res.*, 546: 250–260.

Barber, R.P., Phelps, P.E., Houser, C.R., Crawford, G.D., Salvaterra, P.M. and Vaughn, J.E. (1984) The morphology and distribution of neurons containing choline acetyltransferase in the adult rat spinal cord: an immunocytochemical study. *J. Comp. Neurol.*, 229: 329–346.

Berkowitz, A. and Stein, P.S.G. (1994) Activity of descending propriospinal axons in the turtle hindlimb enlargement during two forms of fictive scratching: broad tuning to regions of the body surface. *J. Neurosci.*, 14: 5089–5104.

Borges, L.F. and Iversen, S.D. (1986) Topography of choline acetyltransferase immunoreactive neurons and fibers in the rat spinal cord. *Brain Res.*, 362: 140–148.

Bregman, B.S., McAtee, M., Dai, H.N. and Kuhn, P.L. (1997) Neurotropic factors increase axonal growth after spinal cord injury and transplantation in the adult rat. *Exp. Neurol.*, 148: 475–494.

Brownstone, R.M. and Hultborn, H. (1992) Regulated and intrinsic properties of the motoneuron: Effect on input–output relations. In: L. Jami, E. Pierrot-Deseilligny and D. Zytnicki (Eds.), *Muscle Afferents and Spinal Control of Movement*. Pergamon Press, Oxford, pp. 175–181.

Carr, P., Huang, A., Noga, B., Dai, X. and Jordan, L.M. (1995) Cytochemical characterization of cat spinal neurons activated during fictive locomotion. *Brain Res. Bull.*, 37: 213–218.

Carr, P.A., Noga, B.R., Nance, D.M. and Jordan, L.M. (1994) Intracellular labelling of cat spinal neurons using a tetramethylrhodamine–dextran amine conjugate. *Brain Res. Bull.*, 34: 447–451.

Cazalets, J.R., Sqalli-Houssaini, Y. and Clarac, F. (1992) Activation of the central pattern generators for locomotion by serotonin and excitatory amino acids in neonatal rat. *J. Physiol. (Lond.)*, 455: 187–204.

Cazalets, J.R., Borde, M. and Clarac, F. (1995) Localization and organization of the central pattern generator for hindlimb locomotion in newborn rat. *J. Neurosci.*, 15: 4943–4951.

Cazalets, J.R., Borde, M. and Clarac, F. (1996) The synaptic drive from the spinal locomotor network to motoneurons in the newborn rat. *J. Neurosci.*, 16: 298–306.

Cheng, H., Cao, Y. and Olson, L. (1996) Spinal cord repair in adult paraplegic rats: partial restoration of hind limb function. *Science*, 273: 510–513.

Cina, C. and Hochman, S. (1998) Serotonin receptor pharmacology of the mammalian locomotor CPG: Activation by a 5-HT receptor agonist in the isolated rat spinal cord. *Soc. Neurosci. Abst.*, 24: 654.24.

Cohen, A.H. and Wallen, P. (1980) The neuronal correlate of locomotion in fish. 'Fictive swimming' induced in an in vitro preparation of the lamprey spinal cord. *Exp. Brain Res.*, 41: 11–18.

Connell, L.A. and Wallis, D.I. (1989) 5-Hydroxytryptamine depolarizes neonatal rat motoneurons through a receptor unrelated to an identified binding site. *Neuropharmacology*, 28: 625–634.

Cornea-Hébert, V., Riad, M., Wu, C., Singh, S.K. and Descarries, L. (1999) Cellular and subcellular distribution of the serotonin 5-HT2A receptor in the central nervous system of adult rat. *J. Comp. Neurol.*, 409: 187–209.

Cowley, K.C. and Schmidt, B.J. (1994) A comparison of motor patterns induced by *N*-methyl-D-aspartate, acetylcholine and serotonin in the in vitro neonatal rat spinal cord. *Neurosci. Lett.*, 171: 147–150.

Cowley, K.C. and Schmidt, B.J. (1995) Effects of inhibitory amino acid antagonists on reciprocal inhibitory interactions during rhythmic motor activity in the in vitro neonatal rat spinal cord. *J. Neurophysiol.*, 74: 1109–1117.

Cowley, K.C. and Schmidt, B.J. (1997) Regional distribution of the locomotor pattern-generating network in the neonatal rat spinal cord. *J. Neurophysiol.*, 77: 247–259.

Cowley, K.C. and Schmidt, B.J. (2000) Characterization of propriospinal coupling between the cervical and lumbar regions during rhythmic motor activity in the in vitro neonatal rat spinal cord. *Soc. Neurosci. Abstr.*, 26: 60.2

Deliagina, T.G., Orlovsky, G.N. and Pavlova, G.A. (1983) The capacity for generation of rhythmic oscillations is distributed in the lumbosacral spinal cord of the cat. *Exp. Brain Res.*, 53: 81–90.

Fedirchuk, B., Nielsen, J., Petersen, N. and Hultborn, H. (1998) Pharmacologically evoked fictive motor patterns in the acutely spinalized marmoset monkey (*Callithrix jacchus*). *Exp. Brain Res.*, 122: 351–361.

Feng-Chen, K.C. and Wolpaw, J.R. (1996) Operant conditioning of H-reflex changes synaptic terminals on primate motoneurons. *Proc. Natl. Acad. Sci. USA*, 93: 9206–9211.

Feraboli-Lohnherr, D., Barthe, J.-Y. and Orsal, D. (1999) Serotonin-induced activation of the network for locomotion in adult spinal rats. *J. Neurosci. Res.*, 55: 87–98.

Fornal, C., Auerbach, S. and Jacobs, B.L. (1985) Activity of serotonin-containing neurons in nucleus raphe magnus in freely moving cats. *Exp. Neurol.*, 88: 590–608.

Fraser, D.D. and MacVicar, B.A. (1996) Cholinergic-dependent plateau potential in hippocampal CA1 pyramidal neurons. *J. Neurosci.*, 16: 4113–4128.

Fyda, D.M., Vriend, J. and Jordan, L.M. (2002) Release of monoamines and related metabolites in the thoracolumbar spinal cord of neonatal rats during brainstem electrically-evoked fictive locomotion. *J. Neurosci.*, submitted.

Gerin, C. and Privat, A. (1998) Direct evidence for the link between monoaminergic descending pathways and motor activity, II. A study with microdialysis probes implanted in the ventral horn of the spinal cord. *Brain Res.*, 794: 169–173.

Gerin, C., Becquet, D. and Privat, A. (1995) Direct evidence for the link between monoaminergic descending pathways and motor activity, I. A study with microdialysis probes implanted in the ventral funiculus of the spinal cord. *Brain Res.*, 704: 191–201.

Giménez y Ribotta, M., Orsal, D., Feraboli-Lohnherr, D. and Privat, A. (1998) Recovery of locomotion following transplantation of monoaminergic neurons in the spinal cord of paraplegic rats. *Ann. N.Y. Acad. Sci.*, 860: 393–412.

Giménez y Ribotta, M., Provencher, J., Feraboli-Lohnherr, D., Rossignol, S., Privat, A. and Orsal, D. (2000) Activation of locomotion in adult chronic spinal rats is achieved by transplantation of embryonic raphe cells reinnervating a precise lumbar level. *J. Neurosci.*, 20: 5144–5152.

Grillner, S. (1974) On the generation of locomotion in the spinal dogfish. *Exp. Brain Res.*, 20: 459–470.

Grillner, S. (1981) Control of locomotion in bipeds, tetrapods, and fish. In: S.R. Geiger, V.B. Brooks, J.M. Brookhart and V.B. Mountcastle (Eds.), *Handbook of Physiology — The Nervous System*, Vol. 2, Part 2. Waverly Press, Baltimore, MD, pp. 1179–1236.

Guertin, P.A. and Hounsgaard, J. (1999) L-type calcium channels but not N-methyl-D-aspartate receptor channels mediate rhythmic activity induced by cholinergic agonist in motoneurons from turtle spinal cord slices. *Neurosci. Lett.*, 261: 81–84.

Guest, J.D., Rao, A., Olson, L., Bartlett Bunge, M. and Bunge, R.P. (1997) The ability of human Schwann cell grafts to promote regeneration in the transected nude rat spinal cord. *Exp. Neurol.*, 148: 502–522.

Hagevik, A. and McClellan, A.D. (1994) Coupling of spinal locomotor networks in larval lamprey revealed by receptor blockers for inhibitory amino acids: neurophysiology and computer modeling. *J. Neurophysiol.*, 72: 1810–1829.

Hasan, S.J., Keirstead, H.S., Muir, G.D. and Steeves, J.D. (1993) Axonal regeneration contributes to repair of injured brainstem–spinal neurons in embryonic chick. *J. Neurosci.*, 13: 492–507.

Heisler, L.K. and Tecott, L.H. (2000) A paradoxical locomotor response in serotonin 5-HT$_{2C}$ receptor mutant mice. *J. Neurosci.*, 20: RC71 (1–5).

Ho, S. and O'Donovan, M.J. (1993) Regionalization and intersegmental coordination of rhythm-generating networks in the spinal cord of the chick embryo. *J. Neurosci.*, 13: 1354–1371.

Hoover, J.E. and Durkovic, R.G. (1992) Retrograde labelling of lumbosacral interneurons following injections of red and green fluorescent microspheres into hindlimb motor nuclei of the cat. *Somatosens. Mot. Res.*, 9: 211–226.

Hounsgaard, J. and Kiehn, O. (1989) Serotonin-induced bistability of turtle motoneurons caused by a nifedipine-sensitive calcium plateau potential. *J. Physiol. (Lond.)*, 414: 265–282.

Hounsgaard, J. and Svirskis, G. (1998) Transmitter regulation of plateau properties in turtle motoneurons. *J. Neurophysiol.*, 79: 45–50.

Houser, C.R., Crawford, G.D., Barber, R.P., Salvaterra, P.M. and Vaughn, J.E. (1983) Organization and morphological characteristics of cholinergic neurons: an immunocytochemical study with a monoclonal antibody to choline acetyltransferase. *Brain Res.*, 266: 97–119.

Huang, A., Noga, B.R., Carr, P., Fedirchuk, B. and Jordan, L.M. (2000) Spinal cholinergic neurons activated during locomotion: immunohistochemical localization and electrophysiological characterization. *J. Neurophysiol.*, 83: 3537–3547.

Iwahara, T., Atsuta, Y., Garcia-Rill, E. and Skinner, R.D. (1991) Locomotion induced by spinal cord stimulation in the neonate rat in vitro. *Somatosens. Mot. Res.*, 8: 281–287.

Jacobs, B.L. and Azmitia, E.C. (1992) Structure and function of brain serotonin system. *Physiol. Rev.*, 72: 165–229.

Jakeman, L.B., Wei, P., Guan, Z. and Stokes, B.T. (1998) Brain-derived neurotrophic factor stimulates hindlimb stepping and sprouting of cholinergic fibers after spinal cord injury. *Exp. Neurol.*, 154: 170–184.

Jiang, Z., Carlin, K.P. and Brownstone, R.M. (1999) An in vitro functionally mature mouse spinal cord preparation for the study of spinal motor networks. *Brain Res.*, 816: 493–499.

Jordan, L.M., Nance, D.M. and Madec, K. (2000) 5-HT7 Receptor immunoreactivity is found in some spinal neurons that express C-FOS following treadmill locomotion in the adult rat. *Soc. Neurosci. Abstr.*, 26: 59.2.

Kazennikov, O.V., Shik, M.L. and Yakovleva, G.V. (1983) Responses of upper cervical spinal neurons in cats to stimulation of the brain-stem locomotor region at different frequencies. *Neurophysiology*, 15: 256–261.

Kazennikov, O.V. and Shik, M.L. (1988) Propagation of activity along the 'stepping strip' of the cat spinal cord. *Neirofiziologiya*, 20: 763–769.

Kiehn, O. and Kjaerulff, O. (1996) Spatiotemporal characteristics of 5-HT and dopamine-induced rhythmic hindlimb activity in the in vitro neonatal rat. *J. Neurophysiol.*, 75: 1472–1482.

Kiehn, O., Sillar, K.T., Kjaerulff, O. and McDearmid, J.R. (1999) Effects of noradrenaline on locomotor rhythm-generating networks in the isolated neonatal rat spinal cord. *J. Neurophysiol.*, 82: 741–746.

Kim, D., Adipudi, V., Shibayama, M., Giszter, S., Tessler, A., Murray, M. and Simansky, K.J. (1999) Direct agonists for serotonin receptors enhance locomotor function in rats that received neural transplants after neonatal spinal transection. *J. Neurosci.*, 19: 6213–6224.

Kjaerulff, O. and Kiehn, O. (1996) Distribution of networks generating and coordinating locomotor activity in the neonatal rat spinal cord in vitro: A lesion study. *J. Neurosci.*, 16: 5777–5794.

Kjaerulff, O. and Kiehn, O. (1997) Crossed rhythmic synaptic

138

input to motoneurons during selective activation of the contralateral spinal locomotor network. *J. Neurosci.*, 17: 9433–9447.

Kremer, E. and Lev-Tov, A. (1997) Localization of the spinal network associated with generation of hindlimb locomotion in the neonatal rat and organization of its transverse coupling system. *J. Neurophysiol.*, 77: 1155–1170.

Kudo, N. and Yamada, T. (1987) *N*-methyl-D,L-aspartate-induced locomotor activity in a spinal cord–hindlimb muscles preparation of the newborn rat studied in vitro. *Neurosci. Lett.*, 75: 43–48.

Kudo, N., Ozaki, S. and Yamada, T. (1991) Ontogeny of rhythmic activity in the spinal cord of the rat. In: M. Shimamura, S. Grillner and V.R. Edgerton (Eds.), *Neurobiological Basis of Human Locomotion*. Japan Scientific Societies Press, Tokyo, pp. 127–136.

Legendre, P., Guzman, A., Dupouy, B. and Vincent, J.D. (1989) Excitatory effect of serotonin on pacemaker neurons in spinal cord cell culture. *Neuroscience*, 28: 201–209.

Li, W., Ochalski, A.Y., Brimijoin, S., Jordan, L.M. and Nagy, J.I. (1995) C-terminals on motoneurons: EM localization of cholinergic markers in adult rats and antibody-induced depletion in neonates. *Neuroscience*, 65: 879–991.

MacLean, J.N. and Schmidt, B.J. (2001) Voltage-sensitivity of motoneuron NMDA receptor channels is modulated by serotonin in the neonatal rat spinal cord. *J. Neurophysiol.*, 86: 1131–1138.

MacLean, J.N., Cowley, K.C. and Schmidt, B.J. (1998) NMDA receptor-mediated oscillatory activity in the neonatal rat spinal cord is serotonin dependent. *J. Neurophysiol.*, 79: 2804–2808.

Magnuson, D.S., Schramm, M.J. and MacLean, J.N. (1995) Long-duration, frequency-dependent motor responses evoked by ventrolateral funiculus stimulation in the neonatal rat spinal cord. *Neurosci. Lett.*, 192: 97–100.

Magnuson, D.S.K. and Trinder, T.C. (1997) Locomotor rhythm evoked by ventrolateral funiculus stimulation in the neonatal rat spinal cord in vitro. *J. Neurophysiol.*, 77: 200–206.

Magnuson, D.S.K., Trinder, T.C., Zhang, Y.P., Burke, D., Morassutti, D.J. and Shields, C.B. (1999) Comparing deficits following excitotoxic and contusion injuries in the thoracic and lumbar spinal cord of the adult rat. *Exp. Neurol.*, 156: 191–204.

Marcoux, J. and Rossignol, S. (2000) Initiating or blocking locomotion in spinal cats by applying noradrenergic drugs to restricted lumbar spinal segments. *J. Neurosci.*, 20: 8577–8585.

McClellan, A.D. (1994) Time course of locomotor recovery and functional regeneration in spinal cord-transected lamprey: in vitro preparations. *J. Neurophysiol.*, 72: 847–860.

Mortin, L.I. and Stein, P.S.G. (1989) Spinal cord segments containing key elements of the central pattern generators for three forms of scratch reflex in the turtle. *J. Neurosci.*, 9: 2285–2296.

Nagy, J.I., Yamamoto, T. and Jordan, L.M. (1993) Evidence for the cholinergic nature of c-terminals associated with subsurface cisterns in alpha-motoneurons of rat. *Synapse*, 15: 17–32.

Nishimaru, H., Takizawa, H. and Kudo, N. (2000) 5-Hydroxytryptamine-induced locomotor rhythm in the neonatal mouse spinal cord in vitro. *Neurosci. Lett.*, 280: 187–190.

Noga, B.R., Kriellaars, D.J. and Jordan, L.M. (1991) The effect of selective brainstem or spinal cord lesions on treadmill locomotion evoked by stimulation of the mesencephalic or pontomedullary locomotor regions. *J. Neurosci.*, 11: 1691–1700.

Noga, B.R., Cowley, K.C., Huang, A., Jordan, L.M. and Schmidt, B.J. (1993) Effects of inhibitory amino acid antagonists on locomotor rhythm in the decerebrate cat. *Soc. Neurosci. Abstr.*, 19: 225.4.

Orsal, D., Barthe, J.-Y., Antri, M., Feraboli-Lohnherr, D., Yakovleff, A., Giménez y Ribotta, M., Privat, A., Provencher, J. and Rossignol, S. (2002) Locomotor recovery in chronic spinal rat; long-term pharmacological treatment or transplantation of embryonic neurons. In: L. McKerracher, G. Doucet and S. Rossignol (Eds.), *Spinal Cord Trauma: Neural Repair and Functional Recovery*. Progress in Brain Research, Vol. 137, Elsevier, Amsterdam, pp. 213–230.

Panchin, Y.V., Perrins, R.J. and Roberts, A. (1991) The action of acetylcholine on the locomotor central pattern generator for swimming in *Xenopus* embryos. *J. Exp. Biol.*, 161: 527–531.

Perrins, R. and Roberts, A. (1995a) Cholinergic and electrical motoneuron-to-motoneuron synapses contribute to on-cycle excitation during swimming in *Xenopus* embryos. *J. Neurophysiol.*, 73: 1005–1012.

Perrins, R. and Roberts, A. (1995b) Cholinergic contribution to excitation in a spinal locomotor central pattern generator in *Xenopus* embryos. *J. Neurophysiol.*, 73: 1013–1019.

Perrins, R. and Roberts, A. (1995c) Cholinergic and electrical synapses between synergistic spinal motoneurons in the *Xenopus laevis* embryo. *J. Physiol. (Lond.)*, 485: 135–144.

Phelps, P.E., Barber, R.P., Houser, C.R., Crawford, G.D., Salvaterra, P.M. and Vaughn, J.E. (1984) Postnatal development of neurons containing choline acetyltransferase in rat spinal cord: An immunocytochemical study. *J. Comp. Neurol.*, 229: 347–361.

Prochazka, A. and Mushahwar, V.K. (1999) Spinal cord microstimulation: activation of contralateral muscles. *Soc. Neurosci. Abstr.*, 25: 2, p. 1152.

Pullen, A.H. and Sears, T.A. (1983) Trophism between c-type axon terminals and thoracic motoneurons in the cat. *J. Physiol. (Lond.)*, 337: 373–388.

Roberts, A. and Khan, J.A. (1982) Intracellular recordings from spinal neurons during 'swimming' in paralysed amphibian embryos. *Philos. Trans. R. Soc. Lond. B. Biol. Sci.*, 296: 213–228.

Rossignol, S., Chau, C., Brustein, E., Belanger, M., Barbeau, H. and Drew, T. (1996) Locomotor capacities after complete and partial lesions of the spinal cord. *Acta Neurobiol. Exp.*, 56: 449–463.

Rossignol, S., Chau, C., Brustein, E., Giroux, N., Bouyer, L., Barbeau, H. and Reader, T.A. (1998) Pharmacological activation and modulation of the central pattern generator for locomotion in the cat. *Ann. N.Y. Acad. Sci.*, 860: 346–359.

Rouse Jr., D.T. and McClellan, A.D. (1997) Descending propriospinal neurons in normal and spinal cord-transected lamprey. *Exp. Neurol.*, 146: 113–124.

Schmidt, B.J. and Jordan, L.M. (2000) The role of serotonin in reflex modulation and locomotor rhythm production in the mammalian spinal cord. *Brain Res. Bull.*, 53: 689–710.

Sherriff, F.E. and Henderson, Z. (1994) A cholinergic propriospinal innervation of the rat spinal cord. *Brain Res.*, 634: 150–154.

Shik, M.L. (1983) Action of the brainstem locomotor region on spinal stepping generators via propriospinal pathways. In: C.C. Kao, R.P. Bunge and P.J. Reier (Eds.), *Spinal Cord Reconstruction*. Raven Press, New York, pp. 421–434.

Sillar, K.T. and Simmers, A.J. (1994) 5-HT induces NMDA receptor-mediated intrinsic oscillations in embryonic amphibian spinal neurons. *Proc. R. Soc. Lond. B. Biol. Sci.*, 255: 139–145.

Smith, J.C. and Feldman, J.L. (1987) In vitro brainstem–spinal cord preparations for study of motor systems for mammalian respiration and locomotion. *J. Neurosci. Methods*, 21: 321–333.

Smith, J.C., Feldman, J.L. and Schmidt, B.J. (1988) Neural mechanisms generating locomotion studied in mammalian brain stem–spinal cord in vitro. *FASEB J.*, 2283-2288.

Steeves, J.D. and Jordan, L.M. (1980) Localization of a descending pathway in the spinal cord which is necessary for controlled treadmill locomotion. *Neurosci. Lett.*, 20: 283–288.

Stelzner, D.J. and Cullen, J.M. (1991) Do propriospinal projections contribute to hindlimb recovery when all long tracts are cut in neonatal or weanling rats? *Exp. Neurol.*, 114: 193–205.

Takahashi, T. and Berger, A.J. (1990) Direct excitation of rat spinal motoneurons by serotonin. *J. Physiol. (Lond.)*, 423: 63–76.

Veasey, S.C., Fornal, C.A., Metzler, C.W. and Jacobs, B.L. (1995) Response of serotonergic caudal raphe neurons in relation to specific motor activities in freely moving cats. *J. Neurosci.*, 15: 5346–5359.

Viala, D. and Buser, P. (1969) The effects of DOPA and 5-HTP on rhythmic efferent discharges in hind limb nerves in the rabbit. *Brain Res.*, 12: 437–443.

Whelan, P., Bonnot, A. and O'Donovan, M.J. (2000) Properties of rhythmic activity generated by the isolated spinal cord of the neonatal mouse. *J. Neurophysiol.*, 84: 2821–2833.

White, S.R. and Fung, S.J. (1989) Serotonin depolarizes cat spinal motoneurons in situ and decreases motoneuron afterhyperpolarizing potentials. *Brain Res.*, 502: 205–213.

White, S.R. and Neuman, R.S. (1980) Facilitation of spinal motoneuron excitability by 5-hydroxytryptamine and noradrenaline. *Brain Res.*, 188: 119–127.

Xu, X.M., Guenard, V., Kleitman, N., Aebischer, P. and Bartlett Bunge, M. (1995) A combination of BDNF and NT-3 promotes supraspinal axonal regeneration into Schwann cell grafts in adult rat thoracic spinal cord. *Exp. Neurol.*, 134: 261–272.

Yamaguchi, T. (1986) Descending pathways eliciting forelimb stepping in the lateral funiculus: experimental studies with stimulation and lesions of the cervical cord in decerebrate cats. *Brain Res.*, 379: 125–136.

Zaporozhets, E. and Schmidt, B.J. (2001) Propriospinal connections mediate bulbospinal activation of locomotor-like activity in the in vitro neonatal rat spinal cord. *Soc. Neurosci. Abstr.*, 27: 297.11.

Zieglgansberger, W. and Reiter, C. (1974) A cholinergic mechanism in the spinal cord of cats. *Neuropharmacology*, 13: 519–527.

Ziskind-Conhaim, L., Seebach, B.S. and Gao, B.X. (1993) Changes in serotonin-induced potentials during spinal cord development. *J. Neurophysiol.*, 69: 1338–1349.

L. McKerracher, G. Doucet and S. Rossignol (Eds.)
Progress in Brain Research, Vol. 137
© 2002 Elsevier Science B.V. All rights reserved

CHAPTER 11

Use of robotics in assessing the adaptive capacity of the rat lumbar spinal cord

Ray D. de Leon [1], David J. Reinkensmeyer [5], Wojciech K. Timoszyk [5], Nicolas J. London [3], Roland R. Roy [2] and V. Reggie Edgerton [2,3,4*]

[1] *Department of Kinesiology and Nutritional Science, California State University, Los Angeles, CA 90032-8162, USA*
[2] *Brain Research Institute, University of California, Los Angeles, CA 90095-1761, USA*
[3] *Department of Physiological Science, University of California, Los Angeles, CA 90095-1527, USA*
[4] *Department of Neurobiology, University of California, Los Angeles, CA 90095-1527, USA*
[5] *Department of Mechanical and Aerospace Engineering, University of California, Irvine, CA 92697, USA*

Abstract: We have developed a robotic device that can record the trajectory of the hindlimb movements in rats. The robotic device can also impose programmed forces on the limbs during stepping. In the present paper we describe experiments using this robotic device, i.e. the rat stepper, to determine whether step training improves the locomotor capacity of adult rats that received complete spinal cord transections as neonates. We also determined to what extent the locomotor patterns can be maintained when the step cycle is physically perturbed by the robotic device. The results of the present study demonstrate that a robotic device can be used effectively to quantify the improvements in the locomotor capacity of spinal transected rats that occurs over a period of step training. The present results also demonstrate that when an external force is imposed to disrupt the step cycle, the spinal cord has the neural control elements necessary to normalize the kinematics over a number of steps, in the face of the disrupted forces.

Introduction

The lumbosacral spinal cord can control full weight-bearing stepping over a range of treadmill speeds (Lovely et al., 1986; Barbeau and Rossignol, 1987; Belanger et al., 1996; de Leon et al., 1998a) and can adjust the step cycle so that stepping can continue uninterrupted even when it is physically perturbed within (Rossignol and Drew, 1986) or over a series of steps (Hodgson et al., 1994). However, it remains unclear as to what parameters are being controlled by the nervous system to execute the kinetic and kinematic complexities associated with locomotion (Windhorst et al., 1989). To address this issue we have developed a robotic device, subsequently called the rat stepper, that consists of two robotic arms that are attached proximal to the ankles of the rat, a motorized body weight support system and a treadmill (Reinkensmeyer et al., 2000; Timoszyk et al., 2002; Edgerton et al., 2001). This device can function in multiple modes, e.g., as a passive device to record the trajectory of the movements of the limbs or as an active device to impose programmed forces on the limbs during selected segments of the step cycle. In the present paper we describe experiments using this robotic device to determine whether step training improves the locomotor capacity of complete spinally transected rats (passive mode) and to determine to what extent the locmotor patterns can be sustained when the step cycle is physically perturbed (active and passive modes).

* Correspondence to: V.R. Edgerton, University of California, Los Angeles, Department of Physiological Science, 1804 Life Sciences, 621 Charles E. Young Drive South, Los Angeles, CA 90095-1527, USA. Tel.: +1-310-825-1910; Fax: +1-310-267-2071; E-mail: vre@ucla.edu

Methods

We established the usefulness of the rat stepper for studying locomotion in an initial series of experiments using rats ($n = 28$) that received a complete spinal cord transection at a mid-thoracic level at five days of age (London et al., 2000). At 25 days of age the rats were assigned randomly and equally to one of two groups: (1) spinal non-trained; or (2) spinal step-trained, i.e. trained to step on a treadmill with the hindlimbs for 10 min/day, 5 days/week for 12 weeks. Bipedal hindlimb stepping performance in the trained rats was assessed before training, and after 6 and 12 weeks of step training. Non-trained rats were tested on the same schedule. During testing, locomotor ability was assessed with the robotic device in a passive mode and with two levels of body weight support, i.e. at a normal load level (50% body weight support) and at half of the normal load level (75% body weight support). The locomotor capacity of the rats also was assessed from video recordings when the robotic devices were not attached.

In the second series of experiments, we used the rat stepper to impose a force field during swing, i.e. an upward force was applied to one ankle whenever the hindlimb moved forward (de Leon et al., 2000). The magnitude of the force field generated was proportional to the forward velocity of the robotic arm during the swing phase (Fig. 1). One hindlimb was perturbed while the contralateral hindlimb was not exposed to the force field. The experiment consisted of executing 20 step cycles without any force field applied, i.e. the robotic arms acting passively, followed by 20 step cycles with the force field applied. This pattern of 20 steps with and 20 steps without a force field was repeated 6 times (a total of 240 steps). Electromyographic signals were recorded from the rectus femoris (a hip flexor, knee extensor) and semitendinosus (a hip extensor and knee flexor) muscles via chronic intramuscular implants as described previously (de Leon et al., 1994).

Results

Experimental series 1

The number of consecutive steps that could be performed within 1 min by each non-trained and trained

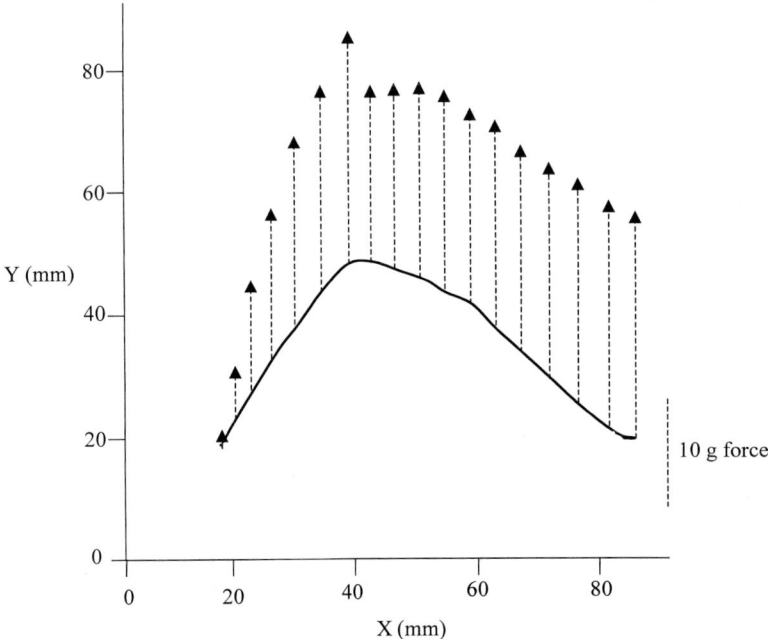

Fig. 1. The rat stepper was used to impose an upward force (arrows) during the swing phase of a step cycle. The vertical force was applied as the hindlimb moved forward. The magnitude of the vertical force (length of the arrows) was proportional to the forward velocity of the robotic arm. Force calibration bar is equal to 10 grams of force.

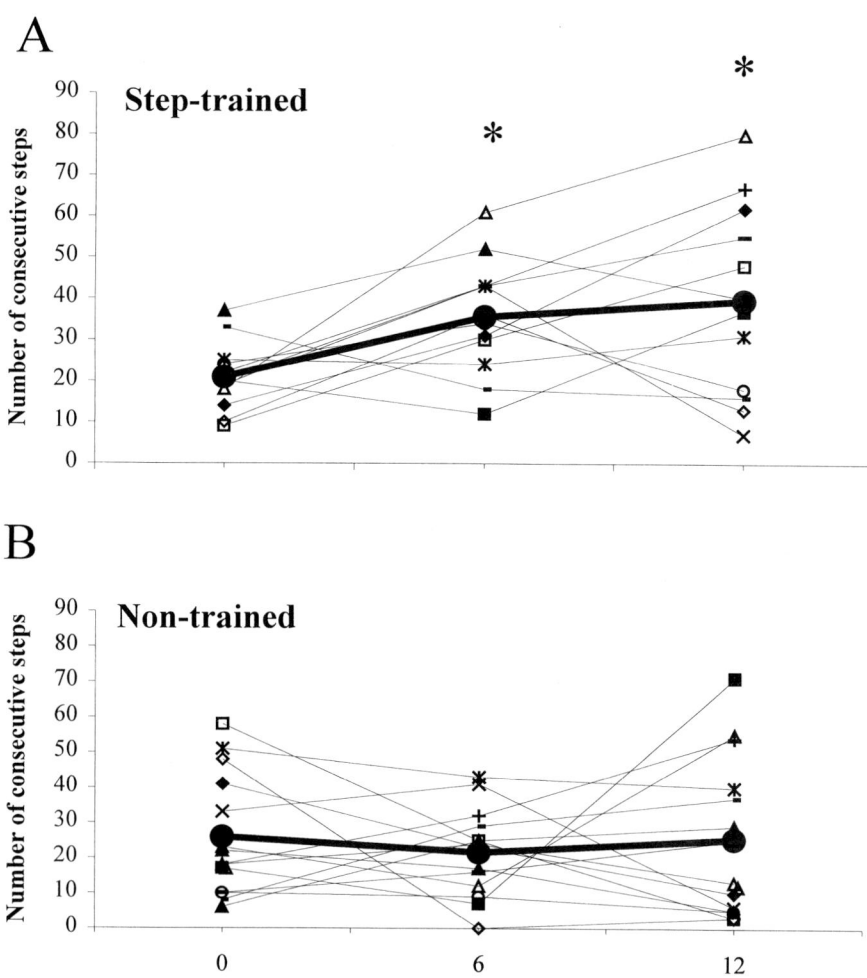

Fig. 2. The maximum number of consecutive steps performed in 1 min by each step-trained (A) and non-trained (B) rat before any training and after 6 and 12 weeks of step training. Only steps that were executed on the plantar surfaces of the paws were counted at a body weight support level of 75%. Each symbol represents an individual rat. The large symbols (circles, thick line) are the means for each time point. *, statistically significant from week 0 ($p < 0.05$). Note that there was improvement in the maximum number of steps taken by the step-trained, but not the non-trained, rats.

spinal rat was measured before and after 6 and 12 weeks of treatment. There was a significant improvement in the mean number of steps performed by the trained rats at both 6 and 12 weeks relative to before training started (see thick line, Fig. 2). In contrast, the stepping ability of the non-trained rats was unchanged over the same time period. The stepping performance was determined from video recordings without the attachment of the robotic arms.

This difference in the ability to consistently execute step cycles was also evident in the trajectories measured by the rat stepper device in trained and non-trained rats. An example of the stepping performance for a step-trained (A) and a non-trained (B) spinal rat with the robotic arms attached in a passive mode is shown in Fig. 3. Although some successful steps were performed during a period of 32 s of recording, the trajectories of the robotic arm attached to the shank of the lower leg of the non-trained rat show more variability than the trajectories

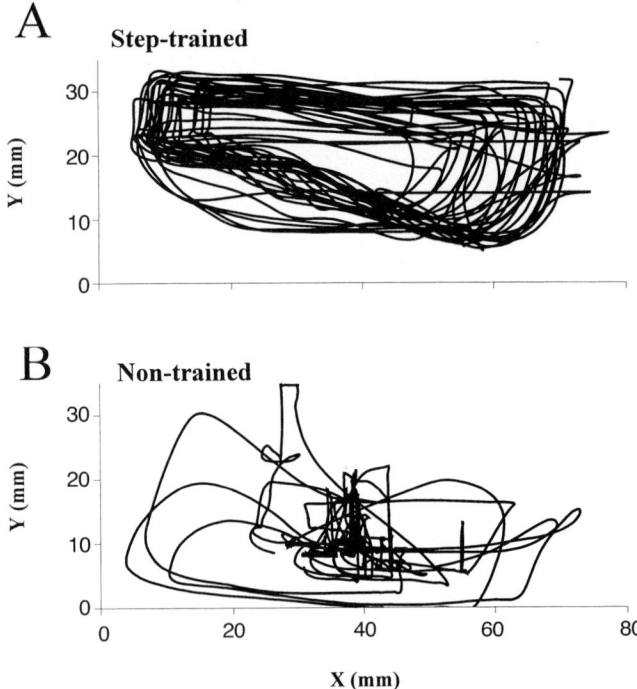

Fig. 3. Scatterplots showing the limb trajectories during stepping (32 s) of a step-trained (A) and a non-trained (B) rat as measured by the robotic arms attached in a passive mode to the ankle of one limb. Note the lower number of steps and the higher variability in the trajectories of the non-trained (B) than the step-trained (A) rat.

in the trained rats (Fig. 3). Based on the trajectory patterns of the shank, more consecutive and consistent steps were observed in the spinal rats that were step trained for 12 weeks than in non-trained rats (Fig. 3).

To more fully analyze the step kinematics based on the trajectories shown in Fig. 3, software was developed to detect specific components of the step cycle. For example, the point at which the paw is lifted from the belt and the phase of the step cycle during which the paw touches the treadmill were defined by a combination of velocity magnitudes in the x and y directions (Fig. 4A,B). The identification of the phases of the step cycle were verified from video recordings made simultaneously with the trajectories of the robotic arms. Based on these detection methods, the trained spinal rats performed a greater number of steps than the non-trained rats (Fig. 4C).

In summary, training in spinal rats transected as neonates: (1) improved locomotor capacity based on the number of successful steps measured from video

recordings; and (2) resulted in a more consistent stepping pattern when tested and measured using the rat stepper. Together, these results demonstrate a clear improvement in the ability of the trained rats to perform weight-bearing stepping compared to the rats that were not trained to step.

Experimental series 2

In the second series of experiments, we examined the adaptive capability of the spinal cord to control the kinematics of the hindlimbs when the swing phase is disrupted by imposing an upward force. The trajectories of one hindlimb during a step taken before the perturbation was induced (Fig. 5A), a step taken during the initial exposure to the perturbation (Fig. 5B) and a step taken when the vertical force field was imposed after multiple exposures to the perturbation (Fig. 5C) are shown in Fig. 5. Compared to the initial control trajectory, the first disruption resulted in a prolonged swing phase and step cycle (compare Fig. 5A and B). After 5 exposures to the pattern of

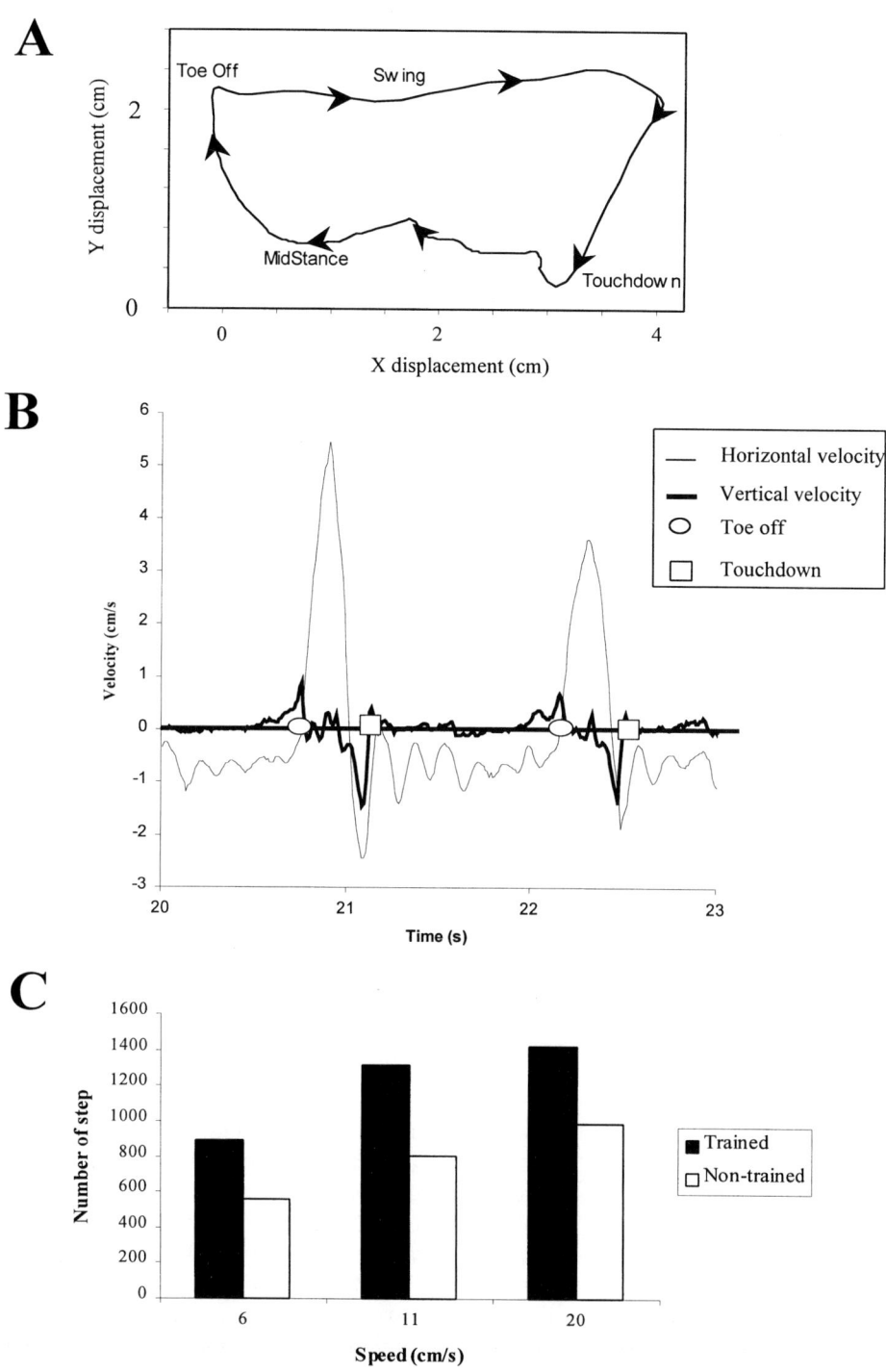

Fig. 4. (A) The determination of the step kinematics, e.g., toe off and touch down, was based on a combination of velocity magnitudes in the x (horizontal) and y (vertical) directions (B). The trajectory shown in (A) corresponds to the scatterplot of the first step depicted in (B). (C) The total number of steps performed by step-trained ($n = 14$) and non-trained ($n = 14$) rats in 1 min at 11 cm/s at 75% body weight support. These data were collected after 8 weeks of training. Note that step-trained rats perform more steps than non-trained rats at each speed tested.

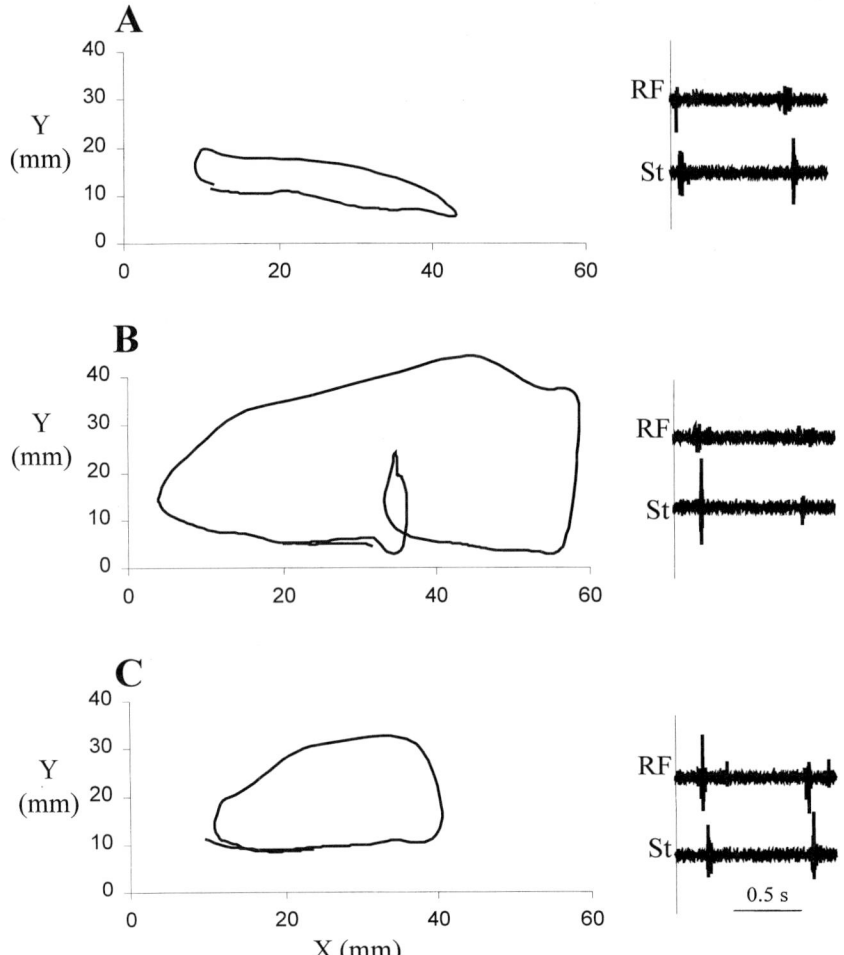

Fig. 5. The limb trajectories (left column) and corresponding EMG activity of the rectus femoris (RF) and semitendinosus (St) muscles (right column) before (A), during the initial exposure to a perturbation (upward force field) during the swing phase of the step (B), and after the fifth exposure to the same perturbation (C) are shown for one representative spinal rat. Note the changes in the limb trajectories and EMG patterns after the first perturbation and the more normal patterns after the fifth exposure. See text for details.

20 steps without and 20 steps with a force field, the spinal cord was able to control the kinematics such that the trajectories were approaching normal in the presence of the force perturbation during the swing phase of the step (compare Fig. 5A and C).

The EMG activity patterns of the rectus femoris and semitendinosus muscles for the same step cycles also are shown in Fig. 5. These data demonstrate that the activation patterns during the step with the initial disruption of the swing differ from those recorded before the perturbation was induced. Furthermore, the results suggest that the EMG patterns further

adjust with repetitive exposure to the disruption, consistent with the changing kinematics (compare Fig. 5B and C).

The effect of the vertical force field on the step cycle during the series of 20 steps with and 20 steps without the perturbation changed dramatically as this series was repeated five times (Fig. 6). The mean swing duration was relatively constant for all of the series of stepping without the force field. The swing duration was elevated more than two-fold during the initial force field series of stepping. However, the length of the swing phase then declined rapidly,

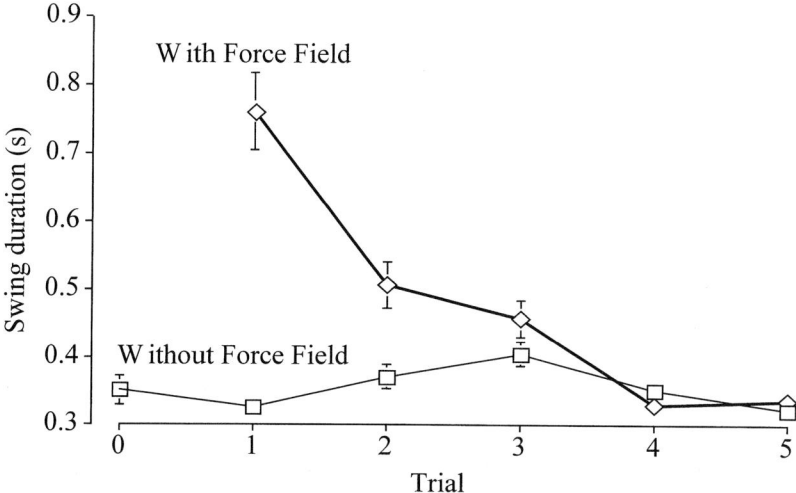

Fig. 6. The changes in swing duration over five trials with and without an imposed perturbation (upward force field) for one representative rat.Note that the swing duration is elevated by more than two-fold during the first perturbation and then quickly returns to levels observed without any perturbation. Swing durations were consistent across trials when the stepping was performed without any force field. Bars are S.E.M.

and there was no obvious difference between the step sequences performed with and those without the force field by the third series.

The results from the force field experiments indicate that the neural control of stepping is designed to regulate the limb kinematics such that the limb trajectory will follow a pattern within some limited 'kinematic envelope' that approximates normal stepping.

Discussion

The feasibility of using robotics to study rat bipedal locomotion is demonstrated

The results of the present study demonstrate that a robotic device can be used effectively to quantify the progression of changes in the locomotor capacity of spinal transected rats that can occur over a period of step training. Spinal rats were trained for 12 weeks with robotic arms attached to their ankles, thus enabling the quantification of stepping ability throughout the entire duration of the experiment. Although the specific data are not included in the present paper, the kinematics of the hindlimbs during stepping with and without the robotic device have been compared in the same rats. The kinematics were not impeded significantly by the attachment of

the robotic arm (unpublished observations). Future experiments, however, will be required to address whether the rat stepper also can be effective in measuring locomotion in normal rats and in assessing locomotor recovery in other models of spinal cord injury, e.g., following a hemisection.

The present results demonstrate the level of detail that can be extracted from the trajectory data obtained from the robotic arms. For example, we show that specific phases of the step cycle can be identified from these trajectories, thus allowing a rapid analysis of hundreds or thousands of step cycles. Finally, the results of these experiments indicate that the robotic device can be used effectively to study a variety of acute interventions to locomotion, such as electrical stimulation of cutaneous nerves, pharmacological manipulations and variations in the levels of loading, with most of the kinematics being available for assessment virtually online.

The fact that the rats learned to step was expected given a previous series of controlled experiments in adult cats designed to differentiate the recovery of stepping that can be attributable to spontaneous recovery vs. that attributable to training of a specific motor task (de Leon et al., 1998a,b, 1999a,b,c). The results from the present series of experiments are consistent with the concept of the specificity of the training, i.e. the type of motor task practiced was the motor task that showed improved function (Edgerton et al., 1997a,b; de Leon et al., 1998a,b, 1999a,b,c). The present results differ from previous studies in that the learning occurred in rats that received complete spinal cord transections at 5 days of age, i.e. before the rats can perform any weight-bearing steps (Altman and Sudarshan, 1975).

The spinal control of locomotion is designed to generate stepping within a well defined 'kinematic window'

The neuromuscular system involved in locomotion seems to be designed to step within a 'kinematic window'. However, the limits of this window are poorly understood as are the neural control mechanisms which can accommodate to disruptions of the step cycle. Somehow this 'kinematic window' must be translated from some neurally-based 'sensorimotor window'. Given that this accommodation occurred in complete spinal rats, it is clear that these sensorimotor pathways must be localized within the lumbosacral spinal networks.

The present results clearly demonstrate that when an external force is imposed to disrupt the step cycle, the spinal cord has the neural control elements necessary to normalize the kinematics, not immediately but over a number of steps, in the face of the disrupted forces. This adaptive ability must encompass some corrective action on the part of the sensory input, on the interneurons which process the sensory information projected to the spinal cord and on the motor components which execute those decisions. Clearly, we do not know how these spinal circuits accommodate to this significant disruption in forces during locomotion since even the nature of the control during stepping in intact animals is poorly understood. Neither is it clear how the spinal cord interprets the imposed disruption and the associated sensory information as being outside the 'kinematic window' nor how motor adjustments are made to return the kinematics back to a more normal pattern. Although some mechanical elements of the limb would seem to play a role in defining this 'kinematic window', it alone cannot explain the accommodations that are made over a series of consecutively disrupted steps. Some insight into this accommodation, however, is suggested by the neural adjustments

reflected by the clear changes in the EMG patterns that occurred during the early and late periods of application of force fields during swing (Fig. 5). The mechanical consequences of these altered EMG patterns and how these changes are accomplished remains to be determined. In addition to the changes in the activation patterns of those motor pools that control the kinematics of stepping, the 'kinematic window' for a given animal is defined to some degree by the functional and structural properties of the limbs that have evolved for a given species.

Acknowledgements

This work was supported in part by NIH Grant NS16333 and Christopher Reeve Paralysis Foundation DA1-9902-2.

References

Altman, J. and Sudarshan, K. (1975) Postnatal development of locomotion in the laboratory rat. *Anim. Behav.*, 23: 896–920.

Barbeau, H. and Rossignol, S. (1987) Recovery of locomotion after chronic spinalization in the adult cat. *Brain Res.*, 412: 84–95.

Belanger, M., Drew, T., Provencher, J. and Rossignol, S. (1996) A. comparison of treadmill locomotion in adult cats before and after spinal transection. *J. Neurophysiol.*, 76: 471–491.

de Leon, R.D., Hodgson, J.A., Roy, R.R. and Edgerton, V.R. (1994) Extensor- and flexor-like modulation within motor pools of the rat hindlimb during treadmill locomotion and swimming. *Brain Res.*, 654: 241–250.

de Leon, R.D., Hodgson, J.A., Roy, R.R. and Edgerton, V.R. (1998a) Locomotor capacity attributable to step training versus spontaneous recovery following spinalization in cats. *J. Neurophysiol.*, 79: 1329–1340.

de Leon, R.D., Hodgson, J.A., Roy, R.R. and Edgerton, V.R. (1998b) Full weight-bearing hindlimb standing following stand training in the adult spinal cat. *J. Neurophysiol.*, 80: 83–91.

de Leon, R.D., Hodgson, J.A., Roy, R.R. and Edgerton, V.R. (1999a) The retention of hindlimb stepping ability in adult spinal cats after the cessation of step training. *J. Neurophysiol.*, 81: 85–94.

de Leon, R.D., Hodgson, J.A., Roy, R.R. and Edgerton, V.R. (1999b) Hindlimb locomotor and postural training modulates glycinergic inhibition in the spinal cord of the adult spinal cat. *J. Neurophysiol.*, 82: 359–369.

de Leon, R.D., London, N., Hodgson, J.A., Roy, R.R. and Edgerton, V.R. (1999c) Failure analysis of stepping in spinal cats. In: M.D. Binder (Ed.), *Peripheral and Spinal Mechanisms in the Neural Control of Movement.* Volume 123, Elsevier, Amsterdam, pp. 341–348.

de Leon, R.D., Timoszyk, W., London, N., Joynes, R.L., Roy, R.R., Reinkensmeyer, D.J. and Edgerton, V.R. (2000) Locomotor adaptations to robot-applied force fields in spinally transected rats. *Soc. Neurosci. Abstr.*, 26: 697.

Edgerton, V.R., de Leon, R.D., Tillakaratne, N., Recktenwald, M.R., Hodgson, J.A. and Roy, R.R. (1997a) Use-dependent plasticity in spinal stepping and standing. In: *Advances in Neurology: Neuronal Regeneration, Reorganization and Repair*. Lippincott-Raven, Philadelphia, pp. 233–247.

Edgerton, V.R., Roy, R.R., de Leon, R., Tillakaratne, N. and Hodgson, J.A. (1997b) Does motor learning occur in the spinal cord? *Neuroscientist*, 3: 287–294.

Edgerton, V.R., de Leon, R.D., Harkema, S.J., Hodgson, J.A., London, N., Reinkensmeyer, D.J., Roy, R.R., Talmadge, R.J., Tillakaratne, N.J., Timoszyk, W. and Tobin, A. (2001) Retraining the injured spinal cord. *J. Physiol. (London)*, 533(N1): 15–22.

Grillner, S. and Rossignol, S. (1978) On the initiation of the swing phase of locomotion in chronic spinal cats. *Brain Res.*, 146: 269–277.

Hodgson, J.A., Roy, R.R., de Leon, R., Dobkin, B. and Edgerton, V.R. (1994) Can the mammalian lumbar spinal cord learn a motor task? *Med. Sci. Sports Exerc.*, 26: 1491–1497.

London, N.J.S., de Leon, R.D., Reinkensmeyer, D.J., Timoszyk, W.K., Roy, R.R. and Edgerton, V.R. (2000) Using Robots to train spinally-transected rats to recover hindlimb stepping. *Soc. Neurosci. Abstr.*, 26: 697.

Lovely, R.G., Gregor, R.G., Roy, R.R. and Edgerton, V.R. (1986) Effects of training on the recovery of full-weight-bearing stepping in the adult spinal cat. *Exp. Neurol.*, 92: 421–435.

Reinkensmeyer, D.J., Timoszyk, W.K., de Leon, R.D., Joynes, R., Kwak, E., Minakata, K. and Edgerton, V.R. (2000) A robotic stepper for retraining locomotion in spinal-injured rodents. *Proceedings of the 2000 IEEE International Conference on Robotics and Automation*, San Francisco, Ca, April, pp. 2889–2894.

Rossignol, S. and Drew, T. (1986). Phasic modulation of reflexes during rhythmic activity. In: S. Grillner, H. Forssberg, P.S. Stein and D. Stuart (Ed.), *Neurobiology of Vertebrate Locomotion*. Macmillan Press, London, pp. 517–534.

Timoszyk, W.K., de Leon, R.D., London, N., Joynes, R., Minakata, K., Edgerton, V.R. and Reinkensmeyer, D.J. (2002) Robot-assisted locomotion training after spinal cord injury: comparison of rodent stepping in virtual and physical treadmill environments. *Robotica*, in press.

Windhorst, U., Hamm, T.M. and Stuart, D.G. (1989) On the function of muscle and reflex partitioning. *Behav. Brain Sci.*, 12: 629–681.

L. McKerracher, G. Doucet and S. Rossignol (Eds.)
Progress in Brain Research, Vol. 137
© 2002 Elsevier Science B.V. All rights reserved

CHAPTER 12

The cat model of spinal injury

S. Rossignol *, C. Chau, N. Giroux, E. Brustein, L. Bouyer, J. Marcoux, C. Langlet,
D. Barthelémy, J. Provencher, H. Leblond, H. Barbeau and T.A. Reader

*Centre de Recherche en Sciences Neurologiques, Faculté de Médecine, Université de Montréal, Pavillon Paul-G.-Desmarais, C.P. 6128,
Succursale Centre-ville, Montreal, QC H3C 3J7, Canada*

Introduction

The evidence provided by different research teams that axons can regrow in the damaged spinal cord under certain conditions raises even more acutely the need to characterize as precisely as possible the functional capacity of the spinal cord when it is isolated from supraspinal structures after complete spinal lesions and in the absence of regenerated axons. It is indeed more and more imperative to differentiate potential functional recovery caused by the regrowth of descending fibres from the recovery of autonomous functions of the spinal cord below the lesion due to the internal reorganization of spinal circuitry. It is finally also crucial, faced with the regeneration of certain identified fibre systems in partial lesion studies, to make sure that the functional recovery observed is really due to the regrowth of fibres of these systems and not of others which are not necessarily labelled or identified. Indeed, the documented regrowth, for instance of corticospinal fibres, does not imply that other systems (e.g. serotonergic sys-

tem) have not also regrown and may be responsible for the observed functional recovery.

Even if the regeneration of axons of various descending systems is successful, such regenerated fibres would have to interface with an already profoundly changed spinal cord. It is thus important to know the characteristics of these changes to understand the specific role played by regenerated fibres. It is therefore necessary to recapitulate some of the work which shows the extent of functional recovery in the isolated spinal cord, particularly in the completely transected adult spinal cat. In the present review, we intend to summarize what changes occurring in the spinal cord may lead to the re-expression of motor patterns such as hindlimb locomotion. We ask the question: why can spinal cats walk? Thus, we will review some aspects of locomotor training with and without the use of drugs, the evolution of pharmacological receptors below the level of lesion, the role of various neurotransmitter systems before and after spinalization, the key role played by certain rostral lumbar segments of the spinal cord in the generation of locomotion and finally the necessity of cutaneous inputs from the pads for the expression of spinal locomotion.

General methodology

Although the specific methodology can be retrieved from the published work of each experimental set as cited in the appropriate sections, we will here

* Correspondence to: S. Rossignol, Centre de Recherche en Sciences Neurologiques, Faculté de Médecine, Université de Montréal, Pavillon Paul-G.-Desmarais, C.P. 6128, Succursale Centre-ville, Montreal, QC H3C 3J7, Canada. Tel.: +1-514-343-6366 or 6371 or 343-6111 ext. 3305; Fax: +1-514-343-6113;
E-mail: serge.rossignol@umontreal.ca

152

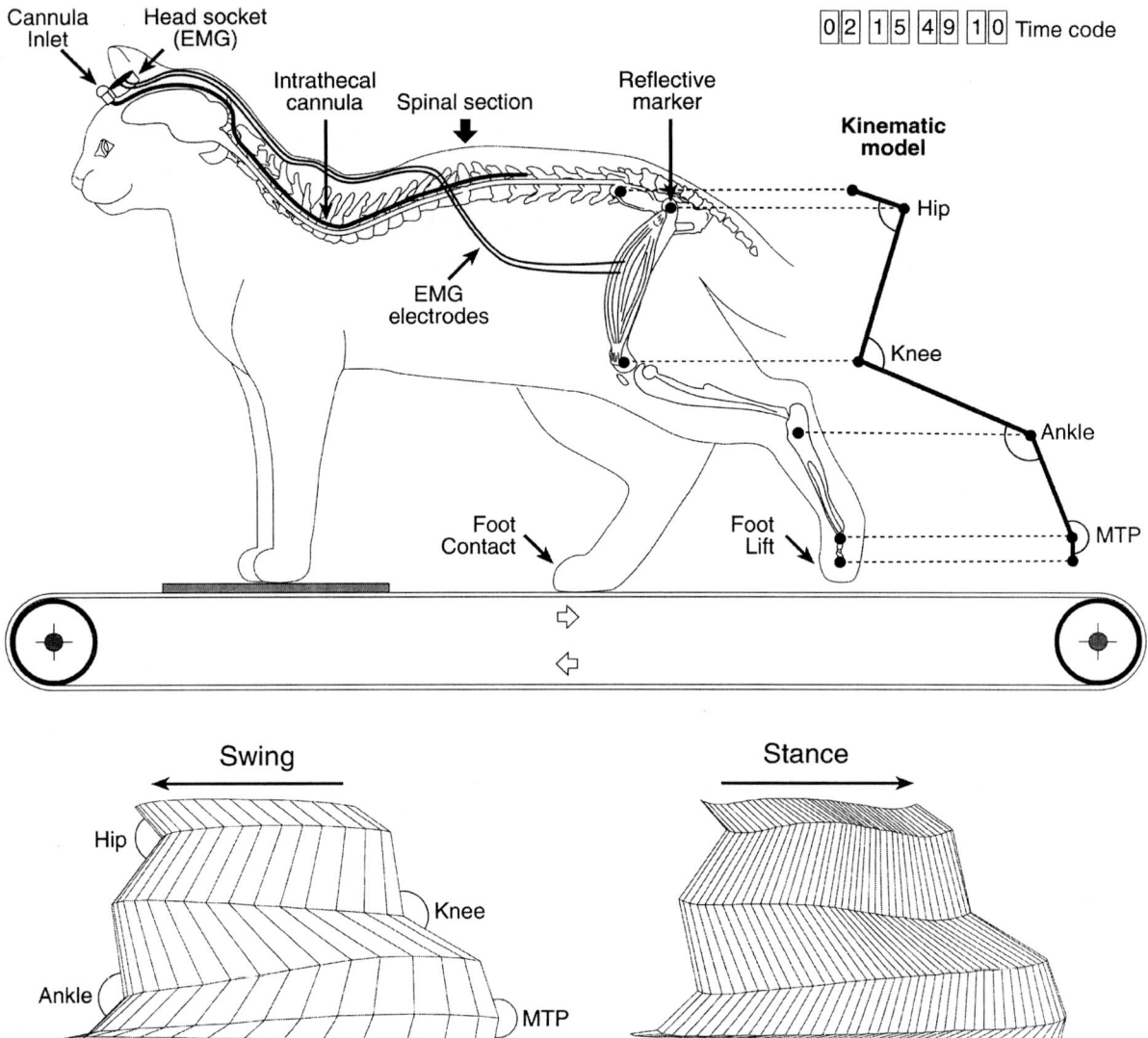

Fig. 1. General methodology to study spinal cats. Cats are placed with their forelimbs standing on a platform while their hindlimbs walk on the treadmill (arrows indicate the direction of the belt). Pairs of EMG wires are implanted in various muscles (only 1 pair represented here) and an intrathecal cannula inserted through the atlanto-occipital ligament down to about L_4. The multipin EMG connector as well as the cannula inlet are cemented to the skull. Reflective markers are placed at various points on the limb and the angle measurements taken with the orientation indicated. For each field (16.7 ms between fields), the coordinates of the reflective markers are obtained and the hindlimb movement reconstructed as indicated by the kinematic model. From such data, the swing and stance phases of each cycle can be reconstructed as shown below. Note that to prevent overlap of the figures, each stick figure is displaced by an amount equal to the displacement of the foot on the horizontal axis. The foot contact and foot lift are also measured to determine cycle length and/or duration and also to synchronize EMG events when needed. The digital SMPTE time code (upper right) is used to synchronize video and EMG recordings. The spinal lesion is made at T_{13}.

briefly summarize the key procedures approved by the Comité de Déontologie pour l'Expérimentation Animale from the Université de Montréal. Fig. 1 gives an overall scheme of the experimental set-up.

Adult cooperative cats were first selected and trained for 3 to 4 weeks to walk steadily at different speeds (0.2–0.8 m/s) on a treadmill. Then, under general anaesthesia (1–3% Isoflurane), they were implanted with chronic electromyographic (EMG) electrodes in hindlimb muscles (Bélanger et al., 1996; Chau et al., 1998a). For this, two 15-pin head connectors previously soldered to insulated stainless steel wires were fixed to the skull with acrylic cement. Each pair of wires was led subcutaneously and inserted within the belly of 7 to 14 muscles.

After the implantation and before any drug injections, recordings of locomotion were done in the intact state as the cat walked freely at different speeds (0.2–0.8 m/s) and tilts (15° up or 15° down) on a treadmill belt. In some cases, the cats were also trained to walk on a horizontal ladder with 8 round rungs (3 cm in diameter) spaced by about 20 cm. The latter task was recorded only on video tape and studied only in the intact state. These recordings served as baseline controls (intact trials).

In some cats, a Teflon tubing (24W) connected to an adaptor (cannula pedestal and dust cap) was fixed to the skull with dental acrylic cement while the other extremity of the tube was led through the subarachnoid space caudally towards L_3–L_4 to deliver drugs intrathecally (i.t.) (Chau et al., 1998a).

After obtaining baseline values for locomotion, drug injection experiments were performed while the spinal cord was still intact. During each drug injection trials, similar recording were done before (pre-drug trial) and at different times after the drug injection (post-drug trial). The α_2-noradrenergic agonist clonidine (2-(2,6-dichlorophenylamino)-2-imidazoline hydrochloride) and the antagonist yohimbine ((16α, 17α)-17-hydroxy yohimbine-16-carboxylic acid methyl ester hydrochloride) were used in these experiments. The drugs were injected as an i.t. bolus of 100 μl and a subsequent bolus of saline (100 μl) was delivered to flush the drug out of the cannula, the dead space of the cannula being about 100 μl.

When all these experiments in the intact state were finished, the cats were then spinalized at T_{13} under general anaesthesia. After surgery, the cats were placed in an incubator until they regained consciousness, and then returned to their individual cages with food and water ad libitum. During the first two and three postoperative days, cats received 0.005–0.01 mg/kg s.c. of Buprenorphine (every 6 h) for analgesia. The floor of the cages was covered with a foam mattress to reduce discomfort and skin ulceration. Cats were attended daily for general inspection, cleaning the head connectors and hindquarters, manual bladder expression and periodically flush the cannula. Thereafter, once the cats had recovered spinal locomotion, the same drugs were re-injected to allow a comparison of the effects of the same drugs in the intact and the spinal states. Overall these experiments lasted for periods ranging from 6 months to 2 years.

The experiments with the spinal cats were made once they had recovered a well-coordinated locomotor pattern of the hindlimbs with full weight support of the hindquarters and plantar foot placement. For spinal locomotion, the forelimbs were placed on a platform located about 2 cm above the treadmill, while the hindlimbs walked on the belt and the tail was held to maintain equilibrium of the hindquarters. A plexiglass separator was placed between the hindlimbs to prevent crossing of the hindlimbs due to increased adductor tonus (Barbeau and Rossignol, 1987).

The EMG signals were differentially amplified (bandwidth of 100 Hz to 3 kHz) and recorded on a 14-channel tape recorder (Vetter Digital, model 4000A PCM recording adapter) with a frequency response of 1.2 kHz per channel. The EMG recordings were synchronized to the video images of the hindlimbs using a digital SMPTE (Society for Motion Picture and Television Engineers) time code. The time code was recorded simultaneously on the EMG tape, the audio channel of the VHF tape as well as into the video image.

Video images of the side view of the left hindlimb during locomotion were captured using a digital camera (Panasonic 5100, shutter speed 1/1000 s) and recorded on a video cassette recorder (Panasonic, AG 7300). Reflective markers were glued to the skin over the bony landmarks (iliac crest, femoral head, knee joint, lateral malleolus, metatarso-phalangeal or MTP joint and the tip of the 4th toe) of the left (ipsilateral) hindlimb.

The kinematic analyses were carried out off-line using a two-dimensional Peak Performance system (Peak Performance Technologies Inc., Englewood, CO). The video images were digitized and the X Y coordinates of different joint markers were obtained at a frequency of 60 fields/s. These coordinates were then used to calculate angular joint movements and

154

could be displayed as continuous angular displacements, or stick diagrams of one step cycle.

At the end of the experimental series, the animals were killed with an overdose of sodium pentobarbital and the spinal cord were removed and divided into blocks of tissue which corresponds to spinal segments were rapidly frozen for autoradiographic analysis in other studies. To assure the completeness of the spinal transection, the segment of the encompassing lesion was completely removed and cut in sagittal 10 μm thick sections that were stained with the Klüver–Barrera method for histological observations.

For the reported acute experiments, cats were spinalized at T_{13} 1 week before the acute experiments. During that week, they were treated as other chronic spinal animals. On the day of the experiment, they were anaesthetized with Isoflurane, their head fixed in a stereotaxic frame and then were decerebrated using an anaemic decerebration method or by removing the brain anterior to a precollicular premammillar section (Marcoux and Rossignol, 2000) after which the gas anaesthesia was discontinued. The blood pressure and end-tidal CO_2 were measured throughout the experiment. Cats were fixed in a spinal fixation unit using three pairs of lateral pins to stabilize the vertebral column. EMG wires were acutely implanted in several muscles and then an extensive laminectomy performed to allow access to the rostral L_3–L_4 segments. The drugs were administered through a 26-gauge needle Hamilton syringe mounted on an electrode holder fixed to the side of the spinal fixation unit. Multiple paramedial injections of 2 μl were made at a depth of 2 mm. EMGs were recorded on-line and video graphic recordings were synchronized to the EMGs using an SMPTE time code.

Locomotor training after spinal cord lesions

As it is well known (Grillner, 1981; Rossignol, 1996, 2000; Rossignol et al., 1996, 2000), adult spinal cats can walk with their hindlimbs on a treadmill after a complete transection. In the spinal state, cats eventually regain plantar foot contact and weight support of the hindquarters. They can walk up to 0.8 m/s on the treadmill and exhibit a good alternation between the two hindlimbs. They have of course lost voluntary control of their gait, have a clearly deficient balance during walking and have to be guided continually so that they do not fall on their side. Fig. 2 compares walking of the same cat in the intact state (Fig. 2A–C) and then in the spinal state (Fig. 2D–F). Note that the kinematic and the EMG timings are quite similar. There is often a tendency to have a foot drag at the onset of swing and a slightly larger knee flexion at the end of swing. The usual delay between St and Srt (see Fig. 2C) is lost after spinalization (see Fig. 2F) and Srt often has a more prolonged discharge. Furthermore, the EMGs are more clonic than in the normal state as revealed by the more spiky aspect of the EMG recordings even after averaging.

In our first extensive study of the recovery of locomotion after a complete spinal transection in adult cats (Barbeau and Rossignol, 1987), we trained the animals for several months and observed that although cats had recovered a good plantar foot contact and weight support by 3–4 weeks, the step cycle duration still increased for the same treadmill speed (0.2 m/s) over a period of 3 months, at which stage most of the parameters of walking stabilized (Fig. 3A,B). Although the rate and the quality of the spontaneous recovery of spinal locomotion varied substantially between spinal animals, almost all the spinal cats used in various studies did indeed recover hindlimb locomotion.

Fig. 2. Comparison between step cycles of the hindlimb (at 0.4 m/s) in the normal and spinal state in the same cat. (A) Stick figures reconstructed from a video sequence of one normal step cycle, displaying separately the swing and the stance phases, with arrows pointing to the direction of motion of the leg. The orientation of joint measurements are given. Note that the calibration in the horizontal is twice that of the vertical because of the foot displacement, as explained in Fig. 1. (B) Angular excursion of the four joints averaged over ten cycles. Flexion always corresponds to downward deflections of the angular traces. The vertical dotted lines separate various epochs (F and E1 constitute swing while E2 and E3 constitute stance) of the step cycle (Philippson, 1905). (C) Average of rectified EMG traces of ten cycles. L = left, R = right. Muscles are: semitendinosus (St, a knee flexor and hip extensor); sartorius, anterior head (Srt,

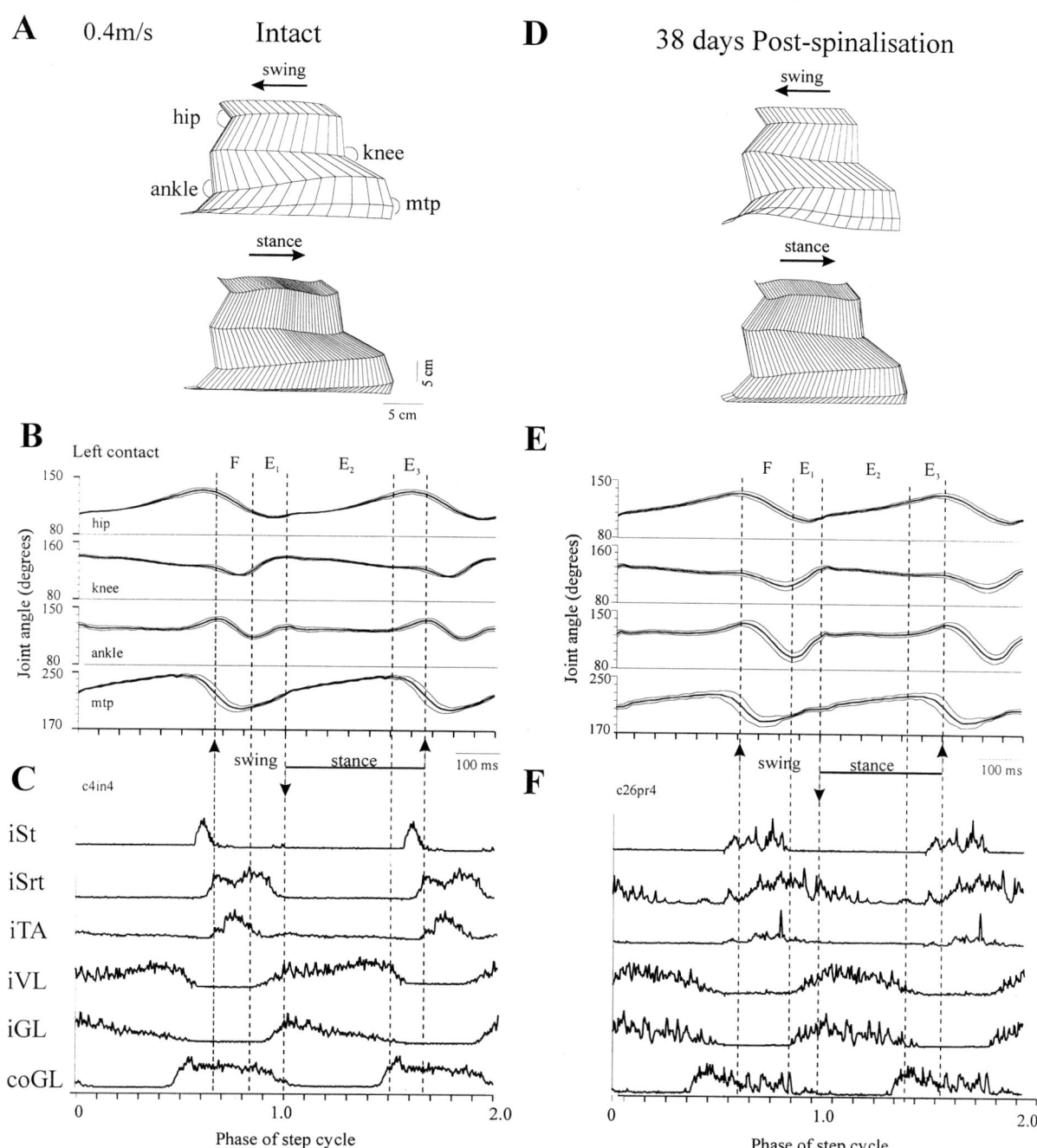

A 0.4m/s   Intact

swing

hip

knee

ankle

mtp

stance

5 cm

5 cm

D 38 days Post-spinalisation

swing

stance

B Left contact

F E₁ E₂ E₃

hip

knee

ankle

mtp

Joint angle (degrees)

150
80
160
80
150
80
250
170

swing stance 100 ms

E

F E₁ E₂ E₃

Joint angle (degrees)

150
80
160
80
150
80
250
170

swing stance 100 ms

C c4in4

iSt
iSrt
iTA
iVL
iGL
coGL

0   1.0   2.0
Phase of step cycle

F c26pr4

iSt
iSrt
iTA
iVL
iGL
coGL

0   1.0   2.0
Phase of step cycle

a hip flexor and knee extensor); tibilais anterior (TA, an ankle flexor); vastus lateralis (VL, a knee extensor); gastrocnemius lateralis (GL, an ankle extensor). The cycle is normalized to 1 and is repeated twice for clarity of illustration at turning points. The average is synchronized on foot contact. (D, E, F) Same format as A, B and C but for a cat spinalized at T_{13}, 38 days previously. Note that the step length is somewhat shortened and therefore there are more steps/min to keep the same walking speed. Note that the time relationship between the muscles is largely preserved (except for the absence of a lag between St and Srt) and the more prolonged Srt burst. The EMGs are more clonic (spiky) than in the control.

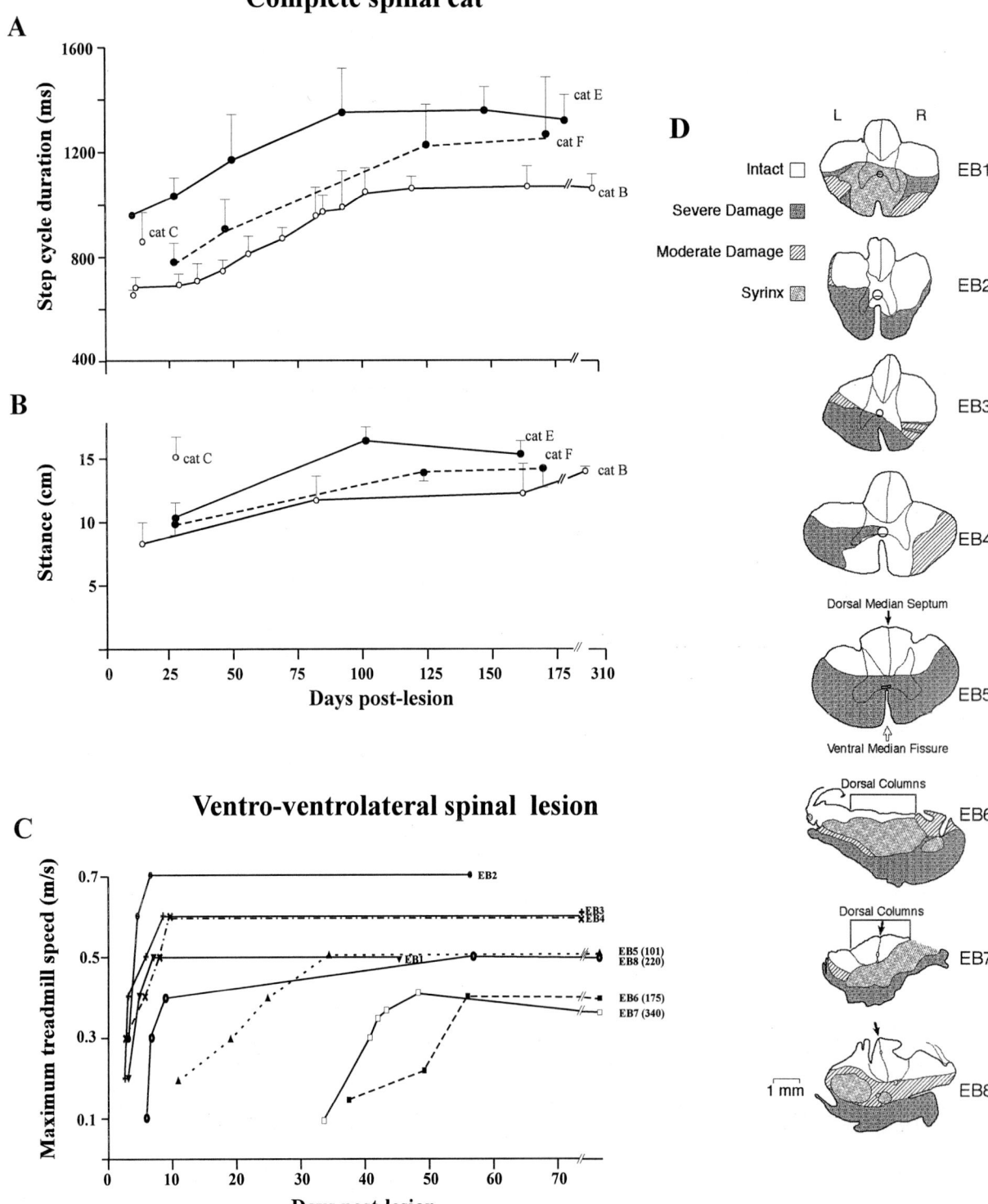

Complete spinal cat

A

Step cycle duration (ms)

cat C
cat E
cat F
cat B

B

Sttance (cm)

cat C
cat E
cat F
cat B

Days post-lesion

Ventro-ventrolateral spinal lesion

C

Maximum treadmill speed (m/s)

EB2
EB3
EB4
EB5 (101)
EB8 (220)
EB1
EB6 (175)
EB7 (340)

Days post-lesion

D

L   R

Intact
Severe Damage
Moderate Damage
Syrinx

EB1

EB2

EB3

EB4

Dorsal Median Septum

EB5

Ventral Median Fissure

Dorsal Columns

EB6

Dorsal Columns

EB7

1 mm

EB8

In another study, we sought to accelerate the rate of locomotor recovery by a daily intrathecal injection of clonidine, an α-2 noradrenergic agonist (Chau et al., 1998b). Clonidine had already been shown to induce locomotion in spinal cats (Forssberg and Grillner, 1973; Barbeau et al., 1987) offering a time window of about 4–6 h to train cats on the treadmill after a single injection. These experiments showed that daily injections of clonidine allowing an early and daily locomotor training resulted in marked improvement of locomotor recovery on the treadmill so that by day 6 to 11, all cats could walk with a plantar foot contact and hindlimb weight support.

In cats with large lesions of the ventral and ventrolateral parts of the spinal cord, the time of recovery of spontaneous quadrupedal locomotion depended on the extent of the lesion (Brustein and Rossignol, 1998). Fig. 3C shows that for the smaller lesions of the ventral/ventrolateral quadrants (EB1–EB4 in Fig. 3D), the recovery time was within a week. With the largest lesions (EB5–EB8 in Fig. 3D), cats behaved initially like complete spinal cats. They walked through the lab with the forelimbs while dragging their hindquarters for several weeks. They were, however, trained to walk also on the treadmill, initially helping them with weight support and eventually (sometimes up to 1–1.5 months) they could walk voluntarily with all four limbs on the ground or on the treadmill.

These findings demonstrate that after a complete spinal transection or a large spinal lesion, the spinal cord and other supraspinal structures can evolve over

several days and weeks to express locomotion and that the underlying mechanisms of plastic changes are accessible to imposed manipulations such as intensive and early locomotor training. Furthermore, Edgerton's group has suggested that, in complete spinal cats, the specificity of training is of paramount importance. Thus spinal cats trained to stand or walk will be better at the trained task suggesting that specific plastic changes may occur within the spinal cord in association with a specific training task (de Leon et al., 1998a,b; see also de de Leon et al., 2002).

The neurochemical and physiological changes underlying this recovery of locomotion have been the subject of a number of more recent studies and some of these will be summarized here.

Pharmacology of locomotion

As already mentioned, the noradrenergic system has been found to have potent effect in eliciting locomotion (Jankowska et al., 1967a,b; Grillner and Zangger, 1979; Grillner, 1981; Barbeau et al., 1987; Barbeau and Rossignol, 1991, 1994; Pearson and Rossignol, 1991; Rossignol et al., 1992, 1998; Rossignol, 1996; Chau et al., 1998b,a). Indeed, the noradrenergic system has been found to be the sole system capable of eliciting locomotion within the first week following the spinal lesion. Although serotonergic agonists were capable of modulating the pattern of locomotion in already well-established spontaneous locomotor pattern, we have been unable

Fig. 3. Time course of recovery after complete or partial spinal section at T_{13}. (A) Step cycle duration of three cats as a function of time after a complete spinalization and always at the same treadmill speed. Each point represents the mean and S.D. of 10–15 cycles. Arrows indicate the day of documented plantigrade placing and weight bearing of each cat. Modified from Barbeau and Rossignol (1987). (B) Stance length measured from video recordings as a function of time after spinalization. Modified from Barbeau and Rossignol (1987). (C) Recovery of treadmill locomotion following spinal lesion for each one of the eight cats shown in D. The graph illustrates the maximal treadmill speed each cat could attain and maintain at least for a few step cycles, as a function of days following spinal lesion. The numbers after the identification of some cats (EB5 to EB8) represent the days for which the last data point is illustrated. Modified from Brustein and Rossignol (1998). (D) Extent of the spinal lesions for all eight cats. The histology of all the cats is based on photomicrographs of the cross-sections taken from the spinal site of lesion, stained with cresyl violet or with Klüver–Barrera, to demonstrate the maximal extent of the lesion. The schematic representations are constructed from observation under the microscope of the site of lesion. For cats EB1–EB5, the total extent of the lesion is projected on a spinal cord section taken more rostrally, after inspecting several consecutive sections, while for cats EB6–EB8 the schemes illustrate the maximal site of lesion to emphasize the deformation of the spinal cord. The various textures identify the extent of damage. *Intact*: myelinated axons (or axonal profiles) appeared normal under the microscope. *Severe damage*: absent or highly fibrotic tissue. *Moderate damage*: some myelinated axons (or axonal profiles) of normal appearance within fibrotic and gliotic tissue. *Syrinx*: cyst. L = left; R = right. Modified from Brustein and Rossignol (1998).

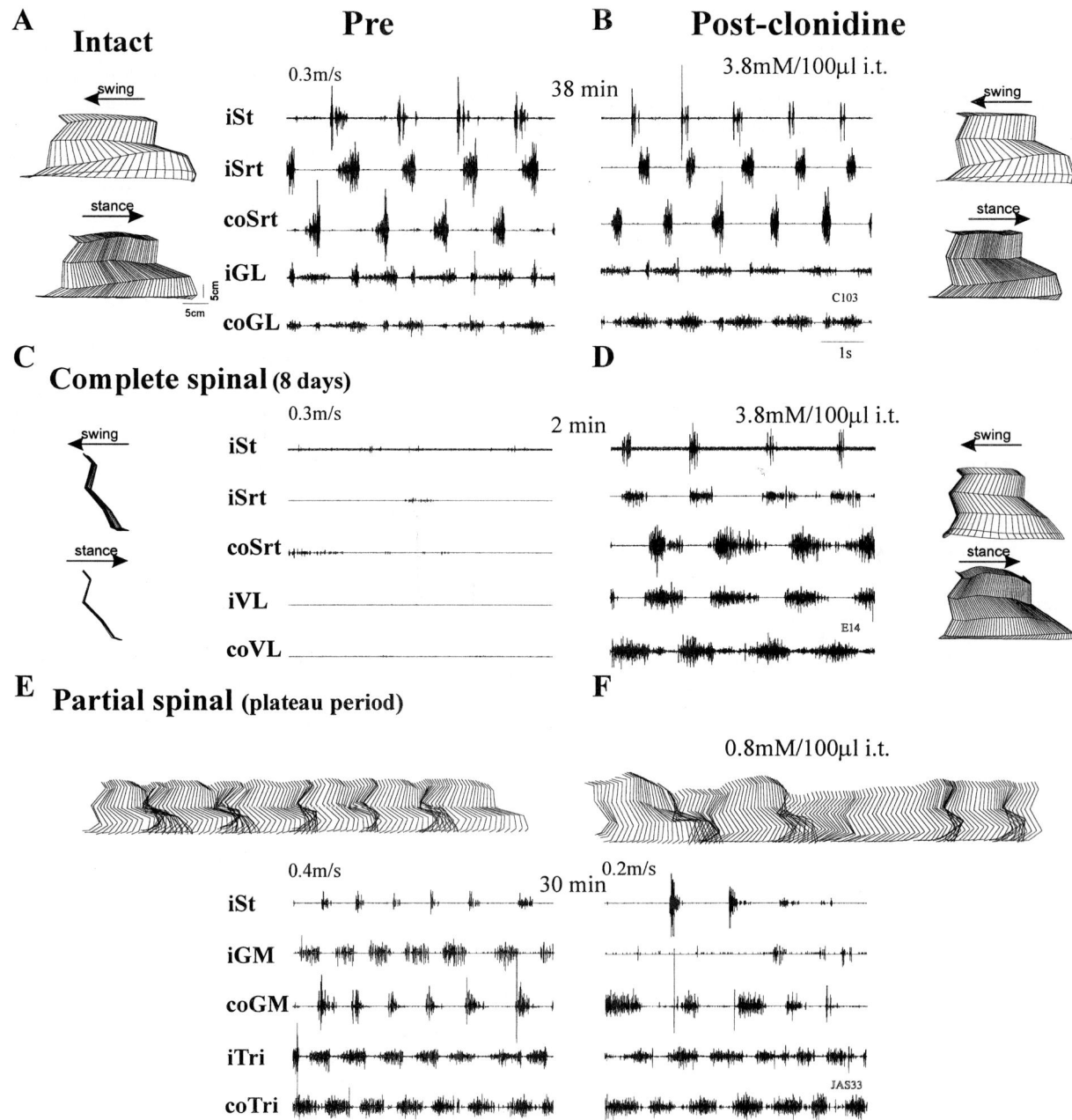

Fig. 4. Locomotor patterns before and after injection of clonidine in intact, complete spinal or after a large lesion of the ventral/ventrolateral quadrants. (A) Kinematics and raw EMGs of intact cat walking at 0.3 m/s. (B) Same cat, 38 min after an intrathecal injection of a bolus of 100 μl of clonidine (3.8 mM). Note that there is almost no effect in the intact state. (C) Kinematic and EMG recordings of a cat 8 days after spinalization. The cat is not walking. (D) Same cat, 2 min after an intrathecal injection of clonidine. The cat steps very well on the treadmill. (E) Stick figures representing five consecutive step cycles and the related raw EMG recordings of cat EB7 (see Fig. 3) taken during a period when the cat had attained a stable locomotor behaviour on the treadmill. (F) 30 min after an intrathecal injection of clonidine, the cat has great difficulty walking; gastrocnemius medialis (GM, an ankle extensor). Figure modified from Giroux et al. (1998).

to trigger locomotion in spinal cats (Barbeau and Rossignol, 1989, 1990). Fig. 4 illustrates the effect of clonidine in three different states. First, in the intact state, clonidine was found to have very little effect on locomotion (Giroux et al., 2001) (Fig. 4A,B). In the spinal state, clonidine can trigger locomotion (Fig. 4C,D). On the other hand, after partial lesion of the ventral/ventrolateral cord, the effect of clonidine on locomotion is seemingly deleterious (Brustein and Rossignol, 1999) (Fig. 4E,F). Indeed, in such cats, clonidine can hamper locomotion dramatically. It is possible that, after a partial spinal lesion, the relative potency of clonidine on pre and post-synaptic receptors might result in a predominant presynaptic effect leading to a decrease in transmitter release. On the other hand, clonidine also exerts a potent effect on the excitability of reflexes, namely cutaneous reflexes (Barbeau et al., 1987; Chau et al., 1998a), and therefore it is likely that a decrease in the excitability of these reflexes may be deleterious in cats because they may rely on them to maintain postural balance during walking.

Since spinalization removes all descending sources of noradrenergic and serotonergic inputs, it is clear that the spontaneous expression of spinal locomotion does not depend on these neurotransmitters. In other words, the fact that agonists such as clonidine acting on noradrenergic receptors can trigger locomotion after spinalization does not mean that these receptors are needed for the spontaneous expression of spinal locomotion, i.e. without drugs. To confirm this, we blocked the noradrenergic receptors by an intrathecal injection of yohimbine which had virtually no effect on spinal locomotion (Fig. 5G,H and I,J) (Giroux et al., 2001). However, yohimbine given i.t. to intact cats did have a significant deleterious effect on the locomotion, especially on interlimb coordination (See Fig. 5 A,B and C,D). This suggests that whereas the stimulation of the noradrenergic receptors may exert a potent modulatory effect on normal locomotion as revealed by this yohimbine effect in intact cats, the stimulation of the noradrenergic system is not essential for the expression of spontaneous spinal locomotion.

In another study, we injected intrathecally a glutamatergic blocker, AP-5, and documented that it could completely block spinal locomotion (Fig. 5K,L) whereas it had only had minor effects (Fig. 5I,J)

on intact locomotion, mainly on the degree of weight support.

Overall, this suggested that although spinal locomotion can be triggered by noradrenergic mechanisms, its spontaneous expression seems to mainly depend on the activation of glutamatergic mechanisms. Thus, these receptors, as was shown in the lamprey (Brodin et al., 1985) and in the neonatal rat (Cazalets et al., 1992; Kiehn et al., 1992) are important for the expression of endogenous rhythmicity even in the cat.

It is intriguing that our initial studies using NMDA did not reveal the ability of NMDA to trigger locomotion (Chau et al., 1994), whereas it did in paralysed decerebrate cats (Douglas et al., 1993). Indeed, injection of NMDA early after spinalization led to an hyperexcitable state characterized by tremor, hyperreflexia and toe fanning. However, later on, when the cat could manifest signs of organized spinal rhythmicity some 5–7 days after the lesion, intrathecal NMDA could trigger a well-developed pattern of locomotion which could be sustained for more than 48 h. At a later stage, after having blocked locomotion with AP-5, locomotion could be reinstated with an injection of NMDA (Chau et al., 1994).

Therefore, it seems very likely that one of the key changes occurring within the spinal cord after a lesion is a reorganization of the balance between neurochemical receptors so that the recovery and expression of spinal locomotion appears to be mainly dependent on the activation of glutamatergic receptors.

The fate of receptors after spinalization

Over the last few years we have also sought to determine the fate of different receptors as a function of time after a spinal transection in cats. Our first study (Giroux et al., 1999) showed that α-1 and α-2 receptors as well as 5-HT1A receptors were up-regulated in the first month after the lesion after which there was a return to control levels. This up-regulation especially occurred in laminae II–IV as well as in lamina IX (α-1) and lamina X (α-2 and 5-HT1A). This is confirmed also in Fig. 6A.

In more recent studies we have also tried to determine the segmental distribution of α-2 adrenergic receptors and AMPA receptors in various segments

Intact

pre-drug

Spinal

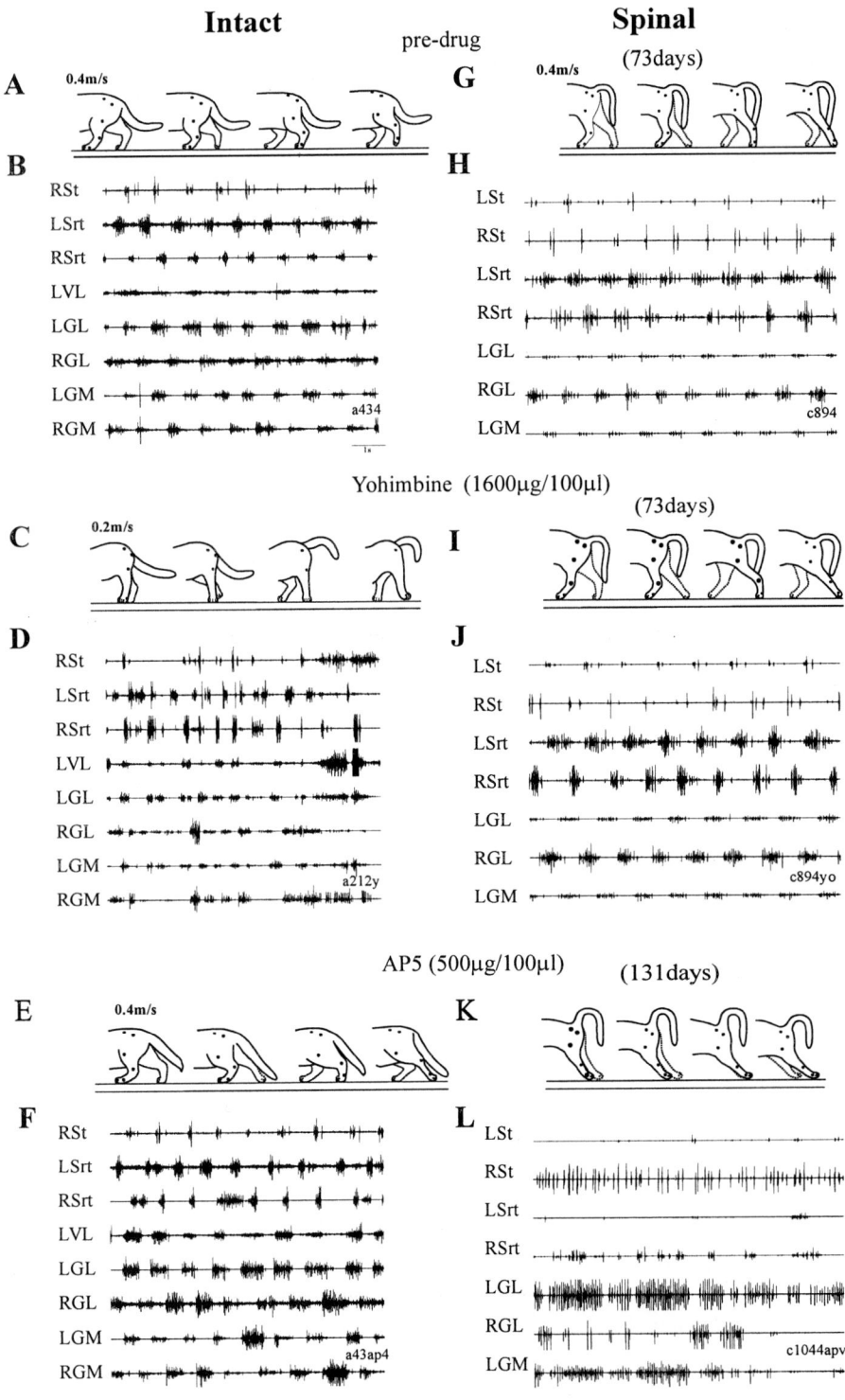

A 0.4m/s

B RSt LSrt RSrt LVL LGL RGL LGM RGM a434

G 0.4m/s

H LSt RSt LSrt RSrt LGL RGL LGM c894

Yohimbine (1600μg/100μl)

(73days)

C 0.2m/s

D RSt LSrt RSrt LVL LGL RGL LGM RGM a212y

I

J LSt RSt LSrt RSrt LGL RGL LGM c894yo

AP5 (500μg/100μl)

(131days)

E 0.4m/s

F RSt LSrt RSrt LVL LGL RGL LGM RGM a43ap4

K

L LSt RSt LSrt RSrt LGL RGL LGM c1044apv

and laminae of the cord in intact cats, short term spinal and long term spinal cats. The α-2 receptors were found to be up-regulated in spinal cats particularly in lumbar segments L_3–L_5 (Fig. 6A), whereas there was a decrease in segments lower than L_7 (only lamina II is shown here). This differential up-regulation of receptors after lesion may suggest that these various segments could play different roles in the expression and in the evolution of locomotion (see below).

Other studies show that glutamate receptors are also up-regulated but, contrary to noradrenergic and serotonergic receptors, their binding densities remained up-regulated even in the long-term spinal cats (see heavy line in Fig. 6B compared to Fig. 6A). Therefore, there is a distinct regulation of receptors after spinalization i.e. noradrenergic and serotonergic receptors are first up-regulated and then return to normal values, whereas NMDA receptors remain up-regulated. This of course corroborates very well the fact that in the chronic stage, locomotion appears to depend critically on NMDA mechanisms as concluded from the work on NMDA blockers reported above.

Segmental organization of spinal locomotion

The above work suggests not only that there is a differential evolution of receptors but also that there is an evolution of the segmental distribution of receptors after a spinal lesion. In a different set of studies, we have investigated whether different spinal segments play a differential role in the expression of locomotion. Experiments in neonatal rats suggest that the upper lumbar segments either drive the lower segments (Cazalets, 2000) or at least are more excitable than lower segments when stimulated by chemicals to induce locomotion (Kjaerulff and

Kiehn, 1996; Kiehn and Kjaerulff, 1998). Experiments in cats (Deliagina et al., 1983) has already suggested that L_3–L_5 segments were very important for another type of rhythmic movement, scratching. The work in the rat suggests that there might be a fine heterogenous distribution of various 5-HT receptor subtypes that may have different effects on locomotion (Jordan and Schmidt, 2002).

In a series of experiments, we have microinjected clonidine in different spinal segments to induce locomotion and we have also tried to block locomotion by local microinjections of yohimbine in spinal cats induced to walk on a treadmill by an i.v. injection of clonidine (Marcoux and Rossignol, 2000). This study has shown that the mid-lumbar segments play a critical role in locomotion because localized injections of clonidine in these segments can trigger a full locomotor pattern while yohimbine in the same segments can block locomotion evoked by clonidine i.v. (See Fig. 7A,B). Furthermore, in these acute experiments, a second transection at the junction of L_3–L_4, or at the junction of L_4–L_5, can completely abolish locomotion. It should be remembered here that according to anatomical work (Vanderhorst and Holstege, 1997) the main hindlimb pools of motoneurones appear at this junction and continue throughout the lumbo-sacral cord. It is therefore most likely that these upper lumbar segments play a major role in the generation of spinal locomotion at a premotoneuronal level.

Very recent work has shown that microinjections of L-DOPA or clonidine in curarized cats were incapable of inducing fictive locomotion in cats spinalized 1 week prior to the acute experiment. However, as was the case for walking cats, yohimbine injected at L_3–L_4 could abolish the fictive locomotor rhythm induced by L-DOPA i.v. (see Fig. 7C,D; Leblond et al., 2001).

Fig. 5. Effects of the noradrenergic antagonist yohimbine and NMDA antagonist AP5 on locomotion in the intact and the spinal state in the same cat (0.4 m/s). (A, C, E, G, I and K) Figurines redrawn from video recordings; from left to right, the hindlimb positions are at left foot contact, onset of right swing, right foot contact, and onset of left swing respectively. (B, D, F, H, J and L) EMGs of the hindlimb muscles during treadmill locomotion in the same sequence. Note that yohimbine has major effects in the intact cat (compare A, B with C, D taken 10 min after the yohimbine injection). The cat had major walking abnormalities characterized by difficulty in maintaining lateral stability of the hindquarters and asymmetry of hindlimb stepping leading to the turning of the hindquarters to one side or the other but there was no effect on the spinal cat (compare G, H with I, J). On the other hand, the NMDA blocker, AP5, has some effect only in the intact cat (cat is more crouched in E, F than in A, B) but virtually blocks locomotion in the spinal state (see K, L). Modified from Rossignol et al. (2001).

162

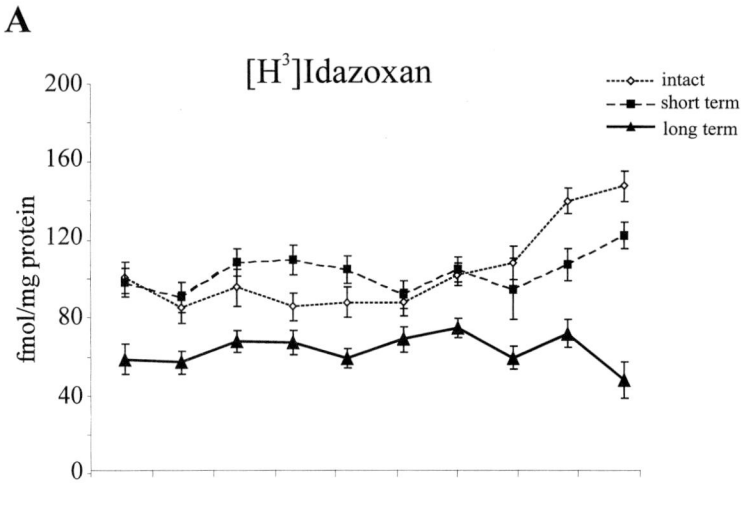

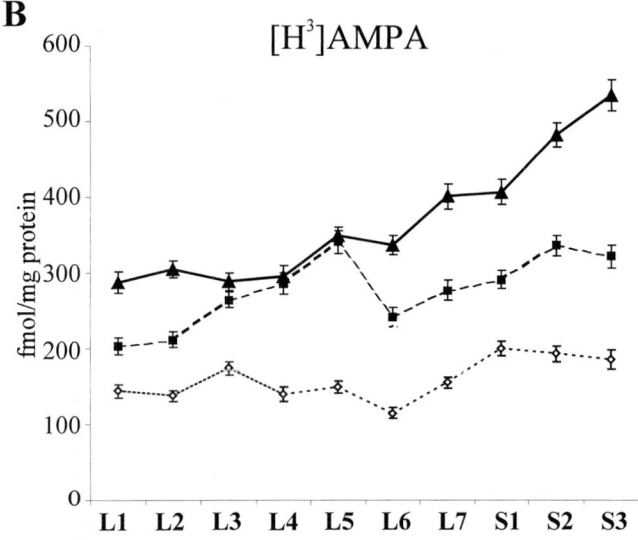

Fig. 6. Laminar and segmental distribution of α2-noradrenergic receptors (labelled with idazoxan) and glutamate receptors of the AMPA subtype in lamina II of control, short-term and long-term and spinal cats. Line graph showing the average amount of specific [3H]idazoxan and [3H]AMPA and binding in lamina II as a function of the lumbosacral spinal segments (L_1–S_3) in two intact, two short-term (30 days) and two long-term (more than 3 months) spinal cats. (A) Note that following spinalization, as indicated by the dotted line, there is an α2-receptor up-regulation measured in the L_2–L_5 segments, while there is a down-regulation from L_7–S_3 segments. In the long-term (thick line), the values obtained were below the values of intact. (B) Note the up-regulation of [3H]AMPA in the short-term spinal cats (dotted line), but also a maintained or further increase in the labelling in the long-term spinal cats (heavy solid line). Note also that the up-regulation appears greater in segments L_3 to L_5, at least for the short-term spinal cats.

We are undertaking a series of experiments in chronically implanted cats to see if a second spinal lesion at L_3–L_4 below the initial T_{13} lesion abolishes spinal locomotion or if cats with an initial lesion at L_3–L_4 can express spinal locomotion. These studies are in progress and we cannot yet reach definitive conclusions. However, this work has shown that a second spinal transection leads, at least initially, to a complete abolition of spinal locomotion. However, some rhythmic activity can be regained at a later stage (C. Langlet and S. Rossignol, unpublished).

Treadmill locomotion

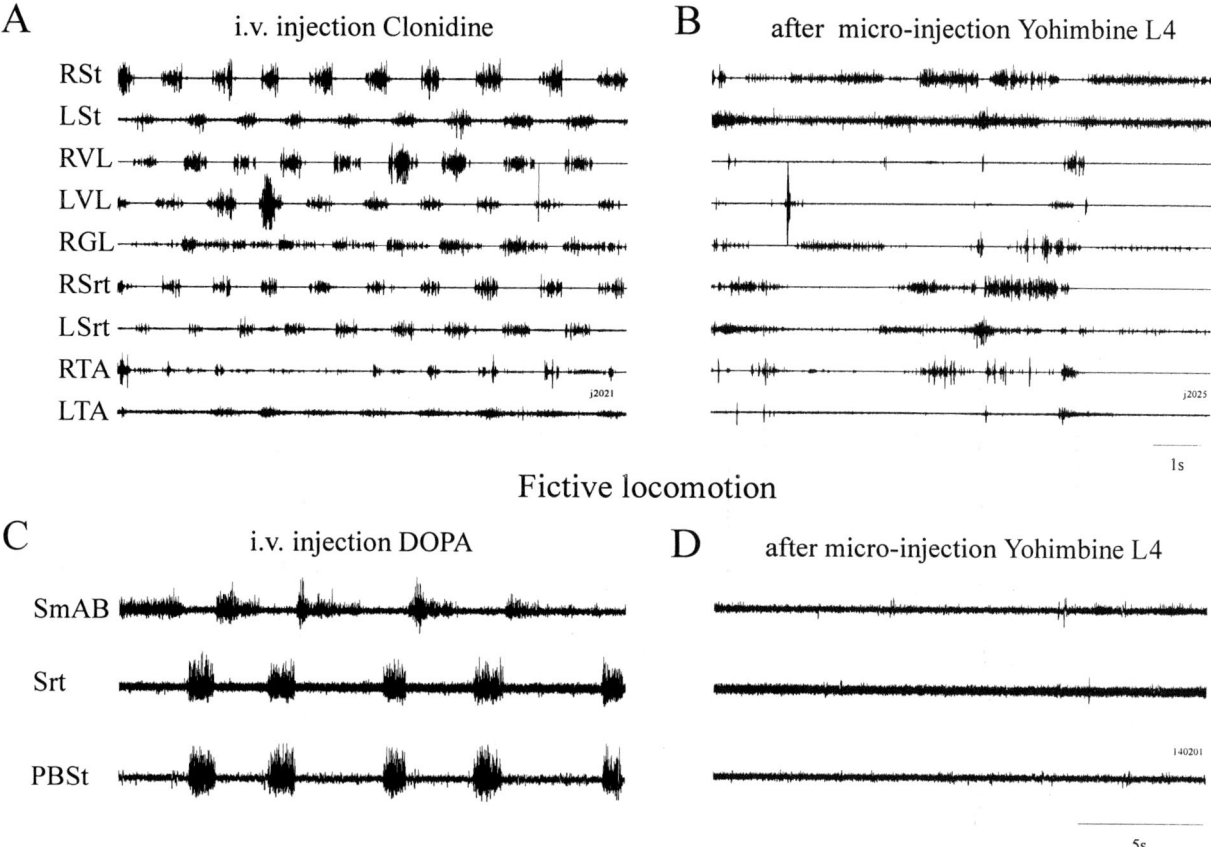

Fig. 7. Initiation and block of locomotion by micro-injections of adrenergic drugs during real treadmill locomotion in a spinal cat and during fictive locomotion. (A) Hindlimb EMG displaying a locomotor pattern 13 min after clonidine i.v. (B) Hindlimb EMG displaying only tonic activity 33 min after nine 2-μl intra-spinal injections of yohimbine (8 mg/ml) at L_4 level and 1 h 25 min after the injection of clonidine i.v. Modified from Marcoux and Rossignol (2000). (C) Fictive locomotion induced by an i.v. injection of L-DOPA (80 mg/kg) in a decerebrate cat spinalized 1 week prior to the decerebration. The cat is paralysed and artificially ventilated. Nerve recordings with cuff electrodes placed on the semimembranosus/anterior biceps nerve (SmAB), Srt nerve and posterior biceps/semitendinosus nerve (PBSt). (D) Similar injections of yohimbine at L_4 block the fictive locomotion (H. Leblond and S. Rossignol, unpublished).

The need for sensory inputs during spinal locomotion

Spinal locomotion is triggered by the movement of the treadmill belt and, early after transection, stimulation of the perineal region and the base of the tail is required to induce stepping. After some weeks, the latter stimulation is no longer required and movement of the belt alone is sufficient to induce locomotion. Various sensory inputs have been studied in relation to their capacity to control parameters of stepping, such as duration of stance or initiation of swing. The position of the hip joint was found to be of importance (Grillner and Rossignol, 1978a) since hip flexion prevents locomotion while extension promotes it (Pearson and Rossignol, 1991). These effects could be due to proprioceptive inputs from muscles acting around the hip or joint afferents (Grillner and Rossignol, 1978b; Rossignol and Julien, 1980). Other proprioceptive inputs have also been found to be important, such as proprioceptors detecting load on ankle extensors (Duysens and Pearson, 1980; see also Gorassini et al., 1994; Hiebert et al., 1994, 1996).

We have studied for many years the role of cutaneous inputs during locomotion. In chronic spinal cats (Forssberg et al., 1977) when the dorsum of the foot is stimulated with a mechanical tapper during swing as if the limb was meeting an obstacle, there is a well-organized response consisting first of a knee flexion, rapidly withdrawing the foot, followed by a flexion of the ankle and hip to step in front of the obstacle. After anaesthesia of the dorsum of the foot, these responses are abolished (Forssberg et al., 1977; Prochazka et al., 1978) and only those responses that were induced by muscle stretch while the foot pushed against the obstacle remain. When the same mechanical stimulus is given during stance, flexor muscles do not respond but on the other hand extensor muscles at the ankle and knee which are already active at that time generate short latency responses.

Cutaneous inputs, during the swing phase, evoke complex organized responses that are well integrated into the step cycle and can recruit flexors and extensors in a very precise sequence. This does not result simply from a greater activation of the ongoing locomotor activity of these muscles (Forssberg et al., 1975; for the forelimbs see also Drew and Rossignol, 1987).

Cutaneous inputs during the stance phase may play different roles depending on their location and strength. Inputs from the pads have a dominant excitatory effects to extensor muscles after a brief inhibitory effect. This appears actually to be the most important effect that could be used to partially regulate stance by providing a positive feedback during stance (phase-promoting reflex) and delaying the onset of swing, perhaps in parallel with muscle proprioceptors of ankle and toe extensors (Duysens and Pearson, 1976). Excitatory responses in extensors, following stimulation of the dorsum of the foot, may serve to shorten the stance and thus minimize the period during which the foot would contact a moving object.

In more recent studies, we have denervated bilaterally the hind-paws by surgical section of all the cutaneous nerves of the foot below the ankle. Although otherwise normal cats display a significant deficit when required to walk on an horizontal ladder or on slippery surface, they can recover treadmill locomotion rapidly within a few days. At that stage, it is nearly impossible to detect any locomotor deficit by kinematic analysis although some changes in flexor muscle discharges are present and persistent. After spinalization, cats which had recovered perfect treadmill locomotion were now unable to place the planta of the foot on the treadmill belt (Bouyer and Rossignol, 1998, 2001). This suggests that although otherwise-normal cats may have the ability to compensate for the missing cutaneous information by using other sensory cues (proprioceptive), the spinal cat needs this cutaneous information to walk properly with plantar foot contact.

It is interesting to speculate that sensory inputs may be necessary to stimulate the locomotor pattern not only for specific controls (step length, foot placement) but also by providing a source of neurochemical excitation through the release of excitatory transmitters, namely glutamate, acting on those receptors that were found to remain up-regulated after spinalization (see above).

Spinal plasticity

We raised above the question of why spinal cats walk. It is quite clear that after spinalization many types of changes occur and we have documented some of them in the above paragraphs: the locomotor pattern changes with time, receptors of neurotransmitters change in the cord and pharmacological responses evolve. Edgerton's group (see de Leon, 1998b) has insisted that there are plastic changes within the cord which are specific to the training of specific tasks (i.e. standing vs locomotion). We have also addressed the question of plasticity in three different paradigms.

In the first set of experiments (Carrier et al., 1997), we neurectomized ankle flexors (tibilais anterior, TA and extensor digitorum levigus, EDL) on one side in normal cats. The kinematics of the recovered locomotion was very similar to control after only a few days. When the cats were spinalized, the stepping became asymmetrical and marked by a large hyperflexion on the denervated side while the other side performed almost normally. Knowing that otherwise-normal cats (not denervated) rapidly recover, symmetrical hindlimb locomotion suggests that the recovery of locomotion after denervation

A. Spinal, before SP section

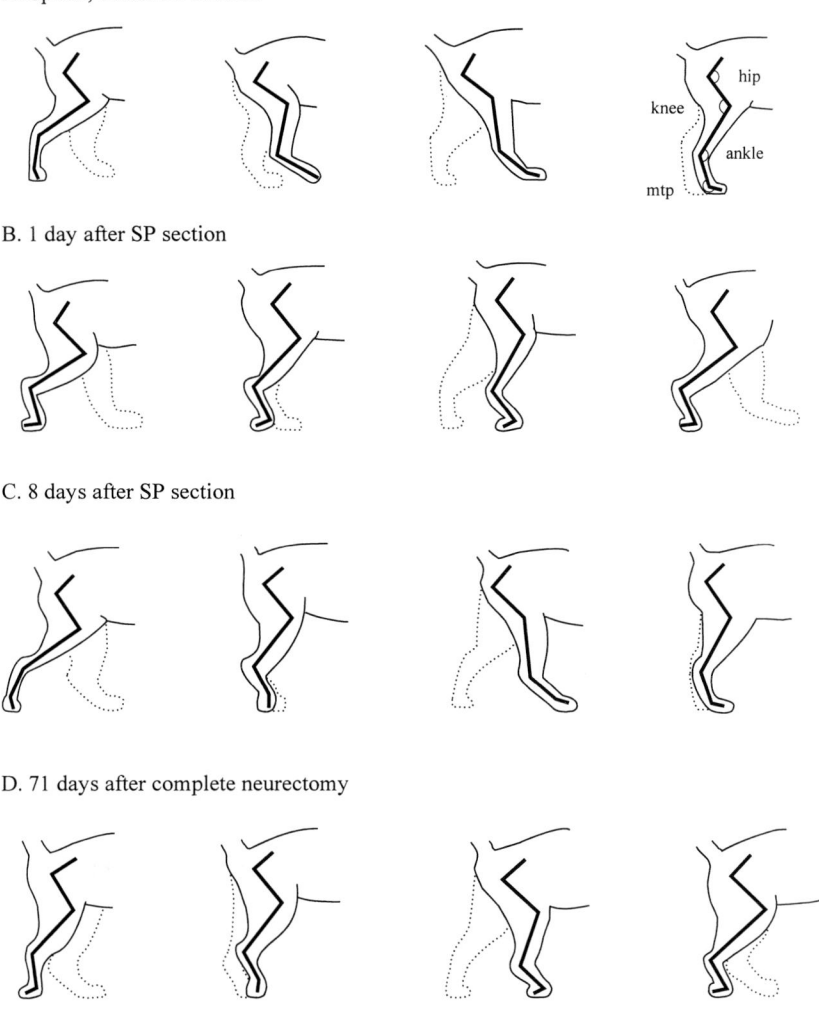

B. 1 day after SP section

C. 8 days after SP section

D. 71 days after complete neurectomy

| foot off | mid swing | foot on | mid stance |

Fig. 8. Adaptation of a spinal cat to a progressive cutaneous denervation of one paw. (A) Walking of a spinal cat 68 days after the spinalization at T_{13} and with a partial denervation of the right hindlimb. The latter involved the sequential neurectomy of the deep peroneal cutaneous branch (28 days before), saphenous nerve (22 days before) and caudal cutaneous sural nerve (7 days before). Despite transient changes occurring for a few hours after each nerve cut, the cat could walk very well as can be seen by the four line drawings reconstructed from video images taken at foot off (beginning of swing), mid swing, foot on (beginning of stance) and mid stance. (B) Day 69; 1 day after cutting the superficial peroneal nerve (SP). The cat basically drags the foot on the dorsum during swing and contacts the treadmill on the dorsum of the foot for the whole stance period. (C) Day 76; after 8 days of treadmill training, the cat improves markedly and lands on the plantar surface of the foot. This adaptation to the partial denervation occurs entirely while the cat is spinal. However, when the last cutaneous nerve is removed (tibial nerve), the cat does not recover a plantigrade walking despite further locomotor training. (D) 71 days after complete neurectomy. The cat drags the foot on the treadmill during swing and keeps contact with the dorsum of the foot on the belt during the whole stance phase. Modified from Rossignol (2000).

probably depends on both supraspinal and spinal mechanisms. Indeed, the abnormal locomotor pattern expressed by the cord alone suggests that changes had occurred within the cord. These intraspinal changes are, however, not sufficient to compensate adequately just by themselves.

In one cat, the neurectomy was performed after the cat had recovered spinal locomotion. For the entire testing period, the cat did not recover ankle flexion but continued to walk symmetrically and it did not display the hyper flexions reported above. This suggests that the changes occurring within the cord are not a consequence of the denervation itself but rather result from the adaptive mechanisms that have taken place before spinalization.

In another study (Bouyer et al., 2001) we lesioned an ankle extensor nerve (lateral gastrocnemius soleus, LGS) on one side in three spinal cats. During the first few days following neurectomy, there was a marked yield at the ankle which was progressively compensated within a week by a persistent change in the activity of the medial gastrocnemius (MG) muscle. Considering that these are spinal cats, this finding suggests that the spinal cord is capable of some remarkable adaptation even without supraspinal systems. How this is achieved still needs to be clarified but it is probable that the spinal cord is capable of modifying the output of its locomotor pattern generator as a function of alterations in the neuromuscular state, either its muscular or sensory component.

The third series of experiments was already mentioned above and consisted in removing the cutaneous inputs from the foot with little or no damage to the motor apparatus, except for some intrinsic foot muscles. Although we reported above that after complete denervation spinal cats were no longer capable of walking on the foot planta, it has been remarkable to observe that after a *partial* skin denervation spinal cats can adapt and recover the normal positioning of the foot. Indeed, when the cutaneous denervation is progressive, the early deficits related to the removal of a nerve are compensated within a few days even in the spinal state. Such compensation could occur only up to the complete removal of all cutaneous inputs. Therefore, even in the spinal state, the animal is capable of achieving a functional compensation after a peripheral lesion (Fig. 8).

Conclusions

These studies indicate that the recovery of locomotion in adult spinal cats is probably the result of numerous plastic changes occurring at the level of the sensory afferents, cellular properties of neurones and receptors for neurotransmitters. These studies also show that the spinal cord is a complex laminar and segmental structure. More needs to be done on this aspect since a better understanding of the segmental spinal organization may simplify the task of stimulating the cord electrically or pharmacologically or even determine the appropriate sites for future grafting. Finally, the objective evidence that the spinal cord possesses some extensive capabilities to adapt its motor output not only to specific sensory phasic inputs but also to tonic permanent changes of the neuromuscular apparatus, definitely raises hopes that various types of manipulation can be used to improve the functional spinal recovery of locomotion. Some work being carried in humans and largely based on cat experiments suggest indeed that the cat model of spinal injury is a useful one.

Acknowledgements

We would like to thank Dr. T. Drew who acted as a special editor for this article as well as several technicians who have participated to this work in various capacities: France Lebel, Claude Gagner, Philippe Drapeau and Claude Gauthier. The authors also wish to express their gratitude to various granting agencies which have supported this work: the Canadian Institute for Health Research (CIHR), the Spinal Cord Research Foundation (SCRF), the Christopher Reeve Paralysis Foundation (CRPF) and the Fonds pour la Formation de Chercheurs et l'Aide à la Recherche (FCAR).

References

Barbeau, H. and Rossignol, S. (1987) Recovery of locomotion after chronic spinalization in the adult cat. *Brain Res.*, 412: 84–95.

Barbeau, H. and Rossignol, S. (1989) Effects of noradrenergic, serotonergic and dopaminergic drugs on the initiation of locomotion in adult spinal cat. *Soc. Neurosci. Abstr.*, 15: 393 No. 160.9.

Barbeau, H. and Rossignol, S. (1990) The effects of serotonergic drugs on the locomotor pattern and on cutaneous reflexes of the adult chronic spinal cat. *Brain Res.*, 514: 55–67.

Barbeau, H. and Rossignol, S. (1991) Initiation and modulation of the locomotor pattern in the adult chronic spinal cat by noradrenergic, serotonergic and dopaminergic drugs. *Brain Res.*, 546: 250–260.

Barbeau, H. and Rossignol, S. (1994) Enhancement of locomotor recovery following spinal cord injury. *Curr. Opin. Neurol.*, 7: 517–524.

Barbeau, H., Julien, C. and Rossignol, S. (1987) The effects of clonidine and yohimbine on locomotion and cutaneous reflexes in the adult chronic spinal cat. *Brain Res.*, 437: 83–96.

Bélanger, M., Drew, T., Provencher, J. and Rossignol, S. (1996) A comparison of treadmill locomotion in adult cats before and after spinal transection. *J. Neurophysiol.*, 76: 471–491.

Bouyer, L. and Rossignol, S. (1998) The contribution of cutaneous inputs to locomotion in the intact and the spinal cat. In: O. Kiehn, R.M. Harris-Warrick, L.M. Jordan, H. Hultborn and N. Kudo (Eds.), *Neuronal Mechanisms for Generating Locomotor Activity*. Annals of the New York Academy of Sciences, New York, pp. 508–512.

Bouyer, L. and Rossignol, S. (2001) Spinal cord plasticity associated with locomotor compensation to peripheral nerve lesions in the cat. In: M.M. Patterson, J.W. Grau, J.R. Wolpaw, W.D.J. Willis and V.R. Edgerton (Eds.), *Spinal Cord Plasticity: Alterations in Reflex Function*. Academic Publishers, New York, pp. 207–224.

Bouyer, L.J.G., Whelan, P., Pearson, K.G. and Rossignol, S. (2001) Adaptive locomotor plasticity in chronic spinal cats after ankle extensors neurectomy. *J. Neurosci.*, 21: 3531–3541.

Brodin, L., Grillner, S. and Rovainen, C.M. (1985) *N*-methyl-D-aspartate (NMDA), kainate and quisqualate receptors and the generation of fictive locomotion in the lamprey spinal cord. *Brain Res.*, 325: 302–306.

Brustein, E. and Rossignol, S. (1998) Recovery of locomotion after ventral and ventrolateral spinal lesions in the cat, I. Deficits and adaptive mechanisms. *J. Neurophysiol.*, 80: 1245–1267.

Brustein, E. and Rossignol, S. (1999) Recovery of locomotion after ventral and ventrolateral spinal lesions in the cat, II. Effects of noradrenergic and serotoninergic drugs. *J. Neurophysiol.*, 81: 1513–1530.

Carrier, L., Brustein, L. and Rossignol, S. (1997) Locomotion of the hindlimbs after neurectomy of ankle flexors in intact and spinal cats: model for the study of locomotor plasticity. *J. Neurophysiol.*, 77: 1979–1993.

Cazalets, J.-R. (2000) Organization of the spinal locomotor network in neonatal rat. In: R.G. Kalb and S.M. Strittmater (Eds.), *Neurobiology of Spinal Cord Injury*. Humana Press, Totowa, NJ, pp. 89–111.

Cazalets, J.R., Sqalli-Houssaini, Y. and Clarac, F. (1992) Activation of the central pattern generators for locomotion by serotonin and excitatory amino acids in neonatal rat. *J. Physiol.*, 455: 187–204.

Chau, C., Barbeau, H. and Rossignol, S. (1998a) Effects of intrathecal α_1- and α_2-noradrenergic agonists and norepinephrine on locomotion in chronic spinal cats. *J. Neurophysiol.*, 79: 2941–2963.

Chau, C., Barbeau, H. and Rossignol, S. (1998b) Early locomotor training with clonidine in spinal cats. *J. Neurophysiol.*, 79: 392–409.

Chau, C., Provencher, J., Lebel, F., Jordan, L., Barbeau, H. and Rossignol, S. (1994) Effects of intrathecal injection of NMDA receptor agonist and antagonist on locomotion of adult chronic spinal cats. *Soc. Neurosci. Abstr.*, 20: 573, No. 214.14.

De Leon, R.D., Hodgson, J.A., Roy, R.R. and Edgerton, V.R. (1998a) Full weight-bearing hindlimb standing following stand training in the adult spinal cat. *J. Neurophysiol.*, 80: 83–91.

De Leon, R.D., Hodgson, J.A., Roy, R.R. and Edgerton, V.R. (1998b) Locomotor capacity attributable to step training versus spontaneous recovery after spinalization in adult cats. *J. Neurophysiol.*, 79: 1329–1340.

De Leon, R.D., Reinkensmeyer, D.J., Timoszyk, W.K., London, N.J., Roy, R.R. and Edgerton, V.R. (2002) Use of robotics in assessing the adaptive capacity of the rat lumbar spinal cord. In: L. McKerracher, G. Doucet and S. Rossignol (Eds.), *Spinal Cord Trauma: Neural Repair and Functional Recovery*. Progress in Brain Research, Vol. 137, Elsevier, Amsterdam, pp. XX–XX.

Deliagina, T.G., Orlovsky, G.N. and Pavlova, G.A. (1983) The capacity for generation of rhythmic oscillations is distributed in the lumbosacral spinal cord of the cat. *Exp. Brain Res.*, 53: 81–90.

Douglas, J.R., Noga, B.R., Dai, X. and Jordan, L.M. (1993) The effects of intrathecal administration of excitatory amino acid agonists and antagonists on the initiation of locomotion in the adult cat. *J. Neurosci.*, 13: 990–1000.

Drew, T. and Rossignol, S. (1987) A kinematic and electromyographic study of cutaneous reflexes evoked from the forelimb of unrestrained walking cats. *J. Neurophysiol.*, 57: 1160–1184.

Duysens, J. and Pearson, K.G. (1976) The role of cutaneous afferents from the distal hindlimb in the regulation of the step cycle of thalamic cats. *Exp. Brain Res.*, 24: 245–255.

Duysens, J. and Pearson, K.G. (1980) Inhibition of flexor burst generation by loading ankle extensor muscles in walking cats. *Brain Res.*, 187: 321–332.

Forssberg, H. and Grillner, S. (1973) The locomotion of the acute spinal cat injected with clonidine i.v. *Brain Res.*, 50: 184–186.

Forssberg, H., Grillner, S. and Rossignol, S. (1975) Phase dependent reflex reversal during walking in chronic spinal cats. *Brain Res.*, 85: 103–107.

Forssberg, H., Grillner, S. and Rossignol, S. (1977) Phasic gain control of reflexes from the dorsum of the paw during spinal locomotion. *Brain Res.*, 132: 121–139.

Giroux, N., Brustein, E., Chau, C., Barbeau, H., Reader, T.A. and Rossignol, S. (1998) Differential effects of the noradrenergic agonist clonidine on the locomotion of intact, partially and completely spinalized adult cats. In: O. Kiehn, R.M. Harris-Warrick, L.M. Jordan, H. Hulborn and N. Kudo (Eds.), *Neuronal Mechanisms for Generating Locomotor Activity*. Annals of the New York Academy of Sciences, New York, pp. 517–520.

Giroux, N., Rossignol, S. and Reader, T.A. (1999) Autoradiographic study of α_1-, α_2-Noradrenergic and Serotonin$_{1A}$ receptors in the spinal cord of normal and chronically transected cats. *J. Comp. Neurol.*, 406: 402–414.

Giroux, N., Reader, T.A. and Rossignol, S. (2001) Comparison of the effect of intrathecal administration of clonidine and yohimbine on the locomotion of intact and spinal cats. *J. Neurophysiol.*, 85: 2516–2536.

Gorassini, M.A., Prochazka, A., Hiebert, G.W. and Gauthier, M.J.A. (1994) Corrective responses to loss of ground support during walking, I. Intact cats. *J. Neurophysiol.*, 71: 603–609.

Grillner, S. (1981) Control of locomotion in bipeds, tetrapods, and fish. In: J.M. Brookhart and V.B. Mountcastle (Eds.), *Handbook of Physiology. The Nervous System II.* American Physiological Society, Bethesda, MD, pp. 1179–1236.

Grillner, S. and Rossignol, S. (1978a) On the initiation of the swing phase of locomotion in chronic spinal cats. *Brain Res.*, 146: 269–277.

Grillner, S. and Rossignol, S. (1978b) Contralateral reflex reversal controlled by limb position in the acute spinal cat injected with clonidine i.v. *Brain Res.*, 144: 411–414.

Grillner, S. and Zangger, P. (1979) On the central generation of locomotion in the low spinal cat. *Exp. Brain Res.*, 34: 241–261.

Hiebert, G.W., Gorassini, M.A., Jiang, W., Prochazka, A. and Pearson, K.G. (1994) Corrective responses to loss of ground support during walking, II. Comparison of intact and chronic spinal cats. *J. Neurophysiol.*, 71: 611–622.

Hiebert, G.W., Whelan, P.J., Prochazka, A. and Pearson, K.G. (1996) Contribution of hind limb flexor muscle afferents to the timing of phase transitions in the cat step cycle. *J. Neurophysiol.*, 75: 1126–1137.

Jankowska, E., Jukes, M.G.M., Lund, S. and Lundberg, A. (1967a) The effect of DOPA on the spinal cord, 5. Reciprocal organization of pathways transmitting excitatory action to alpha motoneurones of flexors and extensors. *Acta Physiol. Scand.*, 70: 369–388.

Jankowska, E., Jukes, M.G.M., Lund, S. and Lundberg, A. (1967b) The effects of DOPA on the spinal cord, 6. Half centre organization of interneurones transmitting effects from the flexor reflex afferents. *Acta Physiol. Scand.*, 70: 389–402.

Jordan, L.M. and Schmidt, B.J. (2002) Propriospinal neurons involved in the control of locomotion: potential targets for repair strategies? In: L. McKerracher, G. Doucet and S. Rossignol (Eds.), *Spinal Cord Trauma: Neural Repair and Functional Recovery.* Progress in Brain Research, Vol. 137, Elsevier, Amsterdam, pp. 125–139.

Kiehn, O. and Kjaerulff, O. (1998) Distribution of central pattern generators for rhythmic motor outputs in the spinal cord of limbed vertebrates. *Ann. N.Y. Acad. Sci.*, 860: 110–129.

Kiehn, O., Iizuka, M. and Kudo, N. (1992) Resetting from low threshold afferents of N-methyl-D-aspartate-induced locomotor rhythm in the isolated spinal cord–hindlimb preparation from newborn rats. *Neurosci. Lett.*, 148: 43–46.

Kjaerulff, O. and Kiehn, O. (1996) Distribution of networks generating and coordinating locomotor activity in the neonatal rat spinal cord *in vitro: a lesion study. J. Neurosci.*, 16: 5777–5794.

Leblond, H., Marcoux, J. and Rossignol, S. (2001) The relative importance of midlumbar segments in real and fictive locomotion in spinal cats. *Soc. Neurosci. Abstr.*, 27: 517.3.

Marcoux, J. and Rossignol, S. (2000) Initiating or blocking locomotion in spinal cats by applying noradrenergic drugs to restricted lumbar spinal segments. *J. Neurosci.*, 20: 8577–8585.

Pearson, K.G. and Rossignol, S. (1991) Fictive motor patterns in chronic spinal cats. *J. Neurophysiol.*, 66: 1874–1887.

Philippson, M. (1905) L'autonomie et la centralisation dans le système nerveux des animaux. *Trav. Lab. Physiol. Inst. Solvay (Bruxelles)*, 7: 1–208.

Prochazka, A., Sontag, K.H. and Wand, P. (1978) Motor reactions to perturbations of gait: proprioceptive and somesthetic involvement. *Neurosci. Lett.*, 7: 35–39.

Rossignol, S. (1996) Neural control of stereotypic limb movements. In: L.B. Rowell and J.T. Sheperd (Eds.), *Handbook of Physiology, Section 12. Exercise: Regulation and Integration of Multiple Systems.* American Physiological Society, Oxford, pp. 173–216.

Rossignol, S. (2000) Locomotion and its recovery after spinal injury. *Curr. Opin. Neurobiol.*, 10: 708–716.

Rossignol, S. and Julien, C. (1980) Crossed hindlimb reflexes during fictive locomotion in acute spinal cats. *Soc. Neurosci. Abstr.*, 6: 392.

Rossignol, S., Barbeau, H., Pearson, K.G., Chau, C. and Provencher, J. (1992) Pharmacology of locomotion in the spinal cat. *Am. Paralysis Assoc.* (Abstr.).

Rossignol, S., Chau, C., Brustein, E., Bélanger, M., Barbeau, H. and Drew, T. (1996) Locomotor capacities after complete and partial lesions of the spinal cord. *Acta Neurobiol. Exp.*, 56: 449–463.

Rossignol, S., Chau, C., Brustein, E., Giroux, N., Bouyer, L., Barbeau, H. and Reader, T. (1998) Pharmacological activation and modulation of the Central Pattern Generator for locomotion in the cat. In: O. Kiehn, R.M. Harris-Warrick, L.M. Jordan, H. Hulborn and N. Kudo (Eds.), *Neuronal Mechanisms for Generating Locomotor Activity.* Annals of the New York Academy of Sciences, New York, pp. 346–359.

Rossignol, S., Bélanger, M., Chau, C., Giroux, N., Brustein, E., Bouyer, L., Grenier, C.-A., Drew, T., Barbeau, H. and Reader, T. (2000) The spinal cat. In: R.G. Kalb and Strittmatter, S.M. (Eds.), *Neurobiology of Spinal Cord Injury.* Humana Press, Totowa, NJ, pp. 57–87.

Rossignol, S., Giroux, N., Chau, C., Marcoux, J., Brustein, E. and Reader, T. (2001) Pharmacological aids to locomotor training after spinal injury in the cat. *J. Physiol. (Lond.)*, 533: 65–74.

Vanderhorst, V.G.J.M. and Holstege, G. (1997) Organization of lumbosacral motoneuronal cell groups innervating hindlimb, pelvic floor, and axial muscles in the cat. *J. Comp. Neurol.*, 382: 46–76.

SECTION III

Neuroprotection and transplantation

L. McKerracher, G. Doucet and S. Rossignol (Eds.)
Progress in Brain Research, Vol. 137
© 2002 Elsevier Science B.V. All rights reserved

CHAPTER 13

Neurotrauma/neurodegeneration and mitochondrial dysfunction

Marina Frantseva [1,2], Jose Luis Perez Velazquez [2], Alexandre Tonkikh [1],
Yana Adamchik [1] and Peter L. Carlen [1,*]

[1] *Toronto Western Research Institute, Room 12-413, 399 Bathurst Street, Toronto, ON M5T 2S8, Canada*
[2] *Hospital for Sick Children, Department of Neurology, 555 University Avenue, Toronto, ON M5T 1X8, Canada*

Introduction

Traumatic brain damage consists in part of mechanical disruption of neuronal and vascular tissue, and much of it could be irreversible. This damage can be viewed as a summation of two processes: the initial traumatic disruption of tissue from direct impact and from shock waves, and the secondary processes set in action subsequent to a primary insult. These secondary processes, which start immediately at the time of insult, are not clinically apparent for hours to days, which may provide a 'window of opportunity' for treatment of one or more of the developing pathophysiological mechanisms. They comprise a complex series of pathophysiological events leading to cellular death of additional tissue originally spared from the primary injury (Braughler and Hall, 1992). Even though there is considerable evidence that the major components of this 'secondary injury' are ischaemia, excitotoxic damage, and free radical generation (Miller, 1985), the precise mechanisms of irreversible cell damage remain unknown. These mechanisms are universal for all types of traumatised

* Correspondence to: P.L. Carlen, Toronto Western Research Institute, Rm. 12-413, 399 Bathurst St., Toronto, ON M5T 2S8, Canada. Tel.: +1-416-6035040; Fax: +1-416-6035745; E-mail: carlen@uhnres.utoronto.ca

brain tissue in all parts of the central nervous system, but the details vary depending on location and tissue type. The actual trauma causes local ischaemia via several mechanisms including disruption of arteries and veins, occlusion of arteries from vasospasm and in situ thrombosis, and blockade of local oxygen transport.

Mechanisms of mitochondrial dysfunction in hypoxia/ischaemia

Hypotheses of brain damage of various origins attribute neurotoxicity to the interplay of excessive cytosolic calcium accumulation and massive free radical production (Choi, 1990). The link between elevation of cytosolic calcium, free radicals, and cell death is being established in several laboratories. Recent evidence indicates that there is a converging event for different molecular routes that lead to cellular death: mitochondrial dysfunction characterised by a calcium-dependent loss of the mitochondrial potential prevented by cyclosporin-A, termed the mitochondrial permeability transition (MPT, reviewed in Zoratti and Szabo, 1995). While the MPT has been documented in a variety of non-neuronal cell systems (Crompton et al., 1987; Crompton and Costi, 1988; Crompton and Andreeva, 1993), clear evidence that the same process takes place in neurons after trauma or ischaemia has not been obtained, even though a number of reports have presented indirect evidence that the MPT occurs in brain tissue, using isolated brain mitochondria and astrocytic cultures exposed to elevated calcium levels (Kristal and Dubinsky, 1997), and in cultured neurons after intense glutamate receptor activation (Schinder et al., 1996; White and Reynolds, 1996). In addition, mitochondria in synaptosomal preparations were shown to depolarise (indicative of mitochondrial deterioration) in response to oxidative stress with hydrogen peroxide (Chinopoulos et al., 1999). All of these above mechanisms can ultimately lead to cell death via apoptosis.

A widely accepted idea is that the MPT represents the opening of a unique molecular entity acting as a pore (the mitochondrial permeability transition pore) in the mitochondrial membrane. However, the concept of the specific pore is still debated, and evidence for its existence in neuronal injury is still circumstantial. Some investigators have proposed an alternative explanation, that the loss of mitochondrial potential that leads to the MPT occurs as a result of aberrant mitochondrial calcium cycling via a specific calcium release pathway which is activated by monoADP-ribosylation of yet unidentified mitochondrial protein(s) (Richter et al., 1983; Weis et al., 1992).

Using our in vitro model of ischaemic injury, which consists of superfusing organotypic cultured hippocampal slices (Stoppini et al., 1991) with glucose-free deoxygenated solution for 8 min (Perez Velazquez et al., 1997) we have demonstrated that after an ischaemic episode, free radicals are produced in pyramidal neurons mostly during reoxygenation and that intracellular calcium levels increase in parallel to free radical generation (Perez Velazquez et al., 1997). Next we obtained evidence for a prolonged mitochondrial depolarisation, indicative of the MPT, during reperfusion in organotypic hippocampal neurons, by using two mitochondrial dyes, rhodamine 123 and JC-1 (Perez Velazquez et al., 1999, 2000). Calcium accumulated in neuronal mitochondria in parallel with the mitochondrial depolarisation after the hypoxic–hypoglycaemic insult (Frantseva et al., 1999a), and both events were arrested by the MPT blocker cyclosporin-A (CsA). Thus, this is important evidence for mitochondrial dysfunction, possibly the MPT, in neurons induced by an ischaemic-like episode. Evidence for large cross-linked protein aggregates of mitochondrial proteins as a result of free radical generation has been obtained by SDS-PAGE using solubilised proteins from mitochondrial membranes exposed to prooxidants (Fagian et al., 1990). However, these high molecular weight protein complexes may or may not be related to the presumed mitochondrial permeability transition pore. We used a blocker of the MPT, cyclosporin-A (CsA), which presumably interacts with the pore and blocks it (Andreeva et al., 1995), to affinity purify the permeability pore. We have made a CsA-affinity column (Nicolli et al., 1996) and have run solubilised mitochondrial proteins from control and ischaemic rat brain tissue (Perez Velazquez et al., 2000). As a positive control, brain mitochondria were exposed to the prooxidant t-butyl-hydroperoxide (t-BuOOH), which causes the MPT and presumably promotes pore formation (Crompton et al., 1987; Fagian et al., 1990; Nieminen et al., 1995). Elution of the proteins retained on the affinity column was achieved with 0.45 mM CsA, and eluted proteins were visualised using SDS-PAGE. The only consistent difference observed between proteins from control mitochondria and those exposed to the prooxidant was a band at 32 kDa in the injured samples. Interestingly, when rat brain slices were subjected to an episode of hypoxia–hypoglycaemia, the same protein band at 32 kDa was present after affinity purification of CsA-binding mitochondrial proteins, suggesting that this protein may be a common occurrence in these two different but related insults. In control and injured samples, CsA eluted a major protein (18 kDa), confirmed to be rat brain cyclophilin as determined by amino-terminal amino acid sequencing. The 32 kDa band was identified as porin (also known as the voltage-dependent anion channel, VDAC) by Western blotting with an anti-porin antibody. Porin is present in the mitochondria outer membrane and makes a pore that allows for the exchange of metabolites across the mitochondrial membrane (reviewed in Kirk and Strange, 1998). Porin is thought to participate in supramolecular complexes such as the mitochondrial benzodiazepine receptor, along with two other proteins of 30 and 18 kDa (McEnery et al., 1992, 1993). Activation of this receptor induces the MPT (Pastorino et al., 1994). We also observed a 30 kDa band using proteins from injured brain tissue in our CsA-affinity column studies, while an 18 kDa band was always present and was confirmed to be cyclophilin as mentioned above, the CsA receptor (Tanveer et al., 1996).

After obtaining biochemical evidence for a possible role of porin in mitochondrial dysfunction, we assessed its functional role. The anti-porin antibody (Calbiochem) we used was shown to be functional (it blocks the pore made by porin) by Szabo et al. (1998). For these experiments, the antibody was injected into individual pyramidal neurons in organotypic slices using the patch-clamp method, and the electrophysiological neuronal characteristics as well as mitochondrial depolarisation after the ischaemic insult were determined by simultaneous fluorescence imaging and whole-cell recordings (Perez Velazquez et al., 1999, 2000). Neurons injected with the antibody did not deteriorate and their mitochondria did not depolarise during ischaemia–reperfusion. We also assessed whether the antibodies prevented cellular death after ischaemia in organotypic hippocampal cultures (Perez Velazquez et al., 1999). Cell death was evaluated by staining the slices with propidium iodide (PI). The antibody was loaded into cells via osmotic lysis of pinocytic vesicles. The results of three experiments confirmed a significant decrease in cellular death after ischaemia–reperfusion by treatment with the anti-porin antibody. In addition, we also obtained preliminary evidence indicating that the antibody attenuates neuronal death in dissociated cultures exposed to NMDA. We should take into consideration that the antibodies may not be very efficiently loaded into cells by the Influx reagent, therefore the protection observed in these experiments with slices and dissociated cultures is very promising. These observations taken together with recent evidence that the pro-apoptotic protein Bax and the anti-apoptotic protein Bcl-2 interact directly with porin, the former promoting the open state of porin and the latter maintaining it closed (Shimizu et al., 1999), strongly suggests that porin plays a crucial role in cellular damage during ischaemia–reperfusion.

MPT and traumatic neurodegeneration

Recent observations provide evidence for alterations of mitochondrial function resulting from traumatic brain injury. Specifically, significant reductions in the rate of mitochondrial respiration and depression of energy metabolism were documented following the experimental brain trauma (Vink et al., 1990; Verweij et al., 1997; Xiong et al., 1997, 1998, 1999; Vagnozzi et al., 1999). Decreased mitochondrial potential (Sullivan et al., 1999) and altered calcium uptake (Verweij et al., 1997; Xiong et al., 1997, 1999), the hallmarks of mitochondrial permeability transition, were documented following traumatic brain injury. In addition, the ability of the classical MPT inhibitor cyclosporin-A to prevent the loss of mitochondrial potential, mitochondrial swelling and neuronal loss, resulting from brain trauma (Shiga et al., 1992; Okonkwo and Povlishock, 1999; Sullivan et al., 1999), indicates that mitochondrial permeability transition is a key event in traumatic neurodegeneration, similar to this resulting from ischaemic/excitotoxic injury.

In order to explore this possibility we performed preliminary experiments using in vitro trauma model developed in our laboratory (Adamchik et al., 2000). We use organotypic hippocampal slice cultures because they offer advantages over dissociated cultures in that they preserve the synaptic and anatomical organisation of the neuronal circuitry and have functional characteristics similar to those found in vivo (Stoppini et al., 1991). To model trauma injury, a weight of 0.137 g is dropped from a height of 5 mm on a localised area of the organotypic slice (Fig. 1B). Our impact injury consistently results in eventual spread of cell death, which is sensitive to neuroprotective strategies (Adamchik et al., 2000; Frantseva et al., 2001). The experiments are carried out after 12–14 days in vitro, and the percentage of cell death is calculated as described (Frantseva et al., 1999b; Adamchik et al., 2000). Our traumatic insult reproduces several of the features found in injuries to the intact brain. For example, in addition to the neuronal loss, as determined by staining with PI or by cresyl violet stained cell counts we also observe a proliferation of astrocytes which reflects the known phenomenon termed reactive gliosis that occurs after traumatic episodes (D'Ambrosio et al., 1999). We also observe a reduction of synaptic function immediately after the impact and a partial recovery 24 h later (Frantseva et al., 2001), similarly to the depression of neuronal activity described in brain trauma in

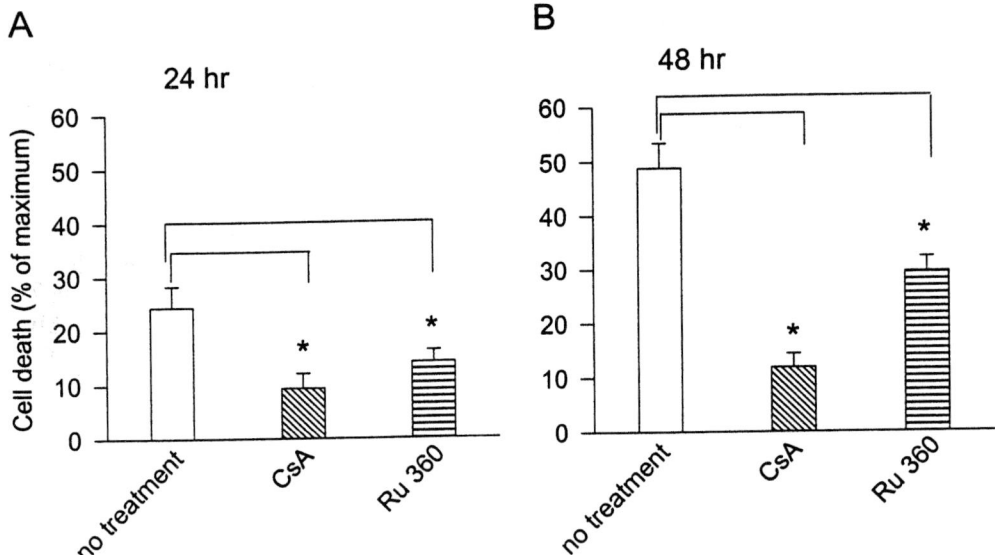

Fig. 1. Prevention of mitochondrial dysfunction decreases the spread of post-traumatic cell death. Graphs represent cell death, measured as percentage (mean ± standard deviation) of maximal cell death. Slices in the continuous presence of 5 μM cyclosporin-A (CsA) or Ru 360 show less cell death 24 and 48 h after the impact injury compared with non-treated controls. Statistical significance is shown with asterisks (unpaired Student's t-test), comparing treated versus non-treated groups.

vivo (Dixon et al., 1987). Field potentials recorded in the CA1 or CA3 areas were absent (neither evoked nor spontaneous activity) in 60% of the slices, which indicates a severe impairment of synaptic function. The abolition of synaptic transmission could be related to the phenomenon of spreading depression, known to occur after ischaemic episodes (Joshi and Andrew, 2001), since a voltage shift of 5 to 15 mV was recorded 2–5 min after the impact.

Consistent with previously published observations, pretreatment with the MPT inhibitor CsA (5 μM) significantly reduced cell death, resulting from the impact injury in our model for up to 48 h (see Fig. 1). An excessive accumulation of mitochondrial calcium, one of the major triggers of MPT, has also been demonstrated to be the primary cause of the excitotoxic cell death (Stout et al., 1998). In order to examine whether or not mitochondrial calcium uptake plays a role in cell death resulting from trauma, impact injury was initiated in slices pretreated with 10 μM of cell-permeable blocker of mitochondrial calcium uptake, Ru 360 (Matlib et al., 1998). Ru 360 greatly diminished cell death 24 and 48 h after the trauma injury when compared with non-treated slices (Fig. 1).

Conclusion

We conclude that mitochondrial dysfunction, which results from several converging deleterious mechanisms, also plays a major role in traumatic cell death. To date mitochondria have been little studied for their involvement in traumatic brain injury, but they could be an important therapeutic target for the early treatment and prevention of secondary brain and spinal cord damage. Specifically, the identification of targets to prevent MPTP opening and free radical formation should provide novel therapeutic strategies for improving recovery after ischaemic or traumatic brain injury.

Acknowledgements

Supported by the Ontario Neurotrauma Foundation.

References

Adamchik, Y., Frantseva, M.V., Weisspapir, M., Carlen, P. and Perez Velazquez, J.L. (2000) Methods to induce primary and secondary traumatic damage in organotypic hippocampal slice cultures. Brain Res. Protoc., 5: 153–158.

Andreeva, L., Tanveer, A. and Crompton, M. (1995) Evidence

for the involvement of a membrane-associated cyclosporin-A-binding protein in the calcium activated inner membrane pore of heart mitochondria. *Eur. J. Biochem.*, 230(3): 1125–1132.

Braughler, J.M. and Hall, E.D. (1992) Central nervous system trauma and stroke. *Free Radic. Biol. Med.*, 6: 289–301.

Chinopoulos, C., Tretter, L. and Adam-Vizi, V. (1999) Depolarization of in situ mitochondria due to hydrogen peroxide-induced oxidative stress in nerve terminals: inhibition of α-ketoglutarate dehydrogenase. *J. Neurochem.*, 73: 220–228.

Choi, D. (1990) Cerebral hypoxia: some new approaches and unanswered questions. *J. Neurosci.*, 10(8): 2493–2501.

Crompton, M. and Andreeva, L. (1993) On the involvement of a mitochondrial pore in reperfusion injury. *Basic Res. Cardiol.*, 88(5): 513–523.

Crompton, M. and Costi, A. (1988) Kinetic evidence for a heart mitochondrial pore activated by calcium, inorganic phosphate and oxidative stress. *Eur. J. Biochem.*, 178: 489–501.

Crompton, M., Costi, A. and Hayat, L. (1987) Evidence for the presence of a reversible calcium dependent pore activated by oxidative stress in heart mitochondria. *Biochem. J.*, 245: 915–918.

D'Ambrosio, R., Maris, D.O., Grady, M.S., Winn, H.R. and Janigro, D. (1999) Impaired K^+ homeostasis and altered electrophysiological properties of post-traumatic hippocampal glia. *J. Neurosci.*, 19: 8152–8162.

Dixon, C.E., Lyeth, B.G., Povlishock, J.T., Findling, R.L., Hamm, R.J., Marmarou, A., Young, H.F. and Hayes, R.L. (1987) A fluid percussion model of experimental brain injury in the rat. *J. Neurosurg.*, 67: 110–119.

Fagian, M.M., Pereira-da-Silva, L., Martins, L.S. and Vercesi, A.E. (1990) Permeabilization of the inner mitochondrial membrane by Ca^{2+} and prooxidants is associated with oxidation of protein thiols forming cross-linked protein aggregates. *J. Biol. Chem.*, 265: 19955–19960.

Frantseva, M.V., Carlen, P.L. and Perez Velazquez, J.L. (1999a) Molecular mechanisms of free radical production and protective efficacies of antioxidants in in vitro ischaemia–reperfusion. *Ann. N.Y. Acad. Sci.*, 893: 286–290.

Frantseva, M.V., Carlen, P.L. and El-Beheiry, H. (1999b) A submersion method to induce hypoxic damage in organotypic hippocampal cultures. *J. Neurosci. Methods*, 89: 25–31.

Frantseva, M.V., Kokarovtseva, L., Carlen, P.L., Naus, C.C.G. and Perez Velazquez, J.L. (2001) Role of specific gap junctions in spreading brain traumatic injury. *J. Neurosci.*, submitted.

Joshi, I. and Andrew, R.D. (2001) Imaging anoxic depolarization during ischemia-like conditions in the mouse hemi-brain slice. *J. Neurophysiol.*, 85: 414–424.

Kiedrowski, L. and Costa, E. (1995) Glutamate induced destabilization of intracellular calcium concentration homeostasis in cultured cerebellar granule cells: role of mitochondria in calcium buffering. *Mol. Pharmacol.*, 47: 140–147.

Kirk, K. and Strange, K. (1998) Functional properties and physiological roles of organic solute channels. *Annu. Rev. Physiol.*, 60: 719–739.

Kristal, B.S. and Dubinsky, J.M. (1997) Mitochondrial permeability transition in the central nervous system: induction by

calcium cycling-dependent and independent pathways. *J. Neurochem.*, 69(2): 524–538.

Matlib, M.A., Zhou, Z., Knight, S., Ahmen, S., Choi, K.M., Krause-Bauer, J., Phillips, R., Altschuld, R.A., Katsube, Y. and Sperekalis, N. (1998) Oxygen-bridged dinuclear ruthenium amine complex specifically inhibits calcium uptake into mitochondria in vitro and in single cardiac myocytes. *J. Biol. Chem.*, 273: 1022–10231.

McEnery, M.W., Snowman, A.M., Trifiletti, R.R. and Snyder, S.H. (1992) Isolation of the mitochondrial benzodiazepine receptor: association with the voltage dependent anion channel and the adenine nucleotide carrier. *Proc. Natl. Acad. Sci. USA*, 89: 3170–3174.

McEnery, M.W., Dawson, T.M., Verma, A., Gurley, D., Colombini, M. and Snyder, S.H. (1993) Mitochondrial voltage-dependent anion channel. *J. Biol. Chem.*, 268(31): 23289–23296.

Miller, J.D. (1985) Head injury and brain ischemia: implications for therapy. *Br. J. Anaesth.*, 57: 120–129.

Nicolli, A., Basso, E., Petronilly, V., Wengers, R. and Bernardi, P. (1996) Interactions of cyclophilin with the mitochondrial inner membrane and regulation of the permeability transition pore, a cyclosporin A-sensitive channel. *J. Biochem.*, 271(4): 2185–2192.

Nieminen, A.L., Saylor, A.K., Tesfai, S.A., Herman, B. and Lemasters, J.J. (1995) Contribution of the mitochondrial permeability transition to lethal injury after exposure of hepatocytes to *t*-butylhydroperoxide. *Biochem. J.*, 307: 99–106.

Okonkwo, D.O. and Povlishock, J.T. (1999) An intrathecal bolus of Cyclosporin A before injury preserves mitochondrial integrity and attenuates axonal dysruption in traumatic brain injury. *J. Cereb. Blood Flow Metab.*, 19: 443–451.

Pastorino, J.G., Simbula, G., Gilfor, E., Hoek, J.B. and Farber, J.L. (1994) Protoporphyrin IX, an endogenous ligand of the peripheral benzodiazepine receptor, potentiates induction of the mitochondrial permeability transition and the killing of cultured hepatocytes by rotenone. *J. Biol. Chem.*, 269(49): 31041–31046.

Perez Velazquez, J.L., Frantseva, M.V. and Carlen, P.L. (1997) In vitro ischemia promotes glutamate-mediated free radical generation and intracellular calcium accumulation in hippocampal pyramidal neurones. *J. Neurosci.*, 17(23): 9085–9094.

Perez Velazquez, J.L., Frantseva, M.V., Huzar, D., Guezurian, C. and Carlen, P.L. (1999) Mitochondrial porin, a novel target to prevent ischaemia-induced neurodegeneration? *Ann. N.Y. Acad. Sci.*, 893: 369–372.

Perez Velazquez, J.L., Frantseva, M.V., Huzar, D. and Carlen, P.L. (2000) Porin required for ischemia-induced mitochondrial dysfunction and neuronal damage. *Neuroscience*, 97(2): 363–369.

Richter, C., Winterhalter, K.H., Baumhuter, S., Lötscher, H.R. and Moser, B. (1983) ADP-ribosylation in the membrane of rat liver mitochondria. *Proc. Natl. Acad. Sci. USA*, 80: 3188–3192.

Schinder, A.F., Olson, E., Spitzer, N.C. and Montal, M. (1996) Mitochondrial dysfunction is a primary event in glutamate neurotoxicity. *J. Neurosci.*, 16(19): 6125–6133.

Shiga, Y., Onodera, H., Matsuo, Y. and Kogure, K. (1992) Cyclosporin A protects against ischemia-reperfusion injury in the brain. *Brain Res.*, 595: 145–148.

Shimizu, S., Narita, M. and Tsujimoto, Y. (1999) Bcl-2 family proteins regulate the release of apoptogenic cytochrome c by the mitochondrial channel VDAC. *Nature*, 399: 483–487.

Stoppini, L., Buchs, L.-A. and Muller, D. (1991) A simple method for organotypic cultures of nervous tissue. *J. Neurosci. Methods*, 37: 173–182.

Stout, A.K., Raphael, H.M., Kanterewicz, B.I., Klann, E. and Reynolds, I.J. (1998) Glutamate-induced neuron death requires mitochondrial calcium uptake. *Nat. Neurosci.*, 1: 366–373.

Sullivan, P.G., Thompson, M.B. and Scheff, S.W. (1999) Cyclosporin A attenuates acute mitochondrial dysfunction following traumatic brain injury. *Exp. Neurol.*, 160: 226–234.

Szabo, I., Bathori, G., Tombola, F., Coppola, A., Schmehl, I., Brini, M., Ghazi, A., DePinto, V. and Zoratti, M. (1998) Double-stranded DNA can be translocated across a planar membrane containing purified mitochondrial porin. *FASEB J.*, 12(6): 495–502.

Tanveer, A., Virji, S., Andreeva, L., Totty, N.F., Hsuan, J.J., Ward, J.M. and Crompton, M. (1996) Involvement of cyclophilin D in the activation of a mitochondrial pore by calcium and oxidant stress. *Eur. J. Biochem.*, 238(1): 166–172.

Vagnozzi, R., Marmarou, A., Tavazzi, B., Signoretti, S., Di Pierro, D., Del Bolgia, F., Amorini, A.M., Fazzina, G., Sherkat, S. and Lazzarino, G. (1999) Changes of cerebral energy metabolism and lipid peroxidation in rats leading to mitochondrial dysfunction after diffuse brain injury. *J. Neurotrauma*, 16(10): 903–913.

Verweij, B.H., Muizelaar, J.P., Vinas, F.C., Peterson, P.L., Xiong, Y. and Lee, C.P. (1997) Mitochondrial dysfunction after experimental and human brain injury and its possible reversal with a selective N-type calcium channel antagonist (SNX-111). *Neurol. Res.*, 19: 334–339.

Vink, R., Head, V.A., Rogers, P.J., McIntosh, T.K. and Faden, A.I. (1990) Mitochondrial metabolism following traumatic brain injury in rats. *J. Neurotrauma*, 7: 21–27.

Weis, M., Kass, G.E., Orrenius, S. and Moldeus, P. (1992) N-acetyl-p-benzoquinone imine induces calcium release from mitochondria by stimulating pyridine nucleotide hydrolysis. *J. Biol. Chem.*, 267(2): 804–809.

White, R.J. and Reynolds, I.J. (1996) Mitochondrial depolarization in glutamate-stimulated neurons: an early signal specific to excitotoxin exposure. *J. Neurosci.*, 16(18): 5688–5697.

Xiong, Y., Gu, Q., Peterson, P.L., Muizelaar, J.P. and Lee, C.P. (1997) Mitochondrial dysfunction and calcium perturbation induced by traumatic brain injury. *J. Neurotrauma*, 14: 23–34.

Xiong, Y., Peterson, P.L., Verweij, B.H., Vinas, F.C., Muizelaar, J.P. and Lee, C.P. (1998) Mitochondrial dysfunction after experimental traumatic brain injury: combined efficacy of SNX-111 and U-101033E. *J. Neurotrauma*, 15: 531–544.

Xiong, Y., Gu, Q., Peterson, P.L. and Lee, C.P. (1999) Effect of N-acetylcysteine on mitochondrial function following traumatic brain injury in rats. *J. Neurotrauma*, 16: 1067–1082.

Zoratti, M. and Szabo, I. (1995) The mitochondrial permeability transition. *Biochem. Biophys Acta*, 1241: 139–176.

L. McKerracher, G. Doucet and S. Rossignol (Eds.)
Progress in Brain Research, Vol. 137

CHAPTER 14

Secondary injury mechanisms of spinal cord trauma: a novel therapeutic approach for the management of secondary pathophysiology with the sodium channel blocker riluzole

Gwen Schwartz and Michael G. Fehlings [*]

The Toronto Western Research Institute, Division of Cell and Molecular Biology and Division of Neurosurgery, University of Toronto, Toronto, Canada

Abstract: Traumatic spinal cord injury is a consequence of a primary mechanical insult and a sequence of progressive secondary pathophysiological events that confound efforts to mitigate neurological deficits. Pharmacotherapy aimed at reducing the secondary injury is limited by a narrow therapeutic window. Thus, novel drug strategies must target early pathological mechanisms in order to realize the promise of efficacy for this form of neurotrauma. Research has shown that an accumulation of intracellular sodium as a result of trauma-induced perturbation of voltage-sensitive sodium channel activity is a key early mechanism in the secondary injury cascade. As such, voltage-sensitive sodium channels are an important therapeutic target for the treatment of spinal cord trauma. This review describes the evolution of acute spinal cord injury and provides a rationale for the clinical utility of sodium channel blockers, particularly riluzole, in the management of spinal cord trauma.

Current understanding and treatment of acute spinal cord injury

The clinical management of spinal cord injury (SCI) has perplexed physicians since the earliest description of this devastating condition by Egyptian physicians ca. 2500 B.C. (Breasted, 1930). Throughout millennia and as recently as 50 years ago, victims of SCI rarely survived their injuries. Late-twentieth-century advances in emergency care, diagnostic techniques, surgical intervention, and rehabilitation of

[*] Correspondence to: M.G. Fehlings, Toronto Western Hospital Research Institute, McLaughlin Pavilion 2-417, 399 Bathurst St., Toronto, ON M5T 2S8, Canada. Tel.: +1-416-603-5627; Fax: +1-416-603-5745; E-mail: michael@uhnres.utoronto.ca

the patient have greatly improved the survival of the victims of SCI. However, even with much-improved medical intervention many people with SCI die before reaching a trauma center and those who do survive the critical insult are left devastated by the life-long physical consequences of their injury.

In North America, an estimated 10,000 new cases of SCI are reported annually mostly as a result of motor vehicle accidents, violent acts, falls, and recreational sporting activities (NSCISC, 1997). More than half of those individuals affected survive the trauma with complete and/or incomplete paraplegia and tetraplegia (DeVivo, 1997). Although the incidence of traumatic SCI is low in comparison to other forms of central nervous system (CNS) trauma it is a leading cause of functional neurological impairment in young adults, affecting those with a mean age at injury of 32 years and a gender ratio slightly higher than 4 : 1 for males versus females (NSCISC, 1997). Thus, in addition to the great personal loss for the victims and their families, the overwhelming financial burden to society can be measured in the millions of dollars, per patient, for long-term medical and rehabilitative care and lost earnings (Tator et al., 1995; Hu et al., 1996).

The clinical and social implications of this form of neurotrauma have stimulated a vast amount of research directed towards reducing neurological impairment following SCI. The last decade realized the first effective therapeutic strategy for victims of acute SCI. In 1990, the National Acute Spinal Cord Injury Study II (NASCIS II), a multicenter clinical trial involving 487 patients presenting with neurologically complete or incomplete lesions at intake, reported that the steroid drug, methylprednisolone sodium succinate (MPSS), when administered within 8 h of injury, improved motor and sensory recovery of patients as compared to those who received naloxone or placebo (Bracken et al., 1990). Evaluation of patients in NASCIS II at 1-year follow-up confirmed the beneficial effects of MPSS (Bracken et al., 1992). Since the publication of the NASCIS II trial results and on the recommendations of NASCIS III, a multicenter clinical trial designed to determine the dose-administration protocol for MPSS (Bracken et al., 1997), the drug has been adopted as a standard of care for acute SCI in most North American centers. Although MPSS is the first accepted treatment strategy for acute SCI, criticisms regarding the drug's therapeutic physiological effects and its appreciable benefits to recipients have been raised (Hurlbert, 2000; Pointillart et al., 2000). In particular, the functional neurological improvement and independence measure scores, reported in NASCIS II and III, respectively, were only modestly enhanced in patients receiving MPSS within 8 h of SCI, suggesting that most victims are still left devastated by the physical impairments of their injury. These criticisms have led to the questioning of MPSS's therapeutic efficacy in the clinical setting and as a result, to the recently disseminated professional guidelines that downgrade the clinical use of this drug from that of a standard of care to an option (AANS/CNS, 2002). Nonetheless, the 'therapeutic window' established by the second NASCIS trial showed conclusively that acute SCI is amenable to drug therapy. Given this window of op-

portunity, improving drug treatment strategies aimed at attenuating early trauma-induced pathophysiology would be of great clinical value for the victims of SCI.

Along these lines, research directed at elucidating the physiological mechanisms underlying pathological alterations to neural tissue following trauma, that is the secondary injury, indicates that the deregulation of sodium ion (Na^+) homeostasis with an accumulation of intracellular sodium ($[Na^+]_i$) is a key early event in the pathogenesis of secondary CNS injury (Stys et al., 1992; Friedman and Haddad, 1994; Xie et al., 1994; Fehlings and Agrawal, 1995; Agrawal and Fehlings, 1996; Calabresi et al., 1999). Accordingly, pharmacological compounds demonstrating a neuroprotective mechanism of action involving the interruption of Na^+-induced secondary injury present a particularly attractive therapeutic strategy for the treatment of traumatic SCI. Recently, we reported that the anticonvulsant Na^+ channel blocker, riluzole, is neuroprotective and promotes functional neurological recovery after traumatic SCI in rodents (Schwartz and Fehlings, 2001). Moreover, the systemic, acute post-injury interval administration protocol employed in our study substantiates the effectiveness of early therapeutic intervention in order to mitigate secondary injury. In the present review, we briefly summarize current concepts of the pathophysiology of acute SCI with an emphasis on the key role of Na^+ channels. We also summarize the data supporting riluzole as an attractive candidate for clinical trials in acute SCI.

The concept of primary and secondary acute spinal cord injury

Neurotrauma is characterized by a primary mechanical injury resulting in focal destruction of neural substrates at the site of insult followed by secondary pathological damage to residual tissue. In the event of acute SCI, neurological dysfunction at the level of the lesion is attributed with and consequent upon the force and nature of the primary insult (Gale et al., 1985; Noble and Wrathall, 1985; Tator and Fehlings, 1991; Behrmann et al., 1992; Blight, 1996). A number of primary mechanisms associated with acute SCI have been documented including spontaneous spinal cord infarction, missile injury-induced laceration of the spinal cord, and acute stretching of the cord as a result of iatrogenic vertebral distraction or abrupt acceleration–deceleration of the spinal column (Fehlings and Tator, 1988). However, the most common underlying mechanism of trauma-induced paralysis results from acute compression or laceration of the spinal cord due to the displacement of bone or disc into the spinal column during fracture-dislocation or burst fracture of the spine (Tator, 1983). Although it is understood that the spinal cord is rarely totally transected even after severe SCI associated with complete paralysis (Kakulas, 1984; Bunge et al., 1993), the initial mechanical impact and subsequent persisting compression on spinal cord tissue initiates secondary pathophysiological alterations, at both the cellular and molecular level, which can induce complete transection-like pathology (Tator and Rowed, 1979).

The sequence of pathological changes in the cord, following the initial trauma, includes hemorrhage, edema, axonal and neuronal necrosis, and demyelination followed by cyst formation and infarction (Allen, 1914; Ducker et al., 1971; Dohrmann et al., 1972; Bresnahan et al., 1976; Sandler and Tator, 1976a; Tator and Rowed, 1979; Blight, 1983; Griffiths and McCulloch, 1983; Kakulas, 1984; Banik et al., 1987; Wallace et al., 1987). The temporal continuum by which these secondary events progress corresponds with early residual gray matter (GM) loss and delayed white matter (WM) degeneration (Balentine, 1978a,b). The developmental progression of this secondary injury is consistent with the gradual expansion of the initial lesion, both radially and longitudinally, from the epicenter of the initial force (Osterholm, 1978; Noble and Wrathall, 1985; Guizar-Sahagun et al., 1994). Subsequently, adjacent spinal segments are recruited into the successive secondary pathophysiological cascade adding to an increase in tissue destruction that ultimately contributes to heightened functional impairment.

Evidence for this post-traumatic autodestruction was first reported by Allen (1914). He theorized that progressive damage to traumatized spinal cord tissue was a result of a noxious 'biochemical factor' present in the hemorrhagic residual tissue. Since Allen's report, numerous clinical and experimental studies have described the contributing role of secondary pathophysiological mechanisms to neuronal

degeneration and the subsequent and persisting neurological dysfunction after acute SCI (Bresnahan et al., 1976; Sandler and Tator, 1976b; Bresnahan, 1978; Tator and Rowed, 1979; Blight, 1983; Kakulas, 1984; Wallace et al., 1987; Tator and Fehlings, 1991; Young, 1993; Fehlings and Tator, 1995; Anthes et al., 1996). In general, it is understood that mechanical disruption of spinal cord tissue, occurring at the moment of trauma, initiates within seconds a cascade of biophysical and neurochemical sequelae that can continue for minutes, days, weeks, and in some cases months after injury (Table I). However, the evolution of secondary injury is best described as a complex interplay of multiple autodestructive mechanisms that are interwoven with positive feedback loops that serve to amplify preceding events. Pathophysiological mechanisms characterized in the acute post-injury phase such as ischemia (Tator and Fehlings, 1991), metabolic perturbations (Anderson et al., 1980), ionic homeostatic deregulation (Stys and Lopachin, 1998; LoPachin et al., 1999), cytotoxic and vasogenic edema (Balentine, 1978b; Narayana et al., 1999), lipid peroxidation and free radical formation (Anderson et al., 1985a), and excitotoxicity (Li et al., 1999) give rise to more delayed secondary injury processes associated with cell-mediated degeneration including induction of pro-inflammatory mediators (Taoka and Okajima, 1998), macrophage invasion (Mabon et al., 2000) and apoptosis (Katoh et al., 1996; Li et al., 1996; Yong et al., 1998).

Mechanisms of action of neuroprotective pharmacotherapy

The complexity and temporal nature of the secondary injury cascade affords the opportunity for pharmacological intervention on several levels. Many pharmacological approaches aimed at attenuating the secondary injury cascade have been documented; however, this brief overview will focus on those agents demonstrating clinical applicability for the management of acute SCI.

Evidence attained from animal studies investigating the physiological mechanisms underlying MPSS's efficacy indicates that the drug may limit post-traumatic alterations of membrane lipid metabolism thereby reducing damage to cellular mem-

TABLE I

Primary and secondary mechanisms of acute spinal cord injury

Primary Injury Mechanisms ⟶		Secondary Injury Mechanisms
Acute Compression Impact Missile Distraction Laceration Shear	**Seconds** **Weeks**	**Vascular Alterations:** • Hemorrhage, Reduced Blood Flow • Systemic Hypotension, Arteriole Vasospasm • Thrombosis, Loss of Microcirculation Metabolic Changes: • Increased Glucose Utilization, Reduced Oxygen Tension • Loss of High Energy Phosphates (ATP), Acidosis Electrolytic Shifts: • Increased $[Na^+]_i$, $[Cl^-]_i$, $[P^{3-}]_i$, $[K^+]_e$, $[Mg^{2+}]_e$ • Increased $[Ca^{2+}]_i$, $[H_2O]_i$ Biochemical Changes: 1. Lipid Peroxidation • Free-Radical and Fatty Acid Production • Arachidonic Acid Release • Prostanoid and Eicosanoid Synthesis 2. Neurotransmitter Accumulation • Excitotoxic Amino Acids, Catecholamines, Endogenous Opioids Edema Cell-Mediated Injury: 1. Inflammation • Polymorphonuclear Neutrophilic Leukocyte Infiltration • Macrophage Invasion • Induction of Reactive Microglia 2. Apoptosis

branes that contributes to neuronal death after injury (Anderson et al., 1985a; Anderson and Means, 1985b; Saunders et al., 1987). Others have suggested that the drug's mechanism of action may reside with its ability to reduce inflammation near the injury and suppress the activation of immune cells that contribute to neuronal damage (Schleimer et al., 1989; Mabon et al., 2000). Suppression of the post-traumatic inflammatory response with prosta-cyclin, gabexate mesilate, and activated protein C (APC) also has been associated with significant attenuation of motor deficits in SCI rats (Taoka and Okajima, 1998). Another agent, GM-1 ganglioside, which has shown effective enhancement of functional recovery after SCI in phase III clinical trials (Geisler et al., 2001), has a mechanism of action attributable to the prevention of more delayed secondary injury processes (Greene et al., 1996). In fact, several neuroprotective agents designed to intervene at various steps along the secondary injury cascade have reached phase III efficacy trials for the treatment of acute ischemic stroke or traumatic brain injury (TBI). Some of these agents may be of benefit for the treatment of acute SCI although, to date, efficacy results have been mixed (Muizelaar et al., 1993; Hickenbottom and Grotta, 1998). Nonetheless, results attained from experimental models of acute traumatic CNS injury have demonstrated conclusively that neuroprotective treatments are maximally effective when instituted within the first hours after injury. Given this narrow therapeutic window, it follows that neuroprotective potential resides with drugs that target the earliest autodestructive mechanisms within the secondary injury cascade, thereby mitigating downstream pathological events and the pathophysiological cycle.

Candidate agents with this neuroprotective potential demonstrate a capacity to inhibit electrolytic homeostatic perturbations. The rationale for this assertion is based on experimental findings demonstrating a correlation between early disruption of subcellular ion distributions and depressed electrophysiological function, swollen axons, and neuroglia and myelin disruption in injured spinal cord tissue (LoPachin et al., 1999). Abnormal calcium ion (Ca^{2+}) homeostasis is understood to be a key cellular process underlying secondary CNS tissue damage following trauma (Tymianski and Tator, 1996). However, Ca^{2+} channel antagonists investigated for clinical applicability have failed to demonstrate improved neurological outcome in phase III trials of acute ischemic stroke (Gelmers and Hennerici, 1990), TBI (Teasdale et al., 1992), or in experimental spinal cord trauma (Cheng et al., 1984; Ford and Malm, 1985; Haghighi et al., 1993).

The reasons behind the lack of neuroprotective efficacy with Ca^{2+} channel antagonists support the involvement of another ion-dependent protagonist in the toxic secondary cascade. Accumulation of $[Na^+]_i$, as a result of trauma-induced activation of voltage-sensitive Na^+ channels, has been associated with an accumulation of $[Ca2^+]_i$ (Stys et al., 1991, 1992; Agrawal and Fehlings, 1996; Zhang and Lipton, 1999). In addition, increased $[Na^+]_i$ stimulates intracellular phospholipase activity (Gusovsky et al., 1986), promotes intracellular acidosis (Haigney et

al., 1994; Reithmeier, 1994), and induces cytotoxic edema (Regan and Choi, 1991) and excitotoxic cell death (Taylor et al., 1992; Li et al., 1999). Importantly, the neuroprotective and functional restorative efficacy from pharmacological blockade of excitatory amino acid-induced excitotoxic secondary injury, as demonstrated following experimental TBI and SCI (von Euler et al., 1994; Wrathall et al., 1994; Alaoui et al., 1995; Agrawal and Fehlings, 1997b; Rosenberg et al., 1999a), is significantly augmented with Na^+ channel blockers, suggesting that reduced excitotoxicity is a consequence of attenuated Na^+-mediated cytotoxicity (Lynch et al., 1995; Okiyama et al., 1995). Thus, pharmacological blockade of voltage-sensitive Na^+ channels is an important therapeutic intervention following CNS trauma.

Therapeutic efficacy of voltage-dependent Na^+ channel blockers

In general, voltage-dependent Na^+ channel blockers can be classified as compounds demonstrating potent physiotoxic activity or into three broad therapeutic categories based on their clinical utility: (1) local anesthetics; (2) antiarrhythmics; and (3) anticonvulsants. In accord with the neuronal theory of experimental traumatic SCI, postulated by Kobrine (1975), both experimental and therapeutic Na^+ channel blockers have been shown to be effective neuroprotective strategies. For instance, application of the potent Na^+ channel neurotoxin, tetrodotoxin (TTX), to the focal lesion following compressive or contusive SCI in rats results in attenuated post-traumatic axonal dysfunction in vitro and improved behavioral recovery and residual WM sparing in vivo (Agrawal and Fehlings, 1996; Teng and Wrathall, 1997; Rosenberg et al., 1999b). Although the neuro- and cardio-toxic side effects of TTX preclude its use as a therapeutic intervention for traumatic SCI in humans, less toxic Na^+ channel blockers have demonstrated similar functional and neuroanatomical protective effects at therapeutically relevant concentrations (Kobrine et al., 1984; Agrawal and Fehlings, 1996, 1997a).

The earliest accounts of neuroprotective efficacy with voltage-sensitive Na^+ channel blockers were demonstrated in cerebral tissue with those agents belonging to the local anesthetic class (Geddes and Quastel, 1956). These compounds also demonstrate neuroprotective efficacy after acute traumatic SCI. Kobrine and colleagues studied the effects of systemically administered lidocaine after experimental acute SCI in cats. They noted that the drug had a marked effect on the restoration of electrophysiological responses 4 h after injury in addition to a neuroanatomical protective effect at the site of injury (Kobrine et al., 1984). In addition, partial preservation of descending motor axons after traumatic SCI has been reported with another local anesthetic, QX-314; however, the neuroprotective effects of this drug were insufficient to result in sustained improvements in functional neurological recovery (Agrawal and Fehlings, 1997a). Anticonvulsant-class Na$^+$ channel blockers also are neuroprotective after traumatic SCI and TBI. The established antiepileptic drug phenytoin (PHT) confers significant cerebroprotection against both anoxic and ischemic injury in vitro and in vivo (Cullen et al., 1979; Taft et al., 1989; Boxer et al., 1990; Fern et al., 1993; Rataud et al., 1994; Probert et al., 1997). In cultured mouse spinal cord neurons and in squid giant axon PHT demonstrates an ability to attenuate sustained high-frequency repetitive firing and to reduce the rate of action potentials during prolonged depolarizing current pulses (Lipicky et al., 1972; McLean and Macdonald, 1983), suggesting that the drug may be effective at attenuating secondary pathophysiological consequences associated with traumatic SCI. Indeed, systemically administered PHT, 15 min after compressive SCI in rats, confers significant long-term neuroanatomical protection of lesion site tissue (Schwartz and Fehlings, 2001). Other PHT-like anticonvulsants, such as the lamotrigine derivatives BW1003C87 and BW619C89, are neuroprotective after lateral fluid percussion TBI, reducing regional brain edema, neuronal loss, and behavioral deficits in treated rats (Okiyama et al., 1995; Sun and Faden, 1995). Novel benzothiazole anticonvulsants also prevent the pathological consequences of excessive Na$^+$ influx after CNS trauma. One such compound, lubelzole, has demonstrated neuroprotective efficacy in in vitro models of cerebral ischemia (Ashton et al., 1997; Culmsee et al., 1998; Wiedemann and Hanke, 1999) and in vivo models of TBI (Kroppenstedt et al., 1999). When systemically administered after experimentally induced cortical infarct, lubeluzole significantly reduced lesion size, rescued sensorimotor hindlimb long-tract neurons, and preserved functional behavior (De Ryck et al., 1996).

The promise of neuroprotective efficacy evidenced with Na$^+$ channel blockers, particularly lubeluzole and fosPHT in preclinical animal models of ischemia, has led to phase II and phase III clinical trials of these agents for the treatment of stroke (Grotta, 1997; Diener, 1998; Hickenbottom and Grotta, 1998). But despite the vast amount of experimental data supporting neuroprotective efficacy in CNS trauma models, surprisingly few therapeutic Na$^+$ channel blockers have been assessed in preclinical trials for TBI and even fewer for SCI. However, riluzole, a benzothiazole anticonvulsant, known to have beneficial effects in chronic, neurodegenerative motoneuron diseases including amyotrophic lateral sclerosis (ALS) and Parkinson's disease (Bensimon et al., 1994; Barneoud et al., 1996; Gurney et al., 1996; Guyot et al., 1997), also has shown great potential as a neuroprotective strategy for both TBI and SCI in rats. Moreover, direct comparison of the pharmacodynamic properties of riluzole, PHT, and lamotrigine has shown the former to have superior inhibitory effects on voltage-dependent inward Na$^+$ conductance (Stefani et al., 1997), a mechanism that may account for riluzole's enhanced neuroprotective effects in trauma states. Thus, riluzole would be an interesting therapeutic candidate to pursue in translational studies of SCI. The rationale for this assumption will be the focus of the remainder of this review.

Neuroprotective effects of riluzole

Riluzole demonstrates potent neuroprotective activity in rodent models of cerebral ischemia both in vitro and in vivo (Pratt et al., 1992; Wahl et al., 1993; Ashton et al., 1997; O'Neill et al., 1997; Ettaiche et al., 1999; Kanthasamy et al., 1999). Riluzole also has been shown to attenuate and prevent ischemia-induced secondary pathophysiology in a rabbit model of spinal cord ischemia (Lang-Lazdunski et al., 1999). In rodent trauma models, riluzole treatment reduces the extent of cellular damage associated with the attenuation of acute and long-term functional neurological deficits sustained after TBI (McIntosh et al., 1996; Wahl et al., 1997). The largest therapeutic window established by the aforementioned trauma studies was 1 to 6 h post-injury with repeated systemic doses ranging from 4 to 8 mg/kg for up to 7 days. However, in a rat model of traumatic SCI, Stutzmann and colleagues demonstrated both anatomical and functional neurological protection with riluzole, at a concentration of 2 mg/kg administered intravenously at 30 min and thereafter twice daily for 10 consecutive days post-trauma. This protocol resulted in a reduction of lesion volume, WM protection, recovery of neuronal somatosensory evoked potentials, and qualitatively assessed functional improvement (Stutzmann et al., 1996).

Although the study by Stutzmann et al. was the first to report riluzole's neuroprotective efficacy in a rodent model of compression-induced trauma of the spinal cord, the benefits of the drug were only assessed in the acute and subacute post-injury period and conclusive motor recovery was not demonstrated. However, as recently reported, the beneficial neurological effects of riluzole can be sustained, resulting in long-term behavioral and neuroanatomical recovery after SCI. These effects were realized in a study designed to assess the effectiveness of riluzole and other Na^+ channel blockers on long-term tissue sparing and functional neurological recovery after traumatic SCI (Schwartz and Fehlings, 2001). In the study, adult rats were subjected to severe compressive cervical SCI. Fifteen minutes post-trauma the animals received a single intraperitoneal injection of either 5 mg/kg riluzole ($n = 13$), 30 mg/kg phenytoin ($n = 13$), 15 mg/kg CNS5546A, a novel pharmacological compound with sodium channel blocking capabilities ($n = 14$), or a vehicle control compound ($n = 14$). Clinical neurological recovery of motor behavior was assessed 1 week post-injury and weekly thereafter for 6 weeks, with 2 behavioral recovery indexes: the Basso, Beattie and Bresnahan (BBB) expanded locomotor rating scale (Basso et al., 1995) and the inclined plane (IP) technique (Rivlin and Tator, 1977). Seven weeks post-injury, digital morphometry of the lesion site and quantitation of neurons in the midbrain and brainstem retrogradely labeled by fluorogold were used to assess the preservation of residual tissue and integrity of descending axons, respectively. In this model of

SCI, all animals were uniformly paraplegic immediately postoperatively. Progressive, partial recovery of hindlimb function was seen over several weeks in all injured animals; however, motor recovery differed significantly among treatment groups across the testing period for both the BBB ($p = 0.0001$) and IP ($p < 0.0001$) (Fig. 1). Post-hoc analyses of the behavioral data revealed that riluzole treatment significantly enhanced the functional recovery of rats on both recovery indexes as compared to the other treatments ($p < 0.05$). Morphologically, all three Na^+ channel blockers significantly enhanced residual tissue area at the injury epicenter compared to the control treatment ($p < 0.0001$) with riluzole having the greatest effect on tissue sparing ($p < 0.05$). Riluzole also significantly reduced tissue loss in rostrocaudal regions surrounding the epicenter, with overall sparing of gray matter ($p < 0.02$) and selective sparing of white matter ($p < 0.05$) (Fig. 2). Counts of neurons in the red nucleus, retrogradely labeled by fluorogold introduced caudal to the injury site 7 weeks after trauma, also were significantly increased in the riluzole group ($p < 0.02$) (Fig. 3A). In particular, large-diameter red nucleus neurons were preferentially spared ($p < 0.05$), indicating a riluzole-induced preservation of rubrospinal tract axons. We also noted a trend toward enhanced sparing of other motor tract associated neurons in the riluzole treated group (Fig. 3B–E). The findings of this study suggest that systemic Na^+ channel blockers, primarily riluzole, can confer significant neuroprotection after in vivo SCI in rats. Moreover these neuroprotective effects were conferred at a concentration significantly less than those reported in other trauma models. Taken together, this study may represent the first step in recognizing riluzole as a clinically applicable therapeutic agent for acute SCI.

Determinants of clinical applicability of riluzole for the treatment of acute spinal cord injury

The pursuit of effective neuroprotective pharmacotherapy for the clinical management of SCI has revealed much about the pathological determinants of this form of neurotrauma. There is much experimental support for the neuroprotective potential of many compounds that target specific steps along the

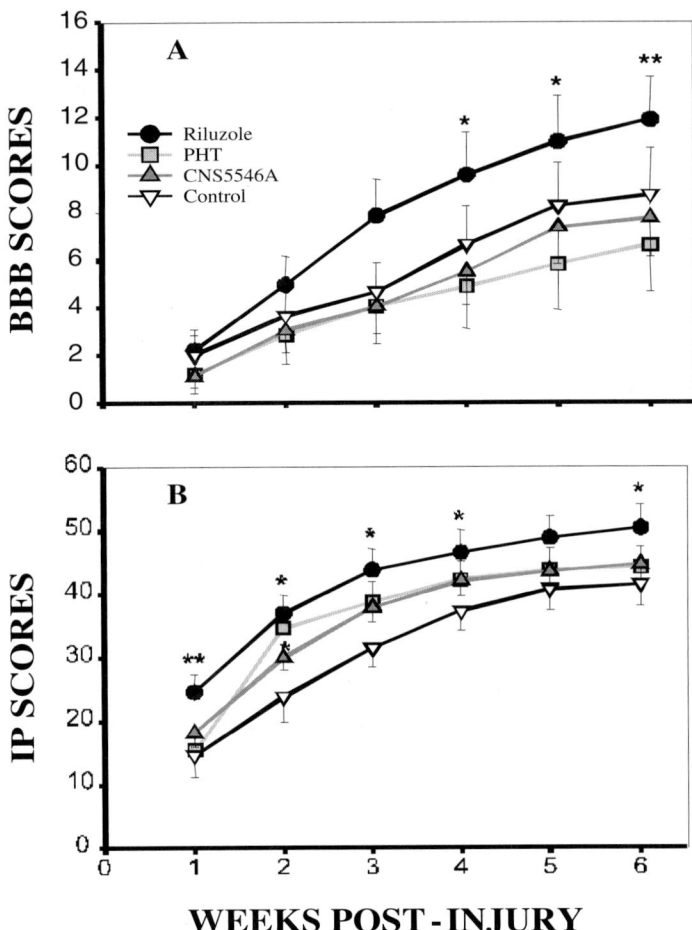

Fig. 1. Functional hindlimb recovery over time after SCI in rats that received either 5 mg/kg riluzole ($n = 13$; •), 30 mg/kg PHT ($n = 13$; ■), 15 mg/kg CNS5546A ($n = 14$; ▲), or 5 mg/kg control ($n = 14$; ▽). (A) Locomotor recovery graded on the BBB scale (Basso et al., 1995), where 0 represents complete paralysis and 21 represents normal hindlimb function. Data points represent group average ± SEM. (B) Inclined plane performance. Data points represent average ± SEM maximum angle at which animals can maintain position for 5 s. Data were analyzed with 2-factor ANOVA, which showed an overall significant main effect of treatment on both BBB and IP performance ($p = 0.0001$ and 1.84×10^{-35}, respectively). Means with single asterisk (*) are significantly different from the PHT-treated group (BBB) or the control-treated group (IP) at specified testing trial by Fisher's LSD test ($p < 0.05$). Two asterisks (**) indicate that means are significantly different from PHT- and CNS5546A-treated groups (BBB), or from control- and PHT-treated groups (IP) at specified time after SCI by Fisher's LSD test ($p < 0.05$). (Modified with permission from Schwartz and Fehlings, 2001.)

secondary injury cascade. However, their efficacy in preclinical trials has failed to provide compelling data to support further examination. Other promising agents have shown cerebroprotective efficacy clinically. Some of these drugs may have utility in the treatment of human SCI, but despite the promise of efficacy in experimental or preclinical animal studies, their beneficial effects have not been translated to the human population. It has been suggested

that this lack of efficacy may reflect a compromise of fundamental experimental design principles that, if adhered to, could ensure successful translation (Hickenbottom and Grotta, 1998). For instance, many experimental neuroprotective agents are beneficial only at dosages beyond tolerable safety and toxicity ranges and those that are tolerable, with respect to the aforementioned, are only beneficial within a given therapeutic window. Thus, careful

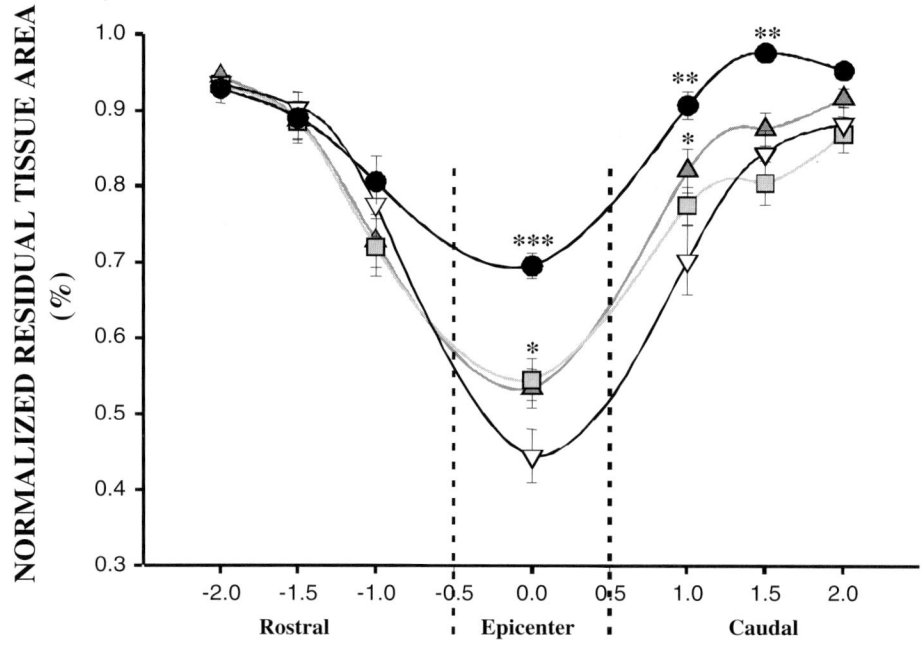

Fig. 2. Effects of Na$^+$ channel blockers on lesion morphometry at 7 weeks after SCI. Normalized residual tissue area (WM and GM combined) in spinal cord sections rostrocaudal (±1.0, 1.5, and 2.0 mm) from injury epicenter (0 ± 0.5 mm). Data represent the average $\pm$ SEM from four rats per group. Where no error bar is shown, the SEM was smaller than the symbol. Groups received 5 mg/kg riluzole (●), 30 mg/kg PHT (■), 15 mg/kg CNS5546A (▲), or 5 mg/kg vehicle-control (▽). There were significant main effects of treatment overall ($p = 3.43 \times 10^{-17}$) and at the epicenter ($p = 1.86 \times 10^{-11}$) (2-factor ANOVA). Single (*), double (**), and triple (***) asterisk(s) indicate that means are significantly different ($p < 0.05$) from control-treated, control- and PHT-treated, or control-, PHT-, and CNS5546A-treated groups, respectively (SNK method). (Modified with permission from Schwartz and Fehlings, 2001.)

examination of a given compound's dose–response characteristics and compliance with preclinically established therapeutic windows is essential in order to assess the promise of pharmacotherapeutic efficacy at the clinical level.

With regard to riluzole's therapeutic potential for the treatment of acute SCI, our study has demonstrated promising preliminary evidence supporting its beneficial effects. Moreover, riluzole is a safe drug that is already in use clinically for the treatment of ALS (Bensimon et al., 1994). However, riluzole's efficacy should further be examined to clarify the therapeutic window as well as the dosage and duration of treatment for SCI. In addition, a combination of riluzole with MPSS or GM-1 ganglioside may enhance the appreciable benefits to victims of SCI, since riluzole's chief neuroprotective mechanism of action, namely trauma-induced Na$^+$ cytotoxicity, precedes those of MPSS or GM-1 gan-

glioside within the secondary injury cascade. Thus, efficient preclinical tests of this nature can ensure a rapid translation to clinical trials for this promising therapy.

Conclusions

The functional neurological deficits sustained after spinal cord trauma are not solely the result of the initial traumatic insult. Rather, it is widely held that the primary injury precipitates complex pathophysiological changes in spinal cord tissue that lead to irreversible sensory and motor deficits. Considerable research aimed at attenuating the secondary injury following trauma has led to the development of several promising drug therapies that target distinct mechanisms within the secondary injury cascade. However, only MPSS is being used clinically for the treatment of patients with acute SCI. Today, some

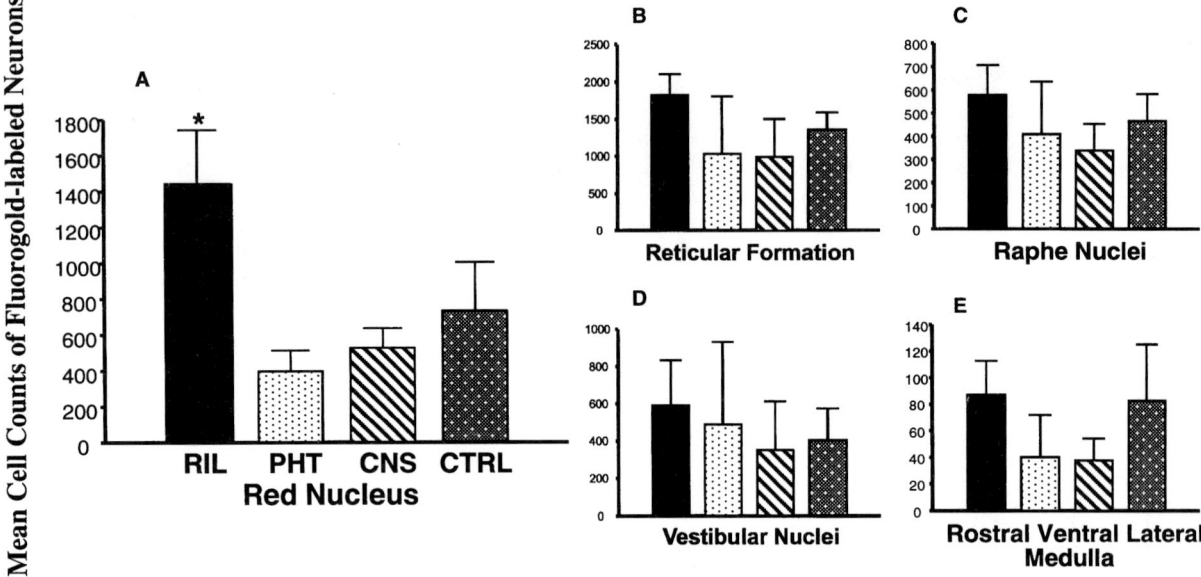

Fig. 3. Mean cell counts of retrograde fluorogold-labeled cells in brainstem nuclei associated with descending motor long tracts in the rat, 7 weeks after severe clip-compression SCI. (A) Red nucleus (rubrospinal tract). * Riluzole (RIL) treatment resulted in significantly greater counts of red nucleus cell bodies as compared to the other treatments (PHT = phenytoin; CNS = CNS5546A) or control (CTRL), $p < 0.02$. (B) Reticular formation (reticulospinal tract). (C) Raphe nuclei (raphespinal tracts). (D) Vestibular nuclei (vestibulospinal tract). (E) Rostral ventral lateral medulla (bulbospinal tract). (Data derived with permission from Schwartz and Fehlings, 2001.)

patients receive MPSS within 3 h after SCI, especially if the injury is severe. This drug's narrow therapeutic window of opportunity establishes the necessity of providing rapid intervention in order to attenuate secondary SCI. As such, new strategies aimed at limiting early secondary pathophysiological mechanisms may enhance the functional outcome for victims of acute SCI. In this review, we have focused on the therapeutic potential of Na^+ channel blockers for the treatment of acute spinal cord trauma because trauma-induced activation of voltage-sensitive Na^+ channels is a primary portal for intracellular accumulation of Na^+, a key early event in the pathogenesis of secondary CNS injury. We have shown that the Na^+ channel blocker riluzole can significantly attenuate motor deficits and enhance the preservation of spinal cord GM and WM after compression trauma of the spinal cord in rats. Although riluzole is a particularly attractive therapeutic candidate for the treatment of acute SCI, further research in order to attain compelling preclinical data is necessary before this drug's neuroprotective benefits can be evaluated in patients with acute SCI.

Acknowledgements

Our work was supported by grants from the Physician Services Incorporated Foundation and the Krembil Chair in Neural Repair and Regeneration. G. Schwartz is supported by the Ontario Neurotrauma Foundation. M.G. Fehlings is an Ontario Ministry of Health Career Scientist.

References

AANS/CNS Section on Disorders of the Spine and Peripheral Nerves (2002). *Neurosurg.*, 50: S63–S72.

Agrawal, S.K. and Fehlings, M.G. (1996) Mechanisms of secondary injury to spinal cord axons in vitro: role of Na^+, Na(+)-K(+)-ATPase, the Na(+)–H^+ exchanger, and the Na(+)–Ca^{2+} exchanger. *J. Neurosci.*, 16: 545–552.

Agrawal, S.K. and Fehlings, M.G. (1997a) The effect of the sodium channel blocker QX-314 on recovery after acute spinal cord injury. *J. Neurotrauma*, 14: 81–88.

Agrawal, S.K. and Fehlings, M.G. (1997b) Role of NMDA and non-NMDA ionotropic glutamate receptors in traumatic spinal cord axonal injury. *J. Neurosci.*, 17: 1055–1063.

Alaoui, F., Pratt, J., Trocherie, S., Court, L. and Stutzmann, J.M.

(1995) Acute effects of irradiation on the rat brain: protection by glutamate blockade. *Eur. J. Pharmacol.*, 276: 55–60.

Allen, A. (1914) Remarks on the histopathological changes in spinal cord due to impact. An experimental study. *J. Nerv. Ment. Dis.*, 41: 141–147.

Anderson, D.K. and Means, E.D. (1985b) Iron-induced lipid peroxidation in spinal cord: protection with mannitol and methylprednisolone. *J. Free Radic. Biol. Med.*, 1: 59–64.

Anderson, D.K., Means, E.D., Waters, T.R. and Spears, C.J. (1980) Spinal cord energy metabolism following compression trauma to the feline spinal cord. *J. Neurosurg.*, 53: 375–380.

Anderson, D.K., Saunders, R.D., Demediuk, P., Dugan, L.L., Braughler, J.M., Hall, E.D., Means, E.D. and Horrocks, L.A. (1985a) Lipid hydrolysis and peroxidation in injured spinal cord: partial protection with methylprednisolone or vitamin E and selenium. *Cent. Nerv. Syst. Trauma*, 2: 257–267.

Anthes, D.L., Theriault, E. and Tator, C.H. (1996) Ultrastructural evidence for arteriolar vasospasm after spinal cord trauma. *Neurosurgery*, 39: 804–814.

Ashton, D., Willems, R., Wynants, J., Van Reempts, J., Marrannes, R. and Clincke, G. (1997) Altered Na(+)-channel function as an in vitro model of the ischemic penumbra: action of lubeluzole and other neuroprotective drugs. *Brain Res.*, 745: 210–221.

Balentine, J.D. (1978a) Pathology of experimental spinal cord trauma, I. The necrotic lesion as a function of vascular injury. *Lab. Invest.*, 39: 236–253.

Balentine, J.D. (1978b) Pathology of experimental spinal cord trauma, II. Ultrastructure of axons and myelin. *Lab. Invest.*, 39: 254–266.

Banik, N.L., Hogan, E.L. and Hsu, C.Y. (1987) The multimolecular cascade of spinal cord injury: studies on prostanoids, calcium, and proteinases. *Neurochem. Pathol.*, 7: 57–77.

Barneoud, P., Mazadier, M., Miquet, J.M., Parmentier, S., Dubedat, P., Doble, A. and Boireau, A. (1996) Neuroprotective effects of riluzole on a model of Parkinson's disease in the rat. *Neuroscience*, 74: 971–983.

Basso, D.M., Beattie, M.S. and Bresnahan, J.C. (1995) A sensitive and reliable locomotor rating scale for open field testing in rats. *J. Neurotrauma*, 12: 1–21.

Behrmann, D.L., Bresnahan, J.C., Beattie, M.S. and Shah, B.R. (1992) Spinal cord injury produced by consistent mechanical displacement of the cord in rats: behavioral and histologic analysis. *J. Neurotrauma*, 9: 197–217.

Bensimon, G., Lacomblez, L. and Meininger, V. (1994) A controlled trial of riluzole in amyotrophic lateral sclerosis. ALS/Riluzole Study Group. *N. Engl. J. Med.*, 330: 585–591.

Blight, A.R. (1983) Cellular morphology of chronic spinal cord injury in the cat: analysis of myelinated axons by line-sampling. *Neuroscience*, 10: 521–543.

Blight, A.R. (1996) An overview of spinal cord injury models. In: R.K. Narayan, J.E. Wilberger Jr. and J.T. Povlishock (Eds.), *Neurotrauma*. McGraw-Hill, Toronto, pp. 1367–1379.

Boxer, P.A., Cordon, J.J., Mann, M.E., Rodolosi, L.C., Vartanian, M.G., Rock, D.M., Taylor, C.P. and Marcoux, F.W. (1990) Comparison of phenytoin with noncompetitive *N*-methyl-D-aspartate antagonists in a model of focal brain ischemia in rat. *Stroke*, 21: 47–51.

Bracken, M.B., Shepard, M.J., Collins, W.F., Holford, T.R., Young, W., Baskin, D.S., Eisenberg, H.M., Flamm, E., Leo-Summers, L. and Maroon, J. et al. (1990) A randomized, controlled trial of methylprednisolone or naloxone in the treatment of acute spinal-cord injury. Results of the Second National Acute Spinal Cord Injury Study. *N. Engl. J. Med.*, 322: 1405–1411.

Bracken, M.B., Shepard, M.J., Collins Jr., W.F., Holford, T.R., Baskin, D.S., Eisenberg, H.M., Flamm, E., Leo-Summers, L., Maroon, J.C. and Marshall, L.F. et al. (1992) Methylprednisolone or naloxone treatment after acute spinal cord injury: 1-year follow-up data. Results of the second National Acute Spinal Cord Injury Study. *J. Neurosurg.*, 76: 23–31.

Bracken, M.B., Shepard, M.J., Holford, T.R., Leo-Summers, L., Aldrich, E.F., Fazl, M., Fehlings, M., Herr, D.L., Hitchon, P.W., Marshall, L.F., Nockels, R.P., Pascale, V., Perot Jr., P.L., Piepmeier, J., Sonntag, V.K., Wagner, F., Wilberger, J.E., Winn, H.R. and Young, W. (1997) Administration of methylprednisolone for 24 or 48 hours or tirilazad mesylate for 48 hours in the treatment of acute spinal cord injury. Results of the Third National Acute Spinal Cord Injury Randomized Controlled Trial. National Acute Spinal Cord Injury Study. *JAMA*, 277: 1597–1604.

Breasted, J.H. (1930) *The Edwin Smith Surgical Papyrus*, Vol. 1. University of Chicago Press, Chicago, pp. 337–342.

Bresnahan, J.C. (1978) An electron-microscopic analysis of axonal alterations following blunt contusion of the spinal cord of the rhesus monkey (*Macaca mulatta*). *J. Neurol. Sci.*, 37: 59–82.

Bresnahan, J.C., King, J.S., Martin, G.F. and Yashon, D. (1976) A neuroanatomical analysis of spinal cord injury in the rhesus monkey (*Macaca mulatta*). *J. Neurol. Sci.*, 28: 521–542.

Bunge, R.P., Puckett, W.R., Becerra, J.L., Marcillo, A. and Quencer, R.M. (1993) Observations on the pathology of human spinal cord injury. A review and classification of 22 new cases with details from a case of chronic cord compression with extensive focal demyelination. *Adv. Neurol.*, 59: 75–89.

Calabresi, P., Marfia, G.A., Centonze, D., Pisani, A. and Bernardi, G. (1999) Sodium influx plays a major role in the membrane depolarization induced by oxygen and glucose deprivation in rat striatal spiny neurons. *Stroke*, 30: 171–179.

Cheng, M.K., Robertson, C., Grossman, R.G., Foltz, R. and Williams, V. (1984) Neurological outcome correlated with spinal evoked potentials in a spinal cord ischemia model. *J. Neurosurg.*, 60: 786–795.

Cullen, J.P., Aldrete, J.A., Jankovsky, L. and Romo-Salas, F. (1979) Protective action of phenytoin in cerebral ischemia. *Anesth. Analg.*, 58: 165–169.

Culmsee, C., Junker, V., Wolz, P., Semkova, I. and Krieglstein, J. (1998) Lubeluzole protects hippocampal neurons from excitotoxicity in vitro and reduces brain damage caused by ischemia. *Eur. J. Pharmacol.*, 342: 193–201.

De Ryck, M., Keersmaekers, R., Duytschaever, H., Claes, C., Clincke, G., Janssen, M. and Van Reet, G. (1996) Lubeluzole protects sensorimotor function and reduces infarct size in a photochemical stroke model in rats. *J. Pharmacol. Exp. Ther.*, 279: 748–758.

DeVivo, M.J. (1997) Causes and costs of spinal cord injury in the United States. *Spinal Cord*, 35: 809–813.

Diener, H.C. (1998) Multinational randomized controlled trial of lubeluzole in acute ischaemic stroke. European and Australian Lubeluzole Ischaemic Stroke Study Group. *Cerebrovasc. Dis.*, 8: 172–181.

Dohrmann, G.J., Wagner Jr., F.C. and Bucy, P.C. (1972) Transitory traumatic paraplegia: electron microscopy of early alterations in myelinated nerve fibers. *J. Neurosurg.*, 36: 407–415.

Ducker, T.B., Kindt, W.K. and Kempe, L.G. (1971) Pathological findings in acute experimental spinal cord trauma. *J. Neurosurg.*, 35: 700–708.

Ettaiche, M., Fillacier, K., Widmann, C., Heurteaux, C. and Lazdunski, M. (1999) Riluzole improves functional recovery after ischemia in the rat retina. *Invest. Ophthalmol. Vis. Sci.*, 40: 729–736.

Fehlings, M.G. and Agrawal, S. (1995) Role of sodium in the pathophysiology of secondary spinal cord injury. *Spine*, 20: 2187–2191.

Fehlings, M.G. and Tator, C.H. (1988) A review of models of acute experimental spinal cord injury. In: L.S. Illis (Ed.), *Spinal Cord Dysfunction: Assessment.* Oxford University Press, Oxford, pp. 3–33.

Fehlings, M.G. and Tator, C.H. (1995) The relationships among the severity of spinal cord injury, residual neurological function, axon counts, and counts of retrogradely labeled neurons after experimental spinal cord injury. *Exp. Neurol.*, 132: 220–228.

Fern, R., Ransom, B.R., Stys, P.K. and Waxman, S.G. (1993) Pharmacological protection of CNS white matter during anoxia: actions of phenytoin, carbamazepine and diazepam. *J. Pharmacol. Exp. Ther.*, 266: 1549–1555.

Ford, R.W. and Malm, D.N. (1985) Failure of nimodipine to reverse acute experimental spinal cord injury. *Cent. Nerv. Syst. Trauma*, 2: 9–17.

Friedman, J.E. and Haddad, G.G. (1994) Anoxia induces an increase in intracellular sodium in rat central neurons in vitro. *Brain Res.*, 663: 329–334.

Gale, K., Kerasidis, H. and Wrathall, J.R. (1985) Spinal cord contusion in the rat: behavioral analysis of functional neurologic impairment. *Exp. Neurol.*, 88: 123–134.

Geddes, I.C. and Quastel, J.H. (1956) Effects of local anesthetics on respiration of rat brain cortex in vitro. *Anesthesiology*, 17: 666–671.

Geisler, F.H., Coleman, W.P., Grieco, G. and Poonian, D. (2001) The Sygen multicenter acute spinal cord injury study. *Spine*, 26(24S): S87–S98.

Gelmers, H.J. and Hennerici, M. (1990) Effect of nimodipine on acute ischemic stroke. Pooled results from five randomized trials. *Stroke*, 21: 81–84.

Greene, K.A., Marciano, F.F. and Sonntag, V.K. (1996) Pharmacological management of spinal cord injury: current status of drugs designed to augment functional recovery of the injured human spinal cord. *J. Spinal Disord.*, 9: 355–366.

Griffiths, I.R. and McCulloch, M.C. (1983) Nerve fibres in spinal cord impact injuries, Part 1. Changes in the myelin sheath during the initial 5 weeks. *J. Neurol. Sci.*, 58: 335–349.

Grotta, J. (1997) Lubeluzole treatment of acute ischemic stroke. The US and Canadian Lubeluzole Ischemic Stroke Study Group. *Stroke*, 28: 2338–2346.

Guizar-Sahagun, G., Grijalva, I., Madrazo, I., Franco-Bourland, R., Salgado, H., Ibarra, A., Oliva, E. and Zepeda, A. (1994) Development of post-traumatic cysts in the spinal cord of rats subjected to severe spinal cord contusion. *Surg. Neurol.*, 41: 241–249.

Gurney, M.E., Cutting, F.B., Zhai, P., Doble, A., Taylor, C.P., Andrus, P.K. and Hall, E.D. (1996) Benefit of vitamin E, riluzole, and gabapentin in a transgenic model of familial amyotrophic lateral sclerosis [see comments]. *Ann. Neurol.*, 39: 147–157.

Gusovsky, F., Hollingsworth, E.B. and Daly, J.W. (1986) Regulation of phosphatidylinositol turnover in brain synaptoneurosomes: stimulatory effects of agents that enhance influx of sodium ions. *Proc. Natl. Acad. Sci. USA*, 83: 3003–3007.

Guyot, M.C., Palfi, S., Stutzmann, J.M., Maziere, M., Hantraye, P. and Brouillet, E. (1997) Riluzole protects from motor deficits and striatal degeneration produced by systemic 3-nitropropionic acid intoxication in rats. *Neuroscience*, 81: 141–149.

Haghighi, S.S., Stiens, T., Oro, J.J. and Madsen, R. (1993) Evaluation of the calcium channel antagonist nimodipine after experimental spinal cord injury. *Surg. Neurol.*, 39: 403–408.

Haigney, M.C., Lakatta, E.G., Stern, M.D. and Silverman, H.S. (1994) Sodium channel blockade reduces hypoxic sodium loading and sodium-dependent calcium loading. *Circulation*, 90: 391–399.

Hickenbottom, S.L. and Grotta, J. (1998) Neuroprotective therapy. *Semin. Neurol.*, 18: 485–492.

Hu, R., Mustard, C.A. and Burns, C. (1996) Epidemiology of incident spinal fracture in a complete population. *Spine*, 21: 492–499.

Hurlbert, R.J. (2000) Methylprednisolone for acute spinal cord injury: an inappropriate standard of care. *J. Neurosurg.*, 93: 1–7.

Kakulas, B.A. (1984) Pathology of spinal injuries. *Cent. Nerv. Syst. Trauma*, 1: 117–129.

Kanthasamy, A.G., Yun, R.J., Nguyen, B. and Truong, D.D. (1999) Effect of riluzole on the neurological and neuropathological changes in an animal model of cardiac arrest-induced movement disorder. *J. Pharmacol. Exp. Ther.*, 288: 1340–1348.

Katoh, K., Ikata, T., Katoh, S., Hamada, Y., Nakauchi, K., Sano, T. and Niwa, M. (1996) Induction and its spread of apoptosis in rat spinal cord after mechanical trauma. *Neurosci. Lett.*, 216: 9–12.

Kobrine, A.I. (1975) The neuronal theory of experimental traumatic spinal cord dysfunction. *Surg. Neurol.*, 3: 261–264.

Kobrine, A.I., Evans, D.E., LeGrys, D.C., Yaffe, L.J. and Bradley, M.E. (1984) Effect of intravenous lidocaine on experimental spinal cord injury. *J. Neurosurg.*, 60: 595–601.

Kroppenstedt, S.N., Stroop, R., Kern, M., Thomale, U.W.,

Schneider, G.H. and Unterberg, A.W. (1999) Lubeluzole following traumatic brain injury in the rat. *J. Neurotrauma*, 16: 629–637.

Lang-Lazdunski, L., Heurteaux, C., Vaillant, N., Widmann, C. and Lazdunski, M. (1999) Riluzole prevents ischemic spinal cord injury caused by aortic crossclamping [see comments]. *J. Thorac. Cardiovasc. Surg.*, 117: 881–889.

Li, G.L., Brodin, G., Farooque, M., Funa, K., Holtz, A., Wang, W.L. and Olsson, Y. (1996) Apoptosis and expression of Bcl-2 after compression trauma to rat spinal cord. *J. Neuropathol. Exp. Neurol.*, 55: 280–289.

Li, S., Mealing, G.A., Morley, P. and Stys, P.K. (1999) Novel injury mechanism in anoxia and trauma of spinal cord white matter: glutamate release via reverse $Na(+)$-dependent glutamate transport. *J. Neurosci.*, 19, RC16.

Lipicky, R.J., Gilbert, D.L. and Stillman, I.M. (1972) Diphenylhydantoin inhibition of sodium conductance in squid giant axon. *Proc. Natl. Acad. Sci. USA*, 69: 1758–1760.

LoPachin, R.M., Gaughan, C.L., Lehning, E.J., Kaneko, Y., Kelly, T.M. and Blight, A. (1999) Experimental spinal cord injury: spatiotemporal characterization of elemental concentrations and water contents in axons and neuroglia. *J. Neurophysiol.*, 82: 2143–2153.

Lynch III, J.J., Yu, S.P., Canzoniero, L.M., Sensi, S.L. and Choi, D.W. (1995) Sodium channel blockers reduce oxygen-glucose deprivation-induced cortical neuronal injury when combined with glutamate receptor antagonists. *J. Pharmacol. Exp. Ther.*, 273: 554–560.

Mabon, P.J., Weaver, L.C. and Dekaban, G.A. (2000) Inhibition of monocyte/macrophage migration to a spinal cord injury site by an antibody to the integrin alphaD: a potential new anti-inflammatory treatment. *Exp. Neurol.*, 166: 52–64.

McIntosh, T.K., Smith, D.H., Voddi, M., Perri, B.R. and Stutzmann, J.M. (1996) Riluzole, a novel neuroprotective agent, attenuates both neurologic motor and cognitive dysfunction following experimental brain injury in the rat. *J. Neurotrauma*, 13: 767–780.

McLean, M.J. and Macdonald, R.L. (1983) Multiple actions of phenytoin on mouse spinal cord neurons in cell culture. *J. Pharmacol. Exp. Ther.*, 227: 779–789.

Muizelaar, J.P., Marmarou, A., Young, H.F., Choi, S.C., Wolf, A., Schneider, R.L. and Kontos, H.A. (1993) Improving the outcome of severe head injury with the oxygen radical scavenger polyethylene glycol-conjugated superoxide dismutase: a phase II trial. *J. Neurosurg.*, 78: 375–382.

Narayana, P., Abbe, R., Liu, S.J. and Johnston, D. (1999) Does loss of gray- and white-matter contrast in injured spinal cord signify secondary injury? In vivo longitudinal MRI studies. *Magn. Reson. Med.*, 41: 315–320.

Noble, L.J. and Wrathall, J.R. (1985) Spinal cord contusion in the rat: morphometric analyses of alterations in the spinal cord. *Exp. Neurol.*, 88: 135–149.

NSCISC (1997) *Spinal Cord Injury: Facts and Figures at a Glance*. University of Alabama at Birmingham, Birmingham, AL.

Okiyama, K., Smith, D.H., Gennarelli, T.A., Simon, R.P., Leach, M. and McIntosh, T.K. (1995) The sodium channel blocker and glutamate release inhibitor BW1003C87 and magnesium attenuate regional cerebral edema following experimental brain injury in the rat. *J. Neurochem.*, 64: 802–809.

O'Neill, M., Bath, C.P., Dell, C.P., Hicks, C.A., Gilmore, J., Ambler, S.J., Ward, M.A. and Bleakman, D. (1997) Effects of Ca^{2+} and Na^{+} channel inhibitors in vitro and in global cerebral ischaemia in vivo. *Eur. J. Pharmacol.*, 332: 121–131.

Osterholm, J.L. (1978) *The Pathophysiology of Spinal Cord Trauma*. Charles C. Thomas, Springfield, IL.

Pointillart, V., Petitjean, M.E., Wiart, L., Vital, J.M., Lassie, P., Thicoipe, M. and Dabadie, P. (2000) Pharmacological therapy of spinal cord injury during the acute phase. *Spinal Cord*, 38: 71–76.

Pratt, J., Rataud, J., Bardot, F., Roux, M., Blanchard, J.C., Laduron, P.M. and Stutzmann, J.M. (1992) Neuroprotective actions of riluzole in rodent models of global and focal cerebral ischaemia. *Neurosci. Lett.*, 140: 225–230.

Probert, A.W., Borosky, S., Marcoux, F.W. and Taylor, C.P. (1997) Sodium channel modulators prevent oxygen and glucose deprivation injury and glutamate release in rat neocortical cultures. *Neuropharmacology*, 36: 1031–1038.

Rataud, J., Debarnot, F., Mary, V., Pratt, J. and Stutzmann, J.M. (1994) Comparative study of voltage-sensitive sodium channel blockers in focal ischaemia and electric convulsions in rodents. *Neurosci. Lett.*, 172: 19–23.

Regan, R.F. and Choi, D.W. (1991) Glutamate neurotoxicity in spinal cord cell culture. *Neuroscience*, 43: 585–591.

Reithmeier, R.A. (1994) Mammalian exchangers and cotransporters. *Curr. Opin. Cell Biol.*, 6: 583–594.

Rivlin, A.S. and Tator, C.H. (1977) Objective clinical assessment of motor function after experimental spinal cord injury in the rat. *J. Neurosurg.*, 47: 577–581.

Rosenberg, L.J., Teng, Y.D. and Wrathall, J.R. (1999a) 2,3-Dihydroxy-6-nitro-7-sulfamoyl-Benzo(f)Quinoxaline reduces glial loss and acute white matter pathology after experimental spinal cord contusion. *J. Neurosci.*, 19: 464–475.

Rosenberg, L.J., Teng, Y.D. and Wrathall, J.R. (1999b) Effects of the sodium channel blocker tetrodotoxin on acute white matter pathology after experimental contusive spinal cord injury. *J. Neurosci.*, 19: 6122–6133.

Sandler, A.N. and Tator, C.H. (1976a) Effect of acute spinal cord compression injury on regional spinal cord blood flow in primates. *J. Neurosurg.*, 45: 660–676.

Sandler, A.N. and Tator, C.H. (1976b) Review of the effect of spinal cord trauma on the vessels and blood flow in the spinal cord. *J. Neurosurg.*, 45: 638–646.

Saunders, R.D., Dugan, L.L., Demediuk, P., Means, E.D., Horrocks, L.A. and Anderson, D.K. (1987) Effects of methylprednisolone and the combination of alpha-tocopherol and selenium on arachidonic acid metabolism and lipid peroxidation in traumatized spinal cord tissue. *J. Neurochem.*, 49: 24–31.

Schleimer, R.P., Freeland, H.S., Peters, S.P., Brown, K.E. and Derse, C.P. (1989) An assessment of the effects of glucocorticoids on degranulation, chemotaxis, binding to vascular endothelium and formation of leukotriene B4 by purified human neutrophils. *J. Pharmacol. Exp. Ther.*, 250: 598–605.

Schwartz, G. and Fehlings, M.G. (2001) Evaluation of the neuroprotective effects of sodium channel blockers after spinal cord injury: improved behavioral and neuroanatomical recovery with riluzole. *J. Neurosurg.*, 94: 245–256.

Stefani, A., Spadoni, F. and Bernardi, G. (1997) Differential inhibition by riluzole, lamotrigine, and phenytoin of sodium and calcium currents in cortical neurons: implications for neuroprotective strategies. *Exp. Neurol.*, 147: 115–122.

Stutzmann, J.M., Pratt, J., Boraud, T. and Gross, C. (1996) The effect of riluzole on post-traumatic spinal cord injury in the rat. *Neuroreport*, 7: 387–392.

Stys, P.K. and Lopachin, R.M. (1998) Mechanisms of calcium and sodium fluxes in anoxic myelinated central nervous system axons. *Neuroscience*, 82: 21–32.

Stys, P.K., Waxman, S.G. and Ransom, B.R. (1991) $Na(+)-Ca^{2+}$ exchanger mediates Ca^{2+} influx during anoxia in mammalian central nervous system white matter. *Ann. Neurol.*, 30: 375–380.

Stys, P.K., Waxman, S.G. and Ransom, B.R. (1992) Ionic mechanisms of anoxic injury in mammalian CNS white matter: role of Na^+ channels and $Na(+)-Ca^{2+}$ exchanger. *J. Neurosci.*, 12: 430–439.

Sun, F.Y. and Faden, A.I. (1995) Neuroprotective effects of 619C89, a use-dependent sodium channel blocker, in rat traumatic brain injury. *Brain Res.*, 673: 133–140.

Taft, W.C., Clifton, G.L., Blair, R.E. and DeLorenzo, R.J. (1989) Phenytoin protects against ischemia-produced neuronal cell death. *Brain Res.*, 483: 143–148.

Taoka, Y. and Okajima, K. (1998) Spinal cord injury in the rat. *Prog. Neurobiol.*, 56: 341–358.

Tator, C.H. (1983) Spine–spinal cord relationships in spinal cord trauma. *Clin. Neurosurg.*, 30: 479–494.

Tator, C.H. and Fehlings, M.G. (1991) Review of the secondary injury theory of acute spinal cord trauma with emphasis on vascular mechanisms. *J. Neurosurg.*, 75: 15–26.

Tator, C.H. and Rowed, D.W. (1979) Current concepts in the immediate management of acute spinal cord injuries. *Can. Med. Assoc. J.*, 121: 1453–1464.

Tator, C.H., Duncan, E.G., Edmonds, V.E., Lapczak, L.I. and Andrews, D.F. (1995) Neurological recovery, mortality and length of stay after acute spinal cord injury associated with changes in management. *Paraplegia*, 33: 254–262.

Taylor, C.P., Geer, J.J. and Burke, S.P. (1992) Endogenous extracellular glutamate accumulation in rat neocortical cultures by reversal of the transmembrane sodium gradient. *Neurosci. Lett.*, 145: 197–200.

Teasdale, G., Bailey, I., Bell, A., Gray, J., Gullan, R., Heiskanan,
O., Marks, P.V., Marsh, H., Mendelow, D.A. and Murray, G. et al. (1992) A randomized trial of nimodipine in severe head injury: HIT I. British/Finnish Co-operative Head Injury Trial Group. *J. Neurotrauma*, 9(Suppl. 2): 545–550.

Teng, Y.D. and Wrathall, J.R. (1997) Local blockade of sodium channels by tetrodotoxin ameliorates tissue loss and long-term functional deficits resulting from experimental spinal cord injury. *J. Neurosci.*, 17: 4359–4366.

Tymianski, M. and Tator, C.H. (1996) Normal and abnormal calcium homeostasis in neurons: a basis for the pathophysiology of traumatic and ischemic central nervous system injury. *Neurosurgery*, 38: 1176–1195.

von Euler, M., Seiger, A., Holmberg, L. and Sundstrom, E. (1994) NBQX, a competitive non-NMDA receptor antagonist, reduces degeneration due to focal spinal cord ischemia. *Exp. Neurol.*, 129: 163–168.

Wahl, F., Allix, M., Plotkine, M. and Boulu, R.G. (1993) Effect of riluzole on focal cerebral ischemia in rats. *Eur. J. Pharmacol.*, 230: 209–214.

Wahl, F., Renou, E., Mary, V. and Stutzmann, J.M. (1997) Riluzole reduces brain lesions and improves neurological function in rats after a traumatic brain injury. *Brain Res.*, 756: 247–255.

Wallace, M.C., Tator, C.H. and Lewis, A.J. (1987) Chronic regenerative changes in the spinal cord after cord compression injury in rats. *Surg. Neurol.*, 27: 209–219.

Wiedemann, M. and Hanke, W. (1999) Lubeluzole shows neuroprotective effects in an 'in-vitro' model for neuronal lesions in the chicken retina. *Brain Res.*, 842: 243–248.

Wrathall, J.R., Choiniere, D. and Teng, Y.D. (1994) Dose-dependent reduction of tissue loss and functional impairment after spinal cord trauma with the AMPA/kainate antagonist NBQX. *J. Neurosci.*, 14: 6598–6607.

Xie, Y., Dengler, K., Zacharias, E., Wilffert, B. and Tegtmeier, F. (1994) Effects of the sodium channel blocker tetrodotoxin (TTX) on cellular ion homeostasis in rat brain subjected to complete ischemia. *Brain Res.*, 652: 216–224.

Yong, C., Arnold, P.M., Zoubine, M.N., Citron, B.A., Watanabe, I., Berman, N.E. and Festoff, B.W. (1998) Apoptosis in cellular compartments of rat spinal cord after severe contusion injury. *J. Neurotrauma*, 15: 459–472.

Young, W. (1993) Secondary injury mechanisms in acute spinal cord injury. *J. Emerg. Med.*, 11: 13–22.

Zhang, Y. and Lipton, P. (1999) Cytosolic Ca^{2+} changes during in vitro ischemia in rat hippocampal slices: major roles for glutamate and Na^+-dependent Ca^{2+} release from mitochondria. *J. Neurosci.*, 19: 3307–3315.

L. McKerracher, G. Doucet and S. Rossignol (Eds.)
Progress in Brain Research, Vol. 137

CHAPTER 15

Strategies for regeneration and repair in spinal cord traumatic injury

Minerva Giménez y Ribotta [1], Manuel Gaviria [1,2], Véronique Menet [1] and
Alain Privat [1,2,*]

[1] *INSERM U. 336, Université Montpellier II, B.P. 106, Place E. Bataillon, 34095 Montpellier Cedex 05, France*
[2] *Centre Propara, Laboratoire de Chirurgie Expérimentale et Laboratoire de Neurophysiologie Clinique, Parc Euromédecine,
34195 Montpellier Cedex 9, France*

Abstract: Spinal cord injury is frequently followed by the loss of supraspinal control of sensory, autonomic and motor functions at the sublesional level. In order to enhance recovery in spinal cord-injured patients, we have developed three fundamental strategies in experimental models. These strategies define in turn three chronological levels of postlesional intervention in the spinal cord. Neuroprotection soon after injury using pharmacological tools to reduce the progressive secondary injury processes that follow during the first week after the initial lesion. This strategy was conducted up to clinical trials, showing that a pharmacological therapy can reduce the permanent neurological deficit that usually follows an acute injury of the central nervous system (CNS). A second strategy, which is initiated not long after the lesion, aims at promoting axonal regeneration by acting on the main barrier to regeneration of lesioned axons: the glial scar. Finally a mid-term substitutive strategy is the management of the sublesional spinal cord by sensorimotor stimulation and/or supply of missing key afferents, such as monoaminergic systems. These three strategies are reviewed. Only a combination of these different approaches will be able to provide an optimal basis for potential therapeutic interventions directed to functional recovery after spinal cord injury.

Introduction

Spinal cord injury (SCI) is a major cause of disability which generally strikes down young and healthy people (55% < 25 years old) (Bracken et al., 1990; Nobunaga et al., 1999). During the latter years, patients have benefited to a large extent from the improvement in the initial care. As a matter of fact, improvement in the treatment of SCI patients has reduced both morbidity and mortality, mostly by preventing secondary trauma complications (DeVivo et al., 1999; McKinley et al., 1999). However, only

very few patients make a major or complete recovery (Bracken et al., 1990). Thus, sequential pathological changes in the basic neurochemistry which begin immediately after SCI (Tator and Fehlings, 1991), absolutely necessitate a rapid intervention to modify the physiopathological activity of potentially neurotoxic molecules and attenuate neuronal damage. Nevertheless, despite the progress in experimental research, no suitable clinical therapy for neurological SCI patient recovery exists at present.

Spinal trauma is followed by alteration or loss of supraspinal motor, sensory and autonomic drive below the level of the lesion. After an acute trauma, the immediate and irreversible primary mechanical injury is followed by the secondary injury caused by a cascade of complex physiopathological reactions, i.e. general and specific vascular, molecular and cellular disturbances (Tator and Fehlings, 1991).

* Correspondence to: A. Privat, INSERM U. 336, Université Montpellier II. B.P. 106. Place E. Bataillon, 34095 Montpellier Cedex 05, France. Tel.: +33-467-143386; Fax: +33-467-143318; E-mail: u336@univ-montp2.fr

Some of these reactions are responsible for accelerating the degeneration of damaged cells and tissues, others might be involved in subsequent repairing mechanisms. Nevertheless, the equilibrium is extremely fragile and loss of cell and tissue autoregulation following injury rapidly transforms the tissue environment into a hostile milieu where the mechanisms of repair are inadequate.

We have developed three lines of research to improve the outcome of traumatic SCI.

Neuroprotection

Early treatment of secondary lesions is possible with several pharmacological molecules. In order to carry out an optimal pharmacological intervention, the targets must be clearly identified, not only as defined static molecular and cellular factors, but as substances and receptors whose concentration and activity changes depend on the length of time from trauma and whose effects on nervous tissue also probably change in a dose-dependent and interaction-dependent manner. A few randomized trials using conventional pharmacological treatments showed that a pharmacological agent can reduce the permanent neurological disability that usually follows an acute SCI (Bracken et al., 1985, 1990, 1997; Geisler et al., 1991). Nevertheless, in spite of optimally designed protocols affecting one specific target of the neurochemical cascade, results are mostly disappointing. Our first strategy is focused on preventing or reducing local and distal neuronal death by counteracting the neurotoxicity of excitatory amino acid (EAA) release (Pencalet et al., 1993).

Regeneration

A second phase postinjury is fundamentally characterized by a glial reaction involving both activated microglia and astroglia, and an important inflammatory response with the recruitment of polymorphonuclear granulocytes and macrophages. Astroglial response to injury is characterized by hyperplasia and hypertrophy of cytoplasmic processes. These changes in number and morphology of astrocytes are correlated with an increase in the expression of glial fibrillary acidic protein (GFAP) and GFAP-mRNA resulting in the formation of a gliotic tissue or glial scar, which constitutes a major impediment to axonal regeneration. However, reactive astrocytes express surface molecules and produce several neurotrophic factors and cytokines, which in turn modulate the production of recognition molecules allowing the support of postlesional axonal regrowth (Ridet et al., 1997). With this in mind, we have developed a second strategy to promote axonal regeneration by modulating the astroglial reaction (Giménez y Ribotta et al., 1995).

Management of sublesional spinal cord

Another issue of major interest for the functional outcome of the lesion is the management of sublesional spinal cord (SC) in order to recover some functions which may be managed independently of the supraspinal control. This includes sensorimotor stimulation by interactive locomotor training (Muir and Steeves, 1997) or pharmacological treatments that control motor functions. We have developed an original alternative strategy by the transplantation of monoaminergic neurons into sublesional cord to supply supraspinal afferents (Privat et al., 1988), which are key elements in the control of locomotion. The combined efforts of physiology, cell biology and gene therapy in the field of sublesional SC management will begin to yield promising openings for a new era of rehabilitation based on the optimal use of spinal circuits controlling important functions such as sensorimotor functions (i.e. locomotion, Giménez y Ribotta et al., 2000) and autonomous functions (i.e. genitourinary functions, Privat et al., 1989).

Thus, an improvement in the disastrous outcome of SC lesions will probably not result from a major breakthrough in basic research, but rather from a combined effort aiming at establishing a rational strategy.

Neuroprotection

During the last decades, numerous studies suggest that one of the main keys in the treatment of traumatic pathologies of the central nervous system (CNS) is the control of post-lesion molecular and cellular changes (Choi, 1992; Faden and Salzman, 1992; McIntosh, 1993; Giménez y Ribotta and

Privat, 1998). Pharmacological intervention for neuroprotection soon after injury represents a promising therapeutic strategy, and some of the principal biochemical targets of the secondary injury mechanism have been identified in experimental models (Bethea et al., 1999; Cauquil-Caubere et al., 1999; Rosenberg et al., 1999; Gaviria et al., 2000a,b). Among these, N-methyl-D-aspartate receptors (NMDA) constitute an excellent therapeutic target.

Acute ischemic experimental SCI

Studies of the microvasculature after acute SCI have shown that one of the main components of secondary lesion is a disorder of the microcirculation. Thus, the infarct model developed by Watson in rats (Watson et al., 1986; Prado et al., 1987; Cameron et al., 1990) and used in our laboratory, has been extremely useful in investigating this component of traumatic SCI (Pencalet et al., 1993; Van Reempts and Borgers, 1994; Bunge et al., 1994; Sampath et al., 1995; Olby and Blakemore, 1996; Gaviria et al., 2000b). In this model, the beam of a xenon lamp conveyed by fiberoptics is focused on the selected irradiation vertebral site, and reacts with the systemically injected dye, Rose Bengal, in the SC microvasculature. The resultant photochemical reaction leads to vascular stasis by releasing free radicals which damage the endothelium of medullary vessels and induce platelet aggregation and thrombosis in the microvasculature.

The release of the EAA neurotransmitter L-glutamate activates a number of neuronal receptors and induces increased cell firing (McLennan, 1983). Thus, L-glutamate mediates physiological responses such as synaptic plasticity and long-term potentiation (Collingridge and Singer, 1990; Zamanillo et al., 1999). A physiopathological condition like ischemia causes a massive increase in the extracellular glutamate concentration (Benveniste et al., 1984; Faden et al., 1989; Nilsson et al., 1990; Katayama et al., 1990; Farooque et al., 1996) and the over-stimulation of glutamate receptors probably triggers cellular processes leading to acute neurodegenerative conditions. The role of the different types of receptors in EAA-mediated neurotoxicity has been extensively studied in vitro (Drian et al., 1991; Choi, 1992; Drian et al., 1999). Thus, NMDA receptors appear primarily responsible for rapidly triggered glutamate-induced cell death, but blockage of non-NMDA ionotropic receptors would also be required to allow survival of neurons subjected to hypoxia and glucose deprivation for a period of time. NMDA receptors are presumed to be responsible for rapidly triggered excitotoxicity mediated by a rapid influx of Ca^{2+} (Siesjo and Wieloch, 1985), and AMPA/kainate receptors for slowly triggered excitotoxicity in which the rate of Ca^{2+} influx is slower, and may involve routes other than receptor-gated channels (Choi, 1992). Evidence of the role of non-NMDA ionotropic receptors in SCI has been reported in several studies using kynuretic acid (Birch et al., 1988) and more recently 2,3-dihydroxy-6-nitro-7-sulfamoyl-benzo(f)quinoxaline (NBQX) (Wrathall et al., 1994; Rosenberg et al., 1999).

Systemic administration of NMDA receptor antagonists such as MK-801 (dizocilpine) or TCP (thienylphencyclidine) has been shown to attenuate the long-term neurological deficit in experimental models of SCI (Faden and Simon, 1988; Pencalet et al., 1993) by preventing the entry of Ca^{2+} into the cell (Tator and Fehlings, 1991). Gacyclidine (GK11, cis-(Pip/Me-1-[1-2-thienyl)-2-methylcyclohexil]piperidine), a molecule structurally derived from TCP (Rondouin et al., 1988; Pencalet et al., 1993) synthesized by Kamenka and co-workers (Kamenka et al., 1982), is highly selective for the phencyclidine PCP1 binding site within the NMDA receptor ion channels. Its binding rate is 2.2 and 8.6 times higher than that of TCP and PCP (phencyclidine), respectively (Vignon et al., 1986). In addition, gacyclidine also possesses some affinity for low affinity PCP binding sites (Hirbec et al., 2000a,b). Neuroprotection afforded by gacyclidine is therefore related to its ability to antagonize glutamate effects at the NMDA receptor (which is the mechanism of the action of other NMDA receptor antagonists), and probably also to its action at 'non-NMDA' binding sites (Hirbec et al., 2001a,b). Its specificity lies in its lack, or low levels, of direct neurotoxicity, which appear in doses that are far higher than those used for neuroprotection and those found with the reference NMDA antagonist MK-801 (Hirbec et al., 2001c).

Gacyclidine has been shown to be neuroprotective in vitro against acute glutamate toxicity to cortical neurons (Chaudieu et al., 1987; Rondouin et al., 1988; Drian et al., 1991; Levallois et al.,

1992; Michaud et al., 1994; Levallois et al., 1995; Drian et al., 1999), strongly suggesting a therapeutic indication in neurotrauma. Timing and doses of gacyclidine have been defined in accordance with previous studies using: (1) MK-801 on experimental cerebral ischemia in the rat (Faden and Simon, 1988); (2) TCP in vitro (Privat et al., 1990) and in vivo (Pencalet et al., 1993). Indeed, TCP protection is most effective during the first 15 min after injury; the massive release of glutamate occurs immediately after trauma and appears to resolve after 60–120 min (Faden et al., 1989; Katayama et al., 1990; Nilsson et al., 1990; Farooque et al., 1996).

Gacyclidine is able to reduce the effects of secondary injury in vivo, following an acute ischemic photochemical lesion of the SC which is reflected by behavioral, electrophysiological and morphological data in animals treated during the first 2 h after SCI (Gaviria et al., 2000b). Moreover, the most significant improvement in neurological status has been observed when treatment is administered early after injury, i.e. 10 min. One of the major findings of gacyclidine's pharmacotherapy in experimental SCI is the apparent limitation of morphological damage above the level of the injury (5.6 mm of the epicenter) in treated groups, which, according to the anatomical characteristics of rats (Hebel and Stromberg, 1986), represents protection of one metameric level and consequently a reduction in the functional deficit. Extension of histological damage has only been observed in untreated animals. The mechanisms of extension of the lesion are probably related to local vascular changes following acute trauma. Gacyclidine appears to limit the failure of autoregulation mechanisms, including loss of microcirculation, probably due to local vasospasm.

Acute contusive experimental SCI

The contusive experimental model of SCI offers the advantage of being clinically pertinent, since the majority of human cord traumas involves damage caused by rapid movements of the vertebral column (acceleration–deceleration) and impact of fractured bone against the SC. The weight-drop method involves dropping a calibrated weight from a specified height down a guide rod in order to strike the surgically exposed SC. This model, originally de-

scribed in dogs (Allen, 1911), was adapted in rats by Wrathall et al. (1985). The rat model of contusion has been shown to provide a reliable and reproducible injury (Black et al., 1988), and some studies have established that the histopathological features are similar to those previously reported in larger species (Bresnahan et al., 1976; Noble and Wrathall, 1985). The model used in our laboratory is a variation of the Wrathall weight-drop model (Gaviria et al., 2000a).

In general, animals receiving a contusive weight-drop injury show a profound neurological impairment immediately after injury, followed by a variable degree of functional recovery up to the next month. The reduction of the effects of secondary injury due to the administration of gacyclidine, are also reflected by behavioral, electrophysiological and morphological data in animals treated during the first 2 h after SCI, particularly in those treated earlier, e.g. 10 min earlier. Moreover, the apparent limitation of the extension of tissular damage above the level of the injury has been confirmed by morphological analyses in treated groups. Thus, gacyclidine is also able to reduce the effects of injury following experimental contusive lesion of the SC where damage involves direct mechanisms, i.e. mechanical disruption of neural pathways, and indirect mechanisms, i.e. delayed neurochemical alterations (Gaviria et al., 2000a).

In view of the encouraging results in animal models, one intriguing question remains, that of the protective effects of gacyclidine within white matter. As a matter of fact, mammalian spinal neurons display a mixture of NMDA and non-NMDA receptor types but NMDA receptors appear to be absent from the white matter (Rosenberg et al., 1999). The mechanisms of extracellular EAA accumulation after SCI may include both increasing release from vesicles, injured cells or blood and decreasing uptake by astrocytes and neurons (Farooque et al., 1996). Protection of gray matter due to gacyclidine effects on NMDA ionotropic receptors could lessen the release of toxic substances that might exacerbate pathology in surrounding white matter. Astrocytes, which play an important role in maintaining ionic homeostasis of the extracellular environment, are apparently modified by glutamate (cytoskeleton changes) and these modifications are prevented by neuroprotectants (Drian et al., 1999). In physiological conditions, astroglial glutamate transporters apparently play a major role in the clearance of the neurotransmitter. Consistently, the re-uptake of extracellular glutamate by astrocytes protects against neurodegeneration due to excitotoxicity. Astroglial cells are thus supposed to play a pivotal role in glutamate homeostasis and thus participate in neuronal protection (Mennerick and Zorumski, 1994; Rothstein et al., 1996; Cauquil-Caubere and Kamenka, 1998). Nevertheless, little is known about the reaction of astrocytes to neurotoxic concentrations of glutamate, apart from the fact that they survive at glutamate concentrations which kill neurons (Drian et al., 1999). Loss of astrocyte function would have detrimental effects on surrounding axons (Sykova et al., 1992). In addition, whereas NMDA receptors are not present on astrocytes, it must be hypothesized that either the astrocyte reaction is a consequence of neuronal death and the subsequent release of a toxic and/or signal substance or that indirect NMDA antagonists may have an influence on astrocytes. It can be speculated that gacyclidine's protection of neurons after SCI may also contribute to the reduction of the extent of the lesion through a more rapid glial-dependent re-establishment of the interaxon ionic homeostasis. On the other hand, it is well documented that glutamate over-stimulation of NMDA receptors results in the production of free radicals in the extracellular milieu in vitro (review Michaelis, 1998) and in vivo (Lancelot et al., 1998; Cauquil-Caubere et al., 1999). These oxidant species are able to kill neuronal or glial cells and particularly oligodendroglia which are very sensitive to radicals because they do not liberate glutathione (Juurlink, 1997). Thus, the inhibition of NMDA Ca^{2+} channels could prevent neighboring cells from extracellular oxidative stress. Alternatively or simultaneously, the white matter can be protected by gacyclidine from radical species released by glutamate over-stimulated neurons.

Clinical trial

Over the last decade, results of clinical trials have raised hopes for a pharmacological treatment of acute spinal injury. Gacyclidine is the first specially designed molecule which completes a clinical trial for the treatment of acute SCI. Preceding randomized trials using conventional pharmacological treatments showed that a pharmacological agent can reduce the permanent neurological disability that usually follows an acute SCI. Nevertheless, in some recent publications the methodology of NASCIS trials has been severely criticized (Coleman et al., 2000; Hurlbert, 2000) and, as a consequence, methylprednisolone has not been officially approved as a medication in SCI in any country. On the other hand, a phase I randomized trial using GM-1 ganglioside (Geisler et al., 1991) has shown a significant improvement of the ASIA motor score in patients treated within 48 h of SCI and continuing for 26 days, but this preliminary report could not be used as evidence for the routine utilization of GM-1 in clinical practice.

Detailed analysis of the different parameters of the gacyclidine's clinical trial shows some differences which, even though they do not attain statistical significance, reveal interesting trends. This is the first time that in a clinical SCI trial, the pharmacological intervention is performed within the first 2 h of the trauma which certainly explains that the overall increase in ASIA motor score in all groups including placebo, is much more marked than in previously published studies (Bracken et al., 1985, 1990, 1997). Analysis of changes in ASIA motor and sensory scores has shown no difference between groups for patients with complete lesions either cervical or thoracic, which is to be expected (Bracken et al., 1990). As a matter of fact, it is known that complete severe lesions are unlikely to show any significant improvement. Conversely, for patients with incomplete cervical lesions, the difference between the placebo group and the group treated with the highest dose of gacyclidine at day 30, corresponds to a difference in gain of more than two SC segments bilaterally. This difference is reduced to 1.5 levels bilaterally at day 365. This important benefit can be related at least partly to the relative ease of the decompression procedure in these patients, and to the good vascularization of the SC at this level (Marsala, 1999), that creates optimized conditions of drug access to the lesion site. Moreover, the better results obtained in incomplete cervical lesions compared with incomplete thoracic lesions would be consistent with the slight different regional distribution of NMDA receptors among spinal levels (Hirbec et al., 2000a,b). Again, in patients with incomplete thoracic lesions, the significant overall treatment effect for ASIA pinprick score at day 365 is consistent with the high density of NMDA receptors in the dorsal horn (lamina I–III) of the cord (Hirbec et al., 2000b). However, the small number of patients concerned (i.e. 25) limits the possibility of concluding on a clinically relevant treatment effect.

The results of this trial give some credit to the strategy of rapid decompression of the cord, recalibration of the vertebral canal and stabilization when comparing the overall improvement with preceding trials (Bracken et al., 1985, 1990, 1997; Geisler et al., 1991). Concerning pharmacological strategies, it is hoped that further basic and clinical studies will lead to significant steps towards the development of new compounds (McIntosh et al., 1998). Pre-clinical and clinical studies to date provide significant evidence of the efficacy of gacyclidine in the development of new and efficient therapeutic strategies. Modeling from experimental animal studies of the secondary injury after a SCI disclosed time-dependent complex neurochemical, cellular and molecular reactions leading to a variable degree of neurological impairment. This clinical trial, optimally designed to aim at one specific target, i.e. the NMDA receptor, has been unable to show a statistically significant improvement. Thus, optimal neuroprotection after SCI will only be achieved by a combination of pharmacological compounds directed to different physiopathological targets: free radical scavengers (Cauquil-Caubere et al., 1999), NMDA antagonists (Pencalet et al., 1993; Gaviria et al., 2000a,b), AMPA-kainate antagonists (Rosenberg et al., 1999), inhibitors or activators of cytokines (Bethea et al., 1998, 1999), taking into account the qualitative and quantitative parameters of specific targets (i.e. receptors) in the human SC.

Regeneration: modulation of the glial scar

The second experimental strategy intended to enhance recovery after SCI consists in promoting axonal regeneration by modulating the glial environment. Indeed, the formation of a glial scar occurs within a few days after the injury (Hatten et al., 1991). It is mainly composed of astrocytes which become hyperplasic and hypertrophic (the so-called 'reactive astrocytes') and also of a heterogeneous assembly of cells including microglia, oligodendrocytes, fibroblasts and other inflammatory cells. All lead to: (1) the formation of a physical barrier; and (2) the emergence of a biochemical barrier by either the down-regulation of growth-promoting or the up-regulation of growth-inhibiting molecules (Ridet et al., 1997; Fitch and Silver, 1999). Thus, the formation of a dense glial scar is one of the major impediments to neural repair (Ramón y Cajal, 1913–1914; Brown and McCough, 1947; Reier et al., 1989; for review see Fawcett and Asher, 1999; Fitch et al., 1999).

Three experimental strategies have been developed to overcome the problem of this non-permissive environment: blockage of glial scar formation, modification of growth-inhibitory molecules, and selective removal of reactive astrocytes. Indeed, rather than applying a single strategy, combined strategies should be devised to ensure robust regeneration and recovery of functions of CNS-lesioned tracts.

Blockage of glial scar formation

One of the most drastic manipulations of the glial environment after an injury aims at blocking the initial formation of the glial scar. Since the reactive gliosis is characterized by a hyperplasia, one interesting experimental method consists of removing all proliferating cells generated in response to CNS injury. This could be achieved by the non-invasive X-ray irradiation approach which disrupts the non-permissive gliotic environment and prevents tissue degeneration around the lesion site (Kalderon and Fuks, 1996a). In a SC transection model, the reduction of the glial scar in the vicinity of the lesion is followed by regeneration of numerous corticospinal axons which is associated with functional motor recovery (Kalderon and Fuks, 1996b). Moreover, we recently showed that early low-dose rather than late high-dose X-ray irradiation improves recovery after SC compression by preventing posttraumatic syringomyelia and gliosis (Ridet et al., 2000).

An alternative approach used to remove proliferating cells consists of injecting ethidium bromide (EtBr) in the lesion area. Indeed, EtBr binds to DNA and RNA and kills the cells by disrupting numerous cell functions. Moon et al. (2000) showed that a region free of cells after EtBr injection supports a robust regeneration of the nigrostriatal axons following nigrostriatal tract transection. However, although this cell-free area induced by EtBr leads temporarily to a permissive environment for axonal regeneration, it is limited by the organization of the CNS macroglia.

Finally, modulation of the glial scar formation can be achieved by injection of specific antibodies (Ridet and Privat, 2000). Indeed, a neutralizing TGFβ-1 antibody administered into the brain of injured rats significantly attenuates the formation of the fibrous scar tissue and the limiting glial membrane (Logan et al., 1994). In addition, the systemic administration of IL-10 (an inhibitor of microglial cytokines synthesis) reduces the inflammatory response and results in a significant attenuation of the astroglial reaction (Balasingam and Yong, 1996), which is correlated with a reduction in neuronal damage after an SCI (Brewer et al., 1999).

Modification of growth-inhibitory molecules

The glial scar is also characterized by an increased deposition of a number of extracellular matrix (ECM) molecules identified as neurite growth-inhibiting molecules. Thus, several experimental manipulations consist in disrupting the ECM to overcome the non-permissive biochemical nature of the scar. One approach aims at reducing the putative inhibitory properties of ECM molecules by applying ECM-degradating enzymes. A characteristic example is the digestion of the glycosaminoglycan side chains of chondroitin sulfate proteoglycans (CSPGs) by chondroitinase ABC. The application of chondroitinase ABC to contused SC decreases the CSPG immunoreactivity (Lemons et al., 1999). In addition, when chondroitinase ABC is placed on top of the interface between the hemisectioned SC and a nerve graft, it enhances axonal growth into the graft (Yick et al., 2000). Another approach consists in interrupting ECM synthesis. Works by Stichel and Muller (1998); Stichel et al. (1999a,b) suggest that the impermeable nature of the scar is principally due to its basal membrane formed of collagen IV and laminin. Reduction of the collagen IV deposition by the iron-chelator 2-2′-dipyridine after a fimbria fornix lesion prevents the formation of a dense collagen network. Moreover, an extensive regeneration of the lesioned axons in the commissural track (Stichel et al., 1999a) is correlated with a reduction of the deposition of potential growth-inhibitoring molecules (Stichel et al., 1999b). However, this treatment is not sufficient to enhance corticospinal regeneration after a mid-thoracic SCI (Weidner et al., 1999).

Finally, numerous studies have dealt with the neuritic growth-inhibitory properties associated with CNS myelin after a CNS traumatism (Caroni and Schwab, 1988). Indeed, the application of a neutralizing antibody (NI-1) aimed at the surface proteins NI-35/250/Nogo-A of oligodendrocytes (Bandtlow and Schwab, 2000) leads to a long-distance regeneration of the corticospinal tractus after a SCI and is associated with some functional recovery (Schnell and Schwab, 1990; Bregman et al., 1995).

Selective removal of reactive astrocytes

Reactive astrocytes are the major cellular components of the glial scar and are considered to play a key role in the CNS regeneration impediment (Reier et al., 1989). Reactive astrocytes are characterized by two parameters: *hyperplasia* and *hypertrophy*, which consist respectively in cell proliferation and over-expression of GFAP, the major structural intermediate filaments (IFs) protein of the astrocyte cytoskeleton. The tightly bound processes of reactive astrocytes constitute a *mechanical* barrier, while their production of growth-inhibiting molecules upregulated following injury induces a *biochemical* barrier to any neuronal repair.

In order to investigate more precisely the roles of reactive astrocytes in the prevention of CNS regeneration, several experimental strategies have been developed.

In a first attempt to reduce the formation of the astrocytic scar, we used a cholesterol derivative, the 7β-hydroxycholesteryl-oleate, known to produce cytotoxic effects on reactive astrocytes (Bochelen et al., 1992). We showed that local administration of that molecule significantly reduces the GFAP-mRNA level and astrocyte proliferation in a hemisection model of the SC in rats. Moreover, this reduction of glial reactivity is correlated with a local increased sprouting of serotonergic axons, below the lesion, from the intact side to the lesioned side. These serotonergic axons establish normal synaptic contacts (Giménez y Ribotta et al., 1995).

These results demonstrate the contribution of the astroglial reactivity in axonal regeneration by showing how the inhibition of astroglial hypertrophy and hyperplasia leads to the removal of physical and chemical barriers to axonal regeneration. However, this experiment could not differentiate the respective roles played by hyperplasia and hypertrophy and the effect was limited to the site of administration. Thus, more specific and widespread tools have to be utilized, on the one hand, to discriminate the potential roles of hyperplasia and hypertrophy, and on the other hand, to interfere with as many reactive astrocytes as possible.

Selective elimination of hyperplasia

An interesting gene therapy tool for interfering with proliferating cells is the herpes simplex virus–thymidine kinase/ganciclovir (HSV–tK/GCV) system. Indeed, in HSV–tK transfected cells, GCV becomes cytotoxic for the cell by blocking the DNA polymerase and thus inducing cell death (Moolten, 1986).

We showed that the HSV–tK/GCV system (transfected with a recombinant replication-deficient adenovirus) is an efficient tool in vitro for killing proliferating astrocytes in primary cultures (Audouy et al., 1999).

To target specifically reactive astrocytes in vivo, Bush et al. (1998) utilized the expression of HSV–tK to astroglial cells using the GFAP promoter in transgenic mice combined with conditionally regulated treatment with GCV (Sofroniew et al., 1999). Indeed, the over-expression of GFAP after a CNS injury is the hallmark of hypertrophy (Bignami and Dahl, 1976; Rataboul et al., 1988; Morin-Richaud et al., 1998).

Using this model, Bush et al. (1999) targeted cell death of reactive proliferative astrocytes and suppressed scar-forming reactive astrocytes after a forebrain lesion (Bush et al., 1998). However, although an increase in axonal sprouting is observed, the entire ablation of reactive astrocytes leads to a failure of blood–brain barrier repair and an increase in leukocyte infiltration, thus underlying the essential role played by astrocytes in maintaining the homeostatic environment in the CNS and limiting the practical use of this approach.

Selective elimination of astrocyte hypertrophy

Hypertrophy is, besides hyperplasia, the main characteristic parameter of reactive astrocytes. It is determined by the over-expression of GFAP and the re-expression of vimentin (Vim), the two major IFs proteins of the astrocytic cytoskeleton. With the aim of inhibiting the hypertrophic aspect of reactive astrocytes, while keeping the cells alive, we took advantage of three transgenic mice, generated by homologous recombination, deficient in Vim (Colucci-Guyon et al., 1994), GFAP (Pekny et al., 1995) and both Vim and GFAP (Ding et al., 1998).

We first performed an in vitro coculture of astrocytes and neurons. The aim of this in vitro approach was: (1) to analyze the possible contribution of the IFs proteins — GFAP and/or Vim — to support neuronal survival and neurite growth; and (2) to determine the expression of extracellular matrix-associated and surface molecules of astrocytes from the three mutants and to compare them with those of astrocytes from wild-type mice (Menet et al., 2001).

We developed a coculture model where wild-type ($+/+$) neocortical neurons (E_{14}) were seeded onto a confluent carpet of SC astrocytes derived from $+/+$, $Vim^{-/-}$, $GFAP^{-/-}$ (Menet et al., 2000) or double knock-out (KO) mice. One interesting characteristic of this heterotopic model is that it mimics what happens during normal CNS development, when neocortical neurons reach their target region (i.e. the spinal cord).

To determine the influence of the absence of GFAP and/or Vim on cocultured neurons, two parameters were evaluated: neuronal survival and neurite growth.

After identification of cocultured neurons by βIII-tubulin immunostaining, neurons growing on $+/+$ SC confluent astrocyte monolayers, as well as neurons growing on $Vim^{-/-}$ SC astrocytes appear isolated and produce very few and short neurites. In contrast, neurons growing on double KO as well as on $GFAP^{-/-}$ astrocytes are more numerous and often clustered, and both develop an important network of neurites. Indeed, neuronal density on $Vim^{-/-}$ SC astrocytes, measured by βIII-tubulin cells/mm^2, is not significantly different from that on $+/+$ SC astrocytes. In contrast, neuronal density on both $GFAP^{-/-}$

and double KO SC astrocytes is almost tripled when compared to that on +/+ SC astrocytes.

Concerning the second parameter evaluated, we demonstrated that the total neurite length per neuron on Vim$^{-/-}$ SC astrocytes is not significantly different from that of neurons grown on +/+ SC astrocyte monolayers whereas total neurite length per neuron is more than doubled on both GFAP$^{-/-}$ and double KO astrocyte monolayers vs. that on +/+ SC astrocytes.

Finally, coculture experiments performed with double KO astrocytes derived from the homotopic region of neurons (i.e. the neocortex) also show an increased permissivity vs. +/+ astrocytes, concerning both neuronal survival and neurite length, when compared to heterotopic cocultures (Menet et al., 2001).

To further delineate the possible influence of soluble factors on both parameters, we realized two additional paradigms: (1) +/+ neurons were plated on a microporous membrane and cocultured over +/+ or double KO SC astrocytes, eliminating all contact between neurons and astrocytes; (2) neurons were grown on +/+ SC astrocytes in the presence of conditioned medium (CM) from double KO SC astrocytes. Our results indicate that soluble factors are partially implicated in the permissivity of double KO SC astrocytes with regard to neuronal survival. However, neurite growth is only increased in a contact-dependent manner (Menet et al., 2001).

Altogether, these results illustrate several interesting points: first, astrocytes totally devoid of intermediate filaments (IFs) proteins (i.e. the double KO astrocytes) are a more permissive substrate for neuronal survival and neurite length than +/+ astrocytes; second, this constitutes a genuine capacity of double KO astrocytes since astrocytes derived from the SC as well as those from the neocortex have the same effects on the two parameters evaluated; third, soluble factors released from double KO astrocytes improve to a limited extent neuronal survival whereas neurite growth is strictly contact-dependent; finally, the sole absence of GFAP, rather than the absence of two IFs proteins, is the key element for the permissivity of astrocytes, whereas the absence of Vim does not appear to interfere with these two parameters (Menet et al., 2001).

To dissect-out the possible mechanisms triggered by the absence of GFAP, we decided to undertake, in the three mutant and +/+ SC astrocytes, an analysis of the expression of key diffusible and/or ECM molecules implicated in neuronal survival and neurite growth. We found that laminin, one of the strongest ECM component promoters for neurite growth during CNS development (Baron van Evercooren et al., 1982; Sanes, 1989; Reichardt and Tomaselli, 1991), is overexpressed in both GFAP$^{-/-}$ and double KO SC astrocytes. In the same way, N-cadherin, a major adhesion molecule involved in neurite growth during development (Neugebauer et al., 1988; Tomaselli et al., 1988; Redies, 2000), is also overexpressed in GFAP$^{-/-}$ and double KO SC astrocytes. Moreover, we found that the organization of the ECM is different in the absence of GFAP. Indeed, laminin expression is restricted to certain groups of cells in wild-type and Vim$^{-/-}$ cultures. Conversely, in both double KO SC and GFAP$^{-/-}$ SC astrocyte monolayers, the laminin staining is uniform, more intense and widespread throughout the culture. Finally, we observed different patterns of fibronectin expression in all the astrocytes cultures. In +/+ astrocytes monolayers, we observed a moderate intracellular staining throughout the cultures and a very limited extracellular staining constituted of thick, fibrous strands. In all mutant astrocyte cultures (Vim$^{-/-}$, GFAP$^{-/-}$ and double KO cultures), the intensity of the immunostaining is enhanced vs. wild-type cultures. In Vim$^{-/-}$ astrocyte cultures, the fibronectin staining is mostly extracellular with a network of thin, packed fibrillar deposits in many areas of the culture. At variance, both GFAP$^{-/-}$ and double KO astrocytes exhibit a different distribution of fibronectin. Although immunostaining for fibronectin is mainly intracellular, some thick fibrillar deposits of fibronectin are already found as described in +/+ astrocyte cultures. Interestingly, most of the extracellular expression of fibronectin appears as in punctuate labeling, which is never observed in +/+ or in Vim$^{-/-}$ astrocyte cultures.

In conclusion, the sole absence of GFAP is correlated, first, with an increased permissivity of astrocytes to neuronal survival and neurite growth, and second, with significant modifications of the expression and the organization of ECM, and of adhesion molecules known to be implicated in the permissive properties of astrocytes. Whether these effects are a direct consequence of the absence of GFAP per se remains to be determined. Interestingly, astrocytes devoid of GFAP can correspond in some respects, to what happens during CNS development. On the one hand, there exists a strong correlation between the differential expression of IFs proteins and the decrease of permissivity (Bovolenta et al., 1984; Liesi et al., 1986). Vim is the IFs protein expressed in highly permissive radial glia and immature astrocytes in embryonic CNS. During the astrocyte differentiation, it is progressively replaced by GFAP (Dahl, 1981; Bignami et al., 1982), which becomes the IFs protein of 'mature' astrocytes. On the other hand, laminin and N-cadherin which are overexpressed in GFAP$^{-/-}$ and double KO SC astrocytes are expressed in immature astrocytes and their expression decreases during maturation of astrocytes (Liesi et al., 1983; Smith et al., 1990).

These promising results led us to carry out in vivo experiments implicating SC lesions. Preliminary results indicate that in the total absence of IFs proteins, Vim and GFAP, a significant modification of astroglial responses to SC hemisection occurs (Giménez y Ribotta et al., 2001), as already demonstrated in another SC lesion model (Pekny et al., 1999). Indeed, in the absence of two IFs proteins, we observed a drastic reduction of the astroglial scar and, below the lesion, an increased axonal sprouting of serotonergic neurons from the intact side to the lesioned side (Menet et al., 1998).

Experiments with single KO mice deficient in GFAP or Vim are currently under way to eventually discriminate the possible contribution of each protein to astroglial reaction and axonal sprouting of supraspinal neurons. Finally, we will correlate the axonal sprouting and/or regeneration with specific motor tasks.

Management of sublesional spinal cord

Management of sublesional SC is based on the reorganization of undamaged neural pathways. SC circuits are capable of a significant reorganization, which is manifested by both activity-dependent and injury-induced plasticity. This plasticity is illustrated in the ability of spinal animals to learn new locomotor tasks (Muir and Steeves, 1997).

Studies in cats and in humans have shown that adult SC can perform, independently of the brain,

many of the functions necessary for walking. These studies have shown that there exists in the SC neuronal circuits which generate a locomotor rhythmic activity, the so-called central pattern generator (CPG) and that this activity is controlled and modulated by supraspinal descending and sensory afferents (Rossignol and Dubuc, 1994; Dimitrijevic et al., 1998). Indeed, the lumbosacral SC in humans, although completely deprived of brain motor control, can respond with a motor pattern underlaid by patterned sensory, phasic inputs from the lower limbs associated with load-bearing stepping (Dietz et al., 1995).

Neurophysiological assessment of subclinical residual motor functions and connections is thus useful in understanding the role of spasticity in SCI patients and in developing more specific restorative training programs (Dietz et al., 1994, 1995). The procedure of electrical SC stimulation of the posterior lumbar structures from the epidural space has become a clinically accepted method for the control of spasticity in subjects with SCI. This procedure is also useful for studying lumbosacral cord mechanisms for locomotion in humans (Dimitrijevic et al., 1998). In this context, the epidural SC stimulation can elicit step-like EMG activity and locomotor synergies in paraplegic subjects (Dimitrijevic et al., 1998). This suggests that spinal circuitry in humans can generate locomotor-like activity even when isolated from brain control.

In this respect, our efforts over the last decade have been directed to an original transplantation strategy: replacement of supraspinal afferents in the sublesional cord by brainstem monoaminergic neurons, which are involved in the activation of the intrinsic SC circuitry that mediates locomotor and autonomic functions (Forssberg and Grillner, 1973; Mas et al., 1985; Rossignol, 1996).

Our experimental paradigm is a complete section of SC at T_8–T_9 level of adult rats. One week later, a cell suspension of raphe from 14-day-old embryos or of locus coeruleus from 13-day-old embryos is injected into the dorsal funiculi, below the section at the T_{11} level. After transection of the cord, all descending monoaminergic fibers below the section degenerate, providing a sublesional SC devoid of supraspinal afferents. Thus, transplanted neurons can easily be identified by immunodetection of serotonin or noradrenaline in the sublesional cord. Moreover, reinnervation coming exclusively from the graft permits good anatomical, biochemical and functional correlations (Giménez y Ribotta et al., 1998).

Anatomical data

Transplanted serotonergic or noradrenergic neurons survive and integrate within the host SC, specifically innervating target regions with a pattern comparable to that of intact animals (Björklund and Skagerberg, 1982; Mansour et al., 1986; Privat et al., 1986, 1988, 1989; Yakovleff et al., 1989, 1995; Roudet et al., 1995; Giménez y Ribotta et al., 1996). Ultrastructural examination shows, in the ventral horn, numerous immunoreactive profiles in the vicinity of motoneurons, although a small number of axosomatic synapses are observed. Axodendritic synapses formed by serotonergic boutons are more numerous and most often located on large dendrites. In addition, some non-synaptic immunoreactive profiles containing small spherical vesicles are observed in single thin sections (Privat et al., 1988, 1989; Yakovleff et al., 1995; Giménez y Ribotta et al., 1996).

When cell suspensions from individual raphe nuclei, i.e. raphe magnus (group B3) or raphe obscurus and pallidus (groups B1–B2) are transplanted in our paradigm of SC transection, the innervation pattern developed is strictly located in the specific natural targets, i.e. B3 neurons develop a dense immunoreactive innervation distributed in the entire dorsal horn, whereas very few serotonergic fibers are observed in the ventral horn. Conversely, B1–B2 neurons develop bundles of serotonergic fibers with a specific segregation in the ventral horn and intermediolateral column, and very few fibers are seen in the dorsal horn (Rajaofetra et al., 1992). In addition, axonal varicosities from B3 neurons frequently do not form typical synapses, similarly to what has been described in intact animals (Marlier et al., 1991a; Ridet et al., 1993). Conversely, transplanted B1–B2 neurons develop classical synapses on dendrites and perikarya of motoneurons and interneurons in the ventral horn, such as is the case in intact animals (Rajaofetra et al., 1992; Ridet et al., 1993).

The re-establishment of specific neural circuitry with a normal pattern of reinnervation and synaptic connectivity is probably not a point-to-point reconstruction of the missing descending pathways. Nevertheless, this precise and remarkable reinnervation of targets must have a repercussion on neural and behavioral functions.

Secondly, we have evaluated the biochemical consequences of this precise restored circuitry.

Biochemical data

It is well known that descending monoaminergic systems regulate sensorimotor and visceral functions involving their specific receptors (Mason and Fibiger, 1979; Connor et al., 1981; Rawlow and Gorka, 1986; Tanabe et al., 1990), which exhibit a well characterized and precise topography in the SC (Young and Kunhar, 1980; Jones et al., 1982; Giron et al., 1985; Roudet et al., 1993, 1994; Marlier et al., 1991b).

In our model of SC transection, a significant increase in the α_1- and α_2-adrenoceptors density has been reported below the section (Roudet et al., 1993, 1994). Because grafted locus coeruleus neurons are able to restore levels of neurotransmitters in chemically depleted cord (Björklund et al., 1986; Moorman et al., 1990), in our transection model, we have investigated whether these noradrenergic neurons are able to normalize the lesion-induced increase in α_1- or α_2-adrenoceptors densities. A quantitative radioautographic study was performed using [^{3}H]prazosin or [^{3}H]rauwolscine as ligands, for which the SC was subdivided into six areas according to the cytoarchitectonic organization of the rat SC (Molander et al., 1984, 1989).

The density of [^{3}H]prazosin binding on α_1-adrenoceptors or of [^{3}H]rauwolscine on α_2-adrenoceptors depends on the level of SC analyzed. In intact and, above the section, in transected and grafted animals, the labeling corresponding to [^{3}H]prazosin binding is homogeneous in the gray matter, and no significant variations are observed in the six areas analyzed. Similar results are observed with [^{3}H]rauwolscine on α_2-adrenoceptors, except in the superficial dorsal horn where a significant increase is observed in grafted animals. At lumbar and sacral levels, in transected animals, the density of [^{3}H]prazosin binding sites is significantly increased compared to values detected in intact animals. The density of [^{3}H]rauwolscine binding sites is also increased within the entire gray matter and in particular in the dorsal horn areas. Interestingly, in grafted animals, at the lumbar level, the density of [^{3}H]prazosin binding sites is similar to that found in intact animals. At variance, at the sacral level, the number of binding sites observed remains significantly increased and is comparable to that found at the same level in transected animals. In contrast, the density of [^{3}H]rauwolscine binding sites is not significantly different from that observed in transected animals at the lumbar level.

Transplanted locus coeruleus neurons are able to develop an axonal outgrowth in the deafferented areas re-establishing the normal terminal innervation pattern, which is visualized up to at least 20 mm rostrocaudally within the SC: the lumbar level is completely reinnervated, whereas the sacral level is not systematically reinnervated by the transplant. Moreover, as in the case of preceding serotonergic neurons, noradrenergic grafted neurons establish synaptic contacts with the host SC. The synaptic contacts observed at the surface of noradrenergic immunoreactive dendritic profiles are mainly of the asymmetric type (Gray's type I). At some distance from the transplant (3–5 mm), noradrenergic immunoreactive profiles generally form synaptic contacts with unlabeled perikarya and dendritic profiles. These immunoreactive varicosities contain round, small, clear vesicles and form type II synapses. Noradrenergic boutons also make synapses with dendritic spines, which appear to be of type II. The frequency of non-synaptic noradrenergic varicosities in single thin sections is similar to that of intact animals. The axosomatic synaptic contacts constitute a small minority and the percentage of axodendritic and axospinous synapses is similar to that of intact animals (Rajaofetra et al., 1992; Giménez y Ribotta et al., 1996).

These results illustrate that the increase in α_1-adrenoceptors densities induced by the lesion returns to normal levels detected in intact animals, in those areas reinnervated by grafted noradrenergic neurons. Although nonspecific mechanisms cannot be excluded, these results suggest that biochemical restoration by monoaminergic innervation is likely to correspond to the presence of adequate quantities of neurotransmitter in a target area rather than to point-to-point connectivity.

In our transplants of raphe or locus coeruleus, not all cells are serotonergic or noradrenergic neurons, nor are all serotonergic or noradrenergic neurons identical. A heterogenous population exists, which can contain other neurotransmitters, stored in the same cell and released even by the same axonal boutons. Such is the case of raphe neurons projecting in the SC (Kachidian et al., 1991). We have confirmed a colocalization in raphe neurons from B1 to B2 nuclei after transplantation in transected SC, where serotonin and substance P coexist in the same terminals of transplanted neurons (Rajaofetra et al., 1991).

In another series of experiments, we evaluated whether transplanted embryonic raphe cells can directly regulate the effectors of autonomic and motor systems in the cord, or if they also regulate the GABAergic phenotype of interneurons in the transected SC of adult rats.

We analyzed the expression of two isoforms of glutamate decarboxylase (GAD), the rate-limiting synthesizing enzyme of GABA. Expression of GAD_{65} and GAD_{67} mRNAs have been analyzed by in situ hybridization procedures using digoxygenin (DIG)-labeled cRNA probes.

The first finding of this study is the detection of numerous GABAergic neurons among the transplanted cells, which show labeling for both GAD mRNAs. Concerning the host SC, the expression of GAD_{67} is highly modified by the transection whereas GAD_{65} remains unaltered.

In transected animals, the number of host neurons expressing GAD_{67} is significantly increased compared to values detected in intact animals. Interestingly, in grafted animals, the number of host neurons expressing GAD_{67} is close to control level. These post-grafting modifications are further associated with increased GABA immunoreactivity in the host tissue. These data illustrate that the graft of embryonic raphe cells also regulates the expression of the GABAergic phenotype in the host SC. This regulation can be mediated by the re-establishment of a local functional reinnervation by both serotonin and GABAergic transplanted neurons (Dumoulin et al., 2000).

Thus, transplantation of embryonic neurons cannot be interpreted only through simple pharmacological interactions. The restitution and balance of neurotransmitters by the graft constitute a complex process by which grafted cells modulate intrinsic circuits which contribute in a still unknown fashion to functional recovery.

Physiological data

We have evidenced in previous studies, the direct implication of medullary monoaminergic systems in locomotion by using microdialysis probes implanted in the ventral funiculus of the rat SC (Gerin et al., 1995). The measurement of local release of monoamines in the ventral funiculus of SC is the most direct evaluation of the function of these systems during motor activity. Thus, we have detected an increase in the release of monoamines during the exercise on a treadmill of rats permanently implanted (Gerin and Privat, 1998). This suggests an activation of monoaminergic systems during locomotor activity, confirming electrophysiological studies concerning the electrical activity of monoaminergic neurons in treadmill-trained cats (Jacobs and Fornal, 1993, 1997).

Thus, in our transplantation paradigm, we have finally analyzed the effect of the transplant on the recovery of motor capacities and especially locomotion in spinal rats.

The locomotor rhythmic activity is generated in SC by a precise neuronal network or CPG. This activity is, however, controlled and modulated by supraspinal descending and sensory afferents (Rossignol and Dubuc, 1994; Dimitrijevic et al., 1998).

After transection of the SC, the supraspinal control is abolished, leaving only the sublesional cord sensory inputs, which are not able to activate the CPG, resulting in a loss of locomotor activity. Transplants of embryonic neurons from raphe nucleus or locus coeruleus in sublesional SC are able to enhance hindlimb flexion reflex (Buchanan and Nornes, 1986) and trigger automatic locomotion in hindlimbs when animals are subjected to a stimulation by treadmill without any pharmacological treatment. Electromyographic recordings (EMG) show in transplanted animals a specific pattern of activation with alternate bursts in homologous muscles of the two hindlimbs, which is not observed in transected animals (Yakovleff et al., 1989, 1995).

In order to eliminate afferent influences on the pattern-generating circuitry, we recorded fictive motor patterns in hindlimb muscle nerves in transected rats grafted with raphe or locus coeruleus neurons. This study revealed an increase in the excitability of locomotor network in transplanted animals with significantly longer locomotor episodes and shorter step cycles than those found in transected animals. In fact, two different fictive motor patterns are identified, one associated with locomotion and the other with hindlimb paw shaking. In these animals, grafted neurons increase the excitability of spinal stepping, whereas neural circuits corresponding paw shaking are not significantly influenced by the transplant (Yakovleff et al., 1995). However, an obvious difference in the characteristics of fictive locomotion cannot be detected between raphe- and locus coeruleus-grafted animals.

Interestingly, a different modulatory effect on locomotion is obtained after pharmacological treatment with noradrenergic or serotonergic agonists. The two types of neurotransmitters may modulate locomotion, in terms of expression of the locomotor pattern. Noradrenergic agonists may markedly increase the duration of the step cycle (Barbeau and Rossignol, 1991; Rossignol et al., 1995), whereas serotonergic agonists may increase the amplitude of the electromyographic activity (Barbeau et al., 1981; Barbeau and Rossignol, 1990, 1991).

The locomotor rhythmic activity developed in transplanted animals by the influence of serotonergic or noradrenergic neurons is well correlated with the identification of an innervation pattern in a normal specific fashion. However, despite the careful microdissection of embryonic tissue to isolate the raphe nuclei or locus coeruleus, in all transplanted animals, the two types of innervation are immunocytochemically detected. This suggests that there exists a combined effect of these two populations on motor activities as evaluated by electrophysiology.

In order to isolate the influence of the serotonergic system on locomotion, we have transplanted raphe cells in our graft-transection paradigm, and 2 months later we removed noradrenergic innervation by intrathecal administration of a specific neurotoxin, 6-hydroxydopamine (6-OHDA). This technical procedure permits the comparison of spinal motor capacities of grafted and grafted-6-OHDA-treated animals with those of transected animals (Feraboli-Lohnherr et al., 1997).

Transected animals move their forelimbs, whereas hindquarters drag over the ground, and occasionally develop some rhythmical flexions and extensions, often alternated in both hindlimbs. However, the posture adopted is an extended position in an almost horizontal plane, even if these animals are stimulated by a treadmill. When the use of the treadmill is associated with tail pinching, flexion and extension movements are limited to proximal joints, but dorsiflexion of the toes is never observed.

On the contrary, grafted animals can stand up and develop typical locomotor patterns, which can be evoked by stimulation of the tail. These rhythmic movements are very similar to those developed by intact animals. Indeed, landing the paw on the ground, which marks the end of the swing phase, is preceded by dorsiflexion of the toes. Such rhythmic activity is identified as a typical locomotor activity. The association of tail pinching with the use of treadmill improves the regularity of the rhythm and the quality of interlimb coordination, suggesting a regulating role for the treadmill, since this latter alone is ineffective.

In grafted 6-OHDA-treated animals, the characteristics of locomotor activity are similar to those detected in grafted animals (Feraboli-Lohnherr et al., 1997). On ultrastructural examination, these animals exhibit a total absence of noradrenergic innervation with few dystrophic and very varicose fibers, and an important and classical serotonin innervation.

Taken together, these results show that serotonergic and, to a lesser extent, noradrenergic neurons transplanted in a SC totally devoid of supraspinal inputs, are able to induce rhythmic motor activities in hindlimbs which are characterized as genuine locomotion. This response is obtained without any pharmacological treatment or training.

In this context, noradrenergic agonists in chronic spinal cats (Rossignol et al., 1986; Barbeau and Rossignol, 1991), and serotonergic agonists in chronic spinal rats (Barbeau et al., 1981) induce hindlimb locomotor movements. Moreover, fictive locomotor activities have also been recorded from the ventral roots of neonatal rat SC with the addition of serotonin (Cazalets et al., 1992).

In order to establish a correlation between the locomotor performance and the reinnervation level of the sublesional SC, we performed a kinematic analysis of locomotion synchronously with an EMG

study of adult paraplegic rats transplanted with embryonic raphe-neurons at two different levels of the cord (Giménez y Ribotta et al., 2000).

After complete transection of SC, wire electrodes are chronically implanted (Chau et al., 1998) in several bilateral flexor and extensor muscles for chronic EMG recording during treadmill locomotion. One week later, a raphe cell suspension was injected in sublesional cord at the T_9 level (T_9 animals) or at T_{11} level (T_{11} animals). The motor activity of these two groups of animals was compared to that of intact and spinal non-transplanted animals.

After a survival time of 2 months, movements of hindlimbs of these four groups of animals were documented by video recording. During these sessions, the hindlimbs are on a treadmill belt while the forelimbs are at rest on a platform spanned over the moving belt. Simultaneous recording of kinematic patterns and EMG signals permits a direct correlation between the analysis of movement and EMG bursts. The treadmill is sometimes associated with a stimulation by tail pinching.

A typical kinematic analysis, in the form of a stick diagram, illustrates the locomotor performance of hindlimbs. During the swing phase, intact animals exhibit a coordinated ankle, knee and hip flexion, elevate the foot to bring it upward and forward. Animals transplanted at T_{11} are capable of standing up, supporting the weight of the hindquarters, and walking on the treadmill with their four limbs when the tail is pinched. Locomotor movements of the hindlimbs resemble globally those of intact animals. The EMG pattern is not very different from that observed in intact animals except for some extra bursts in the knee extensor muscles during the swing phase. Interestingly, a second transection at the site of the original spinal lesion had no effect on the subsequent motor performance, demonstrating that recovery of motor functions occurs at the spinal level and is not due to any regrowth of fibers from supraspinal afferents.

The motor performance of animals transplanted at T_9 does not differ from that of spinal non-transplanted animals. Both cannot stand up and are unable to support the hindquarters. The feet drag on the treadmill belt with all the hindlimb joints in extension. The correlative EMG pattern is very disorganized.

After kinematic and EMG analyses, a blind *post-mortem* immunocytochemical study of the serotonergic reinnervation in the lumbar SC was performed. In transected animals, the sublesional SC is totally devoid of serotonergic immunoreactivity, as expected from the degeneration of all descending pathways. Thus, in the absence of supraspinal control, the pattern-generating circuitry of these animals remains ineffective most likely because of an insufficient activation resulting from the lack of appropriate neurotransmitters or sufficient afferent inputs. In transplanted T_{11} animals, the SC exhibits a well-developed transplant with many serotonergic immunoreactive perikarya. Grafted cells give rise to extensive immunoreactive varicose processes which reinnervate specific targets, preferentially concentrated around motoneurons. The transplant extends rostrocaudally and this innervation pattern becomes gradually more and more sparse at increasing distances from the transplant area, but is well detectable up to 8 mm caudally to the transplant, which corresponds to the L_1–L_2 level. In transplanted T_9 animals, the transplant also develops an extensive network of immunoreactive fibers, which scarcely reach the T_{13} level. No serotonergic fibers are detected at lower levels.

In conclusion, the kinematic patterns of movement and their relationships with the EMG indicate that T_{11} animals can perform walking movements resembling those observed in intact animals, whereas T_9 animals develop very limited movements. However, in both groups of transplanted animals, a specific and remarkable serotonergic reinnervation of targets is developed in the SC. These results suggest that serotonergic reinnervation of the cord at the L_1–L_2 level constitutes a key element in the genesis of locomotor activity, since no serotonergic fibers are detected at this level in T_9 animals. This is particularly interesting, since this region has been claimed to contain a neuronal network for locomotion, the so-called CPG in an in vitro model of neonatal rats (Cazalets et al., 1995). Our results indicate that in adult rats serotonergic innervation at the upper lumbar levels (L_1–L_2) is necessary to activate the CPG for locomotion. Thus, we have shown that precise serotonergic reinnervation specifically activates the circuitry responsible for spinal pattern generation in paraplegic rats, probably by providing an adequate supply of neurotransmitter in a specific site of the SC, thereby triggering a locomotor activity (Giménez y Ribotta et al., 2000).

Anatomical, biochemical and physiological correlations

The high correlation found between the anatomical pattern of innervation with a precise synaptic connectivity and the restoration of α_1-adrenoceptor densities in transplanted animals, and the restoration of locomotor activity, prompted us to investigate a physiological parameter closely linked to the function recovery: the hindlimb muscle phenotypes (Cooper et al., 1996).

We chose a postural tonic muscle, the soleus, and a phasic muscle, the gastrocnemius. In transected animals, the slow type I phenotype in the soleus muscle was transformed (decreased by 94% as compared with intact animals) in a fast type IIa/b phenotype, and it appeared a transitional type IIc fibers (which coexpressed both fast and slow myosin heavy chain isoforms). In grafted animals, however, this transformation was less marked (36%) and the transitional type was also reduced. The observations in the gastrocnemius phenotypes were less marked but significantly different from transected animals. Thus, the partial preservation of the slow type I phenotype in muscles of transplanted animals suggests that a subpopulation of hindlimb motoneurons is tonically activated by the monoaminergic reinnervation of the lumbar cord. Then, small-sized motor units can be excited, preventing their dedifferentiation into type II motor units.

To resume, our experimental paradigm using a complete transection of the cord followed by the transplantation of monoaminergic neurons below the lesion has opened an alternative to regeneration of descending inputs. It has permitted us to confirm and to extend previous evidence for the involvement of monoamines in the control and/or activation of locomotion. Moreover, combined anatomical, biochemical, and functional studies have permitted the establishment of a close correlation between the reinnervation of ventral horn neurons and the restoration of locomotion through the activation of specific receptors. These findings constitute a key element for a future therapeutic strategy in paraplegic patients.

206

In conclusion, we have reviewed here a decade of efforts to elaborate a comprehensive strategy for the treatment of traumatic lesions of the SC. The three lines of research which up to now have been conducted independently from each other will be progressively combined in order to optimize in time and space the care of the lesioned cord. Extensive basic research is still needed to further elucidate the parameters of injury and those of possible recovery. New tools are progressively available for investigation, and transgenic animals are among the most powerful. In parallel, therapeutic tools such as direct and indirect gene therapy are developed, using viral or non-viral vectors which associate a high efficacy of transfection with attenuated toxicity.

Quite obviously, efforts directed at the improvement of the outcome of traumatic spinal cord lesions will benefit other pathologies, such as brain trauma, but also degenerative diseases of the CNS. However, spinal trauma remains an unique paradigm both for its clinical implication and its value as a model for CNS repair.

Acknowledgements

The authors thank Dr. D. Orsal an Dr. S. Rossignol for their contribution in the study of management of sublesional spinal cord. These studies were supported by a France-Québec program, IRME, AFM, Beaufour-Ipsen Pharma and Verticale, and their assistance is gratefully acknowledged.

References

Allen, A.R. (1911) Surgery of experimental lesion of spinal cord equivalent to crush injury of fracture dislocation of spinal column. A preliminary study. *J. Am. Med. Assoc.*, 57: 878–880.

Audouy, S., Mallet, J., Privat, A. and Giménez y Ribotta, M. (1999) Adenovirus-mediated suicide gene therapy in an in vitro model of reactive gliosis. *Glia*, 25: 293–303.

Balasingam, V. and Yong, V.W. (1996) Attenuation of astroglial reactivity by interleukin-10. *J. Neurosci.*, 16: 2945–2955.

Bandtlow, C.E. and Schwab, M.E. (2000) NI-35/250/nogo-a: a neurite growth inhibitor restricting structural plasticity and regeneration of nerve fibers in the adult vertebrate CNS. *Glia*, 29: 175–181.

Barbeau, H. and Rossignol, S. (1990) The effects of serotonergic drugs on the locomotor pattern and on cutaneous reflexes of the adult chronic spinal cat. *Brain Res.*, 514: 55–67.

Barbeau, H. and Rossignol, S. (1991) Initiation and modulation of the locomotor pattern in the adult chronic spinal cat by noradrenergic, serotonergic and dopaminergic drugs. *Brain Res.*, 546: 250–260.

Barbeau, H., Filion, M. and Bédard, P. (1981) Effects of agonists and antagonists of serotonin on spontaneous hindlimb EMG activity in chronic rats. *Neuropharmacology*, 20: 99–107.

Baron van Evercooren, A., Kleinman, H.K., Ohno, S., Marangos, P., Schwartz, J.P. and Dubois-Dalcq, M.E. (1982) Nerve growth factor, laminin, and fibronectin promote neurite growth in human fetal sensory ganglia cultures. *J. Neurosci. Res.*, 8: 179–193.

Benveniste, H., Drejer, J., Schousboe, A. and Diemer, N.H. (1984) Elevation of the extracellular concentrations of glutamate and aspartate in rat hippocampus during transient cerebral ischemia monitored by intracerebral microdialysis. *J. Neurochem.*, 43: 1369–1374.

Bethea, J.R., Castro, M., Keane, R.W., Lee, T.T., Dietrich, W.D. and Yezierski, R.P. (1998) Traumatic spinal cord injury induces nuclear factor-kappaB activation. *J. Neurosci.*, 18: 3251–3260.

Bethea, J.R., Nagashima, H., Acosta, M.C., Briceno, C., Gomez, F., Marcillo, A.E., Loor, K., Green, J. and Dietrich, W.D. (1999) Systemically administered interleukin-10 reduces tumor necrosis factor-alpha production and significantly improves functional recovery following traumatic spinal cord injury in rats. *J. Neurotrauma*, 16: 851–863.

Bignami, A. and Dahl, D. (1976) The astrocytic response to stabbing. Immunofluorescence studies with antibodies to astrocytic-specific protein (GFAP) in mammalian and submammalian vertebrates. *Neuropathol. Appl. Neurobiol.*, 2: 99–110.

Bignami, A., Raju, T. and Dahl, D. (1982) Localization of vimentin, the nonspecific intermediate filament protein, in embryonal glia and in early differentiating neurons. In vivo and in vitro immunofluorescence study of the rat embryo with vimentin and neurofilament antisera. *Dev. Biol.*, 91: 286–295.

Birch, P.J., Grossman, C.J. and Hayes, A.G. (1988) Kynurenate and FG9041 have both competitive and non-competitive antagonist actions at excitatory amino acid receptors. *Eur. J. Pharmacol.*, 151: 313–315.

Björklund, A. and Skagerberg, G. (1982) Descending monoaminergic projections to the spinal cord. In: B. Sjölund and A. Björklund (Eds.), *Brainstem Control of Spinal Mechanisms*. Elsevier, Amsterdam, pp. 55–85.

Björklund, A., Nornes, H. and Gage, F.H. (1986) Cell suspension grafts of noradrenergic locus coeruleus neurons in rat hippocampus and spinal cord: reinnervation and transmitter turnover. *Neuroscience*, 18: 685–698.

Black, P., Markowitz, R.S., Damjanov, I., Finkelstein, S.D., Kushner, H., Gillespie, J. and Feldman, M. (1988) Models of spinal cord injury: Part 3. Dynamic load technique. *Neurosurgery*, 22: 51–60.

Bochelen, D., Eclancher, F., Kupferberg, A., Privat, A. and Mersel, M. (1992) 7 Beta-hydroxycholesterol and 7 beta-hydroxycholesteryl-3-esters reduce the extent of reactive gliosis caused by an electrolytic lesion in rat brain. *Neuroscience*, 51: 827–834.

Bovolenta, P., Liem, R.K. and Mason, C.A. (1984) Development of cerebellar astroglia: transitions in form and cytoskeletal content. *Dev. Biol.*, 102: 248–259.

Bracken, M.B., Shepard, M.J., Hellenbrand, K.G., Collins, W.F., Leo, L.S., Freeman, D.F., Wagner, F.C., Flamm, E.S., Eisenberg, H.M. and Goodman, J.H. et al. (1985) Methylprednisolone and neurological function 1 year after spinal cord injury. Results of the National Acute Spinal Cord Injury Study. *J. Neurosurg.*, 63: 704–713.

Bracken, M.B., Shepard, M.J., Collins, W.F., Holford, T.R., Young, W., Baskin, D.S., Eisenberg, H.M., Flamm, E., Leo-Summers, L. and Maroon, J. et al. (1990) A randomized, controlled trial of methylprednisolone or naloxone in the treatment of acute spinal-cord injury. Results of the Second National Acute Spinal Cord Injury Study. *N. Engl. J. Med.*, 322: 1405–1411.

Bracken, M.B., Shepard, M.J., Holford, T.R., Leo-Summers, L., Aldrich, E.F., Fazl, M., Fehlings, M., Herr, D.L., Hitchon, P.W., Marshall, L.F., Nockels, R.P., Pascale, V., Perot Jr., P.L., Piepmeier, J., Sonntag, V.K., Wagner, F., Wilberger, J.E., Winn, H.R. and Young, W. (1997) Administration of methylprednisolone for 24 or 48 hours or tirilazad mesylate for 48 hours in the treatment of acute spinal cord injury. Results of the Third National Acute Spinal Cord Injury Randomized Controlled Trial. National Acute Spinal Cord Injury Study. *J. Am. Med. Assoc.*, 277: 1597–1604.

Bregman, B.S., Kunkel-Bagden, E., Schnell, L., Dai, H.N., Gao, D. and Schwab, M.E. (1995) Recovery from spinal cord injury mediated by antibodies to neurite growth inhibitors. *Nature*, 378: 498–501.

Bresnahan, J.C., King, J.S., Martin, G.F. and Yashon, D. (1976) A neuroanatomical analysis of spinal cord injury in the rhesus monkey (*Macaca mulatta*). *J. Neurol. Sci.*, 28: 521–542.

Brewer, K.L., Bethea, J.R. and Yezierski, R.P. (1999) Neuroprotective effects of interleukin-10 following excitotoxic spinal cord injury. *Exp. Neurol.*, 159: 484–493.

Brown, J.O. and McCough, G.P. (1947) Abortive regeneration of transected spinal cord. *J. Comp. Neurol.*, 87: 131–137.

Buchanan, J.T. and Nornes, H.O. (1986) Transplants of embryonic brainstem containing the locus coeruleus into spinal cord enhance the hindlimb flexion reflex in adult rats. *Brain Res.*, 381: 225–236.

Bunge, M.B., Holets, V.R., Bates, M.L., Clarke, T.S. and Watson, B.D. (1994) Characterization of photochemically induced spinal cord injury in the rat by light and electron microscopy. *Exp. Neurol.*, 127: 76–93.

Bush, T.G., Savidge, T.C., Freeman, T.C., Cox, H.J., Campbell, E.A., Mucke, L., Johnson, M.H. and Sofroniew, M.V. (1998) Fulminant jejuno-ileitis following ablation of enteric glia in adult transgenic mice. *Cell*, 93: 189–201.

Bush, T.G., Puvanachandra, N., Horner, C.H., Polito, A., Ostenfeld, T., Svendsen, C.N., Mucke, L., Johnson, M.H. and Sofroniew, M.V. (1999) Leukocyte infiltration, neuronal degeneration, and neurite outgrowth after ablation of scar-

forming, reactive astrocytes in adult transgenic mice. *Neuron*, 23: 297–308.

Cameron, T., Prado, R., Watson, B.D., Gonzalez-Carvajal, M. and Holets, V.R. (1990) Photochemically induced cystic lesion in the rat spinal cord. I. Behavioral and morphological analysis. *Exp. Neurol.*, 109: 214–223.

Caroni, P. and Schwab, M.E. (1988) Antibody against myelin-associated inhibitor of neurite growth neutralizes nonpermissive substrate properties of CNS white matter. *Neuron*, 1: 85–96.

Cauquil-Caubere, I. and Kamenka, J.M. (1998) New structures able to prevent the inhibition by hydroxyl radicals of glutamate transport in cultured astrocytes. *Eur. J. Med. Chem.*, 33: 867–877.

Cauquil-Caubere, I., Oxhamre, C., Kamenka, J.M. and Barbanel, G. (1999) Recurrent glutamate stimulations potentiate the hydroxyl radicals response to glutamate. *J. Neurosci. Res.*, 56: 160–165.

Cazalets, J.R., Sqalli-Houssaini, Y. and Clarac, F. (1992) Activation of the central pattern generators for locomotion by serotonin and excitatory amino acids in neonatal rat. *J. Physiol.*, 455: 187–204.

Cazalets, J.R., Borde, M. and Clarac, F. (1995) Localization and organization of the central pattern generator for hindlimb locomotion in newborn rat. *J. Neurosci.*, 15: 4943–4951.

Chau, C., Barbeau, H. and Rossignol, S. (1998) Early locomotor training with clonidine in spinal cats. *J. Neurophysiol.*, 79: 392–409.

Chaudieu, I., Vignon, J., Chicheportiche, M., El Harfi, A., Kamenka, J.M. and Chicheportiche, R. (1987) Comparaison entre les sites de fixation de la [3H]phencyclidine (PCP) et de la [3H](thiényl-2)-1 cyclohexylpipéridine (TCP) dans le système nerveux central de rat. *Eur. J. Med. Chem.*, 22: 359–362.

Choi, D.W. (1992) Excitotoxic cell death. *J. Neurobiol.*, 23: 1261–1276.

Coleman, W.P., Benzel, D., Cahill, D.W., Ducker, T., Geisler, F., Green, B., Gropper, M.R., Goffin, J., Madsen, P.W., Maiman, D.J., Ondra, S.L., Rosner, M., Sasso, R.C., Trost, G.R. and Zeidman, S. (2000) A critical appraisal of the reporting of the National Acute Spinal Cord Injury Studies (II and III) of methylprednisolone in acute spinal cord injury. *J. Spinal Disord.*, 13: 185–199.

Collingridge, G.L. and Singer, W. (1990) Excitatory amino acid receptors and synaptic plasticity. *Trends Pharmacol. Sci.*, 11: 290–296.

Colucci-Guyon, E., Portier, M.M., Dunia, I., Paulin, D., Pournin, S. and Babinet, C. (1994) Mice lacking vimentin develop and reproduce without an obvious phenotype. *Cell*, 79: 679–694.

Connor, H.E., Drew, G.M., Finch, L. and Hicks, P.E. (1981) Pharmacological characteristics of spinal a-adrenoceptors in rats. *J. Auton. Pharmacol.*, 1: 149–156.

Cooper, R., Feraboli-Lohnherr, D., Butler-Browne, G., Orsal, D., Giménez y Ribotta, M. and Privat, A. (1996) Intraspinal injection of embryonic neurons maintains muscle phenotype in adult chronic spinal rats. *J. Neurosci. Res.*, 46: 324–329.

Dahl, D. (1981) The vimentin–GFA protein transition in rat

neuroglia cytoskeleton occurs at the time of myelination. *J. Neurosci. Res.*, 6: 741–748.

DeVivo, M.J., Krause, J.S. and Lammertse, D.P. (1999) Recent trends in mortality and causes of death among persons with spinal cord injury. *Arch. Phys. Med. Rehabil.*, 80: 1411–1419.

Dietz, V., Colombo, G. and Jensen, L. (1994) Locomotor activity in spinal man. *Lancet*, 344: 1260–1263.

Dietz, V., Colombo, G., Jensen, L. and Baumgartner, L. (1995) Locomotor capacity of spinal cord in paraplegic patients. *Ann. Neurol.*, 37: 574–582.

Dimitrijevic, M.R., Gerasimenko, Y. and Pinter, M.M. (1998) Evidence for a spinal central pattern generator in humans. *Ann. New York Acad. Sci.*, 860: 360–376.

Ding, M., Eliasson, C., Betsholtz, C., Hamberger, A. and Pekny, M. (1998) Altered taurine release following hypotonic stress in astrocytes from mice deficient for GFAP and vimentin. *Brain Res. Mol. Brain Res.*, 62: 77–81.

Drian, M.J., Kamenka, J.M., Pirat, J.L. and Privat, A. (1991) Non-competitive antagonists of *N*-methyl-D-aspartate prevent spontaneous neuronal death in primary cultures of embryonic rat cortex. *J. Neurosci. Res.*, 29: 133–138.

Drian, M.J., Kamenka, J.M. and Privat, A. (1999) In vitro neuroprotection against glutamate toxicity provided by novel non-competitive *N*-methyl-D-aspartate antagonists. *J. Neurosci. Res.*, 57: 927–934.

Dumoulin, A., Privat, A. and Giménez y Ribotta, M. (2000) Transplantation of embryonic raphe cells regulates the modifications of the GABAergic phenotype occurring in the injured spinal cord. *Neuroscience*, 95: 173–182.

Faden, A.I. and Salzman, S. (1992) Pharmacological strategies in CNS trauma. *Trends Pharmacol. Sci.*, 13: 29–35.

Faden, A.I. and Simon, R.P. (1988) A potential role for excitotoxins in the pathophysiology of spinal cord injury. *Ann. Neurol.*, 23: 623–626.

Faden, A.I., Demediuk, P., Panter, S.S. and Vink, R. (1989) The role of excitatory amino acids and NMDA receptors in traumatic brain injury. *Science*, 244: 798–800.

Farooque, M., Hillered, L., Holtz, A. and Olsson, Y. (1996) Changes of extracellular levels of amino acids after graded compression trauma to the spinal cord: an experimental study in the rat using microdialysis. *J. Neurotrauma*, 13: 537–548.

Fawcett, J.W. and Asher, R.A. (1999) The glial scar and the central nervous system repair. *Brain Res. Bull.*, 49: 377–391.

Feraboli-Lohnherr, D., Orsal, D., Yakovleff, A., Giménez y Ribotta, M. and Privat, A. (1997) Recovery of locomotor activity in the adult chronic spinal rat after sublesional transplantation of embryonic nervous cells: specific role of serotonergic neurons. *Exp. Brain Res.*, 113: 443–454.

Fitch, M.T. and Silver, J. (1999) Beyond the glial scar. Cellular and molecular mechanisms by which glial cells contribute to CNS regenerative failure. In: M.H. Tuszynski and J.H. Kordower (Eds.), *CNS Regeneration. Basic Science and Clinical Advances*. Academic Press, New York, pp. 55–88.

Fitch, M.T., Doller, C., Combs, C.K., Landreth, G.E. and Silver, J. (1999) Cellular and molecular mechanisms of glial scarring and progressive cavitation: in vivo and in vitro analysis of inflammation-induced secondary injury after CNS trauma. *J. Neurosci.*, 19: 8182–8198.

Forssberg, H. and Grillner, S. (1973) The locomotion of the acute spinal cat injected with clonidine i.v.. *Brain Res.*, 50: 184–186.

Gaviria, M., Privat, A., d'Arbigny, P., Kamenka, J.M., Haton, H. and Ohanna, F. (2000a) Neuroprotective effects of a novel NMDA antagonist, Gacyclidine, after experimental contusive spinal cord injury in adult rats. *Brain Res.*, 874: 200–209.

Gaviria, M., Privat, A., d'Arbigny, P., Kamenka, J.M., Haton, H. and Ohanna, F. (2000b) Neuroprotective effects of gacyclidine after experimental photochemical spinal cord lesion in adult rats: dose-window and time-window effects. *J. Neurotrauma*, 17: 19–30.

Geisler, F.H., Dorsey, F.C. and Coleman, W.P. (1991) Recovery of motor function after spinal-cord injury — a randomized, placebo-controlled trial with GM-1 ganglioside. *N. Engl. J. Med.*, 324: 1829–1838.

Gerin, C. and Privat, A. (1998) Direct evidence for the link between monoaminergic descending pathways and motor activity: II. A study with microdialysis probes implanted in the ventral horn of the spinal cord. *Brain Res.*, 794: 169–173.

Gerin, C., Becquet, D. and Privat, A. (1995) Direct evidence for the link between monoaminergic descending pathways and motor activity. I. A study with microdialysis probes implanted in the ventral funiculus of the spinal cord. *Brain Res.*, 704: 191–201.

Giménez y Ribotta, M. and Privat, A. (1998) Biological interventions for spinal cord injury. *Curr. Opin. Neurol.*, 11: 647–654.

Giménez y Ribotta, M., Rajaofetra, N., Morin-Richaud, C., Alonso, G., Bochelen, D., Sandillon, F., Legrand, A., Mersel, M. and Privat, A. (1995) Oxysterol (7β-hydroxycholesteryl-3-oleate) promotes serotonergic reinnervation in the lesioned rat spinal cord by reducing glial reaction. *J. Neurosci. Res.*, 41: 79–95.

Giménez y Ribotta, M., Roudet, C., Sandillon, F. and Privat, A. (1996) Transplantation of embryonic noradrenergic neurons in two models of adult rat spinal cord injury: ultrastructural immunocytochemical study. *Brain Res.*, 707: 245–255.

Giménez y Ribotta, M., Orsal, O., Feraboli-Lohnherr, D. and Privat, A. (1998) Neuronal mechanisms for generating locomotor activity: recovery of locomotion following transplantation of monoaminergic neurons in the spinal cord of paraplegic rats. *Ann. New York Acad. Sci.*, 860: 393–411.

Giménez y Ribotta, M., Provencher, J., Feraboli-Lohnherr, F., Rossignol, S., Privat, A. and Orsal, D. (2000) Activation of locomotion in adult chronic spinal rats is achieved by transplantation of embryonic raphe cells reinnervating a precise lumbar level. *J. Neurosci.*, 20: 5144–5152.

Giménez y Ribotta, M., Menet, V. and Privat, A. (2001) The role of astrocytes in axonal regeneration in the mammalian CNS. In: B. Castellano Lopez and M. Nieto-Sampedro (Eds.), *Glial Cell Function, Prog. Brain Res.*, Vol. 132, Elsevier, Amsterdam, pp. 587–610.

Giron, L.T., Maccann, S.A. and Crist-Orlando, S.G. (1985) Pharmacological characterization and regional distribution of alpha-noradrenergic binding sites of rat spinal cord. *Eur. J. Pharmacol.*, 115: 285–290.

Hatten, M.E., Liem, R.K.H., Shelanski, M.L. and Mason, C.A. (1991) Astroglia in CNS injury. *Glia*, 16: 779–789.

Hebel, R. and Stromberg, M.W. (1986) *Anatomy and Embryology of the Laboratory Rat.* BioMed Verlag, Wörthsee.

Hirbec, H., Privat, A. and Vignon, J. (2000a) Binding properties of [3H]gacyclidine in the rat central nervous system. *Eur. J. Pharmacol.*, 388: 235–239.

Hirbec, H., Teilhac, J., Kamenka, J., Privat, A. and Vignon, J. (2000b) Binding properties of [3H]gacyclidine (cis(pip/me)-1-[1-(2-thienyl)-2-methylcyclohexyl]piperidine) enantiomers in the rat central nervous system. *Brain Res.*, 859: 177–192.

Hirbec, H., Kamenka, J.M., Privat, A. and Vignon, J. (2001a) Interaction of gacyclidine enantiomers with 'non-NMDA' binding sites in the rat central nervous system. *Brain Res.*, 894: 189–192.

Hirbec, H., Kamenka, J.M., Privat, A. and Vignon, J. (2001b) Characterization of 'non-*N*-methyl-D-aspartate' binding sites for gacyclidine enantiomers in the rat cerebellar and telencephalic structures. *J. Neurochem.*, 77: 190–201.

Hirbec, H., Gaviria, M. and Vignon, J. (2001c) Gacyclidine: a new neuroprotective agent acting at the *N*-methyl-D-aspartate receptor. *CNS Drug*, 7: 172–198.

Hurlbert, R.J. (2000) Methylprednisolone for acute spinal cord injury: an inappropriate standard of care. *J. Neurosurg.*, 93: 1–7.

Jacobs, B.L. and Fornal, C.A. (1993) 5-HT and motor control — a hypothesis. *Trends Neurosci.*, 16: 346–352.

Jacobs, B.L. and Fornal, C.A. (1997) Serotonin and motor activity. *Curr. Opin. Neurobiol.*, 7: 820–825.

Jones, D.J., Kendall, D.E. and Enna, S.J. (1982) Adrenergic receptors in rat spinal cord. *Neuropharmacology*, 21: 191–195.

Juurlink, B.H. (1997) Response of glial cells to ischemia: roles of reactive oxygen species and glutathione. *Neurosci. Biobehav. Rev.*, 21: 151–166.

Kachidian, P., Poulat, P., Marlier, L. and Privat, A. (1991) Immunohistochemical evidence for the coexistence of substance P, thyrotropin-releasing hormone, GABA, methionine-enkephalin, and leucine-enkephalin in the serotonergic neurons of the caudal raphe nuclei: a dual labeling in the rat. *J. Neurosci. Res.*, 30: 521–530.

Kalderon, N. and Fuks, Z. (1996a) Structural recovery in lesioned adult mammalian spinal cord by x-irradiation of the lesion site. *Proc. Natl. Acad. Sci. USA*, 93: 11179–11184.

Kalderon, N. and Fuks, Z. (1996b) Severed corticospinal axons recover electrophysiologic control of muscle activity after x-ray therapy in lesioned adult spinal cord. *Proc. Natl. Acad. Sci. USA*, 93: 11185–11190.

Kamenka, J.M., Chiche, B., Goudal, R., Geneste, P., Vignon, J., Vincent, J.P. and Lazdunski, M. (1982) Chemical synthesis and molecular pharmacology of hydroxylated 1-(1-phenylcyclohexyl-piperidine derivatives. *J. Med. Chem.*, 25: 431–435.

Katayama, Y., Becker, D.P., Tamura, T. and Hovda, D.A. (1990) Massive increases in extracellular potassium and the indis-

criminate release of glutamate following concussive brain injury. *J. Neurosurg.*, 73: 889–900.

Lancelot, E., Revaud, M.L., Boulu, R.G., Plotkine, M. and Callebert, J. (1998) A microdialysis study investigating the mechanisms of hydroxyl radical formation in rat striatum exposed to glutamate. *Brain Res.*, 809: 294–296.

Lemons, M.L., Howland, D.R. and Anderson, D.K. (1999) Chondroitin sulfate proteoglycan immunoreactivity increases following spinal cord injury and transplantation. *Exp. Neurol.*, 160: 51–65.

Levallois, C., Calvet, M.C., Kamenka, J.M., Petite, D. and Privat, A. (1992) TCP enhances the survival of human fetal spinal cord cells in culture. *Brain Res.*, 573: 327–330.

Levallois, C., Calvet, M.C., Kamenka, J.M., Petite, D. and Privat, A. (1995) Primary dissociated cultures of human brainstem cells: a useful tool for their characterization and neuroprotection study. *Cell. Biol. Toxicol.*, 11: 155–160.

Liesi, P., Dahl, D. and Vaheri, A. (1983) Laminin is produced by early rat astrocytes in primary culture. *J. Cell Biol.*, 96: 920–924.

Liesi, P., Kirkwood, T. and Vaheri, A. (1986) Fibronectin is expressed by astrocytes cultured from embryonic and early postnatal rat brain. *Exp. Cell Res.*, 163: 175–185.

Logan, A., Berry, M., Gonzalez, A.M., Frautschy, S.A., Sporn, M.B. and Baird, A. (1994) Effects of transforming growth factor beta 1 on scar production in the injured central nervous system of the rat. *Eur. J. Neurosci.*, 6: 355–363.

Mansour, H., Sandillon, F. and Privat, A. (1986) Transplantation of fetal neurons into the spinal cord after section. *Neurochirurgie*, 32: 507–513.

Marlier, L., Sandillon, F., Poulat, P., Geffard, M. and Privat, A. (1991a) Serotonergic innervation of the dorsal horn of rat spinal cord: light and electron microscopic immunocytochemical study. *J. Neurocytol.*, 20: 310–322.

Marlier, L., Teilhac, J.R., Cerruti, C. and Privat, A. (1991b) Autoradiographic mapping of 5-HT1, 5-HT1A, 5-HT1B and 5-HT2 receptors in the spinal cord. *Brain Res.*, 550: 15–23.

Marsala, M. (1999) Anatomy and physiology of spinal vasculature. In: T.L. Yaksh (Ed.), *Spinal Drug Delivery*. Elsevier, Amsterdam, pp. 145–175.

Mas, M., Zahradnik, M.A., Martino, V. and Davidson, J.M. (1985) Stimulation of spinal serotonergic receptors facilitates seminal emission and suppresses penile erectile reflexes. *Brain Res.*, 342: 128–134.

Mason, S.T. and Fibiger, H.C. (1979) Physiological function of descending noradrenaline projections to the spinal cord: role in post decapitation convulsions. *Eur. J. Pharmacol.*, 57: 29–34.

McIntosh, T.K. (1993) Novel pharmacologic therapies in the treatment of experimental traumatic brain injury: a review. *J. Neurotrauma*, 10: 215–261.

McIntosh, T.K., Juhler, M. and Wieloch, T. (1998) Novel pharmacologic strategies in the treatment of experimental traumatic brain injury. *J. Neurotrauma*, 15: 731–769.

McKinley, W.O., Jackson, A.B., Cardenas, D.D. and DeVivo, M.J. (1999) Long-term medical complications after traumatic spinal cord injury: a regional model systems analysis. *Arch. Phys. Med. Rehabil.*, 80: 1402–1410.

McLennan, H. (1983) Receptors for the excitatory amino acids in the mammalian central nervous system. *Prog. Neurobiol.*, 20: 251–271.

Menet, V., Colucci-Guyon, E., Babinet, C., Privat, A. and Giménez y Ribotta, M. (1998) Astroglial and axonal responses to spinal cord injury in mice deficient for glial fibrillary acidic protein and vimentin. *Abstr. Soc. Neurosci.*, 710.6.

Menet, V., Giménez y Ribotta, M., Sandillon, F. and Privat, A. (2000) GFAP null astrocytes are a favorable substrate for neuronal survival and neurite growth. *Glia*, 31: 267–272.

Menet, V., Giménez y Ribotta, M., Chauvet, N., Drian, M.J., Lannoy, J., Colucci-Guyon, E. and Privat, A. (2001) Inactivation of glial fibrillary acidic protein gene, but not of vimentin, improves neuronal survival and neurite growth by modifying adhesion molecule expression. *J. Neurosci.*, 21: 6147–6158.

Mennerick, S. and Zorumski, C.F. (1994) Glial contributions to excitatory neurotransmission in cultured hippocampal cells. *Nature*, 368: 59–62.

Michaelis, E.K. (1998) Molecular biology of glutamate receptors in the central nervous system and their role in excitotoxicity, oxidative stress and aging. *Prog. Neurobiol.*, 54: 369–415.

Michaud, M., Warren, H. and Drian, M.J. (1994) Homochiral structures derived from 1-[1-(2-thienyl)cyclohexyl]piperudube (TCP) are potent non-competitive antagonists of glutamate at NMDA receptor sites. *Eur. J. Med. Chem.*, 29: 869–876.

Molander, C., Xu, Q. and Grant, G. (1984) The cytoarchitectonic organisation of the spinal cord in the rat. I. The lower thoracic and lumbosacral cord. *J. Comp. Neurol.*, 230: 133–141.

Molander, C., Xu, Q., Rivermelian, C. and Grant, G. (1989) The cytoarchitectonic organization of the spinal cord in the rat. II. The cervical and upper thoracic spinal cord. *J. Comp. Neurol.*, 289: 375–385.

Moolten, F.L. (1986) Tumor chemosensitivity conferred by inserted herpes thymidine kinase genes: paradigm for a prospective cancer control strategy. *Cancer Res.*, 46: 5276–5281.

Moon, L.D.F., Brecknell, J.E., Franklin, R.J.M., Dunnett, S.B. and Fawcett, J.W. (2000) Robust regeneration of CNS axons through a track depleted of CNS glia. *Exp. Neurol.*, 161: 41–69.

Moorman, S.J., Whalen, L.R. and Nornes, H.O. (1990) A neurotransmitter specific functional recovery mediated by fetal implants in the lesioned spinal cord of the rat. *Brain Res.*, 508: 194–198.

Morin-Richaud, C., Feldblum, S. and Privat, A. (1998) Astrocytes and oligodendrocytes reactions after a total section of the rat spinal cord. *Brain Res.*, 783: 85–101.

Muir, G.D. and Steeves, J.D. (1997) Sensorimotor stimulation to improve locomotor recovery after spinal cord injury. *Trends Neurosci.*, 20: 72–77.

Neugebauer, K.M., Tomaselli, K.J., Lilien, J. and Reichardt, L.F. (1988) *N*-cadherin, NCAM, and integrins promote retinal neurite outgrowth on astrocytes in vitro. *J. Cell Biol.*, 107: 1177–1187.

Nilsson, P., Hillered, L., Ponten, U. and Ungerstedt, U. (1990) Changes in cortical extracellular levels of energy-related metabolites and amino acids following concussive brain injury in rats. *J. Cereb. Blood Flow Metab.*, 10: 631–637.

Noble, L.J. and Wrathall, J.R. (1985) Spinal cord contusion in the rat: morphometric analyses of alterations in the spinal cord. *Exp. Neurol.*, 88: 135–149.

Nobunaga, A.I., Go, B.K. and Karunas, R.B. (1999) Recent demographic and injury trends in people served by the Model Spinal Cord Injury Care Systems. *Arch. Phys. Med. Rehabil.*, 80: 1372–1382.

Olby, N.J. and Blakemore, W.F. (1996) Reconstruction of the glial environment of a photochemically induced lesion in the rat spinal cord by transplantation of mixed glial cells. *J. Neurocytol.*, 25: 481–498.

Pekny, M., Leveen, P., Pekna, M., Eliasson, C., Berthold, C.H., Westermark, B. and Betsholtz, C. (1995) Mice lacking glial fibrillary acidic protein display astrocytes devoid of intermediate filaments but develop and reproduce normally. *EMBO J.*, 14: 1590–1598.

Pekny, M., Johansson, C.B., Eliasson, C., Stakeberg, J., Wallen, A., Perlmann, T., Lendahl, U., Betsholtz, C., Berthold, C.H. and Frisen, J. (1999) Abnormal reaction to central nervous system injury in mice lacking glial fibrillary acidic protein and vimentin. *J. Cell Biol.*, 145: 503–514.

Pencalet, P., Ohanna, F., Poulat, P., Kamenka, J.M. and Privat, A. (1993) Thienylphencyclidine protection for the spinal cord of adult rats against extension of lesions secondary to a photochemical injury. *J. Neurosurg.*, 78: 603–609.

Prado, R., Dietrich, W.D., Watson, B.D., Ginsberg, M.D. and Green, B.A. (1987) Photochemically induced graded spinal cord infarction Behavioral, electrophysiological, and morphological correlates. *J. Neurosurg.*, 67: 745–753.

Privat, A., Mansour, H., Pavy, A., Geffard, M. and Sandillon, F. (1986) Transplantation of dissociated foetal serotonin neurons into the transected spinal cord of adult rats. *Neurosci. Lett.*, 66: 61–66.

Privat, A., Mansour, H. and Geffard, M. (1988) Transplantation of fetal serotonin neurons into the transected spinal cord of adult rats: morphological development and functional influence. In: D.M. Gash and J.R. Sladek (Eds.), *Transplantation into the Mammalian Central Nervous System. Progress in Brain Research*, Vol. 78. Elsevier, Amsterdam, pp. 155–166.

Privat, A., Mansour, H., Rajaofetra, N. and Geffard, M. (1989) Intraspinal transplant of serotonergic neurons in the adult rat. *Brain Res. Bull.*, 22: 123–129.

Privat, A., Drian, M.J. and Pirat, J.L. et al. (1990) Protection neurale par les phencyclidines: étude sur des modèles in vitro. *Actual. Chim. Ther.*, 17: 187–200.

Rajaofetra, N., Kachidian, P., Marlier, L., Poulat, P., Konig, N., Geffard, M. and Privat, A. (1991) Electronmicroscopic detection of the axonal coexistence of serotonin and substance-P in B1–B2 raphe cells transplanted into the transected spinal cord of adult rats. *Brain Res.*, 542: 159–162.

Rajaofetra, N., König, N., Poulat, P., Marlier, L., Sandillon, F., Drian, M.J., Geffard, M. and Privat, A. (1992) Fate of B1–B2 and B3 rhombencephalic cells transplanted into the transected spinal cord of adult rats: light and electron microscopic studies. *Exp. Neurol.*, 117: 59–70.

Ramón y Cajal (1913–1914) *Estudios sobre la Degeneración y Regeneración del Sistema Nervioso*. Moya (Ed.), Madrid.

Rataboul, P., Faucon Biguet, N., Vernier, P., De Vitry, F., Boularand, S., Privat, A. and Mallet, J. (1988) Identification of a human glial fibrillary acidic protein cDNA: a tool for the molecular analysis of reactive gliosis in the mammalian central nervous system. *J. Neurosci. Res.*, 20: 165–175.

Rawlow, A. and Gorka, Z. (1986) Involvement of post-synaptic α1 and α2-adrenoceptors in the flexor reflex activity in the spinal rats. *J. Neural Transm.*, 66: 93–105.

Redies, C. (2000) Cadherins in the central nervous system. *Prog. Neurobiol.*, 61: 611–648.

Reichardt, L.F. and Tomaselli, K.J. (1991) Extracellular matrix molecules and their receptors: functions in neural development. *Annu. Rev. Neurosci.*, 14: 531–570.

Reier, P.J., Eng, L.F. and Jakeman, L. (1989) Reactive astrocyte and axonal outgrowth in the injured CNS: Is gliosis really an impediment to regeneration? In: F.J. Seil (Ed.), *Neural Regeneration and Transplantation. Frontiers of Clinical Neuroscience*, Vol. 6. Alan R. Liss, New York, pp. 183–209.

Ridet, J.L. and Privat, A. (2000) Volume transmission. *Trends Neurosci.*, 23: 58–59.

Ridet, J.L., Rajaofetra, N., Teilhac, J.R., Geffard, M. and Privat, A. (1993) Evidence for nonsynaptic serotonergic and noradrenergic innervation of the rat dorsal horn and possible involvement of neuron–glia interaction. *Neuroscience*, 52: 143–157.

Ridet, J.L., Malhotra, S.K., Privat, A. and Gage, F.H. (1997) Reactive astrocytes: cellular and molecular cues to biological function. *Trends Neurosci.*, 20: 570–577.

Ridet, J.L., Pencalet, P., Belcram, M., Giraudeau, B., Chastang, C., Philippon, J., Mallet, J., Privat, A. and Schwartz, L. (2000) Effects of spinal cord X-irradiation on the recovery of paraplegic rats. *Exp. Neurol.*, 161: 1–14.

Rondouin, G., Drian, M.J., Chicheportiche, R., Kamenka, J.M. and Privat, A. (1988) Non-competitive antagonists of *N*-methyl-D-aspartate receptors protect cortical and hippocampal cell cultures against glutamate neurotoxicity. *Neurosci. Lett.*, 91: 199–203.

Rosenberg, L.J., Teng, Y.D. and Wrathall, J.R. (1999) 2,3-Dihydroxy-6-nitro-7-sulfamoyl-benzo(f)quinoxaline reduces glial loss and acute white matter pathology after experimental spinal cord contusion. *J. Neurosci.*, 19: 464–475.

Rossignol, S. (1996) Neural control of stereotypic limb movements. In: L.B. Rowell and J.T. Sheperd (Eds.), *Exercise: Regulation and Integration of Multiple Systems*. American Physiological Society, pp. 173–216.

Rossignol, S. and Dubuc, R. (1994) Spinal pattern generation. *Curr. Opin. Neurobiol.*, 4: 894–902.

Rossignol, S., Barbeau, H. and Julien, C. (1986) Locomotion of the adult chronic spinal cat and its modification by monoaminergic agonists and antagonists. In: M.E. Goldberger, A. Gorio and M. Murray (Eds.), *Development and Plasticity of the Mammalian Spinal Cord*. Fidia Research Series, Vol. III, Liviana Press, Padova, pp. 323–345.

Rossignol, S., Barbeau, H. and Chau, C. (1995) Pharmacology of locomotion in chronic spinal cat. In: A. Taylor, M.H. Gladden and R. Durbaba (Eds.), *Alpha and Gamma Motor Systems*. Plenum Press, New York, pp. 449–455.

Rothstein, J.D., Dykes-Hoberg, M., Pardo, C.A., Bristol, L.A., Jin, L., Kuncl, R.W., Kanai, Y., Hediger, M.A., Wang, Y., Schielke, J.P. and Welty, D.F. (1996) Knockout of glutamate transporters reveals a major role for astroglial transport in excitotoxicity and clearance of glutamate. *Neuron*, 16: 675–686.

Roudet, C., Savasta, M. and Feuerstein, C. (1993) Normal distribution of alpha-1-adrenoceptors in the rat spinal cord and its modification after noradrenergic denervation: a quantitative autoradiographic study. *J. Neurosci. Res.*, 34: 44–53.

Roudet, C., Mouchet, M., Feuerstein, C. and Savasta, M. (1994) Normal distribution of alpha-2 adrenoceptors in the rat spinal cord and its modification after noradrenergic denervation: a quantitative autoradiographic study. *J. Neurosci. Res.*, 39: 319–329.

Roudet, C., Giménez y Ribotta, M., Privat, A., Feuerstein, C. and Savasta, M. (1995) Intraspinal noradrenergic-rich implants reverse the increase of alpha 1 adrenoceptors densities caused by complete spinal cord transection or selective chemical denervation: a quantitative autoradiographic study. *Brain Res.*, 677: 1–12.

Sampath, D., Holets, V. and Perez-Polo, J.R. (1995) Effect of a spinal cord photolesion injury on catalase. *Int. J. Dev. Neurosci.*, 13: 645–654.

Sanes, J.R. (1989) Extracellular matrix molecules that influence neural development. *Annu. Rev. Neurosci.*, 12: 491–516.

Schnell, L. and Schwab, M.E. (1990) Axonal regeneration in the rat spinal cord produced by an antibody against myelin-associated neurite growth inhibitors. *Nature*, 343: 269–272.

Siesjo, B.K. and Wieloch, T. (1985) Cerebral metabolism in ischaemia: neurochemical basis for therapy. *Br. J. Anaesth.*, 57: 47–62.

Smith, G.M., Rutishauser, U., Silver, J. and Miller, R.H. (1990) Maturation of astrocytes in vitro alters the extent and molecular basis of neurite outgrowth. *Dev. Biol.*, 138: 377–390.

Sofroniew, M.V., Bush, T.G., Blumauer, N., Kruger, L., Mucke, L. and Johnson, M.H. (1999) Genetically targeted and conditionally regulated ablation of astroglial cells in the central, enteric and peripheral nervous systems in adult transgenic mice. *Brain Res.*, 835: 91–95.

Stichel, C.C. and Muller, H.W. (1998) Experimental strategies to promote axonal regeneration after traumatic central nervous system injury. *Prog. Neurobiol.*, 56: 119–148.

Stichel, C.C., Hermanns, S., Luhmann, H.J., Lausberg, F., Niermann, H., D'Urso, D., Servos, G., Hartwig, H.G. and Muller, H.W. (1999a) Inhibition of collagen IV deposition promotes regeneration of injured CNS axons. *Eur. J. Neurosci.*, 11: 632–646.

Stichel, C.C., Niermann, H., D'Urso, D., Lausberg, F., Hermanns, S. and Muller, H.W. (1999b) Basal membrane-depleted scar in lesioned CNS: characteristics and relationships with regenerating axons. *Neuroscience*, 93: 321–333.

Sykova, E., Svoboda, J., Simonova, Z. and Jendelova, P. (1992) Role of astrocytes in ionic and volume homeostasis in spinal cord during development and injury. *Prog. Brain Res.*, 94: 47–56.

Tanabe, M., Ono, H. and Fukuda, H. (1990) Spinal alpha 1-

and alpha 2-adrenoceptors mediate facilitation and inhibition of spinal motor transmission respectively. *Jpn. J. Pharmacol.*, 54: 69–77.

Tator, C.H. and Fehlings, M.G. (1991) Review of the secondary injury theory of acute spinal cord trauma with emphasis on vascular mechanisms. *J. Neurosurg.*, 75: 15–26.

Tomaselli, K.J., Neugebauer, K.M., Bixby, J.L., Lilien, J. and Reichardt, L.F. (1988) N-cadherin and integrins: two receptor systems that mediate neuronal process outgrowth on astrocyte surfaces. *Neuron*, 1: 33–43.

Van Reempts, J. and Borgers, M. (1994) Histopathological characterization of photochemical damage in nervous tissue. *Histol. Histopathol.*, 9: 185–195.

Vignon, J., Privat, A., Chaudieu, I., Thierry, A., Kamenka, J.M. and Chicheportiche, R. (1986) [3H]Thienyl-phencyclidine ([3H]TCP) binds to two different sites in rat brain. Localization by autoradiographic and biochemical techniques. *Brain Res.*, 378: 133–141.

Watson, B.D., Prado, R., Dietrich, W.D., Ginsberg, M.D. and Green, B.A. (1986) Photochemically induced spinal cord injury in the rat. *Brain Res.*, 367: 296–300.

Weidner, N., Grill, R.J. and Tuszynski, M.H. (1999) Elimination of basal lamina and the collagen 'scar' after spinal cord injury fails to augment corticospinal tract regeneration. *Exp. Neurol.*, 160: 40–50.

Wrathall, J.R., Pettegrew, R.K. and Harvey, F. (1985) Spinal cord contusion in the rat: production of graded, reproducible, injury groups. *Exp. Neurol.*, 88: 108–122.

Wrathall, J.R., Choiniere, D. and Teng, Y.D. (1994) Dose-dependent reduction of tissue loss and functional impairment after spinal cord trauma with the AMPA/kainate antagonist NBQX. *J. Neurosci.*, 14: 6598–6607.

Yakovleff, A., Roby-Brami, A., Guezard, B., Mansour, H., Bussel, B. and Privat, A. (1989) Locomotion in rats transplanted with noradrenergic neurons. *Brain Res. Bull.*, 22: 115–121.

Yakovleff, A., Cabelguen, J.M., Orsal, D., Giménez y Ribotta, M., Rajaofetra, N., Drian, M.J., Bussel, B. and Privat, A. (1995) Fictive motor activities in adult chronic spinal rats transplanted with embryonic brainstem neurons. *Exp. Brain Res.*, 106: 69–78.

Yick, L.W., Wu, W., So, K.F., Yip, H.K. and Shum, D.K. (2000) Chondroitinase ABC promotes axonal regeneration of Clarke's neurons after spinal cord injury. *NeuroReport*, 11: 1063–1067.

Young, W.S. and Kunhar, M.J. (1980) Noradrenergic a1 and a2 receptors: light microscopic autoradiographic localization. *Proc. Natl. Acad. Sci. USA*, 77: 1696–1700.

Zamanillo, D., Sprengel, R., Hvalby, O., Jensen, V., Burnashev, N., Rozov, A., Kaiser, K.M., Koster, H.J., Borchardt, T., Worley, P., Lubke, J., Frotscher, M., Kelly, P.H., Sommer, B., Andersen, P., Seeburg, P.H. and Sakmann, B. (1999) Importance of AMPA receptors for hippocampal synaptic plasticity but not for spatial learning. *Science*, 284: 1805–1811.

L. McKerracher, G. Doucet and S. Rossignol (Eds.)
Progress in Brain Research, Vol. 137
© 2002 Elsevier Science B.V. All rights reserved

CHAPTER 16

Locomotor recovery in chronic spinal rat: long-term pharmacological treatment or transplantation of embryonic neurons?

D. Orsal [1,*], J.-Y. Barthe [1], M. Antri [1], D. Feraboli-Lohnherr [1], A. Yakovleff [1], M. Giménez y Ribotta [2], A. Privat [2], J. Provencher [3] and S. Rossignol [3]

[1] *Neurobiologie des Signaux Intercellulaires (NSI), Institut de Biologie Intégrative (IFR 83), Université Pierre et Marie Curie, 7 quai Saint Bernard, CNRS UMR 7101, Paris, France*
[2] *DPVSN-EPHE, INSERM U.336, Université Montpellier II, Montpellier, France*
[3] *Centre de Recherches en Sciences Neurologiques (CRSN), Université de Montréal, Montreal, QC, Canada*

Introduction

A complete transverse section of the spinal cord at a thoracic level induces a paraplegic syndrome in which the posture of the hindquarters as well as voluntary and locomotor movements are extensively impaired. At least three experimental strategies have been developed to promote or improve recovery of the lost motor functions (Giménez y Ribotta and Privat, 1998): (1) neuroprotection, aimed at reduction of the progressive secondary injury processes principally due to glutamate toxicity (Pencalet et al., 1993; Gaviria et al., 2000); (2) reconnection, aimed at reestablishment of ascending and descending pathways, and which is based on the promotion of axonal regeneration by various means: trophic factors, inactivation of processes inhibiting axonal growth,

transplantation of stem cells... (Goldberger et al., 1993; Iwashita et al., 1994; Bregman et al., 1995, 1997; Giménez y Ribotta et al., 1995; Cheng et al., 1997; Grill et al., 1997; Li et al., 1997; Ramon-Cueto et al., 1998, 2000); and (3) activation of the sublesional spinal cord circuitry, designed to take advantage of intrinsic spinal capabilities, and mainly based on pharmacological stimulation (Rossignol et al., 1986, 2000; Chau et al., 1998a), transplantation of neurons (Giménez y Ribotta et al., 2000), or of a block of tissue (Slawinska et al., 2000).

The final solution to recovery of function will probably emerge from simultaneous application of several of these strategies. However, at present, some of these approaches appear to be more appropriate to specifically promote the recovery of locomotion, while others are aimed at improving posture and voluntary movements. This statement is based on the fact that locomotion on the one hand and posture and voluntary movements on the other are controlled by neuronal pathways which differ from each other in many aspects. Locomotion is fundamentally a rhythmic automatic motor activity that relies upon contractions of given muscles. The activity of each muscle is precisely coordinated with that of the other

* Correspondence to: D. Orsal, Neurobiologie des Signaux Intercellulaires, CNRS UMR 7101, Institut de Biologie Intégrative (IFR 83), Université Pierre et Marie Curie, 7 quai Saint Bernard, Boite 002, F-75252 Paris, France. Tel.: +33-1-4427-2684; Fax: +33-1-4427-5842; E-mail: didier.orsal@snv.jussieu.fr

muscles acting in the same limb (intralimb coordination) and that of muscles acting in the other limbs (interlimb coordination). This set of muscular activity constitutes what is commonly called the locomotor pattern. This pattern is stereotyped enough to be programmed by specific networks of neurons, the so-called central pattern generators for locomotion (CPGs) which are localized within the spinal cord. However, though stereotyped, the locomotor efferent pattern can be modified in order to take into account external perturbations (slope, bend, obstacle, speed, load. . .). In contrast, most voluntary movements generally use a large variety of muscular coordinations depending on specific goals. Therefore, the motor program generated by the central nervous system for a given voluntary movement is probably significantly different to the one needed for another voluntary movement designed for a different motor task (Georgopoulos and Grillner, 1989) and this program is created mainly by telencephalic structures (Kalaska and Drew, 1993; Grillner et al., 1997).

Nervous control of locomotor activity

Spinal cord

Today, it is well established that thoracic spinal animals in numerous species are able to perform locomotor movements with their hindlimbs when the sublesional spinal cord is properly stimulated. This is interpreted as a clue for the existence of an autonomous spinal CPG for locomotion. For instance, acute spinal cats are able to recover automatic treadmill walking after several weeks of daily training (Barbeau and Rossignol, 1987) suggesting an important role for sensory afferents (Rossignol et al., 1996, 2000). This recovery can also be induced or improved pharmacologically. Thus, locomotor rhythms have been obtained in hindlimbs of several species during the first week following a thoracic section of the spinal cord, after treatment with metabolic precursors of noradrenaline (L-DOPA) (Jankowska et al., 1967a,b; Forssberg and Grillner, 1973; Grillner, 1973, 1975, 1986; Grillner and Zangger, 1979). Similar results have been obtained in acute spinal rabbit, using serotonergic precursors (5-HTP) (Viala and Buser, 1969, 1971). In chronic spinal cats,

when monoaminergic terminals have totally degenerated, metabolic precursors become inefficient and must be replaced by specific noradrenergic agonists (Forssberg and Grillner, 1973; Barbeau et al., 1987; Barbeau and Rossignol, 1990, 1991; Pearson and Rossignol, 1991; Chau et al., 1998b; Marcoux and Rossignol, 2000), acting on postsynaptic specific α_2-receptors, even several months after the lesion. The role of these receptors has recently been confirmed by application of specific antagonists in intact animals such as yohimbine (Giroux et al., 1998, 2001).

Furthermore, a rhythmic pattern generator has been evidenced in numerous in vitro studies of the spinal cord of various vertebrates from cyclostomes (Grillner et al., 1998a,b) to mammalian (Grillner, 1981). In newborn rats, fictive locomotor-like efferent bursts can be evoked on ventral roots of spinal cord isolated in vitro, when serotonin (5-HT) and/or NMA (N-methyl-D/L-aspartate) are bath applied on the upper lumbar segment (Kudo and Yamada, 1987; Cazalets et al., 1990, 1992; Kiehn et al., 1992; Sqalli-Houssaini et al., 1993). Furthermore, in in vitro spinal cord/hindlimb preparations of neonate rats, 5-HT was shown to induce rhythmic coordinated movements in both hindlimbs (Cowley and Schmidt, 1994; Kiehn and Kjaerulff, 1996).

Supraspinal control

Though autonomous, the spinal CPGs are under the control of numerous supraspinal centers and descending pathways involved in the fundamental aspects of the locomotor nervous control: (1) the initiation of locomotor activity when needed by the behavior; (2) the adaptation of the stereotyped efferent locomotor command to particular constraints of the environment. These pathways will only be quoted here (see Fig. 1), since they have been extensively reviewed elsewhere (Arshavsky et al., 1986; Armstrong, 1988; Rossignol, 1996; Armstrong et al., 1997; Grillner et al., 1998b; Jordan, 1998; Matsuyama and Drew, 2000a,b; Rossignol et al., 2000; Prentice and Drew, 2001) (see also Grillner, 2002, this volume).

Activation of locomotion actually involves a complex and indirect pathway (in black in Fig. 1) including motor cortex, basal ganglia and associated structures, mesencephalic locomotor region (MLR)

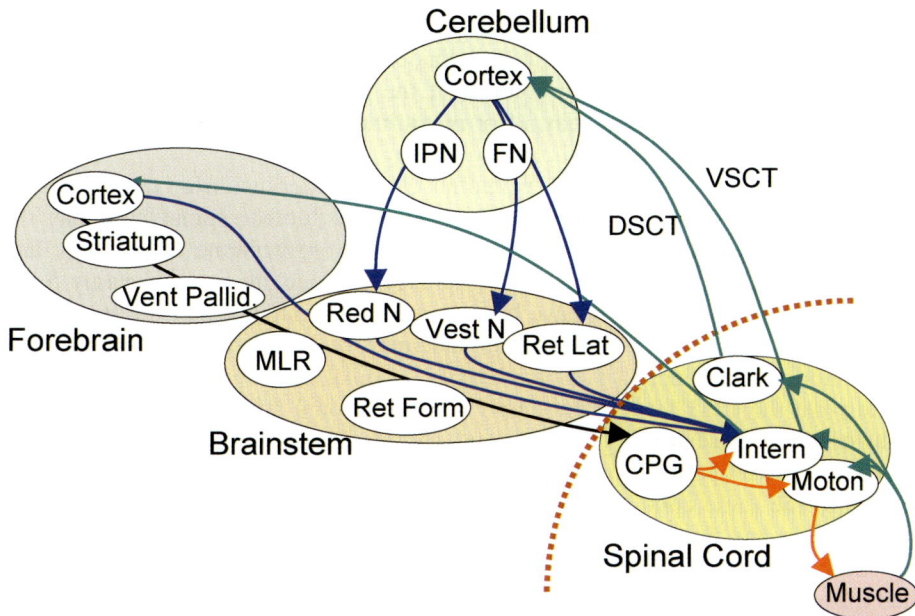

Fig. 1. Main centers and pathways involved in the nervous locomotor control. Spinal cord contains a CPG (itself made of interneurons) for locomotion which acts on motoneurons (Moton) through a premotoneuronal network (Intern). These neurons are locally controlled by afferent systems (in blue). The CPG is activated when needed by a complex descending system (in black) including the cerebral cortex, the striatum, the ventral pallidum, the mesencephalic locomotor region (MLR), and the reticular formation (Ret Form). Another set of descending pathways is designed to adapt the efferent locomotor command. It includes Motor cortex, red nucleus (Red N), vestibular nuclei (Vest N) and lateral reticular nuclei (Ret Lat). These pathways are the efferent parts of regulation loops activated by afferent inputs from the spinal cord via dorsal and ventral spinocerebellar tracts (DSCT, VSCT), cerebellar cortex, interpositus or fastigial nuclei (IPN and FN). The descending neuromodulatory monoaminergic pathways from locus coeruleus and raphe nuclei are not shown.

and reticulospinal pathways (Rossignol, 1996; Jordan, 1998). Adaptation of the locomotor movement and posture during locomotion involves several descending pathways (blue descending pathways in Fig. 1) such as rubrospinal, reticulospinal and vestibulospinal pathways (Matsuyama and Drew, 2000a,b; Prentice and Drew, 2001), which are under control of numerous sensory feedbacks (green ascending pathways in Fig. 1) via ascending spinocerebellar tracts and cerebellum (Arshavsky et al., 1986).

These ascending and descending pathways are definitely cut after complete transverse section of the thoracic spinal cord (red line in Fig. 1).

Spontaneous capabilities of motor recovery in adult spinal rats

In rats spinalized at the thoracic level as adults, most motor activities are drastically impaired, especially locomotion, and spontaneous recovery, al-

though quite limited, is present. Thus, the knowledge of the spontaneous capabilities of locomotor recovery constitutes an essential prerequisite to experimentation designed to improve functional motor recovery.

From the point of view of postural activity, the hindlimbs remain extended, with the feet lying on the ground on the dorsum, and are totally unable to support the weight of hindquarters, even 2 months or more after the lesion. This lack of tonic activity cannot be counteracted by sustained sensory afferent inflow, such as that evoked by tail pinching, which increases the level of excitability of the spinal networks (Grillner and Zangger, 1979; Grillner, 1981).

As far as rhythmic activities are concerned, adult chronic spinal rats can perform several kinds of movements. Some of them are well-coordinated and generally evoked by peripheral stimulation. This is the case of the various forms of paw-shake described in the cat (Smith et al., 1985; Carter and Smith,

1986a,b), which can be evoked in the spinal rat by gentle pinching of the toes (Yakovleff et al., 1995b) or air stepping (Giuliani and Smith, 1985). Some other motor activities appear much less organized, though rhythmic, but with irregular cycle duration, although within the locomotor range of intact rats (Gruner and Altman, 1980; Gruner et al., 1980). Finally, none of these rhythmic activities could be identified as locomotion since neither the movement (Fig. 4B) nor the pattern of EMG activity or the relationship between burst and cycle duration were those conventionally described for locomotion (Giménez y Ribotta et al., 2000), suggesting that the CPG for locomotion is probably not at the origin of these particular motor behaviors, or that its intrinsic properties are hugely impaired. Others came to the same conclusion in the spinal rat (Commissiong and Sauve, 1989) although, astonishingly (Meisel and Rakerd, 1982), in the same model, had an opposite conclusion and suggested that the CPG for locomotion is involved despite description of movements largely abnormal compared to actual locomotor movements. However, these authors did not analyze the temporal characteristics of EMG pattern, which thus appears as a fundamental criterion for identification of the locomotor activity generated by spinal CPGs for locomotion.

It is noteworthy that most of the deficiencies observed in the organization of EMG pattern of activity of chronic spinal rats, such as co-contractions between antagonistic muscles, lack of control of the mean cycle duration by the speed of the treadmill belt, or atypical relationships between bursts and cycle durations, are similar to those described in developing intact rats before postnatal day 14 (Westerga and Gramsbergen, 1990; Westerga and Gramsbergen, 1993), that is before the supraspinal control is completed. This certainly emphasizes, on the one hand, the role of supraspinal descending and ascending pathways in the motor control by spinal networks, and on the other, the markedly different ability of the lumbar spinal cord to recover motor functions in adult and in young spinal animals. For instance, rats spinalized prior to weaning and more precisely, before postnatal day 7, recover the ability to stand up with their hindquarters within a few days (Stelzner et al., 1975; Weber and Stelzner, 1977; Commissiong and Toffano, 1989; Commissiong and Sauve,

1993; Miya et al., 1997). They also recover spontaneous coordinated stepping movements in hindlimbs. In contrast, if the lesion takes place after postnatal day 14 or in adulthood, recovery of motor functions appears to be very weak.

Two points can be underlined from the work mentioned above: (1) the lumbar spinal cord has the endogenous capability to generate locomotion; and (2) in the spinal rat, monoamines and mainly 5-HT have been shown to activate locomotion. In order to stimulate and improve functional recovery of locomotor activity in spinal rats, we developed a strategy to supply the sublesional spinal cord with missing supraspinal neurotransmitters by two different approaches. The first one was through transplantation of embryonic raphe neurons as a continuous and endogenous source of 5-HT, and the second one was through a more classical pharmacological approach.

Transplantation of embryonic raphe neurons: a way to stimulate locomotor endogenous capabilities of the sublesional spinal cord in adult chronic spinal rats

Our first approach to restore permanently 5-HT supply to the lumbar spinal cord after injury has been to transplant embryonic raphe neurons below the lesion in order to compensate partially the postlesional deficit of monoamines. Therefore, in these experiments, no attempt was made to re-establish the supraspinal control of spinal motor system through regeneration.

Methodological considerations

The experimental set-up is schematized in Fig. 2. In the first step, adult rats were spinalized at the T_8 level under general anesthesia. A delay of 7 days was systematically respected before transplantation in order to allow for complete degeneration of monoaminergic pathways descending from the brainstem. Thus, the sublesional spinal cord, totally devoid of supraspinal descending pathways, constitutes an excellent environment for analyzing the influence of transplanted raphe cells on locomotor activity. During this week, all the operated animals appeared totally paralyzed, unable to stand up and to develop any rhythmic movements with their hindlimbs. By

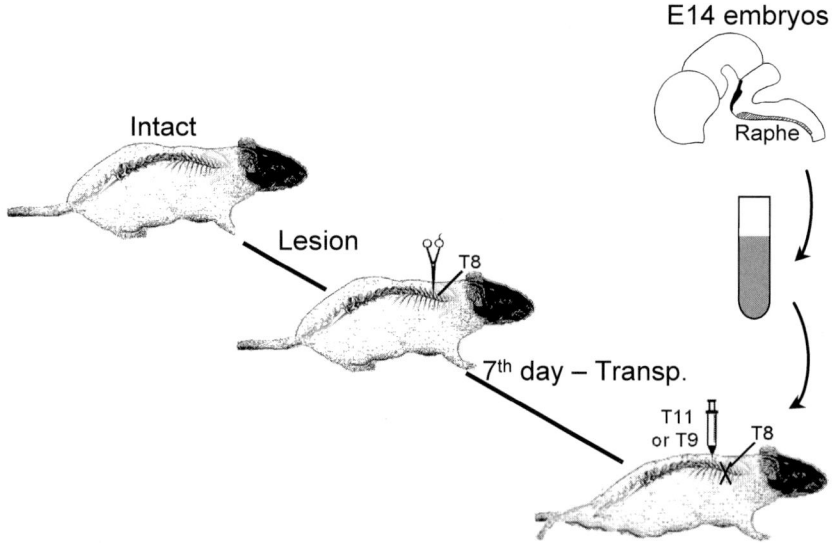

Fig. 2. The protocol of transplantation of monoaminergic embryonic neurons. See text for details.

the morning of the 8th day, a suspension of embryonic cells was prepared from the microdissected raphe nuclei of E14 rat embryos. Five microliters of this suspension, containing about 50,000 cells per μl, were injected using a Hamilton microsyringe, into the dorsal column funiculi, at either the T_{11} (routinely) or T_9 level (in few experiments). In parallel, transected non-transplanted animals were used as control.

Serotonergic reinnervation of the sublesional spinal cord

Early studies by Privat and colleagues illustrated that raphe neurons transplanted in such conditions, survive and reinnervate the main target areas of the sublesional spinal cord (Mansour et al., 1986; Privat et al., 1986, 1988, 1989; Rajaofetra et al., 1992a) (see also Giménez y Ribotta et al., 2002, this volume) developing a synaptic or non-synaptic pattern (Fig. 3D) (Björklund et al., 1986; Privat et al., 1988; Rajaofetra et al., 1992a) similar to that of serotonergic innervation of intact rats (Steinbush, 1981, 1984; Ridet et al., 1993) (Fig. 3C). When injected in T_{11}, the embryonic neurons developed an innervation pattern which became sparser at increasing distance from the site of transplantation and as low as the L_1–L_2 level. When transplanted rostrally, in the T_9 segment, the 5-HT fibers reinnervated cau-

dally the spinal cord reaching only the T_{13} level and did not invade the lumbar enlargement. Finally, in transected non-transplanted rats (Fig. 3B) no 5-HT fibers were detected in sublesional spinal cord even several months after the lesion.

Functional recovery of transplanted animals

Serotonergic reinnervation of the lumbar enlargement is concomitant with the recovery of posture as well as locomotion in the absence of any reconnection of the sublesional spinal cord with the brainstem (Yakovleff et al., 1989, 1995a; Feraboli-Lohnherr et al., 1997; Giménez y Ribotta et al., 2000).

T_{11} transplanted rats adopt a posture similar to that of intact animals at rest (Fig. 4A). The hindlimbs are in a semi-flexed position, the feet contacting the ground on the plantar surface and supporting the hindquarters. Gentle pinching of the tail increases the tonus in extensor muscles which raises the hindquarters. By comparison, in control spinal non-transplanted animals (Fig. 4B), the hindlimbs remain extended, in a position, which is not compatible with the support of the body weight. Stimulation of the tail, even a very strong one, does not induce a supporting reaction.

With respect to locomotion, T_{11} transplanted rats recover hindlimbs weight support and bipedal treadmill locomotion, within the 2 months following

218

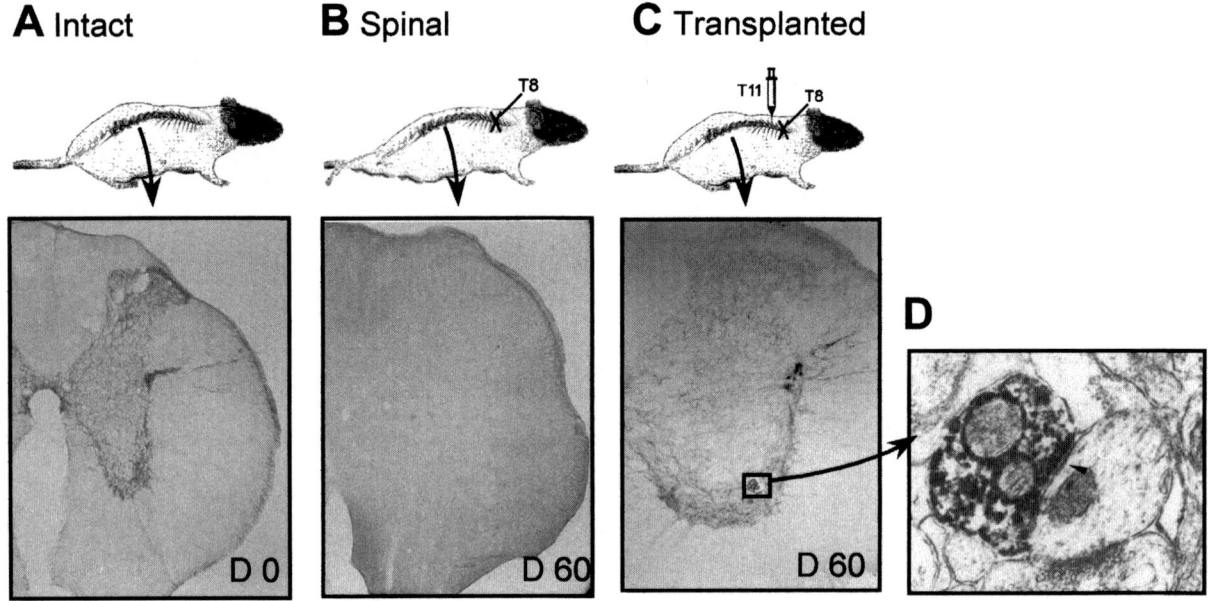

Fig. 3. Immunocytochemical controls of serotonergic terminal in the lumbar spinal cord of different types of adult rats. (A) Intact adult rat. (B) Spinal non-treated adult rat (60 days post-lesion). (C) Spinal and transplanted adult rat (60 days post-lesion). (D) Electron microscopic image of a synapse established between a serotonergic terminal and an host neuron of the ventral horn in the animal C. Note the similar distribution of the serotonergic terminals in intact (A) and transplanted animals (C) and the absence of labeling in spinal animals (B). Rats A and C are able to stand up, but not B.

transplantation (Fig. 4C). Video analyses of the recovered movements allow a clear identification of alternating stance and swing phases (Fig. 5C) comparable to those observed in intact animals (Fig. 5A), though the joint angles remain slightly more extended (Giménez y Ribotta et al., 2000). The pattern of activity in hindlimb muscles and most of the temporal parameters of the motor cycle (Giménez y Ribotta et al., 2000) are quite similar to those described in intact (Gruner and Altman, 1980), thalamic (Goudard et al., 1992) or decerebrate rats (Nicolopoulos-Stournaras and Iles, 1984; Iles and Nicolopoulos-Stournaras, 1996). Furthermore, the cycle duration is in a locomotor range and can be controlled by the velocity of the treadmill belt (Nicolopoulos-Stournaras and Iles, 1984; Yakhnitsa et al., 1985a,b). An important finding is the fact that this recovery is preserved when the spinal cord is cut a second time exactly at the location of the first cut. This suggests that recovery is not a consequence of a possible regrowth of descending serotonergic axons through the glial scar, but is essentially due to endogenous properties of the sublesional spinal cord

stimulated by the transplanted 5-HT neurons. This specific effect was corroborated by the fact that facilitation of serotonergic transmission by zimelidine, a 5-HT reuptake blocker, also facilitates locomotor activity in animals studied in the acute conditions of the so-called 'fictive locomotion' (Fig. 6) (Feraboli-Lohnherr et al., 1997). Incidentally, the fact that this last result was obtained under curare paralysis (the 'fictive locomotion' condition) confirms that generation of locomotor activity observed in our spinal/transplanted model is due to the activity of intrinsic spinal circuitry (the CPG for locomotion) and exclude peripheral sensory loops. Furthermore, the recovered walking does not outlive the selective destruction of transplanted 5-HT neurons by 5,7-dihydroxytryptamine (5,7-DHT) local treatments once recovery of walking was effective. Taken together, these results strongly suggests that 5-HT neurons are the promoters of locomotor recovery.

In contrast, T_9 transplanted animals do not develop a clear authentic locomotor activity and remain definitely in the state described above for spinal non-transplanted animals (see Fig. 4B and Fig. 5B).

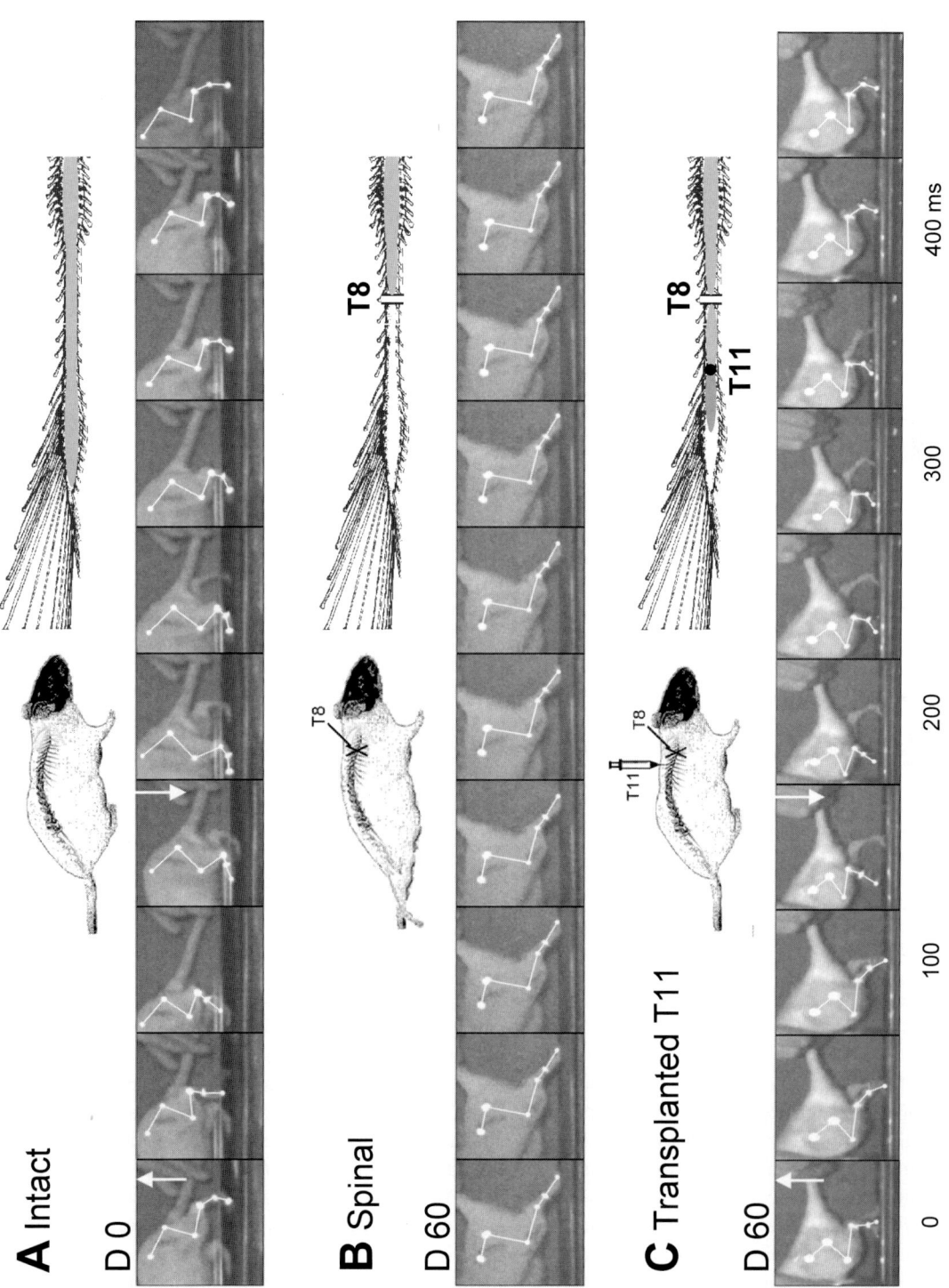

Fig. 4. T₁₁ transplantation of embryonic neurons and functional recovery. Selected frames from video sequences are shown for intact rats (A), spinal rats 2 months after the lesion (B) and transplanted rats 2 months after the lesion (C). The drawings over each series illustrate the usual posture adopted by each type of animal and the extent of the distribution of 5-HT terminals in the spinal cord. Intact animals (A) are able to walk. They have an erect posture, and the spinal cord is totally innervated by serotonergic terminals. Spinal animals are not able to walk on the treadmill, they have no postural behavior and 5-HT terminals are absent in the spinal cord caudal to the lesion. Finally, transplanted animals recover locomotion and posture. Their spinal cord caudal to the lesion is partly reinnervated by serotonergic terminals originating from the transplanted neurons.

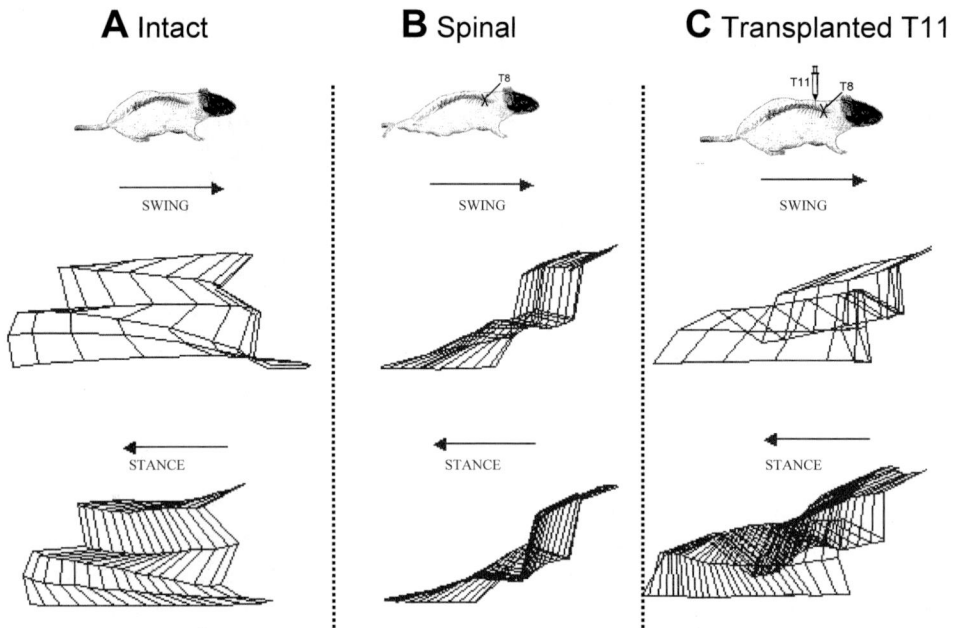

A Intact **B** Spinal **C** Transplanted T11

SWING SWING SWING

STANCE STANCE STANCE

Fig. 5. The rhythmic movements in intact, spinal and transplanted animals. These stick diagrams are a reconstruction from videotapes of rhythmic movements in intact rats (A), spinal rats 2 months after the lesion (B) and transplanted rats 2 months after the lesion (C).

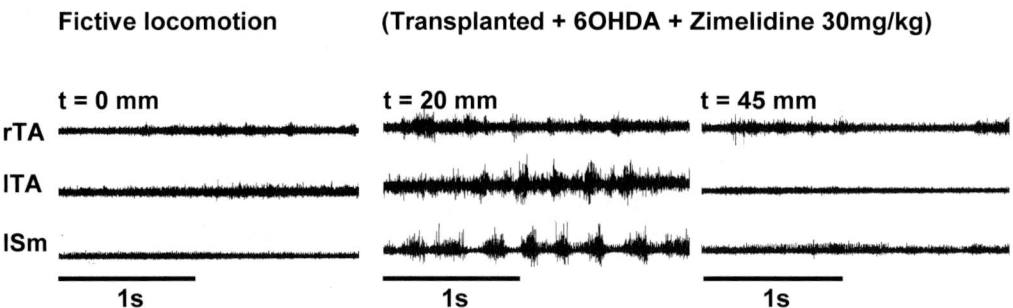

Fictive locomotion **(Transplanted + 6OHDA + Zimelidine 30mg/kg)**

t = 0 mm t = 20 mm t = 45 mm

rTA

lTA

lSm

1s 1s 1s

Fig. 6. Effect of zimelidine on locomotor activity of a transplanted rat. This spinal transplanted adult rats has been treated with 6-OHDA in order to kill noradrenergic neurons (verified postmortem). The spinal cord caudal to the lesion presented serotonergic terminals (verified postmortem). Locomotor activity is studied under flaxedyl paralysis (fictive locomotion). Note that the efferent rhythmic activity is significantly enhanced 20 min after injection of zimelidine, a blocker of 5-HT reuptake.

Importance of the reinnervated spinal segment

Transplantation of 5-HT embryonic neurons does not always lead to functional recovery. In a series of experiments, the transplantation was performed in T_9 instead of T_{11} animals (Giménez y Ribotta et al., 2000). Two months later, the consequence was that the motor capabilities of these T_9 animals did not differ from those of control spinal non-transplanted animals (Fig. 7), although a well-developed graft and a robust serotonergic reinnervation pattern were detected caudally to the transection. However, in these T_9 transplanted animals, the most caudal 5-HT axons could be observed in T_{13} segments only, and none of them was ever seen more caudally. Interestingly, functional motor recovery was observed only when the neo 5-HT axons growing from the graft reinnervated the L_1–L_2 lumbar segments of the sublesional spinal cord. This result is in agreement with data obtained in in vitro studies: locomotor-like

221

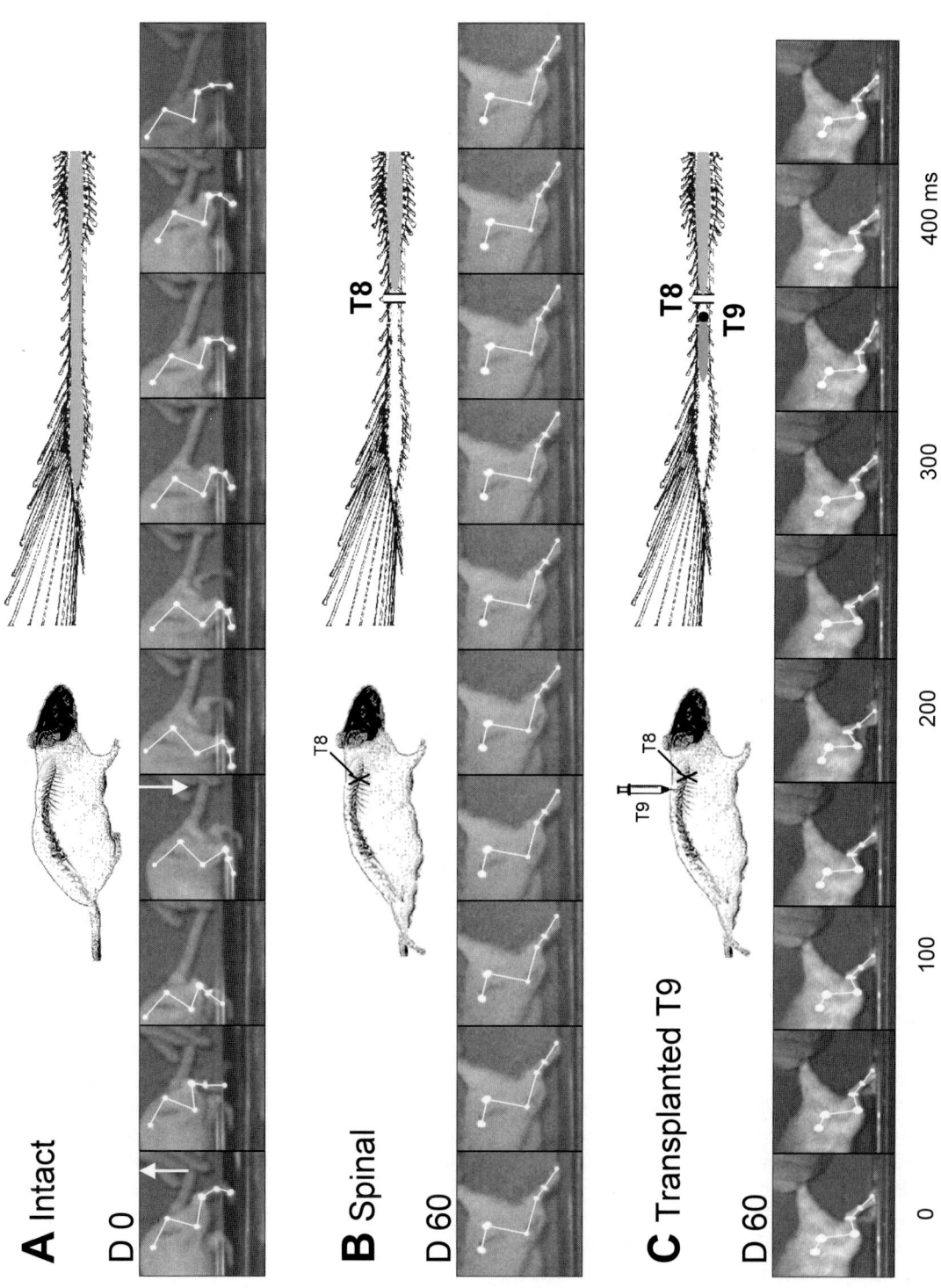

Fig. 7. Effects of T_9 transplantation of embryonic neurons. Same figure as in Fig. 4 except that the transplant was done in the T_9 segment instead of T_{11}. Note in C that the transplanted animal is unable to stand up and walk on the treadmill. However, its spinal cord is immunoreactive for serotonin, but only above the T_{13} segment.

rhythm in ventral roots of neonate spinal cord needs pharmacological stimulation of the L_1–L_2 segments with low doses of 5-HT (Cazalets et al., 1995). This suggests that, with respect to rhythmic motor pattern activation, this region is particularly important as compared to the neighboring segments which are undoubtedly able to generate locomotion but need much more pharmacological stimulation to be activated when disconnected from the L_1–L_2 segments (Kjaerulff and Kiehn, 1996; Cowley and Schmidt, 1997).

This is an important finding which suggests that it is not necessary to reinnervate the whole lumbar spinal cord to obtain significant locomotor recovery with this method. Some strategic targets may be enough.

The spinal CPG for locomotion is involved in this recovery

The implication of the CPG for locomotion can be assessed by the analysis of some parameters that are highly characteristic of its activity. One of the best characteristics is probably the well-known relationship between the duration of the locomotor cycle with the duration of particular phases of the cycle. In intact animals, the duration of the F phase and the related burst in flexor muscles, is relatively independent of the cycle duration, while duration of the stance phase (and more precisely the E3 phase) is definitely correlated with the cycle duration. This relationship is indeed the simple expression of the fact that when the locomotor speed is low (= long cycle duration) the duration of contact of the feet with the ground (= stance phase) is long. This typical relationship has been noticed in transplanted animals 2 months after a T_{11} transplantation. In fact, this relationship appears progressively during the second month following transplantation (Fig. 8). In contrast, this relationship has never been observed in spinal non-transplanted or T_9 transplanted animals.

The time course of recovery of the motor functions seems to fit with the time course of the axonal growth of transplanted neurons. According to Privat et al. (1986), 10 days after spinalization, growth cones immunoreactive for serotonin, could be seen at 15 mm from the transplant site in T_{11}, while 2 months after transplantation, immunoreactive termi-

nals were seen as far as 20 mm from the transplant site (i.e. approximately in L_2). Despite the fact that the density of immunoreactive terminals decreases caudally with respect to the distance from the transplant site, 2 months after transplantation, the spinal segments close to the transplant appear particularly well reinnervated compared to more distant ones.

Pharmacological stimulation of the sublesional spinal cord

Recently, we have investigated whether activation of 5-HT$_2$ receptors could promote recovery of locomotor functions.

Subdural injections of 5-HT in L_1 segment of spinal rats lesioned in T_{11}, activate locomotor activity for about 1 h, with a maximum of effect 30 min postinjection. A similar effect could be obtained with the same timing after i.p. injection of quipazine, a 5-HT$_2$ agonist (Fig. 9C) (Feraboli-Lohnherr et al., 1999). The animal was transiently able to stand up and walk over the treadmill. Astonishingly, this effect has not been confirmed in young rats in the absence of transplantation of embryonic raphe neurons (Kim et al., 1999, 2001). Nevertheless, in adult chronic spinal rats, the locomotor activity was close to that observed in the same conditions of recording in intact animals. However, some characteristics remained abnormal. In particular, the duration of flexor activity which was abnormally long and the duration of extensor activity which was abnormally short. This type of defect has not been observed after transplantation of embryonic 5-HT neurons. This suggests that 5-HT is able to transiently activate the locomotor network through 5-HT$_2$ receptors. But, in order to obtain a normal locomotor pattern, such an acute activation of 5-HT$_2$ receptors is still an incomplete treatment. The time during which the neurotransmitter acts could be of importance. When applied in bolus, the neurotransmitter acts during a short period of time (less than an hour). When applied through transplanted neurons, it is applied during several weeks or months. This long-lasting impregnation could be necessary for a neuromodulatory action.

In order to test this hypothesis, we have submitted the spinal cord over 1 month to continuous injection of quipazine by means of osmotic pumps. This chronic treatment clearly induces a progressive

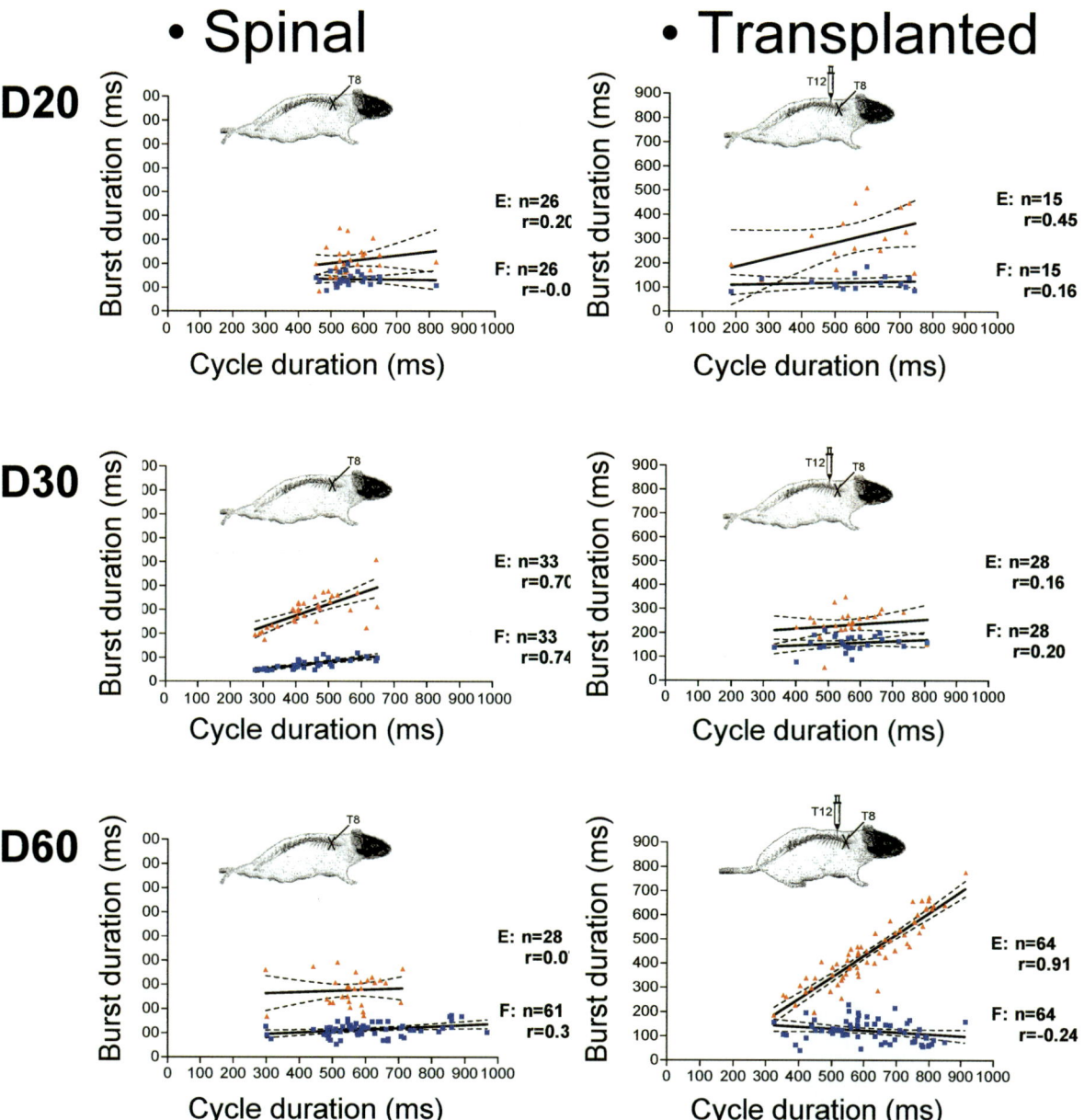

Fig. 8. Timing of the recovery of locomotor function after transplantation of embryonic neurons in adult spinal rats. Burst durations (either flexor or extensor) are plotted versus cycle duration 20, 30 and 60 days after the lesion in spinal (T8) adult rats and spinal (T8) but transplanted in T11 adult rats. A linear regression line has been calculated (coefficients in insert). Note that the relationship between flexor or extensor durations and cycle duration is correct in transplanted animals 2 months after the lesion/transplantation.

improvement of locomotor capabilities from test to test. After 1 month of treatment, a locomotor posture was recovered and the locomotor movement in hindlimbs presented numerous characteristics of

the actual movement in intact animals. However, kinematic analysis pointed out that, although globally typical, the locomotor behavior exhibited some small defects compared to walking of intact animals.

224

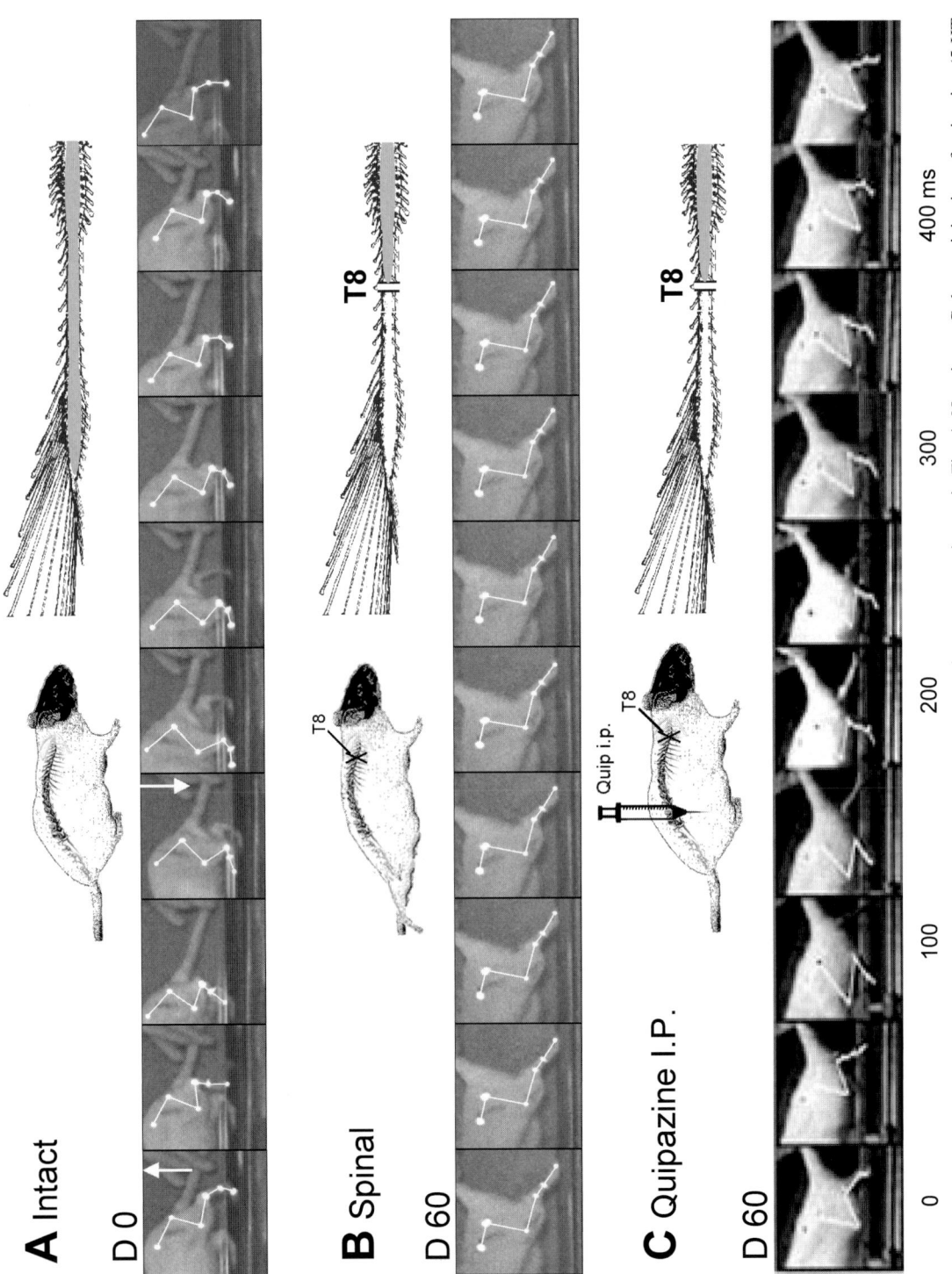

Fig. 9. Motor effects of an i.p. injection of quipazine in a chronic spinal rat. Same presentation as in Fig. 4. Note in rat C that an injection of quipazine (5-HT$_2$ agonist) induces treadmill locomotion and an adequate posture. This effect is maximum 20 min after the injection and disappears after about 1 h. The sublesional spinal cord of this spinal but non-transplanted animal had no 5-HT immunoreactivity.

225

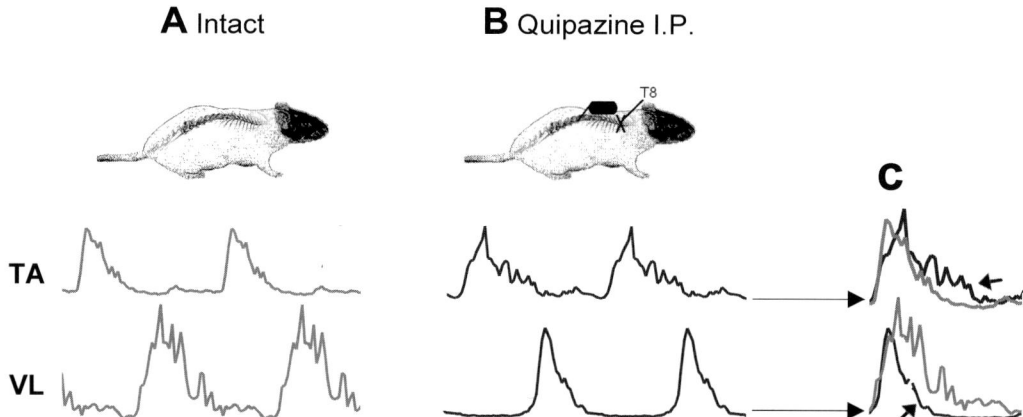

A Intact   **B** Quipazine I.P.   **C**

TA

VL

Fig. 10. Effects of long-term stimulation of the sublesional spinal cord with 5-HT$_2$ agonist. The averaged EMG activity of flexor and extensor muscles of an intact animal (A) are compared to those of a spinal rat (B) after 1 month of continuous quipazine stimulation of the spinal cord caudal to the lesion, by means of an osmotic pump. In C, the average traces are superimposed. Note the lengthening of flexor burst and the shortening of the extensor burst.

These defects concerned either posture (light hyperextension of hindlimbs, belly rubbing the floor. . .) or the locomotor movements themselves (smaller joint excursions, foot placing, defaults in interlimb coordination). For instance, this procedure did not correct the abnormal durations of flexor and extensor activities (Fig. 10) observed by the pharmacological stimulation induced by a bolus of agonist.

Finally, we should note that when the pharmacological treatment was ended, the recovered locomotor activity disappeared within a few days. This suggests that the spinal cord must be continuously stimulated by serotonergic systems (as it is in intact or transplanted animals) in order to be able to generate locomotor command.

Speculative considerations on the possible mechanisms by which the transplant acts

The spinal serotonergic system and its possible function has recently been extensively reviewed (Schmidt and Jordan, 2000; Hochman et al., 2001). These reviews stress the fact that serotonergic system acts mainly through neuromodulatory mechanisms at various levels. In the ventral horn of intact rats, motoneurons are strongly innervated by serotonergic (and noradrenergic terminals) (Björklund and Skagerberg, 1982; Fritschy et al., 1987). Evidence for synapses between transplanted monoaminergic neurons and motoneurons (Rajaofetra et al., 1992b;

Yakovleff et al., 1995b) suggests that transplant may increase the output neuronal networks acting on motoneurons themselves. Serotonin and noradrenaline can evoke long-lasting enhancement of motoneuron excitability by a subthreshold depolarization or induction of plateau properties (White and Neuman, 1980; Kiehn, 1991; White et al., 1991, 1996; Bayliss et al., 1997). The importance of monoaminergic pathways to maintain tonic motor output in the soleus muscle has been stressed in a postural motor task (Kiehn and Kjaerulff, 1996).

However, the role of some other neuroactive substances cannot be excluded. In the spinal cord of adult intact rats, substance P (Chan-Palay et al., 1978; Johansson et al., 1981; Pelletier et al., 1981; Wessendorf and Elde, 1987; Hökfelt et al., 2001) or TRH (Johansson et al., 1981) are known to be colocalized with monoamines in the same terminals. Furthermore, co-localization between serotonin and SP has been evidenced in axons originating from embryonic raphe cell transplanted into the transected spinal cord of adult rats (Rajaofetra et al., 1991). An excitatory effect of substance P (Bédard et al., 1987) and TRH (Barbeau and Bédard, 1981; Bédard et al., 1987; Tremblay and Bédard, 1989; White et al., 1989; Bayliss et al., 1992; Bayliss et al., 1994) on motoneurons of adult rats has been described. Moreover, in neonatal rat spinal cord isolated in vitro (Barthe and Clarac, 1997), substance P was shown to increase excitability of motoneurons and to modulate the networks controlling locomotion at the lumbar level.

Finally, the transplant could also provide some trophic support to injured axons of the sublesional spinal cord, preventing degeneration. Such a trophic effect has been demonstrated in experiments in which a block of embryonic spinal cord tissue was transplanted in the site of lesion of an hemisected spinal cord of rat or cat. In such conditions, a large part of axotomized neurons have been rescued (Bregman and Kunkel-Bagden, 1988; Himes et al., 1994; Miya et al., 1997; Mori et al., 1997).

Conclusions

An important finding with regard to nervous control of locomotion is that locomotor command programming is made by a spinal autonomous neuronal network known as the central pattern generator for locomotion. The localization of this CPG ensures the spinal cord caudal to a complete transversal section, can still exhibit endogenous rhythmogenic properties that can be extensively exploited in a strategy of locomotor function recovery. Indeed, appropriate stimulation of the spinal networks is enough to elicit genuine locomotor command even if the spinal cord remains disconnected from supraspinal structures.

Transplantation of monoaminergic embryonic neurons probably represents one among the most effective means to stimulate the spinal circuitry for a long period of time. The level of locomotor recovery that can be reached using this strategy is high. The way by which the transplant acts enduringly is probably a restoration of the properties of the spinal neurons (excitability, bistable properties, . . .) and, as a result, a reconfiguration of the neural networks in which the neurons are integrated. This neuromodulation is likely due to the activation of various types of receptors, as suggested by experimental data showing that stimulation of one single type of 5-HT receptors (5-HT$_2$), even chronically, leads to a functional recovery which is effective, but which appears significantly of less good quality, as compared to the functional consequences of a transplantation. We probably have to look for the other candidates among the other types of 5-HT receptors, but also among the peptidergic receptors, since serotonin is co-localized with neuropeptides (TRH,

substance P. . .) in a large amount of serotonergic fibers. The noradrenergic system, and especially the α_2-receptors, could be also a good candidate.

The strategy of transplantation of embryonic neurons does not, of course, restore the voluntary control of locomotor movements since the connections between the brain and the CPG remain interrupted. However, it stimulates the spinal cord for a long time and, thus allows triggering of locomotor activity using exteroceptive stimuli. Furthermore, if used together with a strategy of translesion reconnection, it could improve the recovery of voluntary control of locomotor activity.

Acknowledgements

The thesis of M.A. is supported by a grant from Institut pour la Recherche sur la Moelle Épinière (IRME). This work was made possible by the support of the following funding agencies: France-Québec Exchange Program, Institut de Recherche en Santé du Canada (IRSC, Canada), (IRME, France), and Christopher Reeve Paralysis Foundation (CRPF, USA).

References

Armstrong, D.M. (1988) The supra-spinal control of mammalian locomotion. *J. Physiol. (Lond.)*, 405: 1–37.

Armstrong, D.M., Apps, R. and Marple-Horvat, D.E. (1997) Aspects of cerebellar function in relation to locomotor movements. *Prog. Brain Res.*, 114: 401–421.

Arshavsky, Y.I., Gelfand, I.M. and Orlovsky, G.N. (1986) *Cerebellum and Rhythmical Movements*. Springer Verlag, Berlin, pp. 1–166.

Barbeau, H. and Bédard, P.J. (1981) Similar motor effects of 5-HT and TRH in rats following chronic spinal transection and 5-7 dihydroxytryptamine injection. *Neuropharmacology*, 20: 477–481.

Barbeau, H. and Rossignol, S. (1987) Recovery of locomotion after chronic spinalization in the adult cat. *Brain Res.*, 412: 84–95.

Barbeau, H. and Rossignol, S. (1990) The effects of serotonergic drugs on the locomotor pattern and on cutaneous reflexes of the adult chronic spinal cat. *Brain Res.*, 514: 55–67.

Barbeau, H. and Rossignol, S. (1991) Initiation and modulation of the locomotor pattern in the adult chronic spinal cat by noradrenergic, serotonergic and dopaminergic drugs. *Brain Res.*, 546: 250–260.

Barbeau, H., Julien, C. and Rossignol, S. (1987) The effects of clonidine and yohimbine on locomotion and cutaneous reflexes in the adult chronic spinal cat. *Brain Res.*, 437: 83–96.

Barthe, J.Y. and Clarac, F. (1997) Modulation of the spinal network for locomotion by substance P in the neonatal rat. *Exp. Brain Res.*, 115: 485–492.

Bayliss, D.A., Viana, F. and Berger, A.J. (1992) Mechanisms underlying excitatory effects of thyrotrophin-releasing hormone on rat hypoglossal motoneurones in vitro. *J. Neurophysiol.*, 68: 1733–1745.

Bayliss, D.A., Viana, F. and Berger, A.J. (1994) Effects of thyrotropin-releasing hormone on rat motoneurons are mediated by G proteins. *Brain Res.*, 668: 220–229.

Bayliss, D.A., Viana, F., Talley, E.M. and Berger, A.J. (1997) Neuromodulation of hypoglossal motoneurons: cellular and developmental mechanisms. *Respir. Physiol.*, 110: 139–150.

Bédard, P.J., Tremblay, L.E., Barbeau, H., Filion, M., Maheux, R., Richards, C.L. and DiPaolo, T. (1987) Action of 5-hydroxytryptamine, substance P, thyrotropin-releasing hormone and clonidine on motoneurone excitability. *Can. J. Neurol. Sci.*, 14: 506–509.

Björklund, A. and Skagerberg, G. (1982) Descending monoaminergic projections to the spinal cord. In: B. Sjolund and A. Björklund (Eds.), *Brainstem Control of Spinal Mechanisms*. Elsevier, Amsterdam, pp. 55–88.

Björklund, A., Nornes, H., Gage, F.H., Foster, G., Schultzberg, M. and Stenevi, U. (1986) Reinnervation of the denervated spinal cord by grafted noradrenergic and serotonergic brain stem neurons. In: M.E. Goldberger, A. Gorio and M. Murray (Eds.), *Development and Plasticity of the Mammalian Spinal Cord*. Liviana Press, Padova, pp. 291–299.

Bregman, B.S. and Kunkel-Bagden, E. (1988) Effect of target and non-target transplants on neuronal survival and axonal elongation after injury to the developing spinal cord. *Prog. Brain Res.*, 78: 205–212.

Bregman, B.S., Kunkel-Bagden, E., Schnell, L., Dai, H.N., Gao, D. and Schwab, M.E. (1995) Recovery from spinal cord injury mediated by antibodies to neurite growth inhibitors. *Nature*, 378: 498–501.

Bregman, B.S., Diener, P.S., McAtee, M., Dai, H.N. and James, C. (1997) Intervention strategies to enhance anatomical plasticity and recovery of function after spinal cord injury. *Adv. Neurol.*, 72: 257–275.

Carter, M.C. and Smith, J.L. (1986a) Simultaneous control of two rhythmical behaviors. I. Locomotion with paw-shake response in normal cat. *J. Neurophysiol.*, 56: 171–183.

Carter, M.C. and Smith, J.L. (1986b) Simultaneous control of two rhythmical behaviors. II. Hindlimb walking with paw-shake response in the spinal cat. *J. Neurophysiol.*, 56: 184–195.

Cazalets, J.R., Grillner, P., Menard, I., Crémieux, J. and Clarac, F. (1990) Two types of motor rhythm induced by NMDA and amines in an in vitro spinal cord preparation of neonatal rat. *Neurosci. Lett.*, 111: 116–121.

Cazalets, J.R., Sqalli-Houssaini, Y. and Clarac, F. (1992) Activation of the central pattern generators for locomotion by serotonin and excitatory amino acids in neonatal rat. *J. Physiol.*, 455: 187–204.

Cazalets, J.R., Borde, M. and Clarac, F. (1995) Localization and organization of the central pattern generator for hindlimb locomotion in newborn rat. *J. Neurosci.*, 15: 4943–4951.

Chan-Palay, V., Jonsson, G. and Palay, S.L. (1978) Serotonin and substance P coexist in neurons of the rat central nervous system. *Proc. Natl. Acad. Sci. USA*, 75: 1582–1586.

Chau, C., Barbeau, H. and Rossignol, S. (1998a) Early locomotor training with clonidine in spinal cats. *J. Neurophysiol.*, 79: 392–409.

Chau, C., Barbeau, H. and Rossignol, S. (1998b) Effects of intrathecal alpha1- and alpha2-noradrenergic agonists and norepinephrine on locomotion in chronic spinal cats. *J. Neurophysiol.*, 79: 2941–2963.

Cheng, H., Almstrom, S., Gimenez-Llort, L., Chang, R., Ove Ogren, S., Hoffer, B. and Olson, L. (1997) Gait analysis of adult paraplegic rats after spinal cord repair. *Exp. Neurol.*, 148: 544–557.

Commissiong, J.W. and Sauve, Y. (1989) The physiological basis of transplantation of fetal catecholaminergic neurons in the transected spinal cord of the rat. *Comp. Biochem. Physiol. A*, 93: 301–307.

Commissiong, J.W. and Sauve, Y. (1993) Neurophysiological basis of functional recovery in the neonatal spinalized rat. *Exp. Brain Res.*, 96: 473–479.

Commissiong, J.W. and Toffano, G. (1989) Complete spinal cord transection at different postnatal ages: recovery of motor coordination correlated with spinal cord catecholamines. *Exp. Brain Res.*, 78: 597–603.

Cowley, K.C. and Schmidt, B.J. (1994) A comparison of motor patterns induced by N-methyl-D-aspartate, acetylcholine and serotonin in the in vitro neonatal rat spinal cord. *Neurosci. Lett.*, 171: 147–150.

Cowley, K.C. and Schmidt, B.J. (1997) Regional distribution of the locomotor pattern-generating network in the neonatal rat spinal cord. *J. Neurophysiol.*, 77: 247–259.

Feraboli-Lohnherr, D., Orsal, D., Yakovleff, A., Giménez y Ribotta, M. and Privat, A. (1997) Recovery of locomotor activity in the adult chronic spinal rat after sublesional transplantation of embryonic nervous cells: specific role of serotonergic neurons. *Exp. Brain Res.*, 113: 443–454.

Feraboli-Lohnherr, D., Barthe, J.Y. and Orsal, D. (1999) Serotonin-induced activation of the network for locomotion in adult spinal rats. *J. Neurosci. Res.*, 55: 87–98.

Forssberg, H. and Grillner, S. (1973) The locomotion of the acute spinal cat injected with clonidine i.v.. *Brain Res.*, 50: 184–186.

Fritschy, J.-M., Lyons, W.E., Mullen, C.A., Kosofsky, B.E., Molliver, M.E. and Grzanna, R. (1987) Distribution of locus coeruleus axons in the rat spinal cord: a combined anterograde transport and immunohistochemical study. *Brain Res.*, 437: 176–180.

Gaviria, M., Privat, A., d'Arbigny, P., Kamenka, J.M., Haton, H. and Ohanna, F. (2000) Neuroprotective effects of gacyclidine after experimental photochemical spinal cord lesion in adult rats: dose-window and time-window effects. *J. Neurotrauma*, 17: 19–30.

Georgopoulos, A.P. and Grillner, S. (1989) Visuomotor coordination in reaching and locomotion. *Science*, 245: 1209–1210.

Giménez y Ribotta, M. and Privat, A. (1998) Biological interventions for spinal cord injury. *Curr. Opin. Neurol.*, 11: 647–654.

Giménez y Ribotta, M., Rajaofetra, N., Morin-Richaud, C., Alonso, G., Bochelen, D., Sandillon, F., Legrand, A., Mersel, M. and Privat, A. (1995) Oxysterol (7 beta-hydroxycholesteryl-3-oleate) promote serotonergic reinnervation in the lesioned rat spinal cord by reducing glial reaction. *J. Neurosci. Res.*, 41: 79–95.

Giménez y Ribotta, M., Provencher, J., Feraboli-Lohnherr, D., Rossignol, S., Privat, A. and Orsal, D. (2000) Activation of locomotion in adult chronic spinal rats is achieved by transplantation of embryonic raphe cells reinnervating a precise lumbar level [In process citation]. *J. Neurosci.*, 20: 5144–5152.

Giménez y Ribotta, M., Gaviria, M., Menet, V. and Privat, A. (2002) Strategies for regeneration and repair in spinal cord traumatic injury. In: L. McKerracher, G. Doucet and S. Rossignol (Eds.), *Spinal Cord Trauma: Neural Repair and Functional Recovery. Progress in Brain Research*, Vol. 137. Elsevier Science, Amsterdam, pp. 191–212.

Giroux, N., Brustein, E., Chau, C., Barbeau, H., Reader, T.A. and Rossignol, S. (1998) Differential effects of the noradrenergic agonist clonidine on the locomotion of intact, partially and completely spinalized adult cats. *Ann. New York Acad. Sci.*, 860: 517–520.

Giroux, N., Reader, T.A. and Rossignol, S. (2001) Comparison of the effect of intrathecal administration of clonidine and yohimbine on the locomotion of intact and spinal cats. *J. Neurophysiol.*, 85: 2516–2536.

Giuliani, C.A. and Smith, J.L. (1985) Development and characteristics of airstepping in chronic spinal cats. *J. Neurosci.*, 5: 1276–1282.

Goldberger, M.E., Murray, M. and Tessler, A. (1993) Graft and functional recuperation. *Restor. Neurol. Neurosci.*, 7: 69–87.

Goudard, I., Orsal, D. and Cabelguen, J.-M. (1992) An electromyographic study of the hindlimb locomotor movements in the acute thalamic rat. *Eur. J. Neurosci.*, 4: 1130–1139.

Grill, R., Murai, K., Blesch, A., Gage, F.H. and Tuszynski, M.H. (1997) Cellular delivery of neurotrophin-3 promotes corticospinal axonal growth and partial functional recovery after spinal cord injury. *J. Neurosci.*, 17: 5560–5572.

Grillner, S. (1973) Locomotion in the spinal cat. In: P.S.G. Stein, K.G. Pearson, J.L. Smith and J.B. Redford (Eds.), *Control of Posture and Locomotion*. Plenum Press, New York, pp. 515–535.

Grillner, S. (1975) Locomotion in vertebrates central mechanism and reflex interaction. *Physiol. Rev.*, 55: 247–304.

Grillner, S. (2002) The spinal locomotor CPG: a target after spinal cord injury. In: L. McKerracher, G. Doucet and S. Rossignol (Eds.), *Spinal Cord Trauma: Neural Repair and Functional Recovery. Progress in Brain Research*, Vol. 137. Elsevier Science, Amsterdam, pp. 97–108.

Grillner, S. (1981) Control of locomotion in bipeds, tetrapods and fish. In: J.M. Brookhart and V.B. Mountcastle (Eds.), *Handbook of Physiology*. Am. Physiol. Soc., Bethesda, MD, pp. 1179–1236.

Grillner, S. (1986) The effect of L-DOPA on the spinal cord. Relation to locomotion and the half center hypothesis. In: S. Grillner, P.S.G. Stein, D.G. Stuart, H. Forssberg and R.M. Herman (Eds.), *Neurobiology and Motor Control*. MacMillan, London, pp. 311–321.

Grillner, S. and Zangger, P. (1979) On the central generation of locomotion in the low spinal cat. *Exp. Brain Res.*, 34: 241–261.

Grillner, S., Georgopoulos, A.P. and Jordan, L.M. (1997) Selection and initiation of motor behavior. In: P.S.G. Stein, S. Grillner, A.I. Selverston and D.G. Stuart (Eds.), *Neurons, Networks and Motor Behavior*. MIT Press, Cambridge, MA, pp. 3–19.

Grillner, S., Ekeberg, O., El Manira, A., Lansner, A., Parker, D., Tegner, J. and Wallen, P. (1998a) Intrinsic function of a neuronal network — a vertebrate central pattern generator. *Brain Res. Brain Res. Rev.*, 26: 184–197.

Grillner, S., Parker, D. and El Manira, A. (1998b) Vertebrate locomotion — a lamprey perspective. *Ann. New York Acad. Sci.*, 860: 1–18.

Gruner, J.A. and Altman, J. (1980) Swimming in the rat: analysis of locomotor performance in comparison to stepping. *Exp. Brain Res.*, 40: 374–382.

Gruner, J.A., Altman, J. and Spivack, N. (1980) Effects of arrested cerebellar development of locomotion in the rat: electromyographic and cinematographic analysis. *Exp. Brain Res.*, 40: 361–373.

Himes, B.T., Goldberger, M.E. and Tessler, A. (1994) Grafts of fetal central nervous system tissue rescue axotomized Clarke's nucleus neurons in adult and neonatal operates. *J. Comp. Neurol.*, 339: 117–131.

Hochman, S., Garraway, S.M., Machacek, D.W. and Shay, B.L. (2001) 5-HT receptors and the neuromodulatory control of spinal cord function. In: T.C. Cope (Ed.), *Motor Neurobiology of the Spinal Cord*. CRC Press, London, pp. 47–87.

Hökfelt, T., Pernow, B. and Wahren, J. (2001) Substance P: a pioneer amongst neuropeptides. *J. Intern. Med.*, 249(1): 27–40.

Iles, J.F. and Nicolopoulos-Stournaras, S. (1996) Fictive locomotion in the adult decerebrate rat. *Exp. Brain Res.*, 109: 393–398.

Iwashita, Y., Kawaguchi, S. and Murata, M. (1994) Restoration of function by replacement of spinal cord segments in the rat. *Nature*, 367: 167–170.

Jankowska, E., Jukes, M.G.M., Lund, S. and Lundberg, A. (1967a) The effect of DOPA on the spinal cord. VI Half-centre organization of interneurones transmitting effects from flexor reflex afferents. *Acta Physiol. Scand.*, 70: 389–402.

Jankowska, E., Jukes, M.G.M. and Lundberg, A. (1967b) The effect of DOPA on the spinal cord. 5 — Reciprocal organization of pathways transmitting excitatory action to alpha motoneurons of flexors and extensors. *Acta Physiol. Scand.*, 70: 369–388.

Johansson, O., Hökfelt, T., Pentow, B., Jeffcoate, S.L., White, X.X., Steinbush, H.W.M., Verhofstad, A.A.J., Emson, P.C. and Spindle, E. (1981) Immunohistochemical support for three putative transmitters in one neuron: co-existence of 5-

hydroxytryptamine, substance P and thyrotrophin releasing hormone-like immunoreactivity in medullary neurons projecting to the spinal cord. *Neuroscience*, 6: 1857–1882.

Jordan, L.M. (1998) Initiation of locomotion in mammals. *Ann. New York Acad. Sci.*, 860: 83–93.

Kalaska, J.F. and Drew, T. (1993) Motor cortex and visuomotor behavior. *Exerc. Sport Sci. Rev.*, 21: 397–436.

Kiehn, O. (1991) Electrophysiology of 5-HT on vertebrate motoneurones. In: T. Stone (Ed.), *LTP, Galanin, Opioids, Autonomic and 5-HT*. Taylor, London, pp. 527–555.

Kiehn, O. and Kjaerulff, O. (1996) Spatiotemporal characteristics of 5-HT and dopamine-induced rhythmic hindlimb activity in the in vitro neonatal rat. *J. Neurophysiol.*, 4: 1472–1482.

Kiehn, O., Iizuka, M. and Kudo, N. (1992) Resetting from low threshold afferents of *N*-methyl-D-aspartate-induced locomotor rhythm in the isolated spinal cord-hindlimb preparation from newborn rats. *Neurosci. Lett.*, 148: 43–46.

Kim, D., Adipudi, V., Shibayama, M., Giszter, S., Tessler, A., Murray, M. and Simansky, K.J. (1999) Direct agonists for serotonin receptors enhance locomotor function in rats that received neural transplants after neonatal spinal transection. *J. Neurosci.*, 19: 6213–6224.

Kim, D., Murray, M. and Simansky, K.J. (2001) The serotonergic 5-HT(2C) agonist *m*-chlorophenylpiperazine increases weight-supported locomotion without development of tolerance in rats with spinal transections. *Exp. Neurol.*, 169: 496–500.

Kjaerulff, O. and Kiehn, O. (1996) Distribution of networks generating and coordinating locomotor activity in the neonatal rat spinal cord in vitro: a lesion study. *J. Neurosci.*, 16: 5777–5794.

Kudo, N. and Yamada, T. (1987) *N*-Methyl-D,L-aspartate-induced locomotor activity in a spinal cord- hindlimb muscles preparation of the newborn rat studied in vitro. *Neurosci. Lett.*, 75: 43–48.

Li, B., Wang, Z. and Zhu, P. (1997) Changes of BDNF mRNA by molecular hybridization during embryonic spinal cord repairing injury of adult rats. *Chung Hua I. Hsueh Tsa Chih*, 77: 516–520.

Mansour, H., Sandillon, F., Poulat, P. and Privat, A. (1986) Transplantation de neurones foetaux dans la moelle épinière après section. *Neurochirugie*, 32: 507–513.

Marcoux, J. and Rossignol, S. (2000) Initiating or blocking locomotion in spinal cats by applying noradrenergic drugs to restricted lumbar spinal segments. *J. Neurosci.*, 20: 8577–8585.

Matsuyama, K. and Drew, T. (2000a) Vestibulospinal and reticulospinal neuronal activity during locomotion in the intact cat. I. Walking on a level surface. *J. Neurophysiol.*, 84: 2237–2256.

Matsuyama, K. and Drew, T. (2000b) Vestibulospinal and reticulospinal neuronal activity during locomotion in the intact cat. II. Walking on an inclined plane. *J. Neurophysiol.*, 84: 2257–2276.

Meisel, R.L. and Rakerd, B. (1982) Induction of hindlimb stepping movements in rats spinally transected as adults or as neonates. *Brain Res.*, 240: 353–356.

Miya, D., Giszter, S., Mori, F., Adipudi, V., Tessler, A. and

Murray, M. (1997) Fetal transplants alter the development of function after spinal cord transection in newborn rats. *J. Neurosci.*, 17: 4856–4872.

Mori, F., Himes, B.T., Kowada, M., Murray, M. and Tessler, A. (1997) Fetal spinal cord transplants rescue some axotomized rubrospinal neurons from retrograde cell death in adult rats. *Exp. Neurol.*, 143: 45–60.

Nicolopoulos-Stournaras, S. and Iles, J.F. (1984) Hindlimb muscle activity during locomotion in the rat (*Rattus norvegicus*) (Rodent Muridae). *J. Zool. Lond.*, 203: 427–440.

Pearson, K.G. and Rossignol, S. (1991) Fictive motor patterns in chronic spinal cats. *J. Neurophysiol.*, 66: 1874–1887.

Pelletier, G., Steinbush, H.W.M. and Verhofstad, A.A.J. (1981) Immunoreactive substance P and serotonin present in the same densecore vesicles. *Nature*, 293: 71–72.

Pencalet, P., Ohanna, F., Poulat, P., Kamenka, J.M. and Privat, A. (1993) Thienylphencyclidine protection for the spinal cord of adult rats against extension of lesions secondary to a photochemical injury. *J. Neurosurg.*, 78: 603–609.

Prentice, S.D. and Drew, T. (2001) Contributions of the reticulospinal system to the postural adjustments occurring during voluntary gait modifications. *J. Neurophysiol.*, 85: 679–698.

Privat, A., Mansour, H. and Geffard, M. (1988) Transplantation of fetal serotonin neurons into the transected spinal cord of adult rats: morphological development and functional influence. In: D.M. Gash and J.R. Sladek (Eds.), *Transplantation into the Mammalian CNS. Prog. Brain Res.*, vol. 78, Elsevier, Amsterdam, pp. 155–166.

Privat, A., Mansour, H., Pavy, A., Geffard, M. and Sandillon, F. (1986) Transplantation of dissociated foetal serotonin neurons into the transected spinal cord of adult rats. *Neurosci. Lett.*, 66: 61–66.

Privat, A., Mansour, H., Rajaofetra, N. and Geffard, M. (1989) Intraspinal transplants of serotonergic neurons in the adult rats. *Brain Res. Bull.*, 22: 123–129.

Rajaofetra, N., Kachidian, P., Marlier, L., Poulat, P., König, N., Geffard, M. and Privat, A. (1991) Electromicroscopic detection of the axonal coexistence of serotonin and substance P in B1–B2 raphé cells transplanted into the transected spinal cord of adult rats. *Brain Res.*, 542: 159–162.

Rajaofetra, N., König, N., Poulat, P., Marlier, L., Sandillon, F., Drian, M.J., Geffard, M. and Privat, A. (1992a) Fate of B1–B2 and B3 rhombencephalic cells transplanted into the transected spinal cord of adult rats: light and electron microscopic studies. *Exp. Neurol.*, 117: 59–70.

Rajaofetra, N., Poulat, P., Marlier, L., Sandillon, F., Drian, M.J., König, N., Famose, F., Verschuere, B., Gouy, D., Geffard, M. and Privat, A. (1992b) Transplantation of embryonic serotonin immunoreactive neurons into the transected spinal cord of adult monkey (*Macaca fascicularis*). *Brain Res.*, 572: 329–334.

Ramon-Cueto, A., Plant, G.W., Avila, J. and Bunge, M.B. (1998) Long-distance axonal regeneration in the transected adult rat spinal cord is promoted by olfactory ensheathing glia transplants. *J. Neurosci.*, 18: 3803–3815.

Ramon-Cueto, A., Cordero, M.I., Santos-Benito, F.F. and Avila, J. (2000) Functional recovery of paraplegic rats and motor

230

axon regeneration in their spinal cords by olfactory ensheathing glia. *Neuron*, 25: 425–435.

Ridet, J.-L., Rajaofetra, N., Teilhac, J.-R., Geffard, M. and Privat, A. (1993) Evidence for nonsynaptic serotonergic and noradrenergic innervation of the rat dorsal horn and possible involvement of neuron–glia interactions. *Neuroscience*, 52: 143–157.

Rossignol, S. (1996) Neural control of stereotypic limb movements. In: L.B. Rowell and J.T. Sheperd (Eds.), *Exercise: Regulation and Integration of Multiple Systems*. American Physiological Society, Bethesda, MD, pp. 173–216.

Rossignol, S., Barbeau, H. and Julien, C. (1986) Locomotion of the adult chronic spinal cat and its modification by monoaminergic agonists and antagonists. In: M.E. Goldberger, A. Gorio and M. Murray (Eds.), *Development and Plasticity of the Mammalian Spinal Cord*. Liviana Press, Padova, pp. 323–346.

Rossignol, S., Chau, C., Brustein, E., Bélanger, M., Barbeau, H. and Drew, T. (1996) Locomotor capacities after complete and partial lesions of the spinal cord. *Acta Neurobiol. Exp.*, 56: 449–463.

Rossignol, S., Bélanger, M., Chau, C., Giroux, N., Brustein, E., Bouyer, L., Grenier, T., Drew, T., Barbeau, H. and Reader, T.A. (2000) The spinal cat. In: R.G. Kalb and S.M. Strittmatter (Eds.), *Neurobiology of Spinal Cord Injury*. Humana Press, Totowa, pp. 57–87.

Schmidt, B.J. and Jordan, L.M. (2000) The role of serotonin in reflex modulation and locomotor rhythm production in the mammalian spinal cord. *Brain Res. Bull.*, 53: 689–710.

Slawinska U., Majczynski H. and Djavadian, R. (2000) Recovery of hindlimb motor function after spinal cord transection is enhanced by grafts of the embryonic raphe nuclei. *Exp. Brain Res.*, 132: 27–38.

Smith, J.L., Hoy, M.G., Koshland, G.F., Phillips, D.M., Zernicke, R.F. (1985) Intralimb coordination of the paw-shake response: a novel mixed synergy. *J. Neurophysiol.*, 54: 1271–1281.

Sqalli-Houssaini, Y., Cazalets, J.R., Martini, F. and Clarac, F. (1993) Induction of fictive locomotion by sulphur-containing amino acids in an in vitro newborn preparation. *Eur. J. Neurosci.*, 5: 1226–1232.

Steinbush, H.W.M. (1981) Distribution of serotonin-immunoreactivity in the central nervous system of the rat cell bodies and terminals. *Neuroscience*, 6: 557–618.

Steinbush, H.W.M. (1984) Serotonin-immunoreactive neurons and their projections in the CNS. In: A. Björklund, T. Hökfelt and M.J. Kühar (Eds.), *Handbook of Chemical Neuroanatomy*, Vol. 3. Elsevier, Amsterdam, pp. 297–321.

Stelzner, D.J., Ershler, W.B. and Weber, E.D. (1975) Effects of spinal transection in neonatal and weanling rats: survival of function. *Exp. Neurol.*, 46: 156–177.

Tremblay, L.E. and Bédard, P.J. (1989) Chronic administration of thyrotropin-releasing hormone enhances the sensitivity of lumbar motoneurons to 5-hydroxytryptophan in the rat. *Pharmacol. Biochem. Behav.*, 33: 127–130.

Viala, D. and Buser, P. (1969) The effects of DOPA and 5-HTP on rhythmic efferent discharges in hindlimb nerves in the rabbit. *Brain Res.*, 12: 437–443.

Viala, D. and Buser, P. (1971) Modalites d'obtention de rythmes locomoteurs chez le lapin spinal par traitements pharmacologiques (DOPA, 5HTP, D-amphetamine). *Brain Res.*, 35: 151–165.

Weber, E.D. and Stelzner, D.J. (1977) Behavioral effects of spinal cord transection in the developing rat. *Brain Res.*, 125: 241–255.

Wessendorf, M.W. and Elde, T. (1987) The coexistence of serotonin and substance P-like immunoreactivity in the spinal cord of the rat as shown by immunofluorescent double labeling. *J. Neurosci.*, 7: 2352–2363.

Westerga, J. and Gramsbergen, A. (1990) The development of locomotion in the rat. *Dev. Brain Res.*, 57: 163–174.

Westerga, J. and Gramsbergen, A. (1993) Development of locomotion in the rat: the significance of early movements. *Early Hum. Dev.*, 34: 89–100.

White, S.R. and Neuman, R.S. (1980) Facilitation of spinal motoneurone excitability by 5-hydroxytryptamine and noradrenaline. *Brain Res.*, 188: 119–127.

White, S.R., Crane, G.K. and Jackson, D.A. (1989) Thyrotropin-releasing hormone (TRH) effects on spinal cord neuronal excitability. *Ann. New York Acad. Sci.*, 553: 337–350.

White, S.R., Fung, S.J. and Barnes, C.D. (1991) Norepinephrine effects on spinal motoneurons. *Prog. Brain Res.*, 88: 343–350.

White, S.R., Fung, S.J., Jackson, D.A. and Imel, K.M. (1996) Serotonin, norepinephrine and associated neuropeptides: effects on somatic motoneuron excitability. *Prog. Brain Res.*, 107: 183–199.

Yakhnitsa, I.A., Pilyavskii, A.T. and Bulgakova, N.V. (1985a) Comparative analysis of kinematic movements of the rat hindlimbs during different type of locomotion. *Neurophysiology*, 17: 189–198.

Yakhnitsa, I.A., Pilyavskii, A.T. and Bulgakova, N.V. (1985b) Study of different kinds of locomotor movements in rats. *Neurophysiology*, 17: 122–134.

Yakovleff, A., Cabelguen, J.-M., Orsal, D., Giménez y Ribotta, M., Rajaofetra, N., Drian, M.-J., Bussel, B. and Privat, A. (1995a) Fictive motor activities in adult chronic spinal rats transplanted with embryonic brainstem neurons. *Exp. Brain Res.*, 106: 69–78.

Yakovleff, A., Cabelguen, J.M., Orsal, D., Giménez y Ribotta, M., Rajaofetra, N., Drian, M.J., Bussel, B. and Privat, A. (1995b) Fictive motor activities in adult chronic spinal rats transplanted with embryonic brainstem neurons. *Exp. Brain Res.*, 106: 69–78.

Yakovleff, A., Roby-Brami, A., Guezard, B., Mansour, H., Bussel, B. and Privat, A. (1989) Locomotion in the rats transplanted with noradrenergic neurons. *Brain Res. Bull.*, 22: 115–121.

L. McKerracher, G. Doucet and S. Rossignol (Eds.)
Progress in Brain Research, Vol. 137

CHAPTER 17

Spinal cord contusion models

Wise Young [*]

*W.M. Keck Center for Collaborative Neuroscience, Rutgers State University of New Jersey, 604 Allison Rd.,
Piscataway, NJ 08854-8082, USA*

Introduction

Most human spinal cord injuries result from fracture and dislocation of the spinal column. Although penetrating wounds of the spinal cord can result from a knife or gunshot, most human spinal cord injuries are caused by transient compression or contusion of the spinal cord. Scientists have long used animal spinal cord contusion models to study the pathophysiology of spinal cord injury. Contusion models played an important role in the discovery of progressive secondary tissue damage, demyelination, and apoptosis in spinal cord injury. Most therapies that have gone to human clinical trial were first validated in spinal cord contusion models. Spinal cord contusion models have had a significant impact on the field. In this chapter, I will describe the history and practice of animal spinal cord contusion models, with particular emphasis on the Multicenter Animal Spinal Cord Injury Study (MASCIS) Impactor model of rat spinal cord injury.

Early contusion models

In 1911, Reginald Allen described a spinal cord injury model where he dropped a weight onto dog

* Correspondence to: W. Young, W.M. Keck Center for Collaborative Neuroscience, Rutgers State University of New Jersey, 604 Allison Rd., Piscataway, NJ 08854-8082, USA. Tel.: +1-732-445-2061; Fax: +1-732-445-2063; E-mail: young@biology.rutgers.edu

cords exposed by laminectomy (Allen, 1911). In 1914, he reported that midline myelotomy reduced progressive tissue damage in contused spinal cord (Allen, 1914). Unfortunately, Allen died in World War I and his work was lost for nearly 50 years, except for a 1927 study by Ferraro who examined the spinal cord concussion in rabbits (Ferraro, 1927). In 1968, Albin and colleagues (Albin et al., 1968a,b, 1969; White et al., 1969) revived the contusion model when they used a primate spinal cord contusion model to assess hypothermic therapy of spinal cord injury. Ducker and colleagues (Ducker and Assenmacher, 1969; Ducker and Hamit, 1969; Assenmacher and Ducker, 1971; Ducker, 1976) and others subsequently evaluated the effects of corticosteroids (Black and Markowitz, 1971; Green et al., 1980) and hypothermia (Green et al., 1973; Black et al., 1979) on this model. Many investigators described histopathological changes (Goodman et al., 1974; Bresnahan et al., 1976), vascular pathology (Ducker et al., 1971a,b; Ducker and Perot, 1971a,b,c; Tator and Deecke, 1973), blood flow (Kobrine and Doyle, 1976; Kobrine et al., 1976a,b,c,d; Sandler and Tator, 1976a,b,c,d; Bingham et al., 1977; Kobrine et al., 1977a,b, 1980a,b), evoked potentials (Singer et al., 1970), myelin (Horrocks et al., 1973), edema (Green and Wagner, 1973; Yashon et al., 1973), and somatosensory evoked potentials (Cusick et al., 1979) changes in the primate model. Daniell et al. (1975) used force transducer to quantify the spinal cord impact in primate spinal cord.

Several investigators started using the canine

spinal cord contusion model again. Parker and colleagues (Parker et al., 1973; Parker and Smith, 1976) assessed the effects of dexamethasone and chlorpromazine on edema in contused dog spinal cords. Koozekanani et al. (1976) and Gerber and Corrie (1979) examined causes of variability in the model while Griffiths and Miller (Griffiths and Miller, 1974; Griffiths, 1976) and others (Collmann et al., 1978) measured edema and blood flow (Wullenweber et al., 1978) and histopathological changes in contused dog spinal cords (Guth et al., 1977; Ducker et al., 1978a,b,c). Walker et al. (1977, 1979) described the energy metabolism while Clendenon et al. (1978a,b) measured ATPase and hydrolase activities in contused dog spinal cords. Others studied the effects of DMSO (de La Torre et al., 1975a,b; Parker and Smith, 1979; Goodnough et al., 1980), the carotenoid crocetin (Gainer, 1977), hypertension and hypercarbia (Hukuda et al., 1980a,b) on the model. Swaim et al. (1971) and Kadoya et al. (1974) studied respiratory function after cervical spinal cord contusion in dogs. Stokes and Garwood (1982) examined oxygen levels in contused dog spinal cords.

In 1969, Goodkin et al. described progressive tissue damage in the contused cat spinal cord (Goodkin and Campbell, 1969; Goodkin, 1973). Brodkey et al. (1972) and others (Croft et al., 1972; Martin and Bloedel, 1973) assessed evoked potentials while Eidelberg et al. (1975) measured extracellular potassium released after contusion. Several laboratories assessed spinal cord injury therapies (Campbell et al., 1973a,b, 1974; Kajihara et al., 1973; Kuchner and Hansebout, 1976; Brodner and Dohrmann, 1977; Brodner et al., 1977; Flamm et al., 1977), including the effects of angiographic dyes (Fox et al., 1976), the role of cellular immunity (Willenborg et al., 1977), mannitol (Reed et al., 1979) and central nervous depressants (Senter et al., 1979), as well as omentum (Goldsmith et al., 1975) and neuronal transplants (Kao, 1971). Other investigators improved reliability of the cat contusion model (Dohrmann and Panjabi, 1976a,b; Panjabi et al., 1977; Dohrmann et al., 1978; Ikeda and Yamagata, 1978; Ikeda et al., 1978; Hung et al., 1979; Molt et al., 1979).

In 1971, Osterholm and colleagues (Osterholm et al., 1971; Osterholm and Mathews, 1971a,b, 1972a,b; Osterholm, 1974a,b, 1978) proposed that catecholamine accumulation explains the progressive central hemorrhagic necrosis in the contused cat spinal cord. Catecholamines may influence spinal cord blood flow (Alderman et al., 1980a,b; Martinez et al., 1980; McNicholas et al., 1980). Although subsequent studies (Hedeman and Sil, 1974; Hedeman et al., 1974; Naftchi et al., 1974; Torre et al., 1974; Vise et al., 1974; Bingham, 1975; Bingham et al., 1975a,b; Bunegin et al., 1976a,b; Jonsson and Sachs, 1976; Kidman et al., 1976; Schoultz et al., 1976; Brodner and Dohrmann, 1977; Nemecek et al., 1977b; Rawe et al., 1977a,b; Schoultz, 1977) did not confirm the predicted spinal cord catecholamine changes, this was the first excitotoxic theory of neural injury.

Feline spinal cord contusion models

In the 1980s, the feline spinal cord contusion model dominated the field. Several investigators studied biochemical changes (Jones and Keenan, 1982), free radicals (Milvy et al., 1973; Seligman et al., 1977); prostaglandins (Jonsson and Daniell, 1976), calcium-activated proteases (Banik et al., 1979), loss of myelin proteins (Banik et al., 1980), and extracellular potassium (Young et al., 1982a) and calcium (Young et al., 1982b; Young and Koreh, 1986) changes in contused cat spinal cords. Others focused on physiological responses (Greenhoot et al., 1972; Green et al., 1973) to spinal cord injury, including pressor responses (Rawe et al., 1974, 1978; Rawe and Perot, 1979c), peripheral catecholamines (Tibbs et al., 1979a,b), and spontaneous (Molt et al., 1978) and evoked (Benezech et al., 1979) spinal cord potentials, forelimb somatosensory evoked potentials (Katz et al., 1978), and sensitivity of short-range interneurons to trauma (Benoist et al., 1979). Some examined vascular changes (Tator, 1972; Dohrmann and Allen, 1975; Tsubokawa et al., 1975; Griffiths, 1978; Griffiths et al., 1978a,b; Means et al., 1978), edema (Richardson and Nakamaura, 1971; Lewin et al., 1972, 1974; Nemecek et al., 1977a; Shapiro et al., 1977), blood flow (Griffiths, 1973; Senter and Venes, 1978; Senter et al., 1978; Smith et al., 1978; Lohse et al., 1979, 1980; Cawthon et al., 1980; Dow-Edwards et al., 1980), autoregulation (Senter and Venes, 1979), blood–brain barrier breakdown (Beggs and Waggener, 1975, 1979a,b; Stewart and

Wagner, 1979a,b), and progressive tissue damage (Koenig and Dohrmann, 1977; Balentine, 1978a,b; Wagner et al., 1978), mitochondrial dysfunction (Ito et al., 1978), and metabolic changes (Rawe and Perot, 1979a,b,c; Anderson et al., 1980a,b; Rawe et al., 1981). Blight and Decrescito (1986) did the first quantitative morphometric analyses of contused feline cords and demonstrated how contusion selectively damaged larger myelinated axons (Blight, 1988) and that Schwann cells remyelinate axons in the model (Blight and Young, 1989).

The feline contusion model yielded several therapies that went to clinical trial. Early investigators (Campbell et al., 1973a, 1974; Demopoulos et al., 1978, 1982; Green et al., 1980) had reported that methylprednisolone (MP) improved the histological appearance of the spinal cord and scavenged free radicals, leading to the first clinical trial of MP (Bracken et al., 1985). In 1980/1981, Faden et al. (1980b) and Young et al. (1981) found that the opiate receptor antagonist naloxone improved neurological recovery and spinal cord blood flow in cats after spinal cord contusion (Faden et al., 1980a; Holaday and Faden, 1980). In 1982, Young and Flamm reported that higher doses of MP were necessary to improve blood flow and calcium changes in contused cat spinal cords (Young and Flamm, 1982). Hall and Braughler (Braughler and Hall, 1982; Hall and Braughler, 1982a,b) attributed the beneficial effects of high-dose MP to inhibition of lipid peroxidation (Braughler and Hall, 1983a,b, 1984; Faden et al., 1984; Hall et al., 1984). In 1988, Anderson et al. reported beneficial effects of a 21-aminosteroid antioxidant in the feline contusion model. Meanwhile, Blight and Gruner (Blight and Gruner, 1987; Blight, 1989) showed that the potassium channel blocker 4-aminopyridine (4-AP) improved conduction in chronic spinal injured cats.

In 1990, the second National Acute Spinal Cord Injury Study (NASCIS 2) compared naloxone, MP, and placebo treatment of 487 patients with acute spinal cord injury, showing that early therapy (<8 h) with naloxone improves neurological recovery (Flamm et al., 1985) but that very high doses of MP more significantly improved neurological recovery (Bracken, 1991, 2001, 2002; Bracken et al., 1992; Young and Bracken, 1992; Bracken and Holford, 1993). Tirilazad mesylate likewise was studied in

clinical trial (Bracken et al., 1997) and appeared to be beneficial but not better than MP. Several clinical trials (Hansebout et al., 1993; Hayes et al., 1994; Qiao et al., 1997; Segal and Brunnemann, 1997, 1998; Potter et al., 1998a,b; Segal et al., 1999; Darlington, 2000; Wolfe et al., 2001) have suggested that 4-AP improves motor and sensory function in people with chronic spinal cord injury, although one recent trial (van der Bruggen et al., 2001) suggests that 4-AP does not improve motor or sensory function in patients with chronic incomplete spinal cord injury.

Rat spinal contusion models

In 1985, Wrathall and colleagues (Gale et al., 1985; Noble and Wrathall, 1985; Wolf and Hall, 1985; Wrathall et al., 1985) described morphological and behavioral changes in a rat weight-drop contusion model. The weight-drop device (Noble and Wrathall, 1987) was similar to that used for the feline spinal cord contusion model, i.e. a weight dropped on an impounder placed dorsally onto thoracic spinal cord exposed by laminectomy. Wrathall and colleagues (Kerasidis et al., 1987; Wrathall, 1989) developed a combined behavioral score to assess motor, sensory, and reflex recovery in spinal injured rats, correlating these scores with quantitative axonal counts (Rosenberg and Wrathall, 1997), neuronal and glial loss (Grossman et al., 2001b), and evoked potentials (Raines et al., 1988). Wrathall and colleagues have published many studies using this model, including expression of nerve growth factor (Brunello et al., 1990; Bakhit et al., 1991), basic fibroblast growth factor (Follesa et al., 1994; Mocchetti et al., 1996), interleukin (Wang et al., 1997), myelin gene (Wrathall et al., 1998), AMPA (Grossman et al., 1999) and NMDA receptor subunit (Grossman and Wrathall, 2000; Grossman et al., 2001a; Prybylowski et al., 2001), and p75 receptor (Brandoli et al., 2001). They examined bladder function (Pikov et al., 1998; Pikov and Wrathall, 2001, 2002). They have also tested multiple therapies in the model, including fetal neuronal transplants (Hoovler and Wrathall, 1991), the effects of kynurenate (Wrathall et al., 1992a), non-NMDA receptor blockers (Wrathall et al., 1992b, 1997; Follesa et al., 1998; Rosenberg et al., 1999a), and tetrodotoxin (Teng and Wrathall,

234

1997; Rosenberg et al., 1999b; Rosenberg and Wrathall, 2001), and fibroblast growth factor (Teng et al., 1998).

In 1987, Somerson and Stokes described a feedback controlled electromechanical device that indented the spinal cord at a defined force, duration, and extent (Somerson and Stokes, 1987; Beattie, 1992; Stokes et al., 1992). This device has two levels of indentations that caused mild or moderate injury (Behrmann et al., 1994), producing consistent 3-dimensional morphological (Bresnahan et al., 1991) and locomotor changes (Beattie and Bresnahan, 1989). The device was subsequently used to assess the neuroprotective effects of MP (Behrmann et al., 1994) and other drugs (Behrmann et al., 1993). Stokes and colleagues (Stokes and Reier, 1992; Horner and Stokes, 1995), Reier et al. (1992), and Horner et al. (1996a,b) used this model to study fetal transplants to the spinal cord. The model was also used to assess lipid alterations (Murphy et al., 1994), neurotrophin and cytokine expression (McTigue et al., 1998a,b, 2000, 2001; Streit et al., 1998), MHC class II antigen (Popovich et al., 1993), quinolinic acid levels (Popovich et al., 1994), poly-ADR synthetase (Scott et al., 1999), and blood–brain barrier changes (Popovich et al., 1996) in contused rat spinal cords.

In 1989, we developed a rat contusion model at New York University (Kwo et al., 1989). Initially called the 'NYU Impactor', the model uses a weight-drop device (Gruner, 1992) that differs from previous devices in several respects. First, the Impactor drops a steel rod directly onto T_{13} spinal cord exposed by a T_9–T_{10} laminectomy, achieving more consistent contusions. Second, the device used digital optical potentiometers to measure the trajectory of the falling rod with a precision of ± 20 μm and ± 20 μs, providing accurate ($\pm 1\%$) measurements of the delivered trauma. Third, the impactor measured movement of the spinal column at the impact site, subtracting this movement from the cord movement. Fourth, the device was designed to deliver three levels of injury to rat spinal cord by dropping a 10-g rod 12.5, 25.0, or 50.0 mm onto T_{13} spinal cord (T_9–T_{10} bony level), respectively producing mild, moderate, and severe injury with distinct biochemical, histological, and behavioral changes.

The MASCIS impactor

In 1993, NIH funded the Multicenter Animal Spinal Cord Injury Study (MASCIS), a group of eight spinal cord injury laboratories, to validate and standardize the Impactor model. Fig. 1 shows some views of the Impactor device. The group demonstrated that the Impactor produces consistent spinal cord injuries, reflected in a variety of measures, including extracellular potassium (Chesler et al., 1991, 1994) and calcium (Moriya et al., 1994) shifts, blood gas (Huang and Young, 1994) and glucose changes (Sala et al., 1999), evoked responses (Gruner, 1989; Gruner et al., 1993), spinal cord lesion volumes (Kwo et al., 1989), morphological changes (Beattie et al., 1997), and locomotor recovery (Basso et al., 1996a). The model can reliably detect 10% lesion volume changes with seven rats per treatment group (Constantini and Young, 1994). The MASCIS group standardized the ages of the rats (77 ± 1 day), anesthesia (intraperitoneal pentobarbital 45 mg/kg female and 65 mg/kg male), and injury timing (60 ± 5 min after anesthesia induction). Finally, MASCIS (Basso et al., 1996b) validated the Basso–Beattie–Bresnahan (BBB) locomotor score (Basso et al., 1995), a 21-point ordinal behavioral scale that linearly predicts spinal cord histological changes.

Many laboratories studied spinal cord injury mechanisms and responses in the Impactor model. In 1997, three groups reported two waves of apoptosis in contused rat spinal cords (Crowe et al., 1997; Liu et al., 1997; Shuman et al., 1997; Yong et al., 1998), a first wave of neuronal apoptosis at 2–3 days and a second wave involving oligodendroglial cells at 1–3 weeks. Other investigators characterized gliosis (Baldwin et al., 1998a; Grossman et al., 2001b), oligodendroglial (Frei et al., 2000), vascular (Casella et al., 2002), oxidative stress (Baldwin et al., 1998b), cytoskeletal (Zhang et al., 2000), and even anisotrophic magnetic resonance images (Nevo et al., 2001) of the contused rat spinal cord. Some have studied locomotor (van de Meent et al., 1996; Hamers et al., 2001; Lankhorst et al., 2001), skeletal muscle (Hutchinson et al., 2001), and micturation recovery (Pikov and Wrathall, 2002). Several investigators showed the deleterious effects of combining contusion with compression (Dimar et al., 1999), post-traumatic hypoxia (Yanagawa et al., 2001), and hyperthermia (Yu et al., 2001).

In recent years, many investigators assessed gene expression changes in the rat spinal cord contusion model. These include NF-κB (Bethea et al., 1998b), iNOS and nitrotyrosine (Xu et al., 2001b), protein-1 and metalloproteases (de Castro et al., 2000; Xu et al., 2001a), caspases (Citron et al., 2000a), proteases (Citron et al., 2000b), aggrecan (Lemons et al., 2001), BCL-2 (Lou et al., 1998; Qiu et al., 2001), HLH-Id gene family (Tzeng et al., 2001), glutamate receptors (Grossman et al., 1999, 2001a), glucocorticoid receptor (Yan et al., 2001), and Trk receptor (Liebl et al., 2001) expression. Carmel et al. (2001) and Song et al. (2001) carried out the first large-scale gene expression studies in the model.

The model has also been extensively used to test therapies. Lindsey et al. (2000) and Hulsebosch and colleagues (Hulsebosch et al., 2000; Mills et al., 2001b,c) described neuropathic pain behavior and assessed the effects of glutamate receptor blockers (Mills et al., 2001a,d, 2002) and cyclooxygenase inhibitors (Hains et al., 2001) on the neuropathic pain behavior. The model has been used to study cell transplants, including Schwann (Martin et al., 1996), embryonic stem (Liu et al., 2000; Cao et al., 2001) and human fetal cells (Giovanini et al., 1997). Other therapies that have been tested in the model include neutrophil elastase inhibitors (Tonai et al., 2001), IL-6 receptor antagonists (Nesic et al., 2001), hypothermia (Chatzipanteli et al., 2000; Dimar et al., 2000; Yu et al., 2000), riluzole and MP (Mu et al., 2000), VIP and adenyl cyclase activating peptide (Kim et al., 2000), gacyclidine (Feldblum et al., 2000), bFGF (Lee et al., 1999; Rabchevsky et al., 1999, 2000), cyclosporin (Rabchevsky et al., 2001), COX-2 inhibitors (Resnick et al., 1998), progesterone (Thomas et al., 1999), IL-10 (Bethea et al., 1998a, 1999; Plunkett et al., 2001), and myelin-basic protein vaccine (Hauben et al., 2000; Hamers et al., 2001).

Contusion mechanisms

The mechanisms of contusion-induced spinal cord injury are still widely misunderstood. The spinal cord is generally quite tolerant of slow compression and stretching. It can be deformed by a third of its diameter or stretched to a third greater length without significant damage if the deformation is done slowly.

However, prolonged or rapid mechanical deformations of the cord damage the cord. Prolonged (20–30 min) compression causes infarcts in the spinal cord. Rapid indentation or stretching of the spinal cord likewise will damage cells that have been deformed beyond a critical velocity.

Blight (1988) examined the mechanical factors that causes axonal damage in contused spinal cords. He noted that indentation moves the contents of a gel-filled tube longitudinally. The greatest movement centered in the middle of the tube. Blight and Decrescito (1986) had earlier observed that large myelinated axons are most vulnerable to contusion injury and that axons closest to the pial surface are most likely to survive a contusion. This pattern of axonal damage differs significantly from slow compression or ischemia-induced spinal cord injuries that tend to damage small unmyelinated axons and preserve larger myelinated axons.

Myelinated axons are vulnerable to mechanical stretching because the myelin concentrates stretch at the nodes of Ranvier (Maxwell, 1996). Axons break at critical velocities of 0.5–1.0 m/s (Gennarelli et al., 1993). Subcritical velocities also may damage axons by increasing calcium entry through tetrodotoxin-sensitive channels (Wolf et al., 2001) and consequent secondary reactions due to the calcium entry (Maxwell et al., 1997). Microtubule disruptions tend to be localized to the nodal region (Wolf et al., 2001). In contrast, small axons are sensitive to ischemia because they have the largest surface to volume ratio. They are most exposed to extracellular ionic shifts and other toxic effects of ischemia.

Indentation of the spinal cord causes tissue to move rostrally and caudally. Fig. 2 illustrates the tissue movements in a spinal cord contusion. Tissue movements are greatest in the middle of the tube. The movement is less at the surface of the tube and declines with distance from the indentation site. This longitudinal tissue movement shears cells in the gray matter and stretches axons in the white matter. When these longitudinal movements exceed a critical velocity of 0.5–1.0 m/s, large myelinated axons will break at the nodes of Ranvier. This explains the pattern of central hemorrhagic necrosis and progressive centrifugal and longitudinal distribution of tissue damage that occur in contused spinal cord, regardless of the direction of the contusion.

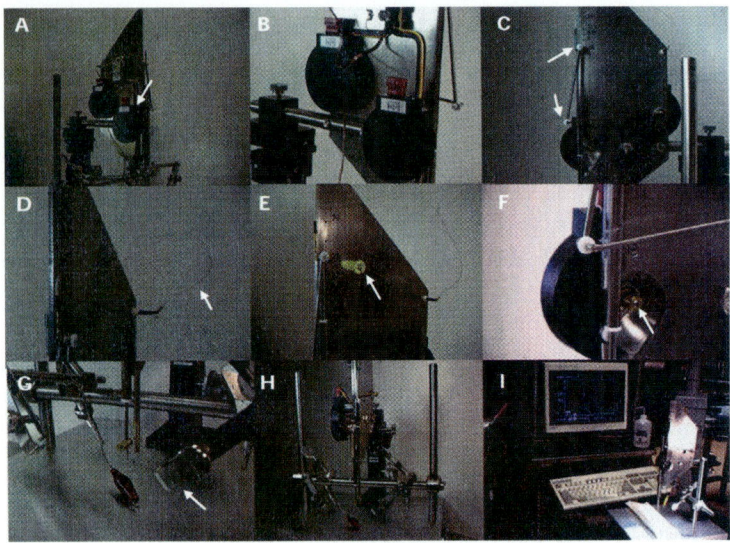

Fig. 1. The Impactor. (A) The digital optical potentiometers (arrow). (B) A close-up of the two digital optical potentiometers. (C) The direct mechanical linkage between the impactor rod and the digital optical potentiometers. (D) The thin wire that completes the circuit when the rod touches the spinal cord. (E) The pin that holds the impactor rod in the 'up' position. (F) The axle for the digital optical potentiometer that senses vertebral movements. (G) The ground clip (red) and one of the vertebral clamps (arrow). (H) The Impactor from the front. (I) The Impactor in the operating room with a graph of the Impactor trajectory on the monitor.

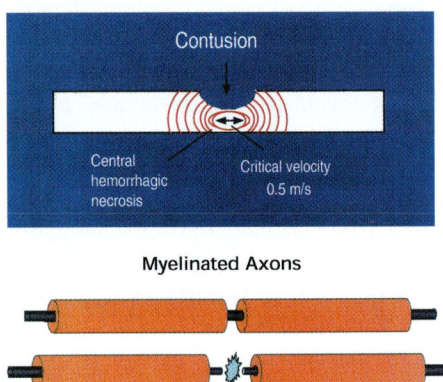

Fig. 2. Spinal cord contusion. When the spinal cord is contused, the tissue can only move longitudinally away from the indentation. The greatest movement is in the center of the cord at the indentation site. When the velocity of the tissue movement exceeds a critical velocity of about 0.5 m/s, cells break, resulting in central hemorrhagic necrosis. The bottom panel shows myelinated axons that the tendency of stretched axons to break at the node of Ranvier, explaining why larger myelinated axons are most vulnerable to contusion injury.

Note that a weight dropped 12.5, 25.0, and 50.0 mm will have terminal velocities close to 0.5, 0.7, and 1 m/s.

Cell volume fraction

To assess the relationship of mechanical parameters and tissue damage, we developed a method to measure cell loss quantitatively and efficiently in rat spinal cords (Constantini and Young, 1994). This method is based on the known distribution of potassium (K) and sodium (Na) ions in nervous tissues. Normally, intracellular K concentration $[K]_i$ is high (124 mM) compared to extracellular K concentration $[K]_e$ (4 mM). In contrast, intracellular Na concentration $[Na]_i$ is low (25 mM) compared to extracellular Na concentration $[Na]_e$ (145 mM). Therefore, highly cellular tissues should have high total K concentrations $[K]_t$ and low total Na concentrations $[Na]_t$. When cells die, they become part of extracellular space and extracellular Na and K equilibrate rapidly with blood and surrounding tissues. Thus, injured tissues should have lower $[K]_t$ and higher $[Na]_t$.

The Na and K levels in tissue are expressed by the following equation:

$$[Na]_t - [K]_t = [Na]_e - [K]_e + 2G \cdot V_i / V_t$$

where $[Na]_t$ and $[K]_t$ are total tissue Na and K concentrations, $[Na]_e$ and $[K]_e$ are extracellular,

$G = [Na]_i - [Na]_e = [K]_e - [K]_i$ or the average ionic gradient across cell members, and V_i/V_t is the ratio of intracellular and tissue volume or the cell volume fraction. The only assumptions used in the derivation of this equation are $[Na]_t + [K]_t = [Na]_e + [K]_e = [Na]_i + [K]_i$, and $V_t = V_i + V_e$. This equation states that the difference of total tissue Na and K concentrations is linearly related to V_i/V_t with a slope of $2G$ and a y-intercept of the difference of extracellular Na and K concentrations. G is approximately -120 mM and since $[Na]_e$ and $[K]_e$ equilibrate rapidly with blood, V_i/V_t can be calculated from $[Na]_t - [K]_t$.

As shown in Fig. 3, impact site Na–K concentrations steadily increased with greater heights of dropping a 10-g rod 12.5, 25.0, 50.0, and 75.0 mm onto the T_{13} spinal cord. The changes were very consistent from rat to rat. Fig. 4 shows a separate experiment where histologically measured tissue damage was correlated with Na–K concentrations in the spinal cord. Histological and ionic cell volume fractions correlated linearly. Measuring tissue Na and K is much more efficient than histological assessments of the spinal cord and provides data that linearly predict tissue damage in the spinal cord.

To estimate spinal cord lesion volumes, we calculate the cell volume fractions of five tissue samples. Each sample is 5-mm long. One sample is centered on the impact site (Imp). P1 and P2 are proximal while D1 and D2 are distal to Imp. The difference in cell volume fraction from normal (0.75) gives the percent loss of cell volume. We then multiply percent cell loss with tissue wet weight in mg, to estimate the volume (μl) of cells lost from each sample. The sum of cell volumes lost from the five samples gives the lesion volume. This approach towards measuring lesion volume is very efficient, requiring measurement of only wet weights and measurements of total Na and K concentrations of five tissue samples.

Impact parameters

The Impactor precisely records the trajectory of a falling rod, estimating the impact velocity from the slope of the trajectory during the 2 ms before the rod contacts the cord. It also measures the cord compression depth (C_d) and the cord compression time (C_t), estimating the average cord compression rate or $C_r = C_d/C_t$. The device also measures the movement of the spinal column at the impact site and corrects the cord compression for vertebral movement. The measurements accurately represent the extent, duration, and rate of cord compression resulting from the weight-drop contusion. Fig. 5 displays the trajectory of the weight drop onto the spinal cord.

The impact velocity represents what the Impactor delivers to the spinal cord. A weight dropped from heights of 12.5, 25.0, and 50.0 mm should achieve impact velocities of about 0.49, 0.70, and 0.97 m/s. Substantial deviations from these velocities would suggest problems with the Impactor. In contrast, C_d, C_t, and C_r reflect the mechanical properties of the spinal cord in addition to the impact velocity. For example, if the impactor is not centered, both C_d and C_t may be shorter. Likewise, if the spinal column is not well clamped, C_t may be longer although C_d may not change much since the Impactor subtracts vertebral movement from the cord movement. Thus, these impact parameters provide a useful and accurate record of trauma delivery to the spinal cord.

The mass of the falling weight has relatively little effect on C_r. The Impactor uses a 10-g rod. A rod mass of 10 g is about 286,000 times greater than the mass of the spinal cord at the impact site (35 mg). The C_r/Imp_V ratio is typically about 0.90. With sufficient mass, C_r should not differ from impact velocity. For example, doubling the mass to 20 g will increase the C_r/Imp_V ratio slightly. However, increasing the mass will increase the cord compression distance (C_d) and time (C_t).

Cord compression rate correlates linearly with behavioral recovery and tissue damage in the spinal cord. Fig. 6 shows an experiment where three groups of seven rats were injured with a 12.5, 25.0, and 50.0 mm weight drop. The rats injured with the 12.5 mm weight drop recovered hindlimb stepping, attaining BBB scores of 14 (hindlimb stepping with one-to-one coordination with forelimb stepping). However, the rats injured with 25.0 and 50.0 mm weight drops had average BBB scores of less than 9 (ability to stand but not step). The BBB scores at 2, 4, and 6 weeks correlated linearly with C_r with correlation coefficients of 0.66–0.79. Likewise, % white matter sparing correlated linearly with C_r with a correlation coefficient of 0.82; % sparing also correlated with BBB scores. Thus, these three parameters linearly predict each other.

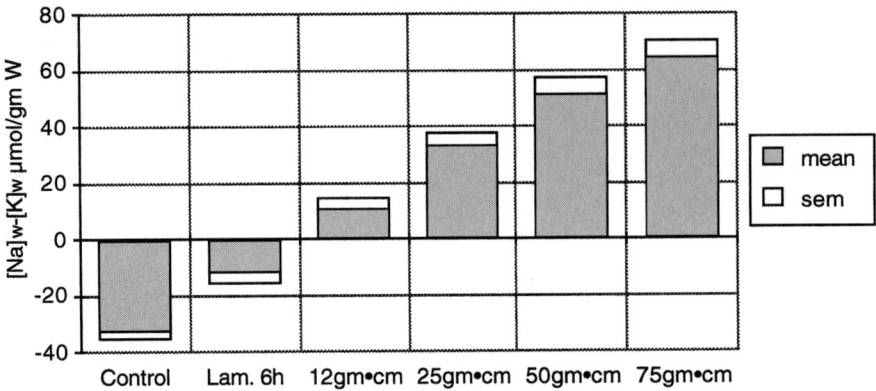

Fig. 3. Na–K concentrations at the T_{13} impact site of uninjured rat spinal cords (Control), 6 h after laminectomy (Lam. 6h), and 6 h after laminectomy and contusion with a 10-g rod dropped 12.5 mm (12 gm·cm), 25.0 mm (25 gm·cm), 50.0 mm (50 gm·cm), and 75.0 mm (75 gm·cm). The values are means from six rats each with standard errors of means (S.E.M.). Note the increasing value of Na–K with greater damage.

Anesthetic considerations

When the Impactor model was first being developed, the MASCIS group had intense debates about which anesthesia to use. Some investigators favored gaseous anesthesia such as halothane and isoflurane while others favored systemically administered drugs such as pentobarbital, ketamine and xylazine, or chloral hydrate. In the end, MASCIS decided to use intraperitoneally administered pentobarbital because dosage of a systematically injected drug is easier to control and monitor than a gaseous anesthesia. We avoided ketamine because it is a glutamate receptor blocker and may have neuroprotective effects. However, it is important to point out all anesthetic agents are likely to affect the response of the animal to spinal cord injury. There is no 'perfect' anesthesia.

Male and female rats require very different doses of pentobarbital. We titrated intraperitoneal doses of pentobarbital required to produce 2–3 h of anesthesia in male and female rats. The effective intraperitoneal doses of pentobarbital were 45 mg/kg for females and 65 mg/kg for male rats. Failure to recognize sex differences in anesthesia dosing has led to overdose of females and inadequate anesthesia of male rats in many laboratories. The protocol allows an additional 5 mg/kg of pentobarbital to be given to rats that are not deeply anesthetized within 5 min after the initial bolus. However, if a rat is still not anesthetized within 10 min after the second dose, they should not be used for the experiment since further doses

will lead to respiratory depression and prolonged anesthesia.

Pentobarbital causes respiratory depression. Arterial blood gases within normal ranges (pO_2 of 60–100 mm Hg, pCO_2 of 25–45 mm Hg, and pH of 7.3–7.4) have little effect on spinal cord lesion volumes (Huang and Young, 1994). However, pH below 7.3 may be associated with significantly smaller lesion volumes, while pO_2 of less than 60 mm Hg may be associated with significantly bigger spinal cord lesion volumes. Both of these conditions can be avoided by observing the color of the rats' feet. As long as they are pink, both arterial blood pH and pO_2 levels were in the normal range. When they are pale or dusky, the rats need tracheal suction to remove secretion and stimulate respiration.

To ensure uniformity of blood pentobarbital levels at the time of injury, the Impactor model stipulates that rats are contused at 60 ± 5 min after induction of anesthesia. In unpublished studies of the effect of injury timing, rats contused with a 25-mm weight at 45 min had a 20% greater lesion volume that rats contused at 75 min. These results are surprising because one might expect anesthesia to depress neurotransmitter release and to be neuroprotective. However, pentobarbital does depress metabolism, blood pressure, blood flow, and other physiological parameters that may influence the response of the spinal cord to contusion.

Anesthesia is an intrinsic part of the spinal cord injury model. Since we cannot avoid anesthesia, our

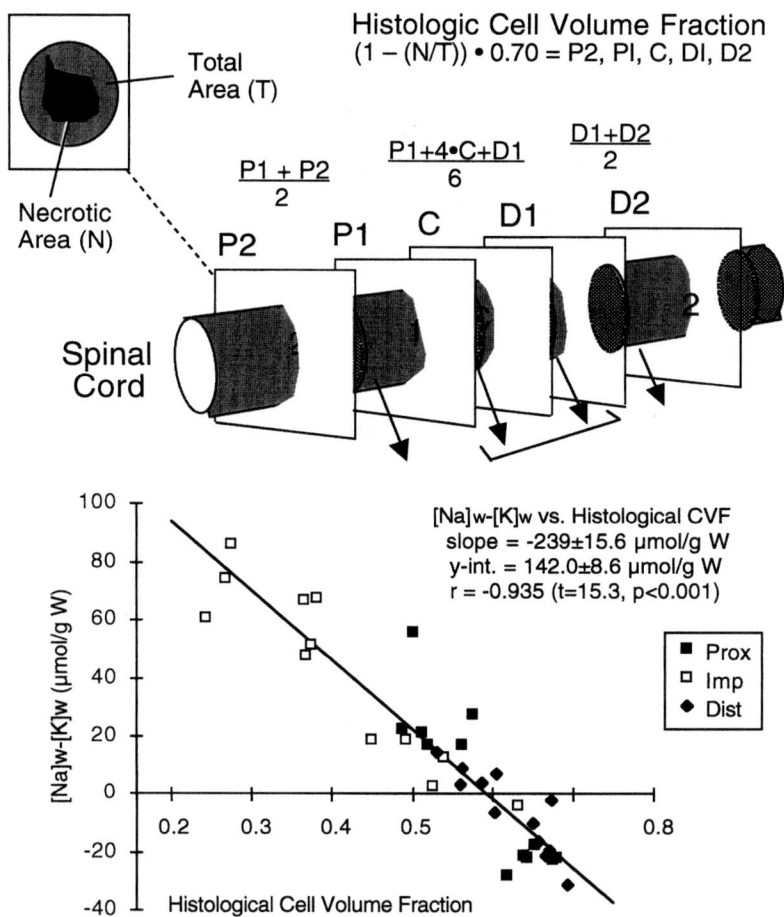

Fig. 4. Ionic and histological cell volume fractions. Three groups of four rats were contused with a 10-g rod dropped 12.5, 25.0 and 50.0 mm on the T_{13} cord. The spinal cords were frozen and coronal sections were obtained at 0, ±2, ±6 and ±10 mm from the impact center. Histological cell volume fractions were estimated from ratios of necrotic (N) to total tissue (T) area in each section, i.e. 1-(N/T) 0.70, averaged, and compared with Na–K measured from tissues between sections. The value of 0.70 is the assumed 'normal' extracellular cell volume fraction in spinal white matter. The two measures correlated well ($r = -0.935$, slope $= -239 \pm 15.6$, y-intercept 142.0 ± 8.6).

goal was to make anesthesia as consistent as possible and to minimize anesthesia side effects. Because response to anesthesia is influenced by sex, the model defines different doses for males and females, based on duration of anesthesia. Finally, although other spinal cord injury models have standardized anesthetic dose, none stipulate timing of the injury after induction of anesthesia.

Age and body weights

Male and female rats grow at different rates, as illustrated in Fig. 7. Although both male and female rats start out at similar body weights at 50 days, males grow 3–4 times faster than females. Linear regression indicates that male rat grows at the rate of about 2 g/day from 50 to 275 days of age while females gained weight at only 0.6 g/day. The females reach a plateau of 340 g between 125 and 275 days old while the male rats continue to grow, reaching 600 g by 200 days. If we select rats by body weight, female rats could be quite old while all the male rats would be young.

Rat spinal cord size varies as a function of rat age and not body weight. To assess spinal cord size, we collected 4-mm spinal cord samples from the

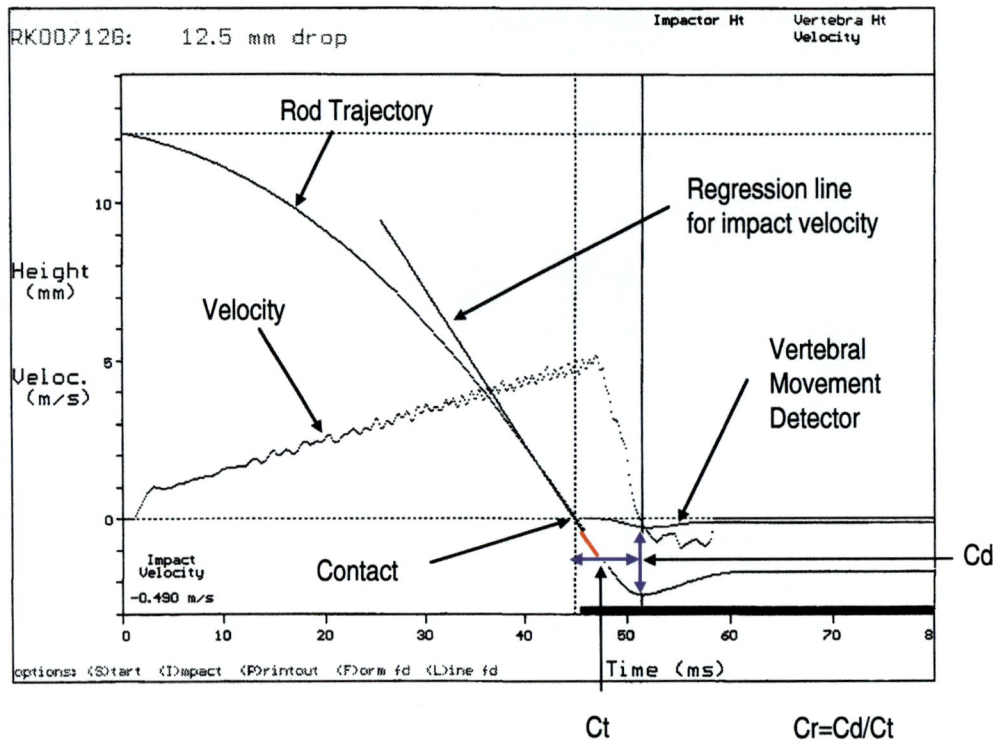

Fig. 5. Impactor trajectory. This picture of a printout from the Impactor shows the trajectory of the 10-g rod falling from 12.5 mm height, hitting a wet sponge at about 45 ms later (Contact), compressing the sponge by about 2.5 mm (Cd) at 7 ms after contact (Ct). The Impactor program automatically does a linear regression from the trajectory 2 ms before contact to obtain the impact velocity (-0.490 m/s).

T_{13} impact site. Since the lengths of the samples were the same, the wet and dry weights of the samples should have reflected changes in the cord size. Typical sample weights ranged from 25–40 mg wet weight and 6–12 mg dry weight. We obtained the latter by drying the tissue samples in a vacuum oven overnight. As shown in Fig. 8, in both male and female rats, cord weights were similar when they were plotted against age but not when they were plotted against body size. Since spinal cord size affects the mechanical characteristics of the spinal cord, we elected to use age as the primary selection criterion for the rats. At 77 days of age, the wet and dry spinal cord sizes in male and females were the most similar.

To assess the effect of spinal cord size, age, sex, and body weight on impact parameters, we studied five groups of rats, summarized in Table I. Group A were young (75 ± 2 days) female rats that weighed 248 ± 2 g. Group B were older (184 ± 7 days) females that weighed 333 ± 2 g. Group C were juvenile (53 ± 1 days) males that weighed 245 ± 2 g. Group D were young (69 ± 2 days) males that weighed 339 ± 2 g. Group E were old (233 ± 9 days) males that weighed 630 ± 8 g. As shown in Fig. 9, the slopes of Imp_V and C_r approached 0.5 in all groups except for E (large and old rats) where the slope was 0.3. Groups A, C, and D showed the best correlation coefficients ($r = 0.88 - 0.91$) between Imp_V and Cr. Groups B and E (older females and males) had worse correlation coefficients ($r = 0.58 - 0.84$).

We thus chose 77 ± 1 days of age as the entry criterion for the model instead of body weight. An age criterion has several other advantages over a body weight criterion. First, a 77-day-old rat is an older juvenile or young adult. The most common age of spinal cord injury in humans is 19 years in the United States. Second, at 77 days, male rats are typically 350 g while females are 250 g. In older animals, at 100 days for example, the body

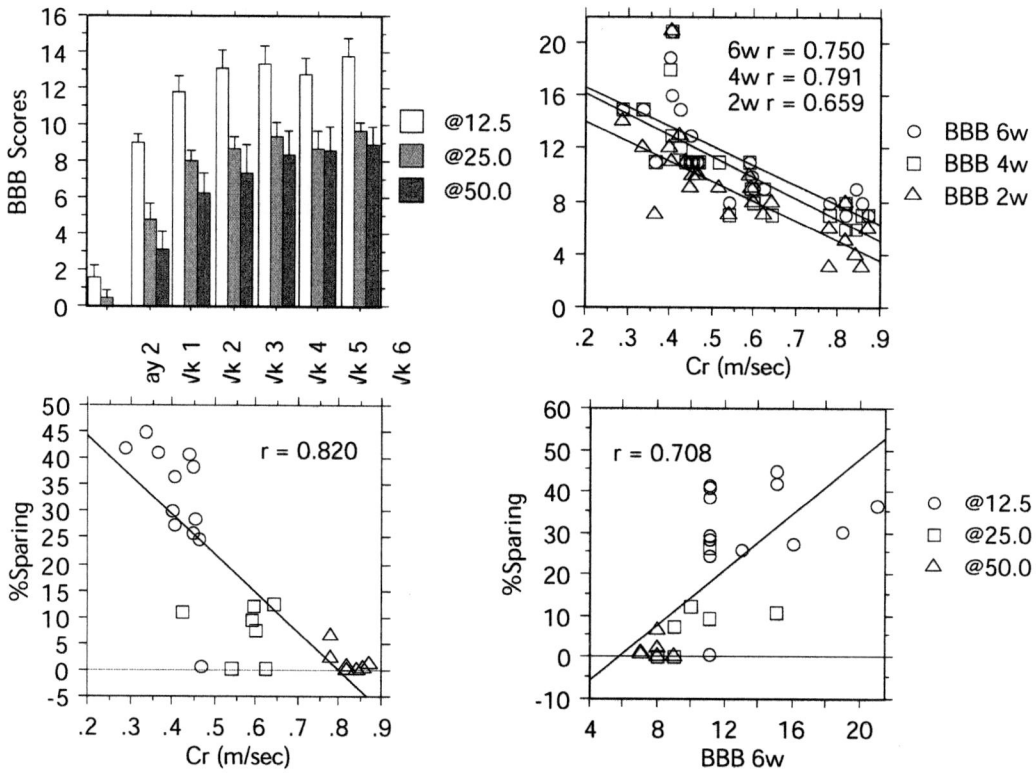

Fig. 6. Three-way correlation between locomotor recovery (BBB Scores), percent white matter sparing (% sparing), and cord compression rate (Cr). The upper left panel shows the mean and standard deviations of 6-week BBB scores from rats injured with a 12.5, 25.0, and 50.0 mm weight drop. Note the big difference between 12.5 and 25.0 mm injuries but not between the 25.0 and 50.0 mm. The BBB score at 2, 4, and 6 weeks correlated linearly with BBB scores (top right panel). % Sparing also correlated linearly with cord compression rate (Cr, m/sec). Likewise, % sparing correlated linearly with 6-week BBB scores.

TABLE I

Preinjury variables

Variables	A	B	C	D	E
n	30	33	30	31	10
Sex (M/F)	F	F	M	M	M
Age (days)	75 ± 2 [b]	184 ± 7 [c]	53 ± 1 [a]	69 ± 2 [b]	233 ± 9 [d]
PreW (g)	248 ± 2 [a]	333 ± 2 [b]	245 ± 2 [a]	339 ± 2 [b]	630 ± 8 [c]
PreBP (mm)	69 ± 4 [b,c]	79 ± 5 [c]	60 ± 3 [a,b]	68 ± 4 [b,c]	48 ± 4 [a]
InjBP (mm)	157 ± 7 [b]	170 ± 8 [b]	132 ± 5 [a]	156 ± 7 [b]	130 ± 6 [a]
PostBP (mm)	96 ± 3 [b,c]	104 ± 4 [c]	83 ± 4 [a,b]	91 ± 6 [a,b,c]	81 ± 6 [a]
pH (log units)	$7.359 \pm .004$ [a]	$7.350 \pm .005$ [a]	$7.394 \pm .006$ [b]	$7.389 \pm .008$ [b]	$7.406 \pm .010$ [b]
PaO_2 (mm)	83.7 ± 1.9 [a]	80.0 ± 1.8 [a]	77.7 ± 2.0 [a]	80.1 ± 2.6 [a]	78.0 ± 3.3 [a]
$PaCO_2$ (mm)	44.9 ± 0.7 [b]	39.8 ± 1.8 [a]	39.7 ± 1.5 [a]	39.0 ± 1.2 [a]	38.6 ± 1.7 [a]
H_2CO_3 (mM)	24.2 ± 0.2 [b]	21.2 ± 0.8 [a]	24.5 ± 0.5 [b]	24.0 ± 0.6 [b]	24.7 ± 0.6 [b]
Base excess	0.37 ± 0.29 [b]	-2.70 ± 0.89 [a]	0.37 ± 0.70 [b]	-0.78 ± 0.76 [a,b]	-0.09 ± 0.83 [b]
$O_{2_{sat}}$ (%)	95.6 ± 0.2 [a]	94.9 ± 0.3 [a]	95.0 ± 0.3 [a]	95.1 ± 0.5 [a]	95.3 ± 0.5 [a]

The mean and standard errors preinjury age (days), body weight (PreW, g), mean arterial pressure (MAP), arterial pH, PaO_2, $PaCO_2$, and H_2CO_3 are listed by group. The lowercase letters indicate significance groupings by Duncan's multiple range test: groups with the same letters do not differ significantly from each other, while groups with different letters differ significantly from each other ($P < 0.05$).

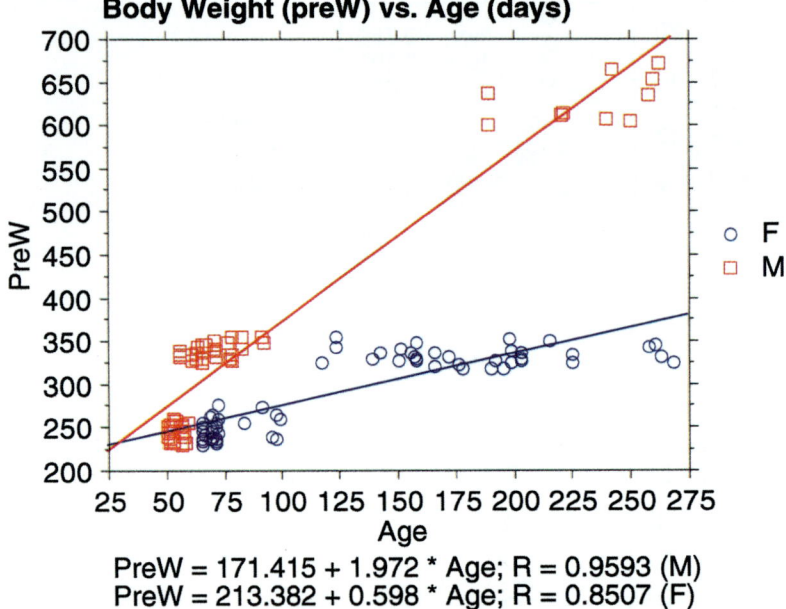

PreW = 171.415 + 1.972 * Age; R = 0.9593 (M)
PreW = 213.382 + 0.598 * Age; R = 0.8507 (F)

Fig. 7. Body weight versus age (days) of Long–Evan hooded rats. Male rats (squares) grow 3–4 times faster than females (circles). Linear regression indicates females have a slope of 0.6 g/day of age while males have a slope of 2.0 g/day.

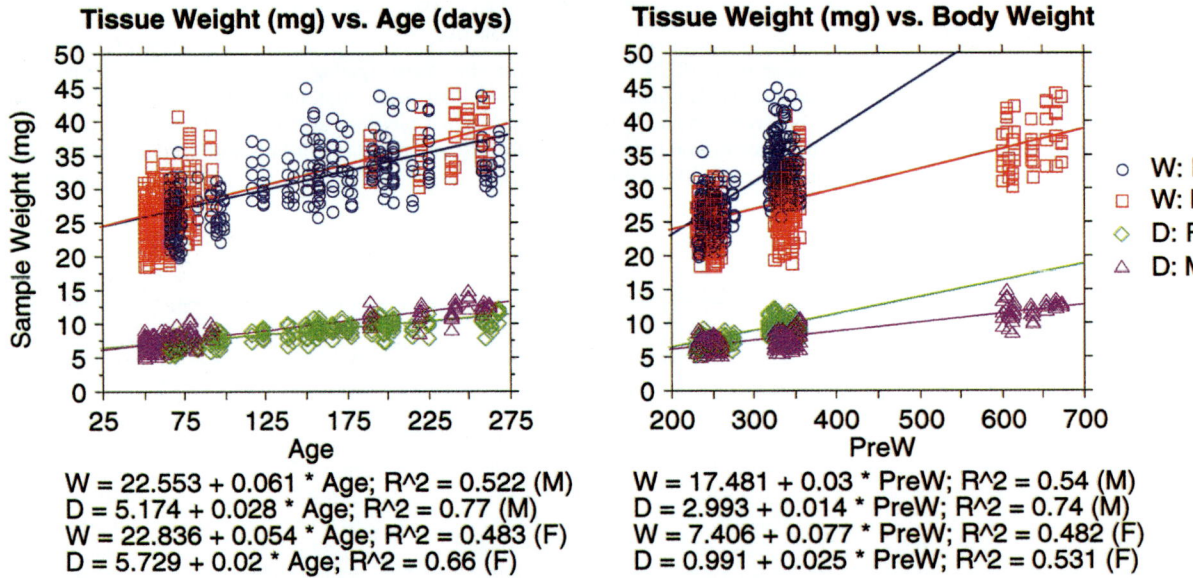

W = 22.553 + 0.061 * Age; R^2 = 0.522 (M)
D = 5.174 + 0.028 * Age; R^2 = 0.77 (M)
W = 22.836 + 0.054 * Age; R^2 = 0.483 (F)
D = 5.729 + 0.02 * Age; R^2 = 0.66 (F)

W = 17.481 + 0.03 * PreW; R^2 = 0.54 (M)
D = 2.993 + 0.014 * PreW; R^2 = 0.74 (M)
W = 7.406 + 0.077 * PreW; R^2 = 0.482 (F)
D = 0.991 + 0.025 * PreW; R^2 = 0.531 (F)

Fig. 8. Spinal cord weight versus age and body weight. The two graphs show the relationship between spinal cord sample wet and dry weight in mg plotted against Age (days) or PreW (body weight, g). The spinal cord samples were obtained from rats that ranged from 50 to 275 days. Each sample was 4 mm in length centered on T_{13}. All the rats received 25 mm weight drop injuries and the samples were obtained at 24 h after injury. Tissue sample dry weights were obtained by drying the samples overnight at 95°C in a vacuum oven.

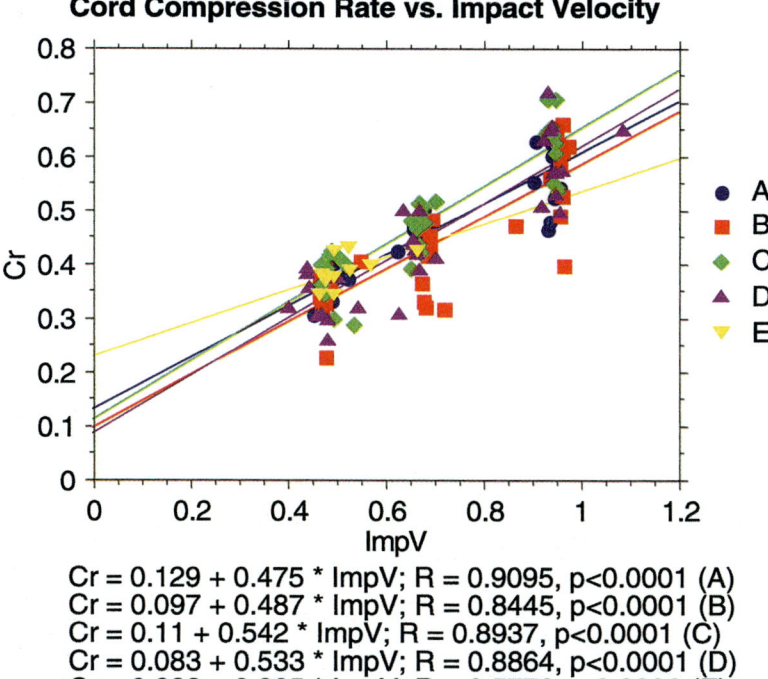

Cord Compression Rate vs. Impact Velocity

Cr = 0.129 + 0.475 * ImpV; R = 0.9095, p<0.0001 (A)
Cr = 0.097 + 0.487 * ImpV; R = 0.8445, p<0.0001 (B)
Cr = 0.11 + 0.542 * ImpV; R = 0.8937, p<0.0001 (C)
Cr = 0.083 + 0.533 * ImpV; R = 0.8864, p<0.0001 (D)
Cr = 0.228 + 0.305 * ImpV; R = 0.5778 p=0.0802 (E)

Fig. 9. Cord compression rate (Cr) and impact velocities (ImpV) from the five groups of rats described in Table I. The rats were contused with a 12.5, 25.0, and 50.0 mm weight drop. Both Cr and ImpV have units of m/s. Linear regression analyses give the slopes and y-intercepts of Cr vs. ImpV.

weights will be much more discrepant. Third, it is easier to plan the experiments around age rather than body weights. Finally, if we choose a body weight criterion of 250 g, males would be too young (50–60 days) while the females would be older (70–100 days). In contrast, a body weight criterion of 350 g may lead to very discrepant ages of males (50–100 days) and females (125–275 days).

Summary and conclusions

Most human spinal cord injuries involve contusions of the spinal cord. Many investigators have long used weight-drop contusion animal models to study the pathophysiology and genetic responses of spinal cord injury. All spinal cord injury therapies tested to date in clinical trial were validated in such models. In recent years, the trend has been towards use of rats for spinal cord injury studies. The MASCIS Impactor is a well-standardized rat spinal cord contusion model that produces very consistent graded spinal cord damage that linearly predicts 24-h lesion volumes, 6-week white matter sparing, and locomotor recovery in rats. All aspects of the model, including anesthesia for male and female rats, age rather than body weight criteria, and arterial blood gases were empirically selected to enhance the consistency of injury.

References

Albin, M.S., White, R.J., Acosta-Rua, G. and Yashon, D. (1968a) Study of functional recovery produced by delayed localized cooling after spinal cord injury in primates. *J. Neurosurg.*, 29: 113–120.

Albin, M.S., White, R.J., Yashon, D. and Massopust Jr., L.C. (1968b) Functional and electrophysiologic limitations of delayed spinal cord cooling after impact injury. *Surg. Forum*, 19: 423–424.

Albin, M.S., White, R.J., Yashon, D. and Harris, L.S. (1969) Effects of localized cooling on spinal cord trauma. *J. Trauma*, 9: 1000–1008.

Alderman, J.L., Osterholm, J.L., D'Amore, B.R. and Williams, H.D. (1980a) Catecholamine alterations attending spinal cord injury: a reanalysis. *Neurosurgery*, 6: 412–417.

Alderman, J.L., Osterholm, J.L., D'Amore, B.R., Williams, H.D. and Irvin, J.D. (1980b) The influence of the adrenal glands upon acute spinal cord injury. *Life Sci.*, 26: 1627–1632.

Allen, A.R. (1911) Surgery of experimental lesion of spinal cord equivalent to crush injury of fracture dislocation of spinal column. A preliminary report. *J. Am. Med. Assoc.*, 57: 878–880.

Allen, A.R. (1914) Remarks on histopathological changes in spinal cord due to impact: an experimental study. *J. Nerv. Ment. Dis.*, 41: 141–147.

Anderson, D.K., Means, E.D. and Waters, T.R. (1980a) Spinal cord energy metabolism in normal and post laminectomy cats. *J. Neurosurg.*, 52: 387–391.

Anderson, D.K., Means, E.D., Waters, T.R. and Spears, C.J. (1980b) Spinal cord energy metabolism following compression trauma to the feline spinal cord. *J. Neurosurg.*, 53: 375–380.

Anderson, D.K., Braughler, J.M., Hall, E.D., Waters, T.R., McCall, J.M. and Means, E.D. (1988) Effects of treatment with u-74006f on neurological outcome following experimental spinal cord injury. *J. Neurosurg.*, 69: 562–567.

Assenmacher, D.R. and Ducker, T.B. (1971) Experimental traumatic paraplegia. The vascular and pathological changes seen in reversible and irreversible spinal cord lesions. *J. Bone Joint Surg. (Am.)*, 53: 671–680.

Bakhit, C., Armanini, M., Wong, W.L., Bennett, G.L. and Wrathall, J.R. (1991) Increase in nerve growth factor-like immunoreactivity and decrease in choline acetyltransferase following contusive spinal cord injury. *Brain Res.*, 554: 264–271.

Baldwin, S.A., Broderick, R., Blades, D.A. and Scheff, S.W. (1998a) Alterations in temporal/spatial distribution of GFAP— and vimentin-positive astrocytes after spinal cord contusion with the New York University spinal cord injury device. *J. Neurotrauma*, 15: 1015–1026.

Baldwin, S.A., Broderick, R., Osbourne, D., Waeg, G., Blades, D.A. and Scheff, S.W. (1998b) The presence of 4-hydroxynonenal/protein complex as an indicator of oxidative stress after experimental spinal cord contusion in a rat model. *J. Neurosurg.*, 88: 874–883.

Balentine, J.D. (1978a) Pathology of experimental spinal cord trauma. I. The necrotic lesion as a function of vascular injury. *Lab. Invest.*, 39: 236–253.

Balentine, J.D. (1978b) Pathology of experimental spinal cord trauma. II. Ultrastructure of axons and myelin. *Lab. Invest.*, 39: 254–255.

Banik, N.L., Powers, J.M. and Smith, K.P. (1979) Ca^{2+} activated neutral proteinase in normal and traumatized spinal cord. *Soc. Neurosci. Abstr.*, 5: 396.

Banik, N.L., Powers, J.M. and Hogan, E.L. (1980) The effects of spinal cord trauma on myelin. *J. Neuropathol. Exp. Neurol.*, 39: 232–244.

Basso, D.M., Beattie, M.S. and Bresnahan, J.C. (1995) A sensitive and reliable locomotor rating scale for open field testing in rats. *J. Neurotrauma*, 12: 1–21.

Basso, D.M., Beattie, M.S. and Bresnahan, J.C. (1996a) Graded histological and locomotor outcomes after spinal cord contusion using the NYU weight-drop device versus transection. *Exp. Neurol.*, 139: 244–256.

Basso, D.M., Beattie, M.S., Bresnahan, J.C., Anderson, D.K., Faden, A.I., Gruner, J.A., Holford, T.R., Hsu, C.Y., Noble, L.J., Nockels, R., Perot, P.L., Salzman, S.K. and Young, W. (1996b) MASCIS evaluation of open field locomotor scores: effects of experience and teamwork on reliability. Multicenter Animal Spinal Cord Injury Study. *J. Neurotrauma*, 13: 343–359.

Beattie, M.S. (1992) Anatomic and behavioral outcome after spinal cord injury produced by a displacement controlled impact device. *J. Neurotrauma*, 9: 157–160.

Beattie, M.S. and Bresnahan, J.C. (1989) Longitudinal assessment of recovery of locomotor function in rats after feedback-controlled spinal cord impact lesions. In: M. Brown and M.E. Goldberger (Eds.), *Criteria for Assessing Recovery of Function: Behavioral Methods*. American Paralysis Association, Springfield, NJ, pp. 16–25.

Beattie, M.S., Bresnahan, J.C., Komon, J., Tovar, C.A., Van Meter, M., Anderson, D.K., Faden, A.I., Hsu, C.Y., Noble, L.J., Salzman, S. and Young, W. (1997) Endogenous repair after spinal cord contusion injuries in the rat. *Exp. Neurol.*, 148: 453–463.

Beggs, J.L. and Waggener, J.D. (1975) Vasogenic edema in the injured spinal cord: a method of evaluating the extent of blood–brain barrier alteration to horseradish peroxidase. *Exp. Neurol.*, 49: 86–96.

Beggs, J.L. and Waggener, J.D. (1979a) The acute microvascular responses to spinal cord injury. *Adv. Neurol.*, 22: 179–189.

Beggs, J.L. and Waggener, J.D. (1979b) Microvascular regeneration following spinal cord injury: the growth sequence and permeability properties of new vessels. *Adv. Neurol.*, 22: 191–206.

Behrmann, D.L., Bresnahan, J.C. and Beattie, M.S. (1993) A comparison of YM-14673, U-50488H, and nalmefene after spinal cord injury in the rat. *Exp. Neurol.*, 119: 258–267.

Behrmann, D.L., Bresnahan, J.C. and Beattie, M.S. (1994) Modeling of acute spinal cord injury in the rat: neuroprotection and enhanced recovery with methylprednisolone, U-74006F and YM-14673. *Exp. Neurol.*, 126: 61–75.

Benezech, J., Flamm, E.S., Frerebeau, P., Privat, J.M. and Gros, C. (1979) Electrophysiological changes in experimental spinal cord trauma. *Acta Neurochir. Suppl.*, 28: 596–598.

Benoist, G., Kausz, M., Rethelyi, M. and Pasztor, E. (1979) Sensitivity of the short range spinal interneurones of the cat to experimental spinal cord trauma. *J. Neurosurg.*, 51: 834–840.

Bethea, J.R., Castro, M., Bricenco, C., Gomez, F., Marcillo, A.E. and Dietrich, D.W. (1998a) Systemically administered interleukin-10 (IL-10) attenuates injury induced inflammation and is neuroprotective following traumatic spinal cord injury. *J. Neurotrauma*, 15: 906.

Bethea, J.R., Castro, M., Keane, R.W., Lee, T.T., Dietrich, W.D. and Yezierski, R.P. (1998b) Traumatic spinal cord injury induces nuclear factor-kappaB activation. *J. Neurosci.*, 18: 3251–3260.

Bethea, J.R., Nagashima, H., Acosta, M.C., Briceno, C., Gomez, F., Marcillo, A.E., Loor, K., Green, J. and Dietrich, W.D.

(1999) Systemically administered interleukin-10 reduces tumor necrosis factor-alpha production and significantly improves functional recovery following traumatic spinal cord injury in rats. *J. Neurotrauma*, 16: 851–863.

Bingham Jr., W.G. (1975) Proceedings: Effect of trauma on spinal cord blood flow in monkeys. *J. Neurol. Neurosurg. Psychiatry*, 38: 411–412.

Bingham, W.G., Goldman, H., Friedman, S.J., Murphy, S., Yashon, D. and Hunt, W.E. (1975a) Blood flow in normal and injured monkey spinal cord. *J. Neurosurg.*, 43: 162–171.

Bingham, W.G., Ruffolo, R. and Friedman, S.J. (1975b) Catecholamine levels in the injured spinal cord of monkeys. *J. Neurosurg.*, 42: 174–178.

Bingham, W.G., Sirinek, L., Crutcher, K. and Mohnacky, C. (1977) Effect of spinal cord injury on cord and cerebral blood flow in monkey. *Acta Neurol. Scand. Suppl.*, 64: 238–239.

Black, P. and Markowitz, R.S. (1971) Experimental spinal cord injury in monkeys: comparison of steroids and local hypothermia. *Surg. Forum*, 22: 409–411.

Black, P., Shepard Jr., R.H. and Markowitz, R.S. (1979) Spinal cord injury in the monkey: rate of cord cooling and temperature gradient during local hypothermia. *Neurosurgery*, 5: 583–587.

Blight, A. (1988) Mechanical factors in experimental spinal cord injury. *J. Am. Paraplegia Soc.*, 11: 26–34.

Blight, A.R. (1989) Effect of 4-aminopyridine on axonal conduction-block in chronic spinal cord injury. *Brain Res. Bull*, 22: 47–52.

Blight, A.R. and Decrescito, V. (1986) Morphometric analysis of experimental spinal cord injury in the cat: the relation of injury intensity to survival of myelinated axons. *Neuroscience*, 19: 321–341.

Blight, A.R. and Gruner, J.A. (1987) Augmentation by 4-aminopyridine of vestibulospinal free fall responses in chronic spinal-injured cats. *J. Neurol. Sci.*, 82: 145–159.

Blight, A.R. and Young, W. (1989) Central axons in injured cat spinal cord recover electrophysiological function following remyelination by Schwann cells. *J. Neurol. Sci.*, 91: 15–34.

Bracken, M.B. (1991) Treatment of acute spinal cord injury with methylprednisolone: results of a multicenter, randomized clinical trial. *J. Neurotrauma*, 8(Suppl. 1): S47–S52.

Bracken, M.B. (2001) Methylprednisolone and acute spinal cord injury: an update of the randomized evidence. *Spine*, 26: S47–S54.

Bracken, M.B. (2002) Methylprednisolone and spinal cord injury. *J. Neurosurg.*, 96: 140–142.

Bracken, M.B. and Holford, T.R. (1993) Effects of timing of methylprednisolone or naloxone administration on recovery of segmental and long-tract neurological function in NASCIS 2 [see comments]. *J. Neurosurg.*, 79: 500–507.

Bracken, M.B., Shepard, M.J., Hellenbrand, K.G., Collins, W.F., Leo, L.S., Freeman, D.F., Wagner, F.C., Flamm, E.S., Eisenberg, H.M., Goodman, J.H., Perot, P.L., Green, B.A., Grossman, R.G., Meagher, J.N., Young, W., Fischer, B., Clifton, G.L., Hunt, W.E. and Rifkinson, N. (1985) Methylprednisolone and neurological function 1 year after spinal cord injury. Results of the National Acute Spinal Cord Injury Study. *J. Neurosurg.*, 63: 704–713.

Bracken, M.B., Shepard, M.J., Collins Jr., W.F., Holford, T.R., Baskin, D.S., Eisenberg, H.M., Flamm, E., Leo-Summers, L., Maroon, J.C. and Marshall, L.F. et al. (1992) Methylprednisolone or naloxone treatment after acute spinal cord injury: 1-year follow-up data. Results of the second National Acute Spinal Cord Injury Study [see comments]. *J. Neurosurg.*, 76: 23–31.

Bracken, M.B., Shepard, M.J., Holford, T.R., Leo-Summers, L., Aldrich, E.F., Fazl, M., Fehlings, M., Herr, D.L., Hitchon, P.W., Marshall, L.F., Nockels, R.P., Pascale, V., Perot Jr., P.L., Piepmeier, J., Sonntag, V.K., Wagner, F., Wilberger, J.E., Winn, H.R. and Young, W. (1997) Administration of methylprednisolone for 24 or 48 hours or tirilazad mesylate for 48 hours in the treatment of acute spinal cord injury. Results of the Third National Acute Spinal Cord Injury Randomized Controlled Trial. National Acute Spinal Cord Injury Study. *J. Am. Med. Assoc.*, 277: 1597–1604.

Brandoli, C., Shi, B., Pflug, B., Andrews, P., Wrathall, J.R. and Mocchetti, I. (2001) Dexamethasone reduces the expression of p75 neurotrophin receptor and apoptosis in contused spinal cord. *Brain Res. Mol. Brain Res.*, 87: 61–70.

Braughler, J.M. and Hall, E.D. (1982) Correlation of methylprednisolone levels in cat spinal cord with its effects on (Na+ + K+)-ATPase, lipid peroxidation, and alpha motor neuron function. *J. Neurosurg.*, 56: 838–844.

Braughler, J.M. and Hall, E.D. (1983a) Lactate and pyruvate metabolism in injured cat spinal cord before and after a single large intravenous dose of methylprednisolone. *J. Neurosurg.*, 59: 256–261.

Braughler, J.M. and Hall, E.D. (1983b) Uptake and elimination of methylprednisolone from contused cat spinal cord following intravenous injection of the sodium succinate ester. *J. Neurosurg.*, 58: 538–542.

Braughler, J.M. and Hall, E.D. (1984) Effects of multi-dose methylprednisolone sodium succinate administration on injured cat spinal cord neurofilament degradation and energy metabolism. *J. Neurosurg.*, 61: 290–295.

Bresnahan, J.C., Beattie, M.S., Stokes, B.T. and Conway, K.M. (1991) Three-dimensional computer-assisted analysis of graded contusion lesions in the spinal cord of the rat. *J. Neurotrauma*, 8: 91–101.

Bresnahan, J.C., King, J.S., Martin, G.F. and Yashon, D. (1976) A neuroanatomical analysis of spinal cord injury in the rhesus monkey (*Macaca mulatta*). *J. Neurol. Sci.*, 28: 521–542.

Brodkey, J.S., Richards, D.E., Blasingame, J.P. and Nulsen, F.E. (1972) Reversible spinal cord trauma in cats. Additive effects of direct pressure and ischemia. *J. Neurosurg.*, 37: 591–593.

Brodner, R.A. and Dohrmann, G.J. (1977) Norepinephrine, dopamine and serotonin in experimental spinal cord trauma: current status. *Paraplegia*, 15: 166–171.

Brodner, R.A., Dohrmann, G.J. and Roth, R.H. (1977) Intramedullary serotonin patters following experimental spinal cord trauma. *Mount Sinai J. Med.*, 44: 213–217.

Brunello, N., Reynolds, M., Wrathall, J.R. and Mocchetti, I.

(1990) Increased nerve growth factor receptor mRNA in contused rat spinal cord. *Neurosci. Lett.*, 118: 238–240.

Bunegin, L., Albin, M.S. and Jannetta, P.J. (1976a) Catecholamine responses to experimental spinal cord impact injury. I. Intrinsic spinal cord synthesis rates. *Exp. Neurol.*, 53: 274–280.

Bunegin, L., Albin, M.S. and Jannetta, P.J. (1976b) Catecholamine responses to experimental spinal cord impact injury. II. Fate of intravenous (3H) norepinephrine. *Exp. Neurol.*, 53: 281–284.

Campbell, J.B., DeCrescito, V., Tomasula, J.J., Demopoulos, H.B., Flamm, E.S. and Ortega, B.D. (1974) Effects of antifibrinolytic and steroid therapy on the contused spinal cord of cats. *J. Neurosurg.*, 40: 726–733.

Campbell, J.B., DeCrescito, V., Tomasula, J.J., Demopoulos, H.B., Flamm, E.S. and Ransohoff, J. (1973a) Experimental treatment of spinal cord contusion in the cat. *Surg. Neurol.*, 1: 102–106.

Campbell, J.B., Tomasula, J.J., DeCrescito, V. and Flamm, E.S. (1973b) Myelotomy. *Proc. Veterans Adm. Spinal Cord Inj. Conf.*, pp. 124–128.

Cao, Q.L., Zhang, Y.P., Howard, R.M., Walters, W.M., Tsoulfas, P. and Whittemore, S.R. (2001) Pluripotent stem cells engrafted into the normal or lesioned adult rat spinal cord are restricted to a glial lineage. *Exp. Neurol.*, 167: 48–58.

Carmel, J.B., Galante, A., Soteropoulos, P., Tolias, P., Recce, M., Young, W. and Hart, R.P. (2001) Gene expression profiling of acute spinal cord injury reveals spreading inflammatory signals and neuron loss. *Physiol. Genomics*, 7: 201–213.

Casella, G.T., Marcillo, A., Bunge, M.B. and Wood, P.M. (2002) New vascular tissue rapidly replaces neural parenchyma and vessels destroyed by a contusion injury to the rat spinal cord. *Exp. Neurol.*, 173: 63–76.

Cawthon, D.F., Senter, H.J. and Stewart, W.B. (1980) Comparison of hydrogen clearance and 14C-antipyrine autoradiography in the measurement of spinal cord blood flow after severe impact injury. *J. Neurosurg.*, 52: 801–807.

Chatzipanteli, K., Yanagawa, Y., Marcillo, A.E., Kraydieh, S., Yezierski, R.P. and Dietrich, W.D. (2000) Posttraumatic hypothermia reduces polymorphonuclear leukocyte accumulation following spinal cord injury in rats. *J. Neurotrauma*, 17: 321–332.

Chesler, M., Sakatani, K. and Hassan, A.Z. (1991) Elevation and clearance of extracellular K+ following contusion of the rat spinal cord. *Brain Res.*, 556: 71–77.

Chesler, M., Young, W., Hassan, A.Z., Sakatani, K. and Moriya, T. (1994) Elevation and clearance of extracellular K+ following graded contusion of the rat spinal cord. *Exp. Neurol.*, 125: 93–98.

Citron, B.A., Arnold, P.M., Sebastian, C., Qin, F., Malladi, S., Ameenuddin, S., Landis, M.E. and Festoff, B.W. (2000a) Rapid upregulation of caspase-3 in rat spinal cord after injury: mRNA, protein, and cellular localization correlates with apoptotic cell death. *Exp. Neurol.*, 166: 213–226.

Citron, B.A., Smirnova, I.V., Arnold, P.M. and Festoff, B.W. (2000b) Upregulation of neurotoxic serine proteases, pro-

thrombin, and protease-activated receptor 1 early after spinal cord injury. *J. Neurotrauma*, 17: 1191–1203.

Clendenon, N.R., Allen, N., Gordon, W.A. and Bingham Jr., W.G. (1978a) Inhibition of Na+-K+-activated ATPase activity following experimental spinal cord trauma. *J. Neurosurg.*, 49: 563–568.

Clendenon, N.R., Allen, N., Ito, T., Gordon, W.A. and Yashon, D. (1978b) Response of lysosomal hydrolases of dog spinal cord and cerebrospinal fluid to experimental trauma. *Neurology*, 28: 78–84.

Collmann, H., Wullenweber, R., Sprung, C. and Duisberg, R. (1978) Spinal cord blood flow after experimental trauma in the dog. II. Early changes of spinal cord blood flow in the surrounding area of a traumatic lesion. *Adv. Neurol.*, 20: 443–450.

Constantini, S. and Young, W. (1994) The effects of methylprednisolone and the ganglioside GM1 on acute spinal cord injury in rats. *J. Neurosurg.*, 80: 97–111.

Croft, T.J., Brodkey, J.S. and Nulsen, F.E. (1972) Reversible spinal cord trauma: a model for electrical monitoring of spinal cord function. *J. Neurosurg.*, 36: 402–406.

Crowe, M.J., Bresnahan, J.C., Shuman, S.L., Masters, J.N. and Beattie, M.S. (1997) Apoptosis and delayed degeneration after spinal cord injury in rats and monkeys. *Nat. Med.*, 3: 73–76.

Cusick, J.F., Myklebust, J.B., Larson, S.J. and Sances Jr., A. (1979) Spinal cord evaluation by cortical evoked responses. *Arch. Neurol.*, 36: 140–143.

Daniell, H.B., Francis, W.W., Lee, W.A. and Ducker, T.B. (1975) A method of quantitating injury inflicted in acute spinal cord studies. *Paraplegia*, 13: 137–142.

Darlington, C. (2000) Fampridine acorda therapeutics. *Curr. Opin. Invest. Drugs*, 1: 375–379.

de Castro Jr., R.C., Burns, C.L., McAdoo, D.J. and Romanic, A.M. (2000) Metalloproteinase increases in the injured rat spinal cord. *NeuroReport*, 11: 3551–3554.

de La Torre, J.C., Johnson, C.M., Goode, D.J. and Mullan, S. (1975a) Pharmacologic treatment and evaluation of permanent experimental spinal cord trauma. *Neurology*, 25: 508–514.

de la Torre, J.C., Kawanaga, H.M., Johnson, C.M., Goode, D.J., Kajihara, K. and Mullan, S. (1975b) Dimethyl sulfoxide in central nervous system trauma. *Ann. New York Acad. Sci.*, 243: 362–389.

Demopoulos, H.B., Yoder, M., Gutman, E., Seligman, M.L., Flamm, E.S. and Ransohof, T. (1978) The fine structure of endothelial surfaces in the microcirculation of experimentally injured feline spinal cords. In: O. Hohari and R.P. Becker (Eds.), *Scanning Electron Microscopy 1978, Vol. II*. Scanning Electron Microscopy Inc., AMF O'Hara, pp. 677–682.

Demopoulos, H.B., Flamm, E.S., Seligman, M.L., Pietronigro, D.D., Tomasula, J. and DeCrescito, V. (1982) Further studies on free-radical pathology in the major central nervous system disorders: effect of very high doses of methylprednisolone on the functional outcome, morphology, and chemistry of experimental spinal cord impact injury. *Can. J. Physiol. Pharmacol.*, 60: 1415–1424.

Dimar II, J.R., Glassman, S.D., Raque, G.H., Zhang, Y.P. and Shields, C.B. (1999) The influence of spinal canal narrowing and timing of decompression on neurologic recovery after spinal cord contusion in a rat model. *Spine*, 24: 1623–1633.

Dimar II, J.R., Shields, C.B., Zhang, Y.P., Burke, D.A., Raque, G.H. and Glassman, S.D. (2000) The role of directly applied hypothermia in spinal cord injury. *Spine*, 25: 2294–2302.

Dohrmann, G.J. and Allen, W.E. (1975) Microcirculation of traumatized spinal cord. A correlation of microangiography and blood flow patterns in transitory and permanent paraplegia. *J. Trauma*, 15: 1003–1013.

Dohrmann, G.J. and Panjabi, M.M. (1976a) 'Standardized' spinal cord trauma: biomechanical parameters and lesion volume. *Surg. Neurol.*, 6: 263–267.

Dohrmann, G.L. and Panjabi, M.M. (1976b) Spinal cord deformation velocity, impulse, and energy related to lesion volume in 'standardized' trauma. *Surg. Forum*, 27: 466–468.

Dohrmann, G.J., Panjabi, M.M. and Banks, D. (1978) Biomechanics of experimental spinal cord trauma. *J. Neurosurg.*, 48: 993–1001.

Dow-Edwards, D., DeCrescito, V., Tomasula, J.J. and Flamm, E.S. (1980) Effect of aminophylline and isoproterenol on spinal cord blood flow after impact injury. *J. Neurosurg.*, 53: 385–390.

Ducker, T.B. (1976) Experimental injury of the spinal cord. In: P.J. Vinken, G.W. Bruyn and R. Braakman (Eds.), *Injuries of the Spine and Spinal Cord, Part I, Handbook of Clinical Neurology* Vol. 25, North Holland Publishing Co., Amsterdam, pp. 9–26.

Ducker, T.B. and Assenmacher, D.R. (1969) Microvascular response to experimental spinal cord trauma. *Surg. Forum*, 20: 428–430.

Ducker, T.B. and Hamit, H.F. (1969) Experimental treatments of acute spinal cord injury. *J. Neurosurg.*, 30: 693–697.

Ducker, T.B. and Perot Jr., P.L. (1971a) Local tissue oxygen and blood flow in the acutely injured spinal cord. *Proc. Veterans Adm. Spinal Cord Inj. Conf.*, 18: 29–32.

Ducker, T.B. and Perot Jr., P.L. (1971b) Spinal cord oxygen and blood flow in trauma. *Surg. Forum*, 22: 413–415.

Ducker, T.B. and Perot, P.L.J. (1971c) Spinal cord blood flow compartments. *Trans. Am. Neurol. Assoc.*, 96: 229–231.

Ducker, T.B., Kindt, G.W. and Kempe, L.G. (1971a) Pathological findings in acute experimental spinal cord trauma. *J. Neurosurg.*, 35: 700–709.

Ducker, T.B., Kindt, G.W. and Kempf, L.G. (1971b) Pathological findings in acute experimental spinal cord trauma. *J. Neurosurg.*, 35: 700–708.

Ducker, T.B., Salcman, M. and Daniell, H.B. (1978a) Experimental spinal cord trauma, III: Therapeutic effect of immobilization and pharmacologic agents. *Surg. Neurol.*, 10: 71–76.

Ducker, T.B., Salcman, M., Lucas, J.T., Garrison, W.B. and Perot Jr., P.L. (1978b) Experimental spinal cord trauma. II: Blood flow, tissue oxygen, evoked potentials in both paretic and plegic monkeys. *Surg. Neurol.*, 10: 64–70.

Ducker, T.B., Salcman, M., Perot Jr., P.L. and Ballantine, D. (1978c) Experimental spinal cord trauma, I: Correlation of blood flow, tissue oxygen and neurologic status in the dog. *Surg. Neurol.*, 10: 60–63.

Eidelberg, E., Sullivan, J. and Brigham, A. (1975) Immediate consequences of spinal cord injury: possible role of potassium in axonal conduction block. *Surg. Neurol.*, 3: 317–321.

Faden, A.I., Jacobs, T.P. and Holaday, J.W. (1980a) Endorphin parasympathetic interaction in spinal shock. *J. Auton. Nerv. Syst.*, 2: 295–304.

Faden, A.I., Jacobs, T.P. and Holaday, J.W. (1980b) Opiate antagonist improves neurologic recovery after spinal injury. *Science*, 211: 493–494.

Faden, A.I., Jacobs, T.P., Patrick, D.H. and Smith, M.T. (1984) Megadose corticosteroid therapy following experimental traumatic spinal injury. *J. Neurosurg.*, 60: 712–717.

Feldblum, S., Arnaud, S., Simon, M., Rabin, O. and D'Arbigny, P. (2000) Efficacy of a new neuroprotective agent, gacyclidine, in a model of rat spinal cord injury. *J. Neurotrauma*, 17: 1079–1093.

Ferraro, A. (1927) Experimental medullary concussion of the spinal cord in rabbits: histologic study of the early stages. *Arch. Neurol. Psychiatry*, 18: 357–373.

Flamm, E.S., Demopoulos, H.B., Seligman, M.L., Tomasula, J.J., De Crescito, V. and Ransohoff, J. (1977) Ethanol potentiation of central nervous system trauma. *J. Neurosurg.*, 46: 328–335.

Flamm, E.S., Young, W., Collins, W.F., Piepmeier, J., Clifton, G.L. and Fischer, B. (1985) A phase I trial of naloxone treatment in acute spinal cord injury. *J. Neurosurg.*, 63: 390–397.

Follesa, P., Wrathall, J.R. and Mocchetti, I. (1994) Increased basic fibroblast growth factor mRNA following contusive spinal cord injury. *Brain Res. Mol. Brain Res.*, 22: 1–8.

Follesa, P., Wrathall, J.R. and Mocchetti, I. (1998) 2,3-Dihydroxy-6-nitro-7-sulfamoyl-benzo(F)-quinoxaline (NBQX) increases fibroblast growth factor mRNA levels after contusive spinal cord injury. *Brain Res.*, 782: 306–309.

Fox, A.J., Kricheff, I.I., Goodgold, J., Spielholz, N. and Tregerman, L. (1976) The effect of angiography on the electrophysiological state of the spinal cord. A study in control and traumatized cats. *Radiology*, 118: 343–350.

Frei, E., Klusman, I., Schnell, L. and Schwab, M.E. (2000) Reactions of oligodendrocytes to spinal cord injury: cell survival and myelin repair. *Exp. Neurol.*, 163: 373–380.

Gainer Jr., J.V. (1977) Use of crocetin in experimental spinal cord injury. *J. Neurosurg.*, 46: 358–360.

Gale, K., Kerasidis, H. and Wrathall, J.R. (1985) Spinal cord contusion in the rat: behavioral analysis of functional neurologic impairment. *Exp. Neurol.*, 88: 123–134.

Gennarelli, T.A., Tipperman, R., Maxwell, W.L., Graham, D.I., Adams, J.H. and Irvine, A. (1993) Traumatic damage to the nodal axolemma: an early, secondary injury. *Acta Neurochir. Suppl. (Wien)*, 57: 49–52.

Gerber, A.M. and Corrie, W.S. (1979) Effect of impounder contact area on experimental spinal cord injury. *J. Neurosurg.*, 51: 539–542.

Giovanini, M.A., Reier, P.J., Eskin, T.A. and Anderson, D.K. (1997) MAP2 expression in the developing human fetal spinal cord and following xenotransplantation. *Cell Transplant*, 6: 339–346.

Goldsmith, H.S., Duckett, S. and Chen, W.F. (1975) Spinal cord vascularization by intact omentum. *Am. J. Surg.*, 129: 262–265.

Goodkin, R. (1973) Sequential pathological changes secondary to impact injury experimental model. *Proc. Veterans Adm. Spinal Cord Inj. Conf.*, pp. 86–100.

Goodkin, R. and Campbell, J.B. (1969) Sequential pathological changes in spinal cord injury: a preliminary report. *Surg. Forum*, 20: 430–432.

Goodman, J.H., Bingham Jr., W.G. and Hunt, W.E. (1974) Edema formation and central hemorrhagic necrosis following impact injury to primate spinal cord. *Surg. Forum*, 25: 440–442.

Goodnough, J., Allen, N., Nesham, M.E. and Clendenon, N.R. (1980) The effect of dimethyl sulfoxide on gray matter injury in experimental spinal cord trauma. *Surg. Neurol.*, 13: 273–276.

Green, B.A. and Wagner, F.C. (1973) Evolution of edema in the acutely injured spinal cord: a fluorescence microscopic study. *Surg. Neurol.*, 1: 98–101.

Green, B.A., Khan, T. and Raimondi, A.J. (1973) Local hypothermia as treatment of experimentally induced spinal cord contusion: quantitative analysis of beneficient effect. *Surg. Forum*, 24: 436–438.

Green, B.A., Kahn, T. and Klose, K.J. (1980) A comparative study of steroid therapy in acute experimental spinal cord injury. *Surg. Neurol.*, 13: 91–97.

Greenhoot, J.H., Shiel, F.O. and Mauck Jr., H.P. (1972) Experimental spinal cord injury. Electrocardiographic abnormalities and fuchsinophilic myocardial degeneration. *Arch. Neurol.*, 26: 524–529.

Griffiths, I.R. (1973) Spinal cord blood flow after impact injury. In: A.M. Harper, W.B. Jennett, J.D. Miller and J.O. Rowan (Eds.), *Blood Flow and Metabolism in the Brain*. Churchill-Livingstone, Edinburgh, pp. 4.27–4.29.

Griffiths, I.R. (1976) Spinal cord blood flow after acute experimental cord injury in dogs. *J. Neurol. Sci.*, 27: 247–259.

Griffiths, I.R. (1978) Ultrastructural changes in spinal gray matter microvasculature after impact injury. *Adv. Neurol.*, 20: 415–422.

Griffiths, I.R. and Miller, R. (1974) Vascular permeability to protein and vasogenic oedema in experiment concussive injuries to the canine spinal cord. *J. Neurol. Sci.*, 22: 291–304.

Griffiths, I.R., Burns, N. and Crawford, A.R. (1978a) Early vascular changes in the spinal grey matter following impact injury. *Acta Neuropathol.*, 41: 33–39.

Griffiths, I.R., McCulloch, M. and Crawford, R.A. (1978b) Ultrastructural appearances of the spinal microvasculature between 12 hours and 5 days after impact injury. *Acta Neuropathol.*, 43: 205–211.

Grossman, S.D. and Wrathall, J.R. (2000) The role of activity blockade on glutamate receptor subunit expression in the spinal cord. *Brain Res.*, 880: 183–186.

Grossman, S.D., Wolfe, B.B., Yasuda, R.P. and Wrathall, J.R. (1999) Alterations in AMPA receptor subunit expression after experimental spinal cord contusion injury. *J. Neurosci.*, 19: 5711–5720.

Grossman, S.D., Rosenberg, L.J. and Wrathall, J.R. (2001a)

Relationship of altered glutamate receptor subunit mRNA expression to acute cell loss after spinal cord contusion. *Exp. Neurol.*, 168: 283–289.

Grossman, S.D., Rosenberg, L.J. and Wrathall, J.R. (2001b) Temporal-spatial pattern of acute neuronal and glial loss after spinal cord contusion. *Exp. Neurol.*, 168: 273–282.

Gruner, J.A. (1989) Comparison of vestibular and auditory startle responses in the rat and cat. *J. Neurosci. Methods*, 27: 13–23.

Gruner, J.A. (1992) A monitored contusion model of spinal cord injury in the rat. *J. Neurotrauma*, 9: 123–128.

Gruner, J.A., Wade, C.K., Menna, G. and Stokes, B.T. (1993) Myoelectric evoked potentials versus locomotor recovery in chronic spinal cord injured rats. *J. Neurotrauma*, 10: 327–347.

Guth, L., Richardson, K.C., Baker, C.A. and Baker, J.H. (1977) Neurohistological and enzyme histochemical staining of adjacent sections in series cut from normal and traumatized spinal cords. *Exp. Neurol.*, 57: 179–191.

Hains, B.C., Yucra, J.A. and Hulsebosch, C.E. (2001) Reduction of pathological and behavioral deficits following spinal cord contusion injury with the selective cyclooxygenase-2 inhibitor NS-398. *J. Neurotrauma*, 18: 409–423.

Hall, E.D. and Braughler, J.M. (1982a) Effects of intravenous methylprednisolone on spinal cord lipid peroxidation and Na+ + K+)-ATPase activity. Dose–response analysis during 1st hour after contusion injury in the cat. *J. Neurosurg.*, 57: 247–253.

Hall, E.D. and Braughler, J.M. (1982b) Glucocorticoid mechanisms in acute spinal cord injury: a review and therapeutic rationale. *Surg. Neurol.*, 18: 320–327.

Hall, E.D., Wolf, D.L. and Braughler, J.M. (1984) Effects of a single large dose of methylprednisolone sodium succinate on experimental posttraumatic spinal cord ischemia. Dose–response and time-action analysis. *J. Neurosurg.*, 61: 124–130.

Hamers, F.P., Lankhorst, A.J., van Laar, T.J., Veldhuis, W.B. and Gispen, W.H. (2001) Automated quantitative gait analysis during overground locomotion in the rat: its application to spinal cord contusion and transection injuries. *J. Neurotrauma*, 18: 187–201.

Hansebout, R.R., Blight, A.R., Fawcett, S. and Reddy, K. (1993) 4-Aminopyridine in chronic spinal cord injury: a controlled, double-blind, crossover study in eight patients. *J. Neurotrauma*, 10: 1–18.

Hauben, E., Butovsky, O., Nevo, U., Yoles, E., Moalem, G., Agranov, E., Mor, F., Leibowitz-Amit, R., Pevsner, E., Akselrod, S., Neeman, M., Cohen, I.R. and Schwartz, M. (2000) Passive or active immunization with myelin basic protein promotes recovery from spinal cord contusion. *J. Neurosci.*, 20: 6421–6430.

Hayes, K.C., Potter, P.J., Wolfe, D.L., Hsieh, J.T., Delaney, G.A. and Blight, A.R. (1994) 4-Aminopyridine-sensitive neurologic deficits in patients with spinal cord injury. *J. Neurotrauma*, 11: 433–446.

Hedeman, L.S. and Sil, R. (1974) Studies in experimental spinal cord trauma. 2. Comparison of treatment with steroids, low molecular weight dextran, and catecholamine blockade. *J. Neurosurg.*, 40: 44–51.

Hedeman, L.S., Shellenberger, M.K. and Gordon, J.H. (1974)

Studies in experimental spinal cord trauma. 1. Alterations in catecholamine levels. *J. Neurosurg.*, 40: 37–43.

Holaday, J.W. and Faden, A.I. (1980) Naloxone acts at central opiate receptors to reverse hypotension, hypothermia and hypoventilation in spinal shock. *Brain Res.*, 189: 295–299.

Hoovler, D.W. and Wrathall, J.R. (1991) Implantation of neuronal suspensions into contusive injury sites in the adult rat spinal cord. *Acta Neuropathol. (Berl.)*, 81: 303–311.

Horner, P.J. and Stokes, B.T. (1995) Fetal transplantation following spinal contusion injury results in chronic alterations in CNS glucose metabolism. *Exp. Neurol.*, 133: 231–243.

Horner, P.J., Popovich, P.G., Mullin, B.B. and Stokes, B.T. (1996a) A quantitative spatial analysis of the blood–spinal cord barrier. II. Permeability after intraspinal fetal transplantation. *Exp. Neurol.*, 142: 226–243.

Horner, P.J., Reier, P.J. and Stokes, B.T. (1996b) Quantitative analysis of vascularization and cytochrome oxidase following fetal transplantation in the contused rat spinal cord. *J. Comp. Neurol.*, 364: 690–703.

Horrocks, L.A., Toews, A., Yashon, D. and Locke, G.E. (1973) Changes in myelin following trauma of the spinal cord in monkeys. *Neurobiology*, 3: 256–263.

Huang, P.P. and Young, W. (1994) The effects of arterial blood gas values on lesion volumes in a graded rat spinal cord contusion model. *J. Neurotrauma*, 11: 547–562.

Hukuda, S., Mochizuki, T. and Ogata, M. (1980a) Effects of hypertension and hypercarbia on spinal cord tissue oxygen in acute experimental spinal cord injury. *Neurosurgery*, 6: 639–643.

Hukuda, S., Mochizuki, T. and Ogata, M. (1980b) Therapeutic trial of combined hypertension and hypercarbia on experimental acute spinal cord injury. *Neurosurgery*, 6: 644–648.

Hulsebosch, C.E., Xu, G.Y., Perez-Polo, J.R., Westlund, K.N., Taylor, C.P. and McAdoo, D.J. (2000) Rodent model of chronic central pain after spinal cord contusion injury and effects of gabapentin. *J. Neurotrauma*, 17: 1205–1217.

Hung, T.K., Lin, H.S., Albin, M.S., Bunegin, L. and Jannetta, P.J. (1979) The standardization of experimental impact injury to the spinal cord. *Surg. Neurol.*, 11: 470–477.

Hutchinson, K.J., Linderman, J.K. and Basso, D.M. (2001) Skeletal muscle adaptations following spinal cord contusion injury in rat and the relationship to locomotor function: a time course study. *J. Neurotrauma*, 18: 1075–1089.

Ikeda, K. and Yamagata, S. (1978) A modified weight-dropping technique for experimental spine and spinal cord injuries. *Neurol. Med.-Chir.*, 18: 129–140.

Ikeda, K., Yamagata, S., Nakano, M. and Tani, E. (1978) Effecting quantitative spine and spinal cord injuries by using a modified weight-dropping technique — a preliminary report (author's translation). *No Shinkei Geka - Neurol. Surg.*, 6: 331–339 (in Japanese).

Ito, T., Allen, N. and Yashon, D. (1978) A mitochondrial lesion in experimental spinal cord trauma. *J. Neurosurg.*, 48: 434–442.

Jones, M. and Keenan, R.W. (1982) A biochemical investigation of spinal cord after contusive injury. *Exp. Neurol.*, 78: 67–82.

Jonsson Jr., H.T. and Daniell, H.B. (1976) Altered levels of

PGF in cat spinal cord tissue following traumatic injury. *Prostaglandins*, 11: 51–61.

Jonsson, G. and Sachs, C. (1976) Regional changes in [3H]-noradrenaline uptake, catecholamines and catecholamine synthetic and catabolic enzymes in rat brain following neonatal 6-hydroxydopamine treatment. *Med. Biol.*, 54: 286–297.

Kadoya, S., Massopust Jr., L.C., Wolin, L.R., Taslitz, N. and White, R.J. (1974) Effect of experimental cervical spinal cord injury on respiratory function. *J. Neurosurg.*, 41: 455–462.

Kajihara, K., Kawanaga, H., De la Torre, J.C. and Mullan, S. (1973) Dimethyl sulfoxide in the treatment of experimental acute spinal cord injury. *Surg. Neurol.*, 1: 16–22.

Kao, C.C. (1971) Neuron transplantation in traumatic cord lesions. *Proc. Veterans Adm. Spinal Cord Inj. Conf.*, 18: 33–34.

Katz, S., Blackburn, J.G., Perot, P.L. and Lam, C.F. (1978) The effects of low spinal injury on somatosensory evoked potentials from forelimb stimulation. *Electroencephalogr. Clin. Neurophysiol.*, 44: 236–238.

Kerasidis, H., Wrathall, J.R. and Gale, K. (1987) Behavioral assessment of functional deficit in rats with contusive spinal cord injury. *J. Neurosci. Methods*, 20: 167–179.

Kidman, A.D., Hinwood, B.G. and Yeo, J.D. (1976) Concentrations of NE and 5-HT in the contused sheep spinal cord: status of the monoamine hypothesis. *J. Neurochem.*, 27: 293–294.

Kim, W.K., Kan, Y., Ganea, D., Hart, R.P., Gozes, I. and Jonakait, G.M. (2000) Vasoactive intestinal peptide and pituitary adenylyl cyclase-activating polypeptide inhibit tumor necrosis factor-alpha production in injured spinal cord and in activated microglia via a cAMP-dependent pathway. *J. Neurosci.*, 20: 3622–3630.

Kobrine, A.I. and Doyle, T.F. (1976) Role of histamine in posttraumatic spinal cord hyperemia and the luxury perfusion syndrome. *J. Neurosurg.*, 44: 16–20.

Kobrine, A.I., Doyle, T.F. and Rizzoli, H.V. (1976a) The effect of antihistamines on experimental posttraumatic edema of the spinal cord. *Surg. Neurol.*, 5: 307–309.

Kobrine, A.I., Doyle, T.F. and Rizzoli, H.V. (1976b) Further studies on histamine in spinal cord injury and post traumatic hyperemia. *Surg. Neurol.*, 5: 101–103.

Kobrine, A.I., Doyle, T.F. and Rizzoli, H.V. (1976c) A method for estimating edema in experimental traumatic spinal cord injury. *Exp. Neurol.*, 50: 240–245.

Kobrine, A.I., Doyle, T.F. and Rizzoli, H.V. (1976d) Spinal cord blood flow as affected by changes in systemic arterial blood pressure. *J. Neurosurg.*, 44: 12–15.

Kobrine, A.I., Evans, D.E. and Rizzoli, H.V. (1977a) The effect of alpha adrenergic blockade on spinal cord autoregulation in the monkey. *J. Neurosurg.*, 46: 336–341.

Kobrine, A.I., Evans, D.E. and Rizzoli, H.V. (1977b) The effects of beta adrenergic blockade on spinal cord autoregulation in the monkey. *J. Neurosurg.*, 47: 57–63.

Kobrine, A.I., Evans, D.E. and Rizzoli, H.V. (1980a) Effects of progressive hypoxia on long tract neural conduction in the spinal cord. *Neurosurgery*, 7: 369–375.

Kobrine, A.I., Evans, D.E. and Rizzoli, H.V. (1980b) Relative

250

vulnerability of the brain and spinal cord to ischemia. *J. Neurol. Sci.*, 45: 65–72.

Koenig, G. and Dohrmann, G.J. (1977) Histopathological variability in 'standardised' spinal cord trauma. *J. Neurol. Neurosurg. Psychiatry*, 40: 1203–1210.

Koozekanani, S.H., Vise, W.M., Hashemi, R.M. and McGhee, R.B. (1976) Possible mechanisms for observed pathophysiological variability in experimental spinal cord injury by the method of Allen. *J. Neurosurg.*, 44: 429–434.

Kuchner, E.F. and Hansebout, R.R. (1976) Combined steroid and hypothermia treatment of experimental spinal cord injury. *Surg. Neurol.*, 6: 371–376.

Kwo, S., Young, W. and Decrescito, V. (1989) Spinal cord sodium, potassium, calcium, and water concentration changes in rats after graded contusion injury. *J. Neurotrauma*, 6: 13–24.

Lankhorst, A.J., ter Laak, M.P., van Laar, T.J., van Meeteren, N.L., de Groot, J.C., Schrama, L.H., Hamers, F.P. and Gispen, W.H. (2001) Effects of enriched housing on functional recovery after spinal cord contusive injury in the adult rat. *J. Neurotrauma*, 18: 203–215.

Lee, T.T., Green, B.A., Dietrich, W.D. and Yezierski, R.P. (1999) Neuroprotective effects of basic fibroblast growth factor following spinal cord contusion injury in the rat. *J. Neurotrauma*, 16: 347–356.

Lemons, M.L., Sandy, J.D., Anderson, D.K. and Howland, D.R. (2001) Intact aggrecan and fragments generated by both aggrecanse and metalloproteinase-like activities are present in the developing and adult rat spinal cord and their relative abundance is altered by injury. *J. Neurosci.*, 21: 4772–4781.

Lewin, M.G., Pappius, H.M. and Hansebout, R.R. (1972) Effects of steroids on edema associated with injury of the spinal cord. In: H. Reulen, J. and K. Schurmann (Eds.), *Steroids and Brain Edema*. Springer-Verlag, Berlin, pp. 101–112.

Lewin, M.G., Hansebout, R.R. and Pappius, H.M. (1974) Chemical characteristics of traumatic spinal cord edema in cats. Effects of steroids on potassium depletion. *J. Neurosurg.*, 56: 106–113.

Liebl, D.J., Huang, W., Young, W. and Parada, L.F. (2001) Regulation of Trk receptors following contusion of the rat spinal cord. *Exp. Neurol.*, 167: 15–26.

Lindsey, A.E., LoVerso, R.L., Tovar, C.A., Hill, C.E., Beattie, M.S. and Bresnahan, J.C. (2000) An analysis of changes in sensory thresholds to mild tactile and cold stimuli after experimental spinal cord injury in the rat. *Neurorehabil. Neural Repair*, 14: 287–300.

Liu, S., Qu, Y., Stewart, T.J., Howard, M.J., Chakrabortty, S., Holekamp, T.F. and McDonald, J.W. (2000) Embryonic stem cells differentiate into oligodendrocytes and myelinate in culture and after spinal cord transplantation. *Proc. Natl. Acad. Sci. USA*, 97: 6126–6131.

Liu, X.Z., Xu, X.M., Hu, R., Du, C., Zhang, S.X., McDonald, J.W., Dong, H.X., Wu, Y.J., Fan, G.S., Jacquin, M.F., Hsu, C.Y. and Choi, D.W. (1997) Neuronal and glial apoptosis after traumatic spinal cord injury. *J. Neurosci.*, 17: 5395–5406.

Lohse, D.C., Senter, H.J., Kauer, J.S. and Collins Jr., W.F. (1979)

Spinal cord blood flow in experimental transient paraplegia. *Surg. Forum*, 30: 450–452.

Lohse, D.C., Senter, H.J., Kauer, J.S. and Wohns, R. (1980) Spinal cord blood flow in experimental transient traumatic paraplegia. *J. Neurosurg.*, 52: 335–345.

Lou, J., Lenke, L.G., Xu, F. and O'Brien, M. (1998) In vivo Bcl-2 oncogene neuronal expression in the rat spinal cord. *Spine*, 23: 517–523.

Martin, D., Robe, P., Franzen, R., Delree, P., Schoenen, J., Stevenaert, A. and Moonen, G. (1996) Effects of Schwann cell transplantation in a contusion model of rat spinal cord injury. *J. Neurosci. Res.*, 45: 588–597.

Martin, S.H. and Bloedel, J.R. (1973) Evaluation of experimental spinal cord injury using cortical evoked potentials. *J. Neurosurg.*, 39: 75–81.

Martinez, L.J., Alderman, J.L., Glaeser, B.S., Hare, T.A. and Osterholm, J.L. (1980) Changes in the free amino acids of the injured spinal cord of the cat. *Brain Res.*, 182: 237–241.

Maxwell, W.L. (1996) Histopathological changes at central nodes of Ranvier after stretch-injury. *Microsc. Res. Tech.*, 34: 522–535.

Maxwell, W.L., Povlishock, J.T. and Graham, D.L. (1997) A mechanistic analysis of nondisruptive axonal injury: a review. *J. Neurotrauma*, 14: 419–440.

McNicholas, L.F., Martin, W.R., Sloan, J.L. and Nozaki, M. (1980) Innervation of the spinal cord by sympathetic fibers. *Exp. Neurol.*, 69: 383–394.

McTigue, D.M., Horner, P.J., Stokes, B.T. and Gage, F.H. (1998a) Neurotrophin-3 and brain-derived neurotrophic factor induce oligodendrocyte proliferation and myelination of regenerating axons in the contused adult rat spinal cord. *J. Neurosci.*, 18: 5354–5365.

McTigue, D.M., Tani, M., Krivacic, K., Chernosky, A., Kelner, G.S., Maciejewski, D., Maki, R., Ransohoff, R.M. and Stokes, B.T. (1998b) Selective chemokine mRNA accumulation in the rat spinal cord after contusion injury. *J. Neurosci. Res.*, 53: 368–376.

McTigue, D.M., Popovich, P.G., Morgan, T.E. and Stokes, B.T. (2000) Localization of transforming growth factor-beta1 and receptor mRNA after experimental spinal cord injury. *Exp. Neurol.*, 163: 220–230.

McTigue, D.M., Wei, P. and Stokes, B.T. (2001) Proliferation of NG2-positive cells and altered oligodendrocyte numbers in the contused rat spinal cord. *J. Neurosci.*, 21: 3392–3400.

Means, E.D., Anderson, D.K., Nicolosi, G. and Gaudsmith, J. (1978) Microvascular perfusion experimental spinal cord injury. *Surg. Neurol.*, 9: 353–360.

Mills, C.D., Fullwood, S.D. and Hulsebosch, C.E. (2001a) Changes in metabotropic glutamate receptor expression following spinal cord injury. *Exp. Neurol.*, 170: 244–257.

Mills, C.D., Grady, J.J. and Hulsebosch, C.E. (2001b) Changes in exploratory behavior as a measure of chronic central pain following spinal cord injury. *J. Neurotrauma*, 18: 1091–1105.

Mills, C.D., Hains, B.C., Johnson, K.M. and Hulsebosch, C.E. (2001c) Strain and model differences in behavioral outcomes after spinal cord injury in rat. *J. Neurotrauma*, 18: 743–756.

Mills, C.D., Xu, G.Y., McAdoo, D.J. and Hulsebosch, C.E.

(2001d) Involvement of metabotropic glutamate receptors in excitatory amino acid and GABA release following spinal cord injury in rat. *J. Neurochem.*, 79: 835–848.

Mills, C.D., Johnson, K.M. and Hulsebosch, C.E. (2002) Role of Group II and Group III Metabotropic Glutamate Receptors in Spinal Cord Injury. *Exp. Neurol.*, 173: 153–167.

Milvy, P., Kakari, S., Campbell, J.B. and Demopoulos, H.B. (1973) Paramagnetic species and radical products in cat spinal cord. *Ann. New York Acad. Sci.*, 222: 1102–1111.

Mocchetti, I., Rabin, S.J., Colangelo, A.M., Whittemore, S.R. and Wrathall, J.R. (1996) Increased basic fibroblast growth factor expression following contusive spinal cord injury. *Exp. Neurol.*, 141: 154–164.

Molt, J.T., Poulos, D.A. and Bourke, R.S. (1978) Evaluation of experimental spinal cord injury by measuring spontaneous spinal cord potentials. *J. Neurosurg.*, 48: 985–992.

Molt, J.T., Nelson, L.R., Poulos, D.A. and Bourke, R.S. (1979) Analysis and measurement of some sources of variability in experimental spinal cord trauma. *J. Neurosurg.*, 50: 784–791.

Moriya, T., Hassan, A.Z., Young, W. and Chesler, M. (1994) Dynamics of extracellular calcium activity following contusion of the rat spinal cord. *J. Neurotrauma*, 11: 255–263.

Mu, X., Azbill, R.D. and Springer, J.E. (2000) Riluzole and methylprednisolone combined treatment improves functional recovery in traumatic spinal cord injury. *J. Neurotrauma*, 17: 773–780.

Murphy, E.J., Behrmann, D., Bates, C.M. and Horrocks, L.A. (1994) Lipid alterations following impact spinal cord injury in the rat. *Mol. Chem. Neuropathol.*, 23: 13–26.

Naftchi, N.E., Demeny, M., DeCrescito, V., Tomasula, J.J., Flamm, E.S. and Campbell, J.B. (1974) Biogenic amine concentrations in traumatized spinal cords of cats. Effect of drug therapy. *J. Neurosurg.*, 40: 52–57.

Nemecek, S., Petr, R., Suba, P., Rozsival, V. and Melka, O. (1977a) Longitudinal extension of oedema in experimental spinal cord injury — evidence for two types of post-traumatic oedema. *Acta Neurochir.*, 37: 7–16.

Nemecek, S., Suba, P. and Cerman, J. (1977b) Serotonin in contused spinal cord. *Acta Neurochir. (Wien)*, 39: 53–58.

Nesic, O., Xu, G.Y., McAdoo, D., High, K.W., Hulsebosch, C. and Perez-Pol, R. (2001) IL-1 receptor antagonist prevents apoptosis and caspase-3 activation after spinal cord injury. *J. Neurotrauma*, 18: 947–956.

Nevo, U., Hauben, E., Yoles, E., Agranov, E., Akselrod, S., Schwartz, M. and Neeman, M. (2001) Diffusion anisotropy MRI for quantitative assessment of recovery in injured rat spinal cord. *Magn. Reson. Med.*, 45: 1–9.

Noble, L.J. and Wrathall, J.R. (1985) Spinal cord contusion in the rat: morphometric analyses of alterations in the spinal cord. *Exp. Neurol.*, 88: 135–149.

Noble, L.J. and Wrathall, J.R. (1987) An inexpensive apparatus for producing graded spinal cord contusive injury in the rat. *Exp. Neurol.*, 95: 530–533.

Osterholm, J.L. (1974a) Noradrenergic mediation of traumatic spinal cord autodestruction [Review]. *Life Sci.*, 14: 1363–1384.

Osterholm, J.L. (1974b) The pathophysiological response to spinal cord injury. The current status of related research. *J. Neurosurg.*, 40: 5–33.

Osterholm, J.L. (1978) *The Pathophysiology of Spinal Cord Trauma*. Charles C. Thomas, Springfield, IL.

Osterholm, J.L. and Mathews, G.J. (1971a) A proposed biochemical mechanism for traumatic spinal cord hemorrhagic necrosis. Successful therapy for severe injuries by metabolic blockade. *Trans. Am. Neurol. Assoc.*, 96: 187–191.

Osterholm, J.L. and Mathews, G.J. (1971b) Treatment of severe spinal cord injuries by biochemical norepinephrine manipulation. *Surg. Forum*, 22: 415–417.

Osterholm, J.L. and Mathews, G.J. (1972a) Altered norepinephrine metabolism following experimental spinal cord injury. 1. Relationship to hemorrhagic necrosis and postwounding neurological deficits. *J. Neurosurg.*, 36: 386–394.

Osterholm, J.L. and Mathews, G.J. (1972b) Altered norepinephrine metabolism, following experimental spinal cord injury. 2. Protection against traumatic spinal cord hemorrhagic necrosis by norepinephrine synthesis blockade with alpha methyl tyrosine. *J. Neurosurg.*, 36: 395–401.

Osterholm, J.L., Mathews, G.J., Irvin, J.D. and Angelakos, E.T. (1971) A review of altered norepinephrine metabolism attending severe spinal injury: results of alpha methyl tyrosine treatment and preliminary histofluorescent studies [Review]. *Proc. Veterans Adm. Spinal Cord Inj. Conf.*, 18: 17–21.

Panjabi, M.M., Dicker, D.B. and Dohrmann, G.J. (1977) Biomechanical quantification of experimental spinal cord trauma. *J. Biomechan.*, 10: 681–687.

Parker, A.J. and Smith, C.W. (1976) Functional recovery from spinal cord trauma following dexamethasone and chlorpromazine therapy in dogs. *Res. Vet. Sci.*, 21: 246–247.

Parker, A.J. and Smith, C.W. (1979) Lack of functional recovery from spinal cord trauma following dimethylsulphoxide and epsilon amino caproic acid therapy in dogs. *Res. Vet. Sci.*, 27: 253–255.

Parker, A.J., Park, R.D. and Stowater, J.L. (1973) Reduction of trauma-induced edema of spinal cord in dogs given mannitol. *Am. J. Vet. Res.*, 34: 1355–1357.

Pikov, V. and Wrathall, J.R. (2001) Coordination of the bladder detrusor and the external urethral sphincter in a rat model of spinal cord injury: effect of injury severity. *J. Neurosci.*, 21: 559–569.

Pikov, V. and Wrathall, J.R. (2002) Altered glutamate receptor function during recovery of bladder detrusor-external urethral sphincter coordination in a rat model of spinal cord injury. *J. Pharmacol. Exp. Ther.*, 300: 421–427.

Pikov, V., Gillis, R.A., Jasmin, L. and Wrathall, J.R. (1998) Assessment of lower urinary tract functional deficit in rats with contusive spinal cord injury. *J. Neurotrauma*, 15: 375–386.

Plunkett, J.A., Yu, C.G., Easton, J.M., Bethea, J.R. and Yezierski, R.P. (2001) Effects of interleukin-10 (IL-10) on pain behavior and gene expression following excitotoxic spinal cord injury in the rat. *Exp. Neurol.*, 168: 144–154.

Popovich, P.G., Streit, W.J. and Stokes, B.T. (1993) Differential expression of MHC class II antigen in the contused rat spinal cord. *J. Neurotrauma*, 10: 37–46.

Popovich, P.G., Reinhard Jr., J.F., Flanagan, E.M. and Stokes, B.T. (1994) Elevation of the neurotoxin quinolinic acid occurs following spinal cord trauma. *Brain Res.*, 633: 348–352.

Popovich, P.G., Horner, P.J., Mullin, B.B. and Stokes, B.T. (1996) A quantitative spatial analysis of the blood–spinal cord barrier. I. Permeability changes after experimental spinal contusion injury. *Exp. Neurol.*, 142: 258–275.

Potter, P.J., Hayes, K.C., Hsieh, J.T., Delaney, G.A. and Segal, J.L. (1998a) Sustained improvements in neurological function in spinal cord injured patients treated with oral 4-aminopyridine: three cases. *Spinal Cord*, 36: 147–155.

Potter, P.J., Hayes, K.C., Segal, J.L., Hsieh, J.T., Brunnemann, S.R., Delaney, G.A., Tierney, D.S. and Mason, D. (1998b) Randomized double-blind crossover trial of fampridine-SR (sustained release 4-aminopyridine) in patients with incomplete spinal cord injury. *J. Neurotrauma*, 15: 837–849.

Prybylowski, K.L., Grossman, S.D., Wrathall, J.R. and Wolfe, B.B. (2001) Expression of splice variants of the NR1 subunit of the *N*-methyl-D-aspartate receptor in the normal and injured rat spinal cord. *J. Neurochem.*, 76: 797–805.

Qiao, J., Hayes, K.C., Hsieh, J.T., Potter, P.J. and Delaney, G.A. (1997) Effects of 4-aminopyridine on motor evoked potentials in patients with spinal cord injury. *J. Neurotrauma*, 14: 135–149.

Qiu, J., Nesic, O., Ye, Z., Rea, H., Westlund, K.N., Xu, G.Y., McAdoo, D., Hulsebosch, C.E. and Perez-Polo, J.R. (2001) Bcl-xL expression after contusion to the rat spinal cord. *J. Neurotrauma*, 18: 1267–1278.

Rabchevsky, A.G., Fugaccia, I., Fletcher-Turner, A., Blades, D.A., Mattson, M.P. and Scheff, S.W. (1999) Basic fibroblast growth factor (bFGF) enhances tissue sparing and functional recovery following moderate spinal cord injury. *J. Neurotrauma*, 16: 817–830.

Rabchevsky, A.G., Fugaccia, I., Turner, A.F., Blades, D.A., Mattson, M.P. and Scheff, S.W. (2000) Basic fibroblast growth factor (bFGF) enhances functional recovery following severe spinal cord injury to the rat. *Exp. Neurol.*, 164: 280–291.

Rabchevsky, A.G., Fugaccia, I., Sullivan, P.G. and Scheff, S.W. (2001) Cyclosporin A treatment following spinal cord injury to the rat: behavioral effects and stereological assessment of tissue sparing. *J. Neurotrauma*, 18: 513–522.

Raines, A., Dretchen, K.L., Marx, K. and Wrathall, J.R. (1988) Spinal cord contusion in the rat: somatosensory evoked potentials as a function of graded injury. *J. Neurotrauma*, 5: 151–160.

Rawe, S. and Perot, P. (1979a) Regional spinal cord glucose utilization following experimental cord injury. *Acta Neurol. Scand.*, 72: 406–407.

Rawe, S.E. and Perot Jr., P.L. (1979b) Hypermetabolism after experimental spinal cord injury. *Surg. Forum*, 30: 459–461.

Rawe, S.E. and Perot Jr., P.L. (1979c) Pressor response resulting from experimental contusion injury to the spinal cord. *J. Neurosurg.*, 50: 58–63.

Rawe, S.E., D'Angelo, C.M. and Collins Jr., W.F. (1974) The pressor response in experimental spinal cord trauma. *Surg. Forum*, 25: 432–433.

Rawe, S.E., Roth, R.H., Boadle-Biber, M. and Collins, W.F. (1977a) Norepinephrine levels in experimental spinal cord trauma. Part 1: Biochemical study of hemorrhagic necrosis. *J. Neurosurg.*, 46: 342–349.

Rawe, S.E., Roth, R.H. and Collins, W.F. (1977b) Norepinephrine levels in experimental spinal cord trauma. Part 2: Histopathological study of hemorrhagic necrosis. *J. Neurosurg.*, 46: 350–357.

Rawe, S.E., Lee, W.A. and Perot Jr., P.L. (1978) The histopathology of experimental spinal cord trauma. The effect of systemic blood pressure. *J. Neurosurg.*, 48: 1002–1007.

Rawe, S.E., Lee, W.A. and Perot, P.L. (1981) Spinal cord glucose utilization after experimental spinal cord injury. *Neurosurgery*, 9: 40–47.

Reed, J.E., Allen, W.E.D. and Dohrmann, G.J. (1979) Effect of mannitol on the traumatized spinal cord. Microangiography, blood flow patterns, and electrophysiology. *Spine*, 4: 391–397.

Reier, P.J., Stokes, B.T., Thompson, F.J. and Anderson, D.K. (1992) Fetal cell grafts into resection and contusion/compression injuries of the rat and cat spinal cord. *Exp. Neurol.*, 115: 177–188.

Resnick, D.K., Graham, S.H., Dixon, C.E. and Marion, D.W. (1998) Role of cyclooxygenase 2 in acute spinal cord injury. *J. Neurotrauma*, 15: 1005–1013.

Richardson, H.D. and Nakamaura, S. (1971) An electron microscopic study of spinal cord edema and the effect of treatment with steroids, mannitol, and hypothermia. *Proc. Veterans Adm. Spinal Cord Inj. Conf.*, 18: 10–16.

Rosenberg, L.J. and Wrathall, J.R. (1997) Quantitative analysis of acute axonal pathology in experimental spinal cord contusion. *J. Neurotrauma*, 14: 823–838.

Rosenberg, L.J. and Wrathall, J.R. (2001) Time course studies on the effectiveness of tetrodotoxin in reducing consequences of spinal cord contusion. *J. Neurosci. Res.*, 66: 191–202.

Rosenberg, L.J., Teng, Y.D. and Wrathall, J.R. (1999a) 2,3-Dihydroxy-6-nitro-7-sulfamoyl-benzo(f)quinoxaline reduces glial loss and acute white matter pathology after experimental spinal cord contusion. *J. Neurosci.*, 19: 464–475.

Rosenberg, L.J., Teng, Y.D. and Wrathall, J.R. (1999b) Effects of the sodium channel blocker tetrodotoxin on acute white matter pathology after experimental contusive spinal cord injury. *J. Neurosci.*, 19: 6122–6133.

Sala, F., Menna, G., Bricolo, A. and Young, W. (1999) Role of glycemia in acute spinal cord injury. Data from a rat experimental model and clinical experience. *Ann. New York Acad. Sci.*, 890: 133–154.

Sandler, A.N. and Tator, C.H. (1976a) Effect of acute spinal compression injury on regional spinal cord blood flow in primates. *J. Neurosurg.*, 45: 660–676.

Sandler, A.N. and Tator, C.H. (1976b) Regional spinal cord blood flow in primates. *J. Neurosurg.*, 45: 647–659.

Sandler, A.N. and Tator, C.H. (1976c) Review of the effect of spinal cord trauma on the vessels and blood flow in the spinal cord. *J. Neurosurg.*, 45: 638–646.

Sandler, A.N. and Tator, C.H. (1976d) Review of the measurement of normal spinal cord blood flow. *Brain Res.*, 118: 181–198.

Schoultz, T.W. (1977) Microscopic analysis of early histopathological spinal cord alterations following trauma in normal and cathecholamine-depleted cats. *J. Neurological Sci.*, 32: 283–295.

Schoultz, T.W., DeLuca, D.C. and Reding, D.L. (1976) Norepinephrine levels in traumatized spinal cord of catecholamine depleted cats. *Brain Res.*, 109: 367–374.

Scott, G.S., Jakeman, L.B., Stokes, B.T. and Szabo, C. (1999) Peroxynitrite production and activation of poly (adenosine diphosphate-ribose) synthetase in spinal cord injury. *Ann. Neurol.*, 45: 120–124.

Segal, J.L. and Brunnemann, S.R. (1997) 4-Aminopyridine improves pulmonary function in quadriplegic humans with longstanding spinal cord injury. *Pharmacotherapy*, 17: 415–423.

Segal, J.L. and Brunnemann, S.R. (1998) 4-Aminopyridine alters gait characteristics and enhances locomotion in spinal cord injured humans. *J. Spinal Cord Med.*, 21: 200–204.

Segal, J.L., Pathak, M.S., Hernandez, J.P., Himber, P.L., Brunnemann, S.R. and Charter, R.S. (1999) Safety and efficacy of 4-aminopyridine in humans with spinal cord injury: a long-term, controlled trial. *Pharmacotherapy*, 19: 713–723.

Seligman, M.L., Flamm, E.S., Goldstein, B.D., Poser, R.G., Demopoulos, H.B. and Ransohoff, J. (1977b) Spectrofluorescent detection of malonaldehyde as a measure of lipid free radical damage in response to ethanol potentiation of spinal cord trauma. *Lipids*, 12: 945–950.

Senter, H.J. and Venes, J.L. (1978) Altered blood flow and secondary injury in experimental spinal cord trauma. *J. Neurosurg.*, 49: 569–578.

Senter, H.J. and Venes, J.L. (1979) Loss of autoregulation and posttraumatic ischemia following experimental spinal cord trauma. *J. Neurosurg.*, 50: 198–206.

Senter, H.J., Burger, D.H. and Metzler, J. (1978) An improved technique for measurement of spinal cord blood flow. *Brain Res.*, 149: 197–203.

Senter, H.J., Venes, J.L. and Kauer, J.S. (1979) Alteration of posttraumatic ischemia in experimental spinal cord trauma by a central nervous system depressant. *J. Neurosurg.*, 50: 207–216.

Shapiro, K., Shulman, K., Marmarou, A. and Poll, W. (1977) Tissue pressure gradients in spinal cord injury. *Surg. Neurol.*, 7: 275–279.

Shuman, S.L., Bresnahan, J.C. and Beattie, M.S. (1997) Apoptosis of microglia and oligodendrocytes after spinal cord contusion in rats. *J. Neurosci. Res.*, 50: 798–808.

Singer, J.M., Russell, G.V. and Coe, J.E. (1970) Changes in evoked potentials after experimental cervical spinal cord injury in the monkey. *Exp. Neurol.*, 29: 449–461.

Smith, A.J., McCreery, D.B., Bloedel, J.R. and Chou, S.N. (1978) Hyperemia, CO2 responsiveness, and autoregulation in the white matter following experimental spinal cord injury. *J. Neurosurg.*, 48: 239–251.

Somerson, S.K. and Stokes, B.T. (1987) Functional analysis of an electromechanical spinal cord injury device. *Exp. Neurol.*, 96: 82–96.

Song, G., Cechvala, C., Resnick, D.K., Dempsey, R.J. and Rao, V.L. (2001) GeneChip analysis after acute spinal cord injury in rat. *J. Neurochem.*, 79: 804–815.

Stewart, W.B. and Wagner, F.C. (1979a) Vascular permeability changes in the contused feline spinal cord. *Brain Res.*, 169: 163–167.

Stewart, W.B. and Wagner, F.C., Jr. (1979b) Fascicular distribution of spinal cord edema following experimental trauma. In: A.J. Popp (Ed.), *Neural Trauma.* Raven Press, New York, pp. 131–135.

Stokes, B.T. and Garwood, M. (1982) Traumatically induced alterations in the oxygen fields in the canine spinal cord. *Exp. Neurol.*, 75: 665–677.

Stokes, B.T. and Reier, P.J. (1992) Fetal grafts alter chronic behavioral outcome after contusion damage to the adult rat spinal cord. *Exp. Neurol.*, 116: 1–12.

Stokes, B.T., Noyes, D.H. and Behrmann, D.L. (1992) An electromechanical spinal injury technique with dynamic sensitivity. *J. Neurotrauma*, 9: 187–195.

Streit, W.J., Semple-Rowland, S.L., Hurley, S.D., Miller, R.C., Popovich, P.G. and Stokes, B.T. (1998) Cytokine mRNA profiles in contused spinal cord and axotomized facial nucleus suggest a beneficial role for inflammation and gliosis. *Exp. Neurol.*, 152: 74–87.

Swaim, S.F., Hoerlein, B.F. and Hankes, G.H. (1971) Injury to the cervical spinal cord in the dog. *J. Am. Vet. Med. Assoc.*, 158: 462–467.

Tator, C.H. (1972) Acute spinal cord injury: a review of recent studies of treatment and pathophysiology. *Can. Med. Assoc. J.*, 107: 143–145.

Tator, C.H. and Deecke, L. (1973) Studies of the treatment and pathophysiology of acute spinal cord injury in primates. *Paraplegia*, 10: 344–345.

Teng, Y.D. and Wrathall, J.R. (1997) Local blockade of sodium channels by tetrodotoxin ameliorates tissue loss and long-term functional deficits resulting from experimental spinal cord injury. *J. Neurosci.*, 17: 4359–4366.

Teng, Y.D., Mocchetti, I. and Wrathall, J.R. (1998) Basic and acidic fibroblast growth factors protect spinal motor neurones in vivo after experimental spinal cord injury. *Eur. J. Neurosci.*, 10: 798–802.

Thomas, A.J., Nockels, R.P., Pan, H.Q., Shaffrey, C.I. and Chopp, M. (1999) Progesterone is neuroprotective after acute experimental spinal cord trauma in rats. *Spine*, 24: 2134–2138.

Tibbs, P.A., Young, B., McAllister, R.G. and Todd, E.P. (1979a) Studies of experimental cervical spinal cord transection. III. Effects of acute cervical spinal cord transection on cerebral blood flow. *J. Neurosurg.*, 50: 633–638.

Tibbs, P.A., Young, B., Ziegler, M.G. and McAllister, R.G. (1979b) Studies of experimental cervical spinal cord transection. II. Plasma norepinephrine levels after acute cervical spinal cord transection. *J. Neurosurg.*, 50: 629–632.

Tonai, T., Shiba, K., Taketani, Y., Ohmoto, Y., Murata, K., Muraguchi, M., Ohsaki, H., Takeda, E. and Nishisho, T. (2001) A neutrophil elastase inhibitor (ONO-5046) reduces neurologic damage after spinal cord injury in rats. *J. Neurochem.*, 78: 1064–1072.

Torre, J.C.D.L., Johnson, C.M., Harris, L.H., Kajihara, K. and Mullan, S. (1974) Monoamine changes in experimental head and spinal cord trauma: failure to confirm previous observations. *Surg. Neurol.*, 2: 5–11.

Tsubokawa, T., Nakamura, S., Hayashi, N., Taguma, N. and Sugawara, T. (1975) The circulatory disturbance of spinal cord injury and its response to local cooling therapy. *Neurol. Med.-Chir.*, 15(1): 87–93.

Tzeng, S.F., Bresnahan, J.C., Beattie, M.S. and de Vellis, J. (2001) Upregulation of the HLH Id gene family in neural progenitors and glial cells of the rat spinal cord following contusion injury. *J. Neurosci. Res.*, 66: 1161–1172.

van de Meent, H., Hamers, F.P., Lankhorst, A.J., Buise, M.P., Joosten, E.A. and Gispen, W.H. (1996) New assessment techniques for evaluation of posttraumatic spinal cord function in the rat. *J. Neurotrauma*, 13: 741–754.

van der Bruggen, M.A., Huisman, H.B., Beckerman, H., Bertelsmann, F.W., Polman, C.H. and Lankhorst, G.J. (2001) Randomized trial of 4-aminopyridine in patients with chronic incomplete spinal cord injury. *J. Neurol.*, 248: 665–671.

Vise, W.M., Yashon, D. and Hunt, W.E. (1974) Mechanisms of norepinephrine accumulation within sites of spinal cord injury. *J. Neurosurg.*, 40: 76–82.

Wagner Jr., F.C., VanGilder, J.C. and Dohrmann, G.J. (1978) Pathological changes from acute to chronic in experimental spinal cord trauma. *J. Neurosurg.*, 48: 92–98.

Walker, J.G., Yates, R.R., O'Neill, J.J. and Yashon, D. (1977) Canine spinal cord energy state after experimental trauma. *J. Neurochem.*, 29: 929–932.

Walker, J.G., Yates, R.R. and Yashon, D. (1979) Regional canine spinal cord energy state after experimental trauma. *J. Neurochem.*, 33: 397–401.

Wang, C.X., Olschowka, J.A. and Wrathall, J.R. (1997) Increase of interleukin-1beta mRNA and protein in the spinal cord following experimental traumatic injury in the rat. *Brain Res.*, 759: 190–196.

White, R.J., Albin, M.S., Harris, L.S. and Yashon, D. (1969) Spinal cord injury: sequential morphology and hypothermic stabilization. *Surg. Forum*, 20: 432–434.

Willenborg, D.O., Staten, E.A. and Eidelberg, E. (1977) Studies on cell-mediated hypersensitivity to neural antigens after experimental spinal cord injury. *Exp. Neurol.*, 54: 383–392.

Wolf, D.L. and Hall, E.D. (1985) Suloctidil treatment prevents the development of post-traumatic feline spinal cord ischemia. *Arch. Int. Pharmacodyn. Ther.*, 274: 139–144.

Wolf, J.A., Stys, P.K., Lusardi, T., Meaney, D. and Smith, D.H. (2001) Traumatic axonal injury induces calcium influx modulated by tetrodotoxin-sensitive sodium channels. *J. Neurosci.*, 21: 1923–1930.

Wolfe, D.L., Hayes, K.C., Hsieh, J.T. and Potter, P.J. (2001) Effects of 4-aminopyridine on motor evoked potentials in patients with spinal cord injury: a double-blinded, placebo-controlled crossover trial. *J. Neurotrauma*, 18: 757–771.

Wrathall, J.R. (1989) Behavioral methods for evaluating rats with contusive spinal cord injury: The combined behavioral score. In: M. Brown and M.E. Goldberger (Eds.), *Criteria for Assessing Recovery of Function: Behavioral Methods.* American Paralysis Association, Springfield, NJ, pp. 26–33.

Wrathall, J.R., Bouzoukis, J. and Choiniere, D. (1992a) Effect of kynurenate on functional deficits resulting from traumatic spinal cord injury. *Eur. J. Pharmacol.*, 218: 273–281.

Wrathall, J.R., Teng, Y.D., Choiniere, D. and Mundt, D.J. (1992b) Evidence that local non-NMDA receptors contribute to functional deficits in contusive spinal cord injury. *Brain Res.*, 586: 140–143.

Wrathall, J.R., Li, W. and Hudson, L.D. (1998) Myelin gene expression after experimental contusive spinal cord injury. *J. Neurosci.*, 18: 8780–8793.

Wrathall, J.R., Pettegrew, R.K. and Harvey, F. (1985) Spinal cord contusion in the rat: production of graded, reproducible, injury groups. *Exp. Neurol.*, 88: 108–122.

Wrathall, J.R., Teng, Y.D. and Marriott, R. (1997) Delayed antagonism of AMPA/kainate receptors reduces long-term functional deficits resulting from spinal cord trauma. *Exp. Neurol.*, 145: 565–573.

Wullenweber, R., Ebhardt, G., Collmann, H. and Duisberg, R. (1978) Spinal cord blood flow after experimental trauma in the dog. I. Morphological findings after standardized trauma. *Adv. Neurol.*, 20: 407–414.

Xu, J., Kim, G.M., Ahmed, S.H., Yan, P., Xu, X.M. and Hsu, C.Y. (2001a) Glucocorticoid receptor-mediated suppression of activator protein-1 activation and matrix metalloproteinase expression after spinal cord injury. *J. Neurosci.*, 21: 92–97.

Xu, J., Kim, G.M., Chen, S., Yan, P., Ahmed, S.H., Ku, G., Beckman, J.S., Xu, X.M. and Hsu, C.Y. (2001b) iNOS and nitrotyrosine expression after spinal cord injury. *J. Neurotrauma*, 18: 523–532.

Yan, P., Li, Q., Kim, G.M., Xu, J., Hsu, C.Y. and Xu, X.M. (2001) Cellular localization of tumor necrosis factor-alpha following acute spinal cord injury in adult rats. *J. Neurotrauma*, 18: 563–568.

Yanagawa, Y., Marcillo, A., Garcia-Rojas, R., Loor, K.E. and Dietrich, W.D. (2001) Influence of posttraumatic hypoxia on behavioral recovery and histopathological outcome following moderate spinal cord injury in rats. *J. Neurotrauma*, 18: 635–644.

Yashon, D., Bingham Jr., W.G., Faddoul, E.M. and Hunt, W.E. (1973) Edema of the spinal cord following experimental impact trauma. *J. Neurosurg.*, 38: 693–697.

Yong, C., Arnold, P.M., Zoubine, M.N., Citron, B.A., Watanabe, I., Berman, N.E. and Festoff, B.W. (1998) Apoptosis in cellular compartments of rat spinal cord after severe contusion injury. *J. Neurotrauma*, 15: 459–472.

Young, W. and Bracken, M.B. (1992) The Second National Acute Spinal Cord Injury Study. *J. Neurotrauma*, 9(Suppl. 1): S397–S405.

Young, W. and Flamm, E.S. (1982) Effect of high-dose corticosteroid therapy on blood flow, evoked potentials, and extracellular calcium in experimental spinal injury. *J. Neurosurg.*, 57: 667–673.

Young, W. and Koreh, I. (1986) Potassium and calcium changes in injured spinal cords. *Brain Res.*, 365: 42–53.

Young, W., Flamm, E.S., Demopoulos, H.B., Tomasula, J.J. and DeCrescito, V. (1981) Effect of naloxone on posttraumatic ischemia in experimental spinal contusion. *J. Neurosurg.*, 55: 209–219.

Young, W., Koreh, I., Yen, V. and Lindsay, A. (1982a) Effect of sympathectomy on extracellular potassium ionic activity and blood flow in experimental spinal cord contusion. *Brain Res.*, 253: 115–124.

Young, W., Yen, V. and Blight, A. (1982b) Extracellular calcium ionic activity in experimental spinal cord contusion. *Brain Res.*, 253: 105–113.

Yu, C.G., Jagid, J., Ruenes, G., Dietrich, W.D., Marcillo, A.E. and Yezierski, R.P. (2001) Detrimental effects of systemic hyperthermia on locomotor function and histopathological outcome after traumatic spinal cord injury in the rat. *Neurosurgery*, 49: 152–159.

Yu, W.R., Westergren, H., Farooque, M., Holtz, A. and Olsson, Y. (2000) Systemic hypothermia following spinal cord compression injury in the rat: an immunohistochemical study on MAP 2 with special reference to dendrite changes. *Acta Neuropathol. (Berl.)*, 100: 546–552.

Zhang, S.X., Underwood, M., Landfield, A., Huang, F.F., Gison, S. and Geddes, J.W. (2000) Cytoskeletal disruption following contusion injury to the rat spinal cord. *J. Neuropathol. Exp. Neurol.*, 59: 287–296.

L. McKerracher, G. Doucet and S. Rossignol (Eds.)
Progress in Brain Research, Vol. 137

Transplants and neurotrophic factors increase regeneration and recovery of function after spinal cord injury

Barbara S. Bregman *, Jean-Valery Coumans, Hai Ning Dai, Penelope L. Kuhn, James Lynskey, Marietta McAtee and Faheem Sandhu

Department of Neuroscience, Georgetown University Medical Center, Washington, DC 20007, USA

Introduction

After axotomy in the mature CNS both intrinsic neuronal and extrinsic environmental factors contribute to the lack of axonal regeneration. The dogma that the adult mammalian central nervous system is hard-wired and incapable of significant plasticity is no longer tenable. It is now clear that reorganization of CNS pathways occurs after injury and contributes to recovery of function. Experimental conditions that alter the intrinsic capacity of mature CNS neurons for growth and those that modify the environment at the injury site increase axonal regeneration and recovery of function. We have shown, for example, that neural tissue transplants (which provide a favorable terrain for axonal elongation at the injury site) and neurotrophic factors (which alter the neuronal capacity for regrowth after injury) increase regeneration after spinal cord injury (Bregman and Bernstein-Goral, 1991; Bernstein-Goral and Bregman, 1993; Bregman et al., 1997a,b; Bregman, 1998; Diener and Bregman, 1998a; Broude et al., 1999). After spinal cord lesions at birth, for example, transplants rescue immature axotomized CNS

* Correspondence to: B.S. Bregman, Department of Neuroscience, Georgetown University, 3970 Reservoir Road NW, Washington, DC 20007, USA. Tel.: +1-202-687-1452; Fax: +1-202-687-0617;
E-mail: bregmanb@georgetown.edu

neurons from retrograde cell death (Bregman and Reier, 1986) and support the regrowth of supraspinal axons into and through the transplants (Bregman and Bernstein-Goral, 1991; Bernstein-Goral and Bregman, 1993). The anatomical reorganization supports recovery of locomotion and skilled forelimb function (Kunkel-Bagden and Bregman, 1990; Diener and Bregman, 1998a,b). After injury in the adult, although supraspinal axons regrow into the transplants, the projection is spatially restricted and axons terminate near the host transplant border (Bregman et al., 1997b). We review here recent work from this laboratory that demonstrates that experimental conditions that alter the intrinsic capacity of mature CNS neurons for growth and those that modify the environment at the injury site increase axonal regeneration and recovery of function. After spinal cord *transection* at T_6, transplants and neurotrophic factors restore supraspinal projections across the injury site and the regrowth contributes to recovery of locomotion (Coumans et al., 2001). Surprisingly, there is greater axonal growth and greater recovery of function if the interventions are delayed by 2–4 weeks than following immediate transplantation (Coumans et al., 2001). The neuronal circuitry underlying skilled reaching, however, is far more complex than that underlying locomotion. After high cervical spinal cord hemisection, transplants and neurotrophic factors support regrowth and recovery of skilled forelimb movement (Lynskey et al., 2001;

Sandhu et al., 2000). We suggest that both regrowth of specific pathways into/through the transplant and re-organization of other CNS pathways above and below the injury site contribute to this recovery.

Normal motor control of locomotion and skilled forelimb movement

The anatomical circuitry underlying rhythmic, alternating stepping movements is intrinsic within the spinal cord and is known as the spinal pattern generator for locomotion (SPGL) (Grillner, 1986, 1996; Grillner and Dubuc, 1988; Grillner and Georgopoulos, 1996; Grillner et al., 1998). Normally, the spinal pattern generator for locomotion is under control and modulation by segmental sensory afferent influences, intersegmental (propriospinal) influences, and descending (suprasegmental) control from brainstem and cortical regions.

Research, largely from studies of normal motor control in mammals, has suggested that although the basic circuitry underlying locomotion lies within the spinal cord, particular pathways contribute particular aspects to the initiation and performance of locomotion (Andersson et al., 1978; Grillner and Rossignol, 1978; Rossignol et al., 1986; Grillner and Dubuc, 1988; Chau et al., 1998a,b). For example, most mammals are capable of goal-directed locomotion, including the ability to avoid obstacles, even in the absence of the cerebral cortex. Under normal conditions, the cortex appears to contribute to fine control and volitional positioning of the limbs during conditions requiring accurate foot placement during locomotion (Grillner and Dubuc, 1988). Corticospinal pathways also make specific contributions to reflex motor control, mediating particular reflex responses such as low-threshold contact-placing responses (Amassian and Ross, 1978; Bregman and Goldberger, 1982, 1983a,b, 1983c). Brainstem–spinal pathways also contribute to the postural support and equilibrium required for locomotor function.

Skilled forelimb movement such as target-directed reaching, however, is not under the influence of pattern generators. The neural circuitry underlying skilled forelimb movement such as reaching may be far more complex than those underlying rhythmic alternating movements such as locomotion. In addition to direct supraspinal input from the cortex to forelimb motorneurons and interneurons to control reaching, supraspinal, intraspinal and segmental pathways and feedback loops are integrated by the propriospinal network. These propriospinal neurons project to forelimb segments to guide target reaching and to hindlimb segments to influence postural adjustments associated with reaching. In normal animals, rubrospinal neurons not only play a major role in the normal motor control involved in locomotion, but also contribute to the control of skilled forelimb movement such as reaching (McKenna and Whishaw, 1999; Rho et al., 1999; Muir and Whishaw, 2000). It is likely that the mechanisms underlying recovery of rhythmic alternating movements such as overground locomotion differ from those underlying target-directed movements such as reaching and grasping or locomotion over difficult terrain. Since the neuronal circuitry underlying stepping is intrinsic within the spinal pattern generators located within the spinal cord (Grillner, 1975, 1996; Grillner and Dubuc, 1988; Pearson, 1995), the recovery of overground locomotion may simply require the re-establishment of some modest level of supraspinal control. Skilled forelimb movement, in contrast, may require more precise restoration of supraspinal input for recovery to occur.

Possible mechanisms underlying recovery of function after spinal cord injury: lesion-induced plasticity

A spinal cord lesion removes the descending suprasegmental and propriospinal control over the spinal cord circuitry either completely (transection) or partially (hemisection, contusion injuries), alters the balance between excitatory and inhibitory influences on the spinal cord circuitry and results in a loss of function caudal to the site of injury. The loss of function after spinal cord injury is invariably followed by some subsequent recovery of function. Since, without other interventions, those pathways that were injured directly (axotomized) do not regenerate, the motor behavior that recovers must be mediated by alterations in the remaining undamaged pathways. There are a number of potential sources of input that may contribute to recovery of function after spinal cord injury. After lesions in the developing or mature nervous system, there is some recovery of function, even *without* any particular intervention (Bregman and Goldberger, 1982, 1983b,c; Goldberger, 1988b,c; Kunkel-Bagden and Bregman, 1990; Bregman et al., 1991; Helgren and Goldberger, 1993; Howland et al., 1995a,b). This recovery is mediated by sources intrinsic to the CNS, such as spared pathways not damaged directly by the lesion. The response of the spared pathways to the loss of other pathways determines both the extent of recovery and the specific functions, which recover (Goldberger, 1988c, 1991; Bregman, 1994).

There are several potential mechanisms that may contribute to naturally occurring recovery of function after spinal cord injury. For example, in the absence of descending input to the SPGL, previously ineffective synapses may be recruited and may contribute to the activation of segmental reflex activity at a spinal cord level. The sensitivity of the neurons composing the SPGL may be altered as a consequence of spinal cord injury. Some of the other intrinsic mechanisms that may contribute to recovery of function after spinal cord injury include behavioral substitution, physiologic recovery and remyelination of injured, but intact axonal pathways. Anatomic sprouting of undamaged pathways has also been implicated in recovery of function after spinal cord injury at birth or at maturity (Goldberger and Murray, 1978; Goldberger, 1988b,c, 1991; Goldberger et al., 1990). These studies have demonstrated that sprouting of undamaged pathways is not a random response to injury, but must be regulated in some manner, such that a hierarchy of pathways that sprout in response to a particular injury exists (Goldberger, 1988a).

While it has been clear for some time that lesion-induced anatomical reorganization occurs after lesions early in development, the existence of such anatomical remodeling after injury in the mature nervous system has been much more controversial. A number of recent studies provide convincing evidence that extensive neural plasticity is not unique to the developing nervous system, but also occurs after injury to the mature CNS. For example, after unilateral sensorimotor cortical injury, there are extensive anatomical changes in the contralateral cortex, including time-dependent increases in dendritic arborization, neuropil volume, synapse to neuron ratios, and in the nature of the synapses (Jones et al.,

1996; Kleim et al., 1998; Jones, 1999; Jones et al., 1999; Bury et al., 2000). While it was generally thought that remodeling in the mature CNS, when it occurs, is restricted to an increased density of existing connections (Goldberger and Murray, 1978), more recent studies indicate substantial remodeling over spatially extensive distances (Jain et al., 2000). After spinal cord lesion, deafferentation, or forelimb amputation in primates, there is substantial functional reorganization within the sensorimotor cortex (Florence and Kaas, 1995; Sengelaub et al., 1997; Florence et al., 1998; Kaas et al., 1999; Jain et al., 2000). Recent studies have demonstrated that this functional recovery is accompanied by substantial remodeling at the level of the dorsal column nuclei (Jain et al., 2000). After these injuries that denervate the dorsal column nuclei, trigeminal primary afferent axons invade the cuneate nucleus (Jain et al., 2000). Thus, after CNS injury in the adult, there is significant remodeling of connections. It is likely that this remodeling contributes to the recovery of function that has been observed.

It is unlikely that when regeneration is induced experimentally, it precludes the intrinsic plasticity that follows CNS lesions. More likely, under experimental conditions that support regeneration, both axonal regeneration of pathways damaged directly and axonal reorganization in pathways not damaged directly occur in parallel and together contribute to the recovery observed.

Effects of transplants and neurotrophic factors on regeneration and recovery of function

Transplants of fetal spinal cord tissue placed into the lesion site in either the neonatal or adult operates increases the extent of recovery beyond that mediated by naturally occurring mechanisms intrinsic to the animal (see Bregman and Kunkel-Bagden, 1994 and Bregman et al., 1997a for reviews). The presence of a transplant of fetal spinal cord tissue at the injury site may restore a more normal balance among the segmental, intersegmental and suprasegmental influences on the spinal pattern generator for locomotion and permit the development or recovery of more normal patterns of locomotor function. In transplantation paradigms, the regrowth of supraspinal axons across the site of the trans-

rovide sufficient input to initiate stepping and provide balance required for overground locomotion. The re-establishment of even moderate amounts of descending control (either directly or by means of a relay) in the presence of a transplant is sufficient to mediate significant improvements in locomotor function (Kunkel-Bagden and Bregman, 1990; Stokes and Reier, 1992; Bregman et al., 1993; Bregman and Kunkel-Bagden, 1994; Howland et al., 1995a,b, 1995c; Ribotta et al., 2000). The extent of recovery is greater in the transplant groups than in the lesion-only groups. Although recovery of function is substantial, permanent deficits persist after spinal cord injury and transplantation in both neonatal and adult operates. The transplants are able to restore some, but not all, of the function lost after spinal cord injury. Combinations of interventions may be required to restore reflex, sensory and locomotor function to more normal levels after spinal cord injury.

After neonatal cervical spinal cord injury, the presence of a transplant at the injury site not only restores rhythmic alternating movements, such as those involved in locomotion, but the neuroanatomical reorganization supported by the transplant is also able to support the development and recovery of skilled forelimb movements involved in target-directed reaching and grooming behaviors (Bregman et al., 1997a; Diener and Bregman, 1998a,b).

After spinal cord lesions and transplants in the *adult*, neurotrophins increase the *density* and *extent* of axonal elongation into transplants of fetal spinal cord tissue and alter the cell body response to injury

The capacity of CNS neurons for axonal regrowth after injury decreases as the age of the animal at time of injury increases (Fig. 1). After spinal cord lesions and transplants at birth, there is extensive regenerative growth into and beyond a transplant of fetal spinal cord tissue placed at the injury site (Bregman, 1987; Bregman et al., 1989; Bernstein-Goral and Bregman, 1993). After injury in the adult, host corticospinal and brainstem–spinal axons project into the transplant. Their distribution, however, is restricted to within 200 μm of the host/transplant border (Bregman et al., 1989, 1997b). The exoge-

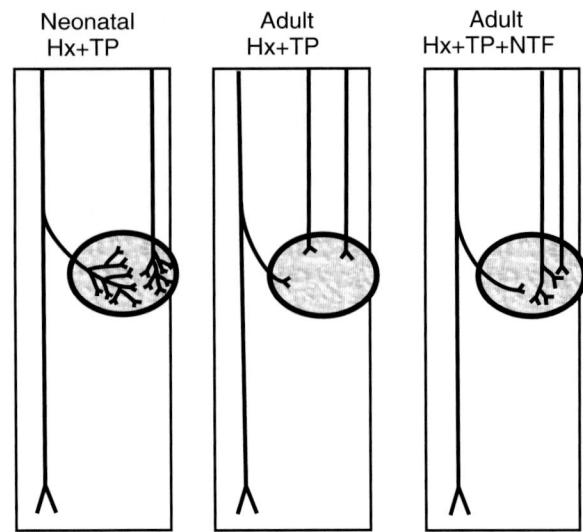

Fig. 1. After spinal cord lesions at birth, transplants of fetal spinal cord tissue support the regrowth of supraspinal axons into and through (not shown) the lesion site. As the age at time of injury increases, the growth of supraspinal axons into the transplant is attenuated. The exogenous administration of neurotrophic factors increases the density and extent of axonal growth within the transplant.

nous administration of neurotrophic factors increases the capacity of mature CNS neurons for regrowth after injury (Bregman et al., 1997b; Broude et al., 1999). Spinal cord over-hemisection lesions were made at T_6 in adult rats. Transplants of E14 fetal spinal cord tissue were placed into the lesion site. BDNF, NT-3, NT-4, CNTF or vehicle alone was administered at the site of the transplant at the time of injury and transplantation (5 μl at 1 μg/μl). After 1–2 months survival, neuroanatomical tracing and immunocytochemical methods were used to examine the growth of host axons within the transplants. BDNF, NT-3, and NT-4 *each* increased both the density and extent of serotonergic axonal ingrowth into the transplants dramatically. In controls (transplant only, no neurotrophin), serotonergic axons terminate at the immediate host: transplant border. In the presence of exogenous neurotrophic support, there is an increase in the distance and density of ingrowth within the transplant tissue. In animals treated with either BDNF or NT-3, there was an increase in corticospinal axonal ingrowth within the transplants, similar to that observed for the serotonergic axons.

Qualitatively, the extent of CS ingrowth was similar with each of the neurotrophins examined (BDNF, NT-3, NT-4). This was surprising in light of previous observations (Schnell and Schwab, 1993; Schnell et al., 1994) that indicated that NT-3 but not BDNF increased the sprouting of corticospinal axons after spinal cord lesion. The influence of the administration of the neurotrophins on the growth of injured CNS axons was not a generalized effect of growth factors per se, since the administration of CNTF had *no effect* on the growth of any of the descending CNS axons tested. These results are important because they indicate that in addition to influencing the survival of developing CNS and PNS neurons, neurotrophic factors are able to exert a *neurotropic* influence on injured mature CNS neurons by increasing their axonal growth within a transplant.

Transplants and neurotrophins support greater axonal regeneration after *chronic* spinal cord transection than after acute injury in adult rats

In studies described above we have shown that after acute spinal cord *hemisection*, the exogenous application of neurotrophic factors in conjunction with the transplants increases the extent of axonal growth within the transplant. Those interventions that increase growth within the transplant also modify the cell body response to injury by up-regulating growth associated cellular programs and preventing the atrophy of the injured neurons (Broude et al., 1997, 1999; Bregman et al., 1998). After partial spinal cord injury, both regenerating and sprouting axons can contribute to the regrowth observed (Bernstein-Goral et al., 1997). In the current study, we have examined the capacity of transplants and neurotrophic factors to influence axonal regeneration across the injury site after acute and chronic spinal cord transection (Fig. 2). Complete spinal cord transections were made at a mid-thoracic level in adult rats. Fetal spinal cord transplants were placed into the lesion cavity either immediately following the transection (acute injury) or after a 2-week delay (which we have defined as chronic injury), and neurotrophic factors were administered exogenously via an implanted minipump. The extent of axonal regrowth of supraspinal axons across the injury site and the extent of recovery of locomotor function were examined. The

exogenous administration of neurotrophins led to increased axonal growth after spinal cord transection and transplantation.

Surprisingly, both the amount of axonal regrowth and the extent of recovery of function were actually greater in the *chronic* injury group than in the acute injury group

Transection alone permanently abolished all supraspinal axonal projections caudal to the transection. After either acute or chronic spinal cord transection (either with or without neurotrophins), the transplants survived, grew and matured to bridge the gap between the rostral and caudal stumps of the host spinal cord. Descending axons from the host CNS grew into transplants after either acute or chronic injury. Supraspinal axons grew *through* the transplant and back into the host spinal cord caudal to the transection in only 55% of the acute group of animals but did so in 89% of the chronic group of animals. In the delayed transplant group, not only was there a greater proportion of animals with growth distal to the transplant in the chronic injury group, the projection was denser and more complex in its pattern, and the axons were located in both gray matter and white matter regions within the host caudal to the transection (Fig. 3). The reasons for the greater axonal growth after chronic as compared to acute injury remain to be determined, but there are several possible candidates that may contribute to this enhanced regrowth. There may be a down-regulation of some of the myelin-associated inhibitors within the spinal cord caudal to the injury at prolonged times after the transection. In the chronic transplantation paradigm, when the lesion site is exposed the glial scar is cleared. This may serve as a conditioning injury that increases the regenerative capacity of the axotomized neurons, as has been described previously for dorsal root ganglion neurons (Richardson and Issa, 1984; Chong et al., 1999; Neumann and Woolf, 1999). The milieu at the injury site may differ between acute and chronic injury time points. For example, we have shown that the expression of pro-inflammatory cytokines is attenuated in the chronic injury group compared to the acute injury group (Nakamura et al., 2001). Neurotrophins themselves, can also alter the response of neurons to myelin. The exogenous

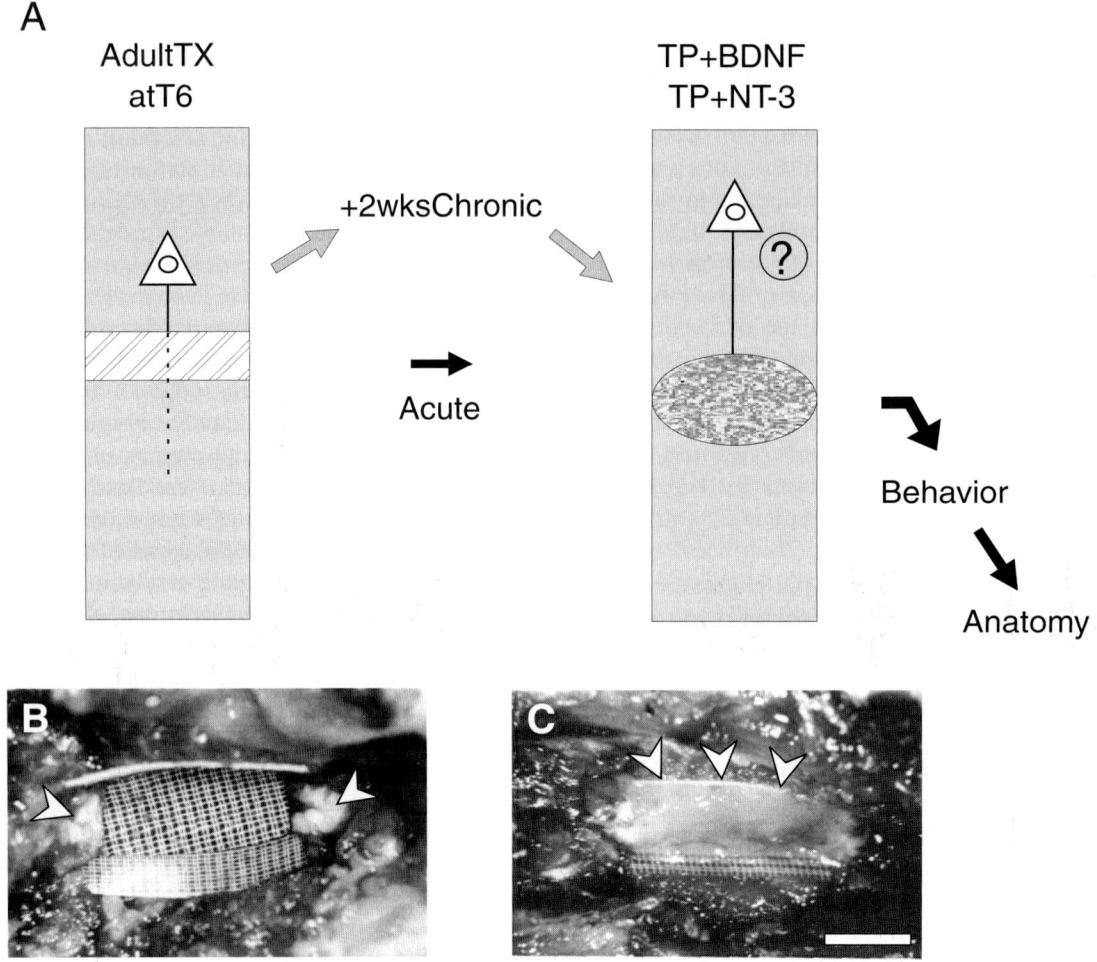

Fig. 2. (A) Experimental model. Complete spinal cord transections were made at T_6 in adult rats. Transplants of fetal spinal cord tissue were placed into the lesion site either immediately (acute) or following a 2 week delay (chronic). Neurotrophic factors BDNF or NT-3 or saline were administered by alzet pump. Animals underwent qualitative and quantitative behavioral analysis prior to anatomical evaluation of axonal growth. (B) Surgical transection site. The cut ends of the cord (arrows) are indicated; typically a 7–9 mm gap separates the rostral and caudal cord stumps. Artificial dura lines the floor and sides of the lesion cavity. (C) Transplant of fetal spinal cord tissue (arrows) is placed into the lesion site, filling the gap. Scale bar = 5 mm for B and C.

administration of neurotrophins in vivo may increase the intrinsic capacity of mature CNS neurons for growth as they do in vitro. Studies by Filbin and colleagues (Cai et al., 1999) show that exposure of neurons to neurotrophins in vitro, before they encounter the inhibitory influence of myelin-associated glycoproteins or myelin, increases the amount of neurite outgrowth, via a cAMP-dependent mechanism.

The growth of chronically injured supraspinal pathways across the transplant and back into the host spinal cord caudal to the transection was also confirmed by retrograde neuroanatomical tracing. Retrograde tracing experiments in transplant and neurotrophin treated animals revealed FluoroGold labeled neurons both within the transplant itself and in the spinal cord rostral to the transplant as well (Fig. 4). In addition, neurons containing Fluoro-Gold were clearly identified within the cortex and in the brainstem nuclei (red nucleus, locus coeruleus, lateral vestibular nucleus, raphe nuclei) of these animals, indicating retrograde transport by supraspinal axons that regenerated through the embryonic trans-

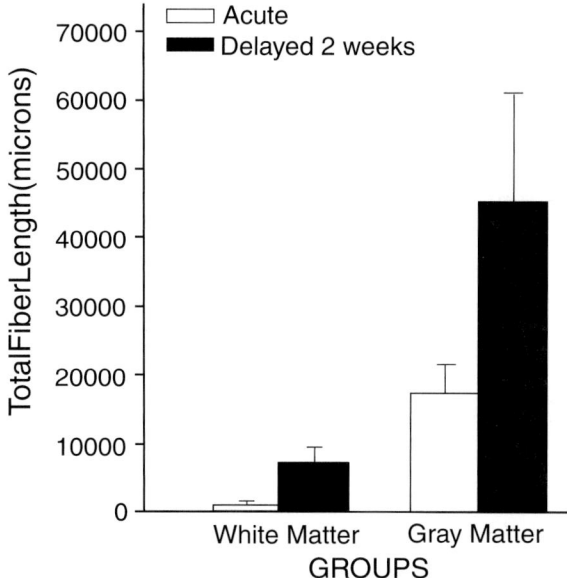

Fig. 3. Serotonergic fiber growth caudal to transection. In animals with transplants and exogenous neurotrophic support there is growth of supraspinal axons across the transplant and back into the host spinal cord. Surprisingly, the amount of growth is significantly greater in the delayed transplantation group. Axonal growth is seen in both gray and white matter regions of the host spinal cord caudal to the TX+TP. (Modified from Coumans, 2001.)

plant into the caudal host cord (Fig. 4). In transection only animals and in animals with transections and transplants (but no neurotrophins), there were no retrogradely labeled neurons in any of the brainstem nuclei or in the host spinal cord rostral to the lesion. Taken together, the anatomical data indicates that after spinal cord lesions in adult rats, the transplants serve both as a bridge and as a relay to restore supraspinal input to the spinal cord circuitry below the level of injury.

Transplants and neurotrophins support recovery of locomotor function after *chronic* spinal cord transection in adult rats

Under experimental conditions as described above, all animals underwent quantitative behavioral analysis (Bregman and Kunkel-Bagden, 1989; Bregman et al., 1993, 1995; Bregman, 1994; Miya et al., 1997) prior to sacrifice, in order to determine if the anatomical re-establishment of supraspinal and propriospinal input improved locomotor function. The animals with transplants and neurotrophins showed greater recovery of locomotor function. On overground and treadmill locomotion, chronic TX+TP+NTF animals exhibited partial hindlimb weight support, with frequent unilateral or bilateral plantar foot placement (Fig. 5). In chronic injury animals with transplant and neurotrophins, extended periods of forelimb–hindlimb coordination during overground walking were seen more frequently than in acute injury animals. Unoperated control animals showed weight-supported stepping in 100% of the steps. Under these testing conditions, transection only animals showed no weight-supported step cycles. In contrast, 45% of the step cycles for chronic injury animals with transplants and neurotrophins were characterized by weight-supported hindlimb steps, frequently with plantar foot placement (Fig. 5). Chronic TX+TP+NTF animals had significantly ($P < 0.001$, ANOVA, Tukey Multiple Comparison Test) more weight-supported steps than did any other experimental group. No weight-supported stepping was observed in transection only (without transplant) or in transplant only (without neurotrophin) animals. Acute TX+TP+NTF animals rarely showed any weight-supported stepping. The chronic injury animals with transplants and neurotrophins displayed similar improvements in motor function during overground locomotor tasks such as stair climbing (Fig. 6); both hindlimbs show good weight support and plantar foot placement. There was reciprocal hindlimb movement during stair-climbing and evidence of fore and hindlimb coordination in ascent. This was observed with a greater frequency in the chronic injury animals than in the acute injury group. Transection only and TX+TP animals without neurotrophins did not use the hindlimbs during stair ascent. The chronic TX+TP+NTF animals showed significantly more hindlimb weight-supported steps during stair-climbing than did transection only animals ($P < 0.001$). Re-transection of the spinal cord rostral to the transplant in the TP+NTF animals abolished the movements that had recovered; there was no subsequent recovery of weight-supported stepping and plantar foot placement on treadmill, overground or on the stairs during the subsequent 5-week observation period. This suggests that at least some of the motor recovery observed was dependent

264

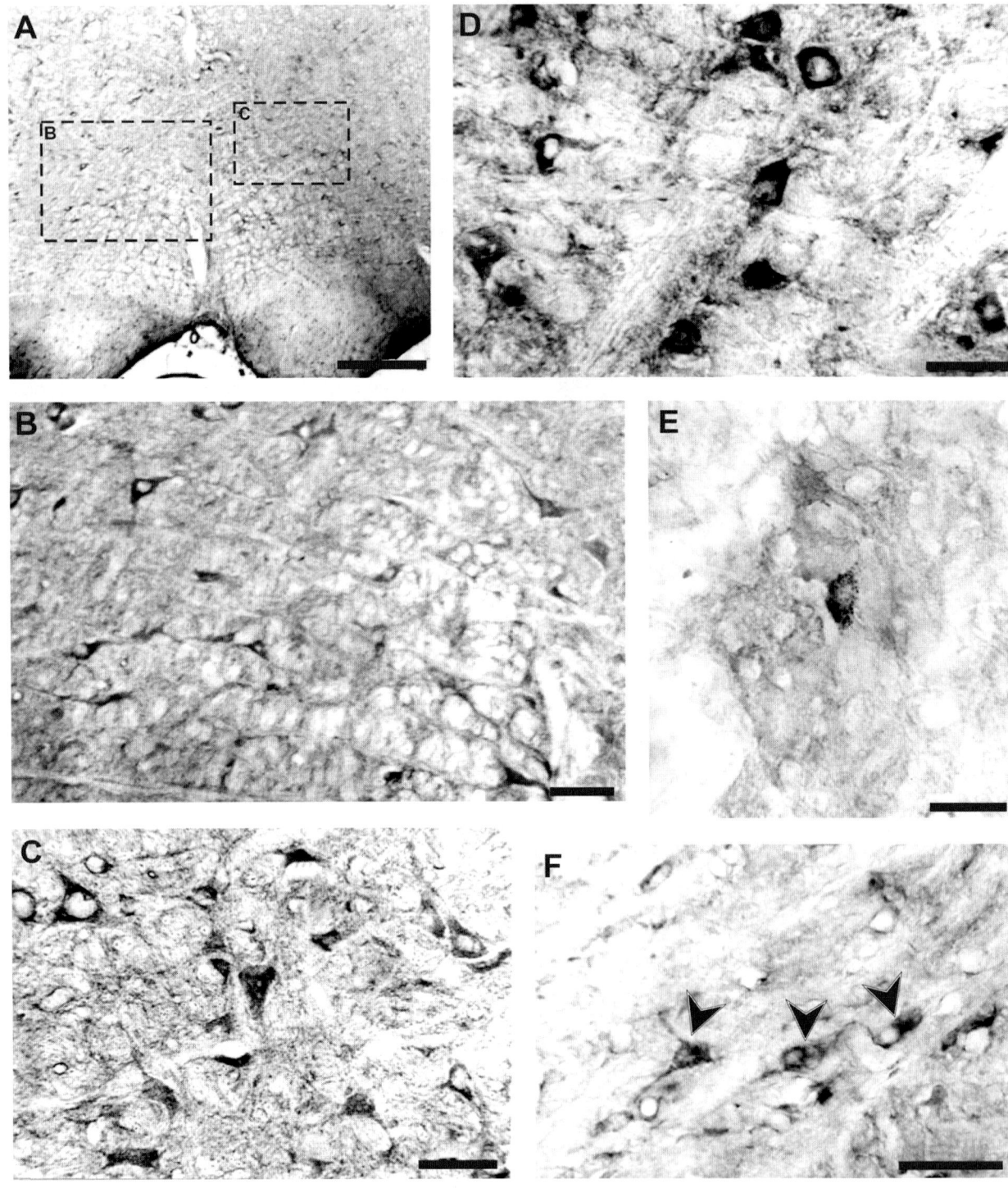

LESION ONLY | TP + NTF

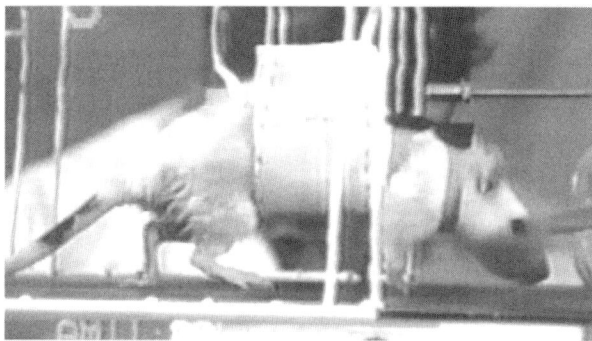

Fig. 5. Transplant plus neurotrophic factor treatment improves locomotion. Lesion only animals fail to establish weight-supported hindlimb stepping during either treadmill or overground locomotion. In contrast TP+NTF animals establish hindlimb weight-supported locomotion with plantar foot placement and sufficient weight support to maintain body weight. Harness in both photos provides postural support for the trunk. Balance remains impaired in both groups of animals.

upon the anatomical connections established through the transplants.

Taken together, these data suggest that after chronic spinal cord injury, transplants and neurotrophic factors can support the regrowth of supraspinal pathways and can re-establish some supraspinal and propriospinal input across the transection site. This regrowth is associated with consistent improvements in hindlimb locomotor function. The findings suggest that CNS neurons with longstanding injuries can re-initiate a growth response leading to improvement in motor function (Coumans et al., 2001). While it is clear that the anatomical connections established across the transplant (in the presence of neurotrophic support) contribute to the recovery of function after complete spinal cord transection, we do not believe that the regeneration is *solely* responsible for the recovery. Rather, we predict that plasticity within the spinal cord caudal to the lesion and plasticity at supraspinal levels also make major contributions to the recovery.

Transplants and exogenous neurotrophic support also modify the anatomical plasticity and recovery of skilled forelimb movement after high cervical spinal cord lesions

The recovery of rhythmic alternating movements involved in locomotion may be a less formidable requirement after spinal cord injury than is the recovery of skilled forelimb movement (Fig. 7). There are substantial deficits in forelimb motor control after spinal cord injury in the adult (Schrimsher and Reier, 1992, 1993), as there are after lesions at birth (Bregman and Goldberger, 1983a,b; Diener and Bregman, 1998b). In a recent series of experiments we have examined the capacity for anatomical plasticity and recovery after cervical spinal cord injury in adult rats. We have demonstrated that fetal spinal cord transplants plus exogenous neurotrophic factors increase supraspinal pathway regeneration and significantly improve functional behavioral recovery in adult rats following cervical spinal cord lesions

Fig. 4. Immunocytochemical visualization of FluoroGold (FG) labeled neurons. FluoroGold was injected into the host spinal cord 10 mm caudal to delayed TP+NTF. (A–C) Raphe nucleus, (D) red nucleus, (E) locus coeruleus, (F) transplant. TX abolishes all supraspinal input to the host spinal cord caudal to the transection. Transplants and neurotrophic factors restore supraspinal input. (A) Low power image through medulla demonstrates retrogradely labeled FG neurons in the raphe nucleus. Areas enlarged in B and C are indicated. (B and C) Raphe nucleus neurons are retrogradely labeled with FG. Corticospinal (data not shown), red nucleus (D) and locus coeruleus neurons (E) are retrogradely labeled with FG after spinal cord TX + delayed TP+NTF. Propriospinal projections are established across the transplant in both acute and delayed transplantation with neurotrophins (data not shown). Neurons within the transplant also project to the host spinal cord and are retrogradely labeled with FG (arrows) following injection into the host spinal cord. Scale bars A = 300 μm, B = 100 μm, C–F = 50 μm.

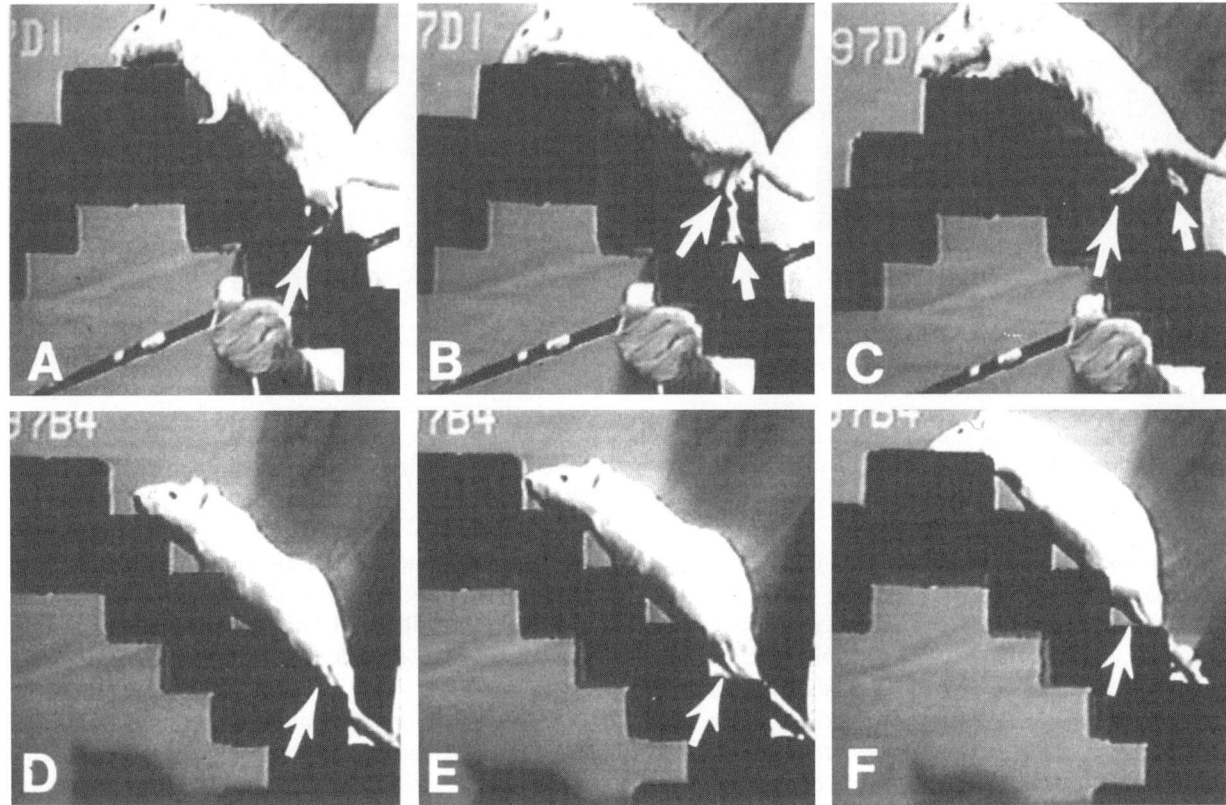

Fig. 6. Stair climbing. Transplant plus neurotrophin-treated animals use weight-supported hindlimb stepping during stair climbing. (A–C) Delayed transplant plus neurotrophic factor, (D–F) transplant only. (A–C) Video frames taken during stair-climbing task. The delayed TX+TP+NTF animals develop the ability to climb stairs with good hindlimb weight support (arrows) and coordination between forelimb and hindlimb movement. (D–F) Video frames from TX+TP only animal. This group of animals (like the TX only animals, do not use the hindlimbs during stair climbing. All propulsion is provided by the forelimbs, and the hindlimbs are dragged passively, without weight support (arrows).

(Lynskey et al., 1999, 2000; Sandhu F.A. et al., 1999; Sandhu et al., 2000). The lesions studied were C_3/C_4 cervical overhemisections, which produced a unilateral lesion disrupting the right rubrospinal tract and damaged the corticospinal tracts bilaterally. Transplantation surgery was performed 2 weeks following the initial spinal cord lesion. Four to six weeks following the transplantation surgery, the anatomical regeneration was evaluated via neuroanatomical tracing experiments and immunohistochemistry. Anterograde tracing of the corticospinal and rubrospinal pathways and dorsal root afferents was conducted using biotin dextran amine (BDA – 10,000, Molecular Probes, Eugene, OR). As we demonstrated above after thoracic hemisection, after cervical hemisection the transplants and neurotrophic factors act syner-

gistically to increase axonal regeneration after spinal cord injury in the adult. Anterograde tracing of corticospinal (Fig. 8A,B,C) and rubrospinal (data not shown) axons using BDA clearly labels the axons in the transplant. While some CST axons grow into the transplant in saline treated animals, the amount of growth is increased with the exogenous administration of neurotrophins. Rubrospinal axons, in contrast, fail to grow into the transplant in saline only animals, but do so with the neurotrophins.

The axonal growth elicited by the transplants and neurotrophic factors permits the recovery of skilled forelimb movement after cervical spinal cord injury in adult rats (Fig. 8D). Prior to any tracing or anatomical analysis, the animals underwent extensive behavioral testing. Animals were trained

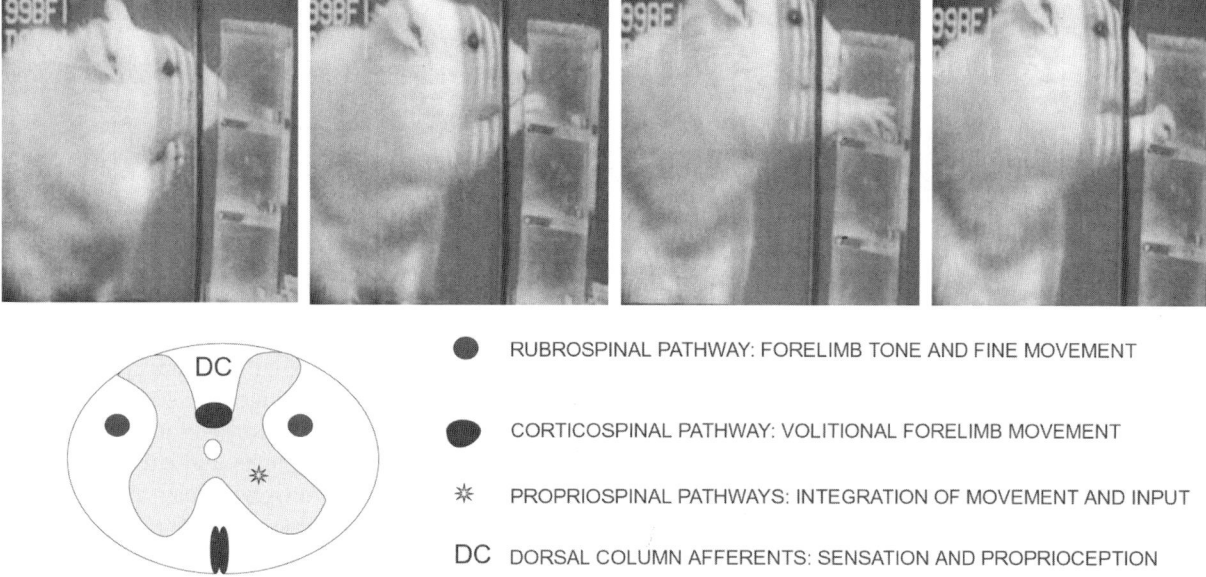

Fig. 7. The neural circuitry underlying skilled reaching is more complex than that underlying locomotion. Normally, corticospinal, rubrospinal, and propriospinal neurons contribute to the descending control of reaching. Video frames of reaching task in a control animal.

and tested on skilled reaching for food, forehead sticker removal, and rearing. Four main effects of the transplants plus exogenous neurotrophic factors were observed. First, transplant plus neurotrophic treated animals demonstrated a greater recovery of skilled target reaching bilaterally. The average number of reaches per trial for each animal was greater for transplant plus neurotrophic factor treated animals for both left and right forelimb reaches as compared to animals treated with transplant plus saline. Second, greater proximal and distal forelimb motor control was observed during skilled target reaching. Only animals treated with transplant plus neurotrophic factors recovered the ability to reach above the first shelf with their right forelimbs (Fig. 8D). Distally, right forepaw digit extension during reaching was closer to normal in transplant plus neurotrophic factor treated animals. Third, multiple characteristics of skilled target reaching of transplant plus neurotrophic factor treated animals resembled the movement seen in normal animals. These characteristics were digit extension, forelimb pronation, bilateral forelimb use during pellet consumption, and the quality and accuracy of successful reaches. These qualitative measurements were performed using a five point scale analyzing each of the ten compo-

nents of a reach, modified from Whishaw (Whishaw et al., 1986, 1993; Whishaw and Kolb, 1988; Diener and Bregman, 1998a). Fourth, the animals treated with transplants plus neurotrophic factors successfully removed the sticker from their forehead a greater percentage of the time. 84% of the transplant plus neurotrophic factors treated animals removed the sticker successfully, whereas only 57% of the animals treated with transplants and saline group removed the sticker. Thus, after chronic cervical spinal cord injury, transplants plus neurotrophins supported recovery of goal directed forelimb movements (toward the body and in space). Both the corticospinal and rubrospinal pathways contribute to skilled forelimb function under normal conditions (Schrimsher and Reier, 1993; Whishaw et al., 1993; McKenna and Whishaw, 1999) and both are disrupted after a cervical spinal cord over-hemisection injury. We suggest that the regrowth of corticospinal and rubrospinal projections contribute to the recovery of both automatic and skilled forelimb movement. While these results have led us to suggest that the increased anatomical regrowth of supraspinal axons contributes to the observed recovery of function. We do not believe, however, that the axonal regrowth within the transplant and within the host spinal cord

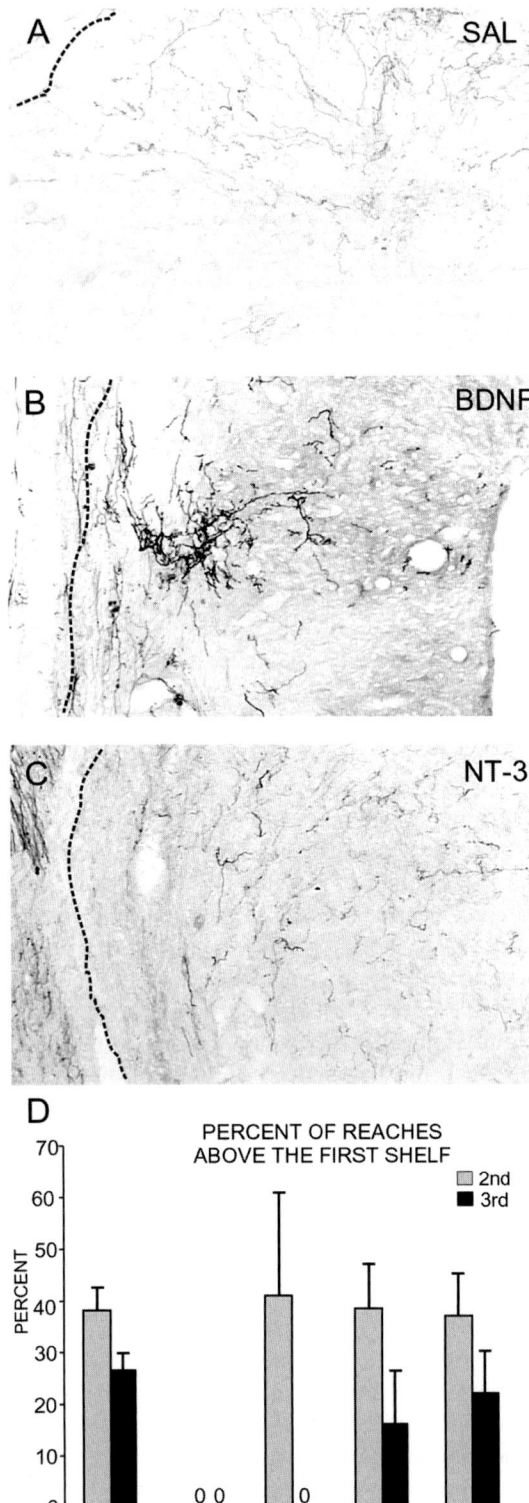

caudal to the transplant is solely responsible for this recovery of function. It is likely that plasticity at multiple levels of the neuraxis contributes to recovery of function.

Summary

Earlier studies suggested that while after spinal cord lesions and transplants at birth, the transplants serve both as a bridge and as a relay to restore supraspinal input caudal to the injury (Bregman, 1994), after injury in the adult the spinal cord transplants serve as a relay, but not as a bridge. We show here, that after complete spinal cord transection in adult rats, delayed spinal cord transplants and exogenous neurotrophic factors, the transplants can also serve as a bridge to restore supraspinal input (Fig. 9). We demonstrate here that when the delivery of transplants and neurotrophins are delayed until 2 weeks after spinal cord transection, the amount of axonal growth and the amount of recovery of function are dramatically increased. Under these conditions, both supraspinal and propriospinal projections to the host spinal cord caudal to the transection are reestablished.

The growth of supraspinal axons across the transplant and back into the host spinal cord caudal to the lesion was dependent upon the presence of exogenous neurotrophic support. Without the neurotrophins, only propriospinal axons were able to re-establish connections across the transplant. Studies using peripheral nerve or Schwann cell grafts have shown that some anatomical connectivity can be restored across the injury site, particularly under the influence of neurotrophins (Xu et al., 1995a,b; Cheng et al., 1996; Ye and Houle, 1997). Without neurotrophin treatment, brainstem axons do not enter

Fig. 8. (A–C) Anterograde labeling of corticospinal axons. Border between host and transplant is indicated by dashed line. After cervical hemisection and delayed transplantation, there is some growth of CST axons into the transplant. The extent of this growth is increased following administration of either BDNF (B) or NT-3 (C). (D) While there is some improvement in skilled reaching in animals with transplants (SAL) compared to lesion only animals (HX), the recovery of skilled reaching is significantly improved following treatment with neurotrophic factors (BDNF, NT-3).

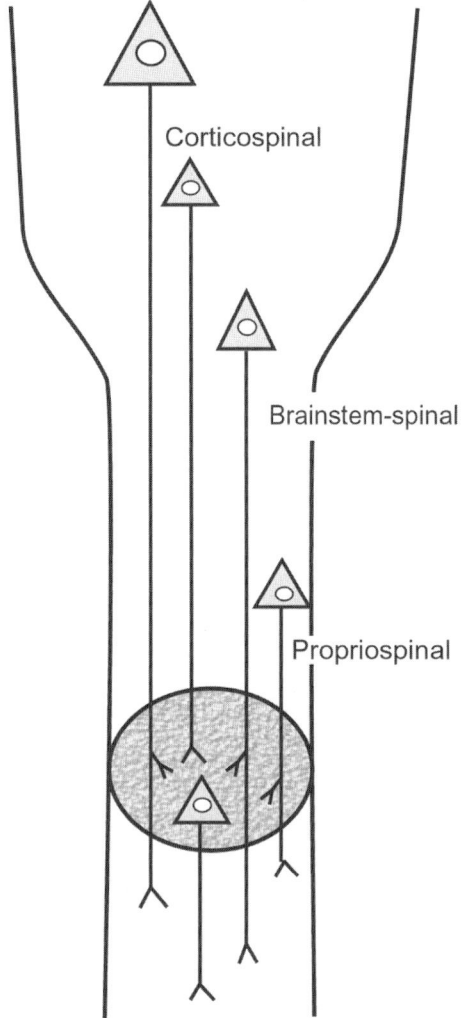

Corticospinal

Brainstem-spinal

Propriospinal

Fig. 9. Schematic diagram demonstrating influence of transplants and neurotrophic factors on anatomical circuitry. (See text for description.)

the graft (Xu et al., 1995a,b; Cheng et al., 1996; Ye and Houle, 1997). Similarly, cells genetically modified to secrete neurotrophins and transplanted into the spinal cord influence the axonal growth of specific populations of spinally projecting neurons (Tuszynski et al., 1996, 1997; Grill et al., 1997; Blesch and Tuszynski, 1997). Taken together, these studies support a role for neurotrophic factors in the repair of the mature CNS.

The regrowth of supraspinal and propriospinal input across the transection site was associated with consistent improvements in hindlimb locomotor function. Animals performed alternating and reciprocal hindlimb stepping with plantar foot contact to the treadmill or stair during ascension. Furthermore, they acquired hindlimb weight support and demonstrated appropriate postural control for balance and equilibrium of all four limbs. After spinal cord injury in the adult, the circuitry underlying rhythmic alternating stepping movements is still present within the spinal cord caudal to the lesion, but is now devoid of supraspinal control.

We show here that restoring even relatively small amounts of input allows supraspinal neurons to access the spinal cord circuitry. Removing the re-established supraspinal input after recovery (by re-transection rostral to the transplant) abolished the recovery and abolished the serotonergic fibers within the transplant and spinal cord caudal to the transplant. This suggests that at least some of the recovery observed is due to re-establishing supraspinal input across the transplant, rather than a diffuse influence of the transplant on motor recovery. It is unlikely, however, that the greater recovery of function in animals that received delayed transplant and neurotrophins is due solely to the restoration of supraspinal input. Recent work by Ribotta et al. (2000) suggests that segmental plasticity within the spinal cord contributes to weight support and bilateral foot placement after spinal cord transection. This recovery of function occurs after transplants of fetal raphe cells into the adult spinal cord transected at T_{11}. Recovery of function appears to require innervation of the L_1–L_2 segments with serotonergic fibers, and, importantly, animals require external stimulation (tail pinch) to elicit the behavior. In the current study, animals with transection only did not develop stepping overground or on the treadmill without tail pinch, although the transplant and neurotrophin-treated groups did so without external stimuli. Therefore both reorganization of the segmental circuitry and partial restoration of supraspinal input presumably interact to yield the improvements in motor function observed.

It is unlikely that the recovery of skilled forelimb movement observed can be mediated solely by reorganization of segmental spinal cord circuitry. We suggest that the restoration of supraspinal input contributes to the recovery observed. It is likely that after CNS injury, reorganization occurs both within the spinal cord and at supraspinal levels, and together contribute to the recovery of automatic and skilled forelimb function and of locomotion. In summary, the therapeutic intervention of tissue transplantation and exogenous neurotrophin support leads to improvements in supraspinal and propriospinal input across the transplant into the host caudal cord and a concomitant improvement in locomotor function. Paradoxically, delaying these interventions for several weeks after a spinal cord transection leads to dramatic improvements in recovery of function and a concomitant restoration of supraspinal input into the host caudal spinal cord. These findings suggest that opportunity for intervention after spinal cord injury may be far greater than originally envisioned, and that CNS neurons with long-standing injuries may be able to re-initiate growth leading to improvement in motor function.

Acknowledgements

Research in my laboratory described in this review has been supported by grants from the National Institutes of Health (NINDS) (NIH NS 19259 and NIH NS 27054) and grants from the International Spinal Research Trust and the Daniel Heumann Fund for Spinal Cord Research. J-VC, JL and FS were supported in part by a training grant (T32 HD 07459) from the National Center for Medical Rehabilitation Research.

References

Amassian, V.E. and Ross, R.J. (1978) Developing role of sensorimotor cortex and pyramidal tract neurons in contact placing in kittens. *J. Physiol.*, 74: 165–184.

Andersson, O., Grillner, S., Lindquist, M. and Zomlefer, M. (1978) Peripheral control of the spinal pattern generators for locomotion in cat. *Brain Res.*, 150: 625–630.

Bernstein-Goral, H. and Bregman, B.S. (1993) Spinal cord transplants support the regeneration of axotomized neurons after spinal cord lesions at birth: a quantitative double-labeling study. *Exp. Neurol.*, 123: 118–132.

Bernstein-Goral, H., Diener, P.S. and Bregman, B.S. (1997) Regenerating and sprouting axons differ in their requirements for growth after injury. *Exp. Neurol.*, 148: 51–72.

Blesch, A. and Tuszynski, M.H. (1997) Robust growth of chronically injured spinal cord axons induced by grafts of genetically modified NGF-secreting cells. *Exp. Neurol.*, 148: 444–452.

Bregman, B.S. (1987) Spinal cord transplants permit the growth of serotonergic axons across the site of neonatal spinal cord transection. *Brain Res.*, 431: 265–279.

Bregman, B.S. (1994) Recovery of function after spinal cord injury: Transplantation strategies. In: S.B. Dunnett and A. Bjorklund (Eds.), *Functional Neural Transplantation*. Raven Press, New York, pp. 489–529.

Bregman, B.S. (1998) Regeneration in the spinal cord. *Curr. Opin. Neurobiol.*, 8: 800–807.

Bregman, B.S. and Bernstein-Goral, H. (1991) Both regenerating and late-developing pathways contribute to transplant-induced anatomical plasticity after spinal cord lesions at birth. *Exp. Neurol.*, 112: 49–63.

Bregman, B.S. and Goldberger, M.E. (1982) Anatomical plasticity and sparing of function after spinal cord damage in neonatal cats. *Science*, 217: 553–555.

Bregman, B.S. and Goldberger, M.E. (1983a) Infant lesion effect: I. Development of motor behavior following neonatal spinal cord damage in cats. *Brain Res.*, 285: 103–117.

Bregman, B.S. and Goldberger, M.E. (1983b) Infant lesion effect: II. Sparing and recovery of function after spinal cord damage in newborn and adult cats. *Brain Res*, 285: 119–135.

Bregman, B.S. and Goldberger, M.E. (1983c) Infant lesion effect: III. Anatomical correlates of sparing and recovery of function after spinal cord damage in newborn and adult cats. *Brain Res.*, 285: 137–154.

Bregman, B.S. and Kunkel-Bagden, E. (1989) Methods of determining development and recovery of motor function after spinal cord lesions and transplants in rats. In: M. Brown and M.E. Goldberger (Eds.), *Criteria for Assessing Recovery of Function: Behavioral Methods*. American Paralysis Association, Springfield, NJ.

Bregman, B.S. and Kunkel-Bagden, E. (1994) Potential mechanisms underlying transplant mediated recovery of function after spinal cord injury. In: J. Marwah, H. Teitelbaum and K. Prasad (Eds.), *Neural Transplantation, CNS Neuronul Injury and Regeneration*. CRC Press, Boca Raton, pp. 81–102.

Bregman, B.S. and Reier, P.J. (1986) Neural tissue transplants rescue axotomized rubrospinal cells from retrograde death. *J. Comp. Neurol.*, 244: 86–95.

Bregman, B.S., Kunkel-Bagden, E., McAtee, M. and O'Neill, A. (1989) Extension of the critical period for developmental plasticity of the corticospinal pathway. *J. Comp. Neurol.*, 282: 355–370.

Bregman, B.S., Bernstein-Goral, H. and Kunkel-Bagden, E. (1991) CNS transplants promote anatomical plasticity and recovery of function after spinal cord injury. *J. Restor. Neurol. Neurosci.*, 2: 327–338.

Bregman, B.S., Kunkel-Bagden, E., Reier, P.J., Dai, H.N., McAtee, M. and Gao, D. (1993) Recovery of function after spinal cord injury: mechanisms underlying transplant-mediated recovery of function differ after spinal cord injury in newborn and adult rats. *Exp. Neurol.*, 123: 3–16.

Bregman, B.S., Kunkel-Bagden, E., Schnell, L., Dai, H.N., Gao, D. and Schwab, M.E. (1995) Recovery from spinal cord injury mediated by antibodies to neurite growth inhibitors. *Nature*, 378: 498–501.

Bregman, B.S., Diener, P.S., McAtee, M., Dai, H.N. and James, C. (1997a) Intervention strategies to enhance anatomical plasticity and recovery of function after spinal cord injury. *Adv. Neurol.*, 72: 257–275.

Bregman, B.S., McAtee, M., Dai, H.N. and Kuhn, P.L. (1997b) Neurotrophic factors increase axonal growth after spinal cord injury and transplantation in the adult rat. *Exp. Neurol.*, 148: 475–494.

Bregman, B.S., Broude, E., McAtee, M. and Kelley, M.S. (1998) Transplants and neurotrophic factors prevent atrophy of mature CNS neurons after spinal cord injury. *Exp. Neurol.*, 149: 13–27.

Broude, E., McAtee, M., Kelley, M.S. and Bregman, B.S. (1997) c-Jun expression in adult rat dorsal root ganglion neurons: differential response after central or peripheral axotomy. *Exp. Neurol.*, 148: 367–377.

Broude, E., McAtee, M., Kelley, M.S. and Bregman, B.S. (1999) Fetal spinal cord transplants and exogenous neurotrophic support enhance c-Jun expression in mature axotomized neurons after spinal cord injury. *Exp. Neurol.*, 155: 65–78.

Bury, S.D., Eichhorn, A.C., Kotzer, C.M. and Jones, T.A. (2000) Reactive astrocytic responses to denervation in the motor cortex of adult rats are sensitive to manipulations of behavioral experience. *Neuropharmacology*, 39: 743–755.

Cai, D., Shen, Y., De Bellard, M., Tang, S. and Filbin, M.T. (1999) Prior exposure to neurotrophins blocks inhibition of axonal regeneration by MAG and myelin via a cAMP-dependent mechanism. *Neuron*, 22: 89–101.

Chau, C., Barbeau, H. and Rossignol, S. (1998a) Early locomotor training with clonidine in spinal cats. *J. Neurophysiol.*, 79: 392–409.

Chau, C., Barbeau, H. and Rossignol, S. (1998b) Effects of intrathecal alpha1- and alpha2-noradrenergic agonists and norepinephrine on locomotion in chronic spinal cats. *J. Neurophysiol.*, 79: 2941–2963.

Cheng, H., Cao, Y. and Olson, L. (1996) Spinal cord repair in adult paraplegic rats: partial restoration of hind limb function. *Science*, 273: 510–513.

Chong, M.S., Woolf, C.J., Haque, N.S. and Anderson, P.N. (1999) Axonal regeneration from injured dorsal roots into the spinal cord of adult rats. *J. Comp. Neurol.*, 410: 42–54.

Coumans, J.V., Lin, T.T.-S., Dai, H.N., McAtee, M., Nash, C. and Bregman, B.S. (2001) Axonal regeneration and functional recovery after complete spinal cord transection in rats by delayed treatment with transplants and neurotrophins. *J. Neurosci.*, 21: 9334–9344.

Diener, P.S. and Bregman, B.S. (1998a) Fetal spinal cord transplants support growth of supraspinal and segmental projections after cervical spinal cord hemisection in the neonatal rat. *J. Neurosci.*, 18: 779–793.

Diener, P.S. and Bregman, B.S. (1998b) Fetal spinal cord transplants support the development of target reaching and coordinated postural adjustments after neonatal cervical spinal cord injury. *J. Neurosci.*, 18: 763–778.

Florence, S.L. and Kaas, J.H. (1995) Large-scale reorganization at multiple levels of the somatosensory pathway follows therapeutic amputation of the hand in monkeys. *J. Neurosci.*, 15: 8083–8095.

Florence, S.L., Taub, H.B. and Kaas, J.H. (1998) Large-scale sprouting of cortical connections after peripheral injury in adult macaque monkeys. *Science*, 282: 1117–1121.

Goldberger, M.E. (1988a) Spared-root deafferentation of a cat's hindlimb: hierarchical regulation of pathways mediating recovery of motor behavior. *Exp. Brain Res.*, 73: 329–342.

Goldberger, M.E. (1988b) Partial and complete deafferentation of cat hindlimb: the contribution of behavioral substitution to recovery of motor function. *Exp. Brain Res.*, 73: 343–353.

Goldberger, M.E. (1988c) Spared-root deafferentation of a cat's hindlimb: hierarchical regulation of pathways mediating recovery of motor behavior. *Exp. Brain Res.*, 73: 329–342.

Goldberger, M.E. (1991) The use of behavioral methods to predict spinal cord plasticity. *J. Restorative Neurol. Neurosci.*, 2: 339–350.

Goldberger, M. and Murray, M. (1978) Axonal sprouting and recovery of function may obey some of the same laws. In: C. Cotman (Ed.), *Neuronal Plasticity*. Raven Press, New York, pp. 73–96.

Goldberger, M.E., Bregman, B.S., Vierck Jr., C.J. and Brown, M. (1990) Criteria for assessing recovery of function after spinal cord injury: behavioral methods. *Exp. Neurol.*, 107: 113–117.

Grill, R., Murai, K., Blesch, A., Gage, F.H. and Tuszynski, M.H. (1997) Cellular delivery of neurotrophin-3 promotes corticospinal axonal growth and partial functional recovery after spinal cord injury. *J. Neurosci.*, 17: 5560–5572.

Grillner, S. (1975) Locomotion in vertebrates: central mechanisms and reflex interaction. *Physiol. Rev.*, 55: 247–304.

Grillner, S. (1986) Locomotion in spinal vertebrates: Physiology and pharmacology. In: M.E. Goldberger, A. Gorio and M. Murray (Eds.), *Development and Plasticity of the Mammalian Spinal Cord*. Liviana Press, Padova, pp. 311–321.

Grillner, S. (1996) Neural networks for vertebrate locomotion. *Sci. Am.*, 274: 64–69.

Grillner, S. and Dubuc, R. (1988) Control of locomotion in vertebrates: Spinal and supraspinal mechanisms. In: S.G. Waxman (Ed.), *Functional Recovery in Neurological Disease*. Raven Press, New York, pp. 425–453.

Grillner, S. and Georgopoulos, A.P. (1996) Neural control. *Curr. Opin. Neurobiol.*, 6: 741–743.

Grillner, S. and Rossignol, S. (1978) On the initiation of the swing phase of locomotion in chronic spinal cats. *Brain Res.*, 146: 269–277.

Grillner, S., Ekeberg, El Manira, A., et al. (1998) Intrinsic function of a neuronal network - a vertebrate central pattern generator. *Brain Res. Brain Res. Rev.*, 26: 184–197.

Helgren, M.E. and Goldberger, M.E. (1993) The recovery of postural reflexes and locomotion following low thoracic hemisection in adult cats involves compensation by undamaged primary afferent pathways. *Exp. Neurol.*, 123: 17–34.

Howland, D.R., Bregman, B.S. and Goldberger, M.E. (1995a) The development of quadrupedal locomotion in the kitten. *Exp. Neurol.*, 135: 93–107.

Howland, D.R., Bregman, B.S., Tessler, A. and Goldberger, M.E.

(1995b) Development of locomotor behavior in the spinal kitten. *Exp. Neurol.*, 135: 108–122.

Howland, D.R., Bregman, B.S., Tessler, A. and Goldberger, M.E. (1995c) Transplants enhance locomotion in neonatal kittens whose spinal cords are transected: a behavioral and anatomical study. *Exp. Neurol.*, 135: 123–145.

Jain, N., Florence, S.L., Qi, H.X. and Kaas, J.H. (2000) Growth of new brainstem connections in adult monkeys with massive sensory loss. *Proc. Natl. Acad. Sci. USA*, 97: 5546–5550.

Jones, T.A. (1999) Multiple synapse formation in the motor cortex opposite unilateral sensorimotor cortex lesions in adult rats. *J. Comp. Neurol.*, 414: 57–66.

Jones, T.A., Kleim, J.A. and Greenough, W.T. (1996) Synaptogenesis and dendritic growth in the cortex opposite unilateral sensorimotor cortex damage in adult rats: a quantitative electron microscopic examination. *Brain Res.*, 733: 142–148.

Jones, T.A., Chu, C.J., Grande, L.A. and Gregory, A.D. (1999) Motor skills training enhances lesion-induced structural plasticity in the motor cortex of adult rats. *J. Neurosci.*, 19: 10153–10163.

Kaas, J.H., Florence, S.L. and Jain, N. (1999) Subcortical contributions to massive cortical reorganizations. *Neuron*, 22: 657–660.

Kleim, J.A., Barbay, S. and Nudo, R.J. (1998) Functional reorganization of the rat motor cortex following motor skill learning. *J. Neurophysiol.*, 80: 3321–3325.

Kunkel-Bagden, E. and Bregman, B.S. (1990) Spinal cord transplants enhance the recovery of locomotor function after spinal cord injury at birth. *Exp. Brain Res.*, 81: 25–34.

Lynskey, J.V., Sandhu, F.A., Dai, H.N., McAtee, M. and Bregman, B.S. (1999) Axonal regeneration and functional recovery after chronic cervical spinal cord injury. *Soc. Neurosci. Abstr.*, 25: 482.

Lynskey, J.V., Sandhu, F.A., Dai, H.N., McAtee, M., Sinha, M. and Bregman, B.S. (2000) Regeneration of rubrospinal tract fibers contributes to functional recovery after chronic cervical spinal cord injury in adult rats. *Soc. Neurosci. Abstr.*, 26: 862.

McKenna, J.E. and Whishaw, I.Q. (1999) Complete compensation in skilled reaching success with associated impairments in limb synergies, after dorsal column lesion in the rat. *J. Neurosci.*, 19: 1885–1894.

Miya, D., Giszter, S., Mori, F., Adipudi, V., Tessler, A. and Murray, M. (1997) Fetal transplants alter the development of function after spinal cord transection in newborn rats. *J. Neurosci.*, 17: 4856–4872.

Muir, G.D. and Whishaw, I.Q. (2000) Red nucleus lesions impair overground locomotion in rats: a kinetic analysis. *Eur. J. Neurosci.*, 12: 1113–1122.

Nakamura, M., Houghtling, R., MacArthur, L., Bayer, B. and Bregman, B. (2001) Changes in cytokine mRNAs and inflammatory responses in adult rat spinal cord after hemisection. Submitted.

Neumann, S. and Woolf, C.J. (1999) Regeneration of dorsal column fibers into and beyond the lesion site following adult spinal cord injury. *Neuron*, 23: 83–91.

Pearson, K.G. (1995) Proprioceptive regulation of locomotion. *Curr. Opin. Neurobiol.*, 5: 786–791.

Rho, M.J., Lavoie, S. and Drew, T. (1999) Effects of red nucleus microstimulation on the locomotor pattern and timing in the intact cat: a comparison with the motor cortex. *J. Neurophysiol.*, 81: 2297–2315.

Ribotta, M.G., Provencher, J., Feraboli-Lohnherr, D., Rossignol, S., Privat, A. and Orsal, D. (2000) Activation of locomotion in adult chronic spinal rats is achieved by transplantation of embryonic raphe cells reinnervating a precise lumbar level. *J. Neurosci.*, 20: 5144–5152.

Richardson, P.M. and Issa, V.M. (1984) Peripheral injury enhances central regeneration of primary sensory neurones. *Nature*, 309: 791–793.

Rossignol, S., Barbeau, H. and Julien, C. (1986) Locomotion of the adult chronic spinal cat and its modification by monoaminergic agonists and antagonists. In: M.E. Goldberger, A. Gorio and M. Murray (Eds.), *Development and Plasticity of the Mammalian Spinal Cord*. Liviana Press, Padova, pp. 323–345.

Sandhu, F.A., Lynskey, J., Dai, H.N., McAtee, M. and BS, Bregman (1999) Fetal transplants and NTFs aid axonal regeneration and functional recovery in adult rats after chronic cervical cord injury. *Eighth Int. Sympos. Neural. Regeneration Abstr.*, 61.

Sandhu, F., Dai, H., McAtee, M. and Bregman, B. (2000) Propriospinal and segmental reorganization following spinal cord injury, delayed fetal transplantation and neurotrophin administration. *Soc. Neurosci. Abstr.*, 26: 862.

Sandhu, F., Lynskey, J., Dai, H., McAtee, M. and Bregman, B. (2002) Delayed fetal transplants and neurotrophins support axonal regeneration after cervical hemisection in adult rats. In review.

Schnell, L. and Schwab, M.E. (1993) Sprouting and regeneration of lesioned corticospinal tract fibres in the adult rat spinal cord. *Eur. J. Neurosci.*, 5: 1156–1171.

Schnell, L., Schneider, R., Kolbeck, R., Barde, Y.A. and Schwab, M.E. (1994) Neurotrophin-3 enhances sprouting of corticospinal tract during development and after adult spinal cord lesion. *Nature*, 367: 170–173.

Schrimsher, G.W. and Reier, P.J. (1992) Forelimb motor performance following cervical spinal cord contusion injury in the rat. *Exp. Neurol.*, 117: 287–298.

Schrimsher, G.W. and Reier, P.J. (1993) Forelimb motor performance following dorsal column, dorsolateral funiculi, or ventrolateral funiculi lesions of the cervical spinal cord in the rat. *Exp. Neurol.*, 120: 264–276.

Sengelaub, D.R., Muja, N., Mills, A.C., Myers, W.A., Churchill, J.D. and Garraghty, P.E. (1997) Denervation-induced sprouting of intact peripheral afferents into the cuneate nucleus of adult rats. *Brain Res.*, 769: 256–262.

Stokes, B.T. and Reier, P.J. (1992) Fetal grafts alter chronic behavioral outcome after contusion damage to the adult rat spinal cord. *Exp. Neurol.*, 116: 1–12.

Tuszynski, M.H., Gabriel, K., Gage, F.H., Suhr, S., Meyer, S. and Rosetti, A. (1996) Nerve growth factor delivery by gene transfer induces differential outgrowth of sensory, motor, and noradrenergic neurites after adult spinal cord injury. *Exp. Neurol.*, 137: 157–173.

Tuszynski, M.H., Murai, K., Blesch, A., Grill, R. and Miller,

I. (1997) Functional characterization of NGF-secreting cell grafts to the acutely injured spinal cord. *Cell Transplant*, 6: 361–368.

Whishaw, I.Q. and Kolb, B. (1988) Sparing of skilled forelimb reaching and corticospinal projections after neonatal motor cortex removal or hemidecortication in the rat: support for the Kennard doctrine. *Brain Res.*, 451: 97–114.

Whishaw, I.Q., O'Connor, W.T. and Dunnett, S.B. (1986) The contributions of motor cortex, nigrostriatal dopamine and caudate- putamen to skilled forelimb use in the rat. *Brain*, 109: 805–843.

Whishaw, I.Q., Pellis, S.M., Gorny, B., Kolb, B. and Tetzlaff, W. (1993) Proximal and distal impairments in rat forelimb use in reaching follow unilateral pyramidal tract lesions. *Behav.*

Brain Res., 56: 59–76.

Xu, X.M., Guenard, V., Kleitman, N., Aebischer, P. and Bunge, M.B. (1995a) A combination of BDNF and NT-3 promotes supraspinal axonal regeneration into Schwann cell grafts in adult rat thoracic spinal cord. *Exp. Neurol.*, 134: 261–272.

Xu, X.M., Guenard, V., Kleitman, N. and Bunge, M.B. (1995b) Axonal regeneration into Schwann cell-seeded guidance channels grafted into transected adult rat spinal cord. *J. Comp. Neurol.*, 351: 145–160.

Ye, J.H. and Houle, J.D. (1997) Treatment of the chronically injured spinal cord with neurotrophic factors can promote axonal regeneration from supraspinal neurons. *Exp. Neurol.*, 143: 70–81.

L. McKerracher, G. Doucet and S. Rossignol (Eds.)
Progress in Brain Research, Vol. 137
© 2002 Elsevier Science B.V. All rights reserved

CHAPTER 19

Bridging the transected or contused adult rat spinal cord with Schwann cell and olfactory ensheathing glia transplants

Mary Bartlett Bunge [*]

The Chambers Family Electron Microscopy Laboratory, The Miami Project to Cure Paralysis, Departments Cell Biology and Anatomy and Neurological Surgery, University of Miami School of Medicine, Miami, FL 33136, USA

Introduction

One of the pathological outcomes of spinal cord injury in humans is the formation of cavities of varying size in the cord interior (Bunge et al., 1993, 1997). Such cavities could be receptacles for cell transplants to promote axonal regeneration across the area of injury to improve function. In this review, our new findings from studies of cell transplantation in a rat contusion model will be compared with those utilizing a complete transection/cellular bridge paradigm. Whereas studying transplantation in a contusion model is clinically relevant, there is the challenge of distinguishing spared and sprouted fibers from fibers that have regenerated. Therefore, to obtain unambiguous results, we initially used a complete transection model, placing a cellular bridge between the stumps of completely transected adult Fischer rat thoracic spinal cord. If fibers were seen below the injury, they clearly had regenerated. The first part of this discussion will focus on findings

_____
[*] Correspondence to: M.B. Bunge, The Miami Project to Cure Paralysis, University of Miami School of Medicine, The Lois Pope LIFE Center, P.O. Box 016960 (R-48) Miami, FL 33101, USA. Tel.: +1-305-243-4596; Fax: +1-305-243-3923; E-mail: mbunge@miami.edu

from the complete transection/cellular bridge model that we developed and a later section will report new results using a contusion model.

Complete transection/cellular bridge model

In the complete transection model, a cable of Schwann cells (SCs) was placed between the stumps, which were inserted about 1 mm into the ends of a polymer channel that enclosed the cellular cable (Xu et al., 1997). SCs were our cells of choice initially for reasons that have been reviewed many times (e.g., Guénard et al., 1993). Nerve fibers regenerate into tunnels of SCs enclosed within a basement membrane in the peripheral nervous system. A large body of tissue culture work has demonstrated that SCs support axonal growth from central neurons. SCs function in the CNS, that is, they form myelin and ensheathe central fibers. They produce growth factors, express cell adhesion molecules and surface integrins, and produce extracellular matrix components, all known to promote nerve fiber growth. In addition, SCs, including human SCs, now can be obtained in very large numbers after a few weeks in culture (Bonamichi et al., 1997; Bunge, 2001). For human SCs, a piece of human peripheral nerve may yield enough SCs to form a graft the diameter of the human cord and several feet long in 5 to 6 weeks.

If this nerve is taken from a spinal cord injured person, then the SCs derived from it could be placed into the site of spinal cord injury, with no concern about immune rejection. While the SCs are being prepared in vitro for transplantation, they could be genetically engineered to provide larger amounts of growth factors.

It is known that large numbers of SCs may enter the lesion in human spinal cord injury (Bruce et al., 2000). This 'Schwannosis' is seen beginning at 4 months after injury. SCs may be found years after injury. Moreover, with appropriate staining it has been demonstrated that there are nerve fibers in association with these SCs. Clearly, then, SCs can survive for long periods of time in the human spinal cord lesion milieu and nerve fibers are in association with them.

Schwann cell bridge

In the Fischer rat complete transection model, (1) axons grew onto the bridge from both stumps, (2) an average of over 1000 spinal cord neurons responded by extending fibers onto the bridge, (3) a mean of about 2000 myelinated axons was found in the bridge (Table I), and (4) eight times more nonmyelinated axons were present in the bridge as well, as demonstrated by electron microscopy (Xu et al., 1997). There was only a very modest growth of serotonergic and noradrenergic fibers a short distance onto the bridge. Cross-sections of the bridge revealed an image similar to peripheral nerve, SCs having formed myelin and ensheathed axons in their typical manner. When a sagittal section of the rostral Schwann cell graft–host cord interface was stained for neurofilaments, axons were seen to extend from the cord onto the bridge, where they became fasciculated by the SCs. Thus, there was substantial regeneration of axons from spinal cord neurons onto the bridge, but there was minimal response from brainstem neurons. This is not surprising, because in peripheral nerve grafting work, it was only when peripheral nerve was inserted at the high cervical level that a response of brainstem neurons to the nerve was seen (Richardson et al., 1984; Houle et al., 1994). Also, fibers in this paradigm, with no additional strategy, did not leave the bridge to enter the contiguous cord.

That the regenerated fibers did not leave the bridge may be due, in part, to an accumulation of inhibitory chondroitin sulfate proteoglycans at the caudal graft–host interface. An immunostaining study by Plant et al. (2001a) revealed that CS-56 antigen, neurocan and phosphacan, all chondroitin sulfate proteoglycans considered to be inhibitory to neurite growth (Fawcett and Asher, 1999; Fitch and Silver, 1999; Lemons et al., 1999), were found in association with astrocytes near the bridge. In comparing the caudal with the rostral graft–cord interface, it was found, with CS-56 and phosphacan antibodies, that there was more accumulation of the proteoglycan at the caudal than at the rostral interface. Moreover, SCs were stained with CS-56 antibody in the caudal but not the rostral region of the bridge. If the stumps alone, the stumps inside an empty polymer channel, or a polymer channel containing only matrigel (without SCs) were immunostained, there was no difference in staining by these antibodies at the two stumps. Apparently, an interaction between the SCs and the caudal stump had occurred that led to greater accumulation of chondroitin sulfate proteoglycan. It is not known how the caudal stump differs from the rostral stump. The caudal stump is always inserted into the channel after the rostral stump; the caudal stump may swell while the rostral stump is being inserted and is, therefore, more damaged by insertion into the channel. Other potential differences between the caudal and rostral stumps are discussed elsewhere (Plant et al., 2001a). A few studies to diminish the amount of chondroitin sulfate proteoglycan to improve regeneration have appeared (Lemons et al., 1999; Yick et al., 2000; Moon et al., 2001).

Schwann cell bridge plus methylprednisolone

In order to encourage growth of axons from brainstem neurons onto the bridge and fiber growth from the bridge into the cord, we initiated combination strategies in the Fischer rat transection/cellular bridge model. One of these strategies involved the administration of the glucocorticoid, methylprednisolone, which is given to some persons within 8 h of spinal cord injury. In comparing animals receiving SC bridges with and without methylprednisolone administration, it was observed that the rostral in-

TABLE I

Numbers of myelinated axons in the SC graft and neurons in the spinal cord that extend axons into the graft in differing transplantation procedures

References	Strategy	Myelinated axons		Responding cord neurons	
		capped [a] channel	open channel	capped [a] channel	open channel
Xu et al. (1995a, 1997)	Rat SC/matrigel (matrigel only)	501 ± 83 (71 ± 25)	1990 ± 594 (3 ± 0.9)	306 ± 69 –	1064 ± 145 –
Chen et al. (1996); Bunge and Kleitman (1999)	Rat SC/matrigel + methylprednisolone (SC/matrigel + vehicle)	1159 ± 308 (335 ± 108)	3237 ± 2478 (1324 ± 342)	1116 ± 113 (284 ± 88)	2083 ± 321 (1064 ± 145)
Xu et al. (1995b)	Rat SC/matrigel + BDNF, NT-3 (SC/matrigel + vehicle)	1523 ± 292 (882 ± 287)	– –	967 ± 104 –	– –

The numbers are means ± SEM. The information in parentheses pertains to control animals. SC = Schwann cell.

[a] Initial experiments were conducted with distally capped channels to focus on responses of descending tracts.

terface appeared very different in these two sets of animals (Chen et al., 1996; Bunge and Kleitman, 1997). In the animals not given methylprednisolone, the interface was much broader and the host cord tissue which had been inserted into the polymer channel had not survived. In contrast, with methylprednisolone, the interface was much narrower and the host cord tissue inserted into the channel survived. In addition, there were more than twice as many myelinated axons (means, 3237 vs 1324) in the SC bridge, twice as many spinal cord neurons (means, 2083 vs 1064) extended axons onto the bridge (Table I), and there was considerable growth of serotonergic and noradrenergic fibers along the bridge. By placing a tracer into the middle of the bridge, an average of 57 brainstem neurons could be labeled. Also, by placing tracer above the bridge, it could be demonstrated that there was a modest number of fibers that left the bridge to enter the cord. Thus, by administering methylprednisolone at the time of SC bridge transplantation, the distance factor between the thoracically placed bridge and the brainstem neurons was overcome to some degree, as was the lack of growth from the bridge into the cord.

Schwann cell bridge plus neurotrophins

Another combination strategy that was tried was the application of neurotrophins, molecules which are known to be key for neuronal survival and outgrowth of their processes. In the first set of experiments, we infused brain-derived neurotrophic factor (BDNF) and neurotrophin-3 (NT-3) into the area around the SC graft inside the polymer channel (Xu et al., 1995b). Both neurotrophins were delivered at 12 µg/day for 14 days; animals were maintained for 1 month. When the neurotrophins were present, twice as many myelinated axons (means, 1523 vs 882) were in the graft, three times more spinal cord neurons (means, 967 vs 306) (Table I) extended into the graft and serotonergic and noradrenergic axons grew into the graft. When a tracer was introduced into the graft, a mean of 92 brainstem neurons (primarily vestibulospinal) were labeled. Again, by adding one more step (neurotrophins) to the SC bridge, the regenerative response was improved, including response from distant brainstem neurons.

Next, we tested delivery of BDNF by genetically engineering SCs to produce human BDNF (Menei et al., 1998). Schwann cells, genetically engineered or not, were placed into a syringe, the needle of which was inserted 5 mm into the caudal stump after complete transection. A 5 mm long trail of 500,000 SCs was deposited upon withdrawal of the syringe needle and then an additional 500,000 SCs were placed in the transection site itself. In this paradigm, there was no cable of SCs, but simply an injection of SCs to form a trail and to fill the transection site. Because the SCs were labeled with Hoechst dye before injection, 1 month later the trail was seen to have remained largely intact. With immunostaining it was seen that nerve fibers were clustered along the length of the trail. In trails of BDNF-SCs, there was evidence for growth of both serotonergic and noradrenergic fibers; these fibers from brainstem neurons had been able to cross the complete transection site and grow along the length of the trail. Tracer injected at the caudal end of the trail allowed counts of labeled brainstem neurons; in some of the animals there was a good response (e.g., in one animal there was a total of 135 labeled neurons) in brainstem nuclei. With untreated SCs there was a far more modest response, and with no SC transplantation there were no labeled neurons above the transection site. In these experiments, then, the genetic engineering of SCs to secrete human BDNF greatly improved the regenerative response, enabling fibers to cross the transection site and grow along the 5 mm long trail and, moreover, to extend from brainstem neurons along this trail.

Schwann cell bridge plus ensheathing glia

Another combination strategy that we tested was the combination of the SC bridge with the introduction of olfactory ensheathing glia (OEG). The use of OEG has intrigued those interested in CNS regeneration because they are found in the area of the olfactory system where fibers grow throughout adulthood, from the periphery into the central nervous system. The transplantation of SCs and OEG has been compared elsewhere (Franklin and Barnett, 1997, 2000; Kleitman and Bunge, 2000; Plant et al., 2001b). The rationale for our strategy was that the OEG could enable fibers to leave the peripheral nerve environment of the bridge and grow into the CNS environment of the cord. Aliquots of 200,000 OEG were injected into the stumps on either side of the SC bridge and, at an appropriate time later, a tracer was introduced into the cervical region to enable visualization of fibers that extended across the bridge and into the distal cord (Ramón-Cueto et al., 1998). There were three major findings from this study. (1) Serotonergic fibers grew in the connective tissue that formed on the outside of the polymer channel and reentered the cord caudal to the bridge, where they regenerated at least 1.5 cm. They chose a milieu of OEG/connective tissue instead of the OEG/SC bridge. (2) Following anterograde tracing with WGA-HRP, labeled fibers were seen to exit

the bridge and enter the distal cord (Fig. 1). Finally, (3) labeled neurons were seen in the lumbar region. Our interpretation was that the fibers of these neurons, severed at the caudal interface, then regenerated across the caudal interface, along the bridge, and then across the rostral interface to enter the cord and extend to the area into which the tracer had been injected, a growth of at least 2.5 cm. Thus, the OEG enabled regenerated fibers to cross the host cord/SC graft interfaces and to grow for considerable distances in the cord.

Contusion lesion/cellular transplant

Most recently, we have compared the transplantation of SCs and OEG into contusion lesions of the adult rat thoracic spinal cord (Bunge et al., 2000, 2001). The NYU impactor was used to induce a moderate contusion injury into which two million SCs or OEG or one million of each in a combination graft were injected in a 6 μl volume at 7 days following the contusion. Purified populations of these cell types were prepared from adult animals. The 7-day time point was chosen because Moonen's group found that SC survival was best when transplanted either immediately or at least 1 week after lesioning compared with 2–4 days (Martin et al., 1993, 1996). Also the immediate excitotoxic response should have subsided somewhat by 7 days (e.g., Panter et al., 1990; Liu et al., 1991; Bethea et al., 1999).

In horizontal sections of the contusion site at 12 weeks, the typical large cavity was seen in control animals injected with culture medium instead of cells. Less cavitation was seen with any type of transplant. The grafts reduced the volume of tissue damage by 80% (SC), 68% (SC/OEG) and 55% (OEG) compared with medium injection only. Antibodies were used to detect SCs, OEG, astrocytes, neurofilaments, GAP-43, and chondroitin sulfate proteoglycan. The p75 low-affinity nerve growth factor receptor antibody, which recognizes both cell types, stained SC transplants intensely and, to a lesser extent, the OEG and SC/OEG transplants. In the control animals, there was some staining in the trabeculae of the contusion cavity, most probably due to host SCs that migrated into these areas. Neurofilament or GAP-43 antibody staining was absent in the contused area (except in trabeculae), but was

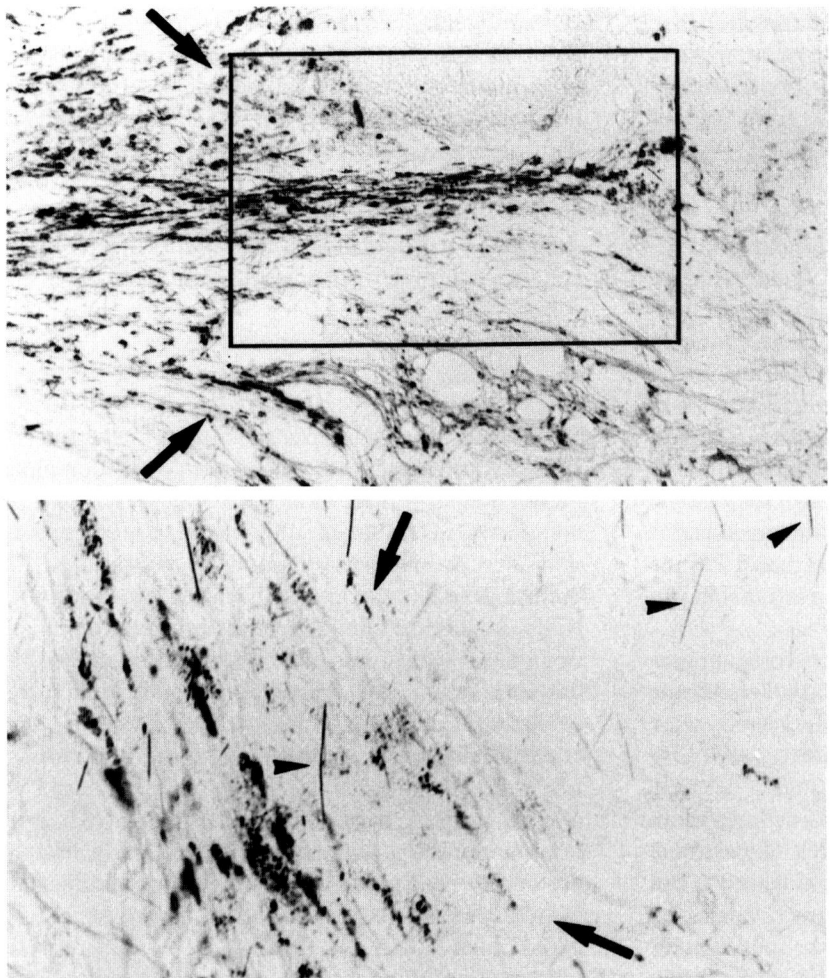

Fig. 1. A tracer, WGA-HRP, was introduced into the cervical region (above the bridge) to detect fibers that exited the Schwann cell bridge to grow into the cord below the bridge. When ensheathing glia were present, tracer-containing fibers (within the box) could be found leaving the distal bridge–cord interface (top panel). The arrows point to the interface between the bridge (left) and the spinal cord (right). In contrast, when ensheathing glia were not injected beside the bridge, there was no evidence of fibers leaving the Schwann cell bridge (bottom panel, distal interface indicated by arrows). (The arrowheads point to non-specific crystals.) Horizontal sections; the bar represents 160 μm (top) or 50 μm (bottom). (From Ramón-Cueto et al., 1998; copyright 1998 by the Society for Neuroscience.)

present in all the transplants, most intense in SC grafts. Typically, there was a bright rim of GFAP staining around the contusion cavity in the control animal group, as reported by others (e.g., Lemons et al., 1999). Most notably, in preliminary findings, the interface between the OEG graft and the host cord was not similarly bright. This was also true for chondroitin sulfate proteoglycan staining; the rim around a small cavity in the section was stained, but the area of the OEG transplant was not, including the interface between the OEG transplant and the

cord. CS-56 antibody stained both SC and SC/OEG transplants.

Tissue was prepared for plastic semi-thin and thin sectioning for examination in the light and electron microscopes. Again, there was more cavitation in the control than in the other three groups. In 1 μm thick sections, in trabeculae in the control animals, SCs related to myelin sheaths were seen. In SC grafted animals, the grafts appeared very healthy and displayed a plethora of SC myelinated axons. Looking at such a transplant in the electron microscope, a striking finding was the lack of fasciculation. When host SCs migrate into a lesion area, they are always attended by cells that form perineurial-like ensheathment. The absence of this in these grafts further confirmed the survival of transplanted SCs. Axonal diameter varied considerably from larger axons surrounded by myelin to very thin axons that were only ensheathed with SC cytoplasm. At the interface between the SC graft and the host cord, there was little astrogliosis in general; only a fine tracery of thin astrocytic processes and basal lamina were visible in many areas. The OEG graft did not contain as much myelin as an SC or an SC/OEG graft; the peripheral type myelin could have been formed by host SCs that migrated into the transplant area. Electron micrographs were studied for potential OEG. Some cells were identified in areas of central myelin near the lesion; they exhibited patches of basal lamina and processes that meandered among axons but did not encircle them as do SCs.

After Fast blue injection into the cord approximately 6 mm caudal to the caudal edge of the contusion injury/transplant, labeled nerve cells were counted at various levels of the cord (C_2, C_6, T_2, T_7–T_8), brainstem, and cortex. The tracing detected three times more propriospinal and two times more brainstem axons projecting to the area of Fast blue injection. No label was seen in cortical neurons. But the terminations of the corticospinal tract, labeled by injection of biotinylated dextran amine into the cortex, were significantly closer to the lesion epicenter when any graft was present compared with control animals, confirming the other tracing results showing that the grafts are neuroprotective. The closer proximity of the corticospinal tract to the epicenter was mostly likely due to tissue sparing rather than regeneration. Tracing of the reticulo- and vestibulospinal tracts revealed fibers in all animals in the spared white matter outside the lesion; they were not evident in the grafts. Finally, the BBB locomotion performance scale (Basso et al., 1995) was modestly, but significantly (12 vs 10.8) improved only when SC-containing grafts were present.

Thus, in our first transplantation experiments utilizing the weight-drop model, we observed that SC, OEG, and SC/OEG grafts filled substantial areas of the contusion lesion, diminished cavitation, were neuroprotective, and supported substantial axonal regeneration into the graft. These axons were primarily propriospinal (and probably sensory which was not investigated); vestibulo-, reticulo- and cortico-spinal fibers were not evident in the grafts, but the first two fiber types were present in the spared white matter. SC grafts were full of myelinated axons and led to an improved locomotion score, primarily better weight support of the hind limbs. More work needs to be done to determine if fibers left the graft to enter the cord.

Comparison of the two models

The contusion injury/transplantation experiments agree with results obtained with the complete transection/SC bridge model in a number of ways. In both cases, SCs support substantial axonal regeneration and myelination in the graft. In neither case do brainstem or cortical axons appear to enter the graft. Regenerated fibers do not exit the bridge without additional strategies; this is clear in the transection/SC bridge paradigm and remains to be determined for SC and OEG grafts in the contusion lesion. Our contusion lesion/transplantation results are similar to those published by Moonen's group (Martin et al., 1991, 1993, 1996), who transplanted SCs into lesions induced by an inflatable balloon. They reported that the grafts filled the lesion, diminished cavitation and astrogliosis, and supported 'massive' axonal ingrowth. Many types of sensory fibers were identified by immunostaining; tracing was not done to identify fibers of spinal cord origin. They found no evidence of corticospinal or monoaminergic fibers in the grafts or evidence of growth from the graft into the cord.

Prospectus

Clearly, successful bridging of a spinal cord injury will require growth of axons from both spinal cord and supraspinal neurons across the injury and into the cord beyond. Schwann cell grafts promote regeneration of spinal cord but not supraspinal axons across the bridge. Additional strategies, such as the introduction of neurotrophins, enable regeneration of brainstem fibers across the bridge. Diminution of chondroitin sulfate proteoglycans at the bridge–cord interfaces or provision of OEG or neurotrophins may also be required to lure regenerated fibers off the bridge. The presence of OEG also leads to lengthier axonal growth along the cord. Overcoming inhibition of axonal growth by myelin-related compounds will also be an important strategy (Schwab, 2002). Whereas cellular grafts help to spare tissue from secondary loss, an effective neuroprotection strategy will be a critical component of a combination strategy to improve outcome after injury. An effective combination strategy may also require additional steps, such as pharmacological intervention to increase the activity of serotonergic and noradrenergic systems, and rehabilitation procedures.

Acknowledgements

Work in the Bunge laboratory cited here was accomplished by Drs. X. Xu, A. Chen, V. Guénard, N. Kleitman, P. Menei, C. Montero-Menei, A. Ramón-Cueto, G. Plant, M. Oudega, T. Takami, A.E. Marcillo and P.M. Wood. Excellent laboratory assistance is gratefully acknowledged in the original papers. R.P. Bunge and S.R. Whittemore served as mentors. Word processing of this review was done by D. Masella and G.M. Escobar. The laboratory has been supported by NS 09923 and PO1 NS 38665, The Miami Project to Cure Paralysis, and the Christopher Reeve Paralysis, Hollfelder and Heumann Foundations. Drs. Xu and Oudega were Werner Heumann Memorial International Scholars, the Meneis were funded by IRME, and Dr. Takami was supported in part by Osaka City University.

References

Basso, D.M., Beattie, M.S. and Bresnahan, J.C. (1995) A sensitive and reliable locomotor rating scale for open field testing in rats. *J. Neurotrauma*, 12: 1–21.

Bethea, J.R., Nagashima, H., Acosta, M.C., Briceno, C., Gomez, F., Marcillo, A.E., Loor, K., Green, J. and Dietrich, W.D. (1999) Systemically administered Interleukin-10 reduces tumor necrosis factor-alpha production and significantly improves functional recovery following traumatic spinal cord injury in rats. *J. Neurotrauma*, 16: 851–863.

Bonamichi, G.T.B., Bunge, R.P., Margitich, I.S., Kleitman, N. and Wood, P.M. (1997) Factors influencing human Schwann cell growth in vitro. *Soc. Neurosci. Abstr.*, 23: 65.

Bruce, J.H., Norenberg, M.D., Kraydieh, S., Puckett, W., Marcillo, A. and Dietrich, D. (2000) Schwannosis: role of gliosis and proteoglycan in human spinal cord injury. *J. Neurotrauma*, 9: 781–788.

Bunge, M.B. (2001) Bridging areas of injury in the spinal cord. *Neuroscientist*, 7: 325–339.

Bunge, M.B. and Kleitman, N. (1997) Schwann cells as facilitators of axonal regeneration in CNS fiber tracts. In: B.H.J. Juurlink, R.M. Devon, J.R. Doucette, A.J. Nazarali, D.J. Schreyer and V.M.K. Verge (Eds.), *Cell Biology and Pathology of Myelin*. Plenum Press, New York, NY, pp. 319–333.

Bunge, M.B. and Kleitman, N. (1999) Neurotrophins and neuroprotection improve axonal regeneration into Schwann cell transplants placed in transected adult rat spinal cord. In: M.H. Tuszynski and J.H. Kordower (Eds.), *CNS Regeneration: Basic Science and Clinical Advances*. Academic Press, New York, NY, pp. 631–646.

Bunge, M.B., Takami, T., Marcillo, A.E. and Oudega, M. (2000) Schwann cell and ensheathing glia implantation in the contused adult rat thoracic spinal cord. *Soc. Neurosci. Abstr.*, 26: 1103.

Bunge, M.B., Takami, T., Wood, P.M., Kleitman, N. and Oudega, M. (2001) Schwann cell and olfactory ensheathing glia transplantation in the moderately contused adult rat thoracic spinal cord, *Soc. Neurosci. Abstr.*, 27: 966.

Bunge, R.P., Puckett, W.R., Becerra, J.L., Marcillo, A. and Quencer, R.M. (1993) Observations on the pathology of human spinal cord injury. A review and classification of 22 new cases with details from a case of chronic cord compression with extensive focal demyelination. In: F.J. Seil (Ed.), *Advances in Neurology*, Vol. 59. Raven Press, New York, NY, pp. 75–89.

Bunge, R.P., Puckett, W.R. and Hiester, E.D. (1997) Observations on the pathology of several types of human spinal cord injury, with emphasis on the astrocyte response to penetrating injuries. In: F.J. Seil (Ed.), *Advances in Neurology, Neuronal Regeneration, Reorganization, and Repair*, Vol. 72. Lippincott-Raven, Philadelphia, PA, pp. 305–315.

Chen, A., Xu, X.M., Kleitman, N. and Bunge, M.B. (1996) Methylprednisolone administration improves axonal regeneration into Schwann cell grafts in transected adult rat thoracic spinal cord. *Exp. Neurol.*, 138: 261–276.

Fawcett, J.W. and Asher, R.A. (1999) The glial scar and central nervous system repair. *Brain Res. Bull.*, 49: 377–391.

Fitch, M.T. and Silver, J. (1999) Beyond the glial scar. Cellular and molecular mechanisms by which glia contributes to CNS regenerative failure. In: M.H. Tuszynski and J.H. Kordower (Eds.), *CNS Regeneration. Basic Science and Clinical Advances*. Academic Press, New York, NY, pp. 55–88.

Franklin, R.J.M. and Barnett, S.C. (1997) Do olfactory glia have advantages over Schwann cells for CNS repair? *J. Neurosci. Res.*, 50: 665–672.

Franklin, R.J.M. and Barnett, S.C. (2000) Olfactory ensheathing cells and CNS regeneration: the sweet smell of success? *Neuron*, 28: 15–18.

Guénard, V., Xu, X.M. and Bunge, M.B. (1993) The use of Schwann cell transplantation to foster central nervous system repair. *Neurosciences*, 5: 401–411.

Houle, J.D., Wright, J.W. and Ziegler, M.K. (1994) After spinal cord injury, chronically injured neurons retain the potential for axonal regeneration. In: H. Teitelbaum and K.N. Prasad (Eds.), *Neural Transplantation, CNS Neuronal Injury, and Regeneration. Recent Advances*. CRC, Boca Raton, FL, pp. 103–118.

Kleitman, N. and Bunge, M.B. (2000) Olfactory ensheathing glia: their application to spinal cord regeneration and remyelination strategies. *Top. Spinal Cord Inj. Rehab.*, 6: 65–81.

Lemons, M.L., Howland, D.R. and Anderson, D.K. (1999) Chondroitin sulfate proteoglycan immunoreactivity increases following spinal cord injury and transplantation. *Exp. Neurol.*, 160: 51–65.

Liu, D., Thangnipon, W. and McAdoo, D.J. (1991) Excitatory amino acids rise to toxic levels upon impact injury to the rat spinal cord. *Brain Res.*, 547: 344–348.

Martin, D., Schoenen, J., Delrée, P., Leprince, P., Rogister, B. and Moonen, G. (1991) Grafts of syngenic cultured, adult dorsal root ganglion-derived Schwann cells to the injured spinal cord of adult rats: preliminary morphological studies. *Neurosci. Lett.*, 124: 44–48.

Martin, D., Schoenen, J., Delrée, P., Rigo, J.-M., Rogister, B., Leprince, P. and Moonen, G. (1993) Syngeneic grafting of adult rat DRG-derived Schwann cells to the injured spinal cord. *Brain Res. Bull.*, 30: 507–514.

Martin, D., Robe, P., Franzen, R., Delrée, P., Schoenen, J., Stevenaert, A. and Moonen, G. (1996) Effects of Schwann cell transplantation in a contusion model of rat spinal cord injury. *J. Neurosci. Res.*, 45: 588–597.

Menei, P., Montero-Menei, C., Whittemore, S.R., Bunge, R.P. and Bunge, M.B. (1998) Schwann cells genetically modified to secrete human BDNF promote enhanced axonal regrowth across transected adult rat spinal cord. *Eur. J. Neurosci.*, 10: 607–621.

Moon, L.D.F., Asher, R.A., Rhodes, K.E. and Fawcett, J.W. (2001) Regeneration of CNS axons back to their target following treatment of adult rat brain with chondroitinase ABC. *Nat. Neurosci.*, 4: 465–466.

Panter, S.S., Yum, S.W. and Faden, A.I. (1990) Alteration in extracellular amino acids after traumatic spinal cord injury.

Ann. Neurol., 27: 96–99.

Plant, G.W., Bates, M.L. and Bunge, M.B. (2001a) Inhibitory proteoglycan immunoreactivity is higher at the caudal than the rostral Schwann cell graft–transected spinal cord interface. *Mol. Cell. Neurosci.*, 17: 471–487.

Plant, G.W., Ramón-Cueto, A. and Bunge, M.B. (2001b) Transplantation of Schwann cells and ensheathing glia to improve regeneration in adult spinal cord. In: N.A. Ingoglia and M. Murray (Eds.), *Axonal Regeneration in the Central Nervous System*. Marcel Dekker, New York, NY, pp. 529–561.

Ramón-Cueto, A., Plant, G., Avila, J. and Bunge, M.B. (1998) Long-distance axonal regeneration in the transected adult rat spinal cord is promoted by olfactory ensheathing glia transplants. *J. Neurosci.*, 18: 3803–3815.

Richardson, P.M., Issa, V.M. and Aguayo, A.J. (1984) Regeneration of long spinal axons in the rat. *J. Neurocytol.*, 13: 165–182.

Schwab, M.E. (2002) Increasing plasticity and functional recovery of the lesioned spinal cord. In: L. McKerracher, G. Doucet and S. Rossignol (Eds.), *Spinal Cord Trauma: Neural Repair and Functional Recovery*. Progress in Brain Research, Vol. 137, Elsevier, Amsterdam, pp. 351–359.

Xu, X.M., Guénard, V., Kleitman, N. and Bunge, M.B. (1995a) Axonal regeneration into Schwann cell-seeded guidance channels grafted into transected adult rat spinal cord. *J. Comp. Neurol.*, 351: 145–160.

Xu, X.M., Guénard, V., Kleitman, N., Aebischer, P. and Bunge, M.B. (1995b) A combination of BDNF and NT-3 promotes supraspinal axonal regeneration into Schwann cell grafts in adult rat thoracic spinal cord. *Exp. Neurol.*, 134: 261–272.

Xu, X.M., Chen, A., Guénard, V., Kleitman, N. and Bunge, M.B. (1997) Bridging Schwann cell transplants promote axonal regeneration from both the rostral and caudal stumps of transected adult rat spinal cord. *J. Neurocytol.*, 26: 1–16.

Yick, L.-W., Wu, W., So, K.-F., Yip, H.K. and Shum, D.K.-Y. (2000) Chondroitinase ABC promotes axonal regeneration of Clarke's neurons after spinal cord injury. *Neuroreport*, 11: 1063–1067.

L. McKerracher, G. Doucet and S. Rossignol (Eds.)
Progress in Brain Research, Vol. 137

CHAPTER 20

Potent possibilities: endogenous stem cells in the adult spinal cord

Adam C. Lipson and Philip J. Horner [*]

Department of Neurological Surgery, University of Washington, Harborview Medical Center, 325 Ninth Avenue, Box 359655, Seattle, WA 98104-2499, USA

Introduction

Stem cells have generated excitement for their application to the study of organ development and disease, and their potential to replace damaged cells. Neuronal and glial cell production has been demonstrated from both neural and non-neural tissues and promises an exciting and novel method for central nervous system (CNS) repair. The expanding body of literature on stem cell transplantation reflects this early enthusiasm, but there remains much to be reconfirmed, and the issues surrounding stem cell grafting are both complex and controversial. A relatively less explored approach for stem cell-mediated repair is the recruitment of endogenous cells without transplantation. In the present review, we will focus on stem cells that reside within the CNS and, in particular, the adult spinal cord. We will discuss the factors that direct stem cell fate in the developing and adult CNS as they may be applied to recruit and direct endogenous repair of the injured spinal cord.

The origin and biology of adult neural stem cells (aNSC) as well as their application to repair has been extensively reviewed in recent years (Cameron and McKay, 1998; Alvarez-Buylla et al., 2000; Gage, 2000; van der Kooy and Weiss, 2000). Within this literature, it is clear that research into the biology of aNSC is accelerating, but there is much to be learned. Indeed, the basic mechanisms underlying aNSC proliferation, migration and differentiation are largely undiscovered. There has been considerably more progress in understanding these processes in stem cells of the developing brain, but there is no clear indication that these events are recapitulated in the aNSC (Temple, 2001). Yet, despite our relatively primitive understanding of the aNSC, there remains considerable basis for optimism. The aNSC is known to be prevalent throughout the CNS and can routinely replace neurons and glia in the adult brain, exhibiting impressive self-renewal and differentiation capabilities both in vivo, and in vitro.

These observations lead us to ask an important question: if stem cells are resident throughout the CNS, why does spontaneous recovery and cell replacement not occur following CNS injury? Current data suggest that self-repair is not a limitation of the aNSC, but rather the lack of pro-regenerative signaling, or the action of inhibitory factors that prevent extensive cell replacement. Understanding the molecular signals which instruct aNSC behavior may help to elucidate the clinical translation of stem cell research to disorders affecting the CNS.

---

[*] Correspondence to: P.J. Horner, Department of Neurological Surgery, University of Washington, Harborview Medical Center, 325 Ninth Avenue, Box 359655, Seattle, WA 98104-2499, USA. Tel.: +1-206-341-5715; Fax: +1-206-341-5804; E-mail: phorner@u.washington.edu

Stem cells of the nervous system

In this review, we will draw upon the developmental literature to compare and contrast what we know about aNSC biology. It is first important to define the aNSC and its progeny within the existing stem cell nomenclature. To earn their title, CNS stem cells must fundamentally demonstrate the capacity to undergo constitutive proliferation, self-renewal and differentiation along all neural lineages to generate mature neurons, astrocytes and oligodendrocytes (Gage, 2000). By definition totipotent stem cells, such as the zygote, are the most primitive population, able to form a full organism. Pluripotent stem cells, such as the embryonic stem (ES) cell derived from the inner cell mass of the blastocyst, can generate precursors across all cell lineages, to form all cell types, but cannot form the organism de novo (Gokhan and Mehler, 2001). Intermediate ES-derived glial (GRP) and neuronal-restricted precursor cells (NRP) continue to self-replicate, but begin to differentiate along lineage-restricted pathways. During development, the stem cells of neuroectodermal origin have been shown to arise from the embryonic and fetal ventricular zone, which is the primary germinal region of the brain (Davis and Temple, 1994). Neural stem cells are prominent during early neural plate formation and demonstrate early positional specification. For example, there is dorsal–ventral patterning during neural induction and temporal specification with the generation of neurons before glia (Temple, 2001). While the aNSC is likely derived from the ES cell, the pathway and phenotypic intermediates are not yet known. The aNSC may give rise to more restricted progeny similar to the GRP and NRP cells found during development, but these progeny are as yet only partially defined, and are referred to as adult neural progenitor cells (aNPC). The aNPC remains multipotent, but is thought to have reduced capacity for self-renewal as compared to the aNSC.

Cells that meet the strict criteria of a stem cell were initially localized to the subependymal zone of the lateral ventricles, also known as the subventricular zone (SVZ), and from the dentate gyrus of the hippocampal formation (reviewed in Momma et al., 2000; Geuna et al., 2001). While the focus of their discovery was originally centered upon the production of neurons, aNSC also demonstrate the capacity to undergo gliogenesis by giving rise to astrocyte and oligodendroglial progenitors (Zhang et al., 1999; Alvarez-Buylla et al., 2000). Regional localization of cells that exhibit stem cell characteristics has expanded in recent years to include regions throughout the CNS, including the spinal cord. A summary of these discoveries is presented in Table I along with factors shown to affect their proliferation, differentiation and migration in vivo.

How are stem cells identified? There are no surface antigens considered unique to the neural stem cell that may be used as a reliable immunochemical marker. Nestin expression and immunoreactivity has been utilized as a cellular marker to facilitate identification of immature cells in vitro and in development (Lendahl et al., 1990), but is not ubiquitous to all stem cell populations, and may be up-regulated by mature glia following injury (Lin et al., 1995). Antibodies directed against the CD133 antigen have allowed for the isolation of adult stem cells by fluorescence-activated cell sorting (Uchida et al., 2000). However, neural stem cells are usually characterized in vivo by identifying their proliferating progeny, initially via ^{3}H-thymidine (Altman and Das, 1965), and subsequently by retroviral and bromodeoxyuridine (BrdU) incorporation during DNA replication. Evidence of cell division has been used to indicate plasticity and along with immunolabeling for progenitor markers has been the most widely accepted method to identify aNPC and their phenotypic fate. However, it is important to recognize the limitations of these techniques particularly for determining the functional fate of aNPC into a differentiated phenotype. Electrophysiology should be utilized to confirm synapse formation in the case of neurogenesis, and to demonstrate myelin formation in the case of oligodendroglial differentiation. The challenging process to validate neurogenesis has been recently reviewed in detail (Svendsen et al., 2001).

Stem cell transplantation into the CNS

Novel sources for neural cell replacement

Recent evidence of transdifferentiation across stem cell lineages, previously thought to be tissue-restricted, may further expand our view of the ther-

TABLE I

A list of mammalian in vivo experiments summarizing the anatomic location of aNSC populations, along with the signals which may influence their proliferation, migration and differentiation in the adult CNS — in comparison to the developing CNS, relatively little is known about the factors that regulate endogenous aNSC fate

Target stem cell population	Mitogen	Migration	Cell phenotype	Reference
Ependymal layer		+	N, A	(Johansson et al., 1999)
Subventricular zone (SVZ)	TGFα	+	N, A, O	(Kuhn et al., 1997; Tropepe et al., 1997; Fallon et al., 2000)
	FGF-2	+	N, A	(Craig et al., 1996)
	EGF	+	A, O	
	Noggin		N	(Lim et al., 2000)
	BMP		O, A	
	EPO	+	N	(Shingo et al., 2001)
Hippocampus	FGF-2	+	N, A	(Eriksson et al., 1998; Gage et al., 1998; Yoshimura et al., 2001)
Olfactory bulb	BDNF	+	N	(Luskin, 1993; Zigova et al., 1998; Pagano et al., 2000)
Striatum			N	(Reynolds and Weiss, 1992)
	BDNF	+		(Pencea et al., 2001)
	FGF-2			(Palmer et al., 1995)
	TGFα			(Fallon et al., 2000)
Septum	BDNF	+	N	(Pencea et al., 2001)
Thalamus				
Hypothalamus				
Cerebral cortex			N, A, O	(Magavi et al., 2000; Gould et al., 2001)
Cerebellum			N, A, O	(Vicario-Abejon et al., 1995; Laywell et al., 2000)
Retina			N	(Tropepe et al., 2000)
Medial ganglionic eminence		+	N	(Wichterle et al., 1999)
Optic nerve			O, A	(Palmer et al., 1995)
Spinal cord	NT-3		O	(McTigue et al., 1998)
	BDNF, FGF-2	+	A, O	(Shihabuddin et al., 1997, 2000)

Legend: N = neuron; A = astrocyte; O = oligodendrocyte; + = the aNSC studied was capable of undergoing migration.

apeutic potential of neural stem cells. In vitro manipulations of stem cells isolated from adult mouse demonstrate their differentiation into skeletal muscle (Galli et al., 2000) and into hematopoietic cell types (Bjornson et al., 1999). Likewise, hematopoietic (Mezey et al., 2000), bone marrow stromal (Brazelton et al., 2000), and dermal (Toma et al., 2001) progenitor cells have been shown to produce neural stem cells. Thus, there may exist non-neuronal sources of stem cells to transplant. One must temper enthusiasm for these transplantation studies, and apply some caution with regards to the heterogeneity of the stem cell sources and culture conditions (Anderson et al., 2001).

Nonetheless, these studies fundamentally challenge our view of potential resources from which neural tissue can be generated. It is possible that stem cells may demonstrate further plasticity than anticipated, crossing the line between lineage- and tissue-restricted boundaries. The observation that committed precursor cells can undergo de-differentiation is noteworthy in this regard. Oligodendroglial precursors can be stimulated in vitro to revert back to a multipotent stem cell state, and subsequently redirected to form astrocytes and neurons (Kondo and Raff, 2000). Similarly, stem cells isolated from non-neurogenic regions of the adult rat brain, such as optic nerve and cerebral cortex, can be stimulated to generate neurons in vitro after exposure to FGF-2, indicating either the recruitment of quiescent stem cells or redirection of glial-restricted progenitor cells down a neuronal lineage (Palmer et al., 1999). Thus, stem and progenitor cells may not be irreversibly committed to one lineage or tissue, and may be reprogrammed or undergo transdifferentiation in response to extracellular signals within their local environment.

These studies also blur the line between stem cell and progenitor cell with regards to their ability to repair the injured spinal cord. It suggests that under the appropriate conditions progenitor cells have sufficient multipotency and proliferation capacity to effectively replace neural cells. Given the prevalence of progenitor cells and the increased number of cellular markers compared to stem cells, aNPC may be particularly interesting for the study of neural repair.

The transplantation of neural and glial progenitor cells as a repair strategy in spinal cord injury

Spinal cord injury produces a complex series of events leading to the loss of motor and sensory function below the level of injury. Secondary injury is associated with microvascular changes, glutamate excitotoxicity, neuronal electrolyte shifts, elaboration of oxygen free radicals and lipid peroxidation, accumulation of serotonin and endogenous opioids, arachidonic acid and eicosanoid release, inflammatory changes involving cytokines, and astrocytic edema (Tator, 1998). These various insults contribute to neuronal necrosis, apoptosis, axonal retraction and demyelination, followed by cyst formation. There is an abortive and occasionally aberrant regenerative effort made by the injured axons, but this has been shown to be limited due to the presence of astroglial scarring, inhibitory myelin-associated glycoproteins and neuronal injury (Behar et al., 2000).

In the context of this pathophysiology, considerable attention has focused on the reconnection of disrupted pathways. Transplantation approaches using artificial and cellular bridges, fetal tissue, fibroblasts or Schwann cells expressing neurotrophins, hybridoma cells expressing myelin inhibitory protein-blocking antibodies, and olfactory ensheathing cells have produced axonal regeneration and/or functional benefit (Olson, 1997; Horner and Gage, 2000).

Stem cells have recently been added to the list of promising spinal cord therapies. For example, behavioral improvement by open field testing has been demonstrated in adult rats receiving transplants of mouse ES cells following spinal cord contusion, with 43% of the cells labeling positive for oligodendrocytes, 19% for astrocytes, and 8% for neurons (McDonald et al., 1999). Spinal cord dorsal column remyelination has been reported using human aNSC (Akiyama et al., 2001) and mouse ES cells (Liu et al., 2000), and has been proposed as a potential mech-

anism for rapid functional recovery following spinal cord injury. Stem cell populations have also been modified in culture to provide for gene-based delivery of growth promoting molecules, such as NT-3, to the spinal cord (Y. Liu et al., 1999). Transplantation of neural stem cells may therefore be utilized to both replace deficient neuronal populations and express foreign genes as they incorporate into the CNS (Flax et al., 1998).

Endogenous stem cells

Stem cells of the embryonic spinal cord

During development, neuroepithelial stem cells are noted along the central canal, within the ventricular zone, generating neuronal precursors. They undergo dorsoventral segmentation and demonstrate discrete progenitor zones defined by different homeodomain transcription factors (Briscoe et al., 2000). Both neuronal-restricted progenitors (NRPs) (Mayer-Proschel et al., 1997) and glial-restricted precursor cells (GRPs) (Rao et al., 1998), have been isolated from the spinal cord of E13.5 rats. The glial-restricted progenitors are tripotent, giving rise to the O-2A progenitor cell, which differentiates into oligodendrocytes and type 2 astrocytes, and to type 1 astrocytes.

Stem cells of the adult spinal cord

Current evidence suggests that there are likely multiple regions where stem cells exist in the spinal cord during adulthood. An adult stem cell population is likely to be localized in or adjacent to the ependymal layer lining the central canal, regionally akin to the SVZ in the cerebrum (Alonso, 1999; Chiasson et al., 1999; Doetsch et al., 1999; Johansson et al., 1999). In addition, aNSC have been isolated from regions of the spinal cord separate from the central canal and its associated ependymal cell lining. Progenitor cells capable of forming neurospheres and able to differentiate into neurons in vitro have been recently reported throughout adult spinal cord parenchyma (Yamamoto et al., 2001a).

A separate population of aNPCs was demonstrated in the adult rodent spinal cord by BrdU labeling in vivo, with few proliferating cells noted in the ependymal layer of the central canal, but numerous cells throughout the outer white matter and in the substantia gelatinosa (Horner et al., 2000). These data revealed two basic progenitor morphologies, with no evidence for migration from the central canal. Many of these BrdU-labeled cells co-localized with oligodendrocyte and astrocyte markers indicating that glial cell production continues in the adult spinal cord. The co-labeling of cells with antibody directed against NG2 chondroitin sulfate, an immature marker believed to be associated with O-2A progenitors, further confirms that these cells proceed towards a glial-restricted lineage. Cells expressing the NG2 proteoglycan co-express the platelet-derived growth factor alpha receptor (PDGFr-α), and represent a major glial cell population thought to represent oligodendrocyte progenitor cells during development and adulthood. One common finding of all proliferation studies in the adult spinal cord is the absence of neurogenesis in vivo. A potential caveat to consider in interpreting these data is the possibility that CNS macrophages may also label with the NG2 marker non-specifically, though the stem cells identified in this study appeared quite different with respect to their morphology, and lack of OX-42 labeling. It is nonetheless important to recognize that the NG2-positive (NG2$^+$) population of dividing cells may represent a heterogeneous mix of progenitor and differentiated phenotypes (Dawson et al., 2000). There is increasing evidence that NG2$^+$ progenitors self-renew and are stem cell-like in character (Dawson et al., 2000; Tang et al., 2001). However, other evidence suggests that these precursor cells may possess an intrinsic timer to undergo cell cycle arrest and differentiation (Durand et al., 1998).

The presence of stem cell populations in the adult spinal cord leads us to inquire how these cells might behave in injurious versus non-injurious states. By defining and understanding the stem cell activities, we may be able to stimulate or inhibit the process as appropriate to direct axonal repair and neuroregeneration. The proliferation of endogenous stem cells can be demonstrated following spinal cord injury (Adrian and Walker, 1962), with an increased formation of neurospheres capable of neurogenesis in vitro (Yamamoto et al., 2001a). Contusion injury to the adult rat spinal cord results in the proliferation of BrdU-labeled dividing cells, mostly microglia

and macrophages during the first week after injury. There is subsequent up-regulation of NG2$^+$ proliferation during the second, third and fourth weeks after injury after a dramatic reduction in oligodendrocyte numbers during the first week (McTigue et al., 2001). Similarly, demyelinating lesions of the spinal cord induce a rapid proliferation of NG2$^+$ cells prior to remyelination, with the obliteration of both the NG2$^+$ progenitor and remyelinating response if the spinal cord and host stem cells are X-irradiated (Keirstead et al., 1998).

Endogenous stem cells are likely significant for investigation of the cellular response to spinal cord injury, but what is the evidence for possible roles mediated by these progenitors during spinal cord injury? NG2$^+$ progenitors may play a role in axonal remyelination. It has been demonstrated that spinal cord neurons and oligodendrocytes undergo apoptosis after spinal cord injury (Liu et al., 1997). This occurs concomitant with the initial loss of myelin and subsequent re-myelination at the site of injury (Griffiths and McCulloch, 1983), which temporally correlates with the expansion in host NG2$^+$ progenitors. While these studies do not prove that the new oligodendrocytes reported are derived from proliferating endogenous progenitors, their results provide some evidence confirming that the NG2-immunoreactive aNPC population is present within the adult spinal cord, and that it can survive and respond to injurious insult.

These insights may also shed further light into current existing treatments for spinal cord injury. It has been observed for example that prolonged corticosterone treatment decreases the proliferation of adult NG2$^+$ progenitors throughout the white and gray matter regions of the adult rat brain except in the SVZ (Alonso, 2000). The administration of glucocorticoids for human spinal cord injury is considered beneficial, though little is known of its effects on the host adult spinal cord stem cells.

Endogenous molecular cues contribute to stem cell fate; lessons from development

Numerous extracellular signals act as stem cell mitogens, influencing aNSC division, expansion and occasionally migration. In vitro studies have demonstrated proliferative effects in multipotential embryonic spinal cord neuroblast progenitors using basic fibroblast growth factor (FGF-2) (Ray and Gage, 1994), and in adult mouse neurospheres using a combination of FGF-2 and epidermal growth factor (EGF) (Weiss et al., 1996). In general, neural stem cells can be isolated from different regions of the CNS using FGF-2 as the mitogen during very early development, and EGF and FGF as the mitogen during later development (Tropepe et al., 1999; Zhu et al., 2000). It is important to remember that these findings are species, age, and in vitro model dependent. The peripheral infusion of insulin-like growth factor-I (IGF-I) also has been shown to enhance neurogenesis in the sub-granular zone of the early post-natal rat hippocampus (Aberg et al., 2000).

Extrinsic factors influence neural stem cell differentiation down neuronal, astroglial or oligodendroglial pathways. *Notch* signaling can promote CNS multipotent neural progenitors to undergo astroglial differentiation (Tanigaki et al., 2001). Likewise, PDGF plays an important role in maintaining the proliferative capacity of oligodendroglial progenitors, which express PDGFr-α (Nishiyama et al., 1996; Calver et al., 1998; Rogister et al., 1999). The withdrawal of PDGF stimulates oligodendrocyte differentiation. Thyroid hormone (TH) and retinoic acid (RA) also signal oligodendrocyte precursor cells to mature and differentiate (Barres et al., 1994). Similarly, *neuregulin* has been shown to act as an axon-associated survival signal and may prevent differentiation of the O-2A glial restricted progenitor cell (Fernandez et al., 2000). In the spinal cord *neuregulin* has been shown to be essential for oligodendrocyte development. Ciliary neurotrophic factor (CNTF) was found to be important for gliogenesis, and induces the differentiation of aNSCs into type 2 astrocytes in the presence of extracellular matrix (Aberg et al., 2001).

Developmental signals known to modulate early neuronal differentiation also play a significant role in regulating stem cell lineage. Spinal cord neuronal precursor cells are responsive to two factors which play a prominent role in the dorsoventral patterning of the neuraxis during early embryogenesis, with bone morphogenetic protein (BMP) acting dorsally and sonic hedgehog (*Snh*) acting ventrally (Tanabe and Jessell, 1996). Applying these factors in vitro to cultured embryonic spinal cord neuronal precursors,

BMP-2 and BMP-4 promoted differentiation and maturation into a heterogeneous population of neurons secreting numerous neurotransmitters, including dopamine, acetylcholine, GABA, and glycine (Kalyani et al., 1998). Accordingly, *Snh*, which normally regulates the induction of motoneurons and ventral interneurons, also exhibits mitogenic effects, maintaining the NRPs in a proliferative, undifferentiated state in vitro (Kalyani et al., 1998), and in vivo, via the *Patched-1* transmembrane receptor and *Gli-1* zinc finger transcription factor (Rowitch et al., 1999). In the latter study the *Wnt-1* enhancer was used to direct transgenic overexpression in the roofplate of the developing mouse spinal cord.

Developmental signals such as BMP may also affect stem cell lineage choice across tissues. For example, in the embryonic spinal cord, neuroepithelial-derived precursor cells have been shown to differentiate into peripheral nervous system (PNS) phenotypes (peripheral neurons, smooth muscle and Schwann cells) and into the low-affinity neurotrophin receptor p75-positive neural crest stem cells which populate the PNS, after BMP-2/4 induction (Mujtaba et al., 1998). Thus, embryonic spinal cord stem cells demonstrate significantly greater plasticity after in vitro manipulation, in being able to populate both the CNS and PNS.

Primarily studied during development, transcription factors have been shown to regulate stem cell differentiation, and contribute significant insight to the molecular cascades impacting stem cell fate. The basic helix–loop–helix (bHLH) transcription factors have been implicated as positive and negative regulators of neuronal differentiation. *Mash1*, *Prox1* (Torii et al., 1999) and *NeuroD* (Miyata et al., 1999) are positive bHLH genes notable for directing early neuronal differentiation during development. Knockout studies indicate that these are required factors for the specification of intermediate neuronal progenitors. *Ngn2* has also been expressed in subsets of neural progenitors in both the developing spinal cord (Yamamoto et al., 2001b). *Olig1* and *Olig2* have been shown to be expressed in oligodendrocytes and their progenitors, with *Olig2* expressed in early spinal cord oligodendroglial progenitors (Zhou et al., 2000).

Alternatively, the negative bHLH factor *Hes1* may contribute to the maintenance of the self-renewing, multipotent state, repressing neurogenesis and migration out of the ventricular zone (Nakamura et al., 2000). Overexpression of *Hes1* and *Hes5* in the developing mouse brain results in the expansion of undifferentiated neural stem cells, and inhibits both neurogenesis and gliogenesis (Ohtsuka et al., 2001). The *Id* (inhibitor of differentiation) family of proteins represents another negative bHLH regulator of stem cell commitment, analogous to *Hes* (Lyden et al., 1999).

Inflammatory cytokines are stem cell modulators. TNFα, believed to be produced by CNS microglia and astrocytes, has been shown to promote the proliferation of NG2$^+$ oligodendrocyte progenitors, signaling via TNF receptor 2, and may have a critical role in nerve myelinogenesis following demyelination (Arnett et al., 2001). However, other studies indicate that TNFα may be cytotoxic to oligodendrocytes and their progenitors (Cammer, 2000). In addition, BMP-2 can redirect the fate of fetal mouse telencephalic NRPs from neuronal to astroglial differentiation (Nakashima et al., 2001), and may act synergistically with leukemia inhibitory factor (LIF) (Nakashima et al., 1999), to induce the expression of negative bHLH proteins for a downstream effect of inhibiting neurogenesis. Interleukin-1β (IL-1β) expression in mice exposed to cuprizone, to produce a demyelinating insult, was found to promote remyelination and NG2$^+$ progenitor differentiation into mature oligodendrocytes, correlating with IGF-I induction in microglia, macrophages and astrocytes (Mason et al., 2001).

Molecular cues that influence the aNSC

In comparison to our understanding of neural progenitor cells in development, little is known about the molecular signals required to differentiate an aNSC into neuronal, astrocytic and oligodendrocytic phenotypes. Those factors demonstrating in vivo effects during adulthood are summarized in Table I. In addition to EGF and FGF-2, transforming growth factor alpha (TGFα), which binds to the EGF tyrosine kinase receptor encoded by the *ErbB* gene, demonstrates mitogenic effects on adult SVZ cells, and in fact has been shown to be required for proliferation (Tropepe et al., 1997).

BMP signaling was shown to promote glial differentiation, and BMP antagonism by *Noggin* expression in ependymal cells was shown to promote neurogenesis in the adult mouse subventricular zone (Lim et al., 2000). aNPCs derived from the spinal cord were recently shown to be restricted in their capacity to differentiate into motoneurons or interneurons in vitro, with *Notch* signaling likely contributing to the inhibition of neuronal differentiation both in vitro and in vivo. Indeed, *Notch1* expression was demonstrated to be enhanced in response to injury indicating that *Notch* may actively suppress neuronal differentiation from endogenous aNPCs and, hence, prevent post-injury neurogenesis (Yamamoto et al., 2001b).

Endogenous induction of aNSCS in the CNS

Given the presence of stem cells throughout the adult CNS, one may obviate the need for a transplantation procedure by manipulating the endogenous stem cells using various developmental factors as outlined above. For example, endogenous FGF-2 expression was shown to significantly influence neuronal differentiation in the dentate gyrus of the adult mouse hippocampus following kainic acid-induced seizure and middle cerebral artery occlusion (Yoshimura et al., 2001). Intraventricular infusion of EGF into the adult mouse (Craig et al., 1996), and either FGF-2 or EGF into the adult rat (Kuhn et al., 1997), resulted in the proliferation and migration of sub-ependymal aNSCs, with EGF favoring gliogenesis, and FGF-2 promoting neurogenesis. In the spinal cord, a combination of EGF and FGF was required to stimulate proliferation of nestin-immunoreactive cells near the ependymal canal (Kojima and Tator, 2000).

Erythropoietin (EPO) infused into the lateral ventricle promotes aNSC migration to the olfactory bulb and an increase in interneuron formation, possibly acting via *NF-κB* and *Mash1* signaling (Shingo et al., 2001). Similarly, infusions of TGFα into the ventricles of Parkinsonian rats stimulates the proliferation of adult SVZ neural stem cells concomitant with EGF receptor up-regulation, migration towards the lesioned striatum, and dopaminergic neuronal differentiation, accompanied by improved behavioral scores (Fallon et al., 2000). Cell-mediated delivery of NT-3 either directly or through the induction of axon growth increases the number of myelin producing cells from mitotically active progenitor cells (McTigue et al., 1998).

These experiments suggest that single factors may have the potential to influence proliferation or even fate choice of aNPCs in the intact and injured CNS. Future work is needed to determine whether these factors induce novel repair pathways or if they are simply hastening the endogenous repair process. Indeed, there is a local response of aNPC to injury in the spinal cord (Johansson et al., 1999; Nakimi and Tator, 1999) but it is not known whether this represents repair, aberrant cell proliferation or a combination of both.

Targets and pitfalls of stem cell-mediated repair

The replacement of neurons, astrocytes or oligodendrocytes may be considered for several proposed targets in spinal cord injury (Fig. 1). These paradigms suggest only a fraction of the potential stem cell targets that apply to many neural injury models. A better understanding of the cellular and molecular framework underlying aNSC interactions will allow us to refine its use in a repair strategy. Considerations of whether to transplant or activate endogenous cells and when to time one's intervention are complex decisions. The choices for spinal cord repair will revolve around their effectiveness to positively impact glial scarring, axonal myelination, local interneuron plasticity, central pattern generator function, and other trauma-related processes. Finally, we must consider that stem cell transplantation or activation carries the potential risk for aberrant cell generation and/or a worsening of outcomes.

Gliogenesis

There is a mosaic of glial reactions to CNS injury that is thought to prevent axonal regeneration (Hoke and Silver, 1996; Fawcett and Asher, 1999). It is not clear what role glial progenitor cells play in the process but there is evidence that NG2 immunoreactive progenitor cells proliferate in response to injury and demyelination. But is $NG2^+$ aNPC proliferation necessarily beneficial for spinal cord recovery? Its role in oligodendrocyte production and potential contribution to remyelination may be helpful in restoring axonal conduction. Additionally, as a glial progenitor, astrocytic differentiation may be protective of the damaged axon and may help to guide the

regenerating axon to its target. However, the NG2 proteoglycan is noted to inhibit neurite outgrowth (Fidler et al., 1999). Indeed, depletion of $NG2^+$ cells in a nigrostriatal injury model using ethidium bromide was associated with the loss of myelin and the absence of the astroglial scar, creating a permissive environment for TH^+ axonal regeneration (Moon et al., 2000). Therefore, there may be potential reasons for reducing or inhibiting certain aspects of the endogenous spinal cord stem cell response following injury.

Neurogenesis

With respect to neuron replacement, there is concern that aberrant reinnervation may worsen the effects of spinal cord injury by inducing spastic or neuropathic changes. Ectopic cell generation or cell overgrowth may contribute to the induction of seizure activity or inappropriate inhibition of surviving pathways (Parent et al., 1997; Scharfman et al., 2000). The latter may be the primary concern for spinal cord injury. There is evidence that remaining signals and circuitry in the injured spinal cord may be sufficient to guide the appropriate reinnervation. For example, the central pattern generator has been implicated in the genesis of locomotor rhythmic activity responsible for gait recovery and may provide a target for stem cell-directed repair. Serotonergic reinnervation of the L_1–L_2 level, accomplished by embryonic raphe transplants into the chronically injured rat spinal cord below the lesion, resulted in the expression of locomotor rhythmic activity as demonstrated by kinematic and electromyographic analysis (Ribotta et al., 2000). Likewise, the functional reinnervation spinal circuitry by corticorubrospinal fibers following pyramidotomy provides some early optimism that even ectopic axonal growth can compensate for lost pathways (Raineteau and Schwab, 2001).

The environment and endogenous induction

There is significant appeal to being able to control in vitro conditions and to isolate and identify a stem or progenitor phenotype that will be ideal for repair. Indeed, recent successes highlighted above indicate the power of stem cell transplantation in models of

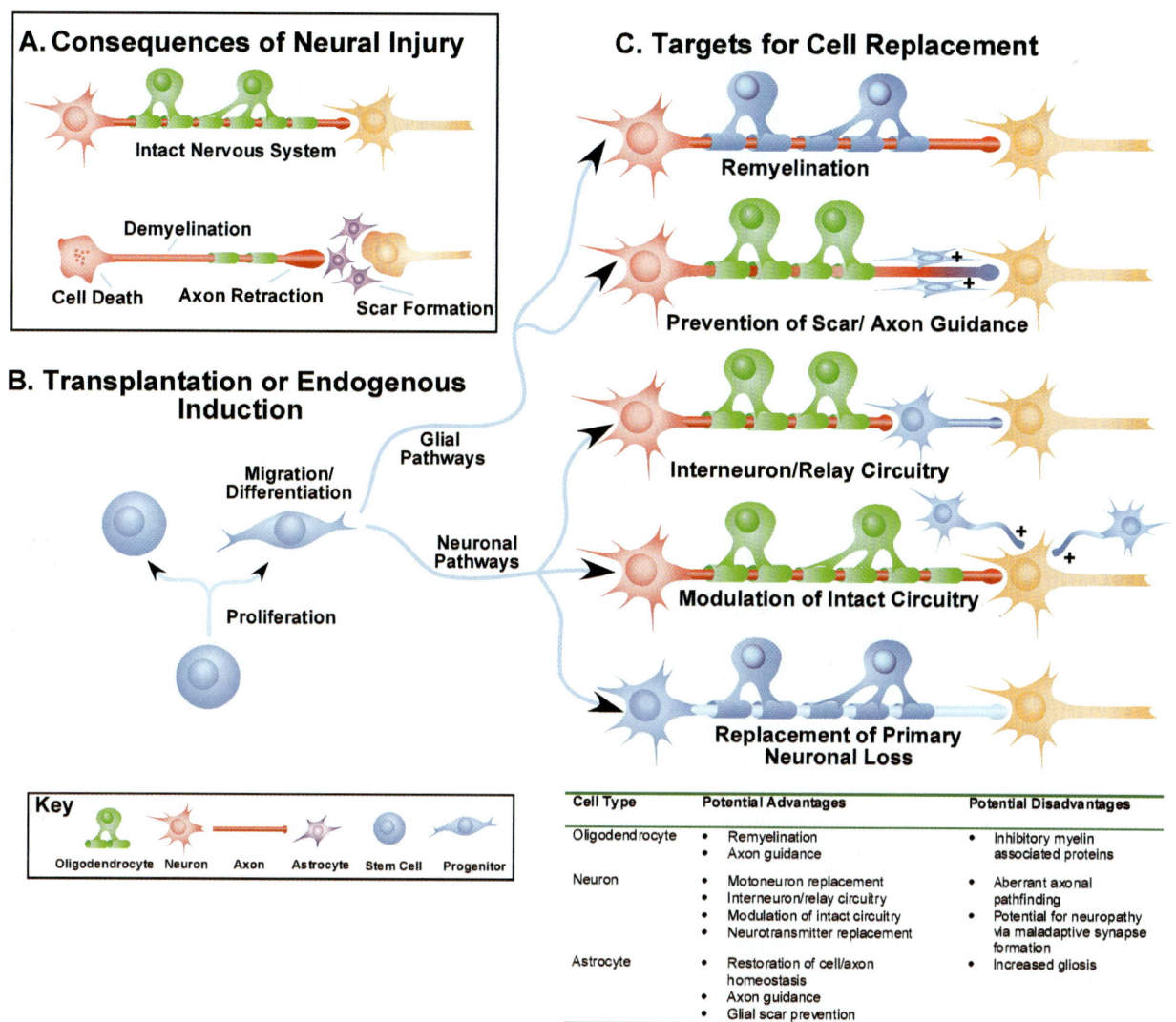

Fig. 1. The consequences of spinal cord injury (A), and hence the targets for repair, are common to many insults of the CNS. Neuronal cell death, axonal retraction, demyelination and scar formation are all features of neural injury that lead to long-term deficits with limited spontaneous repair. Most of the experiments utilizing a stem cell approach in spinal cord repair have been general attempts to determine stem cell survival and differentiation in the lesion environment. Some of these experiments have yielded modest functional improvements. The next challenge is to investigate the mechanism of observed functional changes and determine the optimal source of undifferentiated cells and the appropriate targets for repair. It may not be necessary to select the most immature cell for transplantation or endogenous induction (B). Instead, partial differentiation and selection of stem cell-derived progeny will yield tools with which to test cell replacement hypotheses. For example, more restricted transplantation or endogenous induction of progenitor cells into a glial fate (C) may shed light on the functional benefit of remyelination and axon guidance. Neuronal progenitor cells might be used to create relay circuitry, modulate the excitatory nature of surviving networks or even replace entire pathways. In addition to targeted cell therapy, we must identify the aberrant effects of cell replacement. These may come in the form of increased scar formation or axon mis-targeting. Prevention of these processes will allow us to achieve the highest level of functional improvement.

CNS trauma. However, transplantation carries risks that may or may not be surmountable in the near future. In addition, despite the ability to pre-program immature cells in vitro there may be inherent obstacles within the CNS that significantly reduce cell replacement. These cues are undoubtedly responsible for the lack of complete repair from endogenous cells. For example, although aNSC show considerable plasticity in vitro, their phenotypic fate appears to be restricted by the niche into which they are introduced. Clonal in vitro preparations of adult rat spinal cord stem cells expanded in the presence of FGF-2 generate neurons upon transplantation into the hippocampus, but are restricted to glial phenotypes when the same clonal population is transplanted into the spinal cord (Shihabuddin et al., 2000). Thus, expanded progenitors from an adult non-neurogenic zone such as the spinal cord can integrate and generate region-specific neurons, but only where that differentiated fate is supported by the environment in vivo. The importance of the local milieu on stem cell lineage may be extended to the injury environment as well. For example, pluripotent embryonic and adult SVZ neural stem cells capable of neuronal differentiation in vitro were restricted only to astrocytic differentiation following transplantation into the normal or injured adult rat spinal cord, suggesting that the adult spinal cord environment greatly influences progenitor lineage (Cao et al., 2001).

In spite of the remarkable plasticity reported after in vitro expansion, there is also evidence that stem cells do not behave uniformly within the CNS environment. This is probably a combined function of the heterogeneity of stem cells that are derived from various CNS regions and developmental time-periods, as well as the heterogeneous expression of fate-determining factors within compartments of the CNS. This concept is nicely illustrated in development and recently confirmed for the adult spinal cord. Region-specific expression of transcription factors such as *Sox2* occurs during embryogenesis, such that early differences between telencephalic and spinal cord stem cells are being observed (Zappone et al., 2000). In the adult spinal cord, homeodomain transcription factors expression demonstrates aNSC heterogeneity as well, with Pax6, Pax7, Nkx2.2 being distinctly and differentially expressed, indicating the potential for multiple progenitor subtypes (Yamamoto et al., 2001b). Embryonic neuronal progenitor cells isolated from the spinal cord also differ from SVZ-derived neuronal progenitors in their migration and differentiation properties (Yang et al., 2000). Finally, there is also evidence of differing electrophysiological properties between embryonic

(Kalyani et al., 1998) and adult (R.H. Liu et al., 1999) brain and spinal cord-derived neural progenitors, indicating heterogeneous populations of neural precursor cells.

It is clear that further investigation of the injury-induced factors that regulate stem cell migration, proliferation and differentiation in vivo is important. Application of this knowledge will illuminate targets to unlock the potential of endogenous aNPC to respond to injury. For example, while aNPC do not produce neurons in situ following spinal cord injury, attenuation of *Notch* signaling or forced expression of *Ngn2* promotes the neuronal differentiation of spinal cord aNPCs in vitro (Yamamoto et al., 2001b). Thus, both intrinsic properties of aNPC as well as the injury-induced environmental signals may account for the lack of neuronal replacement from endogenous progenitor cells.

Conclusions

The finding of stem cells resident in the adult spinal cord offers a promising new approach to correcting spinal cord injury. Endogenous activation of these cells represents an exciting alternative to transplantation. Enthusiasm in translating this research must be guided by continued discovery of the basic mechanisms governing stem cell fate as well as an eye to stringent appraisal of experimental results. Future research will continue to be guided by developmental discoveries keeping in mind that clear departures may exist between cells derived from fetal and adult as well as intact and injured CNS. Exploring the role of the post-injury environment in directing cell fate may prove to be of equal or greater importance than choosing the most suitable stem cell for repair. In the future, manipulation of the post-injury milieu with subsequent recruitment of endogenous progenitor cells may prove to be an effective neuroprotective and/or neurorestorative strategy.

Abbreviations

aNPC	adult neural progenitor cell
aNSC	adult neural stem cell
APC	adenomatous polyposis coli tumor suppresser gene
BDNF	brain-derived neurotrophic factor

bHLH	basic helix–loop–helix
BMP	bone morphogenetic protein
BrdU	bromodeoxyuridine
CNTF	ciliary neurotrophic factor
EGF	epidermal growth factor
ES	embryonic stem cell
EPO	erythropoietin
FGF-2	basic fibroblast growth factor
GFAP	glial fibrillary acidic protein
GRP	glial-restricted progenitor
IGF-I	insulin-like growth factor one
IL-1β	interleukin-one beta
LIF	leukemia inhibitory factor
Ngn2	neurogenin 2
NRP	neuronal-restricted progenitor
NT-3	neurotrophin-3
PDGF	platelet-derived growth factor
PDGFr-α	platelet-derived growth factor alpha
SVZ	subventricular zone
TGFα	transforming growth factor alpha
TH	tyrosine hydroxylase
TNFα	tumor necrosis factor alpha

Acknowledgements

The authors would like to thank Don Maris for editorial assistance. PJH receives support from the Christopher Reeve Paralysis Foundation, The Kirsch Foundation, The Glaucoma Research Foundation and the National Institutes of Health (PO1 NS28121-09A1). ACL is supported by an NIH Training Grant (5T32NS07144-23).

References

Aberg, M.A., Aberg, N.D., Hedbacker, H., Oscarsson, J. and Eriksson, P.S. (2000) Peripheral infusion of IGF-I selectively induces neurogenesis in the adult rat hippocampus. *J. Neurosci.*, 20: 2896–2903.

Aberg, M.A., Ryttsen, F., Hellgren, G., Lindell, K., Rosengren, L.E., MacLennan, A.J., Carlsson, B., Orwar, O. and Eriksson, P.S. (2001) Selective introduction of antisense oligonucleotides into single adult CNS progenitor cells using electroporation demonstrates the requirement of STAT3 activation for CNTF-induced gliogenesis. *Mol. Cell. Neurosci.*, 17: 426–443.

Adrian Jr., E.K. and Walker, B.E. (1962) Incorporation of thymidine-H[3] by cells in normal and injured mouse spinal cord. *J. Neuropathol. Exp. Neurol.*, 21: 597–609.

Akiyama, Y., Honmou, O., Kato, T., Uede, T., Hashi, K. and Kocsis, J.D. (2001) Transplantation of clonal neural precursor cells derived from adult human brain establishes functional peripheral myelin in the rat spinal cord. *Exp. Neurol.*, 167: 27–39.

Alonso, G. (1999) Neuronal progenitor-like cells expressing polysialylated neural cell adhesion molecule are present on the ventricular surface of the adult rat brain and spinal cord. *J. Comp. Neurol.*, 414: 149–166.

Alonso, G. (2000) Prolonged corticosterone treatment of adult rats inhibits the proliferation of oligodendrocyte progenitors present throughout white and gray matter regions of the brain. *Glia*, 31: 219–231.

Altman, J. and Das, G.D. (1965) Autoradiographic and histologic evidence of post-natal neurogenesis in rats. *J. Comp. Neurol.*, 124: 319–335.

Alvarez-Buylla, A., Herrera, D.G. and Wichterle, H. (2000) The subventricular zone: source of neuronal precursors for brain repair. *Prog. Brain Res.*, 127: 1–11.

Anderson, D.J., Gage, F.H. and Weissman, I.L. (2001) Can stem cells cross lineage boundaries? *Nat. Med.*, 7: 393–395.

Arnett, H.A., Mason, J., Marino, M., Suzuki, K., Matsushima, G.K. and Ting, J.P. (2001) TNFalpha promotes proliferation of oligodendrocyte progenitors and remyelination. *Nat. Neurosci.*, 4: 1116–1122.

Barres, B.A., Lazar, M.A. and Raff, M.C. (1994) A novel role for thyroid hormone, glucocorticoids and retinoic acid in timing oligodendrocyte development. *Development*, 120: 1097–1108.

Behar, O., Mizuno, K., Neumann, S. and Woolf, C.J. (2000) Putting the spinal cord together again. *Neuron*, 26: 291–293.

Bjornson, C.R., Rietze, R.L., Reynolds, B.A., Magli, M.C. and Vescovi, A.L. (1999) Turning brain into blood: a hematopoietic fate adopted by adult neural stem cells in vivo. *Science*, 283: 534–537.

Brazelton, T.R., Rossi, F.M., Keshet, G.I. and Blau, H.M. (2000) From marrow to brain: expression of neuronal phenotypes in adult mice. *Science*, 290: 1775–1779.

Briscoe, J., Pierani, A., Jessell, T.M. and Ericson, J. (2000) A homeodomain protein code specifies progenitor cell identity and neuronal fate in the ventral neural tube. *Cell*, 101: 435–445.

Calver, A.R., Hall, A.C., Yu, W., Walsh, F.S., Heath, J.K., Betsholtz, C. and Richardson, W.D. (1998) Oligodendrocyte population dynamics and the role of PDGF in vivo. *Neuron*, 20: 869–882.

Cameron, H.A. and McKay, R. (1998) Stem cells and neurogenesis in the adult brain. *Curr. Opin. Neurobiol.*, 8: 677–680.

Cammer, W. (2000) Effects of TNFalpha on immature and mature oligodendrocytes and their progenitors in vitro. *Brain Res.*, 864: 213–219.

Cao, Q.L., Zhang, Y.P., Howard, R.M., Walters, W.M., Tsoulfas, P. and Whittemore, S.R. (2001) Pluripotent stem cells engrafted into the normal or lesioned adult rat spinal cord are restricted to a glial lineage. *Exp. Neurol.*, 167: 48–58.

Chiasson, B.J., Tropepe, V., Morshead, C.M. and van der Kooy, D. (1999) Adult mammalian forebrain ependymal and subependymal cells demonstrate proliferative potential, but only subependymal cells have neural stem cell characteristics. *J. Neurosci.*, 19: 4462–4471.

Clarke, D.L., Johansson, C.B., Wilbertz, J., Veress, B., Nilsson, E., Karlstrom, H., Lendahl, U. and Frisen, J. (2000) Generalized potential of adult neural stem cells. *Science*, 288: 1660–1663.

Craig, C.G., Tropepe, V., Morshead, C.M., Reynolds, B.A., Weiss, S. and van der Kooy, D. (1996) In vivo growth factor expansion of endogenous subependymal neural precursor cell populations in the adult mouse brain. *J. Neurosci.*, 16: 2649–2658.

Davis, A.A. and Temple, S. (1994) A self-renewing multipotential stem cell in embryonic rat cerebral cortex. *Nature*, 372: 263–266.

Dawson, M.R., Levine, J.M. and Reynolds, R. (2000) NG2-expressing cells in the central nervous system: are they oligodendroglial progenitors? *J. Neurosci. Res.*, 61: 471–479.

Doetsch, F., Caille, I., Lim, D.A., Garcia-Verdugo, J.M. and Alvarez-Buylla, A. (1999) Subventricular zone astrocytes are neural stem cells in the adult mammalian brain. *Cell*, 97: 703–716.

Durand, B., Fero, M.L., Roberts, J.M. and Raff, M.C. (1998) p27Kip1 alters the response of cells to mitogen and is part of a cell-intrinsic timer that arrests the cell cycle and initiates differentiation. *Curr. Biol.*, 8: 431–440.

Eriksson, P.S., Perfilieva, E., Bjork-Eriksson, T., Alborn, A.M., Nordborg, C., Peterson, D.A. and Gage, F.H. (1998) Neurogenesis in the adult human hippocampus. *Nat. Med.*, 4: 1313–1317.

Fallon, J., Reid, S., Kinyamu, R., Opole, I., Opole, R., Baratta, J., Korc, M., Endo, T.L., Duong, A., Nguyen, G., Karkehabadhi, M., Twardzik, D., Patel, S. and Loughlin, S. (2000) In vivo induction of massive proliferation, directed migration, and differentiation of neural cells in the adult mammalian brain. *Proc. Natl. Acad. Sci. USA*, 97: 14686–14691.

Fawcett, J.W. and Asher, R.A. (1999) The glial scar and central nervous system repair. *Brain Res. Bull.*, 49(6): 377–391.

Fernandez, P.A., Tang, D.G., Cheng, L., Prochiantz, A., Mudge, A.W. and Raff, M.C. (2000) Evidence that axon-derived neuregulin promotes oligodendrocyte survival in the developing rat optic nerve. *Neuron*, 28: 81–90.

Fidler, P.S., Schuette, K., Asher, R.A., Dobbertin, A., Thornton, S.R., Calle-Patino, Y., Muir, E., Levine, J.M., Geller, H.M., Rogers, J.H., Faissner, A. and Fawcett, J.W. (1999) Comparing astrocytic cell lines that are inhibitory or permissive for axon growth: the major axon-inhibitory proteoglycan is NG2. *J. Neurosci.*, 19: 8778–8788.

Flax, J.D., Aurora, S., Yang, C., Simonin, C., Wills, A.M., Billinghurst, L.L., Jendoubi, M., Sidman, R.L., Wolfe, J.H., Kim, S.U. and Snyder, E.Y. (1998) Engraftable human neural stem cells respond to developmental cues, replace neurons, and express foreign genes. *Nat. Biotechnol.*, 16: 1033–1039.

Gage, F.H. (2000) Mammalian neural stem cells. *Science*, 287: 1433–1438.

Gage, F.H., Kempermann, G., Palmer, T.D., Peterson, D.A. and Ray, J. (1998) Multipotent progenitor cells in the adult dentate gyrus. *J. Neurobiol.*, 36: 249–266.

Galli, R., Borello, U., Gritti, A., Minasi, M.G., Bjornson, C., Coletta, M., Mora, M., De Angelis, M.G., Fiocco, R., Cossu, G. and Vescovi, A.L. (2000) Skeletal myogenic potential of human and mouse neural stem cells. *Nat. Neurosci.*, 3: 986–991.

Geuna, S., Borrione, P., Fornaro, M. and Giacobini-Robecchi, M.G. (2001) Adult stem cells and neurogenesis: historical roots and state of the art. *Anat. Rec.*, 265: 132–141.

Gokhan, S. and Mehler, M.F. (2001) Basic and clinical neuroscience applications of embryonic stem cells. *Anat. Rec.*, 265: 142–156.

Gould, E., Vail, N., Wagers, M. and Gross, C.G. (2001) Adult-generated hippocampal and neocortical neurons in macaques have a transient existence. *Proc. Natl. Acad. Sci. USA*, 98: 10910–10917.

Griffiths, I.R. and McCulloch, M.C. (1983) Nerve fibres in spinal cord impact injuries. *J. Neurol. Sci.*, 58: 335–349.

Hoke, A. and Silver, J. (1996) Proteoglycans and other repulsive molecules in glial boundaries during development and regeneration of the nervous system. *Prog. Brain Res.*, 108: 149–163.

Horner, P.J. and Gage, F.H. (2000) Regenerating the damaged central nervous system. *Nature*, 407: 963–970.

Horner, P.J., Power, A.E., Kempermann, G., Kuhn, H.G., Palmer, T.D., Winkler, J., Thal, L.J. and Gage, F.H. (2000) Proliferation and differentiation of progenitor cells throughout the intact adult rat spinal cord. *J. Neurosci.*, 20: 2218–2228.

Johansson, C.B., Momma, S., Clarke, D.L., Risling, M., Lendahl, U. and Frisen, J. (1999) Identification of a neural stem cell in the adult mammalian central nervous system. *Cell*, 96: 25–34.

Kalyani, A.J., Piper, D., Mujtaba, T., Lucero, M.T. and Rao, M.S. (1998) Spinal cord neuronal precursors generate multiple neuronal phenotypes in culture. *J. Neurosci.*, 18: 7856–7868.

Keirstead, H.S., Levine, J.M. and Blakemore, W.F. (1998) Response of the oligodendrocyte progenitor cell population (defined by NG2 labelling) to demyelination of the adult spinal cord. *Glia*, 22: 161–170.

Kojima, A. and Tator, C.H. (2000) Epidermal growth factor and fibroblast growth factor 2 cause proliferation of ependymal precursor cells in the adult rat spinal cord in vivo. *J. Neuropathol. Exp. Neurol.*, 59: 687–697.

Kondo, T. and Raff, M. (2000) Oligodendrocyte precursor cells reprogrammed to become multipotential CNS stem cells. *Science*, 289: 1754–1757.

Kuhn, H.G., Winkler, J., Kempermann, G., Thal, L.J. and Gage, F.H. (1997) Epidermal growth factor and fibroblast growth factor-2 have different effects on neural progenitors in the adult rat brain. *J. Neurosci.*, 17: 5820–5829.

Laywell, E.D., Rakic, P., Kukekov, V.G., Holland, E.C. and Steindler, D.A. (2000) Identification of a multipotent astrocytic stem cell in the immature and adult mouse brain. *Proc. Natl. Acad. Sci. USA*, 97: 13883–13888.

Lendahl, U., Zimmerman, L.B. and McKay, R.D. (1990) CNS stem cells express a new class of intermediate filament protein. *Cell*, 60: 585–595.

Lim, D.A., Tramontin, A.D., Trevejo, J.M., Herrera, D.G., Garcia-Verdugo, J.M. and Alvarez-Buylla, A. (2000) Noggin antagonizes BMP signaling to create a niche for adult neurogenesis. *Neuron*, 28: 713–726.

Lin, R.C., Matesic, D.F., Marvin, M., McKay, R.D. and Brustle, O. (1995) Re-expression of the intermediate filament nestin in reactive astrocytes. *Neurobiol. Dis.*, 2: 79–85.

Liu, R.H., Morassutti, D.J., Whittemore, S.R., Sosnowski, J.S. and Magnuson, D.S. (1999) Electrophysiological properties of mitogen-expanded adult rat spinal cord and subventricular zone neural precursor cells. *Exp. Neurol.*, 158: 143–154.

Liu, S., Qu, Y., Stewart, T.J., Howard, M.J., Chakrabortty, S., Holekamp, T.F. and McDonald, J.W. (2000) Embryonic stem cells differentiate into oligodendrocytes and myelinate in culture and after spinal cord transplantation. *Proc. Natl. Acad. Sci. USA*, 97: 6126–6131.

Liu, X.Z., Xu, X.M., Hu, R., Du, C., Zhang, S.X., McDonald, J.W., Dong, H.X., Wu, Y.J., Fan, G.S., Jacquin, M.F., Hsu, C.Y. and Choi, D.W. (1997) Neuronal and glial apoptosis after traumatic spinal cord injury. *J. Neurosci.*, 17: 5395–5406.

Liu, Y., Himes, B.T., Solowska, J., Moul, J., Chow, S.Y., Park, K.I., Tessler, A., Murray, M., Snyder, E.Y. and Fischer, I. (1999) Intraspinal delivery of neurotrophin-3 using neural stem cells genetically modified by recombinant retrovirus. *Exp. Neurol.*, 158: 9–26.

Luskin, M.B. (1993) Restricted proliferation and migration of postnatally generated neurons derived from the forebrain subventricular zone. *Neuron*, 11: 173–189.

Lyden, D., Young, A.Z., Zagzag, D., Yan, W., Gerald, W., O'Reilly, R., Bader, B.L., Hynes, R.O., Zhuang, Y., Manova, K. and Benezra, R. (1999) Id1 and Id3 are required for neurogenesis, angiogenesis and vascularization of tumour xenografts. *Nature*, 401: 670–677.

Magavi, S.S., Leavitt, B.R. and Macklis, J.D. (2000) Induction of neurogenesis in the neocortex of adult mice. *Nature*, 405: 951–955.

Mason, J.L., Suzuki, K., Chaplin, D.D. and Matsushima, G.K. (2001) Interleukin-1beta promotes repair of the CNS. *J. Neurosci.*, 21: 7046–7052.

Mayer-Proschel, M., Kalyani, A.J., Mujtaba, T. and Rao, M.S. (1997) Isolation of lineage-restricted neuronal precursors from multipotent neuroepithelial stem cells. *Neuron*, 19: 773–785.

McDonald, J.W., Liu, X.Z., Qu, Y., Liu, S., Mickey, S.K., Turetsky, D., Gottlieb, D.I. and Choi, D.W. (1999) Transplanted embryonic stem cells survive, differentiate and promote recovery in injured rat spinal cord. *Nat. Med.*, 5: 1410–1412.

McTigue, D.M., Horner, P.J., Stokes, B.T. and Gage, F.H. (1998) Neurotrophin-3 and brain derived neurotrophic factor induce oligodendrocyte proliferation and myelination of regenerating axons in the contused rat spinal cord. *J. Neurosci.*, 18: 5354–5365.

McTigue, D.M., Wei, P. and Stokes, B.T. (2001) Proliferation of NG2-positive cells and altered oligodendrocyte numbers in the contused rat spinal cord. *J. Neurosci.*, 21: 3392–3400.

Mezey, E., Chandross, K.J., Harta, G., Maki, R.A. and McKercher, S.R. (2000) Turning blood into brain: cells bearing neuronal antigens generated in vivo from bone marrow. *Science*, 290: 1779–1782.

Miyata, T., Maeda, T. and Lee, J.E. (1999) NeuroD is required

for differentiation of the granule cells in the cerebellum and hippocampus. *Genes Dev.*, 13: 1647–1652.

Momma, S., Johansson, C.B. and Frisen, J. (2000) Get to know your stem cells. *Curr. Opin. Neurobiol.*, 10: 45–49.

Moon, L.D., Brecknell, J.E., Franklin, R.J., Dunnett, S.B. and Fawcett, J.W. (2000) Robust regeneration of CNS axons through a track depleted of CNS glia. *Exp. Neurol.*, 161: 49–66.

Mujtaba, T., Mayer-Proschel, M. and Rao, M.S. (1998) A common neural progenitor for the CNS and PNS. *Dev. Biol.*, 200: 1–15.

Nakamura, Y., Sakakibara, S., Miyata, T., Ogawa, M., Shimazaki, T., Weiss, S., Kageyama, R. and Okano, H. (2000) The bHLH gene hes1 as a repressor of the neuronal commitment of CNS stem cells. *J. Neurosci.*, 20: 283–293.

Nakashima, K., Yanagisawa, M., Arakawa, H., Kimura, N., Hisatsune, T., Kawabata, M., Miyazono, K. and Taga, T. (1999) Synergistic signaling in fetal brain by STAT3–Smad1 complex bridged by p300. *Science*, 284: 479–482.

Nakashima, K., Takizawa, T., Ochiai, W., Yanagisawa, M., Hisatsune, T., Nakafuku, M., Miyazono, K., Kishimoto, T., Kageyama, R. and Taga, T. (2001) BMP2-mediated alteration in the developmental pathway of fetal mouse brain cells from neurogenesis to astrocytogenesis. *Proc. Natl. Acad. Sci. USA*, 98: 5868–5873.

Namiki, J. and Tator, C.H. (1999) Cell proliferation and nestin expression in the ependyma of the adult rat spinal cord after injury. *J. Neuropathol. Exp. Neurol.*, 58: 489–498.

Nishiyama, A., Lin, X.H., Giese, N., Heldin, C.H. and Stallcup, W.B. (1996) Co-localization of NG2 proteoglycan and PDGF alpha-receptor on O2A progenitor cells in the developing rat brain. *J. Neurosci. Res.*, 43: 299–314.

Ohtsuka, T., Sakamoto, M., Guillemot, F. and Kageyama, R. (2001) Roles of the basic helix–loop–helix genes Hes1 and Hes5 in expansion of neural stem cells of the developing brain. *J. Biol. Chem.*, 276: 30467–30474.

Olson, L. (1997) Regeneration in the adult central nervous system: experimental repair strategies. *Nat. Med.*, 3: 1329–1335.

Pagano, S.F., Impagnatiello, F., Girelli, M., Cova, L., Grioni, E., Onofri, M., Cavallaro, M., Etteri, S., Vitello, F., Giombini, S., Solero, C.L. and Parati, E.A. (2000) Isolation and characterization of neural stem cells from the adult human olfactory bulb. *Stem Cells*, 18: 295–300.

Palmer, T.D., Ray, J. and Gage, F.H. (1995) FGF-2-responsive neuronal progenitors reside in proliferative and quiescent regions of the adult rodent brain. *Mol. Cell. Neurosci.*, 6: 474–486.

Palmer, T.D., Markakis, E.A., Willhoite, A.R., Safar, F. and Gage, F.H. (1999) Fibroblast growth factor-2 activates a latent neurogenic program in neural stem cells from diverse regions of the adult CNS. *J. Neurosci.*, 19: 8487–8497.

Pencea, V., Bingaman, K.D., Wiegand, S.J. and Luskin, M.B. (2001) Infusion of brain-derived neurotrophic factor into the lateral ventricle of the adult rat leads to new neurons in the parenchyma of the striatum, septum, thalamus, and hypothalamus. *J. Neurosci.*, 21: 6706–6717.

Raineteau, O. and Schwab, M.E. (2001) Plasticity of motor systems after incomplete spinal cord injury. *Nat. Rev. Neurosci.*, 2: 263–273.

Rao, M.S., Noble, M. and Mayer-Proschel, M. (1998) A tripotential glial precursor cell is present in the developing spinal cord. *Proc. Natl. Acad. Sci. USA*, 95: 3996–4001.

Ray, J. and Gage, F.H. (1994) Spinal cord neuroblasts proliferate in response to basic fibroblast growth factor. *J. Neurosci.*, 14: 3548–3564.

Reynolds, B.A. and Weiss, S. (1992) Generation of neurons and astrocytes from isolated cells of the adult mammalian central nervous system. *Science*, 255: 1707–1710.

Ribotta, M.G., Provencher, J., Feraboli-Lohnherr, D., Rossignol, S., Privat, A. and Orsal, D. (2000) Activation of locomotion in adult chronic spinal rats is achieved by transplantation of embryonic raphe cells reinnervating a precise lumbar level. *J. Neurosci.*, 20: 5144–5152.

Rogister, B., Ben Hur, T. and Dubois-Dalcq, M. (1999) From neural stem cells to myelinating oligodendrocytes. *Mol. Cell. Neurosci.*, 14: 287–300.

Rowitch, D.H., Jacques, B., Lee, S.M., Flax, J.D., Snyder, E.Y. and McMahon, A.P. (1999) Sonic hedgehog regulates proliferation and inhibits differentiation of CNS precursor cells. *J. Neurosci.*, 19: 8954–8965.

Parent, J.M., Yu, T.W., Leibowitz, R.T., Geschwind, D.H., Sloviter, R.S. and Lowenstein, D.H. (1997) Dentate granule cell neurogenesis is increased by seizures and contributes to aberrant network reorganization in the adult rat hippocampus. *J. Neurosci.*, 17: 3727–3738.

Scharfman, H.E., Goodman, J.H. and Sollas, A.L. (2000) Granule-like neurons at the hilar/CA3 border after status epilepticus and their synchrony with area CA3 pyramidal cells: functional implications of seizure-induced neurogenesis. *J. Neurosci.*, 20: 6144–6158.

Shihabuddin, L.S., Ray, J. and Gage, F.H. (1997) FGF-2 is sufficient to isolate progenitors found in the adult mammalian spinal cord. *Exp. Neurol.*, 148: 577–586.

Shihabuddin, L.S., Horner, P.J., Ray, J. and Gage, F.H. (2000) Adult spinal cord stem cells generate neurons after transplantation in the adult dentate gyrus. *J. Neurosci.*, 20: 8727–8735.

Shingo, T., Sorokan, S.T., Shimazaki, T. and Weiss, S. (2001) Erythropoietin regulates the in vitro and in vivo production of neuronal progenitors by mammalian forebrain neural stem cells. *J. Neurosci.*, 21: 9733–9743.

Svendsen, C.N., Bhattacharyya, A. and Tai, Y.T. (2001) Neurons from stem cells: preventing an identity crisis. *Nat. Rev. Neurosci.*, 2: 831–834.

Tanabe, Y. and Jessell, T.M. (1996) Diversity and pattern in the developing spinal cord. *Science*, 274: 1115–1123.

Tang, D.G., Tokumoto, Y.M., Apperly, J.A., Lloyd, A.C. and Raff, M.C. (2001) Lack of replicative senescence in cultured rat oligodendrocyte precursor cells. *Science*, 291: 868–871.

Tanigaki, K., Nogaki, F., Takahashi, J., Tashiro, K., Kurooka, H. and Honjo, T. (2001) Notch1 and Notch3 instructively restrict bFGF-responsive multipotent neural progenitor cells to an astroglial fate. *Neuron*, 29: 45–55.

Tator, C.H. (1998) Biology of neurological recovery and functional restoration after spinal cord injury. *Neurosurgery*, 42: 696–707.

Temple, S. (2001) The development of neural stem cells. *Nature*, 414: 112–117.

Toma, J.G., Akhavan, M., Fernandes, K.J., Barnabe-Heider, F., Sadikot, A., Kaplan, D.R. and Miller, F.D. (2001) Isolation of multipotent adult stem cells from the dermis of mammalian skin. *Nat. Cell Biol.*, 3: 778–784.

Torii, M., Matsuzaki, F., Osumi, N., Kaibuchi, K., Nakamura, S., Casarosa, S., Guillemot, F. and Nakafuku, M. (1999) Transcription factors Mash-1 and Prox-1 delineate early steps in differentiation of neural stem cells in the developing central nervous system. *Development*, 126: 443–456.

Tropepe, V., Craig, C.G., Morshead, C.M. and van der Kooy, D. (1997) Transforming growth factor-alpha null and senescent mice show decreased neural progenitor cell proliferation in the forebrain subependyma. *J. Neurosci.*, 17: 7850–7859.

Tropepe, V., Sibilia, M., Ciruna, B.G., Rossant, J., Wagner, E.F. and van der Kooy, D. (1999) Distinct neural stem cells proliferate in response to EGF and FGF in the developing mouse telencephalon. *Dev. Biol.*, 208: 166–188.

Tropepe, V., Coles, B.L., Chiasson, B.J., Horsford, D.J., Elia, A.J., McInnes, R.R. and van der Kooy, D. (2000) Retinal stem cells in the adult mammalian eye. *Science*, 287: 2032–2036.

Uchida, N., Buck, D.W., He, D., Reitsma, M.J., Masek, M., Phan, T.V., Tsukamoto, A.S., Gage, F.H. and Weissman, I.L. (2000) Direct isolation of human central nervous system stem cells. *Proc. Natl. Acad. Sci. USA*, 97: 14720–14725.

Van der Kooy, D. and Weiss, S. (2000) Why stem cells? *Science*, 25: 1439–1441.

Vicario-Abejon, C., Johe, K.K., Hazel, T.G., Collazo, D. and McKay, R.D. (1995) Functions of basic fibroblast growth factor and neurotrophins in the differentiation of hippocampal neurons. *Neuron*, 15: 105–114.

Weiss, S., Dunne, C., Hewson, J., Wohl, C., Wheatley, M., Peterson, A.C. and Reynolds, B.A. (1996) Multipotent CNS stem cells are present in the adult mammalian spinal cord. *J. Neurosci.*, 16: 7599–7609.

Wichterle, H., Garcia-Verdugo, J.M., Herrera, D.G. and Alvarez-Buylla, A. (1999) Young neurons from medial ganglionic eminence disperse in adult and embryonic brain. *Nat. Neurosci.*, 2: 461–466.

Yamamoto, S.S., Yamamoto, N., Kitamura, T., Nakamura, K. and Nakafuku, M. (2001a) Proliferation of parenchymal neural progenitors in response to injury in the adult rat spinal cord. *Exp. Neurol.*, 172: 115–127.

Yamamoto, S.S., Nagao, M., Sugimori, M., Kosako, H., Nakatomi, H., Yamamoto, N., Takebayashi, H., Nabeshima, Y.Y., Kitamura, T., Weinmaster, G., Nakamura, K. and Nakafuku, M. (2001b) Transcription factor expression and notch-dependent regulation of neural progenitors in the adult rat spinal cord. *J. Neurosci.*, 21: 9814–9823.

Yang, H., Mujtaba, T., Venkatraman, G., Wu, Y.Y., Rao, M.S. and Luskin, M.B. (2000) Region-specific differentiation of neural tube-derived neuronal restricted progenitor cells after heterotopic transplantation. *Proc. Natl. Acad. Sci. USA*, 97: 13366–13371.

Yoshimura, S., Takagi, Y., Harada, J., Teramoto, T., Thomas, S.S., Waeber, C., Bakowska, J.C., Breakefield, X.O. and Moskowitz, M.A. (2001) FGF-2 regulation of neurogenesis in adult hippocampus after brain injury. *Proc. Natl. Acad. Sci. USA*, 98: 5874–5879.

Zappone, M.V., Galli, R., Catena, R., Meani, N., De Biasi, S., Mattei, E., Tiveron, C., Vescovi, A.L., Lovell-Badge, R., Ottolenghi, S. and Nicolis, S.K. (2000) Sox2 regulatory sequences direct expression of a (beta)-geo transgene to telencephalic neural stem cells and precursors of the mouse embryo, revealing regionalization of gene expression in CNS stem cells. *Development*, 127: 2367–2382.

Zhang, S.C., Ge, B. and Duncan, I.D. (1999) Adult brain retains the potential to generate oligodendroglial progenitors with extensive myelination capacity. *Proc. Natl. Acad. Sci. USA*, 96: 4089–4094.

Zhou, Q., Wang, S. and Anderson, D.J. (2000) Identification of a novel family of oligodendrocyte lineage-specific basic helix–loop–helix transcription factors. *Neuron*, 25: 331–343.

Zhu, G., Mehler, M.F., Mabie, P.C. and Kessler, J.A. (2000) Developmental changes in neural progenitor cell lineage commitment do not depend on epidermal growth factor receptor signaling. *J. Neurosci. Res.*, 59: 312–320.

Zigova, T., Pencea, V., Wiegand, S.J. and Luskin, M.B. (1998) Intraventricular administration of BDNF increases the number of newly generated neurons in the adult olfactory bulb. *Mol. Cell. Neurosci.*, 11: 234–245.

L. McKerracher, G. Doucet and S. Rossignol (Eds.)
Progress in Brain Research, Vol. 137
© 2002 Elsevier Science B.V. All rights reserved

CHAPTER 21

Repairing the damaged spinal cord: a summary of our early success with embryonic stem cell transplantation and remyelination

John W. McDonald * and Michael J. Howard

Center for the Study of Nervous System Injury, Spinal Cord Injury Restorative Treatment and Research Program, and Department of Neurology, Washington University School of Medicine, Campus Box 8111, 660 S. Euclid Avenue, St. Louis, MO 63110, USA

Abstract: Demyelination contributes to the loss of function consequent to central nervous system (CNS) injury. Optimizing remyelination through transplantation of myelin-producing cells may offer a pragmatic approach to restoring meaningful neurological function. An unlimited source of cells suitable for such transplantation therapy can be derived from embryonic stem (ES) cells, which are both pluripotent and genetically flexible. Here we review work from our group showing that neural precursor cells can be derived from ES cells and that transplantation of these cells into the injured spinal cord leads to some recovery of function. We have further examined and optimized methods for enriching oligodendrocyte differentiation from ES cells. ES cell-derived oligodendrocytes are capable of rapid differentiation and myelination in mixed neuron/glia cultures. When transplanted into the injured spinal cord of adult rodents, the neural-induced precursor cells are capable of differentiating into oligodendrocytes and myelinating host axons. The role of myelination and remyelination will be discussed in the context of regeneration strategies.

Introduction

Spinal cord injury (SCI) can be a catastrophic event resulting in life-long disability. Traumatic SCI most commonly occurs as a result of motor vehicle accidents (for review see McDonald et al., 1999a; McDonald and Sadowsky, 2002). Injury is seldom due to transection of the spinal cord. Rather, it is usually displaced fragments of fractured vertebrae and soft tissue ligaments that impact the delicate spinal cord. This initial mechanical trauma initiates a cascade of

secondary injury processes, which markedly extends the development of the injury over hours to days. The majority of injury to both neurons and glia is complete within 24 h, but a more delayed protracted wave of oligodendrocyte cell death occurs for several weeks in degenerating white matter tracts. When the injury is complete, the spinal cord is left in a complex state of disarray. At the injury level, a variable donut-shaped rim of white matter typically remains surrounding a fluid filled cyst. Variable loss of neurons and oligodendrocytes with segmental demyelination occurs for several segments above and below the cyst. Only one pharmacological treatment for acute SCI is FDA approved (methylprednisolone), and it must be administered in the first 8 h following injury (for review: Bracken et al., 1990, 1997; McDonald and Sadowsky, 2002). In contrast, there are no FDA approved therapies available to promote regeneration of the injured spinal cord.

* Correspondence to: J. McDonald, Center for the Study of Nervous System Injury, Spinal Cord Injury Restorative Treatment and Research Program, and Department of Neurology, Washington University School of Medicine, Campus Box 8111, 660 S. Euclid Avenue, St. Louis, MO 63110, USA. Tel.: +1-314-454-7510; Fax: +1-314-454-5300; E-mail: mcdonald@neuro.wustl.edu

Repair of the damaged spinal cord is a challenging problem and this complex task will require multi-stage interventions spaced temporally. One early clinical target proving to be a pragmatic approach to SCI repair is remyelination (Waxman, 1992; Bunge et al., 1993; McDonald and Sadowsky, 2002). Demyelination is an important contributor to disability after SCI because it renders axons that remain anatomically intact physiologically nonfunctional due to conduction block at the level of injury. Since each oligodendrocyte myelinates 10–20 different axons, loss of a single oligodendrocyte can cause dysfunction in many different axons. Studies in animal models strongly suggest that dysmyelination and demyelination contribute to neurological dysfunction, but similar studies in humans have not been completed. Such studies require detailed EM work, not possible in most post-mortem human tissues (Bunge et al., 1993). However, studies in non-human primates should be considered and would be a great contribution to the field. The natural reparative response to CNS injury is inadequate for any number of reasons and therefore transplantation of replacement oligodendrocytes is a pragmatic approach to the problem. In the remainder of this chapter we will describe our early success with generating oligodendrocyte precursor cells from embryonic stem (ES) cells and our attempts to remyelinate the injured spinal cord.

Spinal cord repair in perspective

Long-regarded as impossible, spinal-cord repair may soon become an attainable goal of clinical therapeutics. Important concepts to consider in treatment of the injured spinal cord include the following: (1) a complete cure is not required, (2) the goal should be partial repair, (3) functional goal priorities are not walking but restoration of important, limited functions that alter quality of life, and (4) some repair strategies will predictably be more easy to accomplish than others (McDonald and Sadowsky, 2002).

A cure is not required and partial repair should be the goal. Limited repair of the damaged spinal cord can produce disproportionate return of function. In animal models, approximately 10% of the functional connections across the lesion are required to support ambulation (Blight, 1983). Therapeutic goals should

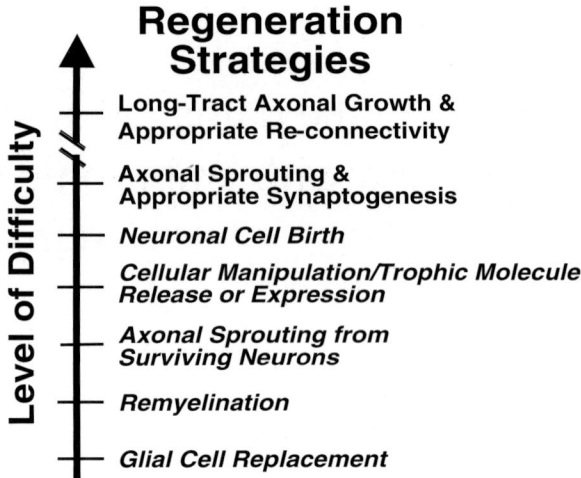

Fig. 1. Hierarchy of scientific feasibility for regenerative strategies. The most difficult goal, recapitulation of long white matter tracts, has not been accomplished in any animal model. However, replacement of glial cells through transplantation or endogenous cell birth has been possible for several years. In fact, it appears that glial cell birth occurs relatively commonly after SCI and inappropriate development may actually need to be limited. Limited remyelination of intact axons by transplanted or endogenous glia has already been demonstrated in animal models and may be the easiest way to achieve meaningful functional recovery. Axons truncated by injury can sprout and extend for short distances, but sprouting occurs in limited areas and has little effect on long-tract-mediated function. Genetic and cellular methods for inducing cells to express and release factors to support cell survival, sprouting and function are currently under development. A more difficult task, but one that is receiving growing attention, is replacement of lost cells, including neurons, from endogenous progenitor cells. Adapted and reprinted from McDonald and Sadowsky, 2002, with permission.

focus on step-wise restoration of function (McDonald and Sadowsky, 2002). The goals should not simply be limited to walking, but should include return of important but limited functions, such as recovery of bowel and bladder control, improved pulmonary function, or improved movement of a limb or a hand. Some reparative strategies will be more feasible than others and Fig. 1 estimates the level of difficulty in achieving each of the current major therapeutic strategies for repair.

Recovery in the damaged spinal cord is hindered by the limited ability of the vertebrate CNS to replace lost cells, repair damaged myelin, regenerate long tract axons and reestablish functional neural connections. Endogenous neural progenitor cells are susceptible to many of the same injury processes as mature cells and the response of endogenous progenitor cells to nervous system injury is inadequate to replace loss tissue. Therefore, an obvious approach for cellular replacement has been transplantation.

Many sources of transplantable cells have been used for the purpose of SCI repair. Mature CNS cells are post-mitotic and do not divide in culture, making it difficult to amass large numbers of cells for transplantation. Primary CNS cells can be induced to re-enter the mitotic cycle by transformation with genes from tumor cells, but transplanting cells containing cancer genes is not ideal. Fetal CNS cells can, on the other hand, be expanded in culture, but the ethical considerations of using fetal tissue in research or clinical trials make the widespread use of fetal cells impractical. A third alternative is to use precursor cells that are present in the mature CNS. The primary drawback to using these cells is that they are present in very small numbers in the adult CNS and methods for large-scale production have not been developed. Recently, a novel source of replenishable pluripotent cells for transplantation has become available through the use of ES cells (for review see McDonald, 2001). This chapter will review work from our group at Washington University developing ES cells as a therapeutic approach to repair of the injured spinal cord.

Embryonic stem cells

ES cells provide a novel source of renewable cells for cellular transplantation. Several unique features of ES cells make them excellent candidates for transplantation. ES cells can replicate indefinitely without aging. They are pluripotent and can give rise to all the cells of the body. ES cells are genetically normal and are also highly genetically manipulable and double allele knock-ins and knock-outs are possible in single cells (for review see McDonald, 2001). The scientific power of ES cells is just beginning to be harnessed at the individual cell level. This potential of ES cells can be realized based on the role of ES cells in the generation of transgenic animals and the impact of transgenic animal technology in the neurosciences.

ES cells are commonly derived through in vitro fertilization. Fertilized eggs are grown to the pre-implantation blastocysts stage. Cells of the inner cell mass can be selectively isolated using immunodissection. Two decades of work have defined methods useful for indefinitely propagating ES cells in an undifferentiated state (for review see McDonald, 2001). ES cells have been successfully derived from multiple vertebrate species, including mice and humans. ES cells have recently been successfully generated by somatic nuclear transfer allowing the therapeutic option for self-transplantation (Kawase et al., 2000; Wakayama et al., 2001).

Differentiation of embryonic stem cells

Differentiation of ES cells is typically initiated by withdrawal of leukemia inhibitory factor (LIF). Our group has had the most experience with a differentiation protocol utilizing exposure to retinoic acid (McDonald, 2001). The $4^-/4^+$ retinoic acid embryoid body protocol for differentiation of ES cells was developed by our colleague, David Gottlieb, and is outlined in Fig. 2 (Bain et al., 1995). Briefly, induction is initiated by withdrawal of LIF and plating of dissociated ES cells in a non-adhesive petri dish. This procedure promotes cell aggregation and formation of floating clumps of cells, termed embryoid bodies. During the last 4 days of the 8-day protocol, 500 nM retinoic acid is added to direct further differentiation down the neural lineage. At the end of this protocol, the majority of the cells contained in the embryoid body are nestin-positive cells representative of the tri-potential (neuron/astrocyte/oligodendrocyte) neural progenitor (Liu et al., 2000). It is this stage of ES cell-derived neural progenitor cells that we have used for culture or transplantation. $4^-/4^+$ embryoid bodies can be dissociated and grown under standard culture conditions, and we have developed conditions that support growth of mixed cultures containing neurons, astrocytes (type I and type II), and oligodendrocytes (Liu et al., 2000). Such ES cell-derived neuronal/glial cultures can be grown that are largely indistinguishable from primary cultures (Fig. 3). Work from our laboratory has shown that multiple phenotypes of neurons can be produced including GABA-, glutamate-, ChAT-, DBH-, CGRP-, Peripherin-, 5-HT-, TH-, and Met-Enk-immunoreactive neuron-like cells (unpublished observations, J.W. McDonald et al.).

In Vitro Neural Differentiation of Embryonic Stem Cells

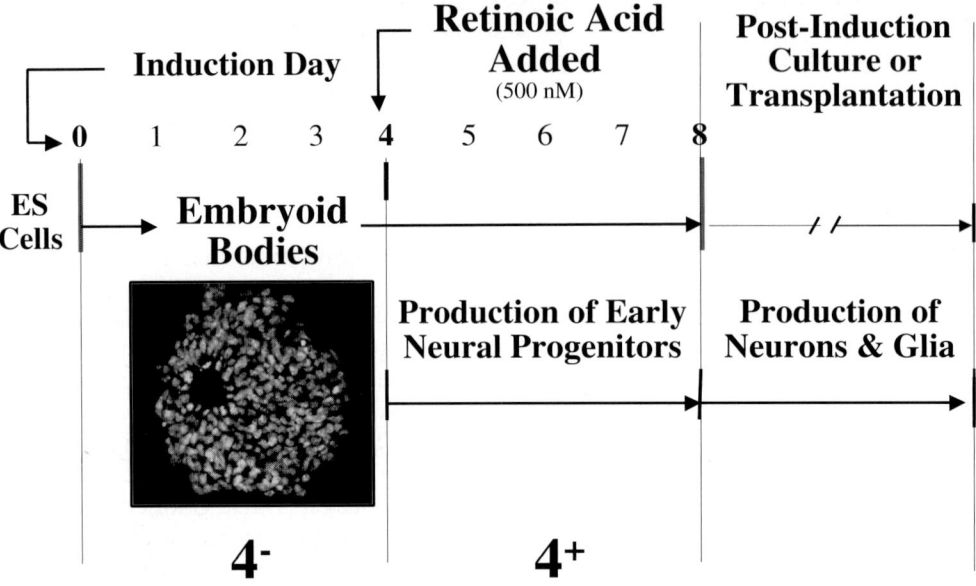

Fig. 2. Schematic depiction of ES cell differentiation. The method of differentiation used in our studies is outlined as originally developed by Bain et al. (1995). ES cells are grown in clusters called embryoid bodies (cell cluster, inset). After 4 days in culture, cells are exposed to retinoic acid for 4 days. This process, termed the $4^-/4^+$ protocol, instructs the ES cells to become neural lineage cells. At the $4^-/4^+$ stage, cells can be either plated in culture or transplanted. Reprinted from McDonald, 2001, with permission.

Myelination and oligodendrocytes derived from embryonic stem cells

A major focus of our laboratory has been a study of myelination and, in particular, derivation of oligodendrocytes from ES cells. We have been using conditions supportive of myelination in previous studies of primary cultures to demonstrate that ES-derived oligodendrocytes can myelinate axons in vitro (Liu et al., 2000). $4^-/4^+$ embryoid bodies were dissociated and grown in SATO defined medium (DMEM plus BSA, progesterone, putrescine, thyroxine, triiodothyronine, apo-transferrin and sodium selenite; for details see Liu et al., 2000) containing 5% horse serum and 5% fetal calf serum for 9 days. Under these conditions, a mixed culture system is generated in which oligodendrocytes and neurons grow on top of an astrocyte monolayer. With these methods, contaminating non-neuronal cells are much less problematic than in primary cultures where fibroblast and macrophage infiltration is prevalent. Large numbers of oligodendrocytes can be observed in these mixed cultures derived from ES cells. The ES cell-derived oligodendrocytes are morphologically similar to cultured primary oligodendrocytes (Fig. 4). In contrast to primary cultures, however, it appears that myelination is more widespread and occurs more rapidly in the ES cell-derived cultures (Liu et al., 2000). Individual ES cell-derived oligodendrocytes can be observed to extend, wrap and myelinate multiple segments of single axons and multiple individual axons. We have used immunohistochemistry, scanning and transmission electron microscopy to demonstrate early forms of axonal myelination achieved within 9 days of culture.

We have developed additional methods to simply and rapidly enrich for oligodendrocytes (Liu et al., 2000). This procedure involves a subsequent culturing step, which leads to development of an oligodendrocyte-enriched stage termed an oligo-

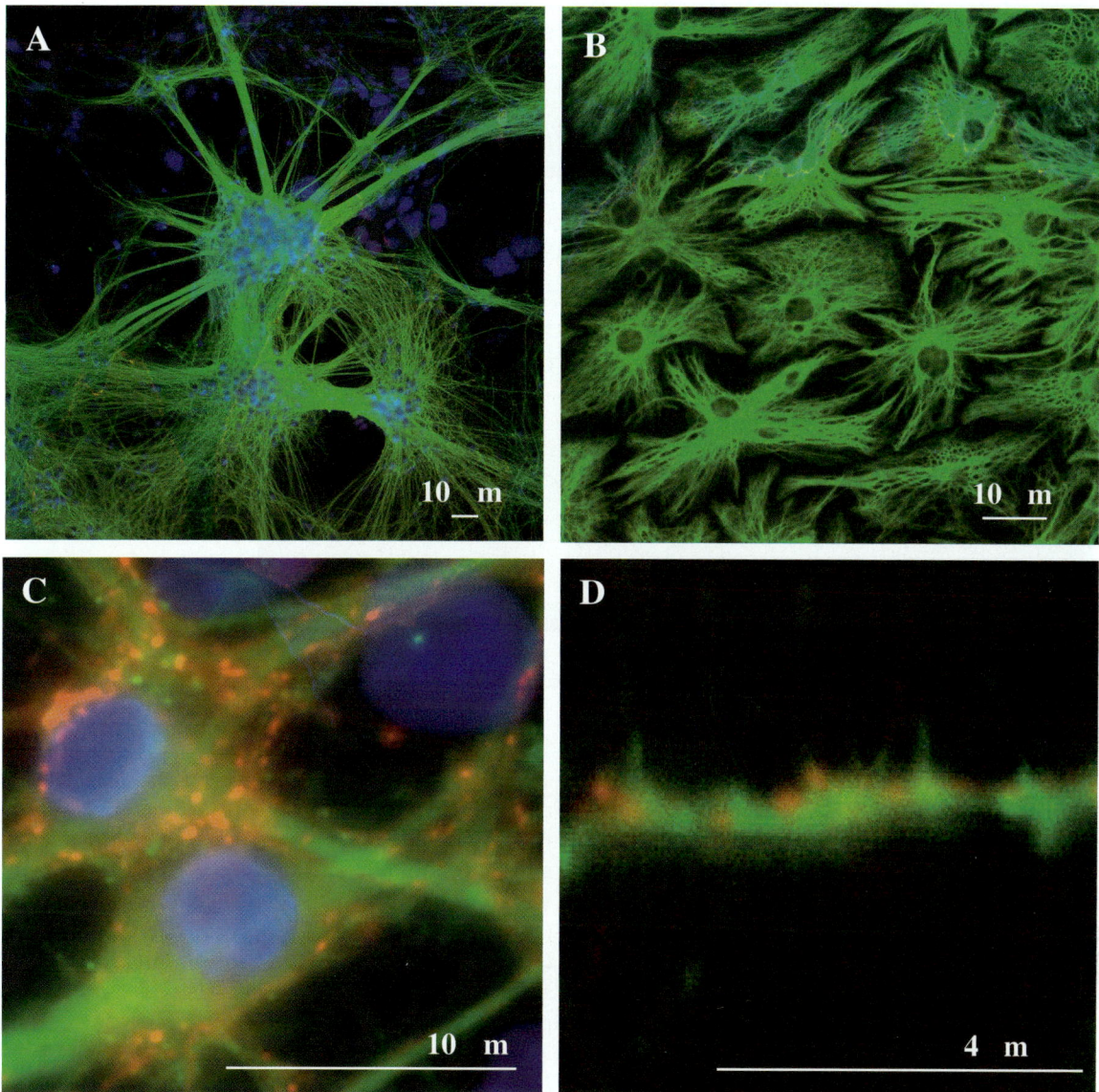

Fig. 3. ES cell-derived neuronal cultures are indistinguishable from cultures of primary cells derived from embryos. (A) Mixed cultures of neuronal networks growing atop an astrocyte monolayer (DIV 9). Green = Tuj1, blue = Hoechst nuclear DNA staining (B) Astrocyte monolayer immunolabeled with anti-GFAP (green). (C,D) Anti-synaptophysin (C) and anti-SV2 (D) immunoreactivity suggests that large numbers of synapses are present in DIV 9 cultures derived from $4^-/4^+$ EBs, and this is consistent with electrophysiological studies previously reported in similar cultures (Bain et al., 1995). In panels C–D, red = synaptophysin/SV2, green = MAP-2, blue = Hoechst nuclear staining.

sphere. Briefly, $4^-/4^+$ embryoid bodies are dissociated and replated in non-adhesive petri dishes containing serum-free SATO medium and bFGF. Under these conditions, floating balls of cells are formed that contain some Nestin+ precursors and later-staged neural stem cells, including a large population of glial progenitor cells. Using this method we have demonstrated that cultures highly enriched for oligodendrocytes (greater than 90% oligodendrocytes) can be easily created. We have used both the

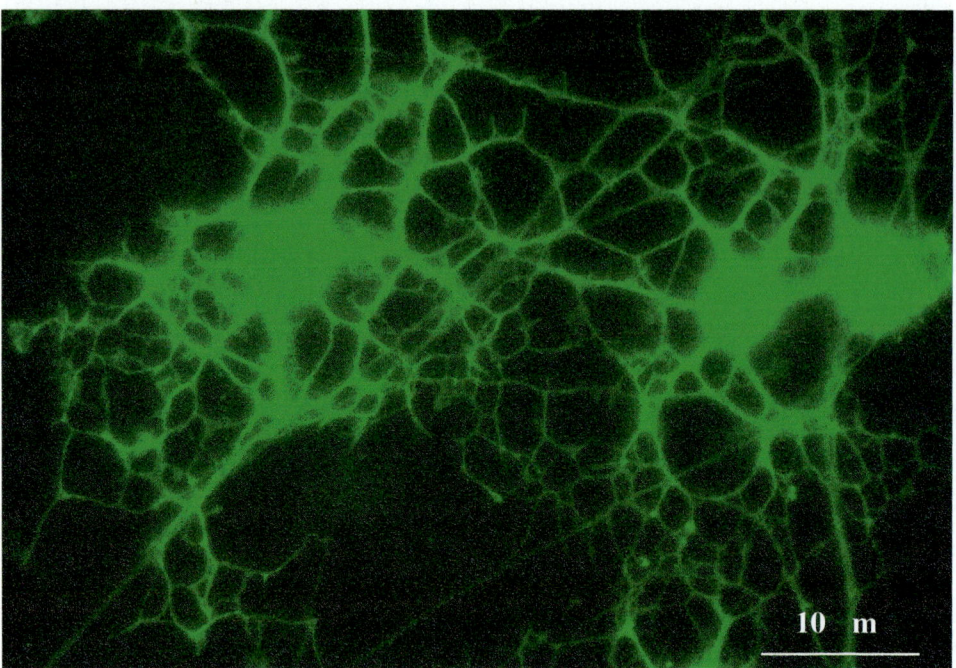

Fig. 4. Oligodendrocytes derived from ES cells are morphologically similar in culture to primary oligodendrocytes harvested from postnatal brain. Shown are two mature ES cell-derived oligodendrocytes growing on top of an astrocyte monolayer. Green immunolabel is for O-1, a marker of mature oligodendrocytes.

$4^-/4^+$ embryoid body and oligospheres to evaluate the role of ES cell-derived neural precursors in repair of the damaged spinal cord following transplantation.

The NYU SCI contusion weight drop injury model was used to evaluate transplantation of $4^-/4^+$ stage ES cell progenitors into injured spinal cord (Gruner, 1992). We chose to transplant 9 days after injury into the forming cyst of female rats subjected to a 25 mm weight drop SCI at T_{10} (McDonald et al., 1999b). This interval was chosen for the following reasons: (1) to avoid potential neuroprotective roles that accompany and complicate acute transplantation, (2) to allow assessment of regeneration, (3) to reduce transplant cell death (the inflammatory cascade is attenuated by 9 days and the blood–brain barrier is mostly intact (Popovich et al., 1996, 1997), (4) to promote regeneration potential of the transplanted ES cells [neurotrophic factor expression is enhanced during the second week after SCI, (McDonald et al., 1999b; Dougherty et al., 2000; Liebl et al., 2001)], and (5) behavioral improvements in locomotion in adult models of SCI had not been demonstrated when the treatment intervention was delayed more than 24 h after injury. Approximately 1 million $4^-/4^+$ stage ES cell progenitors were transplanted in a 5 μl volume directly into the cord cyst. Behavior was assessed using the BBB locomotor rating scale (Basso et al., 1995). Groups of sham transplanted (vehicle culture medium) and ES cell transplanted animals were sacrificed at 2 and 5 weeks after transplantation. Substantial cell death occurs in the first 72 h after transplantation (M.J. Howard and J.W. McDonald, unpublished observations). Histological analysis indicated that this was largely apoptosis, although a great amount of necrosis may occur immediately after injection if the cells are not properly prepared for transplantation. Despite this early death, the remaining ES cell-derived progenitors continued to divide (see below). Histological analysis at 2 weeks revealed extensive growth of ES cells within the injury cavity and long-distance migration, with cells found more than 1 cm from the edge of the cyst (McDonald et al., 1999b). Of the identifiable ES cells, the majority differentiated into oligodendrocytes (60%) followed by astrocytes (30%) and neu-

TABLE I

Types of markers that can be used to identify transplanted ES cells

Marker class	Examples
Genetic	LacZ [a], GFP [b], YFP [c]
Species-specific antibodies	Mouse specific-M2 [d], M6 (EMA) [e], Thy 1.2 [f]
DNA	Y chromosome in situ hybridization [g]
Cell pre-labeling	Paramagnetic markers [h] Cell tracker orange [i] BrdU [j] Hoechst 33342 [k]

Note: male mouse ES cells were transplanted into female rats.
[a] Friedrich and Soriano, 1991. [b] Green fluorescent protein (Hadjantonakis et al., 1998). [c] Yellow fluorescent protein (Hadjantonakis and Nagy, 2000). [d] Lagenaur and Schachner, 1981. [e] Baumrind et al., 1992. [f] Deacon et al., 1998. [g] Wu and Keating, 1993. [h] Bulte et al., 1999. [i] West et al., 2001. [j] Gage et al., 1995. [k] Baron-Van Evercooren et al., 1991.

rons (<10%) (McDonald et al., 1999b). The majority of ES cells distant from the site of transplantation expressed oligodendrocyte phenotypes. ES cell-derived neuron-like cells were evident with long processes that extended beyond the lesion cavity. Overall there was less reactive inflammation in groups receiving ES cell transplantation as measured with GFAP and OX-42 (macrophage marker) immunoreactivity (unpublished observations, J.W. McDonald et al.). Cell counts reveal a greater number of ES cell-derived cells than was originally transplanted, suggesting that the transplanted ES cell-derived progenitors had the capacity to divide. This has been confirmed by co-localization of markers of cellular division with the transplanted ES cells. No abnormal tissue formation has been observed.

One of the limitations in transplant biology is the difficulty of clearly identifying transplanted cells. We used an array of markers to ensure proper identification of transplanted cells and these include the types of markers listed in Table I. No one marker is sufficient, each has its pros and cons, and triple labeling is required for accurate identification; co-localization of the nucleus (e.g. Hoechst), marker of ES cell identity (Table I), and display of the appropriate phenotype (e.g. a neuron must have appropriate structure with processes, a small nucleus, and the immunomarker correctly located in the cell).

By 5 weeks after transplantation, the nuclear density at the site of transplant was reduced, but the extracellular space was filled with extracellular matrix (McDonald et al., 1999b). The extracellular matrix was primarily comprised of laminin and fibronectin, but little chondroitin sulfates were present (unpublished observations, J.W. McDonald). The role of extracellular matrix in survival and migration of transplanted cells is currently being evaluated.

A consistent behavioral improvement was observed in groups receiving ES cell transplantation compared to vehicle medium or adult mouse cortical cell transplantation. Open field volitional locomotion was assessed using the BBB locomotor rating scale (McDonald et al., 1999b). Animals in the control groups demonstrated characteristic spontaneous recovery that plateaued at a BBB score of 8 by 3 weeks following injury. In contrast, animals that received ES cell transplantation demonstrated an average plateau BBB score of 10 (Fig. 5). Although numerically small, this two-point difference represents the difference between weight bearing walking and no weight bearing walking (examples are available on our website: http://www.neuro.wustl.edu/sci). When placed in a glass cylinder, animals that received ES cell transplantation, but not vehicle medium, were capable of rearing and supporting their full weight on their hindlimbs (forelimbs on glass cylinder). Forelimb–hindlimb coordination could not be conclusively demonstrated using the BBB locomotor scale.

We have also examined transplantation into the spinal cord dorsal columns 3 days after chemical demyelination (Liu et al., 2000). $4^-/4^+$ stage ES cells were transplanted and animals examined 7 days later. In contrast to transplantation into the contusion injured spinal cord, preferential differentiation of ES cells into oligodendrocytes was observed; little astrocyte or neuronal immunoreactivity was observed. One possible interpretation of the preferential differentiation is that early $4^-/4^+$ stage ES cells use cues in the injured nervous system to direct their differentiation. Ultrastructural examination using transmission electron microscopy demonstrated early forms of myelin derived from ES cells (Liu et al., 2000).

The capacity of ES cells to myelinate was studied in more detail using the shiverer mouse, a mouse strain that lacks the ability to make myelin basic pro-

306

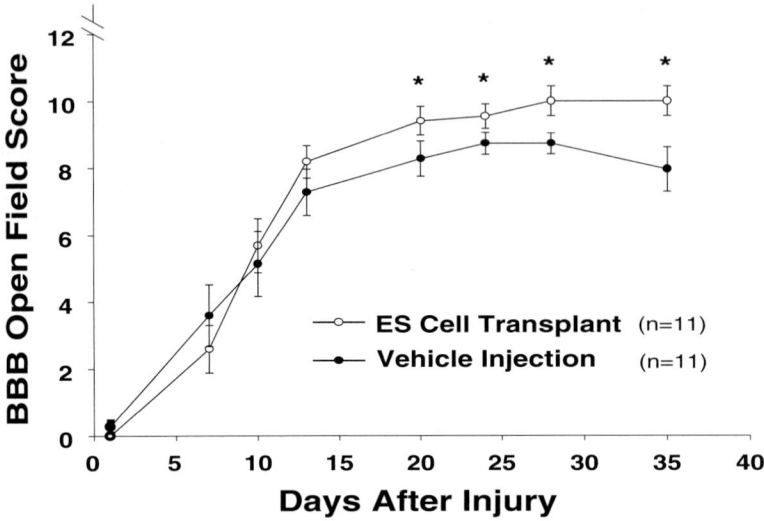

Fig. 5. Transplantation of $4^-/4^+$ ES cells facilitates behavioral recovery after spinal cord contusion injury. Open circles, ES cell transplant group; closed diamonds, vehicle treated group ($n = 11$ per group, mean $\pm$ SEM). * Difference at $P < 0.05$ vs. control at same time point (repeated measures ANOVA with Tukey's test).

tein (MBP), an integral component of myelin (Liu et al., 2000). This makes identification of ES cell-derived myelin simple, since anti-MBP immunoreactivity can be used as an accurate index of transplant-derived myelin. One month after transplantation, MBP immunoreactivity could be observed several millimeters from the transplant site. ES cell-derived oligodendrocytes could be observed that extended processes that appeared to wrap host axons. Ultrastructural examination using transmission EM demonstrated early forms of compact myelin derived from ES cells. The shiverer mice demonstrate a characteristic whole body shiver-like behavior that is highly variable and context dependent. We examined behavior using a sensitive 3-dimensional video-based system, tracking a single point on the mid back and analyzing the frequency and magnitude of the tremor. Extensive intra- and inter-animal variability in shivering was observed and it was concluded that differences in shivering could not accurately be used to assess transplant efficacy.

Mechanism of transplant-associated improvement in locomotor function

These initial studies in the contusion injury model were not designed to test specific mechanisms and currently our data cannot conclude causality based on any one mechanism or set of mechanisms. Based on the preponderance of oligodendrocyte differentiation, their ability to myelinate in vitro and in vivo, the rapid return of function (over 3 weeks) and the fact that the 25 mm weight drop injury spares only a small rim of white matter at the injury level, we are setting out to test the hypothesis that ES cell differentiation into oligodendrocytes and myelination may, in part, be related to recovery. However, multiple mechanisms likely account for the behavior recovery and our data do not distinguish among these possibilities. Determining causality is a problem in the entire field of SCI and at best the field has relied on correlations of anatomical findings with behavior. It has not been possible to more conclusively test hypotheses in vivo. ES cells may provide a unique approach to go one step further. Loss of the recovered function with selective ablation or reduction of function of the transplanted ES cells would provide a better level of proof. The genetic flexibility of ES cells may provide the tools to selectively kill or inactivate only a subset of the transplanted ES cell-derived cells. Conditional expression of sensitivity genes (e.g. thymidine kinase) that make only the ES cell-derived cells vulnerable to agent-induced death would allow proof of principle (see McDonald, 2001). For example, if myelin-producing ES cell-derived oligodendrocytes could be selectively killed by treating an animal with gancyclovir, or inactivated by overexpressing the MBP antisense, then loss of the recovered behavior would provide stronger evidence that myelination was a contributing mechanism. In contrast, if the loss of the cells did not alter behavior, then it would be unlikely that ES cell myelination played a substantial mechanistic role. Our group is working towards such experiments.

Summary, future directions and questions

Our early studies demonstrate that ES cell transplantation is feasible in the injured adult CNS. These studies indicate that transplanted ES cell-derived neural progenitors (1) survive, migrate and differentiate into the three main types of CNS cells, neurons, astrocytes, and oligodendrocytes, (2) migrate substantial distances in the injured adult spinal cord, (3) preferentially differentiate based on cues in their environment, (4) continue to divide in the host cord, (5) reduce the cellular inflammatory reaction, and (6) improve recovery of volitional locomotion even when transplanted 9 days after injury. It is also clear from this work that the injured adult spinal cord is able to support neurogenesis. The neuron-like cells observed after transplantation had to largely be derived from ES cell-derived progenitors. Few differentiated neural cells are observed in the $4^-/4^+$ embryoid bodies and the majority of transplanted cells are nestin immunoreactive, tri-potential progenitor cells (Liu et al., 2000). Such ES cell-derived neurons integrated and extended processes into host tissue. These findings are interesting, since it appears that the normal adult spinal cord is not capable of supporting neurogenesis from endogenous progenitors (Horner et al., 2000), despite those same spinal cord progenitors being able to differentiate into neurons in culture and after transplantation into the hippocampus (Shihabuddin et al., 2000).

These early studies raise important questions and the following are some of our plans for future directions with this work. The ES cell-derived progenitors need to be better characterized. Availability of GFP-expressing ES cell lines will allow much better analysis of ES cell integration and differentiation. Transplantation of select populations of ES cell-derived progenitors will provide a better understanding of which progenitors are related to the improved function observed. Development of genetic selection methods will provide rapid and simple methods for isolating pure populations of ES cell-derived progenitor cells. Currently, many of our studies are limited by the tools we have available for assessment of our results. As additional cell lines become available, using transgenes that enhance ES cell detection, we will be better able to address the fundamental problem of identification of transplanted cells. Better animal models will allow clearer assessment of transplant survival and integration, as variability will decrease and extensive pathophysiology can be better controlled. Better behavioral assessment techniques will allow us to better quantify the behavioral ramifications of our manipulations and to, perhaps, determine the influence of specific white matter tracts in behavioral changes. Better models of demyelination are required, where behavior can be assessed and related to physiology and anatomy. Currently, most models cause axonal injury and death making relations of physiology and behavior difficult. We are working on in vivo models that minimize the inherent variability in injury models. We hope to be able to completely remove segments of defined white matter tracts without substantial alteration of the blood supply or prolonged breakdown of the blood–brain barrier. We are also in the process of adapting the contusion injury model for use in mice, allowing for the use of transgenic animals. Additionally, we are working on methods for assessing behavior to use in concert with the BBB protocol.

Caution is also prudent at this stage. Behavioral findings should be confirmed with multiple cell lines to exclude cell-line-specific effects. Well-defined populations of progenitors need to be studied. The characteristics of such populations need to be carefully considered. The genetic instability of neural progenitors needs to be considered. These are just scratching the surface.

The use of ES cells is an emerging technology. We have just begun to harness the potential of these cells as research tools, or as a realistic option for therapy in the injured or diseased CNS.

Abbreviations

EB   embryoid body
ES   embryonic stem cells

ESIM   embryonic stem cell induction medium
MBP   myelin basic protein
DIV   days in vitro

Acknowledgements

This work was supported by grants from the National Institutes of Health (NS01931, NS37927, NS 40520), the National Football League Charities, the W.M. Keck Foundation, and the Barnes-Jewish Hospital Foundation. We would also like to acknowledge the support and invaluable contributions of the other members of the ES cell Program Project Grant Team: Dennis W. Choi, MD, PhD, Primary Investigator; David I. Gottlieb, PhD; David H. Gutmann, MD, PhD; Chung Y. Hsu, MD, PhD; Mark F. Jacquin, PhD; and Eugene M. Johnson, Jr., PhD.

References

Bain, G., Kitchens, D., Yao, M. and Gottlieb, D.I. (1995) Embryonic stem cells express neuronal properties in vitro. *Dev. Biol.*, 168: 342–357.

Baron-Van Evercooren, A., Ganmuller, A., Clerin, E. and Gumpel, M. (1991) Hoechst 33342 is a suitable fluorescent marker for Schwann cells after transplantation in the mouse spinal cord. *Neurosci. Lett.*, 131: 241–244.

Basso, D.M., Beattie, M.S. and Bresnahan, J.C. (1995) A sensitive and reliable locomotor rating scale for open field testing in rats. *J. Neurotrauma*, 12: 1–21.

Baumrind, N.L., Parkinson, D., Wayne, D.B., Heuser, J.E. and Pearlman, A.L. (1992) EMA: a developmentally regulated cell-surface glycoprotein of CNS neurons that is concentrated at the leading edge of growth cones. *Dev. Dyn.*, 194: 311–325.

Blight, A.R. (1983) Cellular morphology of chronic spinal cord injury in the cat: analysis of myelinated axons by line-sampling. *Neurosciences*, 10: 521–543.

Bracken, M.B., Shepard, M.J., Collins, W.F., Holford, T.R., Baskin, D.S., Eisenberg, H.M., Flamm, E., Leo-Summers, L., Maroon, J., Marshall, L.F., Perot Jr., P.L., Piepmeir, J., Sonntag, V.K.H., Wagner, F.C., Wilberger, J.E. and Winn, H.R. (1990) A randomized, controlled trial of methylprednisolone or naloxone in the treatment of acute spinal-cord injury. Results of the Second National Acute Spinal Cord Injury Study. *N. Engl. J. Med.*, 322: 1405–1411.

Bracken, M.B., Shepard, M.J., Holford, T.R., Leo-Summers, L., Aldrich, E.F., Fazl, M., Fehlings, M., Herr, D.L., Hitchon, P.W., Marshall, L.F., Nockels, R.P., Pascale, V., Perot Jr., P.L., Piepmeir, J., Sonntag, V.K., Wagner, F., Wilberger, J.E., Winn, H.R. and Young, W. (1997) Administration of methylprednisolone for 24 or 48 hours or tirilazad mesylate for 48 hours in the treatment of acute spinal cord injury. Results of the Third National Acute Spinal Cord Injury Randomized Controlled Trial. National Acute Spinal Cord Injury Study. *JAMA*, 277: 1597–1604.

Bulte, J.W.M., Zhang, S.-C., van Gelderen, P., Herynek, V., Jordan, E.K., Duncan, I.D. and Frank, J.A. (1999) Neurotransplantation of magnetically labeled oligodendrocyte progenitors: magnetic resonance tracking of cell migration and myelination. *Proc. Natl. Acad. Sci. USA*, 96: 15256–15261.

Bunge, R.P., Puckett, W.R., Becerra, J.L., Marcillo, A. and Quencer, R.M. (1993) Observations on the pathology of human spinal cord injury. A review and classification of 22 new cases with details from a case of chronic cord compression with extensive focal demyelination. *Adv. Neurol.*, 59: 75–89.

Deacon, T., Dinsmore, J., Costantini, L.C., Ratliff, J. and Isacson, O. (1998) Blastula-stage stem cells can differentiate into dopaminergic and serotonergic neurons after transplantation. *Exp. Neurol.*, 149: 28–41.

Dougherty, K.D., Dreyfus, C.F. and Black, I.B. (2000) Brain-derived neurotrophic factor in astrocytes, oligodendrocytes, and microglia/macrophages after spinal cord injury. *Neurobiol. Dis.*, 7: 574–585.

Friedrich, G. and Soriano, P. (1991) Promotor traps in embryonic stem cells: a genetic screen to identify and mutate developmental genes in mice. *Genes Dev.*, 5: 1513–1523.

Gage, F.H., Coates, P.W., Palmer, T.D., Kuhn, H.G., Fisher, L.J., Suhonen, J.O., Peterson, D.A., Suhr, S.T. and Ray, J. (1995) Survival and differentiation of adult neuronal progenitor cells transplanted to the adult brain. *Proc. Natl. Acad. Sci. USA*, 92: 11879–11883.

Gruner, J.A. (1992) A monitored contusion model of spinal cord injury in the rat. *J. Neurotrauma*, 9: 123–128.

Hadjantonakis, A.-K. and Nagy, A. (2000) FACS for the isolation of individual cells from transgenic mice harboring a fluorescent protein reporter. *Genesis*, 27: 95–98.

Hadjantonakis, A.-K., Gertsenstein, M., Ikawa, M., Okabe, M. and Nagy, A. (1998) Generating green fluorescent mice by germline transmission of green fluorescent ES cells. *Mech. Dev.*, 76: 79–90.

Horner, P.J., Power, A.E., Kempermann, G., Kuhn, H.G., Palmer, T.D., Winkler, J., Thal, L.J. and Gage, F.H. (2000) Proliferation and differentiation of progenitor cells throughout the intact adult rat spinal cord. *J. Neurosci.*, 20: 2218–2228.

Kawase, E., Yamazaki, Y., Yagi, T., Yanagimachi, R. and Pedersen, R.A. (2000) Mouse embryonic stem (ES) cell lines established from neuronal cell-derived cloned blastocysts. *Genesis*, 28: 156–163.

Lagenaur, C. and Schachner, M. (1981) Monoclonal antibody (M2) to glial and neuronal cell surfaces. *J. Supramol. Struct. Cell Biochem.*, 15: 335–346.

Liebl, D.J., Huang, W., Young, W. and Parada, L.F. (2001) Regulation of Trk receptors following contusion of the rat spinal cord. *Exp. Neurol.*, 167: 15–26.

Liu, S., Qu, Y., Stewart, T., Howard, M., Chakrabortty, S., Holekamp, T. and McDonald, J.W. (2000) Embryonic stem cells differentiate into oligodendrocytes and myelinate in culture and after spinal cord transplantation. *Proc. Natl. Acad. Sci. USA*, 97: 6126–6131.

McDonald, J.W. (2001) ES cells and neurogenesis. In: M.S.

Rao (Ed.), *Stem Cells and CNS Development*. Humana Press, Totowa, NJ, pp. 207–261.

McDonald, J.W. and Sadowsky, C. (2002) Spinal cord injury: doable therapeutics. *Lancet*, 359: 417–425.

McDonald, J.W. and the Research Consortium of the Christopher Reeve Paralysis Foundation (1999a) Repairing the damaged spinal cord. *Sci. Am.*, 281: 64–73.

McDonald, J.W., Liu, X.-Z., Qu, Y., Liu, S., Turetsky, D., Mickey, S.K., Gottlieb, D.I. and Choi, D.W. (1999b) Transplanted embryonic stem cells survive, differentiate, and promote recovery in injured rat spinal cord. *Nat. Med.*, 5: 1410–1412.

Popovich, P.G., Horner, P.J., Mullin, B.B. and Stokes, B.T. (1996) A quantitative spatial analysis of the blood–spinal cord barrier, I. Permeability changes after experimental spinal-contusion injury. *Exp. Neurol.*, 142: 258–275.

Popovich, P.G., Wei, P. and Stokes, B.T. (1997) Cellular inflammatory response after spinal cord injury in Sprague–Dawley and Lewis rats. *J. Comp. Neurol.*, 377: 443–464.

Shihabuddin, L.S., Horner, P.J., Ray, J. and Gage, F.H. (2000) Adult spinal cord stem cells generate neurons after transplantation in the adult dentate gyrus. *J. Neurosci.*, 20: 8727–8735.

Wakayama, T., Tabar, V., Rodriguez, I., Perry, A.C., Studer, L. and Mombaerts, P. (2001) Differentiation of embryonic stem cell lines generated from adult somatic cells by nuclear transfer. *Science*, 292: 740–743.

Waxman, S.G. (1992) Demyelination in spinal cord injury and multiple sclerosis: what can we do to enhance functional recovery? *J. Neurotrauma*, 9: S105–117.

West, C.A., He, C., Su, M., Swanson, S.J. and Mentzer, S.J. (2001) Aldehyde fixation of thiol-reactive fluorescent cytoplasmic probes for tracking cell migration. *J. Histochem. Cytochem.*, 49: 511–518.

Wu, D.D. and Keating, A. (1993) Hematopoietic stem cells engraft in untreated transplant recipients. *Exp. Hematol.*, 21: 251–256.

Molecular targets to promote axon regeneration in the CNS

L. McKerracher, G. Doucet and S. Rossignol (Eds.)
Progress in Brain Research, Vol. 137

CHAPTER 22

Chondroitin sulphate proteoglycans in the CNS injury response

Daniel A. Morgenstern, Richard A. Asher and
James W. Fawcett *

Physiological Laboratory and Centre for Brain Repair, Cambridge University, The E.D. Adrian Building, Forvie Site, Robinson Way, Cambridge CB2 2PY, UK

Introduction

A number of explanations have been proposed to account for the failure of CNS neurons to successfully regenerate their axons following injury. These include intrinsic neuronal factors (such as a failure to upregulate expression of the growth-promoting molecules GAP-43 and L1) and inhibitory molecules associated with both normal CNS white matter (such as the recently cloned *Nogo*) and with the glial cell response to injury. CNS injury leads to a complicated cellular response involving a range of glial cells, including astrocytes, oligodendrocyte progenitor cells (OPCs), microglia and meningeal cells. Importantly, this cellular response results in an increase in the synthesis of extracellular matrix components, including chondroitin sulphate proteoglycans (CSPGs), as well as other molecules, such as tenascins and possibly keratan sulphate proteoglycans. Our laboratory has focussed, in particular, on changes in the expression of these axon growth-inhibitory CSPGs.

Chondroitin sulphate proteoglycans

CSPGs represent a varied class of complex extracellular matrix macromolecules. They share a general molecular structure comprising a central core protein with a number of covalently attached carbohydrate chains, known as glycosaminoglycans (GAG). In the case of CSPGs, these sidechains are of chondroitin sulphate. Considerable molecular diversity comes from differences in the core protein, variation in the number, length and pattern of sulphation of the chondroitin sulphate sidechains, and from the addition to the core protein of N- and O-linked oligosaccharides. CSPGs exist as both transmembrane and secreted proteins, and may also undergo proteolytic processing to create additional forms. The details of individual CSPG molecules are considered further below.

Before embarking on such a discussion, let us first consider the evidence that implicates these molecules in the failure of CNS regeneration. There are four relevant findings: firstly, CSPG expression is increased around CNS injuries; secondly, CSPGs form barriers to axons during development; thirdly, CSPGs have been shown to inhibit neurite outgrowth in vitro; and finally, disruption of CSPGs leads to increased neurite outgrowth both in an ex vivo model of the glial scar and in vivo.

―――――――
* Correspondence to: J.W. Fawcett, Physiological Laboratory and Centre for Brain Repair, Cambridge University, The E.D. Adrian Building, Forvie Site, Robinson Way, Cambridge CB2 2PY, UK. Tel.: +44-1223-331160; Fax: +44-1223-331174; E-mail: jf108@cam.ac.uk

Enhanced CSPG expression in response to CNS injury

Many of the experiments to date into CSPG expression have used the monoclonal antibody CS-56 (Avnur and Geiger, 1984), which recognises an epitope on the GAG sidechains of CSPGs. CS-56 recognises chondroitin sulphate types A (C4S) and C (C6S) but not type B (dermatan sulphate). Increased expression of CSPGs has been shown following dorsal root injury (Pindzola et al., 1993), fornix transection (Lips et al., 1995), ex vivo injured striatum (Gates et al., 1996), and cerebral cortex stab wound and spinal cord crush injury (Fitch and Silver, 1997). A membrane-associated CSPG, IMP (injured membrane proteoglycan), is expressed by reactive astrocytes following neurotoxin injury of the rat hippocampus (Bovolenta et al., 1993). This CSPG inhibits neurite outgrowth in vitro, a property which depends on the attached GAG sidechains (Bovolenta et al., 1997).

In two notable studies, Davies et al. have directly demonstrated a correlation between the upregulation of CSPGs and the failure of axonal regeneration. In the first (Davies et al., 1997), microtransplantation techniques were used to implant DRG neurons into the corpus callosum. Perhaps surprisingly, in most cases axons were able to extend for long distances in the normal host CNS white matter tracts. Importantly, in some experiments axonal growth failed and in these cases the transplanted neurons were surrounded by a striking region of upregulated chondroitin sulphate proteoglycans. This result was confirmed in a subsequent study (Davies et al., 1999) in which neurons were transplanted at a distance from a dorsal column spinal cord lesion. Axons were able to regenerate through the white matter tracts, but came to a halt in the CSPG-rich region around the site of injury.

CSPGs as barrier to axons in development

In the developing embryo, the expression of CSPGs can in many cases be correlated with areas avoided by growing axons. Examples include the posterior half-sclerotome (Oakley and Tosney, 1991), dorsal root entry zone (Pindzola et al., 1993), and the roof plate of the developing spinal cord and the midline of the optic tectum (Snow et al., 1990a,b; Hoffman-Kim et al., 1998). CSPGs are also implicated in the patterning of retinal ganglion cell axons to form the optic nerve. In vitro treatment of the retina with chondroitinase to remove CS sidechains leads to disrupted patterning of axons and their more widespread growth (Brittis et al., 1992). In some cases, particular CSPG molecules have been identified. For example, neurocan is implicated in the formation of the thalamocortical projection (Miller et al., 1995; Meyer-Puttlitz et al., 1996; Fukuda et al., 1997).

CSPGs inhibit neurite outgrowth in vitro

A number of experiments have shown that the neurite-inhibitory properties of cultured astrocytes depend on their expression of CSPGs. In cultures of neonatal rat brain astrocytes, neurites avoid patches of cells which express high levels of CSPG and tenascin-C (Grierson et al., 1990; Meiners et al., 1995). In a comparison of a number of astrocyte cell lines with different neurite outgrowth promoting properties, the neurite-inhibitory properties of the least permissive cell line (Neu7) were, at least partly, attributable to the expression of CSPGs (Smith-Thomas et al., 1994, 1995), particularly NG2 (Fidler et al., 1999). Disruption of CSPG synthesis with β-D-xyloside or chlorate, or removal of GAG sidechains with chondroitinase ABC, led to increased neurite outgrowth. Similarly, cultured cortical astrocytes which have been exposed to β-amyloid peptide substrate become 'reactive' and produce a neurite-inhibitory extracellular matrix which contains CSPGs (Canning et al., 1996).

As more has become known about the specific CSPG molecules expressed in the glial scar, additional data have been derived from experiments examining the effects of purified CSPGs on neurite outgrowth. Many of the CSPGs upregulated following CNS injury have been shown to inhibit neurite outgrowth in in vitro assays; these include NG2 (Dou and Levine, 1994), versican (Schmalfeldt et al., 2000), neurocan (Friedlander et al., 1994; Asher et al., 2000), brevican (Yamada et al., 1997) and phosphacan (Grumet et al., 1993; Milev et al., 1994).

Improved neurite outgrowth following disruption of CSPGs

Further important evidence for an inhibitory role for CSPGs comes from an ex vivo model of the glial scar, in which a nitrocellulose filter is implanted into the cerebral cortex of adult rats and later removed to act as substrates for neurite growth in vitro. Insertion of the filter leads to a gliotic reaction, with reactive astrocytes becoming attached to the filter. These nitrocellulose filters contain large amounts of CSPG (McKeon et al., 1991) and represent a very poor substrate for neurite outgrowth (Rudge and Silver, 1990; McKeon et al., 1991). Significantly, treatment of these nitrocellulose filter explants with chondroitinase ABC leads to substantially increased neurite outgrowth (McKeon et al., 1995), indicating that CSPGs contribute substantially to the inhibitory properties of the glial scar. Treatment with chondroitinase ABC has also been shown to increase neurite outgrowth on cryosections of (normal) adult rat spinal cord (Zuo et al., 1998). Similarly, disruption of CSPG synthesis using chlorate renders three-dimensional cultures of astrocytes relatively more permissive for DRG neurites (Smith-Thomas et al., 1995).

Furthermore, there is now evidence for improved axonal regeneration in vivo following disruption of CSPGs with chondroitinase ABC. Yick et al. (2000) used a small piece of gelfoam to apply the enzyme to the lesioned spinal cord, following the implantation of a peripheral nerve graft. They observed substantially increased axonal regeneration of Clarke's nucleus neurons into the PN graft in those animals which received the chondroitinase treatment. This enhanced regeneration was correlated with a decrease in CSPG immunoreactivity (using a pan-CS antibody). Moon et al. (2001) have reported increased regeneration of the lesioned rat nigrostriatal tract following the repeated local infusion of chondroitinase ABC. Again, axonal regeneration occurred in the region in which the enzyme had degraded chondroitin sulphate sidechains. Similarly, chondroitinase treatment of the lesioned rat spinal cord leads to an enhanced regenerative response (Bradbury et al., 2002).

Further investigations

These various lines of investigation provide, therefore, good evidence that CSPGs contribute to the failure of axonal regeneration following CNS injury. However, it is important to note that many of these studies on CSPG distribution have relied on antibodies against the chondroitin sulphate GAG sidechains of CSPGs and do not, therefore provide an indication of which specific molecules are involved. Indeed, an increase in CS-56 immunoreactivity does not necessarily indicate an upregulation in CSPG protein expression, since such an increase is also explicable in terms of an increase in the degree of glycanation (i.e. the addition of GAG chains) alone. Only recently has attention turned towards examining the expression of specific CSPGs. One of the aims of our laboratory has been to identify those molecules, the expression of which is increased following CNS injury.

We have used an experimental model in which the cerebral cortex of adult rats was lesioned using a scalpel blade inserted stereotaxically and vertically through a parasagittal dorsal craniotomy. In this way, we achieved a reproducible lesion in the right cortex, extending through the cortical grey matter into the underlying white matter. In each case, the contralateral side of the brain was left intact and served as a control. Changes in CSPG expression were then assessed by immunohistochemistry of frozen sections or by Western blot analysis of extracts prepared from small pieces of tissue dissected from around the lesion site and from the equivalent region on the control hemisphere. Both sections and blots were probed with antibodies specific to individual CSPG molecules.

Data now exist concerning changes in the expression of a number of CSPGs after CNS injury. These include members of the hyalectan (or lectican) family: aggrecan, versican, neurocan and brevican. These molecules share a common structure comprising an N-terminal hyaluronic acid binding region, a C-terminal with epidermal growth factor (EGF), lectin and complement regulatory protein (CRP) domains and an intervening region to which CS sidechains are attached. Other, structurally unrelated, CSPGs include NG2 and phosphacan — the secreted form of a transmembrane receptor-type tyrosine phosphatase, RPTPβ (Maurel et al., 1994).

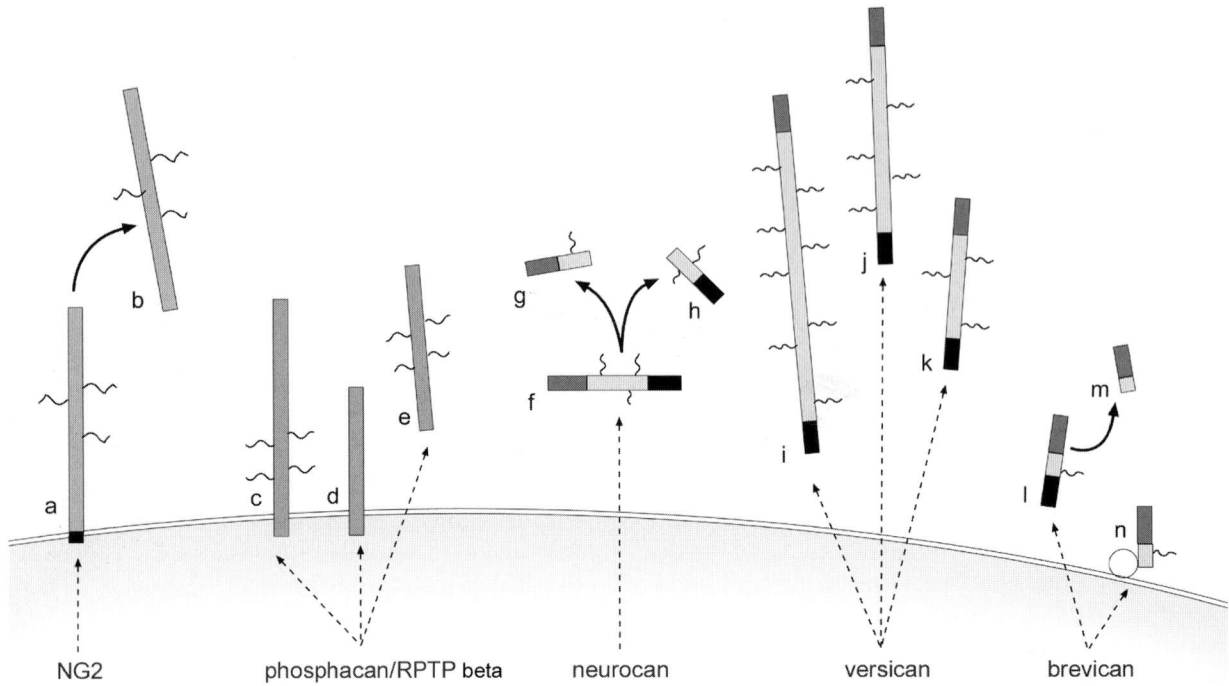

Fig. 1. A number of different CSPGs have been shown to be upregulated following CNS injury. NG2 (a) is synthesised as a transmembrane protein, but also exists in a soluble form (b) following proteolytic cleavage. RPTPβ (c) is another transmembrane CSPG. A splice variant, the short receptor form (d), lacks the CS-binding domain and does not carry GAG sidechains, whilst a third splice variant produces a secreted CSPG, phosphacan (e). Neurocan, versican and brevican are members of the hyalectan family of CSPGs and share a common structure comprising an N-terminal hyaluronic acid binding region (black), a C-terminal which includes a lectin-like domain (dark grey) and an intervening region to which CS sidechains are attached. Neurocan (f) can undergo proteolytic processing to produce neurocan-C (g) and neurocan-N_{130} (h). Versican, by contrast, exists in a number of splice variants, including the full-length versican V_0 (i) and the two shorter forms V_1 (j) and V_2 (k). Brevican (l) can also undergo proteolysis (m), whilst alternative splicing produces a membrane-associated GPI-linked form (n). Bold lines indicate proteolytic events.

Fig. 1 summarises the different molecular forms of these CSPGs.

NG2

NG2 has a primary structure unrelated to other CSPGs. The proteoglycan is synthesised as a transmembrane molecule, but can in vitro undergo proteolytic cleavage to produce a secreted form (Nishiyama et al., 1995). Analysis of CNS extracts has shown that this form also exists in vivo (Morgenstern et al., 1999). Serial extracts prepared from rat cortical tissue, meninges and spinal cord revealed substantial amounts of NG2 in both the initial saline-only extract and following the addition of detergent, confirming for the first time that NG2 in the CNS ex-

ists not just as transmembrane, but also as a soluble, protein (see Fig. 2).

Cellular origin

Within the CNS, NG2 is expressed by oligodendrocyte progenitor cells (OPCs), which represent a fourth major population of glial cells distinct from astrocytes, oligodendrocytes and microglia (Nishiyama et al., 1999), and also by cultured meningeal cells (Morgenstern et al., 1999). Whilst astrocytes in the normal CNS do not express NG2, there are a few reports that suggest that these cells may express NG2 following injury (Grill et al., 1998; Hirsch and Bähr, 1999). It is possible, but by no means confirmed, that these represent astrocytes which have differentiated from

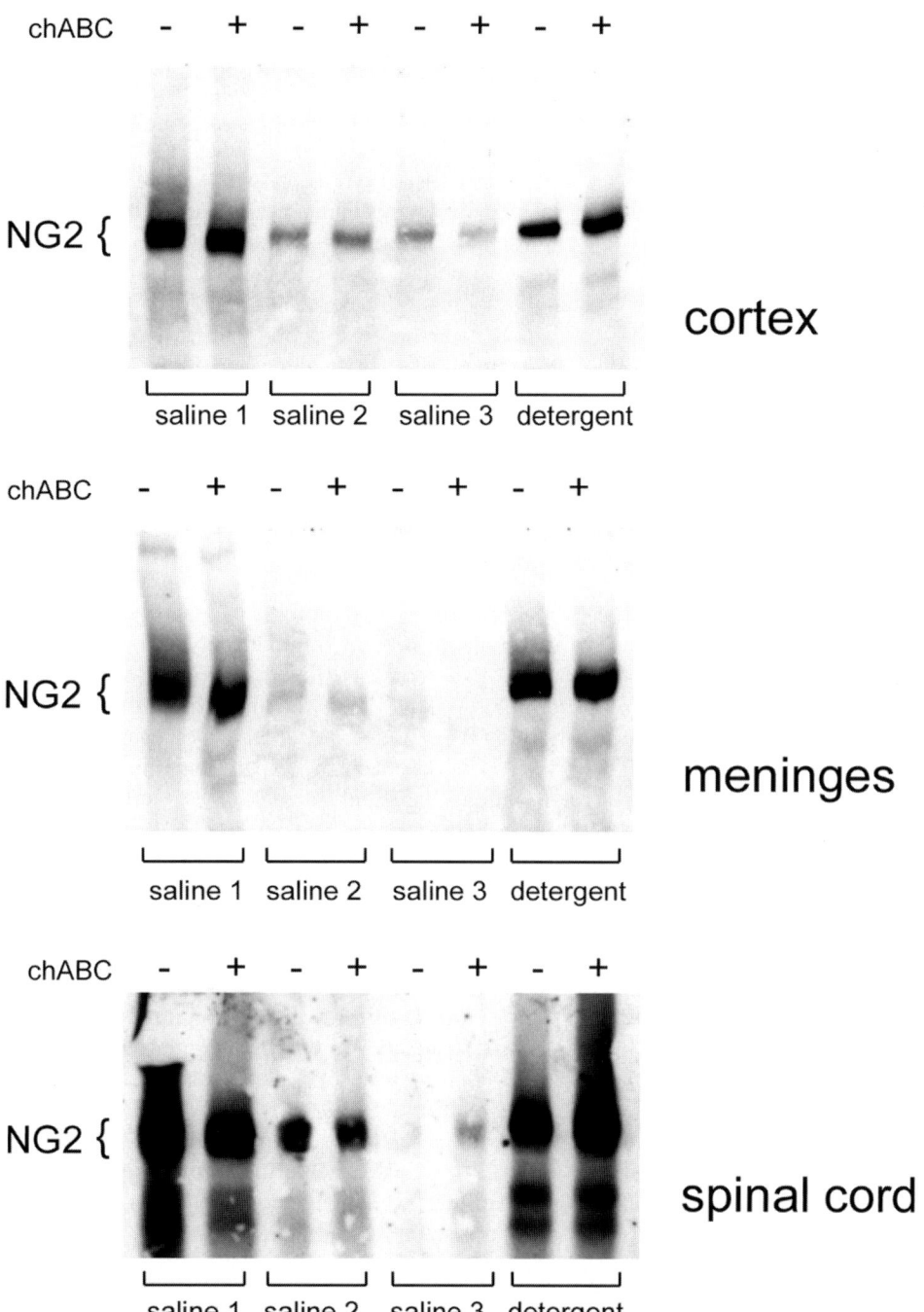

Fig. 2. Comparison of NG2 in serial extracts prepared from rat cortex, meninges and spinal cord. Tissue was extracted three times in Tris-buffered saline and subsequently in the presence of detergent (1% Triton X-100). Samples were left untreated (−) or digested (+) with chondroitinase ABC (chABC), and equal volumes were analysed by Western blotting. Immunoreactive species were visualised using a polyclonal anti-NG2 antibody (kind gift of J.M. Levine). Substantial amounts of NG2 appear in the initial saline extract, and further amounts are subsequently released following the addition of detergent. A similar pattern of extraction is seen in each of the CNS tissues, indicating that they contain both secreted (soluble) and membrane-associated forms of NG2.

the OPC population. Similarly, there is controversy regarding the question of NG2 expression by microglial cells. Immunolabelling studies have indicated that NG2-positive cells are distinct from microglia (Levine, 1994; Nishiyama et al., 1999; Chang et al., 2000), whilst other investigators have reported the co-expression of NG2 and microglial markers (Pouly et al., 1999; Bu et al., 2000).

Inhibition of neurite growth

Dou and Levine (1994) first demonstrated the neurite growth-inhibitory effects of NG2 by culturing cerebellar granule and dorsal root ganglion neurons in vitro. When added to a laminin substrate, NG2 inhibited neurite outgrowth from both neuronal types, whilst in the presence of an L1 substrate, only cerebellar granule neurons were affected. These inhibitory effects were blocked by the addition of rabbit anti-NG2 antibodies. Further evidence comes from a stripe assay comparing membranes from NG2-rich OPCs and Chinese hamster ovary (CHO) cells (which do not express NG2). Cerebellar granule neurons extend axons preferentially on the CHO cell membranes (Chen and Levine, 1999), an effect which is abolished by the addition of rabbit antibodies to NG2. Conversely, neurite outgrowth on membranes from cells transfected to express high levels of NG2 was significantly less than that on untransfected, NG2-negative, cells. Soluble NG2 Fc-fusion proteins have also been demonstrated to cause growth cone collapse (Ughrin and Levine, 1999). Further evidence for the inhibitory properties of NG2 comes from the comparison of two astrocytic cell lines, Neu7 and A7, that are (respectively) inhibitory and permissive for neurite outgrowth (Fidler et al., 1999). Analysis of detergent lysates and conditioned media from cultures of these cells reveal a clear difference in proteoglycan, and in particular NG2, expression. The inhibitory properties of Neu7 cells for DRG and cortical neurites are largely abolished by NG2 antibodies.

Mechanism of neurite inhibition

The mechanism by which NG2 inhibits neurite outgrowth remains to be fully elucidated, but experimental work has indicated a number of possibilities.

Firstly, NG2 may interact directly with growth promoting molecules (such as laminin and L1) to block access by axons to their functional domains, i.e. inhibition by steric hindrance. Secondly, NG2 may exert its inhibitory effect directly via a specific receptor and a pertussis toxin-sensitive G protein intracellular signalling mechanism (Dou and Levine, 1997). Thirdly, NG2 interacts with a variety of molecules (type VI collagen, growth factors, tenascin, etc.) and may modulate the extracellular environment through which neurites must grow. Thus, at least in vivo, NG2 may affect axonal growth indirectly. The degree to which attached (GAG) sidechains contribute to the molecule's inhibitory properties remains to be resolved. In experiments by Dou and Levine (1994) digestion of NG2 with chondroitinase ABC, to remove GAG chains, did not affect the molecule's inhibitory properties, indicating that these are a result of effects mediated by the core alone. This result has been confirmed by more recent experiments using recombinant protein fragments (Ughrin and Levine, 1999). Nevertheless, in other studies, GAG chains on CSPGs have been shown to inhibit neurite outgrowth (Snow et al., 1990a, 1996; McKeon et al., 1991, 1995), and in the experiments outlined above in which Neu7 and A7 cell lines were compared, the inhibitory properties of the Neu7 cells were reduced following chondroitinase ABC digestion or β-D-xyloside treatment of the cells, both of which specifically disrupt GAG sidechains (Smith-Thomas et al., 1995; Fidler et al., 1999). Thus, whilst the core protein of NG2 is clearly sufficient to cause neurite inhibition (in vitro) without the presence of chondroitin sulphate GAG chains, a contribution by these GAG chains to the overall 'character' of the molecule should not be ruled out. The GAG chains may, for example, affect the conformational morphology of NG2 or otherwise determine which regions of the extracellular domain are available to interact with other molecules.

Upregulation following CNS injury

Levine (1994) demonstrated a significant increase in the number of NG2-positive cells and overall NG2 immunoreactivity around a cerebellar puncture wound. This increase in immunoreactivity was accompanied by an upregulation in NG2 mRNA

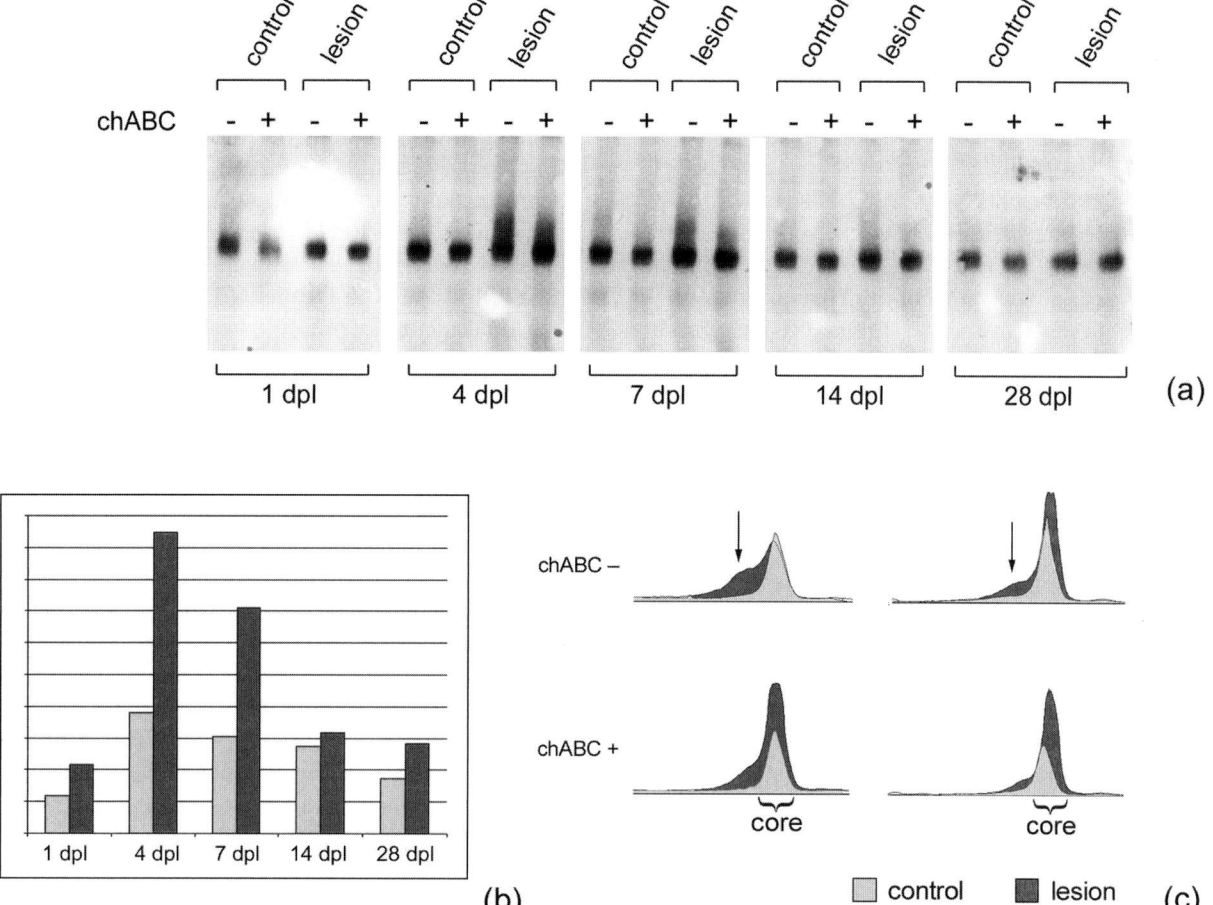

Fig. 3. Timecourse analysis of changes in NG2 expression following cerebral cortex knife-cut injury. Tris-buffered saline extracts were prepared from tissue dissected from the area around the site of the lesion and from the equivalent location in the contralateral uninjured hemisphere which served as a control. Samples were left untreated (−) or digested (+) with chondroitinase ABC (chABC) and equalised for total protein. The blot (a) was probed with anti-NG2 antiserum. Comparison of lesioned and control tissue extracts shows only a slight increase in NG2 expression at 1 dpl, with a clear upregulation at 4 and 7 dpl. By 14 dpl, levels of NG2 expression in the lesioned tissue have essentially returned to normal. The graph (b) illustrates these changes based on quantification of the size/density of the chABC digested bands using NIH image (arbitrary units). Plots of immunoreactivity density at 4 and 7 dpl (c) reveal that not only is there an upregulation in expression of the NG2 core protein, but also of attached chondroitin sulphate sidechains (arrows in c show smear of higher molecular weight species which are removed following chABC digestion). An equivalent pattern of changes in NG2 expression was seen in detergent extracts and in an analysis of a separate series of animals.

synthesis, as demonstrated by in situ hybridisation (Levine, 1994). Direct confirmation of an increase in expression of the NG2 protein has come from experiments conducted in our laboratory (Fig. 3). A comparison by Western blotting of the protein content of injured and control cortical tissue showed an increase in both soluble and membrane-associated NG2 core protein at both 4 and 7 days post-lesion (dpl) with levels returning to normal by 14 dpl. There

was no significant change in the ratio of soluble to membrane-associated forms of NG2 at any of the timepoints following the lesion, indicating that both forms are equally upregulated. Interestingly, these experiments also indicated that, at both 4 and 7 dpl, the amount of glycosaminoglycans carried by the NG2 molecule was increased in the lesioned tissue as compared to control. Examination of tissue at other timepoints revealed a slight increase at 24 h, but no difference between control and lesion extracts at 14 and 28 dpl, confirming, in agreement with Levine (1994), that the increased expression of NG2 is relatively transient.

Regulation of NG2 expression

It is unclear at present how the upregulation in NG2 following CNS injury might be controlled; the increase appears to come about as a result of both an increase in the number of NG2-expressing OPCs around the lesion and an upregulation in their expression of NG2.

Neurocan

Neurocan is a member of the hyalectan family of proteoglycans and shares a common basic structure with the other family members aggrecan, versican and brevican. The molecule is secreted and undergoes proteolytic processing such that in the adult CNS the vast majority of neurocan is found in the form of C- and N-terminal fragments (Meyer-Puttlitz et al., 1995). A single proteolytic cleavage within the central chondroitin sulphate attachment domain is thought to produce a 150 kDa C-terminal fragment, neurocan-C, and a 130 kDa N-terminal fragment, neurocan-N_{130} (Rauch et al., 1992; Matsui et al., 1994). An additional 90 kDa N-terminal fragment has also been described (Meyer-Puttlitz et al., 1995).

Cellular origin

Whilst initially thought to be a product of neurons alone (Engel et al., 1996; Meyer-Puttlitz et al., 1996), it has recently become clear that neurocan is also expressed in vitro by glial cells including both astrocytes (Oohira et al., 1994; Asher et al., 2000) and OPCs (Asher et al., 2000). The expression of neurocan by GFAP-positive astrocytes in vivo has since been confirmed by examination of sections of injured brain (Haas et al., 1999; McKeon et al., 1999).

Inhibition of neurite growth and mechanism of action

Inhibition of neurite outgrowth by neurocan has been demonstrated in stripe assays performed by Braisted

and Levine (Asher et al., 2000) in which L1-coated coverslips were coated with stripes of purified neurocan. Neurites growing from rat P4/P5 cerebellar and P0 cortical explants avoided the neurocan stripes, growing preferentially on the intervening L1. Friedlander et al. (1994) has also demonstrated that neurocan inhibits neuronal attachment to substrates of both L1 and N-CAM, leading to a reduction in L1-mediated neurite outgrowth. Neurocan binds with high affinity to both L1 and N-CAM (Friedlander et al., 1994) and can inhibit the homophilic interactions of these cell adhesion molecules (Grumet et al., 1993); thus neurocan is likely to inhibit neurite outgrowth in vivo by disrupting the interactions between cell adhesion molecules on the growth cone and other cell surfaces. The binding of neurocan to both L1 and N-CAM involves chondroitin sulphate sidechains on the proteoglycan (Friedlander et al., 1994; Oleszewski et al., 2000), and it is likely therefore that CS contributes to the inhibition of L1-mediated neurite outgrowth, although this has not formally been investigated.

In addition to this effect on cell adhesion molecules, neurocan may also exert a direct action on neurons. Neurite outgrowth from PC12D cells is inhibited by a neurocan substrate (Katoh-Semba et al., 1995, 1998). Similarly, neurocan can block neurite outgrowth from embryonic chick CNS neurons when presented as a substrate with anti-Ng-CAM (anti-L1) immunoglobulins, to which it does not bind (Friedlander et al., 1994).

Upregulation following CNS injury

An upregulation of neurocan expression has been demonstrated in a variety of CNS injury models, including our own. Immunohistochemical analysis of frozen sections of brain, at both 7 and 14 days following a cortical knife-cut lesion, shows a clear and substantial increase in neurocan expression around the lesion (Asher et al., 2000). Western blotting of extracts prepared from control and lesioned tissue confirms this result (Asher et al., 2000). In the uninjured adult rat brain amounts of intact neurocan are barely detectable, although there are significant amounts of neurocan-C and neurocan-N_{130}. However, at 7 days following injury there is a very substantial increase in the expression of intact neurocan.

In a separate lesion model in which a nitrocellulose filter is implanted into the cerebral cortex, McKeon et al. (1999) have also demonstrated, by Western blotting of extracts prepared from these filters 14 days after implantation, a clear upregulation in intact neurocan. Immunohistochemistry and in situ hybridisation has confirmed expression by reactive astrocytes which populate the implanted filters.

Finally, in a rather different lesion model, neurocan upregulation has also been reported in the denervated fascia dentata in the hippocampus following entorhinal cortex lesion (Haas et al., 1999). Whilst neurocan was increased at the site of the lesion itself, these data indicate that neurocan expression is also altered at a distance from the injury, with significantly increased expression in the denervated area.

Timecourse of upregulation

A more detailed analysis of the timecourse over which neurocan is upregulated in our CNS injury model has also been undertaken (Fig. 4). Comparison of intact neurocan bands showed little change at 24 h (1 dpl) with a barely detectable difference between control and lesion samples. Thereafter, however, neurocan is massively upregulated, with a clear increase in the expression of intact neurocan at both 4 and 7 dpl. Levels in the lesioned cortex subsequently decline, and whilst still being significantly elevated above control at 14 dpl, by 28 days neurocan levels are almost returned to normal. Importantly, the level of neurocan detected in control extracts remains essentially unchanged (and very low) throughout the course of the experiment. Our results correlate well with those of McKeon et al. (1995) who reported no neurocan immunoreactivity (using mAb 1D1) in nitrocellulose filters 30 days after implantation into the cerebral cortex, whilst showing significant upregulation at 14 days (McKeon et al., 1999).

Regulation of neurocan expression

It is clear, therefore, that neurocan expression is substantially increased in the days following CNS injury, although this upregulation disappears by 28 dpl. It is important therefore to consider what factors might control this response. Cytokines, including in particular TGFβ and TGFα (a member of the EGF family with which it shares the same receptor, EGFR), have been implicated in many aspects of the CNS injury response. Both TGFβ and TGFα are upregulated following CNS injury (Lindholm et al., 1992; Rabchevsky et al., 1998). Infusion of neutralising antibodies to TGFβ leads to an attenuation of the astrocytic response and a reduction in the deposition of extracellular matrix components including CSPGs (Logan and Berry, 1993; Logan et al., 1994, 1999; Griffith and McKeon, 1999). Similarly, TGFα has been implicated in astrogliosis (Rabchevsky et al., 1998). With regard to neurocan expression in particular, both TGFβ and EGF strongly upregulate neurocan expression by cultured astrocytes (Asher et al., 2000) and may therefore play a similar role in vivo.

An additional component of the neurocan upregulation observed following injury is the response of OPCs. Like astrocytes, these cells express neurocan in vitro (Asher et al., 2000) and the increased numbers of these cells around the lesion may therefore contribute to the overall increase in neurocan expression. It would appear, however, that the expression of neurocan by these cells is not significantly affected by cytokines such as TGFβ and TGFα/EGF (R.A. Asher, unpublished observations).

Versican

Like neurocan, versican is a member of the hyalectan family of proteoglycans and shares the same basic structure. However, an important aspect of versican synthesis is structural diversity of the core protein, resulting from the formation of different mRNA splice variants. Four different forms have been reported, resulting from differential splicing of the central part of the versican gene that encodes the GAG attachment region (Ito et al., 1995). This central region is encoded by two exons, GAG-α and GAG-β, and different versican splice variants may contain both, neither or only one of these domains. Thus, the largest versican isoform (V_0) contains both GAG-α and GAG-β and has a molecular mass of approximately 370 kDa; versican V_1 (263 kDa) has only the GAG-β domain, whilst V_2 (180 kDa) has only the smaller GAG-α region; and, finally, the smallest isoform, V_3 (74 kDa) lacks both GAG-α and GAG-β (Dours-Zimmermann and Zimmermann, 1994; Naso et al., 1994; Zako et al., 1995). Different

322

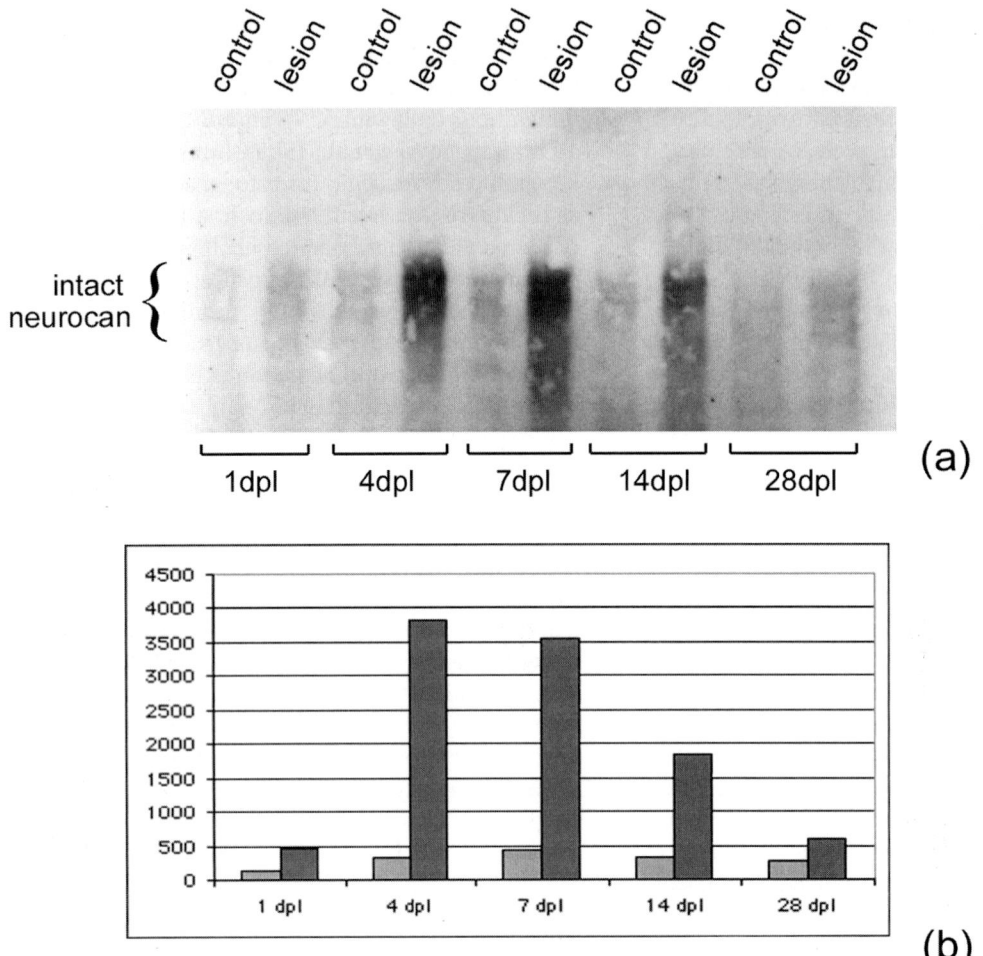

(a)

(b)

Fig. 4. Timecourse analysis of changes in neurocan expression following cortical knife-cut injury. Saline extracts were prepared from control and injured tissue, digested with chABC and reduced with dithiothreitol. Samples were equalised for total protein, separated by SDS–PAGE and blots were probed with mAb 1G2. The blot (a) shows little change in (intact) neurocan expression at 1 dpl. However, by 4 dpl there is a clear upregulation within the lesioned tissue. This is sustained at 7 dpl, but begins to decline by 14 dpl, so that by 28 dpl levels have returned to normal. The graph (b) illustrates these changes based on quantification of the size/density of the chABC digested bands using NIH image (arbitrary units). Similar results were obtained in an analysis of a separate series of animals.

versican isoforms are expressed by different cells and tissues, suggesting that this structural diversity is of functional importance.

Cellular origin

Versican is widely expressed in both neural and non-neural tissues, including connective tissue, cartilage, smooth muscle, blood vessels and skin epidermis. Within these non-neural tissues the major splice variants are V_0 and V_1 (Dours-Zimmermann and Zimmermann, 1994; Lemire et al., 1999), whilst analysis of CNS versican demonstrates that V_2 is by far the most abundant isoform (Paulus et al., 1996; Schmalfeldt et al., 1998, 2000). Within the CNS, versican appears to be mainly a product of cells of the oligodendrocyte lineage. Adult bovine CNS myelin contains versican V_2 (Niederöst et al., 1999), whilst analysis of versican expression by oligodendrocyte lineage cells in vitro reveals that these cells express versican (again V_2) specifically during the early stages of differentiation (Asher et al., 2002).

Thus, within the adult CNS only immature oligodendrocytes appear capable of versican expression. By contrast, neither astrocytes nor microglia synthesise versican (Asher et al., 2002), and whilst cultured meningeal cells do express versican, this is of the V_0 and V_1 isoforms and is therefore distinct from the major V_2 isoform found in the CNS.

Inhibition of neurite growth

A wide range of biological properties have been attributed to versican, including effects on cell migration (Landolt et al., 1995; Henderson et al., 1997; Perissinotto et al., 2000), adhesion (Yamagata et al., 1989; Yang et al., 1999) and proliferation (Zhang et al., 1998; Yang et al., 1999). In addition, brain-derived versican V_2 has recently been shown to exhibit potent neurite growth-inhibitory properties (Schmalfeldt et al., 2000). In these experiments, the authors used a modified Bonhöffer stripe assay, with alternating stripes of laminin alone and mixed laminin and versican V_2. Neurites extending from chick E7 retinal explants, and E12 and E18 dorsal root ganglia, strictly avoided the lanes containing versican, growing exclusively on the stripes coated with laminin alone. The inhibitory properties of versican were reduced, but by no means abolished, after treatment with chondroitinase ABC; thus, neurite growth-inhibition appears to be mediated mainly by the versican V_2 core protein (Schmalfeldt et al., 2000). Nevertheless, attached chondroitin sulphate sidechains appear to make an additional contribution to the neurite growth-inhibitory properties of versican. Versican-expressing oligodendrocytes cause collapse of DRG neurite growth cones when they encounter these cells, an effect which is abolished following β-D-xyloside treatment, which blocks the attachment of GAG sidechains to proteoglycans (Niederöst et al., 1999). Similarly, chondroitinase ABC treatment renders versican-positive differentiating oligodendrocytes more permissive for neurite outgrowth (Asher et al., 2002).

Mechanism of neurite inhibition

The mechanism(s) by which versican exerts its inhibition is not known, although one might speculate that the versican molecule somehow blocks the interaction between the growth cone and its substrate. Like other CSPGs, versican V_2 is a large molecule (potentially highly charged through glycosylation and glycanation) and may therefore block access to growth-promoting substrate molecules through steric hindrance. However, unlike, for example, neurocan, it is unclear to what extent versican binds to such molecules. Braunewell et al. (1995) have reported the binding of a sciatic nerve-derived 'versican-like' molecule to fibronectin (but not to laminin, or type I or type IV collagen). Chick versican (PG-M) has also been shown to bind to fibronectin and type I collagen, although not to laminin or type IV collagen (Yamagata et al., 1986).

Upregulation following CNS injury

Although astrocytes do not express versican, OPCs do express versican in vitro (Asher et al., 2002). Since these cells also form an important part of the CNS response to injury, one might expect this to lead to an increase in versican expression in the region of a CNS lesion. Indeed, immunohistochemistry of frozen sections of injured brains showed a clear increase in versican (mAb 12C5) immunoreactivity around the lesion at both 7 and 14 days after injury (Asher et al., 2002). In control brain, relatively little versican is detectable in the cortical grey matter and is much stronger in the underlying white matter (corpus callosum). However, after injury versican was clearly upregulated in the grey matter around the lesion site. This upregulation has been confirmed by Western blot comparison of extracts prepared from control and injured tissue. These blots showed only a single immunoreactive band, which co-migrates with the major versican isoform found in extracts of control brain and is therefore likely to be versican V_2. A clear upregulation in versican expression (approximately 2–3 fold increase) was seen at both 7 and 14 dpl. Further analysis of samples prepared at 28 dpl indicates that by this timepoint, expression of versican in injured tissue has returned to control levels (Asher et al., 2002).

Regulation of versican expression

The role of cytokines in regulating versican expression is currently unclear. TGFβ has been shown to suppress the proliferation and promote the differentiation of cultured OPCs (McKinnon et al., 1993). Since versican expressed by OPCs (at least in vitro) appears to be linked to both the cessation of proliferation and the onset of differentiation (Asher et al., 2002), the upregulation of TGFβ following CNS injury may therefore play a role in promoting the increase in versican expression.

Brevican

Brevican is the third member of the hyalectan family of proteoglycans for which data concerning post-injury changes in expression are available. The smallest of the hyalectans, the brevican core protein has an apparent molecular weight (on SDS–PAGE) of 145 kDa, although the molecule can also undergo proteolytic processing to produce an 80 kDa band representing the C-terminal fragment of the core protein (Yamaguchi, 1996). There is evidence that the processed fragments (C- and N-termini) may have different biological effects, for example in terms of glioma invasiveness (Matthews et al., 2000). Additional variation comes from alternative splicing producing an isoform which is retained at the cell surface through a glycosylphosphatidylinositol (GPI) anchor rather than being secreted into the extracellular space (Seidenbecher et al., 1995).

Cellular origin

Brevican represents one of the most abundant CSPGs in the adult CNS (Yamada et al., 1997) and is expressed by both astrocytes and cells of the oligodendrocyte lineage. The GPI-linked isoform in particular is expressed by mature white matter oligodendrocytes (Seidenbecher et al., 1995, 1998) and brevican has been isolated from adult bovine CNS myelin (Niederöst et al., 1999).

Inhibition of neurite growth

The neurite inhibitory properties of immunopurified, adult rat brain-derived brevican have been demonstrated by Yamada et al. (1997). Brevican (in a mixture with laminin) was presented to cerebellar granule cells as a substrate and substantially inhibited cell adhesion (as compared to laminin alone or

BSA). Although not rigorously tested in a Bonhöffer stripe assay, neurite outgrowth was inhibited at the border between regions of a brevican-containing and a brevican-free substrate. Significantly, treatment with chondroitinase ABC almost entirely abolished the anti-adhesive and neurite-inhibitory properties of brevican. Thus, in contrast to the neurite-inhibitory effects of versican, which appear to be mediated mainly by both the core protein with some contribution from attached chondroitin sulphate sidechains, those of brevican appear to reside primarily in the GAG component of the molecule. By what mechanism this inhibitory effect is exerted remains, however, to be determined. More recent results have shown that brevican and versican are important constituents of the CSPG fraction of CNS myelin (Niederöst et al., 1999). Immunodepletion of this CSPG fraction with anti-brevican antibodies leads to the loss of some neurite inhibition, confirming the inhibitory properties of this CSPG. Nevertheless, since the neurite-inhibitory properties of this CNS myelin CSPG fraction are relatively resistant to chondroitinase digestion, the authors suggest that versican, rather than brevican, makes the greater contribution (Niederöst et al., 1999).

Changes in expression following CNS injury

Jaworski et al. (1999) have examined changes in brevican expression following a needle stab injury to the mature rat brain. In these experiments, probes specific for the secreted, GPI-linked or both forms of brevican were used for in situ hybridisation studies of brain sections obtained at 2, 4, 7 or 14 days post-lesion. The secreted, but not the GPI-linked, form of brevican mRNA was found to be upregulated at both 4 and 7 dpl. Brevican expression had returned to normal levels by 14 dpl, and no increase in the GPI-linked form was seen at any of the timepoints. This increase in brevican expression was associated with nestin-positive reactive astrocytes along and adjacent to the needle tract.

Jaworski et al. (1999) suggest that the upregulation of brevican might create a "hydrated microenvironment that supports cell proliferation, migration, and glial process outgrowth", or may serve to concentrate growth factors. However, since brevican (like neurocan and versican) has also been shown to be neurite-inhibitory (Yamada et al., 1997), any upregulation of this molecule following CNS injury may also be important in the failure of successful axonal regeneration. It remains to be confirmed whether expression of brevican protein itself is upregulated following injury in line with these increases in mRNA. Similarly, rather little is known at present about what factors might regulate these changes in brevican expression.

Phosphacan

Phosphacan is another secreted nervous system CSPG and represents one of the splice variants of a gene encoding a transmembrane receptor-type tyrosine phosphatase, RPTPβ (Maurel et al., 1994). The full-length molecule (RPTPβ) is synthesised as a transmembrane protein and has three or four attached CS sidechains, whilst the short receptor form lacks this CS attachment domain. Phosphacan (also known as DSD-1 in the mouse) represents a third splice variant encoding the entire extracellular domain of RPTPβ.

Cellular origin

Phosphacan expression is limited to neuronal tissues and is widely expressed within nerve fibre tracts and the parenchyma of the adult CNS (Meyer-Puttlitz et al., 1996). Both astrocytes and OPCs express phosphacan in vitro (Canoll et al., 1996; A. Dobbertin, unpublished observations) and reactive astrocytes have also been shown to express phosphacan in an ex vivo model of the glial scar (McKeon et al., 1999).

Effects on neurite growth

Whilst all of the proteoglycans discussed above have been shown to inhibit neurite outgrowth, the data concerning phosphacan are considerably more difficult to interpret. Indeed, phosphacan has been shown to both inhibit and promote neurite outgrowth. Phosphacan inhibits both the proliferation of, and NGF-induced neurite outgrowth from, PC12D cells in vitro (Oohira et al., 1991; Katoh-Semba and Oohira, 1993, 1998). Phosphacan inhibits both the attachment of and neurite outgrowth from E9 chick cortical neurons on an L1/Ng-CAM substrate (Grumet et al.,

1993; Milev et al., 1994). Neurite outgrowth on an anti-Ng-CAM substrate, to which phosphacan does not bind, is also inhibited by phosphacan suggesting that phosphacan may interact directly with the cell surface to disrupt the interaction with the substrate and thereby inhibit neurite extension (Milev et al., 1994). DSD-1, the mouse homologue of phosphacan, also inhibits DRG neurite outgrowth on a laminin substrate (Garwood et al., 1999). The inhibitory effect is not reduced by removal of CS sidechains with chondroitinase ABC, suggesting that the activity resides in the phosphacan (DSD-1) core protein.

However, in other experiments, phosphacan has been shown to *promote* neurite outgrowth. DSD-1/phosphacan promotes neurite outgrowth from both E14 mesencephalic and E18 hippocampal neurons from rat (Faissner et al., 1994). This effect was abolished by removal of GAG sidechains with chondroitinase ABC, or by addition of mAb 473-HD which binds to an epitope on these sidechains (Faissner et al., 1994). Phosphacan/RPTPβ is also implicated in promoting pleiotrophin-mediated neurite outgrowth from cortical neurons (Maeda et al., 1996) and contactin-mediated outgrowth from tectal neurons (Peles et al., 1995; Sakurai et al., 1997). Neurite outgrowth from embryonic rat cortical neurons sparsely plated onto a poly-L-lysine substrate is also promoted by phosphacan (Maeda and Noda, 1996), an effect which is not reduced by chondroitinase digestion.

Overall, therefore, the effects of phosphacan on neurite outgrowth during both development and regeneration appear somewhat varied. Ultimately, these properties may depend on the following: whether phosphacan is carrying chondroitin sulphate sidechains and the precise molecular nature of these sidechains (e.g. pattern of sulphation); the way in which the molecule is glycosylated; the molecular context (e.g. presence of growth factors, such as pleiotrophin, and other features of the ECM or cell surface); the neuronal type and age; and so on. The inhibitory properties of phosphacan appear to reside in the core protein and probably involve a disruption of the interaction between the neuron and its substrate — phosphacan interacts with both L1/Ng-CAM and N-CAM (Milev et al., 1994). The growth promoting effects of phosphacan appear to involve many regions of the molecule, including GAGs, oligosaccharides and the core protein, effects which are probably mediated by the binding of phosphacan to neurite-promoting molecules, such as pleiotrophin, amphoterin and growth factors, e.g. bFGF.

Changes in expression following CNS injury

The data concerning changes in phosphacan expression following CNS injury are similarly complex. Snyder et al. (1996) have reported a striking upregulation of both RPTPβ and phosphacan mRNAs following hippocampal lesions. This increase was seen at all the timepoints examined: 14, 20, 30 and 45 dpl. Corresponding immunohistochemical analysis for GFAP showed that the region in which RPTPβ and phosphacan were upregulated was one of reactive astrogliosis, implicating astrocytes in this increased phosphacan/RPTPβ expression. RT–PCR analysis of mRNA obtained from the glial scar tissue associated with implanted nitrocellulose filters also reveals an upregulation of phosphacan expression (McKeon et al., 1999). Surprisingly, however, Western blot comparison of protein extracted from the filters (at 14 days post-implantation) and from control cortical tissue did *not* show an upregulation in phosphacan expression. Indeed, amounts of phosphacan within the scar tissue were reduced to approximately 67% of the level in control tissue (McKeon et al., 1999). Our own Western blot analysis of changes in phosphacan expression following cortical injury indicate that this may take the form of a biphasic response (Morgenstern, 2000). Phosphacan expression is initially decreased in injured compared to control tissue at the earliest timepoints (1 and 4 dpl) and is then subsequently upregulated (approximately a 2-fold increase) at later stages (7–14 dpl). Levels of phosphacan expression in injured tissue appear to return to normal by 28 dpl.

Regulation of phosphacan expression

The mechanisms involved in regulating phosphacan expression in the glial scar remain to be determined. However, as with other CSPGs, cytokines are likely to be involved in this regulation and preliminary data indicate that EGF/TGFα upregulates phosphacan expression in cultured astrocytes (A. Dobbertin, personal communication).

Extracellular matrix

In addition to these individual CSPGs, it is important also to consider the overall structure of the glial scar extracellular matrix. The inhibitory CSPGs discussed above do not exist in isolation and their interactions with other ECM molecules may have a significant impact on their properties. In addition to proteoglycans, two other major components of the ECM are hyaluronic acid and the tenascins. Binding to hyaluronic acid of a number of CSPGs, particularly members of the hyalectan family, has been demonstrated both in vitro and in extracts prepared from CNS tissue (Asher et al., 1991; Rauch et al., 1991; LeBaron et al., 1992; Perides et al., 1992; Retzler et al., 1996; Morgenstern, 2000). Tenascins (both -C and -R) represent a further diverse class of neurite inhibitory molecules, the expression of which is also upregulated following CNS injury (reviewed by Faissner, 1997; Pesheva and Probstmeier, 2000). Tenascins have been shown in vitro to interact with a number of CSPGs; for example, tenascin-R and versican coprecipitate from oligodendrocyte conditioned medium (Asher et al., 2002). It is likely, therefore, that within the extracellular matrix of the glial scar, CSPGs form part of a complex network of molecules which also includes hyaluronic acid and tenascins (Fig. 5). Such a complex may form the perineuronal net which surrounds the cell body of some neuronal types (Yamaguchi, 2000). It is unclear at present, however, to what degree different CSPG molecules are bound to this complex matrix and to what extent those that are not directly bound through interactions with hyaluronic acid or tenascins might be free to diffuse within the extracellular space. CSPGs such as NG2 and phosphacan exist in both transmembrane and secreted forms, whilst hyalectans such as neurocan undergo proteolytic processing leading to a separation of the hyaluronic acid and tenascin binding domains.

Summary

As the preceding discussion has demonstrated, experimental data now indicate that the expression of a number of different CSPGs is increased following CNS injury. The hyalectans neurocan, versican and

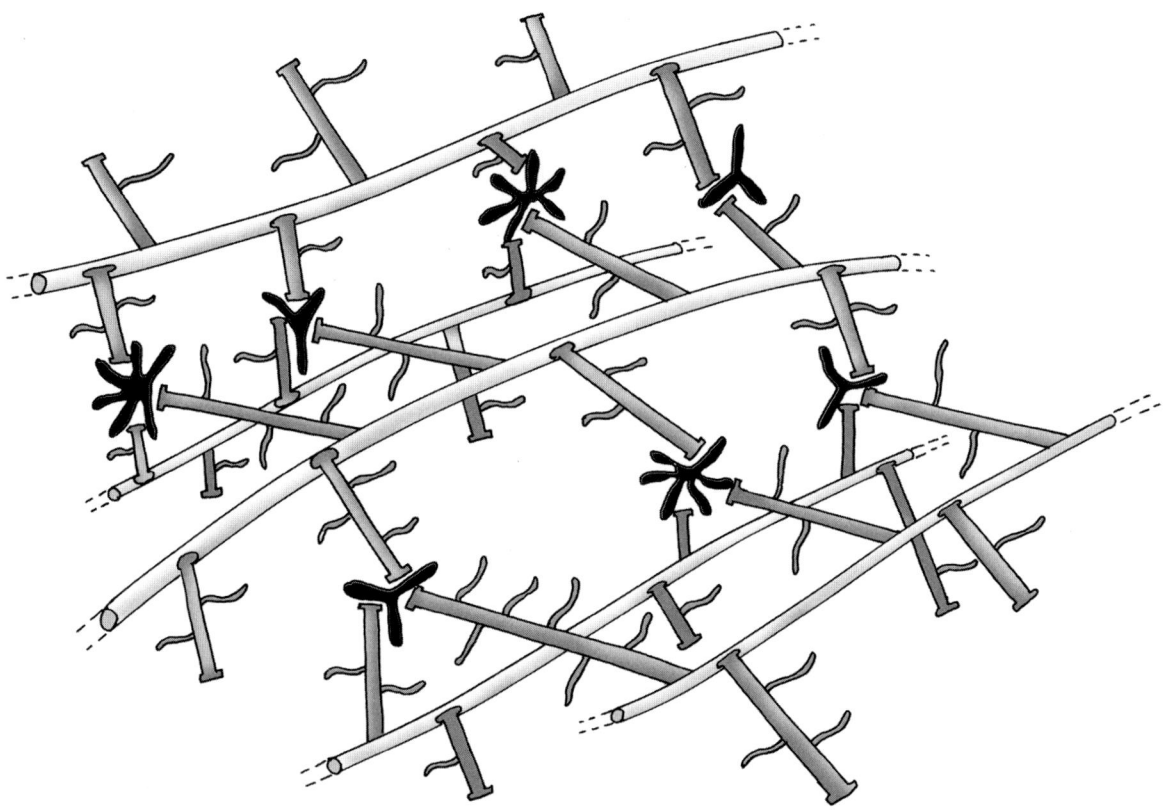

Fig. 5. An impression of the basic structure of the CNS glial scar extracellular matrix. Each long hyaluronic acid (HA) molecule forms the backbone of a complex which includes numerous attached CSPGs. In addition to binding to HA, many of these CSPGs also bind to tenascins (both tenascin-C, which exists as a hexamer of polypeptide chains, and tenascin-R, a trimer). The cross-linking of CSPGs between HA and tenascins leads to the formation of a complex macromolecular matrix.

brevican, plus NG2 and phosphacan are upregulated following injury and all have been shown to exhibit inhibitory effects on neurite outgrowth in vitro. It is likely therefore that the increased expression of these molecules contributes to the non-permissive nature of the glial scar. The relative contributions of individual molecules remain, however, to be determined. It is important to remember also that not only does the glial scar contain many different inhibitory molecules, but that these are the products of a number of different cells, including not just astrocytes, but also oligodendrocyte progenitor and meningeal cells. It is arguable that the latter two cell types make a greater contribution than astrocytes to the inhibitory environment of the injured CNS. Recently, attempts have been made to alter the CSPG component of the glial scar in the hope that this will facilitate improved axonal regeneration. Three studies (Bradbury et al., 2002; Yick et al., 2000; Moon et al., 2001) have reported an improved regenerative response following treatment of the injured CNS with chondroitinase ABC. CSPGs represent a significant source of inhibition within the injured CNS; these studies indicate that successful CNS regeneration may be brought about by interventions which target these molecules and/or the cells which produce them.

Abbreviations

CHO	Chinese hamster ovary
CNS	central nervous system
CS	chondroitin sulphate
CSPG	chondroitin sulphate proteoglycan
dpl	days post-lesion

DRG	dorsal root ganglion
EGF	epidermal growth factor
GAG	glycosaminoglycans
GAP-43	growth-associated protein 43
GFAP	glial fibrillary acid protein
N-CAM	neural cell adhesion molecule
OPC	oligodendrocyte progenitor cell
RPTPβ	receptor-type tyrosine phosphatase β
RT–PCR	reverse transcriptase–polymerase chain reaction
SDS–PAGE	sodium dodecyl sulphate–polyacrylamide gel electrophoresis
TGFα/β	transforming growth factor α/β

Acknowledgements

Original research reported here was supported by the Medical Research Council, International Spinal Research Trust, Wellcome Trust and Action Research. DAM received additional funding from the James Baird Fund.

References

Asher, R.A., Perides, G., Vanderhaeghen, J.-J. and Bignami, A. (1991) Extracellular matrix of central nervous system white matter: demonstration of an hyaluronate–protein complex. *J. Neurosci. Res.*, 28: 410–421.

Asher, R.A., Morgenstern, D.A., Fidler, P.S., Adcock, K.H., Oohira, A., Braisted, J.E., Levine, J.M., Margolis, R.U., Rogers, J.H. and Fawcett, J.W. (2000) Neurocan is upregulated in injured brain and in cytokine treated astrocytes. *J. Neurosci.*, 20: 2427–2438.

Asher, R.A., Morgenstern, D.A., Shearer, M.C., Adcock, K.A., Pesheva, P. and Fawcett, J.W. (2002) Versican is upregulated in CNS injury and is a product of oligodendrocyte lineage cells. *J. Neurosci.*, 22: 2225–2236.

Avnur, Z. and Geiger, B. (1984) Immunocytochemical localization of native chondroitin-sulfate in tissues and cultured cells using specific monoclonal antibody. *Cell*, 38: 811–822.

Bovolenta, P., Wandosell, F. and Nieto-Sampedro, M. (1993) Characterization of a neurite outgrowth inhibitor expressed after CNS injury. *Eur. J. Neurosci.*, 5: 454–465.

Bovolenta, P., Fernaud-Espinosa, I., Mendez-Otero, R. and Nieto-Sampedro, M. (1997) Neurite outgrowth inhibitor of gliotic brain tissue. Mode of action and cellular localization, studied with specific monoclonal antibodies. *Eur. J. Neurosci.*, 9: 977–989.

Bradbury, E.J., Moon, L.D.F., Popat, R.J., King, V.R., Bennett, G.S., Patel, P.N., Fawcett, J.W. and McMahon, S.B. (2002) Chondroitinase ABC promotes functional recovery after spinal cord injury. *Nature*, 416: 636–640.

Braunewell, K.-H., Pesheva, P., McCarthy, J.B., Furcht, L.T., Schmitz, B. and Schachner, M. (1995) Functional involvement of sciatic nerve-derived versican- and decorin-like molecules and other chondroitin sulphate proteoglycans in ECM-mediated cell adhesion and neurite outgrowth. *Eur. J. Neurosci.*, 7: 805–814.

Brittis, P.A., Canning, D.R. and Silver, J. (1992) Chondroitin sulfate as a regulator of neuronal patterning in the retina. *Science*, 255: 733–736.

Bu, J., Akhtar, N. and Nishiyama, A. (2000) NG2 expression by a subpopulation of activated microglia/macrophages in an excitotoxic lesion. *Soc. Neurosci. Abstr.*, 26: 2132.

Canning, D.R., Hoke, A., Malemud, C.J. and Silver, J. (1996) A potent inhibitor of neurite outgrowth that predominates in the extracellular matrix of reactive astrocytes. *Int. J. Dev. Neurosci.*, 14: 153–175.

Canoll, P.D., Petanceska, S., Schlessinger, J. and Musacchio, J.M. (1996) Three forms of RPTP-beta are differentially expressed during gliogenesis in the developing rat brain and during glial cell differentiation in culture. *J. Neurosci. Res.*, 44: 199–215.

Chang, A., Nishiyama, A., Peterson, J., Prineas, J. and Trapp, B.D. (2000) NG2-positive oligodendrocyte progenitor cells in adult human brain and multiple sclerosis lesions. *J. Neurosci.*, 20: 6404–6412.

Chen, Z.J. and Levine, J.M. (1999) Inhibition of axonal outgrowth by oligodendrocyte precursor cells: a role for the NG2 chondroitin sulfate proteoglycan. *Soc. Neurosci. Abstr.*, 25: 748.

Davies, S.J., Fitch, M.T., Memberg, S.P., Hall, A.K., Raisman, G. and Silver, J. (1997) Regeneration of adult axons in white matter tracts of the central nervous system. *Nature*, 390: 680–683.

Davies, S.J., Goucher, D.R., Doller, C. and Silver, J. (1999) Robust regeneration of adult sensory axons in degenerating white matter of the adult rat spinal cord. *J. Neurosci.*, 19: 5810–5822.

Dou, C.-L. and Levine, J.M. (1994) Inhibition of neurite growth by the NG2 chondroitin sulfate proteoglycan. *J. Neurosci.*, 14: 7616–7628.

Dou, C.-L. and Levine, J.M. (1997) Identification of a neuronal cell surface receptor for a growth inhibitory chondroitin sulfate proteoglycan (NG2). *J. Neurochem.*, 68: 1021–1030.

Dours-Zimmermann, M.T. and Zimmermann, D.R. (1994) A novel glycosaminoglycan attachment domain identified in two alternative splice variants of human versican. *J. Biol. Chem.*, 269: 32992–32998.

Engel, M., Maurel, P., Margolis, R.U. and Margolis, R.K. (1996) Cellular sites of synthesis of neurocan and phosphacan. *J. Comp. Neurol.*, 366: 34–43.

Faissner, A. (1997) The tenascin gene family in axon growth and guidance. *Cell Tissue Res.*, 290: 331–341.

Faissner, A., Clement, A., Lochter, A., Streit, A., Mandl, C. and Schachner, M. (1994) Isolation of a neural chondroitin sulfate proteoglycan with neurite outgrowth promoting properties. *J. Cell Biol.*, 126: 783–799.

Fidler, P.S., Schuette, K., Asher, R.A., Dobbertin, A., Thornton,

S.R., Calle-Patino, Y., Muir, E., Levine, J.M., Geller, H.M., Rogers, J.H., Faissner, A. and Fawcett, J.W. (1999) Comparing astrocytic cell lines that are inhibitory or permissive for axon growth: the major axon-inhibitory proteoglycan is NG2. *J. Neurosci.*, 19: 8778–8788.

Fitch, M.T. and Silver, J. (1997) Activated macrophages and the blood–brain barrier: inflammation after CNS injury leads to increases in putative inhibitory molecules. *Exp. Neurol.*, 148: 587–603.

Friedlander, D.R., Milev, P., Karthikeyan, L., Margolis, R.K., Margolis, R.U. and Grumet, M. (1994) The neuronal chondroitin sulfate proteoglycan neurocan binds to the neural cell adhesion molecules Ng-CAM/L1/NILE and N-CAM, and inhibits neuronal adhesion and neurite outgrowth. *J. Cell Biol.*, 125: 669–680.

Fukuda, T., Kawano, H., Ohyama, K., Li, H.P., Takeda, Y., Oohira, A. and Kawamura, K. (1997) Immunohistochemical localization of neurocan and L1 in the formation of thalamocortical pathway of developing rats. *J. Comp. Neurol.*, 382: 141–152.

Garwood, J., Schnadelbach, O., Clement, A., Schutte, K., Bach, A. and Faissner, A. (1999) DSD-1-Proteoglycan is the mouse homolog of phosphacan and displays opposing effects on neurite outgrowth dependent on neuronal lineage. *J. Neurosci.*, 19: 3888–3899.

Gates, M.A., Fillmore, H. and Steindler, D.A. (1996) Chondroitin sulfate proteoglycan and tenascin in the wounded adult mouse neostriatum in vitro: dopamine neuron attachment and process outgrowth. *J. Neurosci.*, 16: 8005–8018.

Grierson, J.P., Petroski, R.E., Ling, D.S. and Geller, H.M. (1990) Astrocyte topography and tenascin cytotactin expression: correlation with the ability to support neuritic outgrowth. *Brain Res. Dev. Brain Res.*, 55: 11–19.

Griffith, R.W. and McKeon, R.J. (1999) Immunoneutralization of TGFbeta attenuates CS-PG synthesis and enhances process outgrowth in vitro and in vivo. *Soc. Neurosci. Abstr.*, 25: 749.

Grill, R.J., Stallcup, W.B. and Tuszynski, M.H. (1998) Temporal upregulation and spatial distribution of putative inhibitory and growth permissive substrate molecules in the injured adult rat spinal cord. *Soc. Neurosci. Abstr.*, 24: 1054.

Grumet, M., Flaccus, A. and Margolis, R.U. (1993) Functional characterization of chondroitin sulfate proteoglycans of brain: interactions with neurons and neural crest adhesion molecules. *J. Cell Biol.*, 120: 815–824.

Haas, C.A., Rauch, U., Thon, N., Merten, T. and Deller, T. (1999) Entorhinal cortex lesion in adult rats induces the expression of the neuronal chondroitin sulfate proteoglycan neurocan in reactive astrocytes. *J. Neurosci.*, 19: 9953–9963.

Henderson, D.J., Ybot-Gonzalez, P. and Copp, A.J. (1997) Overexpression of the chondroitin sulphate proteoglycan versican is associated with defective neural crest migration in the Pax3 mutant mouse (splotch). *Mech. Dev.*, 69: 39–51.

Hirsch, S. and Bähr, M. (1999) Immunocytochemical characterization of reactive optic nerve astrocytes and meningeal cells. *Glia*, 26: 36–46.

Hoffman-Kim, D., Lander, A.D. and Jhaveri, S. (1998) Patterns of chondroitin sulfate immunoreactivity in the developing tec-

tum reflect regional differences in glycosaminoglycan biosynthesis. *J. Neurosci.*, 18: 5881–5890.

Ito, K., Shinomura, T., Zako, M., Ujita, M. and Kimata, K. (1995) Multiple forms of mouse PG-M, a large chondroitin sulfate proteoglycan generated by alternative splicing. *J. Biol. Chem.*, 270: 958–965.

Jaworski, D.M., Kelly, G.M. and Hockfield, S. (1999) Intracranial injury acutely induces the expression of the secreted isoform of the CNS-specific hyaluronan-binding protein BEHAB/brevican. *Exp. Neurol.*, 157: 327–337.

Katoh-Semba, R. and Oohira, A. (1993) Core proteins of soluble chondroitin sulfate proteoglycans purified from the rat brain block the cell cycle of PC12D cells. *J. Cell. Physiol.*, 156: 17–23.

Katoh-Semba, R., Matsuda, M., Kato, K. and Oohira, A. (1995) Chondroitin sulphate proteoglycans in the rat brain: candidates for axon barriers of sensory neurons and the possible modification by laminin of their actions. *Eur. J. Neurosci.*, 7: 613–621.

Katoh-Semba, R., Matsuda, M., Watanabe, E., Maeda, N. and Oohira, A. (1998) Two types of brain chondroitin sulfate proteoglycan: their distribution and possible functions in the rat embryo. *Neurosci. Res.*, 31: 273–282.

Landolt, R.M., Vaughan, L., Winterhalter, K.H. and Zimmermann, D.R. (1995) Versican is selectively expressed in embryonic tissues that act as barriers to neural crest cell migration and axon outgrowth. *Development*, 121: 2303–2312.

LeBaron, R.G., Zimmermann, D.R. and Ruoslahti, E. (1992) Hyaluronate binding properties of versican. *J. Biol. Chem.*, 267: 10003–10010.

Lemire, J.M., Braun, K.R., Maurel, P., Kaplan, E.D., Schwartz, S.M. and Wight, T.N. (1999) Versican/PG-M isoforms in vascular smooth muscle cells. *Arterioscler. Thromb. Vasc. Biol.*, 19: 1630–1639.

Levine, J.M. (1994) Increased expression of the NG2 chondroitin-sulfate proteoglycan after brain injury. *J. Neurosci.*, 14: 4716–4730.

Lindholm, D., Castren, E., Kiefer, R., Zafra, F. and Thoenen, H. (1992) Transforming growth factor-beta 1 in the rat brain: increase after injury and inhibition of astrocyte proliferation. *J. Cell Biol.*, 117: 395–400.

Lips, K., Stichel, C.C. and Muller, H.W. (1995) Restricted appearance of tenascin and chondroitin sulphate proteoglycans after transection and sprouting of adult rat postcommissural fornix. *J. Neurocytol.*, 24: 449–464.

Logan, A. and Berry, M. (1993) Transforming growth factor-beta 1 and basic fibroblast growth factor in the injured CNS. *Trends Pharmacol. Sci.*, 14: 337–342.

Logan, A., Berry, M., Gonzalez, A.M., Frautschy, S.A., Sporn, M.B. and Baird, A. (1994) Effects of transforming growth factor beta 1 on scar production in the injured central nervous system of the rat. *Eur. J. Neurosci.*, 6: 355–363.

Logan, A., Green, J., Hunter, A., Jackson, R. and Berry, M. (1999) Inhibition of glial scarring in the injured rat brain by a recombinant human monoclonal antibody to transforming growth factor-beta2. *Eur. J. Neurosci.*, 11: 2367–2374.

Maeda, N. and Noda, M. (1996) 6B4 proteoglycan/phosphacan

is a repulsive substratum but promotes morphological differentiation of cortical neurons. *Development*, 122: 647–658.

Maeda, N., Nishiwaki, T., Shintani, T., Hamanaka, H. and Noda, M. (1996) 6B4 proteoglycan/phosphacan, an extracellular variant of receptor-like protein-tyrosine phosphatase zeta/RPTPbeta, binds pleiotrophin/heparin-binding growth-associated molecule (HB-GAM). *J. Biol. Chem.*, 271: 21446–21452.

Matsui, F., Watanabe, E. and Oohira, A. (1994) Immunological identification of two proteoglycan fragments derived from neurocan, a brain-specific chondroitin sulfate proteoglycan. *Neurochem. Int.*, 25: 425–431.

Matthews, R.T., Gary, S.C., Zerillo, C., Pratta, M., Solomon, K., Arner, E.C. and Hockfield, S. (2000) Brain-enriched hyaluronan binding (BEHAB)/brevican cleavage in a glioma cell line is mediated by a disintegrin and metalloproteinase with thrombospondin motifs (ADAMTS) family member. *J. Biol. Chem.*, 275: 22695–22703.

Maurel, P., Rauch, U., Flad, M., Margolis, R.K. and Margolis, R.U. (1994) Phosphacan, a chondroitin sulfate proteoglycan of brain that interacts with neurons and neural cell-adhesion molecules, is an extracellular variant of a receptor-type protein tyrosine phosphatase. *Proc. Natl. Acad. Sci. USA*, 91: 2512–2516.

McKeon, R.J., Schreiber, R.C., Rudge, J.S. and Silver, J. (1991) Reduction of neurite outgrowth in a model of glial scarring following CNS injury is correlated with the expression of inhibitory molecules on reactive astrocytes. *J. Neurosci.*, 11: 3398–3411.

McKeon, R.J., Hoke, A. and Silver, J. (1995) Injury-induced proteoglycans inhibit the potential for laminin-mediated axon growth on astrocytic scars. *Exp. Neurol.*, 136: 32–43.

McKeon, R.J., Jurynec, M.J. and Buck, C.R. (1999) The chondroitin sulfate proteoglycans neurocan and phosphacan are expressed by reactive astrocytes in the chronic CNS glial scar. *J. Neurosci.*, 19: 10778–10788.

McKinnon, R.D., Piras, G., Ida Jr., J.A. and Dubois-Dalcq, M. (1993) A role for TGF-beta in oligodendrocyte differentiation. *J. Cell Biol.*, 121: 1397–1407.

Meiners, S., Powell, E.M. and Geller, H.M. (1995) A distinct subset of tenascin/CS-6-PG-rich astrocytes restricts neuronal growth in vitro. *J. Neurosci.*, 15: 8096–8108.

Meyer-Puttlitz, B., Milev, P., Junker, E., Zimmer, I., Margolis, R.U. and Margolis, R.K. (1995) Chondroitin sulfate and chondroitin/keratan sulfate proteoglycans of nervous tissue: developmental changes of neurocan and phosphacan. *J. Neurochem.*, 65: 2327–2337.

Meyer-Puttlitz, B., Junker, E., Margolis, R.U. and Margolis, R.K. (1996) Chondroitin sulfate proteoglycans in the developing central nervous system. II. Immunocytochemical localization of neurocan and phosphacan. *J. Comp. Neurol.*, 366: 44–54.

Milev, P., Friedlander, D.R., Sakurai, T., Karthikeyan, L., Flad, M., Margolis, R.K., Grumet, M. and Margolis, R.U. (1994) Interactions of the chondroitin sulfate proteoglycan phosphacan, the extracellular domain of a receptor-type protein tyrosine phosphatase, with neurons, glia, and neural cell adhesion molecules. *J. Cell Biol.*, 127: 1703–1715.

Miller, B., Sheppard, A.M., Bicknese, A.R. and Pearlman, A.L. (1995) Chondroitin sulfate proteoglycans in the developing cerebral cortex: the distribution of neurocan distinguishes forming afferent and efferent axonal pathways. *J. Comp. Neurol.*, 355: 615–628.

Moon, L.D., Asher, R.A., Rhodes, K.E. and Fawcett, J.W. (2001) Regeneration of CNS axons back to their target following treatment of adult rat brain with chondroitinase ABC. *Nat. Neurosci.*, 4: 465–466.

Morgenstern, D.A. (2000) Chondroitin Sulphate Proteoglycans in the Peripheral and Central Nervous Systems. University of Cambridge, Cambridge, 324 pp.

Morgenstern, D.A., Asher, R.A., Levine, J.M. and Fawcett, J.W. (1999) Expression of the chondroitin sulphate proteoglycan NG2 in normal and regenerating peripheral nerve. *Soc. Neurosci. Abstr.*, 25: 1264.

Naso, M.F., Zimmermann, D.R. and Iozzo, R.V. (1994) Characterization of the complete genomic structure of the human versican gene and functional analysis of its promoter. *J. Biol. Chem.*, 269: 32999–33008.

Niederöst, B.P., Zimmerman, D.R., Schwab, M.E. and Bandtlow, C.E. (1999) Bovine CNS myelin contains neurite growth-inhibitory activity associated with chondroitin sulfate proteoglycans. *J. Neurosci.*, 19: 8979–8989.

Nishiyama, A., Lin, X.-H. and Stallcup, W.B. (1995) Generation of truncated forms of the NG2 proteoglycan by cell surface proteolysis. *Mol. Biol. Cell*, 6: 1819–1832.

Nishiyama, A., Chang, A. and Trapp, B.D. (1999) NG2+ glial cells: a novel glial cell population in the adult brain. *J. Neuropathol. Exp. Neurol.*, 58: 1113–1124.

Oakley, R.A. and Tosney, K.W. (1991) Peanut agglutinin and chondroitin-6-sulfate are molecular markers for tissues that act as barriers to axon advance in the avian embryo. *Dev. Biol.*, 147: 187–206.

Oleszewski, M., Gutwein, P., von Der Lieth, W., Rauch, U. and Altevogt, P. (2000) Characterization of the L1-neurocan binding site. Implications for L1–L1 homophilic binding. *J. Biol. Chem.*, 275: 34478–34485.

Oohira, A., Matsui, F. and Katoh-Semba, R. (1991) Inhibitory effects of brain chondroitin sulfate proteoglycans on neurite outgrowth from PC12D cells. *J. Neurosci.*, 11: 822–827.

Oohira, A., Matsui, F., Watanabe, E., Kushima, Y. and Maeda, N. (1994) Developmentally regulated expression of a brain specific species of chondroitin sulfate proteoglycan, neurocan, identified with a monoclonal antibody IG2 in the rat cerebrum. *Neuroscience*, 60: 145–157.

Paulus, W., Baur, I., Dours-Zimmermann, M.T. and Zimmermann, D.R. (1996) Differential expression of versican isoforms in brain tumors. *J. Neuropathol. Exp. Neurol.*, 55: 528–533.

Peles, E., Nativ, M., Campbell, P.L., Sakurai, T., Martinez, R., Lev, S., Clary, D.O., Schilling, J., Barnea, G. and Plowman, G.D. et al. (1995) The carbonic anhydrase domain of receptor tyrosine phosphatase beta is a functional ligand for the axonal cell recognition molecule contactin. *Cell*, 82: 251–260.

Perides, G., Rahemtulla, F., Lane, W.S., Asher, R.A. and Bignami, A. (1992) Isolation of a large aggregating proteoglycan from human brain. *J. Biol. Chem.*, 267: 23883–23887.

Perissinotto, D., Iacopetti, P., Bellina, I., Doliana, R., Colombatti, A., Pettway, Z., Bronner-Fraser, M., Shinomura, T., Kimata, K., Mörgelin, M., Löfberg, J. and Perris, R. (2000) Avian neural crest cell migration is diversely regulated by the two major hyaluronon-binding proteoglycans PG-M/versican and aggrecan. *Development*, 127: 2823–2842.

Pesheva, P. and Probstmeier, R. (2000) The yin and yang of tenascin-R in CNS development and pathology. *Prog. Neurobiol.*, 61: 465–493.

Pindzola, R.R., Doller, C. and Silver, J. (1993) Putative inhibitory extracellular matrix molecules at the dorsal root entry zone of the spinal cord during development and after root and sciatic nerve lesions. *Dev. Biol.*, 156: 34–48.

Pouly, S., Becher, B., Blain, M. and Antel, J.P. (1999) Expression of a homologue of rat NG2 on human microglia. *Glia*, 27: 259–268.

Rabchevsky, A.G., Weinitz, J.M., Coulpier, M., Fages, C., Tinel, M. and Junier, M.P. (1998) A role for transforming growth factor alpha as an inducer of astrogliosis. *J. Neurosci.*, 18: 10541–10552.

Rauch, U., Gao, P., Janetzko, A., Flaccus, A., Hilgenberg, L., Tekotte, H., Margolis, R.K. and Margolis, R.U. (1991) Isolation and characterization of developmentally regulated chondroitin sulfate and chondroitin/keratan sulfate proteoglycans of brain identified with monoclonal antibodies. *J. Biol. Chem.*, 266: 14785–14801.

Rauch, U., Karthikeyan, L., Maurel, P., Margolis, R.U. and Margolis, R.K. (1992) Cloning and primary structure of neurocan, a developmentally regulated, aggregating chondroitin sulfate proteoglycan of brain. *J. Biol. Chem.*, 267: 19536–19547.

Retzler, C., Wiedemann, H., Kulbe, G. and Rauch, U. (1996) Structural and electron microscopic analysis of neurocan and recombinant neurocan fragments. *J. Biol. Chem.*, 271: 17107–17113.

Rudge, J.S. and Silver, J. (1990) Inhibition of neurite outgrowth on astroglial scars in vitro. *J. Neurosci.*, 10: 3594–3603.

Sakurai, T., Lustig, M., Nativ, M., Hemperly, J.J., Schlessinger, J., Peles, E. and Grumet, M. (1997) Induction of neurite outgrowth through contactin and Nr-CAM by extracellular regions of glial receptor tyrosine phosphatase beta. *J. Cell Biol.*, 136: 907–918.

Schmalfeldt, M., Dours-Zimmermann, M.T., Winterhalter, K.H. and Zimmermann, D.R. (1998) Versican V2 is a major extracellular matrix component of the mature bovine brain. *J. Biol. Chem.*, 273: 15758–15764.

Schmalfeldt, M., Bandtlow, C.E., Dours-Zimmermann, M.T., Winterhalter, K.H. and Zimmermann, D.R. (2000) Brain derived versican V2 is a potent inhibitor of axonal growth. *J. Cell Sci.*, 113: 807–816.

Seidenbecher, C.I., Richter, K., Rauch, U., Fassler, R., Garner, C.C. and Gundelfinger, E.D. (1995) Brevican, a chondroitin sulfate proteoglycan of rat brain, occurs as secreted and cell surface glycosylphosphatidylinositol-anchored isoforms. *J. Biol. Chem.*, 270: 27206–27212.

Seidenbecher, C.I., Gundelfinger, E.D., Bockers, T.M., Trotter, J. and Kreutz, M.R. (1998) Transcripts for secreted and GPI-anchored brevican are differentially distributed in rat brain. *Eur. J. Neurosci.*, 10: 1621–1630.

Smith-Thomas, L.C., Fok-Seang, J., Stevens, J., Du, J.-S., Muir, E., Faissner, A., Geller, H.M., Rogers, J.H. and Fawcett, J.W. (1994) An inhibitor of neurite outgrowth produced by astrocytes. *J. Cell Sci.*, 107: 1687–1695.

Smith-Thomas, L.C., Stevens, J., Fok-Seang, J., Faissner, A., Rogers, J.H. and Fawcett, J.W. (1995) Increased axon regeneration in astrocytes grown in the presence of proteoglycan synthesis inhibitors. *J. Cell Sci.*, 108: 1307–1315.

Snow, D.M., Lemmon, V., Carrino, D.A., Caplan, A.I. and Silver, J. (1990a) Sulfated proteoglycans in astroglial barriers inhibit neurite outgrowth in vitro. *Exp. Neurol.*, 109: 111–130.

Snow, D.M., Steindler, D.A. and Silver, J. (1990b) Molecular and cellular characterization of the glial roof plate of the spinal cord and optic tectum: a possible role for a proteoglycan in the development of an axon barrier. *Dev. Biol.*, 138: 359–376.

Snow, D.M., Brown, E.M. and Letourneau, P.C. (1996) Growth cone behavior in the presence of soluble chondroitin sulfate proteoglycan (CSPG), compared to behavior on CSPG bound to laminin or fibronectin. *Int. J. Dev. Neurosci.*, 14: 331–349.

Snyder, S.E., Li, J., Schauwecker, P.E., McNeill, T.H. and Salton, S.R. (1996) Comparison of RPTP zeta/beta, phosphacan, and trkB mRNA expression in the developing and adult rat nervous system and induction of RPTP zeta/beta and phosphacan mRNA following brain injury. *Mol. Brain Res.*, 40: 79–96.

Ughrin, Y. and Levine, J.M. (1999) Multiple globular domains of the NG2 proteoglycan core protein mediate neurite growth inhibition. *Soc. Neurosci. Abstr.*, 25: 748.

Yamada, H., Fredette, B., Shitara, K., Hagihara, K., Miura, R., Ranscht, B., Stallcup, W.B. and Yamaguchi, Y. (1997) The brain chondroitin sulfate proteoglycan brevican associates with astrocytes ensheathing cerebellar glomeruli and inhibits neurite outgrowth from granule neurons. *J. Neurosci.*, 17: 7784–7795.

Yamagata, M., Yamada, K.M., Yoneda, M., Suzuki, S. and Kimata, K. (1986) Chondroitin sulfate proteoglycan (PG-M-like proteoglycan) is involved in the binding of hyaluronic acid to cellular fibronectin. *J. Biol. Chem.*, 261: 13526–13535.

Yamagata, M., Suzuki, S., Akiyama, S.K., Yamada, K.M. and Kimata, K. (1989) Regulation of cell–substrate adhesion by proteoglycans immobilized on extracellular substrates. *J. Biol. Chem.*, 264: 8012–8018.

Yamaguchi, Y. (1996) Brevican: a major proteoglycan in adult brain. *Perspect. Dev. Neurobiol.*, 3: 307–317.

Yamaguchi, Y. (2000) Lecticans: organizers of the brain extracellular matrix. *Cell. Mol. Life Sci.*, 57: 276–289.

Yang, B.L., Zhang, Y., Cao, L. and Yang, B.B. (1999) Cell adhesion and proliferation mediated through the G1 domain of versican. *J. Cell. Biochem.*, 72: 210–220.

Yick, L.W., Wu, W., So, K.F., Yip, H.K. and Shum, D.K. (2000) Chondroitinase ABC promotes axonal regeneration of Clarke's neurons after spinal cord injury. *Neuroreport*, 11: 1063–1067.

Zako, M., Shinomura, T., Ujita, M., Ito, K. and Kimata, K. (1995) Expression of PG-M(V3), an alternatively spliced form of PG-M without a chondroitin sulfate attachment in region in mouse and human tissues. *J. Biol. Chem.*, 270: 3914–3918.

Zhang, Y., Cao, L., Yang, B.L. and Yang, B.B. (1998) The G3 domain of versican enhances cell proliferation via epidermal growth factor-like motifs. *J. Biol. Chem.*, 273: 21342–21351.

Zuo, J., Neubauer, D., Dyess, K., Ferguson, T.A. and Muir, D. (1998) Degradation of chondroitin sulfate proteoglycan enhances the neurite-promoting potential of spinal cord tissue. *Exp. Neurol.*, 154: 654–662.

L. McKerracher, G. Doucet and S. Rossignol (Eds.)
Progress in Brain Research, Vol. 137

CHAPTER 23

The extracellular matrix in axon regeneration

Barbara Grimpe and Jerry Silver [*]

Case Western Reserve University, School of Medicine, Department of Neurosciences, 10900 Euclid Avenue, Cleveland, OH 44106, USA

Introduction

In the mammalian central nervous system (CNS) dead neurons are usually not replaced and, in the majority of cases, injured axons do not regrow to their original targets. Although there is clear evidence of an age-dependent decrease in the rate of central axonal elongation, as well as variability in the efficiency of growth among various CNS neurons (Vaudano et al., 1989; Snow et al., 1990; Letourneau et al., 1994; Condic, 2001), the failure of CNS neurons to re-establish disrupted connections is also thought to be due to an increasingly inhibitory nature of the mature CNS environment. In this chapter we will focus on a number of the primary extrinsic factors that are believed to play essential roles in the success or failure of CNS axon regeneration.

The differential response to injury in the adult versus embryonic brain appears to be linked to molecular alterations in both astrocytes and oligodendrocytes (Bandtlow et al., 1990). One of the important components of the cell's environment is the extracellular matrix (ECM) which has been shown to contain a mixture of both axon growth-inhibitory and growth-promoting molecules. The balance of these two opposing forces that act upon the cut axon

_____
[*] Correspondence to: J. Silver, Case Western Reserve University, School of Medicine, Department of Neurosciences, 10900 Euclid Avenue, Cleveland, OH, 44106, USA. Tel.: +1-216-368-2150; Fax: +1-216-368-4650; E-mail: jxs10@po.cwru.edu

helps to determine whether or not successful regeneration occurs. One of the major inhibitory molecular families of ECM molecules are the large chondroitin sulfate proteoglycans (CS-PG), sometimes also called the lecticans or hyaluronan-binding proteoglycans, such as aggrecan, versican, neurocan and brevican. Additional members of the CS-PGs are the NG2 proteoglycan and phosphacan. To another ECM proteoglycan family belong the small proteoglycans (decorin, biglycan, fibromodulin and lumican) as well as the cell-surface proteoglycans, the syndecan family (syndecan-1 to syndecan-4) (modified after Lander, 1993). However, the number of identified CS-PGs, especially in the CNS, is still growing and it remains unclear as to which of these many family members contributes to the decrease in axon regeneration potential that occurs as the CNS matures.

Another class of ECM molecules, which contain inhibitory as well as promoting effects, are the tenascins (tenascin-R, tenascin-C and tenascin-X). The members of this family are conserved in all vertebrates and may, therefore, be assumed to have functions that contribute to cell survival (Erickson, 1994) and regeneration. The second class of bifunctional molecules, that both attracts and repels axons, are the netrins (netrin-1 to netrin-3, β-netrin). The netrins are small molecules that are related to laminin. Finally, a family of molecules with activities that are especially relevant for regeneration failure in lesion models which allow for fibroblast migration into the CNS compartment are the semaphorins. However, the semaphorins are not part of the classical ECM family but some members have the ability to bind to the ECM. The semaphorins can exist as secreted, transmembrane or glycosylphosphatidylinositol (GPI)-linked molecules and they are comprised of eight main classes with different numbers of sub-members (semaphorin-1 to 7 plus semaphorin-V) (Pueschel et al., 1995).

A critical growth-promoting molecular family are the 15 so far known laminins (laminin-1 to laminin-15) which are members of one of the best studied, most potent, but least understood neurite outgrowth-promoting families that are believed to function in the CNS. Some members of this family have been shown repeatedly to be essential for growing cultured neurons but their role in vivo remains controversial. A family related to laminin and netrin are the laminets (laminets-1 and laminets-2) which are expressed in the hippocampus. However, a clear function for the newly discovered laminets is not known yet (Ying et al., 2000).

All these aforementioned molecules are hypothesized to be involved with regenerating neurons in the spinal cord as well as in the brain. A reduction of the purported inhibitors coupled with an attempt to stimulate support of a permissive environment for the regenerating neurons is now widely accepted to be an essential part of a strategy for promoting regeneration in the future. In this chapter we do not have enough space to discuss all of the cell types, which express these molecules, as well as all of the molecules that are part of the ECM. However, hopefully, we can give an overview about the most important ones and their function.

Cells during regeneration

Astrocytes

The major component of the glial scar is reactive astroglia, which form as a general reaction of the CNS to essentially any type of insult. It has become clear that the functional state of the reactive glial environment that develops after injury is in large part dictated not only by the state of maturation of the organism but also by the extent of blood brain barrier (BBB) leakage that occurs after the injury. Many types of CNS injuries, even those that are quite substantial, can lead to gliosis far distal to the area of injury that is associated with axonal plastic-

ity (which can be further enhanced with a variety of treatments) (Benowitz et al., 1999; Wenk et al., 1999; Weidner et al., 2001). Also, massive lesions that leave the BBB intact, even in mature animals, can result in axonal plasticity within the lesioned territory itself (e.g., chemical axotomy: Björklund et al., 1973; Nygren and Olson, 1977). Lesions that open the barrier lead to an environment in the territory of blood extravasation that is potently inhibitory (Fitch and Silver, 1997; Moon et al., 2000). The inhibitory state of the astroglial environment might develop because of a failure to synthesize and secrete appropriate growth-promoting ECM constituents and/or the cells may express excesses of growth-inhibitory molecules (Rudge and Silver, 1990; McKeon et al., 1991). It is important to stress that the initial molecular triggers of an inhibitory versus growth-promoting reactive glial environment in vivo are totally unknown. Thus far, only substrate bound β-amyloid (Aβ) has been found to be a potent trigger of the type of reactive extracellular matrix that plays a critical role in creating a functionally inhibitory state of the reactive astrocyte. In Alzheimer's diseased (AD) brain, reactive astrocytes are found in high abundance around molecularly heterogeneous cores of Aβ, which form the senile plaque. This reactive gliosis leads to the deposition of inhibitory molecules, such as sulfated proteoglycans (see below) which may play a role in creating and/or trapping dystrophic neurites within their territory (Canning et al., 1993, 1996; DeWitt and Silver, 1996).

It has now been well documented that proteoglycans within inhibitory reactive astroglial environments in vitro play a critical role in axon regeneration failure. Thus, the environment of three-dimensional cultures of relatively mature astrocytes (so-called 'glial noodles') whose proteoglycan containing ECM is densely packed into a tube via centrifugation does not allow for the penetration of axons (Fawcett et al., 1989; Fawcett and Asher, 1999). This occurs in spite of the fact that mature astrocytes cultured in monolayers, where the PG matrix lies underneath the cells, provide a good substrate for axonal growth (Noble et al., 1984; Smith and Silver, 1988; Fawcett et al., 1989; Smith et al., 1990; Fawcett and Asher, 1999). This suggests that a 3D, wall-like network of PG-rich astrocytes in vitro or those stimulated appropriately in two dimensions to make excesses of proteoglycan containing matrix (e.g., via β-amyloid) can take on functionally inhibitory characteristics that resemble what seems to be happening in the so-called 'glial scar' in vivo. In its final form, the glial scar consists mainly of a meshwork of astrocyte processes tightly interwoven, and bound together by tight and gap junctions that together with its inhibitory ECM might form an extremely potent physical as well as molecular barrier (Rudge and Silver, 1990; Fawcett and Asher, 1999).

Oligodendrocyte precursor cells (OPCs)

The adult CNS contains a continuous network of small cells that stain with an antibody to the proteoglycan NG2. These cells also express receptors for platelet-derived growth factor (PDGF) and basic fibroblast growth factor (bFGF, FGF-2). This combination of antigens identifies these cells as adult oligodendrocyte precursors (OPCs), which under certain circumstances can differentiate into either astrocytes or oligodendrocytes (Wolswijk and Noble, 1989). Therefore, they are widely distributed stem- or stem-like cells. These adult OPCs make up around 5–8% of the glial cell population in the CNS and they are abundant in both gray and white matter areas (Levine et al., 2001). However, they differ in terms of their motility, cell cycle duration and time course of differentiation from perinatal OPCs. Importantly, they are massively recruited to all types of traumatic CNS lesions and, therefore, they participate in the glial injury response. In addition to NG2, these cells also express other inhibitory proteoglycans such as phosphacan, versican and neurocan (Schnaedelbach et al., 1998; Asher et al., 2000). Therefore, oligodendrocyte precursors are identified as a major source of inhibition in the injured CNS.

Fibroblasts

Based on their morphology, spatiotemporal expression pattern and immunohistochemical profile, fibroblasts of meningeal origin are identified as the main nonneural cell types, which are recruited to all kinds of CNS lesions if the BBB is opened. Additionally, they are the main source for the expression of the first discovered member of the semaphorin family, Sema3A. Further molecules, which are expressed by meningeal cells are Sema3B, Sema3C, Sema3E, Sema3F, the V0 form of versican, a CS-PG of the lectican family, tenascin C, NG2 and keratan sulfate PG A (Ajemian et al., 1994; Levin, 1994; Hirsch and Bähr, 1999; Pasterkamp et al., 1999). For a long time, the only source for inhibitory molecules were thought to be oligodendrocytes and astrocytes; however, one must also add fibroblasts to the list.

In addition to scar-associated expression of semaphorins, specific populations of neurons show sustained or elevated semaphorin expression following CNS injury. Therefore, injured neurons may be an additional source of chemorepulsive semaphorins in the CNS. Following injury, damaged as well as intact neurons may release semaphorins at the injury site, thereby further enhancing the nonpermissive properties of CNS tissue (Pasterkamp et al., 1999).

The inhibitory ECM molecules during regeneration

Proteoglycans

The failure of adult mammalian spinal cord to support axonal regeneration has been attributed to an abundance of inhibitory proteoglycans, associated with glial cell surfaces and the surrounding ECM. These proteoglycans can be further grouped into subcategories. These are the heparan sulfate, chondroitin/dermatan sulfate as well as keratan sulfate proteoglycans which are classified as such depending on the configuration of their disaccharide units. Epimerization from the chondroitin sulfate glycosaminoglycan chains (GAGs) forms the dermatan sulfate proteoglycans, which in the form of decorin support the regeneration of axons by binding transforming growth factor-β (TGF-β).

One major group of inhibitory molecules is the chondroitin sulfate proteoglycans (CS-PGs). With their highly sulfated GAG chains, they are particularly abundant in the nervous system and are highly expressed in CNS injury sites during reactive gliosis. Evidence indicates that CSPGs can profoundly influence axonal development and regeneration. Certain CSPGs are growth-inhibitory molecules, which, at high concentrations relative to growth-promoting signals, may suppress axonal growth. Evidence strongly supports the idea that at least one mechanism by which CS-PGs inhibit regeneration is by binding laminin and, thereby, inhibiting laminin's neurite-promoting activity (Burg et al., 1996). This inhibitory mechanism might be an example of how GAG chains may be indirectly responsible for blocking regeneration. It is also possible that proteoglycans entrap regenerating axons by acting directly upon the growth cone to transform it into a dystrophic state.

The cryoculture model can be used as an index of the ability or inability of a given tissue to support axonal regeneration in vivo. In the cryoculture bioassay, neurons are cultured on sections of fresh/frozen tissues, which can be injured in the animal and treated with chondroitinase ABC during culturing. Embryonic dorsal root ganglia (DRGs) showed under such conditions an increase in their neurite outgrowth capacity in the chondroitinase ABC treated normal as well as injured spinal cord cryocultures in comparison to untreated cultures (Zuo et al., 1998).

Moreover, that CS-PGs are inhibitory molecules in vivo has been demonstrated via microtransplantation studies from our lab. Adult DRGs gently microtransplanted into normal or even degenerating white matter of the spinal cord were able to grow robustly until they reached the outer edges of the lesion. The inhibition of outgrowth of the microtransplanted DRGs correlated precisely with the presence of a CS-PG boundary (Davies et al., 1999). A further publication by Plant et al. (2001) showed that when Schwann cells were transplanted into the lesioned spinal cord increases in the expression of CS-PGs occurred at the caudal, in contrast to the rostral, cord–graft interface. Regenerating descending fibers crossed the proximal (rostral) interface into the Schwann cell graft; however, they failed to cross the distal (caudal) interface to enter the cord.

Importantly, recent studies have revealed that CSPG-degrading enzymes markedly increased neuritic regrowth in several models of regeneration failure. Two in vivo models described by Moon et al. (2001) and Bradbury et al. (2002) showed that degradation of CS-PGs using chondroitinase ABC enhanced CNS axon regeneration in the adult lesioned rat nigrostriatal tract and spinal cord. In the first model, severed dopaminergic nigral axons had grown through the injury site and along the course of the original nigrostriatal tract back to their original principal target (the ipsilateral striatum), where they branched. Other axons did not always grow directly toward the target but often grew ectopically, branching extremely frequently. In the second model, intrathecal treatment with chondroitinase ABC of the lesioned spinal cord promoted regeneration of ascending sensory projections and descending corticospinal tract axons with functional improvement. These two models show that degradation of chondroitin sulfate can render the environment of the damaged CNS more permissive to axon regeneration and it confirms that CS-PGs are a significant source of inhibition after CNS injury in vivo.

A further discussion of some specific inhibitory PGs

Aggrecan

Aggrecan belongs to the family of large proteoglycans (lecticans) that has been characterized predominantly as a component of the ECM of cartilage (Doege et al., 1991). Its domain structure is characteristic for the whole family. The N-terminus starts with the signal peptide followed by the Ig-like region and two tandem repeats. The middle part contains a non-homologous region, which varies in length between each member of this family. The C-terminus starts with an EGF-like domain followed by a lectin-like domain and then by a complement-like domain (Fig. 1).

It is now known that aggrecan is present in the developing brain (Schwartz et al., 1993) and it has also been identified recently in the adult brain (Milev et al., 1998). However, the brain-specific form differs from the cartilage form in its concentration of chondroitin sulfate and the absence of keratan sulfate (Krueger et al., 1992). The inhibitory function of aggrecan could be shown in vitro by Condic et al. (1999). Embryonic DRGs showed less profuse outgrowth on laminin with a low amount of aggrecan as a substrate after the first 3 h, in contrast to just laminin, a growth-promoting ECM molecule (which will be described later). The full-length aggrecan protein core is a normal constituent of the rat spinal cord in the embryo and throughout life and it is very similar to aggrecan in the intervertebral disc. Overall, aggrecan core protein content is significantly reduced after spinal cord injury (SCI) and, instead,

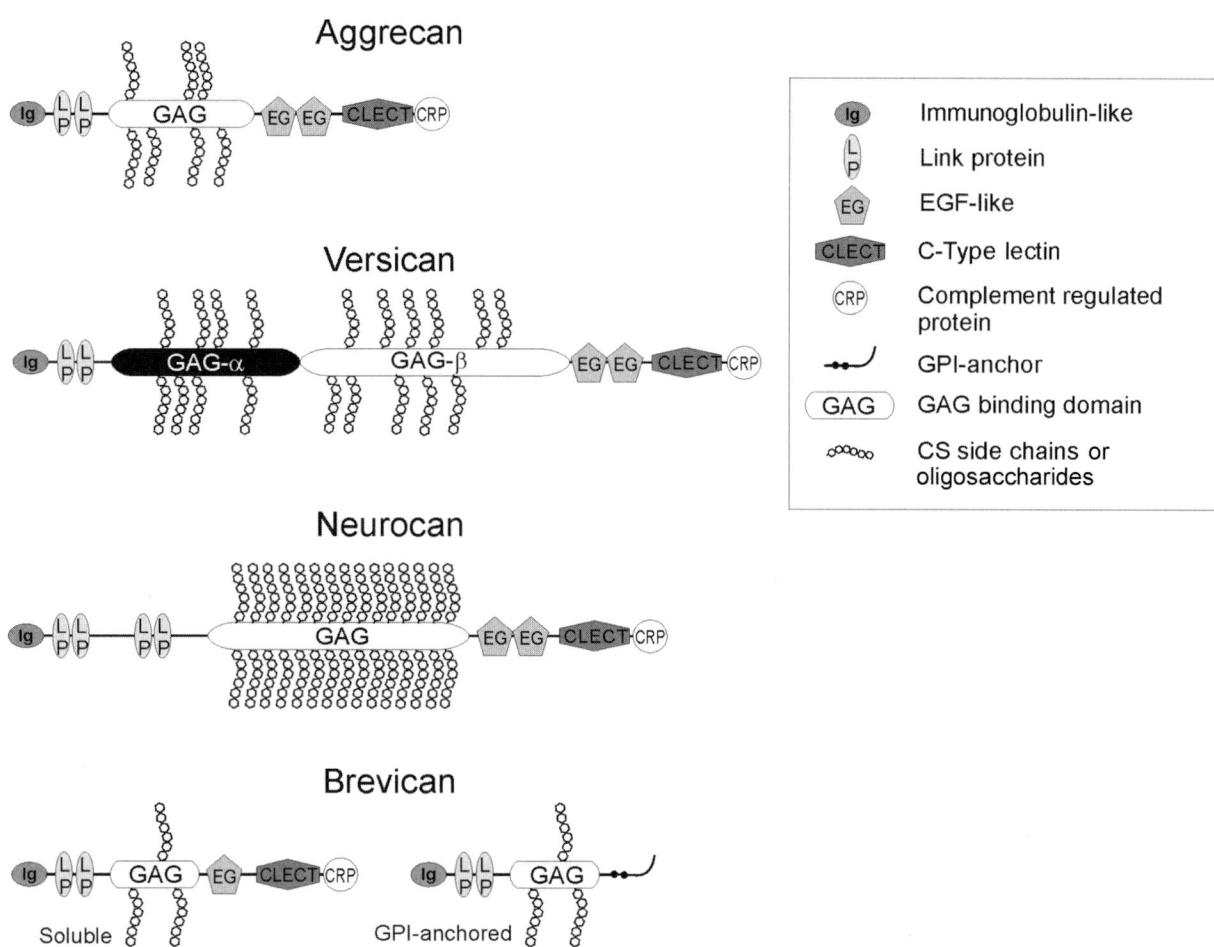

Fig. 1. Schematic presentation of the lectican family, which contains the following molecules: aggrecan, versican, neurocan and brevican. Each member is shown with its representative domains and CS chains. The figure is used with generous permission of Prof. Kuehn (Max Planck Institute, Germany).

fragments of aggrecan are present at 1 and 2 weeks after injury. Full-length aggrecan core protein is consistently undetectable at 1 week after injury. Its fragmentation is the result of an aggrecanase (ADAMTS family = a disintegrin and metalloproteinase with thrombospondin motifs), matrix metalloproteinases (MMP) or Cathepsin B (Cat B). SCI increased the expression of MMP-2 and MMP-9 after injury in vivo by activated microglia. The same MMPs are activated by astrocytes in vitro (Romanic et al., 1998). The increase in these enzymes may further contribute to an extended post-injury degradation of aggrecan. While full-length aggrecan is clearly inhibitory to axonal elongation, the role of aggrecan fragments in axon regeneration or its failure is unknown.

Versican

Versican (PG-M) is the second member of this family discovered in mesenchymal tissue. It exists in four splice forms. Fibroblasts mainly express the V0 form, which contains 31 potential chondroitin sulfate binding sites, nine possible N-glycosylation sites and 45 threonin-O-glycosylation sites. Proliferating keratinocytes express the V1 form (Zimmermann et al., 1994), whereas brain tissue synthesizes the V2 form (Perides et al., 1992). The V2 form is present in the normal CNS in white matter, and is upregulated after injuries (Perides et al., 1995). In vitro it is produced by OPCs, but lost in mature oligodendrocytes. The binding partners of versican are laminin, fibronectin, collagen I and hyaluronic acid. Veriscan's role as an inhibitor to axon regeneration has not yet been resolved. This statement is based on the fact that versican and CS-56 antigen are present on monolayers of the inhibitory astrocyte cell line Neu7 as discontinuous patches. However, growing axons show no sign of avoiding these patches. On the other side of the debate, Niederöst et al. (1999) showed that putative oligodendrocyte inhibitory components other than MAG and bNI-220 of bovine CNS myelin have neurite growth-inhibitory activity and that one of these repulsive activities is via versican V2. It is purported to be one of the main constituents by which oligodendrocytes inhibit neurite outgrowth from cerebellar granule cells and DRG neurons in vitro. Versican V2 is localized on the surface of highly branched oligodendrocytes. These cells have been demonstrated to evoke contact-mediated collapse and retraction of growth cones. Importantly, oligodendrocytes grown in the presence of proteoglycan synthesis inhibitors are less inhibitory for neurite growth than untreated cells. The other inhibitory activity in the bovine CNS myelin fraction is brevican, which will be discussed later.

Neurocan

Neurocan was the first member of this family to be expressed for certain in the CNS. Although initially localized to neurons, neurocan is also expressed by reactive astrocytes (Rauch et al., 1991; Oohira et al., 1994; McKeon et al., 1999) or OPCs (Fawcett and Asher, 1999). The concentration of neurocan in brain increases during late embryonic development but then declines during the early postnatal period together with hyaluronic acid. It interacts with Ng-CAM, N-CAM, tenascin-C and tenascin-R as a binding partner to help form the meshwork of ECM in the CNS. It also binds bFGF (FGF-2) on its core protein and can indirectly contribute to neurite outgrowth, cell migration and differentiation. In 7 day old rats, neurocan is cleaved into ~250 kDa, ~150 kDa, ~130 kDa and ~90 kDa fragments at proteolytic cleavage sites. The ~130 kDa and ~90 kDa fragments are derived from the N-terminus portion of neurocan. The ~150 kDa fragment (also designated as neurocan-C) is the major component in the rat brain after 2 to 3 weeks, even after its mRNA starts to vanish around P14. As one of the major inhibitory

molecules for neurite outgrowth, neurocan plays a role in modulating cell adhesion during development of the CNS. Neurocan first appears in the spinal cord at E16–E19. In adult animals the expression of neurocan in astrocytes after a unilateral knife lesion to the cerebral cortex or after an entorhinal cortex lesion was substantially increased around the lesion or in the fascia dentata in comparison to the uninjured side (Haas et al., 1999; Asher et al., 2000). Also, in the entorhinal cortex lesion model, this upregulation could be already detected after 2 days. Unpublished results from our group confirm an upregulation of neurocan in the spinal cord, two days after injury.

Brevican

Brevican is the smallest member of this family, with a size of 145 kDa. It is only expressed in the CNS (Yamada et al., 1994). Here it participates in forming the ECM. On the other hand, brevican exists as an isoform connected by a GPI anchor to the cell membrane (Seidenbecher et al., 1995). This ECM molecule contains two potential N-glycosylation sites and thirteen potential CS binding sites. In contrast, the GPI-linked cell membrane form lacks the glycosylation sites. Brevican could not be detected in 30-day chronic lesions in the cortex of implanted nitrocellulose membranes. In this particular case reactive astrocytes did not express this molecule. However, others assume that brevican is expressed by glial cells (McKeon et al., 1999) which might be cells from the OPC lineage. In contrast, it could be detected and was upregulated by astrocytes in the fascia dentata, 10 days after entorhinal cortex lesion (Thon et al., 2000). A stab injury to the mature brain leads also to an upregulation of brevican in a subset of reactive astrocytes (Jaworski et al., 1999). While brevican is expressed in the normal mature rat brain as both secreted and cell-surface GPI-anchored isoforms; only the secreted isoform is upregulated during reactive gliosis. The developing and adult spinal cord expresses brevican in the same amount as was shown in the brain. Brevican appears to accumulate with age in the CNS (Milev et al., 1998).

As mentioned earlier, brevican is one of the inhibitory components of the proteoglycan-enriched bovine CNS myelin fraction. Immunodepletion of brevican together with versican V2 resulted in a significant loss of the inhibitory activity in this fraction. Brevican was, like versican V2, expressed by oligodendrocytes. However, chondroitin sulfate glycosaminoglycan (CS-GAG) chains of brevican and versican V2 seem to have only moderate influence on the inhibitory activity (Niederöst et al., 1999).

Phosphacan

Phosphacan, is a CNS-specific CS-PG. However, it is not a member of the lectican family. It exists as an alternative splice variant of the gene that also encodes two isoforms of the receptor tyrosine phosphatase β (RPTP-ζ/β). A third probable splice variant (phosphacan-KS) differs by a deletion in the extracellular region of an 860 amino acid sequence adjacent to the membrane and contains both chondroitin sulfate and keratan sulfate chains in the postnatal rat CNS (Fig. 2). Phosphacan-KS appears to account for some but not all of the detectable keratan sulfates in brain. It also has been shown that

macrophages are a source of KS-PGs (Jones and Tuszynski, 2002). It should be re-emphasized that KS-PGs have also been shown to be potent inhibitors of axon regeneration (Letourneau et al., 1994). As a secreted CS-PG, phosphacan lacks the transmembrane and cytoplasmic domains of the RPTP-ζ/β isoforms and therefore represents the entire extracellular domain of this phosphatase. It is produced by astroglial cells and OPCs in the central nervous system and binds reversibly to N-CAM, Ng-CAM as well as tenascin. Additionally, it can bind bFGF (FGF-2). Phosphacan is a potent inhibitor of neuronal and glial adhesion and of neurite outgrowth. The concentrations of both phosphacan and phosphacan-KS rise steadily after E20 to reach a peak by ~2 weeks postnatal, and remains at these levels through adulthood. In the embryonic CNS the distribution of phosphacan mRNA is primarily present in regions of active cell proliferation. In adult animals after an incision of the cortex with a scalpel blade and insertion of a nitrocellulose membrane, the reactive astrocytes in

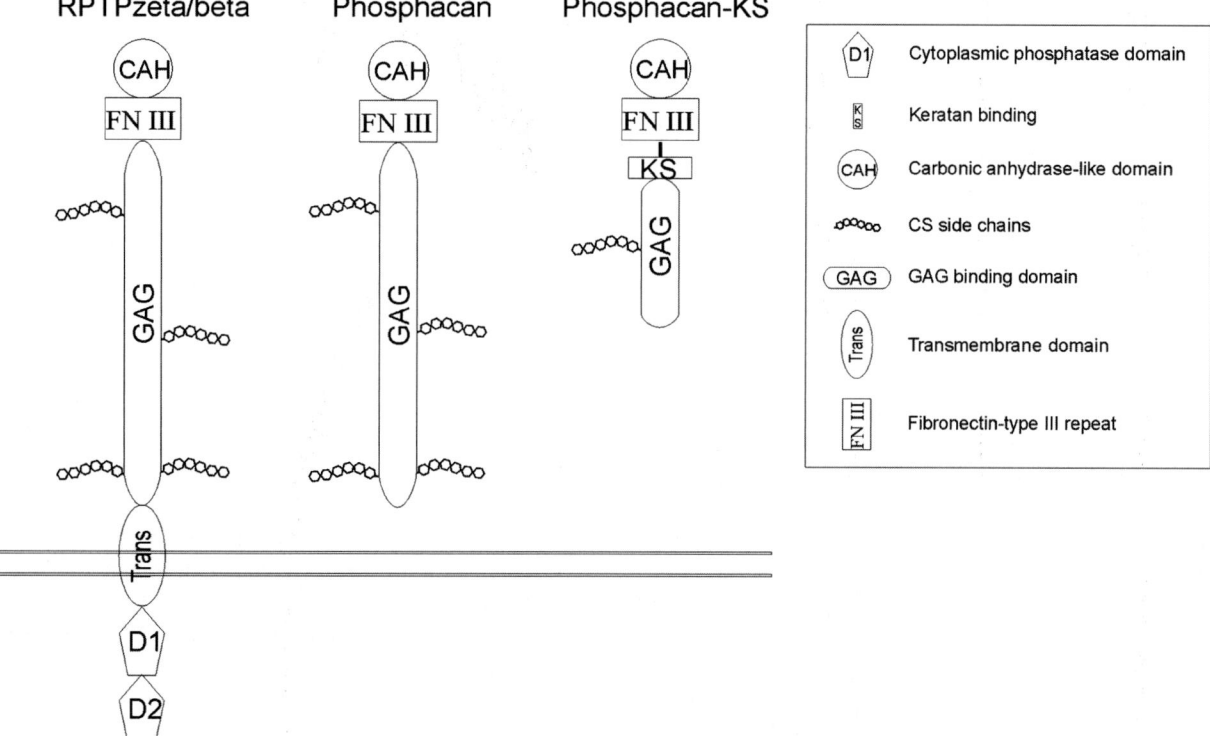

Fig. 2. Schematic presentation of three members of the phosphacan family. Phosphacan and phosphacan-KS are CNS-specific PGs. They are splice variants of RPTP-ζ/β, which is a tyrosine phosphatase.

this chronic CNS glial tissue are a continuing source of phosphacan expression (McKeon et al., 1999).

NG2

NG2 immunoreactive cells are found in large quantities recruited to CNS injury after about 4 days, and these cells are probably OPCs. In addition, astrocytes in spinal cord injuries have been shown to express NG2. Purified NG2 is inhibitory to the growth of both sensory and cerebellar axons. This was shown by an astrocyte cell line, which is inhibitory to axon growth (Neu7). This inhibitory activity was dependent on the production of a CS-PG with laminin-blocking activity (Smith-Thomas et al., 1994). Neutralization of NG2 with a blocking antibody could remove most of the inhibitory activity of the cells. Fractions containing NG2 with CS chains attached showed the inhibitory activity, but fractions containing NG2 without GAG chains were not inhibitory (Fidler et al., 1999).

Decorin

Decorin belongs to the small dermatan sulfate proteoglycans and is secreted in the environment (Fig. 3). It is found as a natural component of the extracellular matrix of most tissues, including those of the CNS. This molecule neutralizes all isoforms of TGF-β by binding the ligand to its core protein (Yamaguchi et al., 1990). TGF-βs have been implicated in numerous CNS pathologies in which fibrosis (i.e., fibroblast invasion) and neural dysfunction are causally associated. For example, decorin is present in posttraumatic brain and spinal cord scarring and hemorrhagic stroke. TGF-βs may also promote development of plaques which are laden with proteoglycans in the reactive glial penumbra of AD and Down's syndrome (DeWitt and Silver, 1996). In all of these conditions, the levels of TGF-β are raised in both the cerebrospinal fluid (CSF) and also locally in damaged neural tissue. Raised levels of TGF-β are correlated with the deposition of fibrotic scar material in brain lesions, while immunoneutralization with TGF-β antibodies markedly inhibits fibrogenic scarring (Logan et al., 1999). After CNS injury, decorin is synthesized by astrocytes in the damaged neuropil (Stichel et al., 1995). There-

fore, rats treated with excesses of decorin, 14 days following lesion of the cerebral cortex, showed an absence of the glia limitans in the scar. Additionally, in the absence of fibroblasts, the numerous activated astroglia neither organized into the expected limiting membrane of the scar nor laid down a laminin-rich basal lamina in the wound. In addition, little or no fibronectin was deposited. In untreated animals the gliotic scars contracted into a dense permanent trilaminar glial/fibrotic complex of fibronectin and collagen. Viable neural tissue was bordered by a laminin-rich basal lamina of the glia limitans. Therefore, decorin is a naturally occurring regulator of TGF-β bioactivity to limit gliosis.

Bi-potential inhibitor and promoter molecules of the ECM

Tenascin

The tenascin family contains three members, tenascin-C (J1, cytotactin, hexabrachion), tenascin-R (J1-160/180, janusin, restrictin) and tenascin-X. Although, tenascin-C is synthesized within the CNS as well as in the periphery, tenascin-R is restricted to the CNS (Fig. 4). The latter is expressed by oligodendrocytes during myelination as well as by neurons during early development when active neurite outgrowth is occurring. The embryonic expression of tenascin-X suggests a role in limb, muscle, and heart development. The tenascins are a large, multi-functional class of six-armed molecules and are distinguished by identical homologue domains. A monomer contains a globular domain on the N-terminus, which is followed by heptad-repeats. Adjacent to these, a variable number of EGF-like domains are followed by fibronectin-type III repeats. The C-terminus contains a fibrinogen-like domain. The tenascin family embodies both stimulatory and anti-adhesive or inhibitory properties for axon growth (Faissner et al., 1994). Indeed, tenascin-R has been shown to be adhesive for astrocytes and repellent towards neurons and growth cones (Pesheva and Probstmeier, 2000).

During development, tenascin-C is predominantly expressed by glia (Bartsch et al., 1992; Zhang et al., 1995), but like tenascin-R also by some neurons (Zhang et al., 1995), and thereafter, glial expression

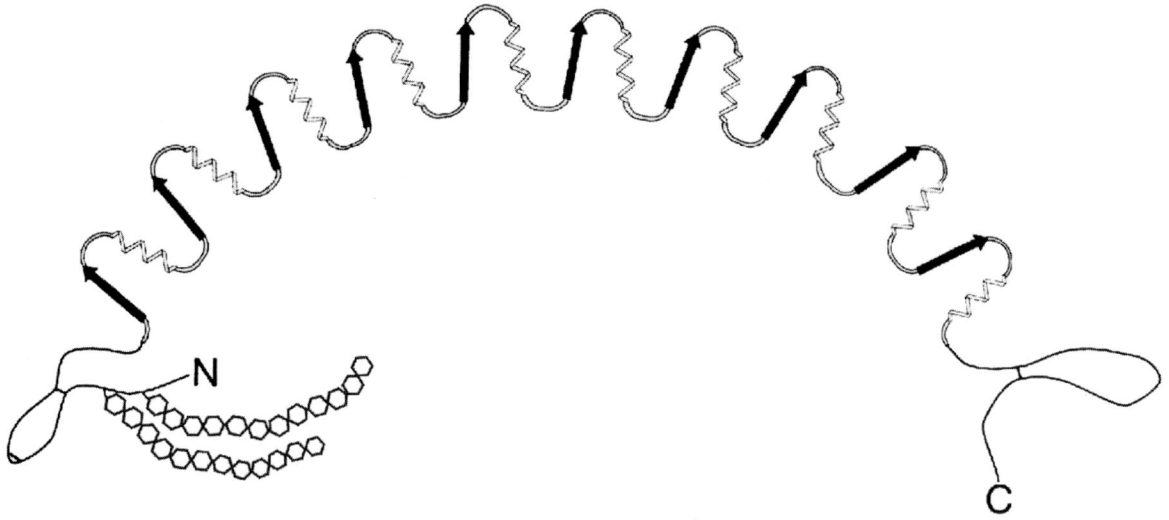

Fig. 3. The decorin molecule belongs to the small CS-PGs and supports the regeneration of neurons in the spinal cord by binding TGFBs. The figure is used with generous permission of Prof. Kuehn (Max Planck Institute, Germany).

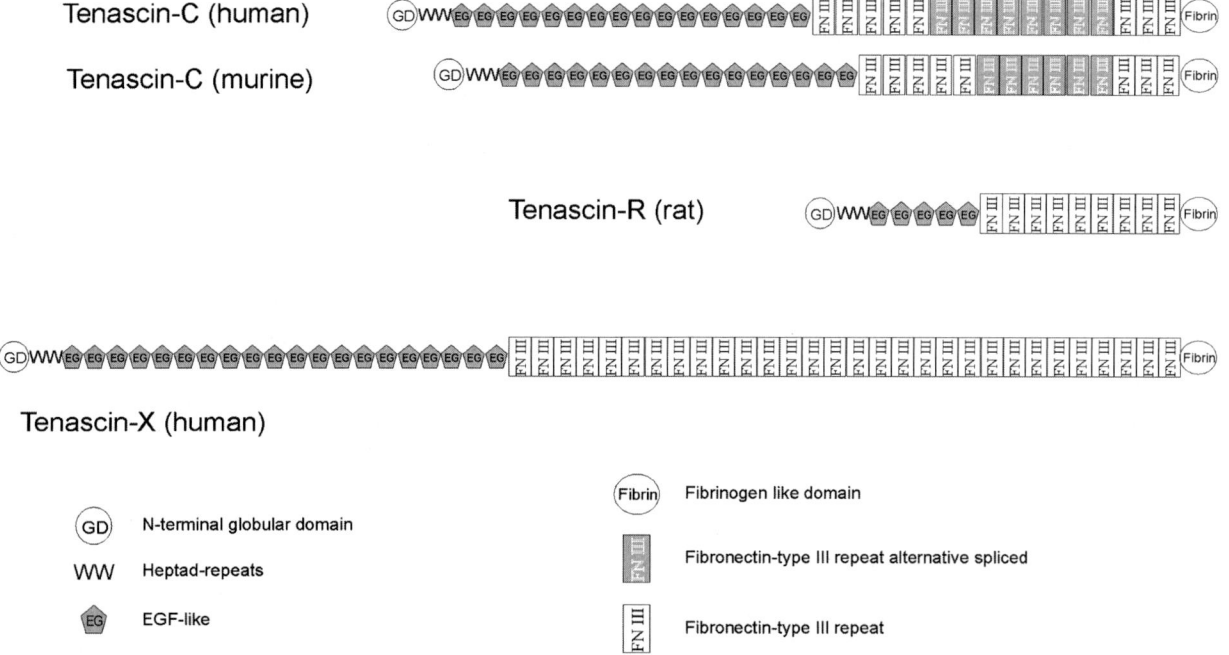

Fig. 4. The tenascin family contains three members in mammals: tenascin-C, tenascin-R and tenascin-X. At the EM level tenascin-C exists as a six-armed molecule which is connected by a central knot of disulfide bridges between the heptad-repeats.

is down-regulated. In contrast, neuronal expression continues to exist into the adult brain. Tenascin-C is reexpressed by astrocytes following injury to some parts of the CNS but only to a limited extent. It is found within and around injuries to the neocortex (McKeon et al., 1991) and the cerebellum (Laywell et al., 1992) always bordering such lesions (Ajemian et al., 1994). When mammalian optic nerve is severed there is little increase of tenascin-C immunore-activity except on leptomeningeal cells and some capillaries (Bartsch et al., 1992). In the intact spinal cord of the rat, tenascin-C is strongly expressed during early postnatal development but in the adult, the protein is confined to irregular patches in the ventral horn around motor neurons, a narrow zone around the central canal, and a thin layer adjacent to the pia mater (Zhang et al., 1995). Following severe dorsal root injury that also slightly damages the cord, tenascin-C is upregulated by astrocytes in the dorsal root entry zone (Pindzola et al., 1993) and in the dorsal column containing axons undergoing Wallerian degeneration (Zhang et al., 1995). Reexpression is rapid, occurring already 1 day after lesion. Additionally, Zhang et al., 1997 could show that most cells that express tenascin-C mRNA in the spinal cord around the lesion and in the degenerating dorsal columns are GFAP[+] astrocytes. All three tenascins were found to be expressed at elevated levels in the spinal cord lesion area. The signal for a splice form of tenascin-R, J1, was clearly elevated at 5 days after the injury and reached a peak 7 days after the lesion. The expression of tenascin-R was confined to a few small cells in the developing scar tissue and reached a maximum about 1 week after the injury. An obvious increase in the signal for tenascin-X, however, was first detected at 7 days after the lesion and a strong expression was maintained at 3 weeks after the operation. The labeling for tenascin-X corresponded to persisting macrophages or invading leptomeningeal cells.

Netrins

The netrins are a family of secreted proteins. The N-termini of netrin-1 to netrin-3 ($\sim$450 amino acids) are related to the N-terminus of the laminin γ1-chain; however, β-netrin, a new member of this family, has a homologous region to the β-chain of laminin. The related subunits include domain VI and the three epidermal growth factor (EGF)-like repeats in domain V of laminin (in netrins called domains V-1, V-2 and V-3). The C-terminal $\sim$159 amino acids domain diverges from laminins (Mitchell et al., 1996)

Netrins are expressed embryonically by the floorplate in vertebrates and were originally identified as diffusible molecules that play a role in guiding commissural axons toward the ventral midline. Additionally, they can form a bound ventral to dorsal gradient in the developing spinal cord. Therefore, netrins are bifunctional in both nematodes and vertebrates, playing roles as chemoattractants for axons extending toward the ventral midline (developing spinal commissural axons) and chemorepellents for axons growing away from it (developing rat trochlear motor neurons) (Manitt et al., 2001).

It is now known that netrin-1 is constitutively expressed by neurons and oligodendrocytes in the adult rat spinal cord. However, the majority of the netrin-1 protein present in the adult spinal cord is not freely soluble but associated with membranes or ECM (Manitt et al., 2001). In a model of the injured adult rat retinal ganglion cells (RGC) the receptor for netrin-1, deleted in colorectal cancer (DCC), was down-regulated after axotomy and during regeneration in a peripheral nerve graft. This suggests that netrin may not contribute to RGC axon regeneration induced by a peripheral nerve graft (Ellezam et al., 2001).

Semaphorins

Semaphorins comprise a large family of secreted and membrane-associated proteins, categorized into eight classes based on distinctive structural features (Fig. 5). The conserved domains include, in addition to the signature semaphorin domain (sema), the N-terminal signal sequence (SS), the immunoglobulin c2-like domain (Ig) of classes 2, 3, 4 and 7, the thrombospondin repeats (TSP), in class 5 of the semaphorins, and the basic domain (BD) of class 3 semaphorins at the C-terminus. The latter might allow the semaphorins to associate with the ECM. It is known that class 3 semaphorins are homodimerized through cysteine disulfide bonds in the carboxyl region and/or through noncovalent interactions (Klostermann et al., 1998; Kopple and Raper, 1998). Dimerization appears to be crucial for the biological activity of semaphorins (Wong et al., 1999). Nowadays, more than 20 different semaphorins have been identified. In addition to domain organization within the primary structure, the semaphorins are classified by the species of origin. Classes 1 and 2 are invertebrate semaphorins, classes 2 through

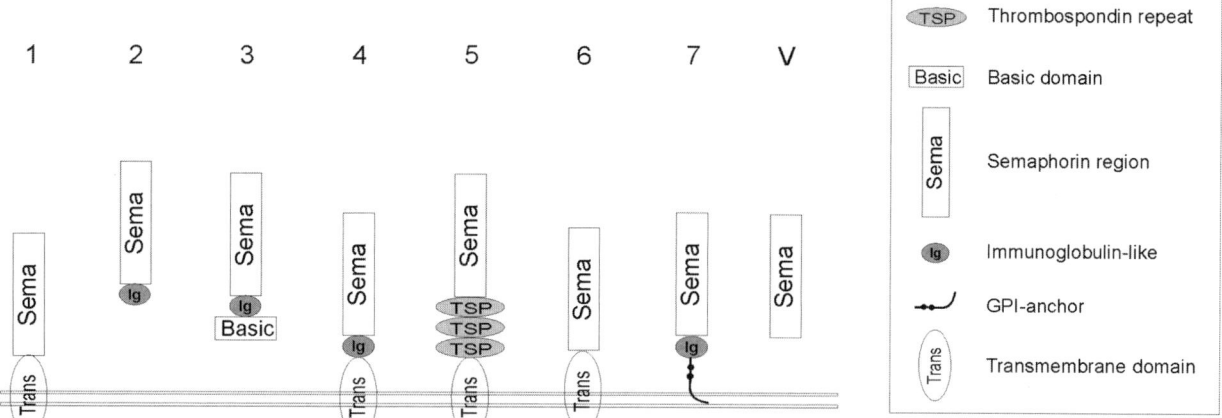

Fig. 5. The semaphorins are a family of eight members, which includes transmembrane, soluble and GPI-anchored forms (V stands for viral).

7 are vertebrate semaphorins, and class V is composed of viral semaphorins. Classes 1, 4, 5, and 6 are membrane-associated and possess transmembrane segments, whereas class 7 has a GPI-anchor motif. In contrast, classes 2, 3, and V are secreted proteins.

During neuroembryogenesis, class 3 semaphorins Sema3A (collapsin-1, semD/III) constitutes chemorepulsive barriers impermeable for axon growth. As development progresses, neural Sema3A mRNA expression declines to become restricted to distinct populations of neurons in the mature nervous system (Giger et al., 1996, 1998). Injury to the mature CNS can induce repulsive boundaries similar to those observed during development.

Stab lesions were performed at different locations in the brain and spinal cord to examine the effect of CNS injuries on the expression of Sema3A. Because of its unique regenerative properties, putative injury-induced alterations of Sema3A mRNA expression were first studied in the mature olfactory system. Olfactory bulbectomy induced the proliferation and migration of fibroblasts, which express high levels of Sema3A mRNA. These fibroblasts occupied the core of the glial scar, tightly encapsulating all bundles of regenerating primary olfactory axons that had grown through the cribriform plate into the lesion site. In contrast to bulbectomy, axotomy of the olfactory nerve only induced local and transient Sema3A mRNA expression at the lesion.

Olfactory axons grew back towards their original targets, carefully circumventing areas of Sema3A in the lesion zone (Pasterkamp et al., 1998). Curiously, the spatial distribution of Sema3A transcripts is different following injuries to the spinal cord and other parts of the CNS. Following brain injuries, Sema3A cells, mostly fibroblasts, occupy most of the lesion site, while following spinal dorsal column transection expression of Sema3A mRNA is restricted to the dorsal and lateral parts of the lesion (Pasterkamp et al., 1998, 1999). This invites the speculation that in the injured spinal cord Sema3A may, instead of blocking axon regrowth across the scar, create an exclusion zone for regenerating dorsal column fibers in the most dorsal and lateral aspects of the lesion site. Such a molecular boundary could prevent dorsal column fibers from growing extensively into nonneuronal structures surrounding the spinal cord. Recently, several other secreted and transmembrane, chemorepulsive semaphorins were detected in the scar, suggesting the involvement of other members of the semaphorin gene family in axon regeneration as well.

The major promoter molecule of the ECM

Laminin

Laminins are a family of large glycoprotein components of the ECM with a potent neurite-promoting

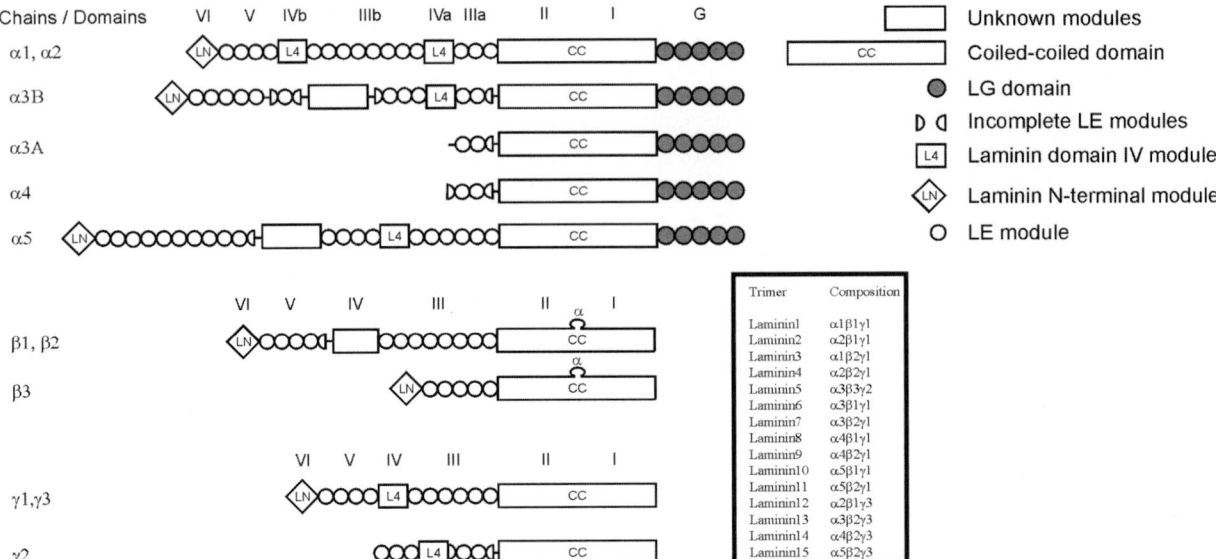

Fig. 6. The laminin family is comprised of a group of molecules, which strongly supports the outgrowth of neurons in vitro, in the peripheral nervous system as well as in the central nervous system. Each of the 15 laminin molecules are comprised of an α-, β- and γ-chain to form a trimer. The possible combinations are shown in the frame at the lower right side of the figure. The Roman numerals are the domain numbers of each chain. The figure is used with generous permission of Prof. Kuehn (Max Planck Institute, Germany).

function (Fig. 6). They play an important role in axonal growth and guidance in the developing nervous system as well as cell attachment and cell proliferation. The prevalence of laminin is also a major determinant of axonal growth in regenerative regions of CNS tissue (Timpl et al., 1979; Liesi, 1985). Each laminin molecule contains an α-, β- and γ-chain. Thus far, five α-chains, three β-chains and three γ-chains are known which form a cruciform structure in each laminin molecule. The γ3-chain was discovered most recently and leads to a tremendous increase in the possible members of this family (Koch et al., 1999). However, over the last decade the source of laminin expression especially in the CNS has been controversial. In nervous tissue, laminin is associated with Schwann and astroglial cells and is detectable primarily in extracellular locations. In astrocytes, there appears to be an interesting and unexpected inverse relationship between the intermediate filament protein, GFAP, and the amount of laminin that is produced (Menet et al., 2001). An intraneuronal localization of laminin has also been reported (Yamamoto et al., 1988; Hagg et al., 1989; Zhou, 1990; Junker et al., 1992), whereas others failed to find laminin-expression in CNS neurons

(Eriksdotter-Nilsson et al., 1986; Hunter et al., 1992; Alonso and Privat, 1993). Additionally, it is now recognized that adult astrocytes can produce the same type of supportive molecules as do young astrocytes, in this case laminin (Liesi et al., 1984). During development of the mouse olfactory nerve, laminin expression is found along the primitive glial fibers and in close spatial and temporal relationship with early growing axons. However, positive staining for laminin in the adult CNS is rare.

Our group has shown that laminin expression is found in the juvenile hippocampus in P4 animals and reduction of the γ1-chain of laminin has a dramatic effect on the regeneration of a particular neuron class, the mossy fibers (Grimpe et al., 2002). The γ1-chain of laminin is part of 10 of the so far known 15 members of this whole family. The pyramidal neurons of the hippocampus at age P4 but also in 1 year old animals express the γ1-chain of laminin and transport this chain in their apical dendrite. Additionally, in adult animals a punctate form of laminin γ1-chain expression could be clearly found in the stratum lucidum. The stratum lucidum is the area that mossy fibers use during their outgrowth in P0 to P21 old animals. To understand the possible function of laminin γ1-chain in axon regeneration within this pathway (and because the corresponding knockout mouse is lethal), we have manipulated laminin synthesis at the mRNA level using antisense technology and DNA enzymes. This was done to alter the γ1-chain in a slice culture model of the lesioned mossy system. In this model, early postnatal mossy fibers severed near the hilus can regenerate robustly across the lesion and elongate rapidly along their proper pathway. However, unlike controls, in the treated lesioned slices, the vast majority of regenerating mossy fibers could not cross the lesion site. The minority of axons that did, were very much shorter than in the mixed base treated or untreated slices and they took a disorganized course. This model offers the possibility to analyze and characterize the function of laminins during juvenile development or early regeneration. Information on the function or expression of laminins with exception of the glia limitans during scar formation in spinal cord is not available.

In summary

This review of ECM molecules shows quite clearly the function of the ECM in development but more importantly in the mature CNS after injury. Most of the proteoglycans, especially the large CS-PGs, are able to inhibit neurite outgrowth and in vivo experiments are now in progress to specifically inhibit these important molecules. The nature of growth promoter ECM molecules in the CNS after injury, either within or distant from the injury is now becoming better appreciated and we suggest that the laminin family should be important targets for exploration. Indeed, a better understanding of the interaction of laminin with those ECM components that are inhibitory is a clear goal for the future. Our ultimate aim must be to change the balance of factors at lesion sites to allow the more permissive environment after CNS injury to predominate.

Abbreviations

Aβ	β-amyloid
AD	Alzheimer disease
ADAMTS	*a d*isintegrin *a*nd *m*etalloproteinase with *t*hrombo*s*pondin motifs
BBB	blood brain barrier
BD	basic domain
CNS	central nervous system
CS	chondroitin sulfate
CSF	cerebrospinal fluid
DCC	deleted in colorectal cancer
DRG	dorsal root ganglion
E	embryonal day
ECM	extracellular matrix
EGF	epidermal growth factor
EM	electron microscope
FGF	fibroblast growth factor (b = basic)
GAG	glycosaminoglycan chains
GFAP	glial fibrillar acidic protein
GPI	glycosylphosphatidylinositol
Ig	immunoglobulin
kDa	kilo dalton
KS	keratan sulfate
LE	laminin-like epidermal growth factor like
LG	laminin G
MMP	matrix metalloproteinase
N-CAM	neuronal cell adhesion molecule
Ng-CAM	neuronal/glial cell adhesion molecule
OPC	oligodendrocyte precursor cell
PDGF	platelet-derived growth factor
PG	proteoglycan
RGC	retinal ganglion cells
RPTP	receptor tyrosine phosphatase
TGF	transforming growth factor
TSP	thrombospondin repeats
SCI	spinal cord injury
SS	signal sequence

References

Ajemian, A., Ness, R. and David, S. (1994) Tenascin in the injured rat optic nerve and in non-neuronal cells in vitro: Potential role in neural repair. *J. Comp. Neurol.*, 340: 233–242.

Alonso, G. and Privat, A. (1993) Reactive astrocytes involved in the formation of lesional scars differ in the mediobasal hypothalamus and in other forebrain regions. *J. Neurosci. Res.*, 34: 523–538.

Asher, R.A., Morgenstern, D.A., Fidler, P.S., Adock, K.H., Oohira, A., Braistead, J.E., Levine, J.M., Margolis, R.U., Rogers, J.H. and Fawcett, J.W. (2000) Neurocan is upregulated in injured brain and in cytokine-treated astrocytes. *J. Neurosci.*, 20: 2427–2438.

Bandtlow, C., Zachleder, T. and Schwab, M.E. (1990) Oligodendrocytes arrest neurite growth by contact inhibition. *J. Neurosci.*, 10: 3837–3848.

Bartsch, U., Bartsch, S., Dörries, U. and Schachner, M. (1992) Immunohistological localization of tenascin in the developing and lesioned mouse optic nerve. *Eur. J. Neurosci.*, 4: 338–352.

Benowitz, L.I., Goldberg, D.E., Madsen, J.R., Soni, D. and Irwin, N. (1999) Inosine stimulates extensive axon collateral growth in the rat corticospinal tract after injury. *Proc. Natl. Acad. Sci. USA*, 96: 13486–13490.

Björklund, A. and Stenevi, U. (1979) Regeneration of monoaminergic and cholinergic neurons in the central nervous system. *Physiol. Rev.*, 59: 62–100.

Björklund, A., Nobin, A. and Stenevi, U. (1973) Regeneration of central serotonin neurons after axonal degeneration induced by 5,6-dihydroxytryptamine. *Brain Res.*, 50: 214–220.

Bradbury, E.J., Moon, L.D., Popat, R.J., King, V.R., Bennett, G.S., Patel, P.N., Fawcett, J.W. and McMahon, S.B. (2002) Chondroitinase ABC promotes functional recovery after spinal cord injury. *Nature*, 416: 636–640.

Burg, M.A., Tillet, E., Timpl, R. and Stallcup, W.B. (1996) Binding of the NG2 proteoglycan to type VI collagen and other extracellular matrix molecules. *J. Biol. Chem.*, 271: 26110–26116.

Canning, D.R., McKeon, R.J., DeWitt, D.A., Perry, G., Wujek, J.R., Frederickson, R.C.A. and Silver, J. (1993) β-amyloid of Alzheimer's disease induces reactive gliosis that inhibits axonal outgrowth. *Exp. Neurol.*, 124: 289–298.

Canning, D.R., Höke, A., Malemud, C.J. and Silver, J. (1996) A potent inhibitor of neurite outgrowth that predominates in the extracellular matrix of reactive astrocytes. *Int. J. Dev. Neurosci.*, 14: 153–176.

Condic, M.L. (2001) Adult neuronal regeneration induced by transgenic integrin expression. *J. Neurosci.*, 21: 4782–4788.

Condic, M.L., Snow, D.M. and Letourneau, P.C. (1999) Embryonic neurons adapt to the inhibitory proteoglycan aggrecan by increasing integrin expression. *J. Neurosci.*, 19: 10036–10043.

Davies, S.J., Goucher, D.R., Doller, C. and Silver, J. (1999) Robust regeneration of adult sensory axons in degenerating white matter of the adult rat spinal cord. *J. Neurosci.*, 19: 5810–5822.

DeWitt, D. and Silver, J. (1996) Regenerative failure: a potential mechanism for neuritic dystrophy in Alzheimer's Disease. *Exp. Neurol.*, 142: 103–110.

Doege, K., Sasaki, M., Horigan, E., Hassell, J.R. and Yamada, Y. (1991) Complete coding sequence and deduced primary structure of the human cartilage large aggregating proteoglycan, aggrecan. Human specific repeats and additional alternatively spliced forms. *J. Biol. Chem.*, 266: 29232–29240.

Ellezam, B., Selles-Navarro, I., Manitt, C., Kennedy, T.E. and McKerracher, L. (2001) Expression of netrin-1 and its receptors DCC and UNC-5H2 after axotomy and during regeneration of adult rat retinal ganglion cells. *Exp. Neurol.*, 168: 105–115.

Erickson, H.P. (1994) Evolution of the tenascin family — implications for function of the C-terminal fibrinogen-like domain. *Perspect. Dev. Neurobiol.*, 2: 9–19.

Eriksdotter-Nilsson, M., Björklund, H. and Olson, L. (1986) Laminin immunohistochemistry: a simple method to visualize and quantitate vascular structure in the mammalian brain. *J. Neurosci. Methods*, 17: 275–286.

Faissner, A., Scholze, A. and Gotz, B. (1994) Tenascin glycoproteins in developing neural tissues: Only decoration? *Perspect. Dev. Neurobiol.*, 2: 53–66.

Fawcett, J.W. and Asher, R.A. (1999) The glial scar and central nervous system repair. *Brain Res. Bull.*, 49: 377–391.

Fawcett, J.W., Housden, E., Smith-Thomas, L. and Meyer, R.L. (1989) The growth of axons in three-dimensional astrocyte cultures. *Dev. Biol.*, 135: 449–458.

Fidler, P.S., Schuette, K., Asher, R.A., Dobbertin, A., Thornton, S.R., Calle-Patino, Y., Muir, E., Levine, J.M., Geller, H.M., Rogers, J.H., Faissner, A. and Fawcett, J.W. (1999) Comparing astrocytic cell lines that are inhibitory or permissive for axon growth: The major axon-inhibitory proteoglycan is NG2. *J. Neurosci.*, 19: 8778–8788.

Fitch, M.T. and Silver, J. (1997) Activated macrophages and the blood–brain barrier: inflammation after CNS injury leads to increase in putative inhibitory molecules. *Exp. Neurol.*, 148: 587–603.

Giger, R.J., Wolfer, D.P., De Wit, G.M.J. and Verhaagen, J. (1996) Anatomy of rat semaphorin III/collapsin mRNA expression and relationship to developing nerve tracts during neuroembryogenesis. *J. Comp. Neurol.*, 375: 378–392.

Giger, R.J., Pasterkamp, R.J., Heijnen, S., Holtmaat, A.J.G.D. and Verhaagen, J. (1998) Anatomical distribution of the chemorepellent semaphorin III/collapsin-1 in the adult rat and human brain: predominant expression in structures of the olfactory–hippocampal pathway and motor system. *J. Neurosci. Res.*, 52: 27–43.

Grimpe, B., Dong, S., Doller, C., Temple, K., Malouf, A.T. and Silver, J. (2002) The critical role of basement membrane-independent laminin gamma 1 chain during axon regeneration in the CNS. *J. Neurosci.*, 22: 3144–3160.

Haas, C.A., Rauch, U., Thon, N., Merten, T. and Deller, T. (1999) Entorhinal cortex lesion in adult rats induces the expression of the neuronal chondroitin sulfate proteoglycan neurocan in reactive astrocytes. *J. Neurosci.*, 19: 9953–9963.

Hagg, T., Muir, D., Engvall, E., Varon, S. and Manthorpe, M. (1989) Laminin-like antigen in rat CNS neurons: distribution and changes upon brain injury and nerve growth factor treatment. *Neuron*, 3: 721–732.

Hirsch, S. and Bähr, M. (1999) Immunocytochemical characterization of reactive optic astrocytes and meningeal cells. *Glia*, 26: 36–46.

Hunter, D.D., Llinas, R., Ard, M., Merlie, J.P. and Sanes, J.R. (1992) Expression of s-laminin and laminin in the developing rat central nervous system. *J. Comp. Neurol.*, 323: 238–251.

Jaworski, D.M., Kelly, G.M. and Hockfield, S. (1999) Intracranial injury acutely induces the expression of the secreted isoform of the CNS-specific hyaluronan-binding protein BEHAB/brevican. *Exp. Neurol.*, 157: 327–337.

Jones, L.L., Tuszynski, M.H. (2002) Spinal cord injury elicits expression of keratan sulfate proteoglycans by macrophages, reactive microglia, and oligodendrocyte progenitors. *J. Neurosci.*, 22: 4611–4624.

Junker, M., Bialobok, P., Hagg, T. and Ingram, D.K. (1992)

Laminin immunohistochemistry in brain is dependent on method of tissue fixation. *Brain Res.*, 586: 166–170.

Klostermann, A., Lohrum, M., Adams, R.H. and Puschel, A.W. (1998) The chemorepulsive activity of the axonal guidance signal semaphorin D requires dimerization. *J. Biol. Chem.*, 273: 7326–7331.

Koch, M., Olson, P.F., Albus, A., Jin, W., Hunter, D.D., Brunken, W.J., Burgeson, R.E. and Champliaud, M.F. (1999) Characterization and expression of the laminin gamma 3 chain: a novel, non-basement membrane-associated, laminin chain. *J. Cell Biol.*, 145: 605–618.

Kopple, A.M. and Raper, J.A. (1998) Collapsin-1 covalently dimerizes, and dimerization is necessary for collapsing activity. *J. Biol. Chem.*, 273: 15708–15713.

Krueger Jr., R.C., Hennig, A.K. and Schwartz, N.B. (1992) Two immunologically and developmentally distinct chondroitin sulfate proteoglycans in embryonic chick brain. *J. Biol. Chem.*, 267: 12149–12161.

Lander, A. (1993) Proteoglycans in the nervous system. *Curr. Opin. Neurobiol.*, 3: 716–723.

Laywell, E.D., Dorries, U., Bartsch, U., Faissner, A., Schachner, M. and Steindler, D.A. (1992) Enhanced expression of the developmentally regulated extracellular matrix molecule tenascin following adult brain injury. *Proc. Natl. Acad. Sci. USA*, 89: 2634–2638.

Letourneau, P.C., Condic, M.L. and Snow, D.M. (1994) Interactions of developing neurons with the extracellular matrix. *J. Neurosci.*, 14: 915–928.

Levin, J.M. (1994) Increased expression of NG2 chondroitin-sulfate proteoglycan after brain injury. *J. Neurosci.*, 14: 4716–4730.

Levine, J.M., Reynolds, R. and Fawcett, J.W. (2001) The oligodendrocyte precursor cell in health and disease. *Trends Neurosci.*, 24: 39–47.

Liesi, P. (1985) Laminin-immunoreactive glia distinguish regenerative adult CNS systems from non-regenerative ones. *EMBO J.*, 4: 2505–2511.

Liesi, P., Kaakkola, S., Dahl, D. and Veheri, A. (1984) Laminin is induced in astrocytes of adult brain by injury. *EMBO J.*, 3: 683–686.

Logan, A., Baird, A. and Berry, M. (1999) Decorin attenuates gliotic scar formation in the rat cerebral hemisphere. *Exp. Neurol.*, 159: 504–510.

Manitt, C., Colicos, M.A., Thompson, K.M., Rousselle, E., Peterson, A.C. and Kennedy, T.E. (2001) Widespread expression of netrin-1 by neurons and oligodendrocytes in the adult mammalian spinal cord. *J. Neurosci.*, 21: 3911–3922.

McKeon, R.J., Schreiber, R.C., Rudge, J.S. and Silver, J. (1991) Reduction of neurite outgrowth in a model of glial scarring following CNS injury is correlated with the expression of inhibitory molecules on reactive astrocytes. *J. Neurosci.*, 11: 3398–3411.

McKeon, R.J., Jurynec, M.J. and Buck, C.R. (1999) The chondroitin sulfate proteoglycans neurocan and phosphacan are expressed by reactive astrocytes in the chronic CNS glial scar. *J. Neurosci.*, 19: 10778–10788.

Menet, V., Ribotta, G.M., Chauvet, N., Drian, M.J., Lannoy, J.,

Colucci-Guyon, E. and Privat, A. (2001) Inactivation of the glial fibrillary acidic protein gene, but not that of vimentin, improves neuronal survival and neurite growth by modifying adhesion molecule expression. *J. Neurosci.*, 221: 6147–6158.

Milev, P., Maurel, P., Chiba, A., Mevissen, M., Popp, S., Yamaguchi, Y., Margolis, R.K. and Margolis, R.U. (1998) Differential regulation of expression of hyaluronan-binding proteoglycans in developing brain: aggrecan, versican, neurocan and brevican. *Biochem. Biophys. Res. Commun.*, 247: 207–212.

Mitchell, K.J., Doyle, J.L., Serafini, T., Kennedy, T.E., Tessier-Lavigen, M., Goodman, C.S. and Dickson, B.J. (1996) Genetic analysis of netrin genes in Drosophila: netrins guide CNS commissural axons and peripheral motor axons. *Neuron*, 17: 203–215.

Moon, L.D.F., Brecknell, J.E., Franklin, R.J.M., Dunnett, S.B. and Fawcett, J.W. (2000) Robust regeneration of CNS axons through a track depleted of CNS glia. *Exp. Neurol.*, 161: 49–66.

Moon, L.D.F., Asher, R.A., Rhodes, K.E. and Fawcett, J.W. (2001) Regeneration of CNS axons back to their target following treatment of adult rat brain with chondroitinase ABC. *Nat. Neurosci.*, 4: 465–466.

Niederöst, B.P., Zimmermann, D.R., Schwab, M.E. and Bandtlow, C.E. (1999) Bovine CNS myelin contains neurite growth-inhibitory activity associated with chondroitin sulfate proteoglycans. *J. Neurosci.*, 19: 8979–8989.

Noble, M., Fok-Seang, J. and Cohen, J. (1984) Glia are a unique substrate for the in vitro growth of central nervous system neurons. *J. Neurosci.*, 4: 1892–1903.

Nygren, L. and Olson, L. (1977) Intracisternal neurotoxins and monoamine neurons innervating the spinal cord: acute and chronic effects on cell and axon counts and verve terminal densities. *Histochemistry*, 52: 281–306.

Oohira, A., Matsui, R., Watanabe, E., Kushima, Y. and Maeda, N. (1994) Developmentally regulated expression of a brain specific species of chondroitin sulfate proteoglycan, neurocan, identified with a monoclonal antibody 1G2 in the rat cerebrum. *Neuroscience*, 60: 145–157.

Pasterkamp, R.J., De Winter, F., Holtmaat, A.J. and Verhaagen, J. (1998) Evidence for a role of the chemorepellent semaphorin III and its receptor neurophilin-1 in the regeneration of primary olfactory axons. *J. Neurosci.*, 18: 9962–9976.

Pasterkamp, R.J., Giger, R.J., Ruitenberg, M.J., Holtmaat, A.J.G.D., De Wit, J., De Winter, F. and Verhaagen, J. (1999) Expression of the gene encoding the chemorepellent semaphorin III is induced in the fibroblast component of neural scar tissue formed following injuries of adult but not neonatal CNS. *Mol. Cell. Neurosci.*, 13: 143–166.

Perides, G., Rahemtulla, F., Lane, W.S., Asher, R.A. and Bignami, A. (1992) Isolation of a large aggregating proteoglycan from human brain. *J. Biol. Chem.*, 267: 23883–23887.

Perides, G., Asher, R.A., Lark, M.W., Lane, W.S., Robinson, R.A. and Bignami, A. (1995) Glial hyaluronate-binding protein: A product of metalloproteinase digestion of versican. *Biochem. J.*, 312: 377–384.

Pesheva, P. and Probstmeier, R. (2000) The yin and yang of

tenascin-R in CNS development and pathology. *Prog. Neurobiol.*, 61: 465–493.

Pindzola, R.R., Doller, C. and Silver, J. (1993) Putative inhibitory extracellular matrix molecules at the dorsal root entry of the spinal cord during development and after root and sciatic nerve lesions. *Dev. Biol.*, 156: 34–48.

Plant, G.W., Bates, M.L. and Bunge, M.B. (2001) Inhibitory proteoglycan immunoreactivity is higher at the caudal than the rostral Schwann cell graft-transected spinal cord interface. *Mol. Cell. Neurosci.*, 17: 471–487.

Pueschel, A.W., Adams, R.H. and Betz, H. (1995) Murine semaphorin D/collapsin is a member of a diverse gene family and creates domains inhibitory for axonal extension. *Neuron*, 14: 941–948.

Rauch, U., Gao, P., Janetzko, A., Flaccus, A., Hilgenberg, L., Tekotte, H., Margolis, R.K. and Margolis, R.U. (1991) Isolation and characterization of developmentally regulated chondroitin sulfate and chondroitin/keratan sulfate proteoglycans of brain identified with monoclonal antibodies. *J. Biol. Chem.*, 266: 14785–14801.

Romanic, A.M., White, R.F., Arleth, A.J., Ohlstein, E.H. and Barone, F.C. (1998) Matrix metalloproteinase expression increases after cerebral focal ischemia in rats: inhibition of matrix metalloproteinase-9 reduces infarct size. *Stroke*, 29: 1020–1030.

Rudge, J.S. and Silver, J. (1990) Inhibition of neurite outgrowth on astroglial scars in vitro. *J. Neurosci.*, 10: 3594–3603.

Schnaedelbach, O., Mandl, C. and Faissner, A. (1998) Expression of DSD-1-PG in primary neural and glial-derived cell line cultures, upregulation by TGF-β, and implications for cell–substrate interactions of the glial cell line Oli-neu. *Glia*, 23: 99–119.

Schwartz, N.B., Henning, A.K., Krueger Jr., R.C., Krzystolik, M., Li, H. and Mangoura, D. (1993) Developmental expression of S103L cross-reacting proteoglycans in embryonic chick. *Prog. Clin. Biol. Res.*, 383B: 505–514.

Seidenbecher, C., Richter, K., Rauch, U., Faessler, R., Garner, C.C. and Gundelfinger, E.D. (1995) Brevican, a chondroitin sulfate proteoglycan of rat brain, occurs as a secreted and cell surface glycosylphosphatidylinositol-anchored isoforms. *J. Biol. Chem.*, 270: 27206–27212.

Smith, G.M. and Silver, J. (1988) Transplantation of immature and mature astrocytes and their effect on scar formation in the lesioned central nervous system. *Prog. Brain Res.*, 78: 353–361.

Smith, G.M., Rutishauser, U., Silver, J. and Miller, R.H. (1990) Maturation of astrocytes in vitro alters the extent and molecular basis of neurite outgrowth. *Dev. Biol.*, 138: 377–390.

Smith-Thomas, L., Fok-Seang, J., Stevens, J., Du, J.-S., Muir, E., Faissner, A., Geller, H.M., Rogers, J.H., Rogers, J.H. and Fawcett, J.W. (1994) An inhibitor of neurite outgrowth produced by astrocytes. *J. Cell Sci.*, 107: 1687–1695.

Snow, D.M., Lemmon, V., Carrino, D.A., Caplan, A.I. and Silver, J. (1990) Sulfated proteoglycans in astroglial barriers inhibit neurite outgrowth in vitro. *Exp. Neurol.*, 109: 111–130.

Stichel, C.C., Kappler, J., Junghans, U., Koops, A., Kresse, H. and Müller, H.W. (1995) Differential expression of the small chondroitin/dermatan sulfate proteoglycan decorin and biglycan after injury of the adult rat brain. *Brain Res.*, 704: 263–274.

Thon, N., Haas, C.A., Rauch, U., Merten, T., Faessler, R., Frotscher, M. and Deller, T. (2000) The chondroitin sulfate proteoglycan brevican is upregulated by astrocytes after entorhinal cortex lesion in adult rats. *Eur. J. Neurosci.*, 12: 2547–2558.

Timpl, R., Rodde, H., Robey, P.G., Rennard, S.I., Foidart, J.-M. and Martin, G.R. (1979) Laminin — a glycoprotein from basement membrane. *J. Biol. Chem.*, 254: 9933–9937.

Vaudano, E., Campbell, G., Hunt, S.P. and Lieberman, A.R. (1989) Axonal injury and peripheral nerve grafting in the thalamus and cerebellum of the adult rat: upregulation of c-jun and correlation with regenerative potential. *Eur. J. Neurosci.*, 10: 2644–2656.

Weidner, N., Ner, A., Salimi, N. and Tuszynski, M.H. (2001) Spontaneous corticospinal axonal plasticity and functional recovery after adult central nervous system injury. *Proc. Natl. Acad. Sci. USA*, 98: 13–18.

Wenk, C.A., Thallmair, M., Kartje, G.L. and Schwab, M.E. (1999) Increased corticofugal plasticity after unilateral cortical lesions combined with neutralization of the IN-1 antigene in adult rats. *J. Comp. Neurol.*, 410: 143–157.

Wolswijk, G. and Noble, M. (1989) Identification of an adult specific glial progenitor cell. *Development*, 105: 387–400.

Wong, J.T., Wong, S.T. and O'Connor, T.P. (1999) Ectopic semaphorin-1a functions as an attractive guidance cue for developing peripheral neurons. *Nat. Neurosci.*, 2: 798–803.

Yamada, H., Watanabe, K., Shimonaha, M. and Yamaguchi, Y. (1994) Molecular cloning of brevican, a novel brain proteoglycan of the aggrecan/versican family. *J. Biol. Chem.*, 269: 10119–10126.

Yamaguchi, Y., Mann, D.M. and Ruoslahti, E. (1990) Negative regulation of transforming growth factor-β by the proteoglycan decorin. *Nature*, 346: 281–284.

Yamamoto, T., Iwasaki, Y., Yamamoto, H., Konno, H. and Isemura, M. (1988) Intraneuronal laminin-like molecule in the central nervous system: demonstration of its unique differential distribution. *J. Neurol. Sci.*, 84: 1–13.

Ying, Y., Miner, J.H., Feng, G. and Sanes, J.R. (2000) Novel laminin-related genes, laminets-1 and -2 are expressed by complementary subsets of adult neurons. *Society for Neuroscience 30th Annual Meeting*, New Orleans, LA, Nov. 4–9, 220.3.

Zhang, Y., Anderson, P.N., Campbell, G., Mohajeri, H., Schachner, M. and Lieberman, A.R. (1995) Tenascin-C expression by neurons and glial cells in the rat spinal cord: Changes during postnatal development and after dorsal root or sciatic nerve injury. *J. Neurocytol.*, 24: 585–601.

Zhang, Y., Winterbottom, J.K., Schachner, M., Lieberman, A.R. and Anderson, P.N. (1997) Tenascin-C expression and axonal sprouting following injury to the spinal dorsal columns in the adult rat. *J. Neurosci.*, 49: 433–450.

Zhou, F.C. (1990) Four patterns of laminin-immunoreactive structure in developing rat brain. *Dev. Brain Res.*, 55: 191–201.

Zimmermann, D.R., Dours-Zimmermann, M.T., Schubert, M. and Bruckner-Trudemann, L. (1994) Expression of the extracellular matrix proteoglycan, versican, in human skin. *J. Cell Biol.*, 124: 817–825.

Zuo, J., Neubauer, D., Dyess, K., Ferguson, T.A. and Muir, D. (1998) Degradation of chondroitin sulfate proteoglycan enhances the neurite-promoting potential of spinal cord tissue. *Exp. Neurol.*, 154: 654–662.

L. McKerracher, G. Doucet and S. Rossignol (Eds.)
Progress in Brain Research, Vol. 137
© 2002 Elsevier Science B.V. All rights reserved

CHAPTER 24

Increasing plasticity and functional recovery of the lesioned spinal cord

Martin E. Schwab [*]

Department of Neuromorphology, Brain Research Institute, University of Zurich and Swiss Federal Institute of Technology, Winterthurerstr. 190, 8057 Zurich, Switzerland

Abstract: In vitro assays have shown that adult CNS tissue, in particular oligodendrocytes and myelin, contains several molecular constituents (Nogo-A/NI-220, MAG, several proteoglycans) which exert neurite growth inhibitory activity. Elimination of oligodendrocytes or myelin, or application of antibodies against some of these constituents enhance regenerative growth and compensatory sprouting of lesioned and unlesioned fiber tracts in spinal cord and brain. Enhanced growth is paralleled by various degrees of functional recovery.

Introduction

The functional outcome of spinal cord lesions varies greatly depending on the extent of the lesion; small lesions have a good prognosis, whereas large destructions of white matter areas in particular lead to life-long paraplegia or tetra-/quadriplegia. The recovery following medium-sized or small lesions probably relies largely on the parallel wiring of the CNS and on processes of compensatory sprouting and new circuit formation (Raineteau and Schwab, 2001). Studies using defined partial white matter lesions in several experimental species as well as in man (e.g. in the context of neurosurgical interventions for intractable pain) have shown that many aspects of motor control can be maintained with as few as 10–15% of the fibers of a particular tract system (Eidelberg et al., 1977; Vilensky et al., 1992;

Nathan, 1994; Raineteau and Schwab, 2001). In cats, classical experiments using transections of the corticospinal tract (CST) in the upper cervical spinal cord showed recovery of precise reaching movements through an indirect pathway involving propriospinal axons (Alstermark et al., 1987), demonstrating that even precision movements can be restored.

Rhythmic movements are well known to depend on spinally located central pattern generators in all tetrapodes including man (Rossignol and Dubuc, 1994; Grillner and Wallen, 1999). Recent studies in paraplegic patients with large lesions and no or very poor ability for spontaneous locomotion have shown that an astonishing degree of functional recovery can occur with specific training of these patients on the treadmill (Dietz et al., 1994; Wernig et al., 1995; Rossignol, 2000; Edgerton et al., 2001). Whereas training effects on the spinal circuitry could even be demonstrated in complete paraplegic patients (Dietz et al., 1994), meaningful functional recovery depended on the existence of functional spared descending fibers. Biologically, the success of this rehabilitation strategy probably depends on the reactivation and consolidation of the spinal locomotor circuitry as well as on the integration of remaining fibers (which may also sprout

---
[*] Correspondence to: M.E. Schwab, Department of Neuromorphology, Brain Research Institute, University of Zurich and Swiss Federal Institute of Technology, Winterthurerstr. 190, 8057 Zurich, Switzerland. Tel.: +41-1-635-3330; Fax: +41-1-635-3303;
E-mail: schwab@hifo.unizh.ch

spontaneously to some extent) into a functional circuitry.

As tragically experienced by patients and therapists in their daily work, however, the capacity of the lesioned adult CNS for self-repair is limited. Understanding the factors and molecular mechanisms responsible for this apparent inability of adult CNS axons to regrow, sprout and reconnect has been a major challenge for neuroscientists over the last 15 years.

The concept of neurite growth inhibitors

Two major theories dominated the field of CNS regeneration until the early 1980s: that of a lack of growth stimulatory factors in the adult CNS tissue (first formulated by Tello, 1911, and Ramon y Cajal, 1928 (see Ramon y Cajal, 1991) and the theory of an intrinsic inability of adult neurons to reactivate their growth program. The latter hypothesis, at least in its absolute formulation, was clearly disproven by the experiments of Albert Aguayo and his group (David and Aguayo, 1981; Richardson et al., 1984; Keirstead et al., 1989) showing that transplants of peripheral nerves of adult rats grafted into the spinal cord, brainstem, or retina induced ingrowth of axons from different types of CNS neurons and elongation over distances of centimeters (see also contribution by Vidal-Sanz et al., 2002, this volume). To test the lack of trophic factor hypothesis, we cocultured explants of adult rat optic nerves and sciatic nerves with dissociated peripheral neurons in the presence of high concentrations of nerve growth factor (NFG) (Schwab and Thoenen, 1985). Abundant ingrowth of axons into the sciatic nerves was in sharp contrast to the absence of axons in the optic nerve explants. The same result occurred when these tissues were previously frozen and thawed several times. We concluded that CNS tissue, in contrast to peripheral nerve, contains potent neurite growth inhibitory constituents (Schwab and Thoenen, 1985). Oligodendrocytes and myelin were subsequently identified as the source of at least part of these inhibitory factors (Schwab and Caroni, 1988). Potent activity was present in a specific high molecular weight band (NI-250 in rat, NI-220 in bovine and human spinal cord; in rat, in addition NI-35) (Caroni and Schwab, 1988b; Spillmann et al., 1997, 1998). Subsequently, myelin-

associated glycoprotein (MAG) (McKerracher et al., 1994; Mukhopadhyay et al., 1994), the proteoglycans brevican and versican V2 (Niederöst et al., 1999) as well as oligodendrocyte and myelin glycoprotein (OMGP/arretin; P.E. Braun, personal communication) were shown to possess neurite growth inhibitory activity at least in vitro.

The neurite growth inhibitory protein Nogo-A

NI-220/250 as a relatively low abundant, high molecular weight membrane protein has only been fully purified and partially sequenced in 1998 (Spillmann et al., 1998). The corresponding cDNA, now called Nogo-A, was cloned in 2000 (Chen et al., 2000; GrandPré et al., 2000; Prinhja et al., 2000). The Nogo gene gives rise to three proteins due to alternative splicing (Nogo-A and -B), and alternative promoter usage (Nogo-C). Nogo-A corresponds to NI-220/250 and is synthesized by oligodendrocytes and localized in myelin in the adult CNS (Chen et al., 2000). Interestingly, Nogo-A in myelin is localized in the innermost, adaxonal and in the outermost myelin membrane, but not in compact myelin (Huber et al., 2002). Nogo-A is also expressed at low level by subpopulations of neurons, including retinal ganglion cells, motoneurons and DRGs. Neuronal expression is higher in development. Nogo-B, which is also expressed outside of the nervous system in a variety of tissues, is localized largely in neurons in the CNS and PNS. Nogo-C is mainly expressed in skeletal muscle. The functions of Nogo-B and Nogo-C as well as the function of Nogo-A in neurons are currently unknown.

All three Nogo forms share a common 188 aa C-terminus containing two long hydrophobic regions. The same 188 aa domain is the only region of the protein with homology to other known genes, i.e. the reticulon proteins (RTN-1, -2, -3) (Chen et al., 2000; GrandPré et al., 2000). RTNs are enriched in the endoplasmic reticulum (like the Nogos), but whether they are also plasma membrane proteins is unknown. Their function is unknown.

Analysis of active fragments of Nogo-A in neurite growth inhibition and growth cone collapse assays have demonstrated the existence of at least two active sites: one in the N-terminal and middle part of Nogo-A and a second, growth cone collapse inducing region in the loop between the two hydrophobic domains (Oertle et al., 2000; Fournier et al., 2001). This loop of 66 aa (Nogo-66) is exposed on the surface of oligodendrocytes (GrandPré et al., 2000) as is the middle and N-terminal domain (Oertle et al., in preparation). Experiments with antibodies against specific domains of Nogo-A in neutralization assays as well as in in vivo regeneration and plasticity studies are currently in progress.

Regeneration by neutralization of myelin-associated growth inhibitors

A series of experiments confirmed the functional importance of myelin-associated growth inhibitory factors for the restriction of axon regrowth in the adult mammalian CNS. Thus, the loss of regenerative growth in specific neuronal systems during postnatal development correlates closely with oligodendrocyte maturation and myelin formation in chicken embryos, and newborn rats and opossums (Hasan et al., 1991; Kapfhammer and Schwab, 1994; Varga et al., 1995). Deletion of oligodendrocytes and prevention of myelin formation allows regenerative growth of transected axons at later, normally non-permissive stages (Savio and Schwab, 1990), and immunocytolysis of myelin in adult rats also restores a regeneration-permissive state (Dyer et al., 1998). A monoclonal antibody (mAB IN-1) raised against the rat 250 kDa inhibitory activity allowed axonal growth on myelin substrates, spinal cord frozen sections or cultured oligodendrocytes in vitro (Caroni and Schwab, 1988a). When hybridoma cells secreting this IN-1 antibody were transplanted as grafts or in millipore filter capsules into the CNS of adult rats, enhanced sprouting and long distance regeneration of lesioned corticospinal tract, optic nerve or cholinergic forebrain fibers could be observed (Schnell and Schwab, 1990; Cadelli and Schwab, 1991; Schnell et al., 1994; Weibel et al., 1994). Regeneration velocities reached 1 mm per day. Similar results were recently obtained with a bacterially produced recombinant Fab fragment of the IN-1 antibody infused by minipumps over spinal cord lesion sites (Brösamle et al., 2000). Regenerated axons were also seen to invade the gray matter of the caudal spinal cord where they formed terminal arbors studded with varicosities.

A similar long distance regeneration of transected corticospinal axons was recently observed in adult mice, immunized with CNS myelin or spinal cord homogenate (Huang et al., 1999). The crucial role of antibodies directed against myelin neurite growth inhibitory constituents in these experiment is underlined by in vitro neutralization of the inhibitory nature of myelin for regenerating neurites by IgGs of these sera, and by pilot studies showing that i.p. injection of such sera induces regeneration in non-immunized spinal cord lesioned rats (David, 2002, this volume).

Scar tissue

In all the regeneration studies discussed above using different experimental approaches and coming from different laboratories, two additional observations were consistently made: (1) the proportion of successfully regenerating axons (as compared to the number of labeled axons in the intact tract rostral to the lesion) was usually relatively small; and (2) large variations exist in a series of animals of a given experiment. The variations correlate in part with the extent of the local tissue destruction. Indeed, many single axons can be observed being seemingly stuck in the scar and debris tissue (Davies et al., 1999; Brösamle et al., 2000). Whether subpopulations of CNS axons and neurons differ in their capability to regenerate is not well studied at present, but is probable (Caroni, 1997). In particular aminergic neurons have been known for a long time to have regeneration and plastic capabilities superior to most other CNS neurons (Schwab and Bartholdi, 1996; Giménez y Ribotta et al., 2000). However, even tracts like the CST, which contains sensory and motor axons of various types (myelinated, unmyelinated, from primary motor cortex or premotor areas etc.), could show differences in the ability to mount a growth response subsequent to a lesion and a particular experimental intervention.

Less debated is the fact that scars are important local barriers for regeneration. Mechanical aspects including dense astrocyte endfeet regions, basement membrane and immigrating meningeal fibroblasts as well as a growing body of evidence indicating the presence of specific growth inhibitory constituents probably play important roles (Schwab and

Bartholdi, 1996; Fitch and Silver, 1997; Fawcett and Asher, 1999). Among the growth inhibitory factors chondroitin sulfate proteoglycans are assigned a crucial role (Fitch and Silver, 1997; Fawcett and Asher, 1999); their removal by chondroitinase infusion enhances sprouting of lesioned nigrostriatal neurites in the hypothalamus, as well as dorsal column axons in the spinal cord (Moon et al., 2001; Morgenstern et al., 2002, this volume).

Myelin-associated neurite growth inhibitors are signaling molecules

Neuronal growth cones collapse and assume a bulbous, immotile morphology upon contact of a few filopodia with co-cultured oligodendrocytes or when treated with NI-35, NI-250, Nogo-66 or MAG. (Bandtlow et al., 1990; Bandtlow et al., 1993; Li et al., 1996; Spillmann et al., 1998; Fournier et al., 2001). Early studies have shown that this response can be abolished by Pertussis toxin and includes a massive elevation of intracellular calcium levels in the affected growth cones (Bandtlow et al., 1993; Igarashi et al., 1993). More recently, cyclic nucleotides were shown to be able to modulate growth cone responses to a variety of attractive as well as repulsive ligands, including MAG and CNS myelin (Cai et al., 1998; Song et al., 1998; Qui et al., 2002, this volume). A further component of the signal transduction pathway of the neurite growth inhibitory signals of CNS myelin is the small GTPase rhoA; rhoA is activated in response to MAG or myelin, and its inactivation prevents growth cone collapse, and enhances neurite outgrowth on myelin protein substrates in vitro and regenerative sprouting in vivo (Lehmann et al., 1999; Ellezam et al., 2002, this volume).

The low concentrations of purified or recombinant Nogo-A, NI-250 or the fragment Nogo-66 required for growth cone collapse or growth inhibition, as well as the presence of defined signal transduction pathways, strongly suggest the existence of specific receptors in the neuronal and growth cone membrane. A first receptor component (for Nogo-66) has recently been cloned and characterized (Fournier et al., 2001). This 473 aa GPI-linked protein has leucin-rich repeats, and when transfected into nonresponsive young embryonic neurons renders them responsive to Nogo-66. As guidance molecules like

the semaphorins, netrins or ephrins, all have multiple receptors, compound receptor complexes, perhaps also mediating multiple functions, may well exist also for Nogo. The receptor for MAG has remained elusive up to now.

Functional outcome in spinal cord lesioned, mAB IN-1-treated adult rats

Fibers that are induced by experimental manipulations to grow in the adult spinal cord could hypothetically have different functional consequences: (1) none, if they are unable to find targets and form synapses; (2) malfunctions due to the formation of wrong or random synaptic connections; and (3) functional improvements if meaningful connections can be established. The latter possibility could be due to the persistence or the re-expression of axonal guidance and target recognition cues and/or an activity-dependent stabilization of functionally meaningful connections. A first analysis using footprints, horizontal grids and the placing reflex in response to light skin stimulation of the hindpaw in overhemisected, mAB IN-1-treated rats showed a very significant recovery of locomotory functions (Bregman et al., 1995). This was recently confirmed in a broad behavioral and electrophysiological study where significant improvements were seen in the BBB open field locomotion score, gridwalk and beam crossing paradigms, and in the EMG pattern of hindlimb muscle activation, in particular with regard to regularity of the flexor/extensor and left/right alterations (Merkler et al., 2001). Co-contractions and spasticity-like activation patterns disappeared along with the normalization of the locomotor function and hindlimb weight bearing in the mAB IN-1 animals. Importantly, pain tests showed no difference between mAB IN-1- and control AB-treated animals, demonstrating that the antibody treatment had not induced random growth and wrong connections of sensory fibers (Merkler et al., 2001).

Functional improvements were also seen in experiments where mice were immunized against myelin and/or spinal cord extract (Huang et al., 1999; David, 2002, this volume). Studies in which antibodies against recombinant Nogo-A are infused by minipumps into spinal cord lesioned rats are currently in progress in our laboratory.

Compensatory sprouting and plasticity as a mechanism for functional recovery in the spinal cord

Voluntary, fine hand or forepaw movements are known to crucially depend on the corticospinal tract (CST) in species as diverse as man, monkeys, cats and rats (Lemon, 1999; Iwaniuk and Whishaw, 2000). Transections of all components of the CST, e.g. by a lesion in the caudal medulla oblongata rostral to the pyramidal decussation in adult rats or hamsters lead to long-lasting severe impairments of skilled reaching movements (Reh and Kalil, 1982; Thallmair et al., 1998). Compensation is poor, also several months after the operation. Interestingly, a recent study shows that much better compensation occurs after a lesion of the dorsal CST in the spinal cord, probably by sprouting of ventral, intact CST fibers (Weidner et al., 2001).

In two experimental paradigms, we studied functional recovery and compensatory sprouting in response to pyramidal CST lesions (transecting *all* components of the CST) in adult rats. In the first series of experiments, the pyramidal tract was transected unilaterally (Thallmair et al., 1998; Z'Graggen et al., 1998). When the cortex corresponding to the transected tracts was traced with biotin dextran amine sprouting was minimal at the transection site and also in the two important brainstem target areas, the red nucleus and the basilar pontine nuclei. Lesion-only animals were not different from rats with a graft of control antibody secreting hybridoma cells in the contralateral hippocampus. In contrast, rats with the same lesions and grafts of mAB IN-1 secreting cells showed pronounced sprouting at the lesion site with innervation of the surrounding brainstem including the contralateral dorsal column nuclei (Raineteau et al., 1999). However, very few of these fibers managed to navigate successfully through the pyramidal decussation into the spinal cord. Surprisingly, pronounced sprouting also occurred on the level of the pons and the red nucleus; fibers crossed the midline and terminated in appropriate, i.e. forelimb-specific areas of the contralateral nuclei (which were, themselves, normally innervated by the intact tract of the contralateral side) (Z'Graggen et al., 1998). In the spinal cord, tracing of the non-lesioned CST showed

the appearance of sprouts crossing the midline and branching in the denervated dorsal and ventral part of the spinal cord (Fig. 1A–C; Thallmair et al., 1998). Such a sprouting occurred on all levels, cervical, thoracic and lumbar. Interestingly, a detailed behavioral analysis, in particular of forelimb reaching for food pellets through a window in a plexiglas box, and of rope climbing showed an almost full restitution of hand and forelimb functions in these mAB IN-1-treated rats, in contrast to the severely impaired controls (Thallmair et al., 1998). As improvements also occurred in the sensory-motor sticky paper test, sprouting of tracts other than the CST may also be involved.

To study the possible contribution of different tract systems in functional recovery after CST lesions, the tract was lesioned bilaterally in 2-month-old rats (Raineteau et al., 2001). Again, lesion-only or control antibody-treated animals showed long-lasting, severe deficits in food pellet reaching. mAB IN-1-treated rats showed an almost full recovery. When the rubrospinal tract was traced, a doubling of the number of collaterals emerging from the tract and entering the gray matter was observed in the cervical spinal cord (Fig. 1D,E). Even more surprising was the finding that some of these fibers grew into the deep ventral horn where they contacted motoneurons of proximal forelimb muscles, a target which is normally not innervated by rubrospinal axons (in contrast to CST axons!) (Raineteau and Schwab, submitted). Electrophysiological experiments confirmed the establishment of a new pathway from the primary motor cortex to the spinal cord in these mAB IN-1-treated animals: low threshold stimulation of the motor cortex, which induces a fast biceps muscle EMG response in intact animals, did not lead to detectable muscle responses in the lesioned, control antibody-treated animals. In contrast, lesioned mAB IN-1-treated rats showed pronounced EMG responses with, however, longer latencies (Raineteau et al., 2001). Injections of the GABA receptor agonist muscimol into the red nucleus abolished these EMG responses. We hypothesize that the experimental interruption of the direct corticospinal connection can be compensated by an indirect corticorubro- and rubrospinal pathway under experimental conditions (mAB IN-1) which allow enhanced growth and plasticity in the adult CNS.

356

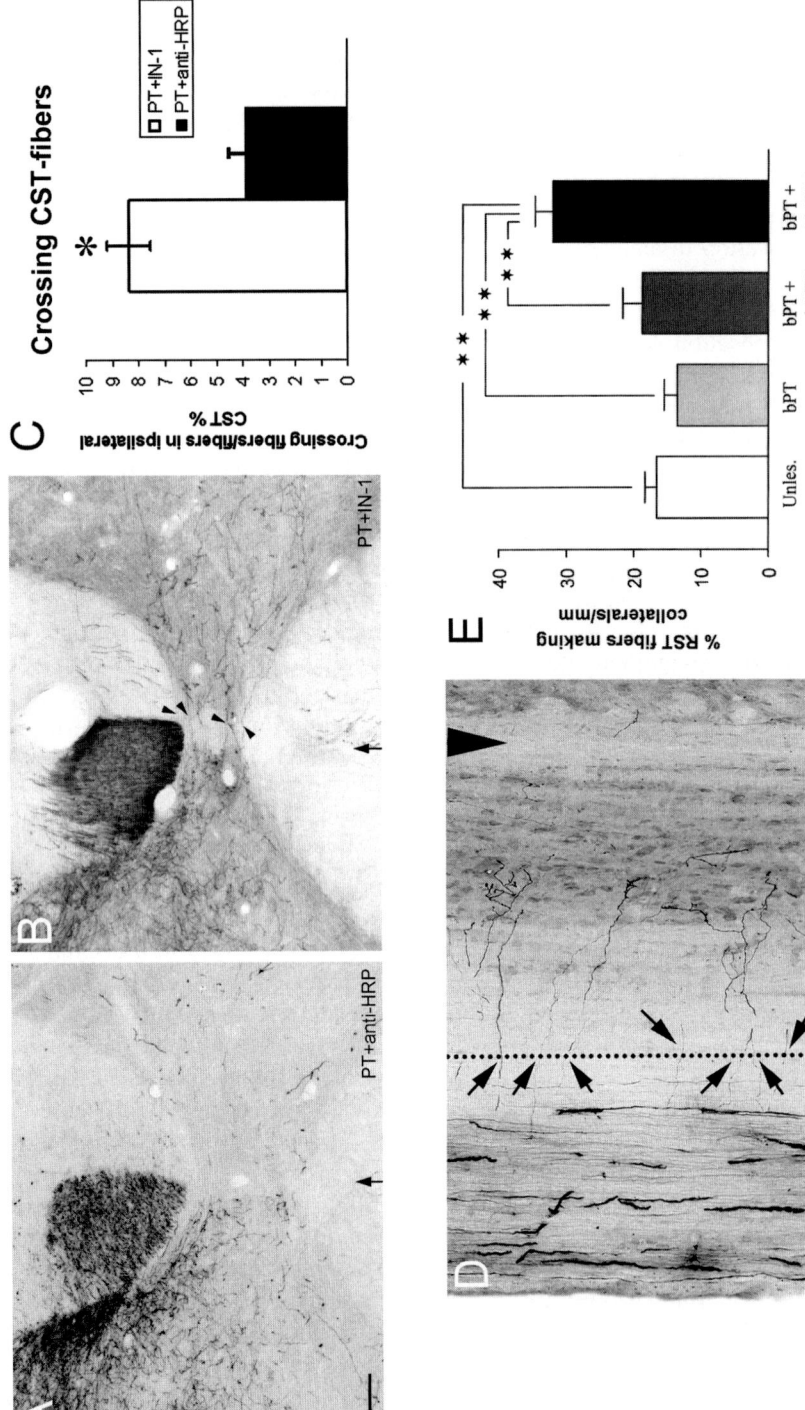

Fig. 1. Compensatory sprouting of corticospinal (A–C) or rubrospinal (D,E) fibers in the adult rat spinal cord following pyramidal tract lesions. (A–C) The pyramidal tract was completely transected unilaterally (PT); 2 weeks later fibers of the contralateral, spared corticospinal tract (CST) showed a normal distribution in untreated or control antibody (anti-HRP)-treated rats (A,C), whereas pronounced sprouting (arrowheads in B) occurred across the midline (arrows) into the denervated half of the spinal cord in mAB IN-1-treated animals (B,C). (D,E) The pyramidal tract was transected completely and bilaterally (bPT). Longitudinal sections of the spinal cord after 2 weeks show enhanced sprouting of rubrospinal axons (arrows) in mAB IN-1-treated animals (D,E), but not in unlesioned, bPT-only or control (anti-HRP) antibody controls (E). Stippled line in D: white matter–gray matter boundary. A–C are from Thallmair et al., 1998; D and E are from Raineteau et al., 2001, with permission.

A most relevant finding of all these experiments as well as of several regeneration experiments reported by various laboratories over the last 5–7 years is the fact that functional improvements of a high degree are observed without indications for malfunctions. This observation strongly suggests that treatments enhancing growth and regeneration in the adult CNS can be used by the system in a meaningful way leading to restitution of lost functions.

References

Alstermark, B., Lundberg, A., Pettersson, L.-G., Tantisira, B. and Walkowska, M. (1987) Motor recovery after serial spinal cord lesions of defined descending pathways in the cats. *Neurosci. Res.*, 5: 68–73.

Bandtlow, C.E., Zachleder, T. and Schwab, M.E. (1990) Oligodendrocytes arrest neurite growth by contact inhibition. *J. Neurosci.*, 10: 3837–3848.

Bandtlow, C.E., Schmidt, M.F., Hassinger, T.D., Schwab, M.E. and Kater, S.B. (1993) Role of intracellular calcium in NI-35-evoked collapse of neuronal growth cones. *Science*, 259: 80–83.

Bregman, B.S., Kunkel-Bagden, E., Schnell, L., Dai, H.N., Gao, D. and Schwab, M.E. (1995) Recovery from spinal cord injury mediated by antibodies to neurite growth inhibitors. *Nature*, 378: 498–501.

Brösamle, C., Huber, A.B., Fiedler, M., Skerra, A. and Schwab, M.E. (2000) Regeneration of lesioned corticospinal tract fibers in the adult rat induced by a recombinant, humanized IN-1 antibody fragment. *J. Neurosci.*, 20: 8061–8068.

Cadelli, D. and Schwab, M.E. (1991) Regeneration of lesioned septohippocampal acetylcholinesterase-positive axons is improved by antibodies against the myelin-associated neurite growth inhibitors NI-35/250. *Eur. J. Neurosci.*, 3: 825–832.

Cai, D., Shen, Y., De Bellards, M.E., Tang, S. and Filbin, M.T. (1998) Prior exposure to neurotrophins blocks inhibition of axonal regeneration by MAG and myelin via a cAMP-dependent mechanism. *Neuron*, 22: 89–101.

Caroni, P. (1997) Intrinsic neuronal determinants that promote axonal sprouting and elongation. *Bioessays*, 19: 767–775.

Caroni, P. and Schwab, M.E. (1988a) Antibody against myelin-associated inhibitor of neurite growth neutralizes nonpermissive substrate properties of CNS white matter. *Neuron*, 1: 85–96.

Caroni, P. and Schwab, M.E. (1988b) Two membrane protein fractions from rat central myelin with inhibitory properties for neurite growth and fibroblast spreading. *J. Cell Biol.*, 106: 1281–1288.

Chen, M.S., Huber, A.B., van der Haar, M.E., Frank, M., Schnell, L., Spillmann, A.A., Christ, F. and Schwab, M.E. (2000) Nogo-A is a myelin-associated neurite outgrowth inhibitor and an antigen form monoclonal antibody IN-1. *Nature*, 403: 434–439.

David, S. (2002) Recruiting the immune response to promote long distance axon regeneration after spinal cord injury. In: L. McKerracher, G. Douchet and S. Rossignol (Eds.), *Spinal Cord Trauma: Neural Repair and Functional Recovery. Progress in Brain Research*, Vol. 137. Elsevier Science, Amsterdam, pp. 407–414.

David, S. and Aguayo, A.J. (1981) Axonal elongation into peripheral nervous system 'bridges' after central nervous system injury in adult rats. *Science*, 214: 931–933.

Davies, S.J.A., Goucher, D.R., Doller, C. and Silver, J. (1999) Robust regeneration of adult sensory axons in degenerating white matter of the adult rat spinal cord. *J. Neurosci.*, 19: 5810–5822.

Dietz, V., Colombo, G. and Jensen, L. (1994) Locomotor activity in spinal man. *Lancet*, 344: 1260–1263.

Dyer, J.K., Bourque, J.A. and Steeves, J.D. (1998) Regeneration of brainstem-spinal axons after lesion and immunological disruption of myelin in adult rat. *Exp. Neurol.*, 154: 12–22.

Edgerton, V.R., Leon, R.D., Harkema, S.J., Hodgson, J.A., London, N., Reinkensmeyer, D.J., Roy, R.R., Talmadge, R.J., Tillakaratne, N.J., Timoszyk, W. and Tobin, A. (2001) Retraining the injured spinal cord. *J. Physiol.*, 533: 15–22.

Eidelberg, E., Straehley, D., Erspamer, R. and Watkins, C.J. (1977) Relationship between residual hindlimb-assisted locomotion and surviving axons after incomplete spinal cord injuries. *Exp. Neurol.*, 56: 312–322.

Ellezam, B., Dubreuil, C., Winton, M., Loy, L., Dergham, P., Sellés-Navarro, I. and McKerracher, L. (2002) Inactivation of intracellular Rho to stimulate axon growth and regeneration. In: L. McKerracher, G. Douchet and S. Rossignol (Eds.), *Spinal Cord Trauma: Neural Repair and Functional Recovery. Progress in Brain Research*, Vol. 137. Elsevier Science, Amsterdam, pp. 371–380.

Fawcett, J.W. and Asher, R.A. (1999) The glial scar and central nervous system repair. *Brain Res. Bull.*, 49: 377–391.

Fitch, M.T. and Silver, J. (1997) Glial cell extracellular matrix: boundaries for axon growth in development and regeneration. *Cell Tissue Res.*, 290: 379–384.

Fournier, A.E., GrandPre, T. and Strittmatter, S.M. (2001) Identification of a receptor mediating Nogo-66 inhibition of axonal regeneration. *Nature*, 409: 341–346.

Giménez y Ribotta, M., Provencher, J., Feraboli-Lohnherr, D., Rossignol, S., Privat, A. and Orsal, D. (2000) Activation of locomotion in adult chronic spinal rats is achieved by transplantation of embryonic raphe cells reinnervating a precise lumbar level. *J. Neurosci.*, 20: 5144–5152.

GrandPré, T., Nakamura, F., Vartanian, T. and Strittmatter, S.M. (2000) Identification of the Nogo inhibitor of axon regeneration as a reticulon protein. *Nature*, 403: 439–444.

Grillner, S. and Wallen, P. (1999) On the cellular bases of vertebrate locomotion. *Prog. Brain Res.*, 123: 297–309.

Hasan, S.J., Nelson, B.H., Valenzuela, J.I., Keirstead, H.S., Shull, S.E., Ethell, D.W. and Steeves, J.D. (1991) Functional repair of transected spinal cord in embryonic chick. *Rest. Neurol. Neurosci.*, 2: 137–154.

Huang, D.W., McKerracher, L., Braun, P.E. and David, S. (1999) A therapeutic vaccine approach to stimulate axon regeneration in the adult mammalian spinal cord. *Neuron*, 24: 639–647.

358

Huber, A.B., Weinmann, O., Brösamle, C., Oertle, T. and Schwab M.E. (2002) Patterns of Nogo mRNA and protein expression in the developing and adult rat and after CNS lesions. *J. Neurosci.*, 22: 3553–3567.

Igarashi, M., Strittmatter, S.M., Vartanian, T. and Fishman, M.C. (1993) Mediation by G proteins of signals that cause collapse of growth cones. *Science*, 259: 77–79.

Iwaniuk, A.N. and Whishaw, I.Q. (2000) On the origin of skilled forelimb movements. *Trends Neurosci.*, 23: 372–376.

Kapfhammer, J.P. and Schwab, M.E. (1994) Increased expression of the growth-associated protein GAP-43 in the myelin-free rat spinal cord. *Eur. J. Neurosci.*, 6: 403–411.

Keirstead, S.A., Rasminsky, M., Fukuda, Y., Carter, D.A., Aguayo, A.J. and Vidal-Sanz, M. (1989) Electrophysiologic responses in hamster superior colliculus evoked by regenerating retinal axons. *Science*, 246: 255–257.

Lehmann, M., Fournier, A., Selles-Navarro, I., Dergham, P., Sebok, A., Lerclerc, N., Tigyi, G. and McKerracher, L. (1999) Inactivation of Rho signaling pathway promotes CNS axon regeneration. *J. Neurosci.*, 19: 7537–7547.

Lemon, R.N. (1999) Neural control of dexterity: what has been achieved? *Exp. Brain Res.*, 128: 6–12.

Li, M., Shibata, A., Li, C., Braun, P.E., McKerracher, L., Roder, J., Kater, S.B. and David, S. (1996) Myelin-associated glycoprotein inhibits neurite/axon growth and causes growth cone collapse. *J. Neurosci. Res.*, 46: 404–414.

McKerracher, L., David, S., Jackson, D.L., Kottis, V., Dunn, R.J. and Braun, P.E. (1994) Identification of myelin-associated glycoprotein as a major myelin-derived inhibitor of neurite growth. *Neuron*, 13: 805–811.

Merkler, D., Metz, G.A.S., Raineteau, O., Dietz, V., Schwab, M.E. and Fouad, K. (2001) Locomotor recovery in spinal cord-injured rats treated with an antibody neutralizing the myelin-associated neurite growth inhibitor Nogo-A. *J. Neurosci.*, 21: 3665–3673.

Moon, L.D., Asher, R.A., Rhodes, K.E. and Fawcett, J.W. (2001) Regeneration of CNS axons back to their target following treatment of adult rat brain with chondroitinase ABC. *Nat. Neurosci.*, 4: 465–466.

Morgenstern, D.A., Asher, R.A. and Fawcett, J.W. (2002) Chondroitin sulfate proteoglycans in the CNS injury response. In: L. McKerracher, G. Douchet and S. Rossignol (Eds.), *Spinal Cord Trauma: Neural Repair and Functional Recovery. Progress in Brain Research*, Vol. 137. Elsevier Science, Amsterdam, pp. 313–332.

Mukhopadhyay, G., Doherty, P., Walsh, F.S., Crocker, P.R. and Filbin, M.T. (1994) A novel role of myelin-associated glycoprotein as an inhibitor of axonal regeneration. *Neuron*, 13: 1–20.

Nathan, P.W. (1994) Effects on movement of surgical incisions into the human spinal cord. *Brain*, 117: 337–346.

Niederöst, B., Zimmermann, D.R., Schwab, M.E. and Bandtlow, C.E. (1999) Bovine CNS myelin contains neurite growth-inhibitory activity associated with chondroitin sulfate proteoglycan. *J. Neurosci.*, 19: 8979–8989.

Oertle, T., Bandtlow, C.E. and Schwab, M.E. (2000) Charac-terization of the gene structure and the inhibitory regions of Nogo/RTN4. *Soc. Neurosci. Abstr.*, 26: 573.

Prinhja, R., Moore, S.E., Vinson, M., Blake, S., Morrow, R., Christie, G., Michalovich, D., Simmons, D.L. and Walsh, F.S. (2000) Inhibitor of neurite outgrowth in humans. *Nature*, 403: 383–384.

Qui, J., Cai, D. and Filbin, M.T. (2002) A role for cAMP in regeneration during development and after injury. In: L. McKerracher, G. Douchet and S. Rossignol (Eds.), *Spinal Cord Trauma: Neural Repair and Functional Recovery. Progress in Brain Research*, Vol. 137. Elsevier Science, Amsterdam, pp. 381–387.

Raineteau, O. and Schwab, M.E. (2001) Plasticity of motor systems after incomplete spinal cord injury. *Nat. Rev. Neurosci.*, 2: 263–274.

Raineteau, O., Z'Graggen, W.J., Thallmair, M. and Schwab, M.E. (1999) Sprouting and regeneration after pyramidotomy and blockade of the myelin-associated neurite growth inhibitors NI-35/250 in adult rats. *Eur. J. Neurosci.*, 11: 1486–1490.

Raineteau, O., Fouad, K., Noth, P., Thallmair, M. and Schwab, M.E. (2001) Functional switch between motor tracts in the presence of the mAB IN-1 in the adult rat. *Proc. Natl. Acad. Sci. USA*, 98: 6929–69341.

Ramon y Cajal, S. (1991) Degeneration and regeneration of the nervous system. In: J. De Felipe and E.G. Jones (Eds.), *Cajal's Degeneration and Regeneration of the Nervous System*, translated by R.M. May. Oxford Univ. Press, Oxford, New York.

Reh, T. and Kalil, K. (1982) Functional role of regrowing pyramidal tract fibers. *J. Comp. Neurol.*, 211: 276–283.

Richardson, P.M., Issa, V.M.K. and Aguayo, A.J. (1984) Regeneration of long spinal axons in the rat. *J. Neurocytol.*, 13: 165–182.

Rossignol, S. (2000) Locomotion and its recovery after spinal injury. *Curr. Opin. Neurobiol.*, 10: 708–716.

Rossignol, S. and Dubuc, R. (1994) Spinal pattern generation. *Curr. Opin. Neurobiol.*, 4: 894–902.

Savio, T. and Schwab, M.E. (1990) Lesioned corticospinal tract axons regenerate in myelin-free rat spinal cord. *Proc. Natl. Acad. Sci. USA*, 87: 4130–4133.

Schnell, L. and Schwab, M.E. (1990) Axonal regeneration in the rat spinal cord produced by an antibody against myelin-associated neurite growth inhibitors. *Nature*, 343: 269–272.

Schnell, L., Schneider, R., Kolbeck, R., Barde, Y.-A. and Schwab, M.E. (1994) Neurotrophin-3 enhances sprouting of corticospinal tract during development and after adult spinal cord lesion. *Nature*, 367: 170–173.

Schwab, M.E. and Bartholdi, D. (1996) Degeneration and regeneration of axons in the lesioned spinal cord. *Physiol. Rev.*, 76: 319–370.

Schwab, M.E. and Caroni, P. (1988) Oligodendrocytes and CNS myelin are nonpermissive substrates for neurite growth and fibroblast spreading in vitro. *J. Neurosci.*, 8: 2381–2393.

Schwab, M.E. and Thoenen, H. (1985) Dissociated neurons regenerate into sciatic but not optic nerve explants in culture irrespective of neurotrophic factors. *J. Neurosci.*, 5: 2415–2423.

Song, H., Ming, G., He, Z., Lehmann, M., McKerracher, L., Tessier-Lavigne, M. and Poo, M.-M. (1998) Conversion of neuronal growth cone responses from repulsion to attraction by cyclic nucleotides. *Science*, 281: 1515–1518.

Spillmann, A.A., Amberger, V.R. and Schwab, M.E. (1997) High molecular weight protein of human central nervous system myelin inhibits neurite outgrowth: an effect which can be neutralized by the monoclonal antibody IN-1. *Eur. J. Neurosci.*, 9: 549–555.

Spillmann, A.A., Bandtlow, C.E., Lottspeich, F., Keller, F. and Schwab, M.E. (1998) Identification and characterization of a bovine neurite growth inhibitor (bNI-220). *J. Biol. Chem.*, 273: 19283–19293.

Tello, F. (1911) La influencia del neurotropismo en la regeneracion de los centros nerviosos. *Trab. Lab. Invest. Biol.*, 9: 123–159.

Thallmair, M., Metz, G.A.S., Z'Graggen, W.J., Raineteau, O., Kartje, G.L. and Schwab, M.E. (1998) Neurite growth inhibitors restrict plasticity and functional recovery following corticospinal tract lesions. *Nat. Neurosci.*, 1: 124–131.

Varga, Z.M., Bandtlow, C.E., Erulkar, S.D., Schwab, M.E. and Nicholls, J.G. (1995) The critical period for repair of CNS of neonatal opossum (*Monodelphis domestica*) in culture: correlation with development of glial cells, myelin and growth inhibitory molecules. *Eur. J. Neurosci.*, 7: 2119–2129.

Vidal-Sanz, M., Aviles-Trigueros, M., Whitely, S.J.O., Sauvé, Y. and Lund, R.D. (2002) Reinnervation of the pretectum in adult rats by regenerated retinal ganglion cell axons: anatomical and functional studies. In: L. McKerracher, G. Douchet and S. Rossignol (Eds.), *Spinal Cord Trauma: Neural Repair and Functional Recovery. Progress in Brain Research*, Vol. 137. Elsevier Science, Amsterdam, pp. 443–452.

Vilensky, J.A., Moore, A.M., Eidelberg, E. and Walden, J.G. (1992) Recovery of locomotion in monkeys with spinal cord lesions. *J. Motor Behav.*, 24: 288–296.

Weibel, D., Cadelli, D. and Schwab, M.E. (1994) Regeneration of lesioned rat optic nerve fibers is improved after neutralization of myelin-associated neurite growth inhibitors. *Brain Res.*, 642: 259–266.

Weidner, N., Ner, A., Salimi, N. and Tuszynski, M.H. (2001) Spontaneous corticospinal axonal plasticity and functional recovery after adult central nervous system injury. *Proc. Natl. Acad. Sci. USA*, 98: 3513–3518.

Wernig, A., Müller, S., Nanassy, A. and Cagol, E. (1995) Laufband therapy based on 'rules of spinal locomotion' is effective in spinal cord injured persons. *Eur. J. Neurosci.*, 7: 823–829.

Z'Graggen, W.J., Metz, G.A.S., Kartje, G.L., Thallmair, M. and Schwab, M.E. (1998) Functional recovery and enhanced corticofugal plasticity after unilateral pyramidal tract lesion and blockade of myelin-associated neurite growth inhibitors in adult rats. *J. Neurosci.*, 18: 4744–4754.

L. McKerracher, G. Doucet and S. Rossignol (Eds.)
Progress in Brain Research, Vol. 137
© 2002 Elsevier Science B.V. All rights reserved

CHAPTER 25

Nogo and the Nogo-66 receptor

Alyson E. Fournier, Tadzia GrandPré, Graham Gould, Xingxing Wang and
Stephen M. Strittmatter [*]

*Department of Neurology and Section of Neurobiology, Yale University School of Medicine, P.O. Box 208018,
New Haven, CT 06510, USA*

Abstract: Nogo has been identified as a component of central nervous system (CNS) myelin preventing axonal regeneration in the adult vertebrate CNS. Our previous analysis of Nogo-A demonstrated that an axon-inhibiting 66 aa domain is expressed at the extracellular surface and the endoplasmic reticulum lumen of transfected cells and oligodendrocytes. We have identified a brain-specific, leucine-rich repeat protein with high affinity for soluble Nogo-66. Cleavage of the Nogo-66 receptor from axonal surfaces renders neurons insensitive to Nogo-66. Nogo-66 receptor expression is sufficient to impart Nogo-66 axonal inhibition to unresponsive neurons. With identified ligand and receptor components, structure–function determinants for inhibition of axon regeneration can now be mapped. The relative contribution of Nogo, myelin-associated glycoprotein, chondroitin sulfate proteoglycan and oligodendrocyte myelin glycoprotein to myelin inhibition can be assessed. Blockade of Nogo-66 interaction with its receptor provides one potential avenue to promote axonal regeneration after adult mammalian CNS injury.

Introduction

The inability of neurons in the adult central nervous system (CNS) to spontaneously regenerate following injury has devastating clinical consequences. Lack of spontaneous regeneration is specific to the CNS since neurons in the adult peripheral nervous system (PNS) are capable of long distance regeneration mediating functional recovery. Regenerative failure is also developmentally restricted since injured neurons in the embryonic CNS can regrow. While it was once hypothesized that adult CNS neurons may be intrinsically incapable of regenerative growth, landmark experiments by Aguayo and colleagues (David and

Aguayo, 1981) demonstrated that injured CNS neurons are capable of regenerating when provided with a growth permissive peripheral nerve environment. These experiments initiated a field of regenerative research attempting to define what prevents an adult CNS neuron from regenerating. Initial research focused on the lack of growth promoting cues, such as neurotrophic factors, required for neurite outgrowth. However, the field was transformed when it was discovered that the adult CNS environment was actively inhibitory for regenerative growth following CNS injury. Two major sources of inhibition exist in the injured CNS environment. An astroglial scar rich in inhibitory molecules such as chondroitin sulfate proteoglycans (CSPGs) and tenascin, and CNS myelin that contains multiple neurite outgrowth inhibitors. The lack of regeneration in the CNS is most certainly due to a combination of insufficient positive cues and of multiple inhibitory influences. This review will focus on arguably the most potent myelin-derived inhibitor, Nogo. Nogo activity was

---

[*] Correspondence to: S.M. Strittmatter, Department of Neurology, Yale University School of Medicine, P.O. Box 208018, New Haven, CT 06510, USA. Tel.: +1-203-785-4878; Fax: +1-203-785-5098;
E-mail: stephen.strittmatter@yale.edu

first identified over 10 years ago by Schwab and colleagues in myelin fractionation experiments (Caroni and Schwab, 1988a). A major advance in the field was achieved last year when three groups independently cloned the Nogo gene, and again this year with the cloning of a Nogo receptor. This review will focus on our current understanding of Nogo, its relationship with the Nogo receptor, and how it may signal to mediate neurite outgrowth inhibition.

Nogo

Nogo activity was originally characterized by Schwab and colleagues through size fractionation experiments of adult CNS myelin (Caroni and Schwab, 1988a). From myelin, two membrane-bound protein fractions of relative molecular masses 35 and 250 kDa were identified to be inhibitory for neurite outgrowth. These two protein fractions came to be known collectively as NI-35/250 (for neurite growth inhibitors). The NI-35/250 proteins are enriched in CNS myelin and analogous fractions from PNS myelin had no inhibitory characteristics (Caroni and Schwab, 1988a). Following the publication of six partial peptide sequences derived from a proteolytic digest of the bovine homologue of rat NI-250 (Nogo-A) (Spillmann et al., 1998), three groups independently cloned the NI-250 gene, termed Nogo (Chen et al., 2000; GrandPre et al., 2000; Prinjha et al., 2000). The cloning of Nogo was met with great excitement in the field primarily due to intriguing results previously achieved with a monoclonal antibody IN-1 (inhibitor neutralization). IN-1 was directed against the rat CNS myelin 250 kDa inhibitory protein fraction (Caroni and Schwab, 1988b) and recognizes both the NI-35 and NI-250 (Nogo-A) proteins. IN-1 antibody treatment in vitro can overcome oligodendrocyte-mediated inhibition of 3T3 fibroblast spreading and axonal outgrowth (Caroni and Schwab, 1988b). In vivo, IN-1 producing hybridoma cells implanted into the cortex of young rats significantly increased the distance of axonal regeneration of corticospinal tract (CST) axons in rats (Schnell and Schwab, 1990). In addition to these anatomical observations, Bregman et al. (1995) demonstrated that chronic exposure to IN-1 improved both sensorimotor reflex and locomotor function following bilat-

eral transection of the CSTs and the dorsal columns in adult rats. While results with the IN-1 antibody are very exciting, it is clear that in addition to binding Nogo, the IN-1 antibody recognizes several other proteins in spinal cord extracts (Spillmann et al., 1998). The cloning of Nogo now makes it possible to investigate the ability of Nogo-specific antibodies to mediate anatomical and behavioral recovery following spinal cord lesions. Experiments with Nogo-specific reagents will facilitate an understanding of Nogo function and its mechanism of action. In addition, specific antagonists can now be generated in an attempt to disrupt Nogo inhibition.

Three major transcripts (Nogo-A, -B, and -C) originate from the Nogo gene by both alternative promoter usage and alternative splicing (Fig. 1). Nogo-A is a 1192 residue protein containing all six peptide sequences derived from the proteolytic digest of the bovine homologue of NI-250 and appears to correspond to NI-250. Nogo-B (373 amino acids) and Nogo-C (199 amino acids) are shorter splice variants of full length Nogo-A. Nogo-B may correspond to NI-35. The three transcripts have a common C-terminal domain of 188 amino acids, and this region is homologous to members of the reticulon (Rtn) or neuroendocrine-specific protein (NSP) gene family (Chen et al., 2000; GrandPre et al., 2000; Prinjha et al., 2000). The function of the Rtn protein family is unknown, but it has been hypothesized to regulate protein sorting or other aspect of endoplasmic reticulum (ER) function due to its association with the ER (van de Velde et al., 1994). A second possibility is that Rtns may play a general role in mRNA trafficking due to the asymmetric distribution of their mRNA (Baka et al., 1996).

As one would anticipate for a CNS inhibitory molecule, Nogo-A RNA is expressed at high levels in adult CNS tissues with little to no expression in peripheral tissues and the sciatic nerve of the PNS (GrandPre et al., 2000). By in situ hybridization Nogo mRNA expression is detected in oligodendrocytes and in subsets of neurons. The mRNA expression parallels Nogo protein expression in oligodendrocytes. Using an antiserum generated against Nogo, a significant portion of Nogo protein was detected on the cell surface of oligodendrocytes (GrandPre et al., 2000). Nogo was also associated with the ER membrane in both oligodendrocytes,

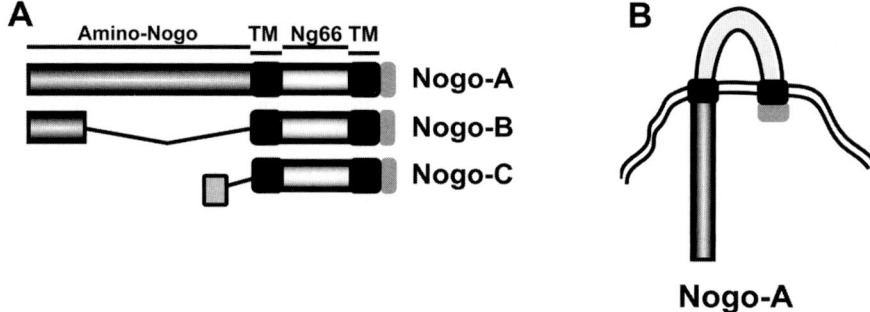

Fig. 1. Nogo structure and topology. (A) Three forms of Nogo, Nogo-A, -B, and -C share a common carboxy terminal domain containing two transmembrane (TM) regions separated by a 66 amino acid segment (Nogo-66). Nogo-A has a 1024 residue amino terminal domain (Amino-Nogo). (B) Immunostaining of transfected 293T cells and oligodendrocytes (GrandPre et al., 2000) demonstrated that the 66 amino acid portion of Nogo between two transmembrane segments (Nogo-66) is extracellular while the amino and carboxy terminal portion of the protein are intracellular.

and to a large extent in transfected 293T cells (Chen et al., 2000; GrandPre et al., 2000). This is consistent with its membership in the reticulon protein family, and with the presence of an ER-retention signal in the C-terminus of Nogo.

The C-terminal domain of Nogo contains two transmembrane domains, separated by a 66 amino acid hydrophilic region. Immunohistologic staining of epitope tags located at the amino or carboxyl termini of Nogo-A or antiserum developed against the Nogo-66 domain suggests that the amino terminus and carboxyl terminus of Nogo are likely to be intracellular while the Nogo-66 domain projects extracellularly (GrandPre et al., 2000) (Fig. 1B). In this conformation (Fig. 1B), axons would be exposed to Nogo-66 in the uninjured state and would only be exposed to Amino-Nogo following injury when oligodendrocyte membrane integrity is compromised. While there is strong evidence that this conformation exists, there is some suggestion that Nogo may be capable of existing in additional conformations within the membrane (Huber and Schwab, 2000). Some indirect evidence for a second topology is presented by Buffo et al. (2000) who demonstrated that application of antiserum 472 raised against a peptide sequence in the amino terminal portion of Nogo-A enhances sprouting of Purkinje cells in the uninjured adult cerebellum. This suggests that Purkinje cells may be exposed to and inhibited by Amino-Nogo in the uninjured state. Such an activity would require Amino-Nogo to be localized extracellularly in CNS white matter.

Functional analysis of Nogo-A in vitro demonstrates that the protein has potent growth inhibitory activity. In both a 3T3 fibroblast spreading assay (Chen et al., 2000), and in E12 chick dorsal root ganglia (DRG) growth cone collapse (GrandPre et al., 2000), Nogo-A demonstrates potent inhibitory activity. Similar to myelin-associated glycoprotein (MAG) (Mukhopadhyay et al., 1994; Bartsch et al., 1995), sensitivity to Nogo appears to be developmentally regulated as E10 chick DRGs are less responsive than E12 DRGs in growth cone collapse assays (GrandPre et al., 2000). Interestingly, two separate domains of Nogo-A can inhibit neurite outgrowth independently. Both the amino terminal portion of Nogo-A (Amino Nogo, Fig. 1A), and the 66 amino acid stretch of Nogo in the carboxy terminal region of the protein (Nogo-66) have growth inhibitory activity. Residues 1–1024 (Amino-Nogo) of Nogo-A inhibit cerebellar neurite outgrowth in a dose dependent manner when presented as an Fc fusion protein (Prinjha et al., 2000). Further, treatment with an antiserum (AS472) directed against a synthetic peptide corresponding to residues 623–640 of Nogo-A promotes rat DRG neurite outgrowth on inhibitory adult rat optic nerve substrates (Chen et al., 2000). Nogo-66 also has potent inhibitory activity and this was originally demonstrated in both growth cone collapse and neurite outgrowth assays of E12 chick DRG neurons (GrandPre et al., 2000). A direct comparison of soluble recombinant Amino-Nogo and Nogo-66 fragments (Fournier et al., 2001) confirmed that both domains possess inhibitory activity, however the activities have unique characteristics raising the possibility that the two domains may act synergistically (Fournier et al., 2001).

To directly compare the two protein domains, glutathione-*S*-transferase (GST) Nogo-66 was prepared in *Escherichia coli* and Amino-Nogo was expressed as a MycHis-tagged protein in HEK293T cells. When coated as tissue culture substrates both Amino-Nogo and Nogo-66 inhibited E12 DRG neurite outgrowth, but only Amino-Nogo prevented the fibroblast-like cells in the DRG culture or cultured 3T3 fibroblasts from spreading. Nogo-66 effects are therefore neuronal specific, while the highly acidic Amino-Nogo may mediate more general effects. When presented in soluble form, GSTNogo-66 collapsed E12 DRG growth cones at 100 nM, and potently inhibited axonal extension while soluble Amino-Nogo protein was inactive. When Amino-Nogo was aggregated with anti-myc and anti-mouse IgG antibodies, Amino-Nogo significantly reduced both DRG and cerebellar axon outgrowth. Similarly inhibition of cerebellar granule neurons required Amino-Nogo to be presented as an Fc fusion protein — presumably in dimeric form (Prinjha et al., 2000). Nogo-66 is therefore a highly potent, neuronal specific inhibitor that is active as a soluble monomeric ligand. Amino-Nogo activity requires dimerization or clustering and has more widespread inhibitory effects on both neuronal and non-neuronal cells. The relative contribution of the two domains to Nogo-A inhibitory activity remains to be determined.

Relative contribution of Nogo to myelin inhibition

While Nogo is clearly a potent neurite outgrowth inhibitor any strategy to overcome inhibition will have to consider that several neurite outgrowth inhibitors exist in myelin. Biochemical fractionation of myelin coupled to neurite outgrowth assays have identified MAG (McKerracher et al., 1994; Mukhopadhyay et al., 1994), CSPGs (Niederost et al., 1999), and arretin/oligodendrocyte myelin glycoprotein (Xiao et al., 1997; Kottis et al., 2001) as additional inhibitory components in myelin.

While MAG has clear inhibitory activity in vitro (McKerracher et al., 1994; Mukhopadhyay et al., 1994), studies performed in MAG null mutant mice showed small (Li et al., 1996; Shen et al., 1998)

or no (Bartsch et al., 1995) improvements in outgrowth on MAG$^{-/-}$ myelin suggesting that the contribution of MAG to overall myelin inhibition may be minimal. The relative contribution of CSPGs to myelin-inhibition has not been clearly defined. CSPG-expressing reactive astrocytes are clearly inhibitory in vitro (McKeon and Silver, 1995; Fawcett and Asher, 1999) and CSPGs are expressed in abundance at the glial scar (Asher et al., 1995; Bode-Lesniewska et al., 1996; Meyer-Puttlitz et al., 1996; Levine, 1998). However, in addition to their presence in the glial scar, brevican and the brain-specific versican V2 splice variant are expressed in myelin (Niederost et al., 1999). Immunodepletion of these CSPGs from myelin reduced the inhibitory activity of the myelin fraction as assayed by neurite outgrowth of cerebellar granule cells. The contribution of a fourth myelin-derived inhibitor originally defined as arretin (Xiao et al., 1997) and more recently identified as oligodendrocyte myelin glycoprotein (OMGp) (Kottis et al., 2001) is yet to be defined. While these myelin components have clear inhibitory activity, their contribution to myelin inhibitory activity may be minor relative to Nogo. Results from the IN-1 antibody strongly suggest that Nogo represents the predominant neurite outgrowth inhibitory signal in CNS myelin. The full extent of Nogo inhibition can now be addressed with Nogo-specific reagents.

Nogo receptor

The multiple inhibitory domains of Nogo raise the possibility that multiple receptors may exist, and certainly these receptors will have to be identified to achieve a full understanding of the mechanism of Nogo action. Indeed, further insight into this question came with the cloning of a receptor for Nogo-66 (Fournier et al., 2001). The receptor was expression cloned using an alkaline phosphatase (AP) fusion protein assay developed by Flanagan and Leder (1990). Nogo-66 was expressed as a placental AP fusion protein Nogo-66-AP (Flanagan and Leder, 1990) which was able to bind to saturable, high affinity binding sites on E12 chick DRG neurons. The biological activity of Nogo-66-AP was verified in growth cone collapse assays where the protein was even more potent than GSTNogo-66 (EC$_{50}$ of 1 and 50 nM, respectively). The Nogo-66-AP fusion

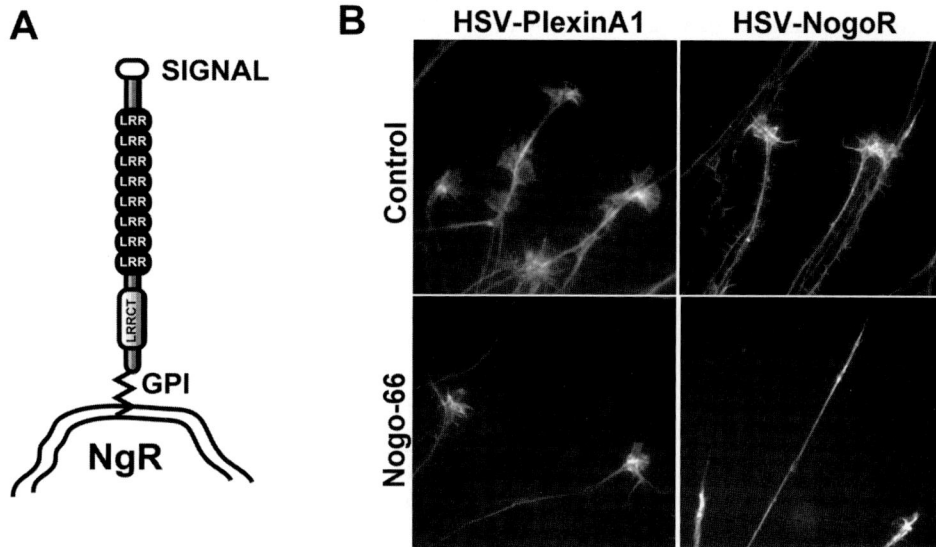

Fig. 2. NgR structure and function. (A) Nogo-66 receptor (NgR) is a 473 amino acid protein with a signal sequence (SIGNAL), 8 leucine rich repeat (LRR) domains, a leucine-rich repeat carboxy terminal (LRRCT) domain, a unique region, and a glycosylphosphatidylinositol (GPI) anchor domain. (B) E7 chick retinal neurons were infected with recombinant control HSVPlexinA1 virus or HSVNgR virus for 24 h, then exposed to 500 nM GSTNogo-66 for 30 min and assayed for growth cone collapse. Control growth cones infected with the plexinA1 virus do not respond to Nogo-66 while NgR-infected cells undergo growth cone collapse.

protein was used to screen COS-7 cells transfected with pools of cDNA from a mouse brain cDNA library. Using this approach, a novel 473 amino acid protein termed the Nogo-66 receptor (NgR) was cloned. NgR contains a signal sequence followed by eight leucine-rich-repeat (LRR) domains, an LRR carboxy-terminal flanking domain that is cysteine rich, a unique region and a glycosylphosphatidylinositol (GPI) anchorage site (Fig. 2A). In addition, a human homologue of the mouse NgR cDNA that shares 89% amino acid identity was identified. The exons of the human NgR gene are located on chromosome 22q11.

NgR mRNA is detected predominantly in brain as one would predict for a functional Nogo receptor. By Northern blot analysis a single 2.3-kb transcript can be detected in adult brain with low levels of mRNA in heart and kidney, but not in other peripheral tissues. Within the brain, NgR RNA is expressed in a variety of neuronal cell types including cerebral cortical neurons, hippocampal neurons, cerebellar Purkinje cells and pontine neurons. NgR mRNA is not expressed in white matter where Nogo-A is expressed by oligodendrocytes. Furthermore, in spinal cord cultures, a reciprocal pattern of NgR protein

and oligodendrocytes is evident. NgR protein is expressed on axons extending from the explants and is absent from Nogo-66-expressing oligodendrocytes in the culture (GrandPre et al., 2000; Fournier et al., 2001). Notably, NgR RNA is expressed in those cerebral cortex pyramidal neurons whose regeneration is enhanced by IN-1 treatment (Schnell and Schwab, 1990), and in cerebellar Purkinje neurons whose sprouting is increased by anti-Nogo-A antibody (Buffo et al., 2000).

The NgR protein was shown to directly bind GSTNogo-66 in a pull down assay and its ability to function as a viable receptor for Nogo-66 was demonstrated in both gain of function and loss of function assays. These experiments took advantage of the differential response of E12 chick DRG neurons and E7 chick retinal ganglion cell (RGC) neurons to Nogo-66. E12 chick DRG neurons respond strongly to Nogo-66 in growth cone collapse assays (GrandPre et al., 2000), while E7 chick RGCs are unresponsive (Fournier et al., 2001). This response correlates with the NgR protein expression profile in the two tissues. A NgR antiserum generated against a GSTNgR fusion protein purified from E. coli detected NgR expression in E12 DRGs, but not E7 RGCs. Nogo-66 sensitivity was lost in E12 DRGs pre-treated with phosphatidylinositol-specific phospholipase C (PI-PLC) to remove NgR from the cell surface. While this result correlates the Nogo-66 response to NgR expression, PI-PLC treatment removes many GPI linked proteins in addition to the NgR from the cell surface. Therefore, gain of function experiments were performed to demonstrate that Nogo-66 sensitivity could be conferred to E7 RGCs in a growth cone collapse assay by expressing NgR. E7 retinal cultures were infected with a recombinant herpes simplex virus (HSV) NgR viral preparation for 24 h, then exposed to Nogo-66 and scored for growth cone collapse (Fig. 2B). NgR expressing RGCs collapsed their growth cones in response to Nogo-66 while RGCs infected with a plexinA1 control virus remained unresponsive. The NgR is therefore capable of mediating both Nogo binding and of mediating the inhibitory activity of Nogo. The ability of HSVNgR-infected E7 RGCs to transduce Nogo-66 signals indicates that E7 RGCs express the necessary signal transducing components and intracellular machinery to mediate Nogo-66 signals. However, NgR-infected E7 RGCs required a higher dose of Nogo-66 than E12 DRGs. This may reflect limited NgR protein expression in infected cultures due to the limits of the HSV infection system or it may reflect reduced levels of other Nogo-66 receptor signaling components.

NgR domains

The NgR protein has several conserved domains including LRR domains and a GPI anchor domain. The LRR domains of the NgR share moderate amino acid sequence similarity (up to 35% amino acid identity) to many other LRR-containing proteins. Because LRR-containing proteins serve a wide variety of functions (Buchanan and Gay, 1996) they offer little insight into the mechanism of NgR signaling. The greatest sequence similarity in the LRR region exists with slit 1–3 and the acid-labile subunit of the insulin-like growth-factor-binding protein complex. Slits are a family of extracellular matrix proteins that are expressed at the CNS midline and repel neurons that express receptors of the Roundabout (Robo) family (Brose et al., 1999; Zinn and Sun, 1999). Recent evidence demonstrates that Robo function is

intricately regulated by both ligand and receptor interactions to facilitate its role in axon pathfinding at the midline (Stein and Tessier-Lavigne, 2001). As with many receptors mediating growth cone guidance, Robo likely signals to the growth cone cytoskeleton to affect changes in axonal guidance. This is supported by evidence that the cytoplasmic domain of Robo interacts with Abl tyrosine kinase and Ena (Bashaw et al., 2000), two proteins involved in modifying the growth cone's actin cytoskeleton. While it remains to be determined if NgR may interact with Robo or utilize common intracellular signaling substrates to modulate neurite outgrowth, the idea is intriguing.

The GPI anchor of the NgR may offer more insight into its mechanism of action. The GPI linkage was verified by demonstrating a shift in protein localization from particulate to soluble fractions of NgR-transfected 293T cells following PI-PLC treatment. Because NgR alone cannot transmit ligand-binding information intracellularly through its GPI linkage, it is likely that a second signal transducing protein exists in a receptor-signaling complex. While the transducing protein has not yet been identified, other GPI-linked receptor proteins form such signaling complexes with intracellular transducing proteins. For example the GPI-anchored receptors $GFR\alpha_1-\alpha_4$ each bind to specific glial cell line derived neurotrophic factor (GDNF) family ligands (GFLs), and all interact with a common receptor tyrosine kinase, RET (Tansey et al., 2000). In this case, $GFR\alpha_1-\alpha_4$ are responsible for providing high affinity binding sites and for mediating binding specificity for the multiple ligands of the GDNF family while RET tyrosine kinase signals intracellularly via its cytoplasmic domain. The GPI anchor plays a critical role in the GFL signaling pathway by restricting $GFR\alpha_1$ protein to lipid rafts and recruiting RET to the lipid raft after GDNF binding (Tansey et al., 2000). $GFR\alpha_1$-mediated RET recruitment to the lipid raft is critical for efficient GFL signaling. Lipid rafts are thought to represent specialized signaling compartments within the plasma membrane because of the enrichment of Src family kinases and other signaling proteins that localize to the intracellular leaflet of lipid rafts (Anderson, 1998). Future studies will examine if the GPI anchor of NgR restricts protein localization within the plasma membrane and if this may be important for efficient Nogo signaling.

A second possibility is that the GPI anchor allows NgR to be cleaved resulting in release of soluble NgR from the cell surface. Soluble NgR could subsequently bind to Nogo and activate a signal-transducing component on another cell in trans. Alternatively, the cell could use protein cleavage as a regulatory mechanism to release NgR and attenuate Nogo signaling.

Identification of the NgR provides a new target to attempt to disrupt Nogo-mediated inhibition. Furthermore, assuming Amino-Nogo cannot mediate inhibition via the NgR, NgR disruption will help to determine the relative contribution of Amino-Nogo and Nogo-66 to Nogo-A inhibitory activity. To this end, we have begun to analyze NgR structure to elucidate what receptor domains are responsible for Nogo-66 binding and signaling. Analysis of Nogo-66-AP binding to cells transfected with various NgR deletion mutants demonstrates that Nogo-66 binding is restricted to NgR LRR domains (AF, GG, SMS, unpublished observations). Ultimately, blockade of Nogo-66 interaction with its receptor may improve axonal regeneration after adult mammalian CNS injury.

NgR intracellular signaling

The intracellular signaling pathways downstream of NgR are not yet known. Certainly calcium represents one candidate-signaling molecule since calcium influx is observed during NI-250 signaling, and blockade of this influx attenuates NI-250 growth cone collapse (Loschinger et al., 1997). The cAMP–PKA pathway represents another candidate pathway since it has been implicated in MAG/myelin-dependent inhibition (Cai et al., 1999). Priming neurons with neurotrophins activates the cAMP–PKA pathway and allows neurons to grow on myelin and MAG substrates.

It is reasonable to speculate that the final target of Nogo will be the neuronal cytoskeleton. One common theme in axon repulsion and neurite outgrowth inhibition is the involvement of rho family small GTPases which act as molecular switches to control growth cone actin dynamics (Hall, 1994; Mackay et al., 1996). Inhibition of RhoA by C3 transferase blocks CNS myelin induced growth cone collapse

(Jin and Strittmatter, 1997) and MAG-dependent outgrowth inhibition (Lehmann et al., 1999). Furthermore, activated rac can protect motor neurons from myelin-induced collapse (Kuhn et al., 1999). Further studies will be required to elucidate the role of small GTPases in modulating Nogo inhibition. Identification of intracellular substrates for NgR will lead to new targets to disrupt Nogo-mediated inhibition. Furthermore, because myelin contains multiple inhibitory proteins, intracellular proteins utilized by multiple myelin-derived inhibitors represent good targets to overcome myelin inhibition.

Development of strategies to promote regenerative growth and functional recovery following CNS injury is a complex problem. Multiple issues must be addressed, including neuronal cell survival, axonal regrowth, guidance to appropriate targets and re-establishment of synaptic connections. The identification of Nogo and NgR represents a significant advance in our understanding of how we may promote axonal regrowth by neutralizing neurite outgrowth inhibition. Blockade of Nogo, NgR or intracellular signaling substrates of NgR may ultimately improve axonal regeneration after adult mammalian CNS injury.

Abbreviations

AP	alkaline phosphatase
CNS	central nervous system
DRG	dorsal root ganglia
ER	endoplasmic reticulum
GDNF	glial cell line derived neurotrophic factor
GFLs	glial cell line derived neurotrophic factor family ligands
GPI	glycosylphosphatidylinositol
GST	glutathione-S-transferase
HSV	herpes simplex virus
LRR	leucine-rich repeat
MAG	myelin-associated glycoprotein
NgR	Nogo-66 receptor
Nogo-66-AP	Nogo-66-alkaline phosphatase
NSP	neuroendocrine specific protein
OMGp	oligodendrocyte myelin glycoprotein
PI-PLC	phosphatidylinositol-specific phospholipase C

368

PNS	peripheral nervous system
RGC	retinal ganglion cell
Rtn	reticulon
Robo	Roundabout

Acknowledgements

This work was supported by grants to S.M.S. from the National Institutes of Health and the Christopher Reeve Paralysis Foundation and The Catherine and Patrick Donaghue Foundation for Medical Research.

References

Anderson, R.G.W. (1998) The caveolae membrane system. *Annu. Rev. Biochem.*, 67: 199–225.

Asher, R.A., Scheibe, R.J., Keiser, H. and Bignami, A. (1995) On the existence of a cartilage-like proteoglycan and link proteins in the central nervous sytem. *Glia*, 13: 294–308.

Baka, I.D., Ninkina, N.N., Pinon, L.G., Adu, J., Davies, A.M., Georgiev, G.P. and Buchman, V.L. (1996) Intracellular compartmentalization of two differentially spliced s-rex/NSP mRNAs in neurons. *Mol. Cell. Neurosci.*, 7: 289–303.

Bartsch, U., Bandtlow, C.E., Schnell, L., Bartsch, S., Spillmann, A.A., Rubin, B.P., Hillenbrand, R., Montag, D., Schwab, M.E. and Schachner, M. (1995) Lack of evidence that myelin-associated glycoprotein is a major inhibitor of axonal regeneration in the CNS. *Neuron*, 15: 1375–1381.

Bashaw, G.J., Kidd, T., Murray, D., Pawson, T. and Goodman, C.S. (2000) Repulsive axon guidance: Abelson and Enabled play opposing roles downstream of the roundabout receptor. *Cell*, 101: 703–715.

Bode-Lesniewska, B., Dours-Zimmermann, D., Odermatt, B.F., Briner, J., Heitz, P.U. and Zimmermann, D.R. (1996) Distribution of the large aggregating proteoglycan versican in adult human tissues. *J. Histochem. Cytochem.*, 44: 303–312.

Bregman, B., Kunkeel-Bagden, E., Schnell, L., Dai, H.N., Gao, D. and Schwab, M.E. (1995) Recovery from spinal cord injury mediated by antibodies to neurite growth inhibitors. *Nature*, 378: 498–501.

Brose, K., Bland, K.S., Wang, K.H., Arnott, D., Henzel, W., Goodman, C.S., Tessier-Lavigne, M. and Kidd, T. (1999) Slit proteins bind robo receptors and have an evolutionarily conserved role in repulsive axon guidance. *Cell*, 96: 795–806.

Buchanan, S.G.S.C. and Gay, N.J. (1996) Structural and functional diversity in the leucine-rich repeat family of proteins. *Prog. Biophys. Mol. Biol.*, 65: 1–44.

Buffo, A., Zagrebelsky, M., Huber, A.B., Skerra, A., Schwab, M.E., Strata, P. and Rossi, F. (2000) Application of neutralizing antibodies against NI-35/250 myelin-associated neurite growth inhibitory proteins to the adult rat cerebellum induces sprouting of uninjured purkinje cell axons. *J. Neurosci.*, 20: 2275–2286.

Cai, D., Shen, Y., De Bellard, M., Tang, S. and Filbin, M.T.

(1999) Prior exposure to neurotrophins blocks inhibition of axonal regeneration by MAG and myelin via a cAMP-dependent mechanism. *Neuron*, 22: 89–101.

Caroni, P. and Schwab, M.E. (1988a) Two membrane protein fractions from rat central myelin with inhibitory properties for neurite growth and fibroblast spreading. *J. Cell Biol.*, 106: 1281–1288.

Caroni, P. and Schwab, M.E. (1988b) Antibody against myelin-associated inhibitor of neurite growth neutralizes nonpermissive substrate properties of CNS white matter. *Neuron*, 1: 85–96.

Chen, M.S., Huber, A.B., van der Haar, M.E., Frank, M., Schnell, L., Spillmann, A.A., Christ, F. and Schwab, M.E. (2000) Nogo-A is a myelin-associated neurite outgrowth inhibitor and an antigen for monoclonal antibody IN-1. *Nature*, 403: 434–439.

David, S. and Aguayo, A.J. (1981) Axonal elongation in peripheral nervous system bridges after central nervous system injury in adult rats. *Science*, 214: 391–393.

Fawcett, J.W. and Asher, R.A. (1999) The glial scar and central nervous system repair. *Brain Res. Bull.*, 49: 377–391.

Flanagan, J.G. and Leder, P. (1990) The kit ligand: a cell surface molecule altered in steel mutant fibroblasts. *Cell*, 63: 185–194.

Fournier, A.E., GrandPre, T. and Strittmatter, S.M. (2001) Identification of a receptor mediating Nogo-66 inhibition of axonal regeneration. *Nature*, 409: 341–346.

GrandPre, T., Nakamura, F., Vartanian, T. and Strittmatter, S.M. (2000) Identification of the Nogo inhibitor of axon regeneration as a Reticulon protein. *Nature*, 403: 439–444.

Hall, A. (1994) Small GTP-binding proteins and the regulation of the actin cytoskeleton. *Annu. Rev. Cell Biol.*, 10: 31–54.

Huber, A.B. and Schwab, M.E. (2000) Nogo-A, a potent inhibitor of neurite outgrowth and regeneration. *Biol. Chem.*, 381: 407–419.

Jin, Z. and Strittmatter, S.M. (1997) Rac1 mediates collapsin-1-induced growth cone collapse. *J. Neurosci.*, 17: 6256–6263.

Kottis, V., Zhang, R., Xiao, Z.C., Gravel, M. and Braun, P.E. (2001) Identification of OMGp as a putative, myelin-associated inhibitor of neurite outgrowth. Abstracts of the XXIIIrd Annual Symposium of the Centre de recherche en science neurologiques, Universite de Montreal. [Online]: http://www.crsn.umontreal.ca/XXIIIs/home.html, PDF document, p. 66.

Kuhn, T.B., Brown, M.D., Wilcox, C.L., Raper, J.A. and Bamburg, J.R. (1999) Myelin and collapsin-1 induce motor neuron growth cone collapse through different pathways: inhibition of collapse by opposing mutants of Rac1. *J. Neurosci.*, 19: 1965–1975.

Lehmann, M., Fournier, A., Selles-Navarro, I., Dergham, P., Sebok, A., Leclerc, N., Tigyi, G. and McKerracher, L. (1999) Inactivation of Rho signaling pathway promotes CNS axon regeneration. *J. Neurosci.*, 19: 7537–7547.

Levine, J. (1998) Increased expression of the NG2 chondroitin-sulfate proteoglycan after brain injury. *J. Neurosci.*, 14: 4716–4730.

Li, M., Shibata, A., Li, C., Braun, P.E., McKerracher, L., Roder, J., Kater, S.B. and David, S. (1996) Myelin-associated glycoprotein inhibits neurite/axon growth and causes growth cone collapse. *J. Neurosci. Res.*, 46: 404–414.

Loschinger, J., Bandtlow, C.E., Jung, J., Klostermann, S., Schwab, M.E., Bonhoeffer, F. and Kater, S.B. (1997) Retinal axon growth cone responses to different environmental cues are mediated by different second-messenger systems. *J. Neurobiol.*, 33: 825–834.

Mackay, D.J.G., Nobes, C.D. and Hall, A. (1996) The Rho's progress: a potential role during neuritogenesis for the Rho family GTPases. *Trends Neurosci.*, 18: 496–501.

McKeon, R.J. and Silver, J. (1995) Injury-induced proteoglycans inhibit the potential for laminin-mediated axon growth on astrocytic scars. *Exp. Neurol.*, 136: 32–43.

McKerracher, L., David, S., Jackson, J.L., Kottis, V., Dunn, R. and Braun, P.E. (1994) Identification of myelin-associated glycoprotein as a major myelin-derived inhibitor of neurite outgrowth. *Neuron*, 13: 805–811.

Meyer-Puttlitz, B., Junker, E., Margolis, R.U. and Margolis, R.K. (1996) Chondroitin sulfate proteoglycans in the developing central nervous system II. Immunocytochemical localization of neurocan and phosphocan. *J. Comp. Neurol.*, 366: 44–54.

Mukhopadhyay, G., Doherty, P., Walsh, F.S., Crocker, P.R. and Filbin, M.T. (1994) A novel role for myelin-associated glycoprotein as an inhibitor of axonal regeneration. *Neuron*, 13: 805–811.

Niederost, B.P., Zimmerman, D.R., Schwab, M.E. and Bandtlow, C.E. (1999) Bovine CNS myelin contains neurite growth-inhibitory activity associated with chondroitin sulfate proteoglycans. *J. Neurosci.*, 19: 8979–8989.

Prinjha, R., Moore, S.E., Vinson, M., Blake, S., Morrow, R., Christie, G., Michalovich, D., Simmons, D.L. and Walsh, F.S. (2000) Inhibitor of neurite outgrowth in humans. *Nature*, 403: 383–384.

Schnell, L. and Schwab, M.E. (1990) Axonal regeneration in the rat spinal cord produced by an antibody against myelin-associated neurite growth inhibitors. *Nature*, 343: 269–272.

Shen, Y.J., DeBellard, M.E., Salzer, J.L., Roder, J. and Filbin, M.T. (1998) Myelin-associated glycoprotein in myelin and expressed by Schwann cell inhibits axonal regeneration and branching. *Mol. Cell Neurosci.*, 12: 79–91.

Spillmann, A.A., Bandtlow, C.E., Lottspeich, F., Keller, F. and Schwab, M.E. (1998) Identification and characterization of a bovine neurite growth inhibitor (bNI-220). *J. Biol. Chem.*, 73: 19283–19293.

Stein, E. and Tessier-Lavigne, M. (2001) Hierarchical organization of guidance receptors: silencing of netrin attraction by Slit through a Robo/DCC receptor complex. *Science*, 291: 1928–1938.

Tansey, M.G., Baloh, R.H., Milbrandt, J. and Johnson, E.M.J. (2000) GFRalpha-mediated localization of RET to lipid rafts is required for effective downstream signaling, differentiation, and neuronal survival. *Neuron*, 25: 611–623.

van de Velde, H.J., Roebroek, A.J., Senden, N.H., Ramaekers, F.C. and Van de Ven, W.J. (1994) NSP-encoded reticulons, neuroendocrine proteins of a novel gene family associated with membranes of the endoplasmic reticulum. *J. Cell Sci.*, 107: 2403–2416.

Xiao, Z.-C., David, S., Braun, P.E. and McKerracher, L. (1997) Characterization of a new myelin-derived growth inhibitory activity. *Soc. Neurosci. Abstr.*, 23: 1994.

Zinn, K. and Sun, Q. (1999) Slit branches out: a secreted protein mediates both attractive and repulsive axon guidance. *Cell*, 97: 1–4.

L. McKerracher, G. Doucet and S. Rossignol (Eds.)
Progress in Brain Research, Vol. 137

CHAPTER 26

Inactivation of intracellular Rho to stimulate axon growth and regeneration

Benjamin Ellezam [1], Catherine Dubreuil [1], Matthew Winton [1], Leanna Loy [1],
Pauline Dergham [1], Inmaculada Sellés-Navarro [2] and Lisa McKerracher [1,*]

[1] *Département de Pathologie et Biologie Cellulaire et Centre de Recherche en Sciences Neurologiques, Université de Montréal,
Montreal, PQ H3T 1J4 Canada*
[2] *Laboratorio de Oftalmologia Experimental, Facultad de Medicina, Universidad de Murcia, Murcia, Spain*

Introduction

Damage to neuronal function following spinal cord injury (SCI) arises from a complex series of reactions. A key determinant of functional loss after SCI is axon injury at the lesion site. Projection neurons that extend long axons within the spinal tracts are crucial for motor and sensory function, and their axons do not regenerate following transection, even though their cell bodies may remain alive for many years. This regenerative failure is explained in part by the presence of growth inhibitory proteins. These molecules repress axon regeneration by severely limiting the ability of growth cones to extend forward. Most known growth inhibitory molecules are concentrated in myelin, the white matter territory where projection neurons extend long axons. Other inhibitory proteins such as proteoglycans are expressed by cells that form the scar directly at the lesion site. Therefore, one challenge to stimulate axon regeneration after injury is to overcome the neuronal response to the diverse types of inhibitory proteins that are expressed in the CNS.

As in development, growing axons in regeneration require the formation of a growth cone, the sensory and mobile apparatus that forms at the proximal tip of a cut axon soon after injury. Regrowth of a cut axon depends on the coordinated assembly, disassembly and contraction of the actin cytoskeleton in the growth cone, and this process is responsible for the extension and retraction of the axon in response to positive and negative extracellular cues. In the mammalian CNS, it is thought that negative cues that limit regeneration have a stronger influence or are in greater abundance than the positive cues, which explains why axons fail to extend very far. In tissue culture, the response of growth cones to inhibitory molecules is to collapse, and growth cone collapse depends on the balance of inhibitory to growth-promoting cues (David et al., 1995; Wenk et al., 2000).

Actin-mediated cell motility is regulated in all cells by the Rho family of GTPases. In neurons, intracellular Rho GTPases regulate the response of growth cones to both chemorepulsive guidance cues and growth inhibitory proteins (Jin and Strittmatter, 1997; Kuhn et al., 1999; Lehmann et al., 1999; Wahl et al., 2000; Dickson, 2001). Growth inhibitory proteins that induce growth cone collapse activate Rho,

* Correspondence to: L. McKerracher, Département de Pathologie et Biologie Cellulaire et Centre de Recherche en Sciences Neurologiques, Université de Montréal, Montreal, PQ H3T 1J4 Canada.
E-mail: mckerral@patho.umontreal.ca

and molecules that promote neurite growth inactivate Rho (Lehmann et al., 1999; Wahl et al., 2000; Wenk et al., 2000). We have investigated whether targeting Rho GTPase activity in neurons can allow them to ignore growth inhibitory signaling and grow directly on inhibitory substrates. The inactivation of Rho not only allows axon growth on myelin and chondroitin sulfate proteoglycan (CSPG) substrates, but also allows axon regeneration after injury in the CNS. Moreover, recent studies suggest that the inactivation of Rho may also have neuroprotective effects (Trapp et al., 2001).

Regulation of Rho GTPases

GTPases bind and hydrolyse GTP and cycle between active and inactive states. They are active when bound to GTP and lose their activity upon hydrolysis to GDP (Bishop and Hall, 2000; Schwartz and Shattil, 2000). To date, more than ten mammalian Rho family members have been identified, and each Rho family member has several isoforms. Rho, Rac and Cdc42 were the first identified and are the best characterized of the Rho family GTPases. Isoforms of the Rho group include RhoA, RhoB and RhoC (Takai et al., 2001). PC12 cells express RhoA, RhoB, RhoC and one unidentified Rho isoform (Lehmann et al., 1999) that may be RhoE, a Rho family protein that shares the effector domain of RhoA, B and C and promotes motility through actin reorganization. Unlike RhoA and RhoB, RhoE is not affected by C3-transferase, an inhibitor of Rho activity (Guasch et al., 1998; Wilde et al., 2001). In neurons, Rho and Rac have opposing effects: active Rho inhibits growth and active Rac stimulates it (Lin et al., 1994; van Leeuwen et al., 1997). Interestingly, it was shown that the effect of neurotrophins on promoting neurite outgrowth is mediated through the p75 receptor by Rho inactivation (Yamashita et al., 1999). Other studies examining the cross talk between different GTPases show that neurotrophins also activate Rac (Yamaguchi et al., 2001). In vivo, GTPases may affect both axons and dendrites differently (Luo et al., 1996; Ruchhoeft et al., 1999), and one consistent finding is that Rho is important in regulating growth cone motility. In the CNS, there is recent evidence that one isoform of Rho, RhoB, is up-regulated after ischemia suggesting that this GTPase may play

a role in the neuronal response to injury (Trapp et al., 2001). Moreover, we have preliminary evidence that an imbalance in Rho expression and activity occurs after SCI, a change that could contribute to the failure of axons to regrow. While the coordinated regulation of the different GTPases remains to be elucidated in regenerating axons, it is clear that the different Rho family GTPases regulate the initiation, growth and guidance of both axons and dendrites, presumably by acting on the actin cytoskeleton in response to diverse extracellular signals.

While Rho GTPases act as molecular switches cycling between active GTP bound and inactive GDP bound states, this switching is catalyzed by other proteins. The guanine exchange factors (GEFs) promote GTP binding to small GTPases. The GTPase activating proteins (GAPs) hydrolyse GTP, pushing the GTPase into the inactive GDP bound state. While Rho is expressed in all cell types, GEFs may exhibit cell-type specificity. Several GEFs that are known to play an important role in axon formation and guidance include Trio, a GEF for Rac, Rho and Cdc42 (Lin and Greenberg, 2000) and Tiam1, a GEF specific for Rac (Kunda et al., 2001). Once activated, the Rho GTPases bind and activate different effector proteins. A principal effector of activated Rho is Rho-associated kinase (ROK), a serine threonine kinase that is activated by Rho-GTP (Matsui et al., 1996). Microinjection of the catalytic domain of ROK into neurons induces neurite retraction, and inhibition of ROK with Y27632, a specific ROK inhibitor, promotes neurite outgrowth (Katoh et al., 1998). Therefore, inhibiting either Rho or its effector ROK is sufficient to promote neurite outgrowth in tissue culture.

Rho GTPases play an important role in integrating different signaling pathways that influence growth cone morphology and collapse (Fig. 1). Recently, Wahl et al. (2000) demonstrated that ephrin-A5, a known inhibitory molecule and ligand of the Eph tyrosine kinase receptors, causes the collapse of growth cones by activating RhoA and downregulating Rac1. This induced collapse was significantly reduced when the cultures were pretreated with the Rho inhibitor C3-transferase, or the ROK inhibitor Y27632. Consistent with these findings, a newly discovered Rho family GEF, ephexin, mediates Eph/ephrin receptor complex to intracellular

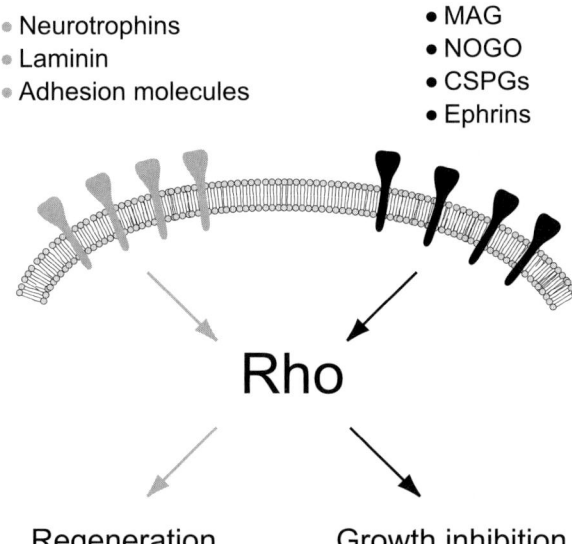

- Neurotrophins
- Laminin
- Adhesion molecules

- MAG
- NOGO
- CSPGs
- Ephrins

Rho

Regeneration   Growth inhibition

Fig. 1. Schematic diagram of multiple growth signals converging to Rho. The activity state of Rho is influenced by extracellular cues through both positive and negative receptor-mediated signaling.

signaling by Rho GTPases to influence growth cone collapse. Ephexin can strongly activate both RhoA and Cdc42, but can only weakly activate Rac1. These studies provide strong evidence for a direct link between extracellular growth inhibitory cues and Rho GTPases. Although there is little information on how extracellular guidance cues control cytoskeleton dynamics and growth cone motility in neurons, there is growing evidence that GTPases in non-neuronal cells are directly modulated by many different extracellular cues. A signaling cascade between integrin signaling and Rho has been demonstrated in fibroblasts (Adams and Schwartz, 2000; Wenk et al., 2000), and integrin binding to laminin is well known to promote neurite outgrowth (David et al., 1995). Therefore, Rho appears to integrate diverse positive and negative signals in axon regeneration.

Extracellular cues can affect many other aspects of cellular regulation, particularly the levels of intracellular cAMP. There is an interesting correlation between Rho signaling and cAMP levels. Increased cAMP levels allow neurons to extend neurites on inhibitory substrates (Cai et al., 1999), and it is thought that endogenous cAMP levels determine the regenerative capacity of a neuron (Qiu et al., 2002,

this volume). Increases in cAMP levels are known to inactivate Rho (Lang et al., 1996), and changes brought about by increasing cAMP levels can be counteracted by Rho activation and by ROK (Dong et al., 1998). Either cAMP or Rho can be manipulated to promote neurite outgrowth in the presence of growth inhibitory molecules (Song et al., 1998; Lehmann et al., 1999). Thus, the Rho pathway appears to act downstream of cAMP, and Rho represents a specific and important target to promote axon growth.

While Rho is best known for regulating the actin cytoskeleton (Mackay and Hall, 1998), more recent evidence implicates activation of Rho in apoptosis. An upregulation of RhoB occurs in ischemia-injured neurons, and stabilization of the actin cytoskeleton helps protect neurons from ischemic cell death (Trapp et al., 2001). In non-neuronal cells, RhoB is required for apoptosis and regulates the apoptotic response of neoplastic cells to DNA damage (Liu et al., 2001). Therefore, inactivation of Rho should not only promote axon regeneration, but also limit cell death after injury.

Inactivation of Rho by C3-transferase promotes neurite growth

C3-ADP ribosyltransferase is a 24-kDa exoenzyme synthesized by *Clostridium botulinum* that specifically ADP ribosylates the RhoA, B, and C isoforms, but not any other members of the Rho families (Wilde et al., 2001). We used recombinant C3-transferase to test if the inactivation of Rho would allow axons to grow on complex myelin and proteoglycan growth inhibitory substrates. The cDNA encoding C3 was cloned into a pGex2T vector (Amersham Pharmacia, Quebec, Canada) that has a glutathione-*S*-transferase (GST) tag. The recombinant C3 protein was produced in *Escherichia coli* and purified by affinity purification with glutathione-agarose beads. Thrombin was used to cleave the GST tag from the purified protein, and *p*-aminobenzamidine agarose beads were used to remove thrombin. Purified C3 was then centrifuged to remove the beads, concentrated, desalted, and stored at $-80°C$.

To test the ability of C3 to promote neurite growth on inhibitory substrates, we have examined two types of primary neuronal cells isolated from early postna-

374

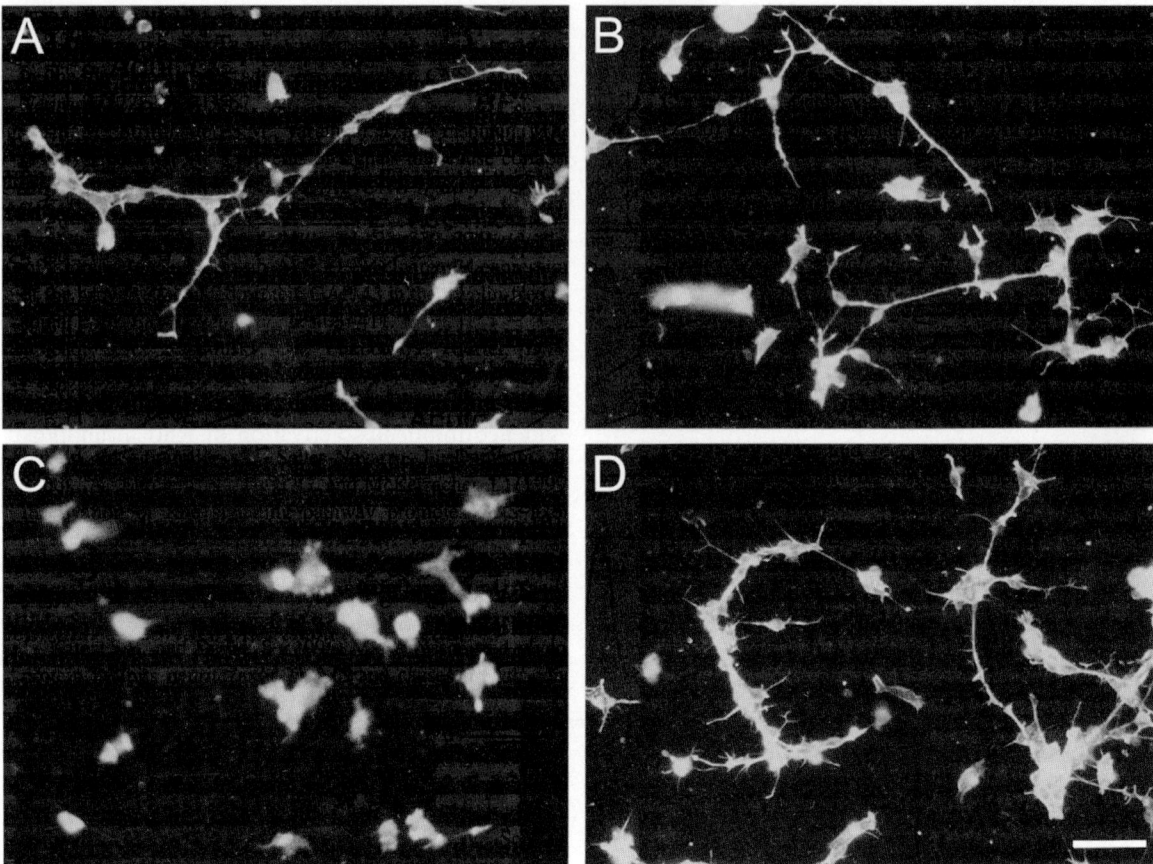

Fig. 2. Treatment of cerebellar granule cells with C3 promotes neurite outgrowth. (A,B) Dissociated cerebellar neurons treated with (A) buffer or (B) C3 and plated on laminin. (C,D) Neurons treated with (C) buffer or (D) C3 and plated on MAG. Treatment of neurons with C3 potentiated neurite growth on laminin, and allowed neurons to extend neurites on a growth inhibitory substrate. Scale bar: 50 μm.

tal rats: retinal neurons and cerebellar granule cells. Retinal neurons were dissociated and plated on inhibitory substrates made of either MAG, myelin or chondroitin sulfate proteoglycans. Addition of C3 allowed retinal neurons to grow neurites on all three inhibitory substrates, and brought an increase in both the number of neurons extending neurites and the average neurite length. Cerebellar neurons were dissociated, prelabeled with DiI, and triturated with C3 (25–50 μg/ml) or buffer, then plated on laminin as a growth-promoting substrate (Fig. 2A,B), or on myelin-associated glycoprotein (MAG) as growth inhibitory substrate (Fig. 2C,D). With cerebellar neurons, C3 treatment allowed neurite outgrowth on MAG (Fig. 2D), and potentiated neurite outgrowth on laminin (Fig. 2B). Untreated cerebellar neurons plated on MAG did not extend neurites (Fig. 2C).

Although C3 is a very effective way to inactivate Rho and stimulate neurite outgrowth, it is not very cell permeable. Thus, trituration of primary neurons was necessary to enable C3 to enter the cell and allow neurites to grow on inhibitory substrates. To improve delivery of C3, we have developed permeable forms that allow us to simply add it to the cell culture medium. Experiments using our new C3-like constructs give the same results as those with C3, the advantage being that lower doses are required.

Inactivation of Rho is sufficient to promote neurite growth on inhibitory substrates

To verify that inactivation of Rho was sufficient to allow neurons to extend neurites on inhibitory substrates, we examined the ability of PC12 cells transfected with dominant negative RhoA (N19TRhoA) to grow on recombinant MAG substrates. Transfected N19TRhoA cells and mock-transfected PC12 cells were tested for their ability to extend neurites when plated on inhibitory MAG substrates. Inactivation of RhoA by dominant negative mutation was sufficient to allow N19TRhoA cells plated on MAG substrates to extend neurites, and by contrast, mock transfected cells were unable to grow on the same substrates (Lehmann et al., 1999). It is not known if dominant negative mutations of Rho expressed in vivo by gene therapy techniques would allow regeneration after axonal injury. In this case, the dominant negative Rho expressed in the cell body would have to be transported to the tip of the transfected axon to be effective. It would be useful to know if this transport occurs at the slow or fast rates of axonal transport, and if direct delivery of dominant negative Rho to a neuronal cell body could stimulate the growth of an axon cut many centimeters away.

The optic nerve microcrush model to study in vivo axon regeneration

Aguayo and colleagues first showed that adult RGC axons could regenerate if they were provided with an alternative environment such as a peripheral nerve graft (So and Aguayo, 1985; Vidal-Sanz et al., 1987). It is now apparent that RGCs can regenerate in their native optic nerve environment if given trophic support (Berry et al., 1996, 1999; Leon et al., 2000), if the optic nerve environment is modified by cell transplantation (Lazarov-Spiegler et al., 1996), or if growth inhibitory myelin proteins are blocked (Weibel et al., 1994; Ellezam and McKerracher, 2000). To develop those strategies, investigators have relied on optic nerve crush to unequivocally axotomize all RGCs and yet preserve tissue integrity between proximal and distal segments. Standard crush lesions cause less cell death and optic nerve damage than complete transection of the optic nerve (Berkelaar et al., 1994; Kiernan, 1985). However, crushing the nerve with forceps creates an area of cavitation with a poorly delimited injury site that makes quantitation of axon regeneration difficult (Giftochristos and David, 1988; Weibel et al., 1994; Zeng et al., 1994; Berry et al., 1996). Therefore, we developed a new type of lesion, where complete axotomy is

achieved by constricting the optic nerve with 10-0 sutures for 60 s (Lehmann et al., 1999). This microcrush lesion results in a clear and defined injury site that is suitable for precise anatomical studies of axon retraction and regeneration (Selles-Navarro et al., 2001).

In characterizing this microlesion model, we found that as early as 6 h following the microcrush, anterogradely labeled RGC axons retract up to 200 μm from the lesion site, and, in the following week, sprout back toward the site of lesion where they abruptly stop (Selles-Navarro et al., 2001). This initial growth response is consistent with the early sprouting observed by Zeng et al. (1994) using electron microscopy. After 2 weeks, very few axons have grown past the injury site, most of them still remaining on the proximal side (Fig. 3C). As for the non-neuronal response, it is similar to that observed after typical optic nerve crush made with forceps (Berry et al., 1996), although constrained to a smaller lesion area. Immediately after injury (24 h), there is a GFAP-negative region, while CSPGs detected with CS56 antibody are expressed along a discrete injury line (Selles-Navarro et al., 2001). CSPG immunoreactivity remains detectable for at least 2 weeks, indicating formation of a persistent glial scar. In fact, it might be more appropriate to refer to the glial scar as the lesion scar since invading meningeal cells contribute importantly to its formation (Selles-Navarro et al., 2001). Indeed, a network of newly formed blood vessels quickly fills the injury site and appears to form a tight physical barrier.

Studying the microcrush lesion model has provided us with some insight on the reason for RGC regeneration failure. Anterograde tracing examination clearly showed that, early after the lesion, adult RGCs have retained their potential to regenerate, since they can regrow for up to 200 μm following the initial retraction. However, without any treatment, the vast majority of axons stop abruptly at the C556 immunoreactive lesion barrier. Yet, despite the presence of a barrier, some axons do cross the lesion site, but only grow for very short distances within the myelin-rich white matter. More often, these axons will either be contained outside the nerve and along the sheath, or in the first 50 μm past the lesion site, within the limits of the myelin-free zone (Lehmann et al., 1999; Selles-Navarro et al., 2001) confirm-

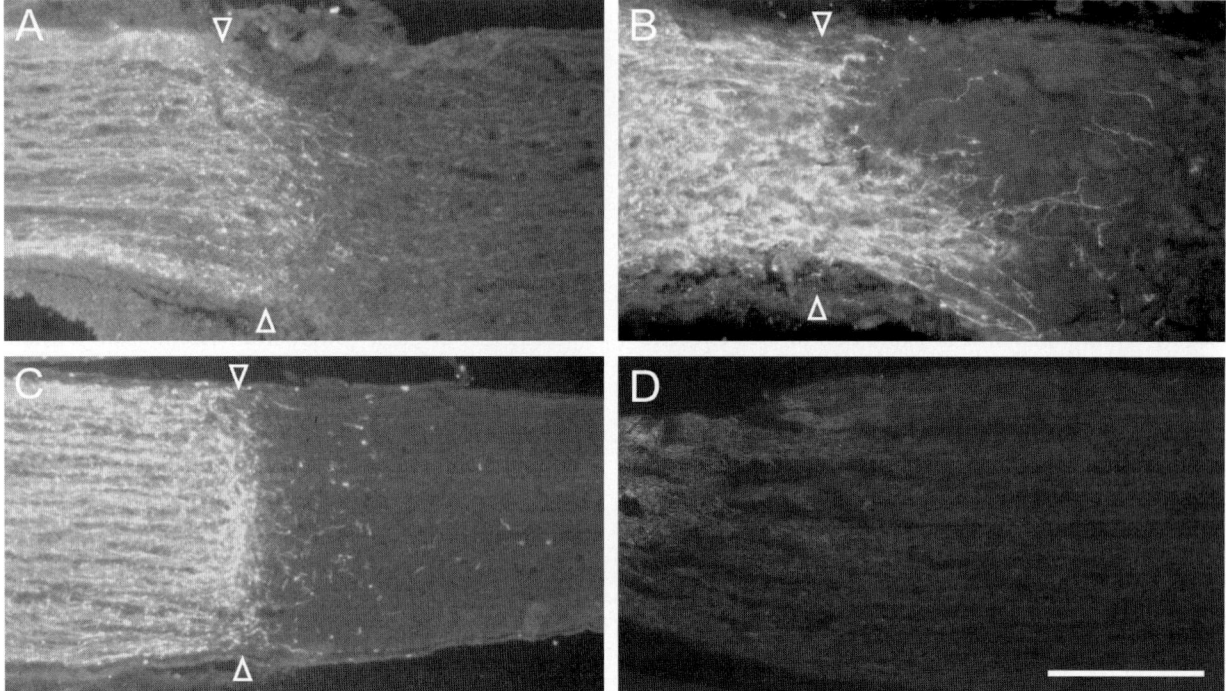

Fig. 3. Regeneration of retinal ganglion cells axons after injury and treatment with C3. (A) Seven days after injury and C3 treatment many axons cross the lesion site as compared to animals treated with buffer alone where axons stop abruptly at the lesion site. (B) Two weeks after C3 treatment, many axons cross the lesion scar (arrowheads) to grow in the distal white matter. (C) Control animal treated with buffer in the Gelfoam and Elvax 7 days after injury and treatment. (D) Normal optic nerve showing that cholera toxin β subunit, used as the anterograde tracer in these studies, does not accumulate when there is no lesion. Scale bar: 250 μm.

ing the importance of myelin inhibitors in blocking regeneration. Moreover, when myelin inhibitors are blocked without any additional intervention, significant regeneration is observed (Weibel et al., 1994), a regrowth most likely driven by the initial sprouting reaction seen after injury. Thus, both the lesion scar and myelin inhibitors contribute to the lack of significant RGC regeneration after optic nerve injury.

Another possible explanation for RGC regenerative failure is the delayed apoptosis that follows axotomy. Indeed, 5 days after optic nerve injury, RGCs rapidly start to die (Berkelaar et al., 1994). However, 1 week after microlesion about 60% of RGCs are still alive (Selles-Navarro et al., 2001), and their axons can actively transport the anterograde tracer cholera toxin β. Moreover, 1 week after optic nerve injury, most surviving cells have a normal morphology when observed after Fluorogold labeling and do not show signs of impending apoptosis (Kikuchi et al., 2000). Yet, all those surviving RGCs typically

do not extend an axon farther than the lesion site. Therefore, the poor regeneration observed at 7 days cannot be accounted for by poor cell survival alone, making growth inhibition an essential target for new regeneration strategies.

C3 promotes axon regeneration of retinal ganglion cell axons in vivo

To test if blocking Rho signaling could promote axon regeneration in vivo, we studied the effect of C3 on RGC regeneration after optic nerve microcrush (Lehmann et al., 1999). Immediately after lesioning, we applied C3 to the lesion site as a 2 mg/ml solution absorbed in Gelfoam, and then wrapped the Gelfoam around the nerve at the site of the crush. In addition, two 3-mm-long tubes of Elvax, a slow release polymer loaded with 20 μg C3, were inserted in the Gelfoam near the nerve for continued slow release of C3. For controls, phosphate-buffered saline (PBS) was used in the Gelfoam and Elvax implants. Seven days or 2 weeks after the nerve crush, RGC axons were anterogradely labeled with cholera toxin β subunit injected into the vitreous. The animals were then fixed by perfusion with 4% paraformaldehyde, and longitudinal cryostat sections of the optic nerve were processed for immunoreactivity to cholera toxin β subunit. Two C3-treated animals and four controls were examined 7 days after lesion. Two weeks post lesion, 16 animals treated with C3, 10 with buffer alone, and 4 subjected to the microcrush only were examined. The number of anterogradely labeled axons per section were counted by light microscopy at distances of 100, 250, and 500 μm from the microcrush. At least four sections per animal were analyzed.

After treatment with C3, large numbers of axons extended through the site of the crush to grow in the distal optic nerve. Seven days after lesion, many axons had grown past the region of the lesion scar (Fig. 3A). In control animals, axons had sprouted to the lesion site by 7 days, but the vast majority stopped abruptly at the crush (Fig. 3C). Most of our observations were made 2 weeks after lesion, when the results were even more dramatic. In C3-treated animals, many axons extended 500 μm past the lesion site by 2 weeks, and axons that extended in the distal optic nerve showed a twisted path of growth, supporting their identification as regenerating axons (Fig. 3B). In control animals, only a few axons were able to grow past the lesion at 1 week, and growth was not observably further at the 2-week time point. To rule out the possibility that some of the fibers observed beyond the lesion site are actually axons spared at the time of injury, the anterograde tracer was injected in the vitreous of untreated animals with intact optic nerves and allowed the same amount of time to be transported before perfusion. Longitudinal sections of those nerves did not show axon profiles past the lamina cribosa (Fig. 3D). Although RGC somata showed accumulation of the tracer (data not shown), axons in turn did not retain it, most likely because the tracer accumulated at their target region. These experiments rule out the possibility that spared fibers were detected after microlesion and C3 treatment.

To quantitatively examine the differences between C3 and buffer-treated animals, we counted the number of axons in each section at distances of 100, 250, and 500 μm past the lesion site. A significantly greater number of axons extended beyond the lesion in the C3-treated animals than in the microcrush lesion or buffer-treated controls. Therefore, C3 applied to injured RGC axons can enter axotomized axons and promote robust axon regeneration in the inhospitable growth environment of the optic nerve. Our current investigations are determining to what extent the new permeable forms of C3 will further augment this regeneration response after injury.

In vivo spinal cord injury experiments

We have also begun a series of experiments to test the ability of C3 to promote regeneration and functional recovery after spinal cord injury. For these studies, we have used a dorsal over-hemisection of the mouse spinal cord. We chose this model because we have previously used it to test a therapeutic vaccine to promote axon regeneration (Huang et al., 1999) and because it is highly suitable to study the regeneration of corticospinal tract fibers by anterograde tracing. In considering the various in vivo models of spinal cord injury, it is important to keep in mind that each model has distinct advantages and disadvantages. The contusion model is believed to most closely resemble human SCI (Bresnahan et al., 1987; Gruner, 1992; Wrathall et al., 1985), and recovery of hindlimb movement can be measured with the BBB scale (Basso et al., 1996). However, after contusion there is a rim of spared tissue, and therefore, this model is unsuitable for the unequivocal histological determination of successful axon regeneration.

We lesioned the spinal cord at the T_7 level by cutting past the central canal with microscissors, then re-cutting with a surgical knife. One month later, wheat germ agglutinin–horse radish peroxidase (WGA–HRP) was injected into several sites of the motor cortex. Two days after the WGA–HRP injections, the animals were fixed by perfusion, and longitudinal cryostat sections of the spinal cord were obtained and reacted for HRP enzymatic activity. The sections were also counterstained with neutral red. This staining allowed us to confirm that the lesion scar extended past the central canal. In control animals, the bundle of CST axons had retracted from the lesion site, as previously observed (Li et al.,

1996; Huang et al., 1999). In mice treated with C3, many axons extended into the lesion site and some axons were able to grow distances as great as 10 mm. Therefore, as in injured optic nerve, inactivation of Rho by C3 can promote axon regeneration in the injured adult spinal cord.

We have also studied recovery of hindlimb movement and walking in C3-treated mice. These mice showed an improvement in locomotion within 24 h. This rapid recovery may be due to neuroprotection, which is known to improve functional outcomes (Giménez y Ribotta et al., 2002, this volume). The activation of Rho has been implicated in cell death after ischemia in the CNS (Trapp et al., 2001), and thus, the inactivation of Rho by C3 may be neuroprotective. Moreover, treated mice showed recovery of walking with hindlimb–forelimb coordination. Control mice recovered walking, but did not recover coordination between hindlimbs and forelimbs.

At this stage of the research, we cannot correlate the observed functional recovery with axon regeneration. Improvement in the BBB openfield locomotor test cannot be correlated with the regeneration of specific tracts, and adaptive plasticity of preserved tracts is likely to contribute to recovery. In our studies, the putative neuroprotective effects of C3 could play an important role in improved recovery, and therefore, it is not clear to what extent improvements in the BBB score reflect the observed regeneration. While the late recovery of hindlimb–forelimb coordination observed at 1 month was consistent with regeneration of cut fibers, it is well documented that reorganization of collateral CST fibers occurs after SCI (Weidner et al., 2001); this process could indeed be enhanced by C3 treatment which may enhance spontaneous plasticity of axons and dendritic remodelling. After incomplete SCI, there is plasticity of motor systems attributed to cortical and subcortical levels, including spinal cord circuitry (reviewed by Raineteau and Schwab, 2001). This plasticity may be attributed to axonal or dendritic sprouting of collaterals and synaptic strengthening or weakening. Additionally, it has been shown that sparing of a few ventrolateral fibers may translate into significant differences in locomotor performance (Brustein and Rossignol, 1998), since these fibers are important in the initiation and control of locomotor pattern through spinal central pattern generators (re-

viewed by Rossignol, 2000). Moreover, the spinal cord devoid of supraspinal input but with peripheral afferents is in and of itself capable of generating hindlimb locomotion through central pattern generators (Rossignol, 2000). Therefore, many factors may contribute to functional recovery. Nonetheless, treatments that stimulate functional recovery in animal models give hope that effective treatment for spinal cord injury will be developed in the foreseeable future. Towards this end, we are developing more effective recombinant Rho antagonists that have increased cell permeability and that can stimulate spinal cord repair at lower doses. This strategy to improve recovery after spinal cord injury is simple: a single recombinant protein given once soon after injury. Further research with different animal models is needed to more directly compare C3-induced functional recovery with the recovery observed with other strategies described in this volume.

Summary

Our studies indicate that the small GTPase Rho is an important intracellular target for promoting axon regrowth after injury. In tissue culture, inactivation of the Rho signaling pathway is effective in promoting neurite growth on growth inhibitory CNS substrates by two different methods: inactivation of Rho with C3 transferase, and inactivation by dominant negative mutation of Rho. In vivo, we have documented the regeneration of transfected axons after treatment with C3 in two different animals models, microcrush lesion of the adult rat optic nerve, and over-hemisection of adult mouse spinal cord. Mice treated with C3 after SCI showed impressive functional recovery, notwithstanding the fact that mice differ from rats in their response to spinal cord injury, especially in the extent of cavitation at the lesion site (Steward et al., 1999). It remains to be determined to what extent the regeneration of specific descending and ascending spinal axons contribute to the recovery, and whether inactivation of Rho enhances the spontaneous plasticity of axonal and dendritic remodeling after SCI. Inactivation of Rho with C3 to promote regeneration and functional recovery after SCI is simple, and our studies reveal the potential for a new, straightforward technique to promote axon regeneration.

References

Adams, J.C. and Schwartz, M.A. (2000) Stimulation of fascin spikes by thrombospondin-1 is mediated by the GTPases Rac and Cdc42. *J. Cell Biol.*, 150: 807–822.

Basso, D.M., Beattie, M.S. and Bresnahan, J.C. (1996) Graded histological and locomotor outcomes after spinal cord contusion using the NYU weight-drop device versus transection. *Exp. Neurol.*, 139: 244–256.

Berkelaar, M., Clarke, D.B., Wang, Y.C., Bray, G.M. and Aguayo, A.J. (1994) Axotomy results in delayed death and apoptosis of retinal ganglion cells in adult rats. *J. Neurosci.*, 14: 4368–4374.

Berry, M., Carlile, J. and Hunter, A. (1996) Peripheral nerve explants grafted into the vitreous body of the eye promote the regeneration of retinal ganglion cell axons severed in the optic nerve. *J. Neurocytol.*, 25: 147–170.

Berry, M., Carlile, J., Hunter, A., Tsang, W., Rosustrel, P. and Sievers, J. (1999) Optic nerve regeneration after intravitreal peripheral nerve implants: trajectories of axons regrowing through the optic chiasm into the optic tracts. *J. Neurocytol.*, 28: 721–741.

Bishop, A.L. and Hall, A. (2000) Rho GTPases and their effector proteins. *Biochem. J.*, 348(2): 241–255.

Bresnahan, J.C., Beattie, M.S., Todd III, F.D. and Noyes, D.H. (1987) A behavioral and anatomical analysis of spinal cord injury produced by a feedback-controlled impaction device. *Exp. Neurol.*, 95: 548–570.

Brustein, E. and Rossignol, S. (1998) Recovery of locomotion after ventral and ventrolateral spinal lesions in the cat. I. Deficits and adaptive mechanisms. *J. Neurophysiol.*, 80: 1245–1267.

Cai, D., Shen, Y., DeBellard, M.E., Tang, S. and Filbin, M.T. (1999) Prior exposure to neurotrophins blocks inhibition of axonal regeneration by MAG and myelin via a cAMP-dependent mechanism. *Neuron*, 22: 89–101.

David, S., Braun, P.E., Jackson, J.L., Kottis, V. and McKerracher, L. (1995) Laminin overrides the inhibitory effects of PNS and CNS myelin-derived inhibitors of neurite growth. *J. Neurosci. Res.*, 42: 594–602.

Dickson, B.J. (2001) Rho GTPases in growth cone guidance. *Curr. Opin. Neurobiol.*, 11: 103–110.

Dong, J.-M., Leung, T., Manser, E. and Lim, L. (1998) cAMP-induced morphological changes are counteracted by the activated RhoA small GTPase and the Rho kinase ROKα. *J. Biol. Chem.*, 273: 22554–22562.

Ellezam, B. and McKerracher, L. (2000) Testing a therapeutic vaccine to stimulate axon regeneration after microcrush of the optic nerve in adult rats. *Soc. Neurosci. Abstr.*, 26: 612.

Giftochristos, N. and David, S. (1988) Laminin and heparin sulfate proteoglycan in the lesioned adult mammalian central nervous system and their possible relationship to axonal sprouting. *J. Neurocytol.*, 17: 385–397.

Giménez y Ribotta, M., Gaviria, M., Menet, V. and Privat, A. (2002) Strategies for regeneration and repair in spinal cord traumatic injury. In: L. McKerracher, G. Douchet and S. Rossignol (Eds.), *Spinal Cord Trauma: Neural Repair and Functional Recovery. Progress in Brain Research*, Vol. 137. Elsevier Science, Amsterdam, pp. 191–212.

Gruner, J.A. (1992) A monitored contusion model of spinal cord injury in the rat. *J. Neurotrauma*, 9: 123–128.

Guasch, R.M., Scambler, P., Jones, G.E. and Ridley, A.J. (1998) RhoE regulates actin cytoskeleton organization and cell migration. *Mol. Cell. Biol.*, 18: 4761–4771.

Huang, D.W., McKerracher, L., Braun, P., McKerracher, L. and David, S. (1999) A therapeutic vaccine approach to stimulate axon regeneration in the adult mammalian spinal cord. *Neuron*, 24: 639–647.

Jin, Z. and Strittmatter, S.M. (1997) Rac1 mediates collapsin-1-induced growth cone collapse. *J. Neurosci.*, 17: 6256–6263.

Katoh, H., Aoki, J., Ichikawa, A. and Negishi, M. (1998) p160 RhoA-binding kinase ROKα induces neurite retraction. *J. Biol. Chem.*, 273: 2489–2492.

Kiernan, J.A. (1985) Axonal and vascular changes following injury to the rat's optic nerve. *J. Anat.*, 141: 139–154.

Kikuchi, M., Tenneti, L. and Lipton, S.A. (2000) Role of p38 mitogen-activated protein kinase in axotomy-induced apoptosis of rat retinal ganglion cells. *J. Neurosci.*, 20: 5037–5044.

Kuhn, T.B., Brown, M.D., Wilcox, C.L., Raper, J.A. and Bamburg, J.R. (1999) Myelin and collapsin-1 induce motor neuron growth cone collapse through different pathways: inhibition of collapse by opposing mutants of rac1. *J. Neurosci.*, 19: 1965–1975.

Kunda, P., Paglini, G., Quiroga, S., Kosik, K. and Caceres, A. (2001) Evidence for the involvement of Tiam1 in axon formation. *J. Neurosci.*, 21: 2361–2372.

Lang, P., Gesbert, F., Delespine-Carmagnat, M., Stancou, R., Pouchelet, M. and Bertoglio, J. (1996) Protein kinase A phosphorylation of RhoA mediates the morphological and functional effects of cyclic AMP in cytotoxic lymphocytes. *EMBO J.*, 15: 510–519.

Lazarov-Spiegler, O., Solomon, A., Zeev-Bran, A.B., Hirschberg, D.L., Lavie, V. and Schwartz, M. (1996) Transplantation of activated macrophages overcomes central nervous system regrowth failure. *FASEB J.*, 110: 1296–1302.

Lehmann, M., Fournier, A., Selles-Navarro, I., Dergham, P., Sebok, A., Leclerc, N., Tigyi, G. and McKerracher, L. (1999) Inactivation of rho signaling pathway promotes CNS axon regeneration. *J. Neurosci.*, 19: 7537–7547.

Leon, S., Yin, Y., Nguyen, J., Irwin, N. and Benowitz, L.I. (2000) Lens injury stimulates axon regeneration in the mature rat optic nerve. *J. Neurosci.*, 20: 4615–4626.

Li, M., Shibata, A., Li, C., Braun, P.E., McKerracher, L., Roder, J., Kater, S.B. and David, S. (1996) Myelin-associated glycoprotein inhibits neurite/axon growth and causes growth cone collapse. *J. Neurosci. Res.*, 46: 404–414.

Lin, M.Z. and Greenberg, M.E. (2000) Orchestral maneuvers in the axon: trio and the control of axon guidance. *Cell*, 101: 239–242.

Lin, C.H., Thompson, C.A. and Forscher, P. (1994) Cytoskeletal reorganization underlying growth cone motility. *Curr. Opin. Neurobiol.*, 4: 640–647.

Liu, A.X., Cerniglia, G.J. and Prendergast, G.C. (2001) RhoB is required to mediate apoptosis in neoplastically transformed

380

cells after DNA damage. *Proc. Natl. Acad. Sci. USA*, 98: 6192–6197.

Luo, L., Hensch, T.K., Ackerman, L., Barbel, S. and Jan, Y.N. (1996) Differential effects of the Rac GTPase on Purkinje cell axons and dendritic trunks and spines. *Nature*, 379: 837–840.

Mackay, D.J. and Hall, A. (1998) Rho GTPases. *J. Biol. Chem.*, 273: 20685–20688.

Matsui, T., Amano, M., Yamamoto, T., Chihara, K., Nakafuku, M., Ito, M., Nakano, T., Okawa, K., Iwamatsu, A. and Kaibuchi, K. (1996) Rho-associated kinase, a novel serine/threonine kinase, as a putative target for small GTP binding protein Rho. *EMBO J.*, 15: 2208–2216.

Qiu, J., Cai, D. and Filbin, M.T. (2002) A role for cAMP in regeneration during development and after injury. In: L. McKerracher, G. Douchet and S. Rossignol (Eds.), *Spinal Cord Trauma: Neural Repair and Functional Recovery. Progress in Brain Research*, Vol. 137. Elsevier Science, Amsterdam, pp. 381–387.

Raineteau, O. and Schwab, M.E. (2001) Plasticity of motor systems after incomplete spinal cord injury. *Nat. Rev. Neurosci.*, 2: 263–273.

Rossignol, S. (2000) Locomotion and its recovery after spinal injury. *Curr. Opin. Neurobiol.*, 10: 708–716.

Ruchhoeft, M.L., Ohnuma, S.-I., Holt, C.E. and Harris, W. (1999) The neuronal architecture of *Xenopus* retinal ganglion cells is sculpted by Rho-family GTPases in vivo. *J. Neurosci.*, 19: 8454–8463.

Schwartz, M.A. and Shattil, S.J. (2000) Signaling networks linking integrins and rho family GTPases. *Trends Biochem. Sci.*, 25: 388–391.

Selles-Navarro, I., Ellezam, B., Fajardo, R., Latour, M. and McKerracher, L. (2001) Retinal ganglion cell and nonneuronal cell responses to a microcrush lesion of adult rat optic nerve. *Exp. Neurol.*, 167: 282–289.

So, K.F. and Aguayo, A.J. (1985) Lengthy regrowth of cut axons from ganglion cells after peripheral nerve transplantation into the retina of adult rats. *Brain Res.*, 328: 349–354.

Song, H.-j., Ming, G.-i., He, Z., Lehmann, M., McKerracher, L., Tessier-Lavigne, M. and Poo, M.-M. (1998) Conversion of growth cone responses from repulsion to attraction by cyclic nucleotides. *Science*, 281: 1515–1518.

Steward, O., Schauwecker, P.E., Guth, L., Zhang, Z., Fujiki, M., Inman, D., Wrathall, J., Kempermann, G., Gage, F.H., Raghupathi, R. and McIntosh, T. (1999) Genetic approaches to neurotrauma research: opportunities and potential pitfalls of murine models. *Exp. Neurol.*, 157: 19–42.

Takai, Y., Sasaki, T. and Matozaki, T. (2001) Small GTP-binding proteins. *Physiol. Rev.*, 81: 153–208.

Trapp, T., Olah, L., Holker, I., Besselmann, M., Tiesler, C., Maeda, K. and Hossmann, K.-A. (2001) GTPase RhoB: an early predictor of neuronal death after transient focal ischemia in mice. *Mol. Cell. Neurosci.*, 17: 883–894.

van Leeuwen, F.N., Kain, H.E.T., van der Kammen, R.A., Michiels, F., Kranenburg, O.W. and Collard, J.G. (1997) The guanine nucleotide exchange factor Tiam1 affects neuronal morphology; opposing roles for the small GTPases Rac and Rho. *J. Cell Biol.*, 139: 797–807.

Vidal-Sanz, M., Bray, G.M., Villegas-Perez, M.P., Thanos, S. and Aguayo, A.J. (1987) Axonal regeneration and synapse formation in the superior colliculus by retinal ganglion cells in the adult rat. *J. Neurosci.*, 7: 2894–2909.

Wahl, S., Barth, H., Ciossek, T., Aktories, K. and Mueller, B.K. (2000) Ephrin-A5 induces collapse of growth cones by activating Rho and Rho kinase. *J. Cell Biol.*, 149: 263–270.

Weibel, D., Cadelli, D. and Schwab, M.E. (1994) Regeneration of lesioned rat optic nerve fibers is improved after neutralization of myelin-associated neurite growth inhibitors. *Brain Res.*, 642: 259–266.

Weidner, N., Ner, A., Salimi, N. and Tuszynski, M.H. (2001) Spontaneous corticospinal axonal plasticity and functional recovery after adult central nervous system injury. *Proc. Natl. Acad. Sci. USA*, 98: 3513–3518.

Wenk, M.B., Midwood, K.S. and Schwarzbauer, J.E. (2000) Tenascin-C suppresses Rho activation. *J. Cell Biol.*, 150: 913–920.

Wilde, C., Chhatwal, G.S., Schmalzing, G., Aktories, K. and Just, I. (2001) A novel C3-like ADP-ribosyltransferase from *Staphylococcus aureus* modifying RhoE and Rnd3. *J. Biol. Chem.*, 276: 9537–9542.

Wrathall, J.R., Pettegrew, R.K. and Harvey, F. (1985) Spinal cord contusion in the rat: production of graded, reproducible, injury groups. *Exp. Neurol.*, 88: 108–122.

Yamaguchi, Y., Katoh, H., Yasui, H., Mori, K. and Negishi, M. (2001) RhoA inhibits the nerve growth factor-induced Rac1 activation through Rho-associated kinase-dependent pathway. *J. Biol. Chem.*, 276: 18977–18983.

Yamashita, T., Tucker, K.L. and Barde, Y.A. (1999) Neurotrophin binding to the p75 receptor modulates Rho activity and axonal outgrowth. *Neuron*, 24: 585–593.

Zeng, B.Y., Anderson, P.N., Campbell, G. and Lieberman, A.R. (1994) Regenerative and other responses to injury in the retinal stump of the optic nerve in adult albino rats: transection of the intraorbital optic nerve. *J. Anat.*, 185: 643–661.

L. McKerracher, G. Doucet and S. Rossignol (Eds.)
Progress in Brain Research, Vol. 137

CHAPTER 27

A role for cAMP in regeneration during development and after injury

Jin Qiu, Dongming Cai and Marie T. Filbin [*]

Biology Department, Hunter College, City University of New York, 695 Park Avenue, New York, NY 10021, USA

Introduction

Axons of the mature, mammalian central nervous system (CNS) do not regenerate after injury. However, a number of studies show that adult CNS neurons have not lost the intrinsic ability to regenerate as they are able to extend axons into grafts of peripheral nerve (Richardson et al., 1980; David and Aguayo, 1981). However, the regenerating axons fail to leave the peripheral graft and stop abruptly upon encountering host CNS. These observations led to the suggestion that, first, the PNS environment is more conducive to axonal growth than the CNS and, second, that CNS axons are capable of long-distance regeneration under certain conditions. If the CNS environment is an obstacle to nerve regeneration then the question raised is what components are responsible for the inhibitory effect. One major source of inhibition is CNS myelin. If CNS myelin is removed by either killing the dividing oligodendrocyte precursor cells by X-irradiation of newborn rats (Savio and Schwab, 1990) or by immunocytolysis in chick (Keirstead et al., 1992), elongation of axons over long distance was observed. Importantly, it was

shown recently that immunization of mice with CNS myelin prior to lesioning of dorsal column axons resulted in extensive axonal regeneration accompanied by partial functional recovery (Huang et al., 1999). This study provides strong, direct evidence that inhibitors in CNS myelin prevent regeneration immediately after injury. Another source of inhibition results from the astrocytic responses to injury and the subsequent formation of the glial scar.

Although the damaged, adult CNS environment is inhibitory to nerve regeneration, embryonic neurons, when transplanted into injured spinal cord, are able to regenerate over long distances (Li and Raisman, 1993). Presumably, embryonic neurons are intrinsically different from their adult counterparts and have a higher growth capacity. It appears, then, that the intrinsic state of the neuron dictates its response to the inhibitory factors in the adult CNS. This is supported by the recent study of Neumann and Woolf (1999), who demonstrated that transection of the sciatic nerve resulted in regeneration of subsequently lesioned dorsal column axons of the same dorsal root ganglion (DRG) neurons, without the addition of any agents that block myelin and glial scar inhibitors. It is conceivable that a prior lesion to the peripheral branch of the DRG increased the growth capacity of these neurons, and conditioned the central axons to overcome the inhibition of the CNS environment.

These studies indicate that two approaches are potentially effective in improving nerve regeneration in the adult CNS. One would be to identify and block

* Correspondence to: M.T. Filbin, Biology Department, Hunter College, City University of New York, 695 Park Avenue, New York, NY 10021, USA. Tel.: +1-212-772-5270; Fax: +1-212-772-4489;
E-mail: filbin@genectr.hunter.cuny.edu

individually all inhibitors in CNS myelin and glial scar. Alternatively, a general mechanism could be devised to enable neurons to overcome all inhibitors simultaneously by increasing their growth capacity.

Here, we present evidence to support the suggestion that neuronal cAMP levels are a key element dictating the regenerative capacity of neurons. First, exposure of neurons to neurotrophins prior to their encounter with myelin inhibitors overcomes the inhibition, and this is mediated by elevation of neuronal cAMP levels. Second, there is a developmentally regulated decrease in the endogenous neuronal cAMP levels, which marks the developmental loss of the regenerative capacity of neurons. Finally, transection of sciatic nerve leads to an elevation of the cAMP levels in DRG neurons, which underlies the molecular mechanism of the conditioning effect.

Myelin-associated glycoprotein

Myelin-associated glycoprotein (MAG) is a well characterized, myelin-specific component that has a profound effect on axonal regeneration (Johnson et al., 1989; McKerracher et al., 1994; Mukhopadhyay et al., 1994; Turnley and Bartlett, 1998). It is a member of the immunoglobulin (Ig) super family and contains five Ig-like domains in its extracellular sequence (Lai et al., 1987; Salzer et al., 1987). It has been reported that, depending on the age of neurons, MAG can either promote or inhibit axonal growth (DeBellard et al., 1996; Cai et al., 2001). For retinal ganglion (RG) neurons and spinal neurons, the switch has occurred by birth; neurite outgrowth of embryonic RG and spinal neurons is promoted by MAG, whereas postnatal axonal growth is potently inhibited (Johnson et al., 1989; DeBellard et al., 1996; Turnley and Bartlett, 1998; Cai et al., 2001). For DRG neurons, the switch occurs postnatally with a sharp transition from promotion to inhibition by MAG by postnatal day 3–4 (P3–4) (DeBellard et al., 1996; Cai et al., 2001). Thus, MAG is a bifunctional molecule with its role being predominantly inhibitory to nerve regeneration in the adult CNS.

Although MAG is normally inserted in the myelin sheath, a soluble form of MAG, dMAG, also exists in vivo. dMAG is a proteolytic fragment of MAG and contains the entire extracellular domain, cleaved just before it enters the membrane. It is present in

normal human tissue but is more abundant in tissue from patients with neurological disorders (Sato et al., 1984a,b; Stebbins et al., 1997). Recently, it was found that dMAG is released in abundance from damaged white matter and spinal cord, and can potently inhibit neurite outgrowth. This strongly suggests that MAG is, indeed, an inhibitory molecule rather than a nonpermissive substrate for neurite growth (Tang et al., 1997). Furthermore, the proteolytic form of MAG, when released from damaged myelin after injury, could exert an immediate inhibitory effect over a distance.

Priming neurons with neurotrophins overcomes the inhibition by MAG and myelin

As mentioned earlier, CNS neurons are able to regenerate into the grafts of peripheral nerve tissue but the regenerating axons fail to grow into the host white matter beyond the lesion (Richardson et al., 1980; David and Aguayo, 1981). Similar results were obtained with embryonic transplants by Bregman and her colleagues (Bregman, 1998). However, they found that, when either brain-derived neurotrophic factor (BDNF) or neurotrophic factor-3 (NT-3) was pumped into the implanted tissue, the injured spinal axons not only grew into the embryonic tissue, but they also extended long processes into the white matter beyond (Bregman, 1998). Similarly, Berry and coworkers showed that if an explant of peripheral nerve tissue was placed in the retina after a lesion was created in the optic nerve, optic nerve axons grew extensively into the white matter, distal to the lesion site (Berry et al., 1996). The unexpected results from both these studies suggest that the neurotrophins used for the spinal cord study and some component secreted from the peripheral nerve explants affects how the growing axon responds to myelin, even to the extent of neutralizing its ability to inhibit axonal regrowth.

To test if neurotrophins can indeed overcome inhibition by MAG and myelin, a variety of neurotrophins were tested individually with neuronal cultures. When added directly to the cultures, none of the neurotrophins had an effect. However, if cerebellar neurons were first cultured overnight (priming) with BDNF or glial-derived neurotrophic factor (GDNF), in the absence of MAG and myelin,

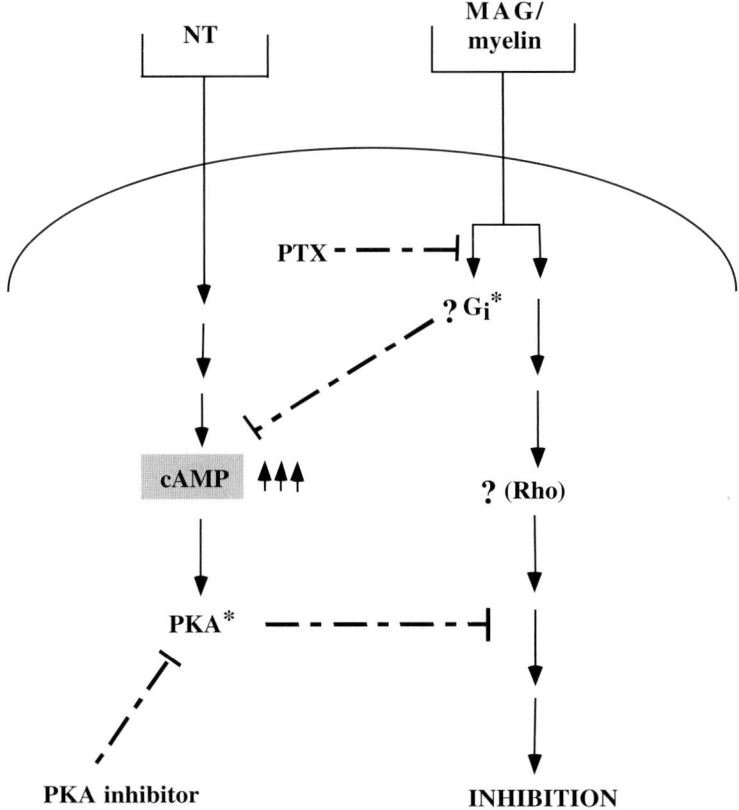

Fig. 1. Model to explain how priming with neurotrophins blocks inhibition by MAG and myelin. During priming, neurotrophins (NT) interact with a surface neuronal receptor and lead to an increase in neuronal cAMP levels, which in turn activates protein kinase A (PKA). Activation of PKA or some as yet unidentified downstream effector molecule then blocks subsequent inhibition by MAG or myelin, perhaps by inactivating the small GTPase, Rho. If, however, neurotrophin is added to the neuron at the same time as the exposure to MAG or myelin, the increase in the cAMP levels is prevented by MAG/myelin activation of a pertussis toxin (PTX)-sensitive G protein (G_i^*) and thus inhibition of axonal regeneration is not blocked. Activation of G protein by MAG or myelin has no direct effect on inhibition of axonal regeneration by MAG or myelin. Adapted from Cai et al., 1999.

and then transferred onto MAG-expressing cells or a myelin substrate, the growth inhibition by MAG and myelin was completely blocked. For DRG neurons, inhibition by MAG and myelin is blocked when the neurons are primed with BDNF, GDNF or nerve growth factor (NGF). The priming effect of neurotrophins was both time- and dose-dependent. A clue to the molecular mechanism whereby neurotrophins block inhibition by MAG and myelin came from in vitro studies of growth cone motility. A number of neurotrophins and axon guidance molecules have been shown to have chemotactic effects on axons. For example, a gradient of netrin-1 normally triggers an attractive turning response of growth cones of cultured *Xenopus* spinal neurons

(Ming et al., 1997). Interestingly, this chemoattractive effect of netrin-1 can be switched to a repulsive one if a competitive analog of cAMP or an inhibitor of protein kinase A (PKA) is included in the culture (Ming et al., 1997). Conversely, a soluble recombinant form of MAG repels these *Xenopus* growth cones, but the repulsion is switched to attraction by addition of a cAMP agonist to the culture media (Song et al., 1998). These studies imply that the intracellular cAMP levels may dictate the neuronal response to a particular guidance cue or myelin protein. If this is the case and if neurotrophins are able to alter the neuronal response to MAG and myelin, then the question is whether this switch is dependent on intracellular cAMP levels. Indeed, we found that neurotrophins increased neuronal cAMP levels, and this increase was prevented if MAG was also present. Further, if neurons were primed with neurotrophins in the presence of a PKA inhibitor, the block of MAG and myelin inhibition was completely abrogated. Moreover, artificial elevation of cAMP levels with an analogue of cAMP, dibutyryl cAMP, also blocked the inhibition by MAG or myelin. Finally, the need to prime was abrogated if neurons were exposed simultaneously to neurotrophins and MAG or myelin in the presence of the G protein inhibitor, pertussis toxin, inhibition is blocked by neurotrophins without priming. Taken together, these results indicate that increased cAMP levels and activation of the PKA pathway can overcome the inhibitory effects of MAG and myelin. The elevation of intracellular cAMP levels in the neuron is prevented by MAG or myelin, which, by binding to the neuron, activates an inhibitory G protein that blocks any increase in cAMP (Fig. 1; Cai et al., 1999).

Developmentally regulated neuronal cAMP levels and the loss in regenerative capacity

When transplanted into the adult CNS, embryonic neurons are able to regenerate over long distances (Li and Raisman, 1993). In addition, the response of a number of different neurons to MAG is switched from promotion to inhibition during development. For RG and spinal neurons, the switch has occurred by birth; embryonic RG and spinal neurons are promoted by MAG, while postnatal axonal growth is inhibited (Johnson et al., 1989; DeBellard et al., 1996; Turnley and Bartlett, 1998; Cai et al., 2001). For DRG neurons, the switch occurs postnatally with a sharp transition from promotion to inhibition by MAG at P3–4 (DeBellard et al., 1996; Cai et al., 2001). Thus, young neurons are intrinsically different from their older counterparts, and are not inhibited by MAG and myelin. The question is, then, what are the intrinsic differences between young and old neurons that determines their response to MAG and myelin? Since elevation of neuronal cAMP levels by priming with neurotrophins is able to block the inhibitory effect by MAG and myelin, we asked if the endogenous cAMP levels in neurons are regulated during development. Indeed, we found that endogenous levels of cAMP was high in embryonic and

neonatal neurons and decreased with age (Fig. 2). PKA inhibitors attenuated the growth from young neurons promoted by MAG and myelin, whereas an analogue of cAMP, db-cAMP, blocked the inhibitory effect of MAG and myelin on older neurons (Fig. 3). Importantly, developmental plasticity of spinal tract axons in neonatal rat pups in vivo is dramatically reduced by inhibition of PKA. Thus, the switch of neuronal response from promotion to inhibition of neurite outgrowth by MAG and myelin, which marks the developmental loss of regenerative capacity, is mediated by a developmentally regulated decrease in endogenous neuronal cAMP levels (Cai et al., 2001).

Elevation of endogenous cAMP levels underlies the molecular mechanisms of the conditioning effect of sciatic nerve transection on dorsal column axonal regeneration

It is known that dorsal column axons do not regenerate in the adult spinal cord after injury, although they do grow into an implanted graft of the peripheral nerve tissue (Richardson and Issa, 1984). If the dorsal column injury is preceded by a primary lesion in the peripheral branch of the same DRG neurons, much more extensive growth was observed into the peripheral nerve grafts (Richardson and Issa, 1984; Neumann and Woolf, 1999). It appears that the conditioning peripheral lesion somehow encourages the majority of lesioned spinal axons to grow towards the most distal edge of the graft but still not into the host CNS tissue beyond. Presumably, myelin-specific inhibitors, along with a glial scar at the graft–host border ultimately halt axonal growth. Recently, a study by Neumann and Woolf (1999) demonstrated that injuring the dorsal column and simultaneously transecting the sciatic nerve resulted in extensive regeneration, in the absence of a peripheral nerve graft, into the lesion site but not beyond. However, when the sciatic nerve was transected 1 week before the dorsal column lesion, about 50% of the animals showed axonal regeneration into the lesion site and beyond, mostly through the gray matter but with considerable regeneration also observed in the white matter. A less effective conditioning effect was observed when the sciatic nerve was transected at the same time as the dorsal column is lesioned or 2 weeks before. What makes this study different and

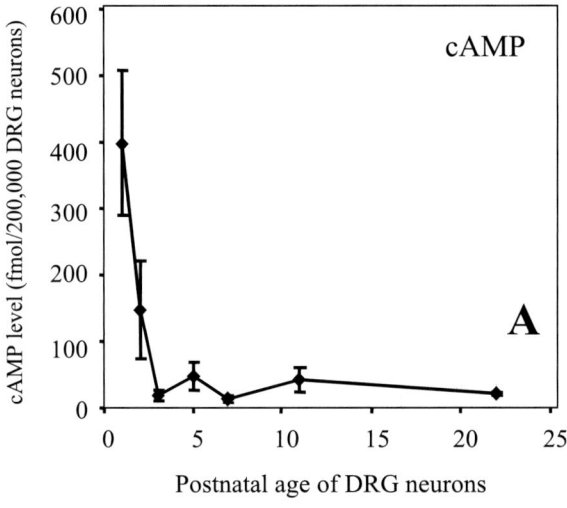

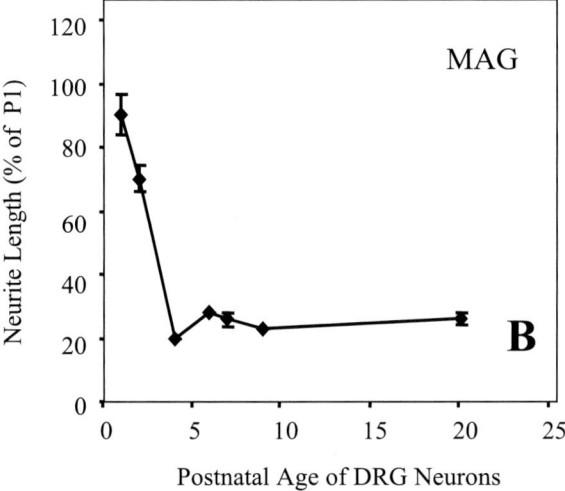

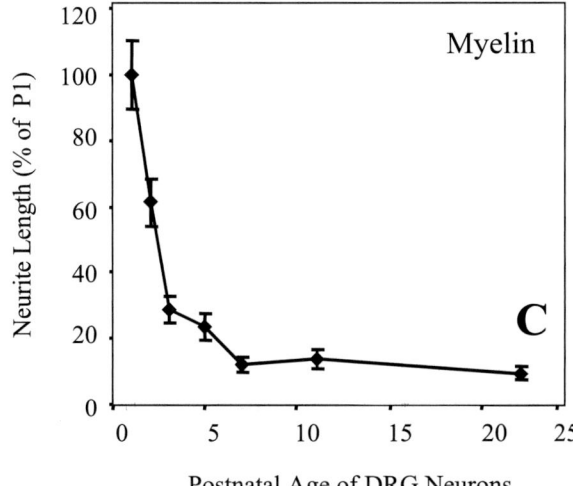

important is not the substantial distance traversed by the regenerating dorsal column axons, nor the possibly greater number of regenerating axons compared to other studies, but rather that no tissue implant was used and nor was any agent that blocks myelin and glial scar inhibitors. Regeneration occurred into what is, by all previous criteria, the highly nonpermissive environment of the damaged spinal cord. It appears that the conditioning lesion in the sciatic nerve increases the growth capacity of the DRG neurons, and allows the central branch to overcome the inhibition of the CNS environment and regenerate. Understanding the molecular changes in the DRG neurons as a result of the conditioning lesion should have significant therapeutic implication in improving nerve regeneration in the adult CNS.

As intracellular cAMP levels play an important role in dictating the neuronal response to myelin components, we asked whether they are also involved in the improved growth of the dorsal column axons after a conditioning lesion (Qui et al., 2002). It was found that 1 day after transection of the sciatic nerve cAMP levels in the DRG were elevated by about three-fold compared to the uninjured control. Furthermore, the growth of DRG neurons on MAG and myelin was significantly increased, and this improvement of growth could be blocked by PKA inhibitors. One week after transection of the sciatic nerve, the cAMP levels in the DRG have dropped back to control levels, but the growth of the DRG neurons on MAG and myelin was even better than after 1 day. However, this increased growth was now insensitive to PKA inhibitors, indicating that PKA independent pathways had been activated. These results indicate that a conditioning lesion leads to a transient increase in cAMP levels in the DRG, which sets off a cascade of events leading to increased growth capacity on MAG and myelin. The improved growth is initially directly dependent on PKA activity that subsequently triggers and activates other pathways. This hypothesis is supported by the

Fig. 2. The cAMP levels in neonatal DRG neurons are high and decrease with age. The decrease in neuronal cAMP levels correlates with the regenerative ability of the DRG neurons to grow on MAG or myelin in vitro.

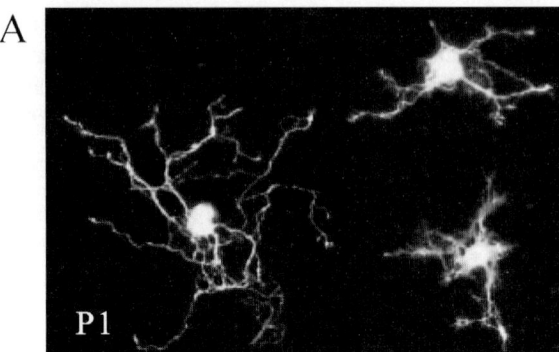

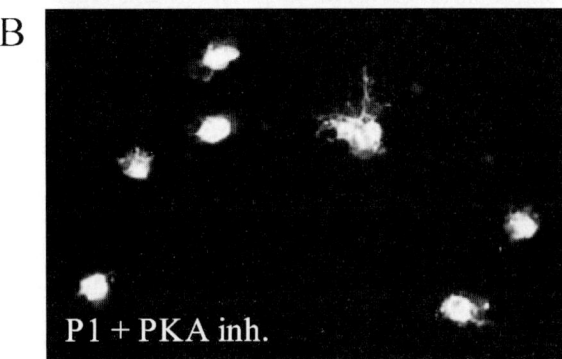

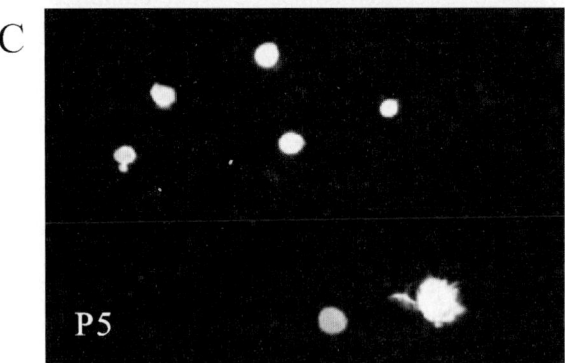

Fig. 3. In vitro growth of P1 DRG neurons on a myelin substrate is much more extensive than that of their P5 counterpart, and can be blocked by PKA inhibitors.

finding that, when a PKA inhibitor, H89, is intrathecally applied around the lumbar DRG, the improved growth 1 day after the conditioning lesion was completely blocked. In addition, intrathecal application of H89 for the entire week after sciatic nerve lesion attenuated the improved growth on MAG and myelin. Importantly, improved growth of DRG neurons on MAG and myelin was observed 1 day and

1 week after an analogue of cAMP, db-cAMP, was directly injected into the DRG in the absence of a peripheral lesion. Most significantly, direct injection of db-cAMP into the DRG mimicked the conditioning effect on regeneration of lesioned dorsal column fibers, resulting in significant axonal regrowth into the lesion site and beyond. Together, it was demonstrated that transection of the sciatic nerve resulted in an elevation of the cAMP levels in the DRG, which increased the growth capacity of the DRG neurons and was responsible for the regeneration of subsequently lesioned dorsal column axonal fibers.

Conclusions

In conclusion, endogenous cAMP levels dictate the neuronal response to the CNS environment. Cyclic AMP levels in younger neurons are high but these levels decrease with age. This decrease in cAMP levels parallels the developmental loss of regenerative capacity of the neuron. In adult neurons, an elevation in cAMP results in increased growth capacity and overcomes the inhibition by MAG and myelin. Thus, manipulation of neuronal cAMP levels is likely to have significant therapeutic implications in improving nerve regeneration in the adult CNS after injury.

Acknowledgements

This work was supported by grants from the National Multiple Sclerosis Society (NMSS), the National Institutes of Health (NIH) (NS 37060 and SNRP 41407), and a core facility grant from the Research Centers for Minorities Institute-NIH. J.Q. is a fellow of the NMSS.

References

Berry, M., Carlile, J. and Hunter, A. (1996) Peripheral nerve explants grafted into the vitreous body of the eye promote the regeneration of retinal ganglion cell axons severed in the optic nerve. *J. Neurocytol.*, 25: 147–170.

Bregman, B.S. (1998) Regeneration in the spinal cord. *Curr. Opin. Neurobiol.*, 8: 800–807.

Cai, D., Shen, Y., De Bellard, M., Tang, S. and Filbin, M.T. (1999) Prior exposure to neurotrophins blocks inhibition of axonal regeneration by MAG and myelin via a cAMP-dependent mechanism. *Neuron*, 22: 89–101.

Cai, D., Qiu, J., Cao, Z., McAtee, M., Bregman, B.S. and Filbin, M.T. (2001) Neuronal cyclic AMP controls the developmental loss in ability of axons to regenerate. *J. Neurosci.*, 21: 4731–4739.

David, S. and Aguayo, A.J. (1981) Axonal elongation into peripheral nervous system 'bridges' after central nervous system injury in adult rats. *Science*, 214: 931–933.

DeBellard, M.E., Tang, S., Mukhopadhyay, G., Shen, Y.J. and Filbin, M.T. (1996) Myelin-associated glycoprotein inhibits axonal regeneration from a variety of neurons via interaction with a sialoglycoprotein. *Mol. Cell. Neurosci.*, 7: 89–101.

Huang, D.W., McKerracher, L., Braun, P.E. and David, S. (1999) A therapeutic vaccine approach to stimulate axon regeneration in the adult mammalian spinal cord. *Neuron*, 24: 639–647.

Johnson, P.W., Abramow-Newerly, W., Seilheimer, B., Sadoul, R., Tropak, M.B., Arquint, M., Dunn, R.J., Schachner, M. and Roder, J.C. (1989) Recombinant myelin-associated glycoprotein confers neural adhesion and neurite outgrowth function. *Neuron*, 3: 377–385.

Keirstead, H.S., Hasan, S.J., Muir, G.D. and Steeves, J.D. (1992) Suppression of the onset of myelination extends the permissive period for the functional repair of embryonic spinal cord. *Proc. Natl. Acad. Sci. USA*, 89: 11664–11668.

Lai, C., Brow, M.A., Nave, K.A., Noronha, A.B., Quarles, R.H., Bloom, F.E., Milner, R.J. and Sutcliffe, J.G. (1987) Two forms of 1B236/myelin-associated glycoprotein, a cell adhesion molecule for postnatal neural development, are produced by alternative splicing. *Proc. Natl. Acad. Sci. USA*, 84: 4337–4341.

Li, Y. and Raisman, G. (1993) Long axon growth from embryonic neurons transplanted into myelinated tracts of the adult rat spinal cord. *Brain Res.*, 629: 115–127.

McKerracher, L., David, S., Jackson, D.L., Kottis, V., Dunn, R.J. and Braun, P.E. (1994) Identification of myelin-associated glycoprotein as a major myelin-derived inhibitor of neurite growth. *Neuron*, 13: 805–811.

Ming, G.L., Song, H.J., Berninger, B., Holt, C.E., Tessier-Lavigne, M. and Poo, M.M. (1997) cAMP-dependent growth cone guidance by netrin-1. *Neuron*, 19: 1225–1235.

Mukhopadhyay, G., Doherty, P., Walsh, F.S., Crocker, P.R. and Filbin, M.T. (1994) A novel role for myelin-associated glycoprotein as an inhibitor of axonal regeneration. *Neuron*, 13: 757–767.

Neumann, S. and Woolf, C.J. (1999) Regeneration of dorsal column fibers into and beyond the lesion site following adult spinal cord injury. *Neuron*, 23: 83–91.

Qiu, J., Cai, D., Dai., H., McAtee, M., Hoffman, P.N., Bregman, B.S. and Filbin, M.T. (2002) Spinal axon regeneration induced by elevation of cyclic AMP. *Neuron*, 34: 1–9.

Richardson, P.M. and Issa, V.M. (1984) Peripheral injury enhances central regeneration of primary sensory neurones. *Nature*, 309: 791–793.

Richardson, P.M., McGuinness, U.M. and Aguayo, A.J. (1980) Axons from CNS neurons regenerate into PNS grafts. *Nature*, 284: 264–265.

Salzer, J.L., Holmes, W.P. and Colman, D.R. (1987) The amino acid sequences of the myelin-associated glycoproteins: homology to the immunoglobulin gene superfamily. *J. Cell Biol.*, 104: 957–965.

Sato, S., Yanagisawa, K. and Miyatake, T. (1984a) Conversion of myelin-associated glycoprotein (MAG) to a smaller derivative by calcium activated neutral protease (CANP)-like enzyme in myelin and inhibition by E-64 analogue. *Neurochem. Res.*, 9: 629–635.

Sato, S., Quarles, R.H., Brady, R.O. and Tourtellotte, W.W. (1984b) Elevated neutral protease activity in myelin from brains of patients with multiple sclerosis. *Ann. Neurol.*, 15: 264–267.

Savio, T. and Schwab, M.E. (1990) Lesioned corticospinal tract axons regenerate in myelin-free rat spinal cord. *Proc. Natl. Acad. Sci. USA*, 87: 4130–4133.

Song, H., Ming, G., He, Z., Lehmann, M., McKerracher, L., Tessier-Lavigne, M. and Poo, M. (1998) Conversion of neuronal growth cone responses from repulsion to attraction by cyclic nucleotides. *Science*, 281: 1515–1518.

Stebbins, J.W., Jaffe, H., Fales, H.M. and Moller, J.R. (1997) Determination of a native proteolytic site in myelin-associated glycoprotein. *Biochemistry*, 36: 2221–2226.

Tang, S., Woodhall, R.W., Shen, Y.J., deBellard, M.E., Saffell, J.L., Doherty, P., Walsh, F.S. and Filbin, M.T. (1997) Soluble myelin-associated glycoprotein (MAG) found in vivo inhibits axonal regeneration. *Mol. Cell. Neurosci.*, 9: 333–346.

Turnley, A.M. and Bartlett, P.F. (1998) MAG and MOG enhance neurite outgrowth of embryonic mouse spinal cord neurons. *NeuroReport*, 9: 1987–1990.

L. McKerracher, G. Doucet and S. Rossignol (Eds.)
Progress in Brain Research, Vol. 137

CHAPTER 28

Inosine stimulates axon growth in vitro and in the adult CNS

Larry I. Benowitz *, David E. Goldberg and Nina Irwin

Children's Hospital, Laboratories for Neuroscience Research in Neurosurgery, Harvard Medical School, Program in Neuroscience and Department of Surgery, 300 Longwood Avenue, Boston, MA 02115, USA

Abstract: Unlike mammals, lower vertebrates can regenerate their optic nerves and certain other CNS pathways throughout life. To identify the molecular bases of this phenomenon, we developed a cell culture model and found that goldfish retinal ganglion cells will regenerate their axons in response to the purine nucleoside inosine. Inosine acts through a direct intracellular mechanism and induces many of the changes in gene expression that underlie regenerative growth in vivo, e.g., upregulation of GAP-43, Tα-1 tubulin, and the cell-adhesion molecule, L1. N-kinase, a 47–49-kDa serine-threonine kinase, may mediate the effects of inosine and serve as part of the modular signal transduction pathway that controls axon growth. In vivo, inosine stimulates extensive axon growth in the mature rat corticospinal tract. Following unilateral transection of the corticospinal tract, inosine applied to the intact sensorimotor cortex stimulated layer 5 pyramidal cells to upregulate GAP-43 expression and to sprout axon collaterals. These collaterals crossed the midline at the level of the cervical enlargement and reinnervated regions whose normal connections had been severed. Further understanding of the molecular changes that lie upstream and downstream of N-kinase may lead to new insights into the control of axon growth and to novel methods to improve functional outcome in patients with CNS injury.

Introduction

Following injury in the adult central nervous system (CNS), severed axons show a limited amount of local sprouting, but no long-distance regrowth (Ramon y Cajal, 1928). This situation has devastating consequences for victims of CNS injury, stroke, or neurodegenerative diseases. Regenerative failure has generally been attributed to an insufficiency of trophic factors, the scar that forms at the injury site, inhibitory influences of CNS glia, or other axon-

repellant cues. In the past 20 years, however, numerous studies have shown that some degree of axon regeneration can be achieved by manipulating neurons' intra- or extracellular milieu. Clearly, as we learn more and more about the biology of axon growth and synapse formation, we are likely to come closer to achieving the goal of improving functional outcome in patients who have sustained CNS injury. This chapter highlights the use of purine nucleosides to restore neurons to the growth state, providing a novel approach to stimulating CNS regeneration.

Goldfish retinal ganglion cells as a model system

Unlike mammals, fish and amphibia can regenerate injured optic nerves throughout life (Sperry, 1963; Jacobson, 1991). This phenomenon has been widely studied for insights into the factors that determine regenerative success or failure. In cell culture, explants

---

* Correspondence to: L.I. Benowitz, Children's Hospital, Laboratories for Neuroscience Research in Neurosurgery, Harvard Medical School, Program in Neuroscience and Department of Surgery, 300 Longwood Avenue, Boston MA 02115, USA. Tel.: +1-617-355-6368; Fax: +1-617-734-1646; E-mail: larry.benowitz@tch.harvard.edu

390

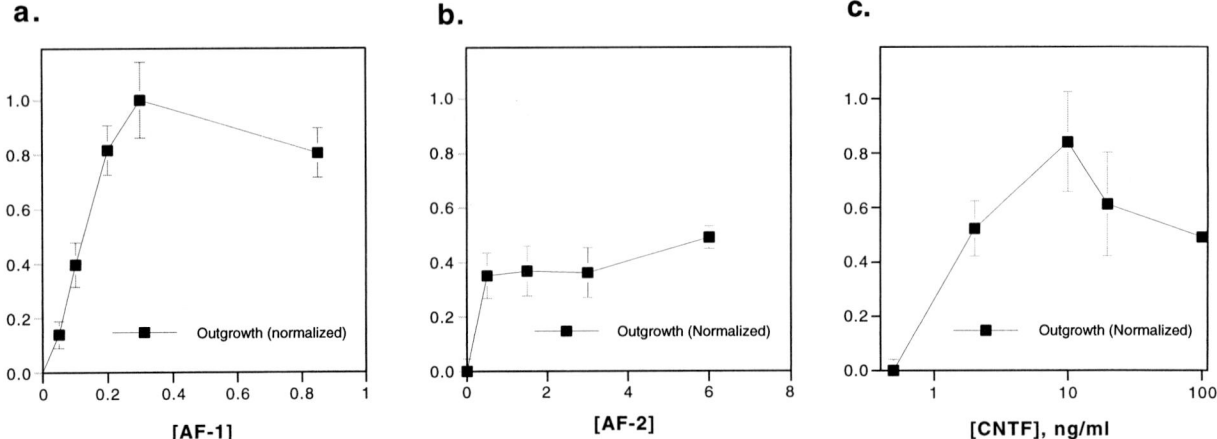

Fig. 1. Goldfish RGCs extend axons in response to several trophic agents. (a) AF-1, a low molecular weight factor derived from optic nerve glia, induces 30–40% of RGCs to extend axons $\geq$ 5 cell diameters in length by 6 days. The net growth in these cells, obtained by subtracting the growth in negative controls grown in defined media (ca. 4%), is used to normalize the data in each experiment. AF-1 induces maximal growth at concentrations $\geq$ 20% (relative to its concentration in optic nerve-conditioned media). (b) The high molecular weight fraction from optic nerve-conditioned media contains a 70-kDa neurite-promoting factor. At concentrations > 0.5×, partially purified AF-2 induces a maximal response equal to about 35% that of AF-1. (c) Recombinant rat CNTF, at concentrations $\geq$ 2 ng/ml, induces 50–70% the level of growth seen with AF-1. (From Schwalb et al., 1995; Petrausch et al., 2000.)

of goldfish retina will extend axons only if the regenerative process had been initiated in vivo by optic nerve injury 1–2 weeks prior to explanting (Landreth and Agranoff, 1976). This observation suggested to us that the program for axon regeneration is not cell-autonomous, and requires factors that are available to retinal ganglion cells (RGCs) in vivo during the priming period. To identify these factors, we cultured dissociated goldfish retinal ganglion cells in defined media and found that they will regenerate their axons in response to two factors that are secreted by optic nerve glia. Far and away the more potent of the two is a small molecule (M_r < 1 kDa) that we refer to as axogenesis factor-1 (AF-1). Axogenesis factor-2 (AF-2) is a 70-kDa polypeptide with considerably lower potency (Schwalb et al., 1995, 1996). Because AF-1 and AF-2 are available to RGC axons at the right time and place after injury, and because they appear to be essential for outgrowth in cell culture, it seems likely that they are important for axon regeneration in vivo. In addition to AF-1 and AF-2, recombinant rat ciliary neurotrophic factor (CNTF) stimulates a level of axon growth intermediate between the levels induced by AF-1 and AF-2 (Petrausch et al., 2000) (Fig. 1).

Purine nucleosides stimulate axon regeneration

In the course of screening candidate molecules for AF-1, we discovered that the purine nucleosides adenosine and guanosine, when present at concentrations $\geq$ 10 µM, stimulated dramatic axon outgrowth (Fig. 2). Pyrimidine nucleosides (cytidine, uridine, thymidine), in contrast showed little activity. We ruled out the possibility that adenosine was acting as an agonist to P_1 purinergic receptors by showing that its effects were not blocked by a P_1 antagonist (8-sulfophenyltheophylline) nor mimicked by a P_1 agonist, the non-hydrolyzable adenosine analog 2-chloroadenosine. The possible involvement of P_2 (purine nucleotide) receptors was excluded by the relative inactivity of the nucleotide derivatives of adenosine and guanosine (e.g., adenosine monophosphate, adenosine diphosphate, ATP). We also ruled out the possibility that adenosine or guanosine were acting via intracellular conversion to the common second messengers cAMP or cGMP, because non-hydrolyzable, membrane-permeable analogs of these cyclic nucleotides were inactive (Fig. 2: Benowitz et al., 1998).

The failure of the non-hydrolyzable adenosine analog 2-chloroadenosine to stimulate growth sug-

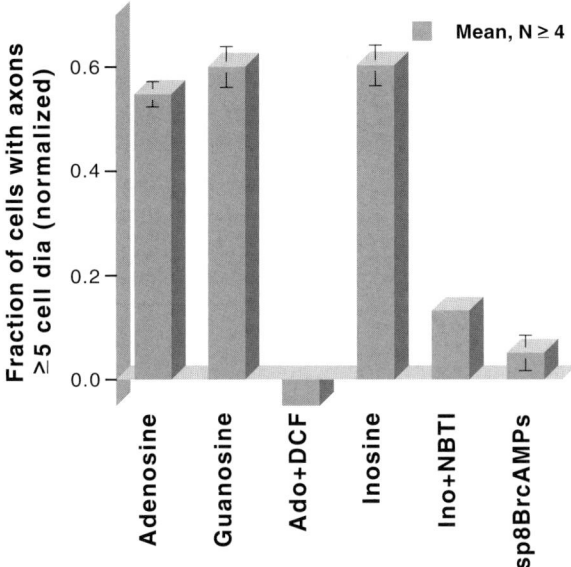

Fig. 2. Purinergic effects on axon outgrowth. The purine nucleosides adenosine (lane 1) and guanosine (lane 2) stimulate goldfish RGCs to regenerate their axons. Adenosine is only active after being hydrolyzed, since its effects are blocked by deoxycoformycin (DCF), an inhibitor of adenosine deaminase (lane 3). Inosine, the product of adenosine hydrolysis, is highly active (ED$_{50}$ = 11 μM: lane 4). Inosine acts through an intracellular mechanism: its effects are blocked by nitrobenzylthioinosine (NBTI), an inhibitor of purine transport (lane 5). Membrane-permeable, non-hydrolyzable analogs of cAMP (sp8BrcAMPs shown in lane 6) or cGMP (not shown) were inactive, indicating that the effects of inosine and guanosine are unrelated to the activities of cyclic nucleotides. All compounds were tested at concentrations of 1–1000 μM; results shown here are at 100 μM. Data are normalized to the level of growth induced by AF-1. (From Benowitz et al., 1998.)

gested an alternative explanation for adenosine's action, i.e., that it must undergo hydrolysis in order to be active. This possibility was verified by experiments showing that deoxycoformycin, an inhibitor of the enzyme which converts adenosine to inosine (adenosine deaminase), blocked the axon-promoting effects of adenosine (Fig. 2). As expected from this result, inosine proved to be highly effective in stimulating axon outgrowth (ED$_{50}$ = 11 μM). Hypoxanthine, the product of inosine's further hydrolysis, showed little activity. The bioactivity of guanosine noted earlier can probably be ascribed to its structural similarity to inosine, differing only by the presence of an NH$_2$ group in position 2 (Fig. 3a). Inosine has previously been shown to stimulate phe-

notypic differentiation in sympathetic neurons (Zurn and Do, 1988), and both inosine and guanosine augment the neuritogenic effects of nerve growth factor in PC12 cells (Braumann et al., 1986; Gysbers and Rathbone, 1996).

Mechanism of purine nucleoside action

Neither inosine nor guanosine is known to act through any extracellular receptors, suggesting that they induce growth through a direct intracellular mechanism. This was verified using nitrobenzylthioinosine, a drug that inhibits the transport of purine nucleosides into the cell. Nitrobenzylthioinosine completely blocked the effects of inosine (Fig. 2) and guanosine on axon growth (Benowitz et al., 1998). The next question, then, is what is the intracellular target upon which inosine and guanosine act? In PC12 cells, nerve growth factor binds to trkA and activates signaling cascades that involve MAP kinases, PI3 kinase, and phospholipase C-γ (Segal and Greenberg, 1996; Chao et al., 1998; Kaplan, 1998). In addition to these, NGF and certain other growth-promoting factors (e.g., FGF-2) rapidly activate a 47–49-kDa serine-threonine kinase referred to as N-kinase (Rowland et al., 1987; Rowland-Gagne and Greene, 1990). The purine analog 6-thioguanine (6-TG), when used at low micromolar concentrations, blocks N-kinase activity and neurite outgrowth in parallel, while not affecting cell survival nor the activity of many other signal transduction molecules (Volonte et al., 1989; Greene et al., 1990; Batistatou et al., 1992; Volonte and Greene, 1992). Thus, N-kinase may be part of a modular signaling cascade that is specific to neurite outgrowth. In view of the structural similarities among 6-TG, inosine and guanosine (Fig. 3a), it occurred to us that the latter two might function as N-kinase agonists.

As a first step in testing whether axon outgrowth in goldfish RGCs is mediated via N-kinase, we investigated whether 6-TG would block outgrowth stimulated by AF-1, AF-2, or CNTF. As shown in Fig. 3b, 6-TG prevents all of these factors from inducing axon growth; cell survival is unaltered (not shown). Next, if inosine is an N-kinase agonist, we would expect it to reverse the inhibitory effects of 6-TG in a competitive fashion. As shown in Fig. 3c, inosine overcomes the inhibitory effects of 6-TG in a dose-dependent manner, suggesting that inosine functions as a competitive agonist at the same site where 6-TG acts, i.e., N-kinase. This hypothesis is further supported by preliminary studies showing that inosine stimulates the activity of N-kinase in vitro (N. Irwin, J. Shieh and L. Benowitz, unpublished observations). In contrast to inosine, the effects of other growth factors are blocked by 6-TG non-competitively (Petrausch et al., 2000).

The purine-sensitive mechanism controls the expression of genes associated with axon growth

During the course of optic nerve regeneration, goldfish retinal ganglion cells exhibit marked changes in their program of gene expression. Foremost among these is a massive induction of the growth-associated protein GAP-43 (Benowitz et al., 1981; Heacock and Agranoff, 1982; Benowitz and Lewis, 1983; Perrone-Bizzozero and Benowitz, 1987; LaBate and Skene, 1989). Changes of a somewhat lesser magnitude are seen for particular cell surface glycoproteins (Bastmeyer et al., 1990; Paschke et al., 1992; Schulte et al., 1997; Ankerhold et al., 1998), cytoskeletal components (Heacock and Agranoff, 1976; Quitschke et al., 1980; Glasgow et al., 1992; Bormann et al., 1998) and certain other proteins (Perry et al., 1987; Ballestero et al., 1995). The purine-sensitive pathway regulates many of these changes. Through immunohistochemistry, we found that inosine induced a 4-fold increase in the number of RGCs that express detectable levels of GAP-43, and a 6-fold increase in the number of cells in which the immunoglobulin superfamily cell adhesion molecule L1 could be detected; DM-GRASP showed a lesser fold-increase, perhaps because its basal level of expression is higher than that of the other two proteins to start with (Figs. 4 and 5). By Western blotting

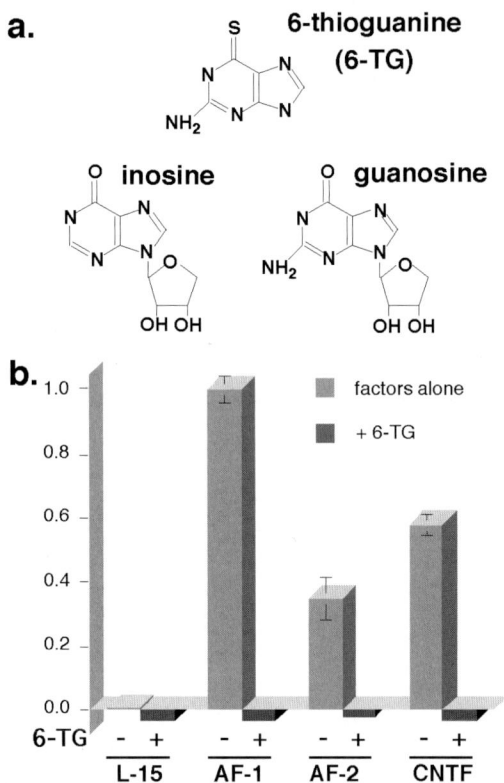

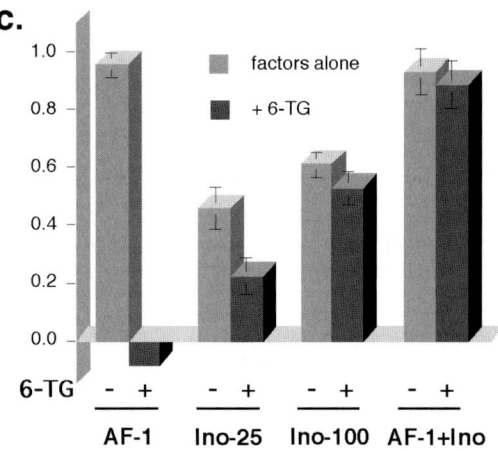

Fig. 3. Inosine and 6-thioguanine act competitively to regulate axon growth. (a) 6-Thioguanine (6-TG) blocks growth and inhibits N-kinase. Its purine structure resembles those of inosine and guanosine except for the substitution of a sulfhydryl for oxygen in position 6. Note the structural similarity between inosine and guanosine, which differ only by the amino group in position 2. (b) In goldfish RGCs, 6-TG (10 μM) completely blocks axon outgrowth induced by AF-1, AF-2, or CNTF. (c) Inosine and 6-TG act competitively. Outgrowth induced by 25 μM inosine is only partly diminished by 10 μM 6-TG, while outgrowth stimulated by 100 μM inosine is unaffected. Inosine (100 μM) restores the full level of growth induced by AF-1 in the presence of 10 μM 6-TG. (From Benowitz et al., 1998; Petrausch et al., 2000.)

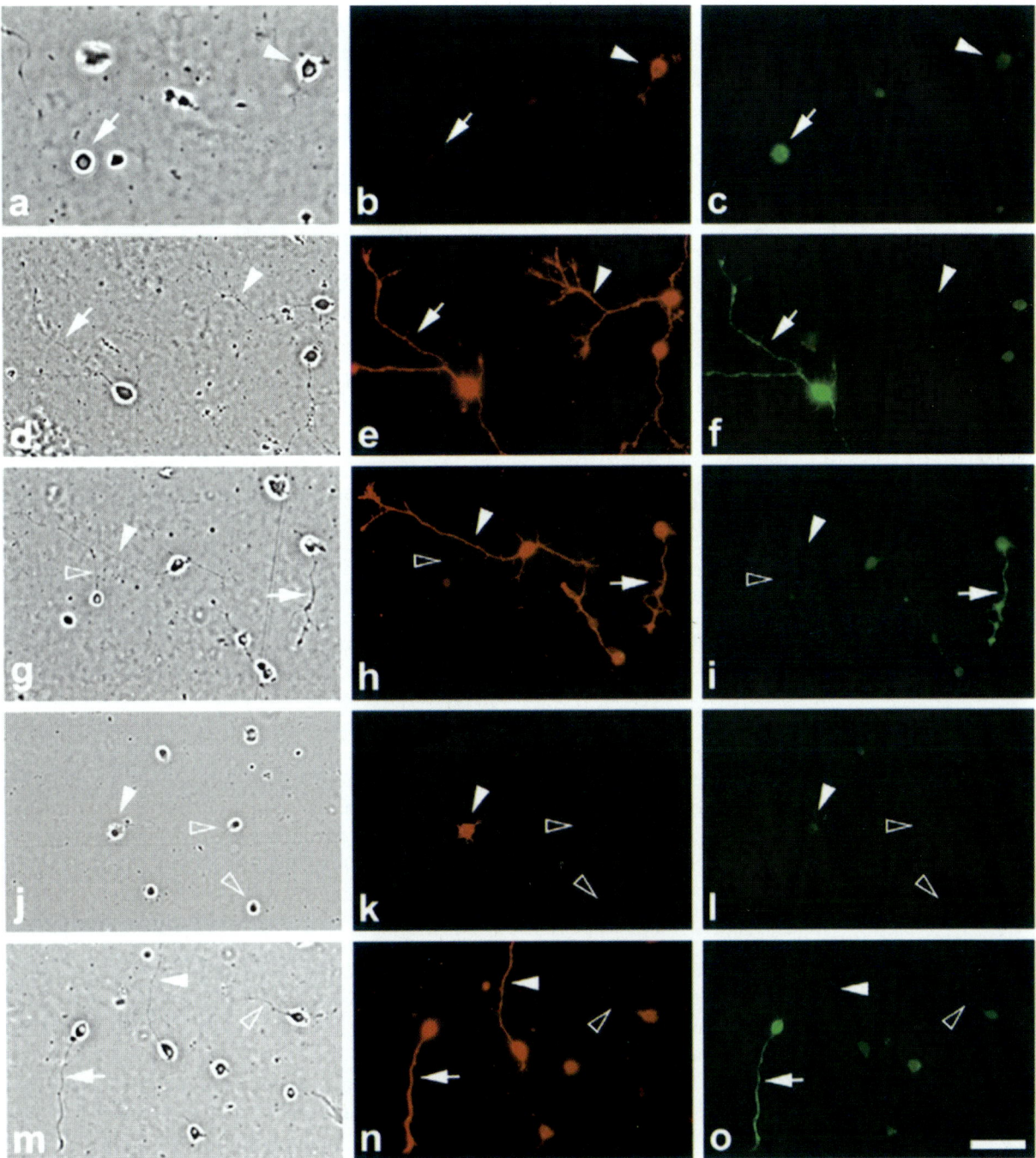

Fig. 4. Purinergic control of growth-associated proteins. Goldfish RGCs were grown in culture with either defined media alone (a–c), AF-1 (d–f), inosine (g–i), AF-1 + 6-TG (j–l) or AF-1 + 6-TG + inosine (m–o). After 6 days, cells were immunostained with antibodies to one of three developmentally regulated proteins: GAP-43 (b,e,h,k,n), L1 (c,f,l), or neurolin (DM-GRASP: i,o). Immunoreactivity was detected with rhodamine or fluorescein-conjugated secondary antibodies. AF-1 and inosine induced expression of all three proteins, whereas 6-TG suppressed their expression (j–l). Inosine acted competitively with 6-TG to restore gene expression (m–o). Thus, several gene products involved in axon growth are regulated through the purine-sensitive pathway. (From Petrausch et al., 2000.)

394

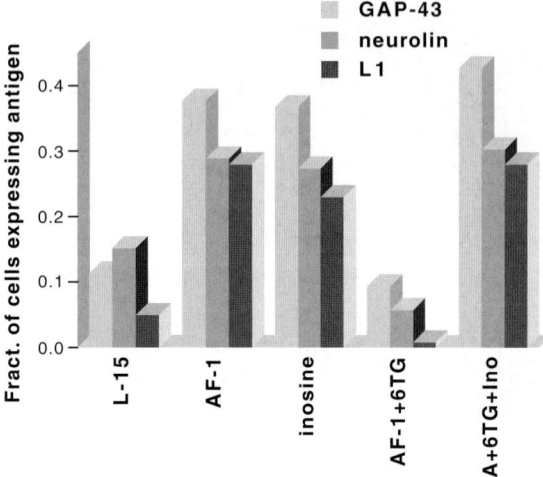

Fig. 5. Quantitation of protein expression. Levels of GAP-43, neurolin (DM-GRASP), and L1 immunostaining were assessed in quadruplicate cultures, counting the number of cells showing moderate-to-high levels of fluorescence. As described in Fig. 3, AF-1 and inosine induced expression of all three proteins; 6-TG suppressed their expression, whereas inosine competitively restored gene expression (A + 6TG + Ino). The number of cells showing GAP-43 labeling increased ca. 4-fold in the presence of AF-1 or inosine, and decreased below baseline in the presence of 6-TG; L1 expression showed an even greater degree of regulation (ca. 10-fold variation), whereas neurolin showed less. (From Petrausch et al., 2000.)

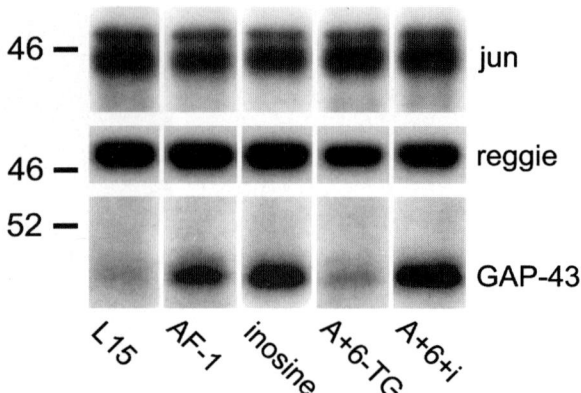

Fig. 6. Selectivity of purinergic effects on gene expression. Levels of Jun family transcription factors ($M_r = 48$ kDa, 45 kDa) were elevated under all conditions, and were not affected by AF-1 or by purinergic manipulations. A similar lack of regulation was seen for the protein reggie. In contrast, GAP-43 levels were strongly regulated by AF-1 and by purinergic manipulations. (From Petrausch et al., 2000.)

(Fig. 6), the overall increase in GAP-43 expression appears to be much greater than estimated by cell staining, probably because, in addition to increasing the number of cells that express detectable levels of the protein, inosine significantly increases GAP-43 levels per cell. Fig. 6 also illustrates the specificity of inosine's actions: axotomy alone induces the expression of jun family transcription factors and the cell surface protein reggie. Unlike the case for GAP-43, the former changes are unaltered by purinergic manipulations. In further studies, we used retinal ganglion cells from transgenic zebrafish which express green fluorescent protein (EGFP) linked to the α_1-tubulin promoter (provided by Daniel Goldman, University of Michigan). α_1-Tubulin expression increases when neurons are growing axons (Miller and Geddes, 1990; Tetzlaff et al., 1991; Hieber et al., 1998), and hence these transgenic cells enabled us to determine whether inosine induces α_1-tubulin expression along with the other molecular changes. As shown in Fig. 7, inosine increased the number

of RGCs expressing α_1-tubulin-EGFP, as did AF-1. 6-TG blocked α_1-tubulin-EGFP induction along with all of the other changes stimulated by AF-1, causing their expression to fall below baseline (Fig. 5); again, the specificity of these effects is demonstrated by the fact that 6-TG did not alter expression of certain other gene products (Fig. 6). Paralleling the effects of purines on axon growth, high concentrations of inosine blocked 6-TG inhibition and restored the expression of GAP-43, α_1-tubulin, and the other purine-sensitive genes (Figs. 4 and 5). These findings suggest, then, that the program of gene expression associated with axon outgrowth is regulated through a purine-sensitive mechanism, presumably via N-kinase activation (Petrausch et al., 2000). Fig. 8 summarizes our working model of the mechanisms through which inosine and growth factors work.

Inosine stimulates extensive axon growth in the injured rat spinal cord

In the rat, the corticospinal tract (CST) is required for fine, learned movements of the paws and digits. This pathway originates in the layer 5 pyramidal cells of the sensorimotor cortex and descends through the ventral pons and medulla; most CST fibers decussate in the caudal medulla and then assume their final

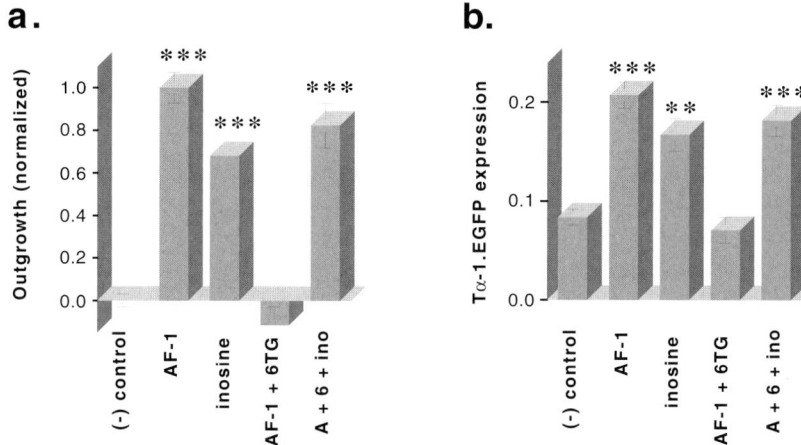

Fig. 7. Regulation of Tα-1 tubulin expression. Transgenic zebrafish RGCs (tg zfRGCs) harbored a reporter construct expressing a Tα-1–EGFP fusion protein driven by the Tα-1 promoter (courtesy of Daniel Goldman, University of Michigan). (a) tg zfRGCs respond in culture similarly to goldfish RGCs, i.e., axon growth is stimulated by AF-1 and inosine, inhibited by 6-TG, and restored by inosine. (b) Expression of Tα-1 is regulated through a purine-sensitive mechanism and parallels axon outgrowth ($^{***}P < 0.001$, $^{**}P < 0.01$ comparing reporter expression with negative controls). (From Petrausch et al., 2000.)

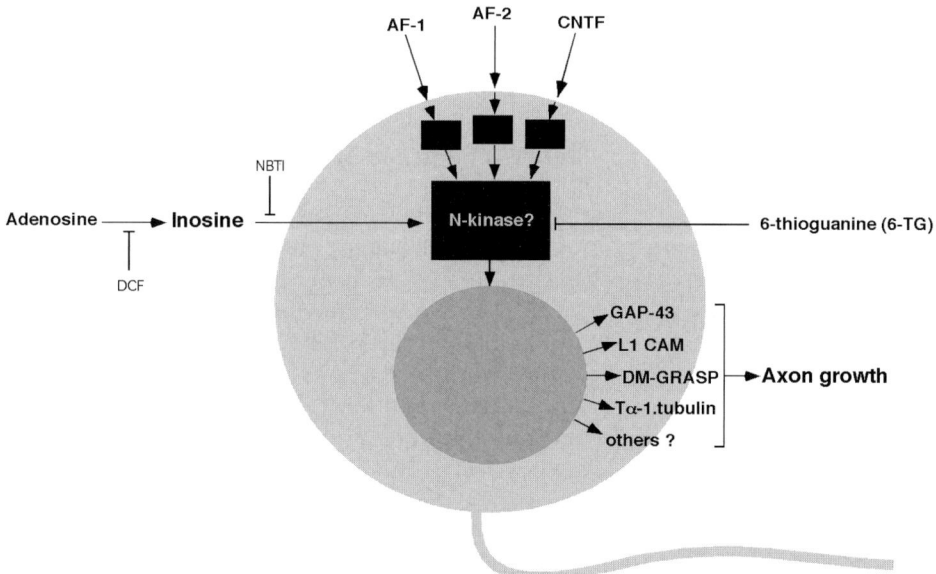

Fig. 8. Proposed mechanism of inosine's action. Inosine, a product of adenosine hydrolysis, is transported across the cell membrane via facilitated diffusion and may act as an N-kinase agonist. Activation of N-kinase leads to changes in gene expression that culminate in axon outgrowth. Multiple growth factors (AF-1, AF-2, CNTF) stimulate axon outgrowth and the underlying program of gene expression via N-kinase activation; their effects can all be blocked by the purine analog 6-TG. Inosine acts competitively with 6TG, and at increasing concentrations, restores growth. Deoxycoformycin inhibits adenosine hydrolysis and renders adenosine inactive; NBTI inhibits purine nucleoside transport across the cell membrane and prevents inosine (or guanosine) from stimulating growth.

position in the dorsal funiculus in the contralateral half of the spinal cord, synapsing primarily upon interneurons that secondarily innervate motor neurons. Although damage to the rat's CST has only limited effects, injury to the homologous pathway in humans has profound consequences. Hence, the development of methods to restore CST functions is very important clinically.

To investigate whether inosine could stimulate axon growth in the CST, we used an experimental model similar to one recently described by Schwab and co-workers (Z'Graggen et al., 1998). In that study, the CST was transected unilaterally through a ventral surgical approach in the medulla (rostral to the decussation) and the IN-1 antibody was administered to neutralize the myelin protein NI-250 (Nogo-A). This treatment stimulated a limited number of axons from the *non-transected* side to sprout collateral branches that crossed over to the denervated side of the spinal cord. In our studies, we likewise transected the CST unilaterally (in the left ventral medulla in mature rats) and applied inosine to pyramidal cells of the normal (right) sensorimotor cortex using a minipump (Alzet). After 2 weeks of delivering inosine or phosphate-buffered saline (PBS) (as a vehicle control), pumps were removed and the trajectories of CST axons were traced by injecting biotin dextran amine (BDA) into the normal (right) sensorimotor cortex.

Inosine induced numerous axon collaterals to sprout from the intact CST, cross the midline, and run through the denervated side of the spinal cord (Fig. 9a: Benowitz et al., 1999). Quantitation of this phenomenon revealed that, at the level of the cervical enlargement, inosine-treated animals had up to 2500 crossed axons per section, with a median value of ca. 500. In comparison, control animals treated with PBS showed, on the average, 30 crossed axons per section. Crossed, BDA-labeled fibers were occasionally observed leaving the white matter and coursing into the denervated gray matter, and preliminary studies indicate that these crossed fibers form synapses in the appropriate laminae on the denervated side of the spinal cord (D. Goldberg, P. Shah, C. Aoki, L. Benowitz, unpublished data).

As an alternative way of evaluating the effects of inosine on CST growth, we used immunohistochemistry to visualize changes in expression of the growth-associated protein, GAP-43. Normally, GAP-43 is expressed at high levels in the developing CST and then declines as the tract matures, persisting at low levels in the adult (Kalil and Skene, 1986; Gorgels et al., 1987); the normal level of GAP-43 in the adult CST can be visualized in Fig. 9d.

In animals treated only with PBS after a unilateral transection of the CST, GAP-43 immunostaining declined on the denervated side (Fig. 9e). Following inosine treatment, we would expect that both the intact side and the denervated side might show increases in GAP-43, since the parent axons, as well as their collateral branches that have crossed over to the denervated side, should both be in a growth state. This prediction was borne out in the results shown in Fig. 9f. Note that the position of the GAP-43-labeled axons on the denervated (right) side of the cord are concentrated in the same medial position visualized by BDA labeling (cf. Fig. 9c).

We have also tested the ability of inosine to enhance sprouting from *transected* axons. Such experiments are generally somewhat difficult to interpret, due to the problem of distinguishing regenerating axons from fibers that were never injured in the first place. Nevertheless, our preliminary studies suggest that inosine does stimulate axotomized pyramidal cells to extend new terminal branches that grow around the lesion (D. Goldberg and L. Benowitz, unpublished data).

Summary and conclusions

Inosine acts intracellularly to induce the expression of GAP-43 and other proteins important for axon outgrowth. The mediator of inosine's actions appears to be N-kinase, a serine-threonine kinase that functions as a 'master switch' in the modular signaling pathway which controls axon growth. Cloning the N-kinase gene and further characterization of its properties is therefore a high priority for understanding axon growth. The purine analog 6-TG is an antagonist of this kinase and acts in the opposite fashion from inosine, blocking axon growth and the underlying pattern of gene induction. Following unilateral transections of the corticospinal tract in rats, inosine applied to the intact sensorimotor cortex stimulated layer 5 pyramidal neurons to upregulate GAP-43 expression and to sprout axon collaterals that grew into regions of the cervical spinal cord which had lost their normal afferents. From a basic neuroscience perspective, it will be important to define the signal transduction steps that lie upstream from N-kinase activation, and this may provide additional targets for drug development. It will also be important to define

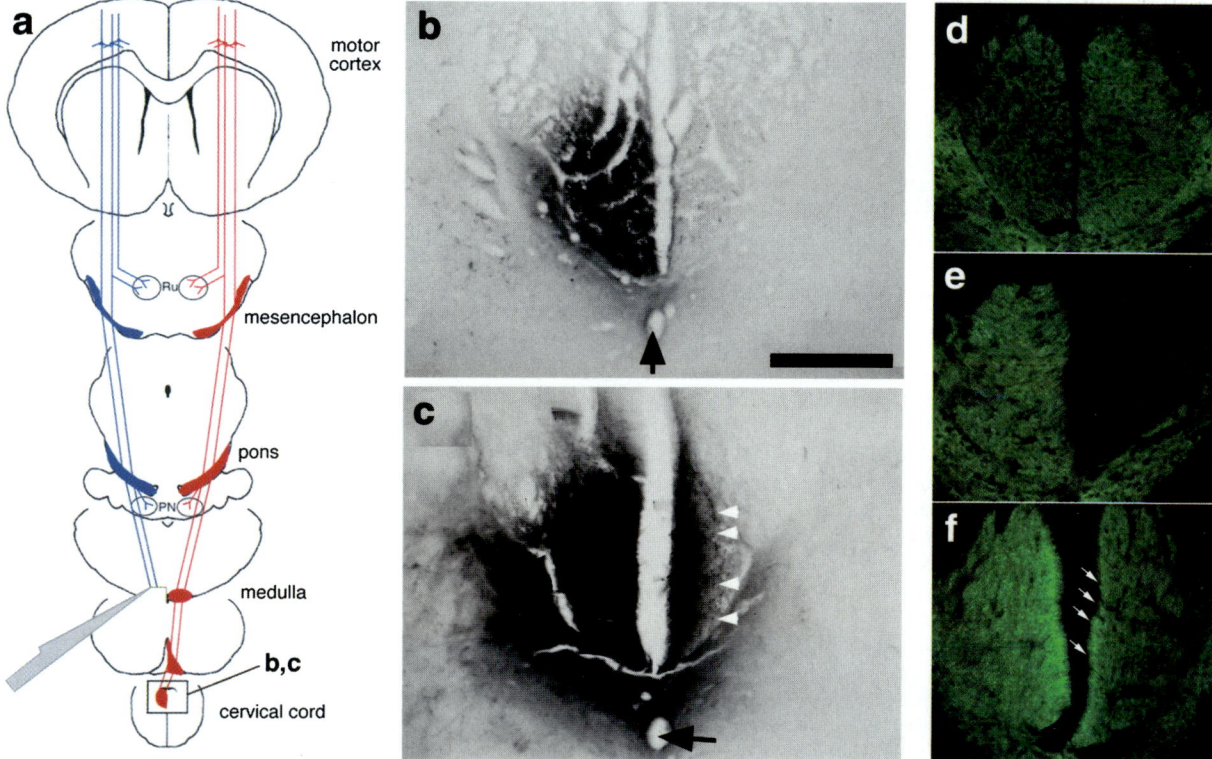

Fig. 9. Inosine stimulates axon growth in the rat corticospinal tract (CST). (a) The rat's CST originates in layer 5 pyramidal cells of the sensorimotor cortex, descends through the brainstem, and courses along the ventromedial medulla, where we transect it unilaterally (blue). Inosine was applied via minipump for 2 weeks to the non-axotomized sensorimotor cortex. Trajectories of inosine-treated CST axons (red) were traced by injecting BDA into the treated (non-axotomized) sensorimotor cortex. (b) In the cervical enlargement of controls treated with PBS, all BDA-labeled fibers (black) remain on the left side, i.e., contralateral to the intact cortex, as expected. (c) In inosine-treated cases, hundreds, and in some cases thousands, of CST fibers crossed over from the intact side to the denervated (right) side of the cord (white arrows). The increased labeling on the left side compared with the control suggests that axon sprouting also occurs on the intact side. Black arrows point to the central canal, a marker for the midline. Scale bar in b is 500 μm. (d–f) Axon growth visualized by GAP-43 immunofluorescence. (d) At the mid-cervical level, modest levels of GAP-43 immunoreactivity (IR) appear bilaterally in the dorsal funiculi, reflecting the continued presence of the protein in the normal adult rat CST. (e) In control animals treated only with vehicle (PBS) after unilateral CST transections, GAP-43 IR disappears from the denervated (right) dorsal funiculus. (c) In animals with unilateral CST injury and inosine treatment, intense GAP-43 IR appears on the intact (left) dorsal funiculus and in many fibers on the denervated (right) side (white arrows show crossed fibers near the midline) (Benowitz et al., 1999).

better the changes in gene expression that lie downstream from N-kinase activation, particularly for proteins involved in axon elongation and pathfinding. Finally, from a clinical perspective, we need to explore the potential benefits of activating this pathway in patients who have sustained CNS injury.

Abbreviations

6-TG	6-thioguanine
AF-1, -2	axogenesis factor-1, -2
BDA	biotinylated dextran amine
CNTF	ciliary neurotrophic factor
CST	corticospinal tract
DCF	deoxycoformycin
EGFP	enhanced green fluorescent protein
NBTI	nitrobenzylthioinosine
NGF	nerve growth factor
ONCM	optic nerve conditioned media
PBS	phosphate-buffered saline
RGC	retinal ganglion cell
tg	transgenic

References

Ankerhold, R., Leppert, C.A., Bastmeyer, M. and Stuermer, C.A. (1998) E587 antigen is upregulated by goldfish oligodendrocytes after optic nerve lesion and supports retinal axon regeneration. *Glia*, 23: 257–270.

Ballestero, R.P., Wilmot, G.R., Leski, M.L., Uhler, M.D. and Agranoff, B.W. (1995) Isolation of cDNA clones encoding RICH: a protein induced during goldfish optic nerve regeneration with homology to mammalian 2′,3′-cyclic-nucleotide 3′-phosphodiesterases. *Proc. Natl. Acad. Sci. USA*, 92: 8621–8625.

Bastmeyer, M., Schlosshauer, B. and Stuermer, C.A. (1990) The spatiotemporal distribution of N-CAM in the retinotectal pathway of adult goldfish detected by the monoclonal antibody D3. *Development*, 108: 299–311.

Batistatou, A., Volonte, C. and Greene, L.A. (1992) Nerve growth factor employs multiple pathways to induce primary response genes in PC12 cells. *Mol. Biol. Cell*, 3: 363–371.

Benowitz, L.I. and Lewis, E.R. (1983) Increased transport of 44,000- to 49,000-dalton acidic proteins during regeneration of the goldfish optic nerve: a two-dimensional gel analysis. *J. Neurosci.*, 3: 2153–2163.

Benowitz, L.I., Shashoua, V.E. and Yoon, M.G. (1981) Specific changes in rapidly transported proteins during regeneration of the goldfish optic nerve. *J. Neurosci.*, 1: 300–307.

Benowitz, L.I., Jing, Y., Tabibazar, R., Rosenberg, P.A., Jo, S., Petrausch, B., Stuermer, C. and Irwin, N. (1998) Axonal regeneration is regulated by an intracellular purine-sensitive mechanism in retinal ganglion cells. *J. Biol. Chem.*, 273: 29626–29634.

Benowitz, L.I., Goldberg, D.E., Madsen, J.R., Soni, D. and Irwin, N. (1999) Inosine stimulates extensive axon collateral growth in the rat corticospinal tract after injury. *Proc. Natl. Acad. Sci. USA*, 96: 13486–13490.

Bormann, P., Zumsteg, V.M., Roth, L.W. and Reinhard, E. (1998) Target contact regulates GAP-43 and alpha-tubulin mRNA levels in regenerating retinal ganglion cells. *J. Neurosci. Res.*, 52: 405–419.

Braumann, T., Jastorff, B. and Richter-Landsberg, C. (1986) Fate of cyclic nucleotides in PC12 cell cultures: uptake, metabolism, and effects of metabolites on nerve growth factor-induced neurite outgrowth. *J. Neurochem.*, 47: 912–919.

Chao, M., Casaccia-Bonnefil, P., Carter, B., Chittka, A., Kong, H. and Yoon, S.O. (1998) Neurotrophin receptors: mediators of life and death. *Brain Res. Rev.*, 26: 295–301.

Glasgow, E., Druger, R.K., Levine, E.M., Fuchs, C. and Schechter, N. (1992) Plasticin, a novel type III neurofilament protein from goldfish retina: increased expression during optic nerve regeneration. *Neuron*, 9: 373–381.

Gorgels, T.G., Oestreicher, A.B., de Kort, E.J. and Gispen, W.H. (1987) Immunocytochemical distribution of the protein kinase C substrate B-50 (GAP43) in developing rat pyramidal tract. *Neurosci. Lett.*, 83: 59–64.

Greene, L.A., Volonte, C. and Chalazonitis, A. (1990) Purine analogs inhibit nerve growth factor-promoted neurite outgrowth by sympathetic and sensory neurons. *J. Neurosci.*, 10: 1479–1485.

Gysbers, J.W. and Rathbone, M.P. (1996) Neurite outgrowth in PC12 cells is enhanced by guanosine through both cAMP-dependent and -independent mechanisms. *Neurosci. Lett.*, 220: 175–178.

Heacock, A.M. and Agranoff, B.W. (1976) Enhanced labeling of a retinal protein during regeneration of optic nerve in goldfish. *Proc. Natl. Acad. Sci. USA*, 73: 828–832.

Heacock, A.M. and Agranoff, B.W. (1982) Protein synthesis and transport in the regenerating goldfish visual system. *Neurochem. Res.*, 7: 771–788.

Hieber, V., Dai, X., Foreman, M. and Goldman, D. (1998) Induction of alpha1-tubulin gene expression during development and regeneration of the fish central nervous system. *J. Neurobiol.*, 37: 429–440.

Jacobson, M. (1991) *Developmental Neurobiology*, 3rd edn. Plenum, New York.

Kalil, K. and Skene, J.H. (1986) Elevated synthesis of an axonally transported protein correlates with axon outgrowth in normal and injured pyramidal tracts. *J. Neurosci.*, 6: 2563–2570.

Kaplan, D.R. (1998) Studying signal transduction in neuronal cells: the Trk/NGF system. *Prog. Brain Res.*, 117: 35–46.

LaBate, M.E. and Skene, J.H. (1989) Selective conservation of GAP-43 structure in vertebrate evolution. *Neuron*, 3: 299–310.

Landreth, G.E. and Agranoff, B.W. (1976) Explant culture of adult goldfish retina: effect of prior optic nerve crush. *Brain Res.*, 118: 299–303.

Miller, F.D. and Geddes, J.W. (1990) Increased expression of the major embryonic alpha-tubulin mRNA, T alpha 1, during neuronal regeneration, sprouting, and in Alzheimer's disease. *Prog. Brain Res.*, 86: 321–330.

Paschke, K.A., Lottspeich, F. and Stuermer, C.A. (1992) Neurolin, a cell surface glycoprotein on growing retinal axons in the goldfish visual system, is reexpressed during retinal axonal regeneration. *J. Cell Biol.*, 117: 863–875.

Perrone-Bizzozero, N.I. and Benowitz, L.I. (1987) Expression of a 48-kilodalton growth-associated protein in the goldfish retina. *J. Neurochem.*, 48: 644–652.

Perry, G.W., Burmeister, D.W. and Grafstein, B. (1987) Fast axonally transported proteins in regenerating goldfish optic axons. *J. Neurosci.*, 7: 792–806.

Petrausch, B., Tabibiazar, R., Roser, T., Jing, Y., Goldman, D., Stuermer, C.A., Irwin, N. and Benowitz, L.I. (2000) A purine-sensitive pathway regulates multiple genes involved in axon regeneration in goldfish retinal ganglion cells. *J. Neurosci.*, 20: 8031–8041.

Quitschke, W., Francis, A. and Schechter, N. (1980) Electrophoretic analysis of specific proteins in the regenerating goldfish retinotectal pathway. *Brain Res.*, 201: 347–360.

Ramon y Cajal, S. (1928) *Degeneration and Regeneration in the Nervous System* (Translated by J. DeFilipe and E.G. Jones). Oxford University Press, NY, 1991.

Rowland, E.A., Muller, T.H., Goldstein, M. and Greene, L.A. (1987) Cell-free detection and characterization of a novely nerve growth factor-activated protein kinase in PC12 cells. *J. Biol. Chem.*, 262: 7504–7513.

Rowland-Gagne, E. and Greene, L.A. (1990) Multiple pathways of N-kinase activation in PC12 cells. *J. Neurochem.*, 54: 423–433.

Schulte, T., Paschke, K.A., Laessing, U., Lottspeich, F. and Stuermer, C.A. (1997) Reggie-1 and reggie-2, two cell surface proteins expressed by retinal ganglion cells during axon regeneration. *Development*, 124: 577–587.

Schwalb, J.M., Boulis, N.M., Gu, M.F., Winickoff, J., Jackson, P.S., Irwin, N. and Benowitz, L.I. (1995) Two factors secreted by the goldfish optic nerve induce retinal ganglion cells to regenerate axons in culture. *J. Neurosci.*, 15: 5514–5525.

Schwalb, J.M., Gu, M.F., Stuermer, C., Bastmeyer, M., Hu, G.F., Boulis, N., Irwin, N. and Benowitz, L.I. (1996) Optic nerve glia secrete a low-molecular-weight factor that stimulates retinal ganglion cells to regenerate axons in goldfish. *Neuroscience*, 72: 901–910.

Segal, R.A. and Greenberg, M.E. (1996) Intracellular signaling pathways activated by neurotrophic factors. *Annu. Rev. Neurosci.*, 19: 463–489.

Sperry, R.W. (1963) Chemoaffinity in the orderly growth of nerve fiber patterns and connections. *Proc. Natl. Acad. Sci. USA*, 50: 703–710.

Tetzlaff, W., Alexander, S.W., Miller, F.D. and Bisby, M.A. (1991) Response of facial and rubrospinal neurons to axotomy: changes in mRNA expression for cytoskeletal proteins and GAP-43. *J. Neurosci.*, 11: 2528–2544.

Volonte, C. and Greene, L.A. (1992) 6-Methylmercaptopurine riboside is a potent and selective inhibitor of nerve growth factor-activated protein kinase N. *J. Neurochem.*, 58: 700–708.

Volonte, C., Rukenstein, A., Loeb, D.M. and Greene, L.A. (1989) Differential inhibition of nerve growth factor responses by purine analogues: correlation with inhibition of a nerve growth factor-activated protein kinase. *J. Cell Biol.*, 109: 2395–2403.

Z'Graggen, W.J., Metz, G.A., Kartje, G.L., Thallmair, M. and Schwab, M.E. (1998) Functional recovery and enhanced corticofugal plasticity after unilateral pyramidal tract lesion and blockade of myelin-associated neurite growth inhibitors in adult rats. *J. Neurosci.*, 18: 4744–4757.

Zurn, A. and Do, K. (1988) Purine metabolite inosine is an adrenergic neurotrophic substance for cultured chicken sympathetic neurons. *Proc. Natl. Acad. Sci. USA*, 85: 8301–8305.

L. McKerracher, G. Doucet and S. Rossignol (Eds.)
Progress in Brain Research, Vol. 137
© 2002 Elsevier Science B.V. All rights reserved

CHAPTER 29

T cell-based therapeutic vaccination for spinal cord injury

Michal Schwartz * and Ehud Hauben

Department of Neurobiology, The Weizmann Institute of Science, 76100 Rehovot, Israel

Abstract: Spinal cord injury results in a massive loss of neurons, due not only to the direct effects of the primary injury but also to self-destructive processes triggered by the insult. Our group has recently reported that traumatic injury of the central nervous system (CNS) spontaneously evokes a purposeful T cell-mediated autoimmune response that reduces the injury-induced degeneration in the CNS; in its absence, the outcome of the injury is worse. Using a rat model of spinal cord contusion, we show here that this autoimmune protection can be induced and/or boosted by post-traumatic immunization with CNS myelin-associated self antigens such as myelin basic protein (MBP). In an attempt to reduce the risk of pathogenic autoimmunity while retaining the benefit of the immunization, we immunized spinally injured rats with MBP-derived peptides with attenuated pathogenic properties created by replacement of one amino acid in the T cell receptor-binding site. Immunization with these altered peptide ligands immediately after spinal cord contusion resulted in a significant improvement in recovery, assessed by locomotor activity in an open field. The feasibility of T cell-based vaccination, as opposed to vaccination mediated by antibodies for the treatment of nerve trauma, is further suggested by the relatively rapid onset of the T cell response following immunization. Such cell-mediated therapy is not only a way to evoke and boost a physiological remedy; it also has the advantage of being mediated by mobile cells, which can produce a variety of neurotrophic factors and cytokines in accordance with the tissue needs. T cells can also regulate other immune cells in a way that favors tissue maintenance and repair.

Background

Spinal cord injury, like any other injury to the central nervous system (CNS), leads to an immediate degeneration of the injured axons with consequent death of their cell bodies (Kalb, 1995; Schwab and Bartholdi, 1996; Crowe et al., 1997). In the absence of therapeutic intervention, the damage propagates both laterally and longitudinally via a process termed secondary degeneration, causing the inevitable loss of additional neurons (Faden, 1993; Povlishock and Jenkins, 1995; Yoles and Schwartz, 1998a). Attempts to halt the progression of damage have focused on pharmacological approaches, such as neutralizing

some of the harmful compounds involved (Panter et al., 1990), or supplying growth factors and cytokines that can change the resistance of the remaining neurons (Blesch and Tuszynski, 1997; Bregman, 1998; Houweling et al., 1998; Franzen et al., 1999; Houle and Ye, 1999; Rabchevsky et al., 1999).

We recently demonstrated that passive transfer of T cells directed against myelin basic protein (MBP) (but not of T cells directed against the exogenous antigen ovalbumin), before or immediately after incomplete spinal cord injury (ISCI) in rats, can reduce the injury-induced neuronal loss (Hauben et al., 2000a,b). We further demonstrated that this autoimmune T cell-mediated neuroprotection is physiologically evoked, with the injury itself acting as the stimulus (Yoles et al., 2001). However, the ability to mount a protective T cell-mediated response was found to be limited to individuals or strains that are genetically endowed with the ability to resist development of CNS autoimmune disease (Kipnis et al.,

---

* Correspondence to: M. Schwartz, Department of Neurobiology, The Weizmann Institute of Science, 76100 Rehovot, Israel. Tel.: +972-8-934-2467; Fax: +972-8-934-4131; E-mail: michal.schwartz@weizmann.ac.il

2001). As both the passive immunization and the endogenous protective immunity were found to be associated with myelin antigens, our interpretation of these findings was that passive immunization is a way to induce and boost an endogenous remedy, with a therapeutic window of at least 1 week (Hauben et al., 2000a). Since the T cell response to active immunization is known to mature within 3–5 days, we envisaged the development of a therapeutic vaccination as a treatment modality for ISCI. Accordingly, we proposed that boosting the self-protective mechanism, using safe (i.e., non-pathogenic) peptides which cross-react with the relevant endogenous proteins, might be the ultimate therapeutic modality for neuronal rescue, and is likely to yield effective neuroprotection with minimal side effects (Hauben et al., 2001a,b).

Autoimmune response evoked by spinal cord injury

'Inflammation' is the term used to describe the accumulation of cells of the immune system in a certain tissue or organ. In the CNS, inflammation is often associated with the innate immune response to injury (manifested by activation of tissue-resident microglia and invasion of blood-borne macrophages). The role of these immune cells in determining the fate of damaged CNS tissue has been the subject of a long-standing debate, with conflicting conclusions (Prewitt et al., 1997; Franzen et al., 1998; Rapalino et al., 1998; Popovich et al., 1999). The activity of immune-derived cells after spinal cord injury was widely considered as deleterious, and indeed inflammation has acquired a bad reputation in the context of CNS injuries in general.

However, during the course of studies aimed at defining the possible contribution of individual pro-inflammatory or anti-inflammatory cytokines on the injured CNS, it became clear that no single effect can be attributed to any particular cytokine, as the effect may vary with the post-injury degeneration phase. Thus, for example, IL-10 was beneficial in spinally injured rats when administered soon after injury, but destructive when administered later (Bethea et al., 1999). These and other variable observations prompted our group to re-examine the role of immune cells in the injured CNS. Initial studies

were conducted in the crush-injured optic nerve of the rat, a useful model for axonal injury (Hirschberg et al., 1994; Yoles and Schwartz, 1998b). Using this model, it was demonstrated that T cells accumulate in the injured optic nerve, but to a significantly lesser extent than in injured peripheral nerves (Moalem et al., 1999a,b, 2000a,b).

Endeavoring to augment the accumulation of CNS myelin-associated T cells at the site of the injury, we subjected rats with crush-injured optic nerves to passive immunization with MBP-reactive T cells. This maneuver, when carried out in spinally injured rats before or up to 1 week after the injury, resulted in a significant decrease in neuronal loss, whereas similar immunization with T cells directed against a non-self antigen (ovalbumin) had no effect (Hauben et al., 2000a). Protection was not observed when the T cells were injected 2 weeks after injury. These results suggest the therapeutic time window for T cell-mediated attenuation of secondary degeneration after spinal injury in rats to be at least 1 week (Hauben et al., 2000a).

The observation that MBP-reactive T cells can promote recovery of rats with spinal cord damage appears to conflict with the finding by Popovich and his colleagues that blood-derived T cells isolated from spinally injured Lewis rats, when transferred, following many cycles of MBP expansion in vitro to naïve Lewis rats, induced a disease known as experimental autoimmune encephalomyelitis (EAE) (Popovich et al., 1996). This apparent discrepancy between finding a T cell-induced autoimmune disease and finding a T cell-induced neuroprotection appears to be resolved by our observation that spontaneously evoked protective autoimmunity is strain-specific (Kipnis et al., 2001). EAE-susceptible strains, such as Lewis rats, which develop an autoimmune disease in response to active vaccination with myelin antigens, are inherently incapable of spontaneously mounting a beneficial autoimmune response, whereas strains that are resistant to EAE development (such as SPD) are inherently capable of sustaining a protective autoimmune response (Kipnis et al., 2001; Schori et al., 2001a). The strain-related difference in response can be illustrated by reviewing uninjured rats injected with splenocytes which were isolated from spinally injured rats 1 week after the injury. While splenocytes transferred from spinally injured Lewis rats can induce EAE in uninjured Lewis recipients, splenocytes transferred from spinally injured SPD rats (which are constitutionally resistant to autoimmune disease) into uninjured SPD recipients did not induce EAE. We concluded that CNS insults evoke a T cell-dependent response, which is beneficial in animals that are genetically endowed with resistance to EAE, but not in animals that are inherently susceptible to EAE. Susceptible strains may even develop a predisposition toward autoimmune disease.

The above studies prompted us to formulate the concept, which is gaining increasingly wide recognition that protective autoimmunity is a physiological response to trauma (Yoles et al., 2001). In this context, it is important to draw a clear distinction between autoimmunity and autoimmune disease. The former refers to a physiological phenomenon, whereas the latter describes a pathological situation. It is important to note, however, that despite a significantly better outcome of CNS injury in EAE-resistant strains, these strains nevertheless undergo substantial secondary degeneration. The challenge, therefore, is not only to induce beneficial autoimmunity in susceptible strains, but also to boost it in resistant strains, so as to rescue as many neurons as possible from secondary degeneration, without incurring the risk of autoimmune disease (Schwartz and Kipnis, 2001).

Therapeutic T cell-based vaccination for inducing and boosting physiological immune neuroprotection

As indicated above, traumatic insult to the spinal cord evokes what appears to be a purposeful T cell-mediated response in the form of protective autoimmunity (Schwartz, 2000; Schwartz and Cohen, 2000). Some individuals may be capable of spontaneously mounting such a response, and may benefit from boosting of the response; in others, induction of protective autoimmunity may require therapeutic assistance. In all individuals, the major challenge is to find a 'safe' antigen, which will simulate an endogenous myelin-associated immune response but will not induce an autoimmune disease. This task was addressed in our recent work (Hauben et al., 2001). First, we confirmed that immunization with a self-antigen could indeed evoke a beneficial response.

We found that immunization of spinally injured rats with MBP or spinal cord homogenate emulsified in complete Freund's adjuvant resulted in better recovery than no immunization or injection of saline or adjuvant only (Fig. 1). We then selected antigens that mimic myelin antigenicity but do not cause an autoimmune disease, such as MBP peptide fragments modified to diminish their encephalitogenicity (collectively termed altered peptide ligands, APLs or a Nogo-A-derived peptide; Gaur et al., 1997; Hauben et al., 2001b). Just as vaccination with attenuated pathogenic microorganisms can lead to immunity with minimal or no symptoms of the disease, vaccination with an attenuated self-antigen (a peptide with no encephalitogenicity) was found to lead to protective autoimmunity without autoimmune disease. Achievement of the most effective post-injury immunization within the therapeutic window is critically dependent on the choice of a potent adjuvant containing the optimal concentration of microbacteria.

The ability to promote better recovery by active vaccination following the injury raises hopes for the therapeutic feasibility of this approach. The term 'therapeutic vaccination' refers to inoculation with an agent or agents designed to protect against progressive degeneration of neurons that escaped the primary injury (Fig. 1). In our experiments on rats and mice, vaccination with individual peptides selected from a battery of peptides, derived from or cross-reactive with myelin-associated peptides yielded similar results to those obtained with the myelin-associated peptides themselves. These results suggest that the T cells in these animals were performing their immunological tasks in the CNS, as they do in any other tissue following activation with their specific antigen (in the context of MHC II) at the site of injury (Hauben et al., 2001a,b).

In all experiments, the post-injury course of events in the vaccinated rats was reminiscent of recovery of spared neurons, and not regeneration of severed axons. We do however have evidence for sprouting in addition to the protection (Butovsky et al., unpublished data). Further studies should be conducted to determine whether or not such sprouting, provided it occurs, contributes to the observed functional recovery. It is important to emphasize that the vaccination was beneficial both in strains

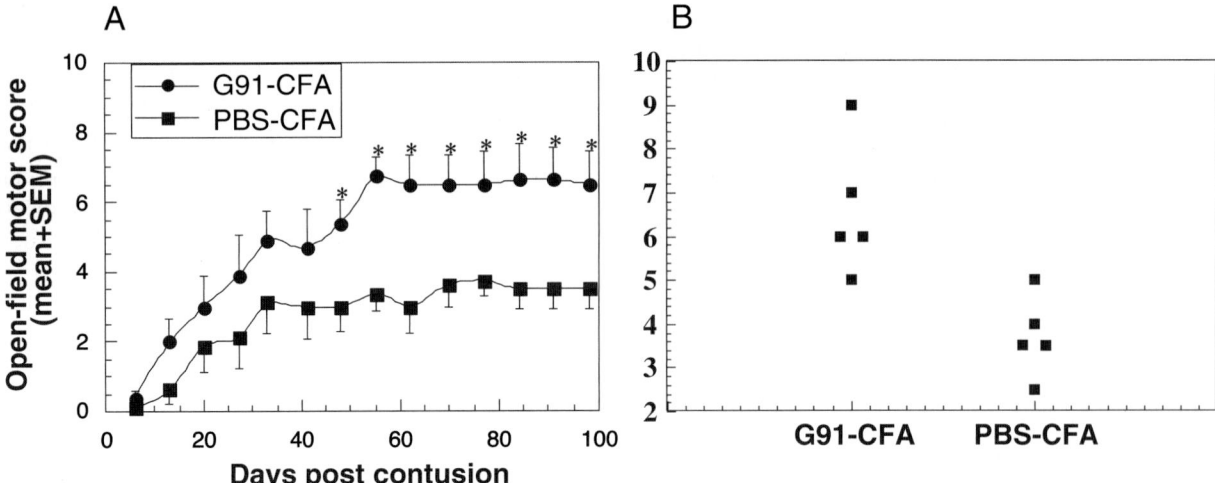

Fig. 1. Immunization with a 'safe', non-encephalitogenic, modified MBP peptide can promote recovery from spinal cord contusion. Five female Lewis rats were immunized at the base of their tail, immediately after spinal cord contusion, with G91 peptide (amino acids 87–99 of MBP, lysine residue 91 replaced with glycine;100 µg/rat) emulsified in CFA (containing 0.5 mg/ml bacteria). Five female littermates were subjected to spinal cord contusion and immediately injected with PBS in the same adjuvant. (A) Significantly better functional recovery was observed in the immunized rats than in the PBS-treated controls ($P < 0.05$, 2-way ANOVA with replications; [*]$P < 0.05$, 2-tailed Student's t-test). (B) BBB open-field motor scores of the 10 rats 77 days after the injury.

that are capable of exhibiting a spontaneous beneficial autoimmune response and in those that are not (Hauben et al., 2001).

Vaccination as a therapeutic approach for CNS degenerative diseases

In any neurodegenerative disorder, at any time, there are neurons which, though located in an environment conducive to degeneration, are still viable, making them suitable candidates for neuroprotection (Schwartz et al., 1999; Schwartz and Kipnis, 2001). Since the therapeutic activity of the T cell-based vaccination is manifested as neuroprotection (Moalem et al., 1999a; Hauben et al., 2000a,b; Kipnis et al., 2000; Schori et al., 2001b), it can presumably also be beneficial for neurodegenerative disorders. In fact, our research group has recently shown that this strategy can be successfully adapted to a neurodegenerative disease such as glaucoma (an optic neuropathy) using a model of chronically elevated intraocular pressure in rats (Schori et al., 2001b). The antigen of choice for different disorders might vary, but the mechanism underlying the protective effect would be the same. The observed effect might be a result of maintenance and repair of the damaged CNS tissue

by immune cells that were recruited to the site of degeneration by an abundance of vaccinated peptides at that site.

Some recent studies have referred to the possible use of another treatment modality using therapeutic vaccination for the treatment of neurodegenerative disorders, based on the use of antibodies acting as receptor antagonists (in the case of cytotoxicity) or as blockers of plaque formation. The concept underlying the therapeutic harnessing of antibodies is based on the ability of antibodies to act as blockers of receptors or as neutralizing agents of plaque-forming proteins. It was reported, for example, that vaccination with amyloid β-peptide could dramatically reduce amyloid deposition in a transgenic mouse model of Alzheimer's disease (Schenk et al., 1999). More recently, Morgan and colleagues showed that a similar immunization protocol can protect transgenic mice from the age-related learning and memory deficits that normally occur in this mouse Alzheimer model (Morgan et al., 2000). These and other authors therefore suggest that vaccination with amyloid β-related peptides might be developed into a therapeutic approach for the treatment, and possibly the prevention, of Alzheimer's disease. It was further suggested that the effect of the vaccination is mediated through antibodies against amyloid β-peptide, which were detected in a serological analysis of the vaccinated mice (Morgan et al., 2000; Frenkel et al., 2001). The role played by T cells in neurodegenerative disorders has recently been discussed (Schwartz and Kipnis, 2001; Schwartz and Kipnis, 2002).

Conclusions

Since neuronal degeneration is a multi-faceted process, we believe that the protection of injured nerves should be multifactorial, involving numerous factors acting in concert. Harnessing of the immune system implies recruitment of the most professional cellular players for the task. Immune cells are endowed with the capacity for self-regulation and self-limitation, and they act in accordance with the tissue needs. Our experiments on the harnessing of protective autoimmunity, and the consequent deduction of a positive view of autoimmunity, is a novel approach, which invites a comprehensive re-evaluation of the role of the immune system in general and of autoimmunity in particular.

Our findings in the context of neuroprotective immunity can be summarized as follows:

- The conviction of autoimmunity as universally harmful is incorrect.
- The substantial loss of neurons following traumatic injury to the spinal cord is a result of secondary degeneration. Protection of neurons that escaped the primary insult should therefore be viewed as an attainable major goal.
- Immune intervention may provide the means for inducing or boosting a self-regulating response to a multi-factorial disease process.
- Vaccination with a 'safe' CNS self-peptides, with the object of directing a cell-mediated autoimmune response to the damaged CNS, should be developed as a therapeutic approach for CNS injuries and degenerative diseases.

References

Bethea, J.R., Nagashima, H., Acosta, M.C., Briceno, C., Gomez, F., Marcillo, A.E., Loor, K., Green, J. and Dietrich, W.D. (1999) Systemically administered interleukin-10 reduces tumor necrosis factor-alpha production and significantly improves functional recovery following traumatic spinal cord injury in rats. *J. Neurotrauma*, 16: 851–863.

Blesch, A. and Tuszynski, M.H. (1997) Robust growth of chronically injured spinal cord axons induced by grafts of genetically modified NGF-secreting cells. *Exp. Neurol.*, 148: 444–452.

Bregman, B.S. (1998) Regeneration in the spinal cord. *Curr. Opin. Neurobiol.*, 8: 800–807.

Crowe, M.J., Bresnahan, J.C., Shuman, S.L., Masters, J.N. and Beattie, M.S. (1997) Apoptosis and delayed degeneration after spinal cord injury in rats and monkeys [published erratum appears in Nat. Med. 1997 Feb; 3(2): 240]. *Nat. Med.*, 3: 73–76.

Faden, A.I. (1993) Experimental neurobiology of central nervous system trauma. *Crit. Rev. Neurobiol.*, 7: 175–186.

Franzen, R., Schoenen, J., Leprince, P., Joosten, E., Moonen, G. and Martin, D. (1998) Effects of macrophage transplantation in the injured adult rat spinal cord: a combined immunocytochemical and biochemical study. *J. Neurosci. Res.*, 51: 316–327.

Franzen, R., Martin, D., Daloze, A., Moonen, G. and Schoenen, J. (1999) Grafts of meningeal fibroblasts in adult rat spinal cord lesion promote axonal regrowth. *NeuroReport*, 10: 1551–1556.

Frenkel, D., Kariv, N. and Solomon, B. (2001) Generation of auto-antibodies towards Alzheimer's disease vaccination. *Vaccine*, 19: 2615–2619.

Gaur, A., Boehme, S.A., Chalmers, D., Crowe, P.D., Pahuja, A., Ling, N., Brocke, S., Steinman, L. and Conlon, P.J. (1997) Amelioration of relapsing experimental autoimmune encephalomyelitis with altered myelin basic protein peptides involves different cellular mechanisms. *J. Neuroimmunol.*, 74: 149–158.

Hauben, E., Butovsky, O., Nevo, U., Yoles, E., Moalem, G., Agranov, E., Mor, F., Leibowitz-Amit, R., Pevsner, E., Akselrod, S., Neeman, M., Cohen, I.R. and Schwartz, M. (2000a) Passive or active immunization with myelin basic protein promotes recovery from spinal cord contusion. *J. Neurosci.*, 20: 6421–6430.

Hauben, E., Nevo, U., Yoles, E., Moalem, G., Agranov, E., Mor, F., Akselrod, S., Neeman, M., Cohen, I.R. and Schwartz, M. (2000b) Autoimmune T cells as potential neuroprotective therapy for spinal cord injury. *Lancet*, 355: 286–287.

Hauben, E., Agranov, E., Gothilf, A., Nevo, U., Cohen, A., Smirnov, I., Steinman, L. and Schwartz, M. (2001) Vaccination after spinal cord injury prevents complete paralysis: Autoimmunity without risk of autoimmune disease. *J. Clin. Invest.*, 108: 591–599.

Hauben, E., Ibarra, I., Mizrahi, T., Barouch, R., Agranov, E. and Schwartz, M. (2001b) Vaccination with a Nogo-A-derived peptide after incomplete spinal cord injury promotes recovery via a T-cell-mediated neuroprotective response: Comparison with other myelin antigens. *Proc. Natl. Acad. Sci. USA*, 98: 15173–15178.

Hirschberg, D.L., Yoles, E., Belkin, M. and Schwartz, M. (1994) Inflammation after axonal injury has conflicting consequences for recovery of function: rescue of spared axons is impaired but regeneration is supported. *J. Neuroimmunol.*, 50: 9–16.

Houle, J.D. and Ye, J.H. (1999) Survival of chronically injured neurons can be prolonged by treatment with neurotrophic factors. *Neuroscience*, 94: 929–936.

Houweling, D.A., Bar, P.R., Gispen, W.H. and Joosten, E.A. (1998) Spinal cord injury: bridging the lesion and the role of neurotrophic factors in repair. *Prog. Brain Res.*, 117: 455–471.

Kalb, L.Y.a.R.G. (1995) Recovery from spinal cord injury: New approaches. *Neuroscientist*, 1: 321–327.

Kipnis, J., Yoles, E., Porat, Z., Cohen, A., Mor, F., Sela, M., Cohen, I.R. and Schwartz, M. (2000) T cell immunity to copolymer 1 confers neuroprotection on the damaged optic nerve: possible therapy for optic neuropathies. *Proc. Natl. Acad. Sci. USA*, 97: 7446–7451.

Kipnis, J., Yoles, E., Schori, H., Hauben, E., Shaked, I. and Schwartz, M. (2001) Neuronal survival after CNS insult is determined by a genetically encoded autoimmune response. *J. Neurosci.*, 21: 4564–4571.

Moalem, G., Leibowitz-Amit, R., Yoles, E., Mor, F., Cohen, I.R. and Schwartz, M. (1999a) Autoimmune T cells protect neurons from secondary degeneration after central nervous system axotomy. *Nat. Med.*, 5: 49–55.

Moalem, G., Monsonego, A., Shani, Y., Cohen, I.R. and Schwartz, M. (1999b) Differential T cell response in central and peripheral nerve injury: connection with immune privilege. *FASEB J.*, 13: 1207–1217.

Moalem, G., Leibowitz-Amit, R., Yoles, E., Muller-Gilor, S., Mor, F., Cohen, I.R. and Schwartz, M. (2000a) Autoimmune T cells retard the loss of function in injured rat optic nerves. *J. Neuroimmunol.*, 106: 189–197.

Moalem, G., Gdalyahu, A., Shani, Y., Otten, U., Lazarovici, P., Cohen, I.R. and Schwartz, M. (2000b) Production of neurotrophins by activated T cells: implications for neuroprotective autoimmunity. *J. Autoimmun.*, 15: 331–345.

Morgan, D., Diamond, D.M., Gottschall, P.E., Ugen, K.E., Dickey, C., Hardy, J., Duff, K., Jantzen, P., DiCarlo, G., Wilcock, D., Connor, K., Hatcher, J., Hope, C., Gordon, M. and Arendash, G.W. (2000) A beta peptide vaccination prevents memory loss in an animal model of Alzheimer's disease. *Nature*, 408: 982–985.

Panter, S.S., Yum, S.W. and Faden, A.I. (1990) Alteration in extracellular amino acids after traumatic spinal cord injury. *Ann. Neurol.*, 27: 96–99.

Popovich, P.G., Stokes, B.T. and Whitacre, C.C. (1996) Concept of autoimmunity following spinal cord injury: possible roles for T lymphocytes in the traumatized central nervous system. *J. Neurosci. Res.*, 45: 349–363.

Popovich, P.G., Guan, Z., Wei, P., Huitinga, I., van Rooijen, N. and Stokes, B.T. (1999) Depletion of hematogenous macrophages promotes partial hindlimb recovery and neuroanatomical repair after experimental spinal cord injury. *Exp. Neurol.*, 158: 351–365.

Povlishock, J.T. and Jenkins, L.W. (1995) Are the pathobiological changes evoked by traumatic brain injury immediate and irreversible? *Brain Pathol.*, 5: 415–426.

Prewitt, C.M., Niesman, I.R., Kane, C.J. and Houle, J.D. (1997) Activated macrophage/microglial cells can promote the regeneration of sensory axons into the injured spinal cord. *Exp. Neurol.*, 148: 433–443.

Rabchevsky, A.G., Fugaccia, I., Fletcher-Turner, A., Blades, D.A., Mattson, M.P. and Scheff, S.W. (1999) Basic fibroblast growth factor (bFGF) enhances tissue sparing and functional recovery following moderate spinal cord injury. *J. Neurotrauma*, 16: 817–830.

Rapalino, O., Lazarov-Spiegler, O., Agranov, E., Velan, G.J., Yoles, E., Fraidakis, M., Solomon, A., Gepstein, R., Katz, A., Belkin, M., Hadani, M. and Schwartz, M. (1998) Implantation of stimulated homologous macrophages results in partial recovery of paraplegic rats. *Nat. Med.*, 4: 814–821.

Schenk, D., Barbour, R., Dunn, W., Gordon, G., Grajeda, H., Guido, T., Hu, K., Huang, J., Johnson-Wood, K., Khan, K., Kholodenko, D., Lee, M., Liao, Z., Lieberburg, I., Motter, R., Mutter, L., Soriano, F., Shopp, G., Vasquez, N., Vandevert, C., Walker, S., Wogulis, M., Yednock, T., Games, D. and Seubert, P. (1999) Immunization with amyloid-beta attenuates Alzheimer-disease-like pathology in the PDAPP mouse. *Nature*, 400: 173–177.

Schori, H., Yoles, E. and Schwartz, M. (2001a) Autoimmunity counteracts the potential toxicity of physiological compounds in the central nervous system. *J. Neuroimmunol.*, in press.

Schori, H., Kipnis, J., Yoles, E., WoldeMussie, E., Ruiz, G., Wheeler, L.A. and Schwartz, M. (2001b) Vaccination for protection of retinal ganglion cells against death from glutamate cytotoxicity and ocular hypertension: implications for glaucoma. *Proc. Natl. Acad. Sci. USA*, 98: 3398–3403.

Schwab, M.E. and Bartholdi, D. (1996) Degeneration and regeneration of axons in the lesioned spinal cord. *Physiol. Rev.*, 76: 319–370.

Schwartz, M. (2000) Beneficial autoimmune T cells and post-traumatic neuroprotection. *Ann. New York Acad. Sci.*, 917: 341–347.

Schwartz, M. and Cohen, I.R. (2000) Autoimmunity can benefit self-maintenance. *Immunol. Today*, 21: 265–268.

Schwartz, M. and Kipnis, J. (2001) Protective autoimmunity: regulation and prospects for vaccination after brain and spinal cord injuries. *Trends Mol. Med.*, 7: 252–258.

Schwartz, M. and Kipnis, J. (2002) Prospects for therapeutic vaccination with glatiramer acetate for neurodegenerative diseases such as Alzheimerźs disease. *Drug Dev. Res.*, in press.

Schwartz, M., Moalem, G., Leibowitz-Amit, R. and Cohen, I.R. (1999) Innate and adaptive immune responses can be beneficial for CNS repair. *Trends Neurosci.*, 22: 295–299.

Yoles, E. and Schwartz, M. (1998a) Potential neuroprotective therapy for glaucomatous optic neuropathy. *Surv. Ophthalmol.*, 42: 367–372.

Yoles, E. and Schwartz, M. (1998b) Evidence for secondary degeneration of spared neurons following partial white matter lesion: implications for optic nerve neuropathies. *Exp. Neurol.*, 153: 1–7.

Yoles, E., Hauben, E., Palgi, O., Agranov, E., Gothilf, A., Cohen, A., Kuchroo, V., Cohen, I.R., Weiner, H. and Schwartz, M. (2001) Protective autoimmunity is a physiological response to CNS trauma. *J. Neurosci.*, 21: 3740–3748.

L. McKerracher, G. Doucet and S. Rossignol (Eds.)
Progress in Brain Research, Vol. 137

CHAPTER 30

Recruiting the immune response to promote long distance axon regeneration after spinal cord injury

Samuel David [*]

Centre for Research in Neuroscience, McGill University Health Centre, Montreal General Hospital Research Institute,
1650 Cedar Avenue, Montreal, QC H3G 1A4, Canada

Introduction

Multiple factors are responsible for the loss of function after injury to the adult mammalian spinal cord. In the early phase, the paramount need is to protect neural tissue at and near the injury site from the direct effects of trauma. This involves preventing the progressive tissue necrosis that results in damage to neurons and glia at the site of contusion injury. Overlapping with this phase and extending beyond it is the period in which axon regeneration should be stimulated. Successful regeneration and functional recovery after trauma to the central nervous system (CNS) also require maintenance of the viability of the injured neurons throughout this period.

One of the major reasons for the loss of motor and sensory function after spinal cord injury is the failure of damaged axons of the long fiber tracts in the spinal cord to regenerate for long distances beyond the injury site. Although damaged neurons are unable to regenerate their axons through CNS tissue, earlier work has shown that neurons in the mature CNS are indeed capable of long distance axon regeneration if they are provided with a suitable

non-CNS environment such as a peripheral nerve graft (David and Aguayo, 1981; Vidal-Sanz et al., 1987).

Since mature CNS neurons can regenerate their axons for long distances through peripheral nerve grafts, the early efforts to find the cause of the failure of axon regeneration in the CNS were focused on the cellular and molecular environment of the CNS through which axons have to regenerate. This resulted in the discovery over the past few years of several axon growth inhibitors associated with CNS glia. These inhibitors include molecules expressed by oligodendrocytes and present in the myelin they elaborate, and others expressed by astrocytes and found in the astrocytic scar they produce. One of the factors that has long been suggested as preventing axon regeneration is the astroglial scar (Ramon y Cajal, 1928; Berry et al., 1983). Numerous studies have characterized the cellular and molecular changes that lead to the formation of the glial scar (Berry et al., 1983; Pindzola et al., 1993; Ajemian et al., 1994; McKeon et al., 1995). In addition, to the astrocytic component of the scar, a fibroblast component also exists, especially in cases of penetrating wounds or wounds which cause a breach in the glia limitans (Ajemian et al., 1994; Logan et al., 1994; Li and David, 1996). The astroglial/fibrotic scar that develops at the site of such injuries results in the reformation of the glia limitans, which can then form an additional barrier to axon growth. More recently, the molecules in the astroglial scar that

_____
[*] Correspondence to: S. David, Centre for Research in Neuroscience, Montreal General Hospital Research Institute, 1650 Cedar Ave., Montreal, QC H3G 1A4, Canada. Tel.: +1-514-937-6011 (4240); Fax: +1-514-934-8265; E-mail: sdavid11@po-box.mcgill.ca

inhibit axon growth have been identified as chondroitin sulfate proteoglycans (Pindzola et al., 1993; Ajemian et al., 1994; McKeon et al., 1995; Davies et al., 1997, 1999; Ness and David, 1997). The inhibitory effects of the scar may be overcome by either preventing its formation (Li and David, 1996), neutralizing the inhibitory molecules expressed in the scar (Moon et al., 2001) or stimulating axons to regenerate across the lesion before the scar fully forms. Astroglial scars and their role in the failure of regeneration are discussed in greater detail in this volume (Grimpe and Silver, 2002; Morgenstern et al., 2002).

The other major contributors to axon growth inhibition are the inhibitors associated with myelin. The main focus of this article will be the ways in which the immune system can be recruited to neutralize these myelin-associated inhibitors to promote long distance axon regeneration after spinal cord injury.

Axon growth inhibitory effects of myelin

Axon growth inhibitors in myelin

Over the past 12 years, several inhibitors in myelin have been identified. These include Nogo, a member of the reticulon family of proteins (Bandtlow and Schwab, 2000), myelin-associated glycoprotein (MAG) a member of the immunoglobulin superfamily (Filbin, 1995; David and McKerracher, 2001), and various proteoglycans (Niederost et al., 1999). Other inhibitory activities have also been detected in fractions obtained from ion exchange chromatography of purified myelin (McKerracher et al., 1994; Li et al., 1996) for which candidate molecules have yet to be identified.

In vivo evidence that myelin is inhibitory

Although peripheral nerves regenerate robustly after injury, peripheral nerve myelin is as inhibitory for neurite growth in vitro as CNS myelin (Bahr and Przyrembel, 1995; David et al., 1995). One reason why peripheral nerves regenerate well might be the rapidity with which myelin is cleared from damaged peripheral nerves distal to the injury, i.e., from areas undergoing Wallerian degeneration. Macrophages enter peripheral nerves 3 days after injury and clear the myelin debris by 10 days. The removal of myelin along with the axon growth inhibitors associated with it is likely to transform the nerve into a permissive terrain for axon regeneration. Strong support for this possibility comes from experiments done on the C57BL/Wld^S mouse. In this mutant mouse, there is a marked delay in the recruitment of macrophages into damaged peripheral nerves resulting in a severe delay in Wallerian degeneration and clearance of myelin and axonal debris (Brown et al., 1992). This delay in myelin clearance is accompanied by a corresponding delay in axon regeneration in these peripheral nerves (Bisby and Chen, 1990; Brown et al., 1992). Evidence that the inhibitors in myelin are involved in the failure of injured peripheral nerves of C57BL/Wld^S mice to regenerate was obtained from experiments in which this mutant was cross-bred with the MAG null mutant (Schafer et al., 1996). In this double mutant mouse, axon regeneration occurred despite the failure of myelin to be removed after peripheral nerve injury. Removal of MAG, an axon growth inhibitor, from the myelin was sufficient to convert the peripheral nerve myelin to a less inhibitory state. In contrast to this, very little, if any, axon regeneration occurs in the CNS of MAG null mice (Bartsch et al., 1995; Li et al., 1996) pointing to the need to block several of the inhibitors in CNS myelin in order to achieve axon regeneration.

Neutralizing the inhibitory effects of myelin

We are studying two different approaches to neutralize the inhibitory effects of myelin. (1) One approach is based on the finding that Wallerian degeneration, which removes myelin from regions distal to the injury, occurs very slowly in the CNS (4–12 weeks in rodents) as compared to peripheral nerves (7–10 days). Therefore, understanding the cellular and molecular mechanisms underlying Wallerian degeneration may aid in developing strategies to enhance this process in the CNS. (2) The second approach is to specifically target the axon growth inhibitors in myelin and block their function using antibodies. In an effort to do this, we have tried to recruit the animal's own immune system to produce antibodies against these inhibitors and thus enable the body to heal itself.

Stimulating rapid myelin clearance in the injured CNS

Wallerian degeneration in the CNS takes 1–3 months in rodents and years in humans (Perry et al., 1987; Miklossy and Van der Loos, 1991; George and Griffin, 1994), but occurs in 7–10 days in peripheral nerves. The work on the C57BL/Wld^S mutant shows that the rapid clearance of myelin by Wallerian degeneration converts the non-permissive peripheral nerve environment into a permissive one for axon regeneration. We provided one of the earliest in vitro evidence that macrophages can also convert the non-permissive nature of the CNS white matter to a permissive state for neurite growth (David et al., 1990). Subsequently, other groups showed that transplanting activated macrophages into the injured spinal cord can improve axon regeneration (Lazarov-Spiegler et al., 1996; Prewitt et al., 1997; Rabchevsky and Streit, 1997).

We have focused our recent efforts to understanding the immune cell responses and the molecular triggers that control macrophage activation in the CNS that lead to rapid myelin phagocytosis. It has been suggested that the poor immune cell response in the CNS after CNS injury might be due to the presence in the CNS of inhibitors of immune activation. Our recent studies indicate, however, that if such inhibitors are present, they can be readily overridden as evidenced by the rapid myelin phagocytosis induced by lysophosphatidylcholine (LPC) (Ousman and David, 2000). We have shown that microinjection of LPC into the mouse spinal cord induces immune cell responses that lead to remarkable myelin clearance and demyelination within 4 days (Ousman and David, 2000). Surprisingly, Mac-1$^+$ monocytes enter the spinal cord parenchyma near the injection site in both the LPC- and PBS-injected controls. However, the activated forms of Mac-1$^+$ cells including phagocytic macrophages were only seen in the CNS parenchyma of LPC-injected mice. These cells were seen as early as 24 h post-LPC injection but not in PBS-injected controls. Interestingly, LPC induced a rapid influx of T cells and neutrophils into the CNS within hours and their numbers peaked 6 h post-LPC injection. These rapid immune cell responses were accompanied by opening of the blood–brain barrier and increases in expression of VCAM-1 and ICAM-1, two cell adhesion molecules involved in immune cell extravasation (Ousman and David, 2000).

It is likely that influx of T cells and/or neutrophils may be required for activation of monocytes, which may then in turn activate resident microglia. This of course is a double-edged sword because abnormal activation of T cells can lead to inflammatory disease and tissue damage such as that seen in EAE. One critical difference in the T cell responses seen after LPC injection and in EAE is the rapid and transient influx of these cells in response to LPC. These studies show that it is indeed possible to stimulate a rapid immune cell response in the adult CNS that leads to the clearance of CNS myelin within 4 days, which is even faster than the time course of Wallerian degeneration in the injured peripheral nerve. Identification of the molecular mechanisms that underlie these responses could help in the development of treatment strategies to stimulate rapid Wallerian degeneration in the CNS to promote axon regeneration.

In an effort to identify the molecular switches that trigger macrophage activation and myelin clearance after LPC injection into the spinal cord, we assessed the expression of ten chemokines and cytokines by RT-PCR (Ousman and David, 2001). Four of these (MCP-1, MIP-1α GM-CSF and TNFα) were expressed at higher levels after LPC injection than in controls within 30 min to 6 h. A series of function-blocking antibody experiments showed that these chemokines (MCP-1, MIP-1α and GM-CSF) and the cytokine TNFα mediate the rapid macrophage activation and myelin clearance induced in the CNS by LPC (Ousman and David, 2000, 2001). An interesting fact to note is that MCP-1, MIP-1α and TNF-α have also been implicated in the destructive immune responses induced in EAE (Karpus et al., 1995; Kennedy et al., 1998). Yet tissue damage is minimal after LPC injection, in which macrophages strip the myelin leaving the axons undamaged (Triarhou and Herndon, 1985; Jeffery and Blakemore, 1995). The essential difference in these two models may lie in the time course of the expression of these molecules. Unlike the prolonged expression seen in EAE, LPC induces a rapid and very transient expression. The latter is also accompanied by the expression of anti-inflammatory cytokines such as IL-10 and TGF-β (Ousman and David, 2001) that may help to control the inflammatory response. The challenge now is to determine the role of these molecules in Wallerian degeneration and how they can be used to enhance myelin clearance after CNS injury to promote axon regeneration in vivo.

Antibody-mediated blocking of myelin-associated axon growth inhibitors

The second approach that we are working on to neutralize the activity of myelin-associated axon growth inhibitors is a vaccine technique. Studies with the IN-1 monoclonal antibody provided the first evidence that an antibody-mediated approach could be used to block the axon growth inhibitors associated with myelin (Schnell and Schwab, 1990). Implantation into the CNS of the hybridoma cells that produce this antibody resulted in long distance regeneration of a small number of axons after spinal cord injury. Given the evidence that there are several inhibitors in myelin, it is likely that more than one of these inhibitors may have to be blocked to achieve regeneration of substantial numbers of axons. In an attempt to accomplish this we tested a vaccine approach in which the animal's own immune system was harnessed to generate antibodies against the inhibitors in myelin using purified myelin or myelin-rich tissue as the immunogen (Huang et al., 1999).

Two important issues that determine the success of using purified myelin as a vaccine are: (1) how can one prevent the induction of an autoimmune response against myelin antigens that could lead to inflammatory disease such as EAE?; and (2) will circulating anti-myelin antibodies cross the blood–brain barrier to enter the CNS parenchyma to block the inhibitors in myelin? Both these issues were addressed in the experiments we have done. Experimental allergic encephalomyelitis is a T cell-mediated disease which can be induced in naïve animals by passive transfer of T cells obtained from an animal with EAE (Zamvil et al., 1985). EAE can also induced by immunizing animals with certain encephalitogenic proteins in myelin (such as myelin basic protein, proteolipid protein or myelin-oligodendrocyte glycoprotein) mixed with complete Freund's adjuvant (Truagott et al., 1985; Goverman et al., 1997). Interestingly, EAE can be prevented

by immunizing the mice first with myelin or myelin antigens mixed with incomplete Freund's adjuvant (IFA) (O'Niell et al., 1992; Tonegawa, 1997). Immunizing with IFA prevents EAE by pushing the T cell response from a Th1 toward a Th2 response (Rivero et al., 1997; Tonegawa, 1997). Th2 T cells produce anti-inflammatory cytokines that prevent EAE and are usually seen during the remission phase of the disease, while T cells that induce an acute episode of EAE are Th1 T cells that produce pro-inflammatory cytokines.

We therefore immunized mice with myelin or myelin-rich tissue mixed with IFA. These mice produced antibodies against myelin as determined by enzyme-linked immunosorbant assay (ELISA) (Huang et al., 1999). Earlier studies also showed that anti-myelin antibodies are generated by immunizing with spinal cord homogenate or purified myelin with IFA as the adjuvant (Rodriguez et al., 1987; Rivero et al., 1997). Studies by Rodriguez et al. (1987) also showed that a monoclonal antibody generated by such an immunization procedure was effective in inducing remyelination in vivo (Rodriguez et al., 1987). In our experiments we assessed if immunization with myelin and IFA could result in the generation of function-blocking antibodies against the axon growth inhibitors in myelin and promote long distance axon regeneration after spinal cord injury.

The other important factor that could influence the success of the vaccine approach is the requirement that antibodies in the circulation be able to cross the blood–brain barrier and enter the CNS parenchyma. We were able to detect using immunohistochemistry for mouse immunoglobulins that the blood–brain barrier was leaky around the site of lesion for distances of several millimeters. The blood–brain barrier has been reported to open for distances of greater the 20 mm after contusion injury to the rat spinal cord (Popovich et al., 1996). Furthermore, the blood–brain barrier of degenerating white matter pathways become leaky for immunoglobulin as the macrophages in the pathway become activated (Jensen et al., 1997). Therefore, the nature of the injury and the degeneration that occurs in the damaged CNS pathways could help to direct antibodies in the circulation to the damaged and degenerating areas of the CNS, i.e., to places where the antibodies are needed and not indiscriminately to all regions of the CNS.

We have shown that mice immunized with either myelin-rich CNS tissue homogenate or purified myelin showed a substantial amount of axonal regeneration after spinal cord hemisection. Anterograde neuronal labeling with wheatgerm-conjugated horseradish peroxidase (WGA–HRP) revealed that the lesioned corticospinal tract axons regenerated for distances of 5–11 mm past the spinal cord lesion. Retrograde double labeling experiments were done in which fluorogold was applied to the lesion site to label the cut axons, and fluororuby injected into the spinal cord 5 mm caudal to the spinal hemisection to label axons of the corticospinal tract. Axons that were cut and regenerated would be double-labeled by both fluorescent markers, while spared axons that extended 5 mm caudal to the lesion would only be labeled by fluororuby. Control experiments indicated that in our model, flurogold only labeled damaged axons and retrogradely labeled neurons from the terminal field (i.e., from the site of termination of the corticospinal tract fibers in the spinal cord gray matter). We also found that, in unlesioned mice, only about 5% of the fibers that normally terminate at the spinal level at which the hemisections were made, also projected collaterals to a distance of 5 mm caudally. If this number is excluded from the number of double-labeled neurons seen in mice immunized with myelin, the percentage of neurons that regenerated ranged from about 20 to 70%. These results confirmed that a large proportion of damaged axons in the corticospinal tracts regenerated after immunization with myelin. We have also found that ascending dorsal column fibers also regenerate robustly after immunization with purified myelin in IFA (Ousman et al., 2000).

In vitro work showed that the serum from mice immunized with myelin was able to neutralize the neurite growth inhibitory effects of myelin. Additional studies in which the immunoglobulins were immunodepleted from these sera demonstrated that the serum effects were mediated by antibodies (Huang et al., 1999).

In more recent work, it has become clear that in addition to the antibody-mediated effects, immunization with myelin also results in an increased influx of T cells and activated macrophages at the site of spinal cord hemisection (Kuo et al., 2001). The latter responses may lead to an increased clearance of myelin after injury. Therefore, both antibody-mediated blocking of the axon growth inhibitors and clearance of myelin by activated macrophages may contribute to the remarkable degree of regeneration seen after myelin-vaccine treatments.

Recent work has also shown that T cells directed against certain myelin antigens can provide a neuroprotective effect after CNS injury (Moalem et al., 1999; Hauben et al., 2000). In our vaccine experiments, we have shown that myelin-reactive antibodies are generated, they cross the blood–brain barrier, bind to myelin and are able to neutralize the inhibitory effects of myelin. Moreover, axon regeneration was shown to occur. Since the purified myelin used in our experiments would contain the antigens needed to obtain T cells that are neuroprotective, our vaccine approach would be expected to have effects on neuroprotection. In fact in recent work Hauben et al. (2001) showed that immunizing rats with spinal cord homogenate in IFA results in increased sparing of spinal cord tissue at the site of spinal cord contusion injury. It is therefore possible that the myelin-vaccine approach may influence recovery after spinal cord injury by recruiting B cell, macrophage and T cell responses (Fig. 1).

Concluding comments

The inhibitors that damaged axons first encounter are likely to be those associated with myelin which will be exposed immediately at the site of injury. Subsequently, after a variable degree of delay after the injury, the inhibitors associated with the scar are expressed and will begin to exert their influence. One likely reason for the remarkable effectiveness of the myelin vaccine treatment after spinal cord hemisection may be the antibody-mediated blocking of many of the myelin-associated inhibitors immediately after the injury. Thus permitting the axons to regenerate across the lesion before the scar-associated inhibitors are fully expressed and become effective. Our recent work indicates that axons grow very rapidly across the lesion immediately after the hemisection in immunized mice (Sicotte and David, 2001). Furthermore axon regeneration failed in animals in which there were large scars at the site of

412

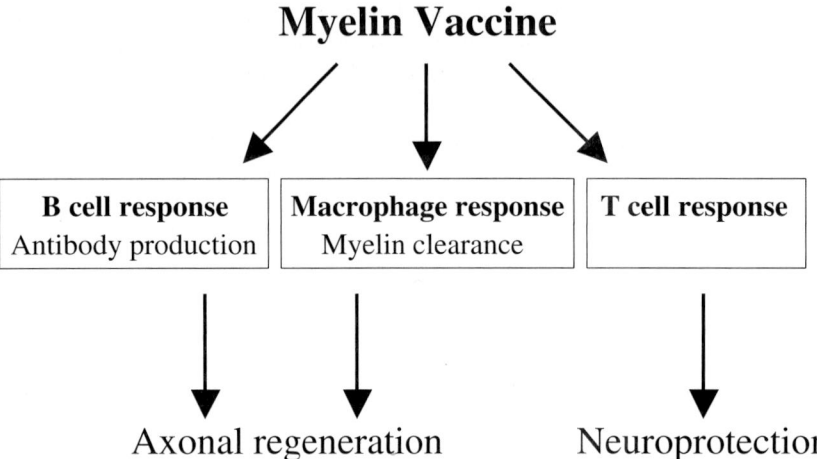

Myelin Vaccine

B cell response	Macrophage response	T cell response
Antibody production	Myelin clearance	

Axonal regeneration   Neuroprotection

Fig. 1. Several possible ways in which myelin vaccine treatments could effect recovery after CNS injury.

hemisection. We chose to work on mice (Balb/c) which rarely develop cysts at the site of hemisection as compared to rats, which often develop cysts. Furthermore the hemisection lesions were done in such a way as to minimize the development of large glial scars. Large scars that often accompany cysts will present another inhibitory barrier to axon regeneration. In addition, development of a fibrotic/glial scar and the formation of a new glial limitans at the site of penetrating injuries will also prevent regeneration even if myelin inhibitors are blocked. Such fibrotic/glial scars form especially well after complete transection of the spinal cord, and in such a model blocking myelin inhibitors alone will not be expected to result in axon regeneration. One will have to combine the myelin vaccine-mediated blocking strategy with cellular or non-cellular transplants to bridge the severed ends of the spinal cord, and possibly also neutralize scar-associated inhibitors to achieve regeneration across complete spinal cord transection.

In the myelin vaccine treatments, mice were immunized for 3 weeks prior to making the lesion. This was done to maximize the conditions for success, i.e., to allow sufficient time for a good antibody response. Our more recent work indicates that regeneration also occurs if anti-myelin serum generated using similar immunization are administered to mice within 30 min after a spinal cord hemisection (Huang et al., 2000). Therefore, a combination of passive immunization with anti-myelin antibodies along with

active immunization with myelin antigens could be effectively developed to treat spinal cord injuries.

Acknowledgements

The work on the chemokines and cytokines involved in myelin clearance was done by Shalina Ousman, and the regeneration work done by Da Wei Huang, S. Ousman, Maryline Sicotte and David Kuo. I would also like to acknowledge collaborations with Drs. L. McKerracher and P.E. Braun. Supported by grants from the Canadian Institutes of Health Research.

References

Ajemian, A., Ness, R. and David, S. (1994) Tenascin in the injured rat optic nerve and in non-neuronal cells in vitro: potential role in neural repair. *J. Comp. Neurol.*, 340: 233–242.

Bahr, M. and Przyrembel, C. (1995) Myelin from peripheral and central nervous system is a non-permissive substrate for retinal ganglion cell axons. *Exp. Neurol.*, 134: 87–93.

Bandtlow, C.E. and Schwab, M.E. (2000) NI-35/250/Nogo-A: a neurite growth inhibitor restricting structural plasticity and regeneration of nerve fibers in the adult vertebrate CNS. *Glia*, 29: 175–181.

Berry, M., Maxwell, W.L., Logan, A., Mathewson, A., McConnell, P., Ashhurst, D.E. and Thomas, G.H. (1983) Deposition of scar tissue in the central nervous system. *Acta Neuropathol. Suppl.*, 32: 31–53.

Bartsch, U. et al. (1995) Lack of evidence that myelin-associated glycoprotein is a major inhibitor of atonal regeneration in the CNS. *Neuron*, 15: 1375–1381.

Bisby, M.A. and Chen, S. (1990) Delayed Wallerian degeneration in sciatic nerves of C57BL/Ola mice is associated with impaired regeneration of sensory axons. *Brain. Res.*, 530: 117–120.

Brown, M.C., Lunn, E.R. and Perry, V.H. (1992) Consequences of slow Wallerian degeneration for regenerating motor and sensory axons. *J. Neurobiol.*, 23: 5221–5236.

David, S. and Aguayo, A.J. (1981) Axonal elongation into peripheral nervous system 'bridges' after central nervous system injury in adult rats. *Science*, 214: 931–933.

David, S. and McKerracher, L. (2001) Inhibition of axon growth by myelin-associated glycoprotein. In: N.A. Ingoglia and M. Marion (Eds.), *Axonal Regeneration in the Central Nervous System*. Marcel Dekker, New York, pp. 425–446.

David, S., Bouchard, C., Tsatas, O. and Giftochristos, N. (1990) Macrophages can modify the non-permissive nature of the adult mammalian central nervous system. *Neuron*, 5: 463–469.

David, S., Braun, P.E., Jackson, D.L., Kottis, V. and McKerracher, L. (1995) Laminin overrides the inhibitory effects of peripheral nervous system and central nervous system myelin-derived inhibitors of neurite growth. *J. Neurosci. Res.*, 42: 594–602.

Davies, S.J.A. et al. (1997) Regeneration of adult axons in white matter tracts of the central nervous system. *Nature*, 390: 680–683.

Davies, S.J.A., Goucher, D.R., Doller, C. and Silver, J. (1999) Robust regeneration of adult sensory axons in degenerating white matter of the adult rat spinal cord. *J. Neursci.*, 19: 5810–5822.

Filbin, M.T. (1995) Myelin-associated glycoprotein: a role in myelination and in the inhibition of axonal regeneration. *Curr. Opin. Neurobiol.*, 5: 588–595.

George, R. and Griffin, J.W. (1994) Delayed macrophage responses and myelin clearance during Wallerian degeneration in the central nervous system: the dorsal radiculotomy model. *Exp. Neurol.*, 129: 225–236.

Grimpe, B. and Silver, J. (2002) The extracellular matrix in axon regeneration. In: L. McKerracher, G. Douchet and S. Rossignol (Eds.), *Spinal Cord Trauma: Neural Repair and Functional Recovery. Progress in Brain Research*, Vol. 137. Elsevier Science, Amsterdam, pp. 333–349.

Goverman, J., Brabb, T., Paez, A., Harrington, C. and van Dassow, P. (1997) Initiation and regulation of CNS autoimmunity. *Crit. Rev. Immunol.*, 17: 469–480.

Hauben, E., Butovsky, O., Nevo, U., Yoles, E., Moalem, G., Agranov, E., Mor, F., Leibowitz-Amit, R., Pevsner, E., Akselrod, S., Neeman, M., Cohen, I.R. and Schwartz, M. (2000) Passive or active immunization with myelin basic protein promotes recovery from spinal cord contusion. *J. Neurosci.*, 20: 6421–6430.

Hauben, E., Agranov, E., Gothilf, A., Nevo, U., Cohen, A., Smirnov, I., Steinman, L. and Schwartz, M. (2001) Post-traumatic therapeutic vaccination with modified myelin self-antigen prevents complete paralysis while avoiding autoimmune disease. *J. Clin. Invest.*, 108: 591–599.

Huang, D.W., McKerracher, L., Braun, P.E. and David, S. (1999) A therapeutic vaccine approach to stimulate axon regeneration in the adult mammalian spinal cord. *Neuron*, 24: 639–647.

Huang, D.W., Tsatas, O. and David, S. (2000) Passive immunization with anti-myelin antiserum promotes regeneration of corticospinal tract fibers. *Soc. Neurosci. Abstr.*, 26: 612.

Jeffery, S.D. and Blakemore, W.F. (1995) Remyelination of mouse spinal cord axons demyelinated by local injection of lysolecithin. *J. Neurocytol.*, 24: 775–781.

Jensen, M.B., Finsen, B. and Zimmer, J. (1997) Morphological and immunophenotypic microglial changes in the denervated fascia dentata of adult rats: correlation with blood–brain barrier damage and astroglial reactions. *Exp. Neurol.*, 143: 103–116.

Karpus, W.J., Lukas, N.W., McRae, B.L., Streiter, R.M., Kunkel, S.L. and Miller, S.D. (1995) An important role for the chemokine macrophage inflammatory protein-1 in the pathogenesis of the T cell-mediated autoimmune disease experimental allergic encephalomyelitis. *J. Immunol.*, 155: 5003–5010.

Kennedy, K.J., Streiter, R.M., Kunkel, S.L., Lukas, N.W. and Karpus, W.J. (1998) Acute and relapsing experimental allergic encephalomyelinitis are regulated by differential expression of the CC chemokines macrophage inflammatory protein-1α and monocyte chemotactic protein-1. *J. Neuroimmunol.*, 92: 98–108.

Kuo, D., Ousman, S., Sicotte, M., Tsatas, O. and David, S. (2001) Treatment with a myelin vaccine stimulates rapid T cell and macrophage responses. *Soc. Neurosci. Abstr.*, 27: 698.2.

Lazarov-Spiegler, O., Solomon, A.S., Zeev-Brann, A.B., Hirschberg, D.L., Lavie, V. and Schwartz, M. (1996) Transplantation of activated macrophages overcomes central nervous system regrowth failure. *FASEB J.*, 10: 1296–1302.

Li, M. and David, S. (1996) Topical glucocorticoids modulate the lesion interface after cerebral cortical stab wounds in adult rats. *Glia*, 18: 306–318.

Li, M., Shibata, A., Li, C., Braun, P.E., McKerracher, L., Roder, J., Kater, S.B. and David, S. (1996) Myelin-associated glycoprotein inhibits neurite/axon growth and causes growth cone collapse. *J. Neurosci. Res.*, 46: 404–414.

Logan, A., Berry, M., Gonzalez, A.M., Frautschy, S.A., Sporn, M.B. and Baird, A. (1994) Effects of transforming growth factor beta 1 on scar production in the injured central nervous system of the rat. *Eur. J. Neurosci.*, 6: 355–363.

McKeon, R.J., Hoke, A. and Silver, J. (1995) Injury-induced proteoglycans inhibit the potential for laminin-mediated axon growth on astrocyte scars. *Exp. Neurol.*, 136: 32–43.

McKerracher, L., David, S., Jackson, D., Kottis, V., Dunn, R. and Braun, P.E. (1994) Identification of myelin-associated glycoprotein as a major myelin-derived inhibitor of neurite growth. *Neuron*, 13: 805–811.

Miklossy, J. and Van der Loos, H. (1991) The long-distance effects of brain lesions: visualization of myelinated pathways in the human brain using polarizing and fluorescence microscopy. *J. Neuropathol. Exp. Neurol.*, 50: 1–15.

Moalem, G., Leibowitz-Amit, R., Yoles, E., Mor, F., Cohen, I.R. and Schwartz, M. (1999) Autoimmune T cells protect neurons from secondary degeneration after central nervous system axotomy. *Nat. Med.*, 5: 49–55.

Moon, L.D., Asher, R.A., Rhodes, K.E. and Fawcett, J.W. (2001)

Regeneration of CNS axons back to their target following treatment of adult rat brain with chondroitinase ABC. *Nat. Neurosci.*, 4: 465–466.

Morgenstern, D.A., Asher, R.A. and Fawcett, J.W. (2002) Chondroitin sulfate proteoglycans in the CNS injury response. In: L. McKerracher, G. Douchet and S. Rossignol (Eds.), *Spinal Cord Trauma: Neural Repair and Functional Recovery. Progress in Brain Research*, Vol. 137. Elsevier Science, Amsterdam, pp. 313–332.

Ness, R. and David, S. (1997) Leptomeningeal cells modulate the neurite growth promoting properties of astrocytes in vitro. *Glia*, 19: 47–57.

Niederost, B.P., Zimmermann, D.R., Schwab, M.E. and Bandtlow, C.E. (1999) Bovine CNS myelin contains neurite growth-inhibitory activity associated with chondroitin sulfate proteoglycans. *J. Neurosci.*, 19: 8979–8989.

O'Niell, J.K., Baker, D. and Turk, J.L. (1992) Inhibition of chronic experimental allergic encephalomyelitis in the Biozzi AB/H mouse. *J. Neuroimmunol.*, 41: 177–187.

Ousman, S. and David, S. (2000) Lysophosphatidylcholine induces rapid recruitment and activation of macrophages in the adult mouse spinal cord. *Glia*, 30: 92–104.

Ousman, S. and David, S. (2001) MIP-1α, MCP-1, GM-CSF, and TNF-α control the immune cell response that mediates rapid phagocytosis of myelin from the adult mouse spinal cord. *J. Neurosci.*, 21: 4649–4656.

Ousman, S., Huang, D.W., Tsatas, O. and David, S. (2000) Regeneration of sensory dorsal column fibers in mice treated with a myelin vaccine to block axon growth inhibitors. *Soc. Neurosci. Abstr.*, 26: 612.

Perry, V.H., Brown, M.C. and Gordon, S. (1987) The macrophage response to central and peripheral nerve injury. A possible role for macrophages in regeneration. *J. Exp. Med.*, 165: 1218–1223.

Popovich, P.G., Horner, P.J., Mullin, B.B. and Stokes, B.T. (1996) A quantitative spinal analysis of the blood–spinal cord barrier. *Exp. Neurol.*, 142: 258–275.

Pindzola, R.R., Doller, C. and Silver, J. (1993) Putative inhibitory extracellular matrix molecules at the dorsal root entry zone of the spinal cord during development and after root and sciatic nerve lesions. *Dev. Biol.*, 156: 34–48.

Prewitt, C.M., Niesman, I.R., Kane, C.J. and Houle, J.D. (1997) Activated macrophage/microglial cells can promote the regeneration of sensory axons into the injured spinal cord. *Exp. Neurol.*, 148: 433–443.

Rabchevsky, A.G. and Streit, W.J. (1997) Grafting of cultured microglial cells into the lesioned spinal cord of adult rats enhances neurite outgrowth. *J. Neurosci. Res.*, 47: 34–48.

Ramon y Cajal, S. (1928) *Degeneration and Regeneration of the Nervous System*. (Translated by M. May), Oxford University Press, London.

Rivero, V.E., Maccioni, M., Bucher, A.E., Roth, G.A. and Riera, C.M. (1997) Suppression of experimental autoimmune encephalomyelitis (EAE) by intraperitoneal administration of soluble myelin antigens in Wistar rats. *J. Neuroimmunol.*, 72: 3–10.

Rodriguez, M., Lennon, V.A., Benveniste, E.N. and Merrill, J.E. (1987) Remyelination by oligodendrocytes stimulated by antiserum to spinal cord. *J. Neuropathol. Exp. Neurol.*, 46: 84–95.

Schafer, T. et al. (1996) Disruption of the myelin-associated glycoprotein (MAG) gene improves atonal regeneration in C57BL/Wld^S mice. *Neuron*, 16: 1170–1183.

Schnell, L. and Schwab, M.E. (1990) Axonal regeneration in the rat spinal cord produced by an antibody against myelin-associated neurite growth inhibitors. *Nature*, 343: 269–272.

Selmaj, K.W. and Raine, C.S. (1988) Tumor necrosis factor mediates myelin and oligodendrocyte damage in vitro. *Ann. Neurol.*, 23: 339–346.

Sicotte, M. and David, S. (2001) Further evidence that myelin-vaccine treatment promotes long distance axon regeneration in the injured spinal cord. *Soc. Neurosci. Abstr.*, 27: 698.1.

Triarhou, L.C. and Herndon, R.M. (1985) Effects of macrophage inactivation on the neuropathology of lysolecithin-induced demyelination. *Br. J. Exp. Pathol.*, 66: 293–301.

Tonegawa, S.M.S. (1997) Tolerance induction and autoimmune encephalomyelitis amelioration after administration of myelin basic protein-derived peptide. *J. Exp. Med.*, 186: 507–517.

Truagott, U., Raine, C.S. and McFarlin, D.E. (1985) Acute experimental allergic encephalomyelitis in the mouse: immunopathology of the developing lesion. *Cell. Immunol.*, 91: 240–254.

Vidal-Sanz, M., Bray, G.M., Villegas-Perez, M.P., Thanos, S. and Aguayo, A.J. (1987) Axonal regeneration and synapse formation in the superior colliculus by retinal ganglion cells in the adult rat. *J. Neurosci.*, 7: 2894–2909.

Zamvil, A., Nelson, P., Trotter, J., Mitchell, D., Knobler, R. and Steinman, L. (1985) T cell clones specific for myelin-basic protein induce chronic replasing paralysis and demyelination. *Nature*, 317: 355–358.

L. McKerracher, G. Doucet and S. Rossignol (Eds.)
Progress in Brain Research, Vol. 137
© 2002 Elsevier Science B.V. All rights reserved

CHAPTER 31

Spontaneous and neurotrophin-induced axonal plasticity after spinal cord injury

Armin Blesch [1] and Mark H. Tuszynski [1,2,*]

[1] *Department of Neurosciences-0626, University of California, San Diego, La Jolla, CA 92093, USA*
[2] *Veterans Administration Medical Center, San Diego, CA 92165, USA*

Introduction

Injury in the adult central nervous system of mammals often leads to permanent functional deficits. The persistence of such functional deficits has been attributed to the lack of regeneration in the adult central nervous system and the inability to sufficiently reorganize the remaining circuitry. Different factors such as the intrinsic inability of neurons to regenerate, the presence of inhibitory myelin-associated factors, inhibitory extracellular matrix molecules and the absence of sufficient growth stimulating cues intrinsic and extrinsic to injured neurons may contribute to the failure of morphological and functional recovery.

Fortunately, it has become clear that the capacity of neurons and their axons to regrow in response to appropriate stimuli, a prerequisite for the reestablishment of functional connections, is extensively preserved throughout adulthood. Supporting this observation is the fact that experimental manipulations of the environment of an injured neuron or its lesioned axon can prevent cell death and induce axonal growth to a degree not normally observed in the adult CNS. The provision of neurotrophic factors to a spinal cord lesion site is one example of a manipulation that can promote axonal growth and, in some cases, generate partial functional recovery.

However, even without treatment, and despite the presence of axonal growth-inhibitory molecules at a lesion site, approximately 40% of patients who sustain a spinal cord injury exhibit limited (and occasionally striking) degrees of spontaneous improvement over extended time periods of weeks to months. It has been known for some time, and has recently become clearer, that in addition to compensatory behavioral strategies, spontaneous injury-induced structural rearrangements (plasticity) in the adult CNS can occur over protracted time courses and can correlate with functional recovery. A thorough investigation and potential enhancement of such mechanisms might lead to new therapeutic strategies after CNS injury. These topics will be discussed in the following sections.

Spontaneous plasticity after spinal cord injury

Injury in the neonatal animal is often followed by substantial recovery of function (Bregman and Goldberger, 1982, 1983; Bregman et al., 1993), although the degree to which this functional recovery is mediated by axonal regeneration, sprouting of spared axonal systems, or compensation by unlesioned sys-

* Correspondence to: M.H. Tuszynski, Department of Neurosciences-0626, 9500 Gilman Drive, University of California, San Diego, La Jolla, CA 92093-0626, USA. Tel.: +1-858-534-8857; Fax: +1-858-534-5220; E-mail: mtuszyns@ucsd.edu

tems remains incompletely understood. Morphological responses to injury are much more limited in the adult, thus injury-induced deficits tend to persist. Yet spontaneous neuronal reorganization after injury has been described in the adult CNS in the hippocampus, sensory cortex and red nucleus, and even in intrinsic spinal cord circuitry (Raisman, 1969; Cotman et al., 1973; Tsukahara et al., 1975; Steward, 1976; Lynch et al., 1977; Blight, 1983; Merzenich et al., 1984; Jones et al., 1996). For example, after unilateral cortical lesions, the intact motor cortex contralateral to the lesioned hemisphere undergoes adaptive neural plasticity (Jones and Schallert, 1994; Jones, 1999) in the form of increases in dendritic arborization and actual synaptogenesis. These changes are use-dependent in nature, and rehabilitative training using a complex motor task can enhance such neural plasticity (Jones et al., 1999). Although injury-induced axonal sprouting at sites of spinal cord lesions has been identified for some time, these changes had not been strictly correlated with functional improvement.

Recently, potential mechanisms underlying spontaneous recovery after spinal cord injury in the adult rat have been investigated in more detail using defined lesions of sub-components of the corticospinal tract (CST) (Weidner et al., 2001). In the rat, the corticospinal tract mediates an important role in fine motor control and its function can be quantified using a skilled forelimb pellet retrieval task (Whishaw et al., 1993). The majority of CST axons in the rat are located in the dorsal column (95%). Roughly 3% reside in the ventral ipsilateral CST and less than 2% are located laterally and dorsolaterally (Vahlsing and Feringa, 1980; Joosten et al., 1992; Brösamle and Schwab, 1997). By lesioning sub-components of the corticospinal tract, the contribution of each component to overall skilled motor function can be investigated.

After cervical lesions of the dorsal component of the CST that disrupt 95% of all CST fibers, there is an early significant decline in fine motor function that gradually improves over a 4-week period (Weidner et al., 2001). Because lesioned corticospinal axons do not spontaneously regenerate, we investigated whether either: (1) an unlesioned sub-component of the CST; or (2) a different axonal population altogether, compensated for the loss of 95% of corticospinal axons. Specifically placed lesions indicated

that functional recovery was in fact mediated by the ventral component of the CST: lesions of both the dorsal and ventral components of the CST simultaneously, or lesions of most of the corticospinal projection prior to its decussation in the medulla, resulted in persistent functional impairments that did not recover over time. Further, functional recovery after dorsal CST lesions could be abolished by subsequent lesions of the ventral component of the CST, clearly establishing a role of the ventral corticospinal tract in functional recovery (Weidner et al., 2001).

Anterograde tracing of corticospinal axons in these experiments confirmed that the majority of corticospinal axons in the rat project to lamina II–VII of the spinal gray matter and do not directly project to motor neurons (unlike the primate). However, some ventral corticospinal axons do project directly to ventromedial spinal motor neurons. Notably, the number of these direct projections to ventral motor neurons significantly changed after injuries of the dorsal CST. Following lesions of the dorsal CST, animals with remaining ventral corticospinal projections exhibited a significant 330% increase in the number of projections of BDA labeled ventral corticospinal axons to medial motor neurons in the ventral spinal cord, compared to unlesioned control animals. This increase was not observed if lesions also included the ventral CST (Weidner et al., 2001).

Thus, substantial *spontaneous* structural plasticity occurred in the spinal cord after CST lesions. The loss of the dorsal CST resulted in an increased number of ventral CST–motor neuron contacts, and this spontaneous structural rearrangement was accompanied by recovery of skilled forelimb movement. Although it is unclear what exact mechanisms account for the spontaneous formation of these new CST axon–motor neuron contacts, these findings indicate that some intrinsic mechanisms exist in the adult spinal cord that can react to injury and compensate for the loss of axonal input.

Treatments aimed at enhancing this inherent spinal cord plasticity may be a means of promoting further recovery. Some neurotrophic factors are naturally upregulated after injury (Nakamura and Bregman, 2001; Widenfalk et al., 2001), and the exogenous application of neurotrophic factors at sites of spinal cord injury can promote growth of axons, sprouting and functional recovery. Thus, injury-induced changes in the expression and localization of neurotrophic factors could be a mechanism underlying spontaneous morphological and functional effects, and the therapeutic delivery of enhanced amounts of growth factors might amplify recovery by promoting sprouting independently of axonal regeneration.

Neurotrophin-induced axonal plasticity

In the last two decades, neurotrophic factors have received substantial interest due to their ability to promote neuronal survival in models of CNS trauma and neurodegenerative disease. More importantly, the ability of trophic molecules to enhance axonal growth have made them potential candidates for promoting morphological and functional recovery after spinal cord injury. Studies of the developing CNS, wherein axonal growth and the formation of mature neuronal connections are influenced by the expression of target-derived neurotrophic factors, further support a rationale for the use of these substances to promote adult CNS regeneration. The increasing knowledge about the receptor expression of neurotrophic factors and their distribution has contributed to the characterization of growth responses of injured axons to neurotrophin delivery. Notably, these studies have also made it clear that at least some growth factor receptors (e.g., trkB) are very widely expressed within the CNS and thus localized delivery might be necessary to prevent unwanted side effects. Both ex vivo gene therapy using grafts of genetically modified cells, and in vivo gene therapy using replication-incompetent recombinant viral vectors, have the capacity to deliver neurotrophic factors in a very specific and well-restricted manner into the CNS.

After spinal cord injury, axonal disruption is often accompanied by the formation of cysts at the lesion site. Thus, axonal growth stimulating factors such as neurotrophins and a suitable substrate molecule for axonal elongation might be necessary to 'bridge' the rostral and caudal 'stumps' of an injured cord. Grafts of genetically modified cells can provide both a cellular substrate for axonal attachment and growth, and can serve as biological mini-pumps for the localized delivery of growth factors.

Cell types used for ex vivo genetic modification and transplantation into the injured spinal cord include fibroblasts, Schwann cells and neural stem cells. Fibroblasts have some properties that make them attractive candidates to investigate neurotrophic factor responses in the injured spinal cord, even though they are a non-neural cell type: fibroblasts can be easily obtained from a skin biopsy, cultivated, and genetically modified in vitro; they survive post-grafting in the lesioned CNS; and they produce extracellular matrix molecules like collagen, fibronectin and laminin, that might be favorable for axonal growth.

Several studies have investigated axonal growth responses to neurotrophin delivery by genetically modified cells producing nerve growth factor (NGF) (Tuszynski et al., 1994, 1996; Grill et al., 1997b; Weidner et al., 1999), brain-derived growth factor (BDNF) (McTigue et al., 1998; Menei et al., 1998; Liu et al., 1999; Lu et al., 2001), neurotrophin-3 (NT-3) (Grill et al., 1997a; McTigue et al., 1998), NT-4/5 (Blesch et al., 1999a), glial cell line-derived neurotrophic factor (GDNF) (Blesch and Tuszynski, 2001) and leukemia inhibitory factor (LIF) (Blesch et al., 1999b) in the injured spinal cord (Table I, Fig. 1). These studies as well as numerous other studies have highlighted some important aspects of cell transplantation and neurotrophic factor delivery in the injured spinal cord.

Axonal growth substrate

As mentioned above, the provision of suitable growth substrates at a lesion site might be important to bridge the rostral and caudal injured segments. However, the preferences of different axonal populations for substrate molecules can differ. Thus, the substrate provided at a lesion site can influence the responses of certain axonal populations.

For example, after delivery of NT-3 by genetically modified fibroblasts in the spinal cord, corticospinal axons show enhanced growth up to 8 mm distal to the lesion site compared to animals with control grafts after dorsal hemisection lesions at midthoracic level in adult rats (Grill et al., 1997a). Yet this growth is restricted to the host gray matter rather than the graft itself. Thus, corticospinal axons seem to prefer the host gray matter as an axonal growth substrate. Alternatively, extracellular matrix molecules expressed at the host graft interface might

TABLE I

Neurotrophic factors and their effects on axonal growth in the injured spinal cord

Neurotrophic factor	Axonal populations	References
NGF	Sensory, coerulospinal	Tuszynski et al., 1994, 1996, 1997, 1998; Grill et al., 1997b
BDNF	Sensory, motor, coerulospinal, rubrospinal, other brainstem-derived axons, propriospinal	Xu et al., 1995; Ye and Houle, 1997; Jakeman et al., 1998; McTigue et al., 1998; Menei et al., 1998; Liu et al., 1999; Bamber et al., 2001; Lu et al., 2001
NT-3	Corticospinal, propriospinal, sensory	Schnell et al., 1994; Grill et al., 1997a; Bradbury et al., 1998; McTigue et al., 1998; Oudega and Hagg, 1999; Blits et al., 2000; Bamber et al., 2001
NT-4/5	Sensory, motor, coerulospinal	Blesch et al., 1999a
GDNF	Sensory, motor	Blesch et al., 1998; Blesch and Tuszynski, 2001
LIF	Corticospinal	Blesch et al., 1999b

inhibit growth into the graft. Whereas corticospinal axons cannot penetrate fibroblast grafts producing different growth factors after midthoracic spinal cord lesions (Grill et al., 1997a; Blesch et al., 1999b; Lu et al., 2001), other axonal phenotypes robustly penetrate neurotrophin-producing grafts. For example NGF-secreting fibroblast grafts induce growth of sensory and noradrenergic axons (Tuszynski et al., 1994, 1996; Grill et al., 1997b). These axons are chemotropically attracted by the grafted NGF-producing cells and densely penetrate the graft.

Thus, neurotrophin-induced axonal growth is dependent on the provision of a suitable substrate molecule and might also be modulated by inhibitory extracellular matrix molecules. Differential preferences for axonal growth substrates and differences in the sensitivity to inhibitory extracellular matrix molecules between neuronal populations may influence the response to a neurotrophin delivery.

Neurotrophism versus neurotropism

For the successful therapeutic application of growth factors in the injured CNS, neurotrophins need to be delivered in a timely and spatially accurate manner. Effects on neuronal survival (neurotrophism) and axonal growth (neurotropism) may depend on the site of delivery, especially after spinal cord injury when the cell bodies of supraspinal neurons and their injured axons are usually distant from one another. Further, neurotrophic factors that promote the survival of a specific neuronal population may or may not induce axonal growth of the same neurons. A comparison of BDNF-mediated responses of injured rubrospinal and corticospinal neurons can illustrate these differences.

Rubrospinal neurons undergo severe atrophy after cervical spinal cord lesions. Infusions of BDNF in the proximity of the cell body prevent many of the degenerative changes of the cell body. Concurrently, the same treatment also enhances growth of the injured axons into peripheral nerve grafts in the cervical spinal cord (Kobayashi et al., 1997). Growth of rubrospinal axons is also promoted if BDNF is delivered by genetically modified fibroblasts at the lesion site in the cervical spinal cord (Liu et al., 1999). Thus, BDNF influences both neuronal survival and axonal growth of rubrospinal neurons and the growth promoting properties are not dependent on the site of delivery.

The same does not appear to be true of corticospinal neurons. Whereas infusions of BDNF (Giehl and Tetzlaff, 1996) or grafts of BDNF-secreting fibroblasts (Lu et al., 2001) close to the cell bodies in the sensorimotor cortex can prevent lesion-induced degeneration of corticospinal neurons, the same BDNF-producing cells fail to induce corticospinal axon growth into or around a BDNF-secreting cell graft in the host gray matter after midthoracic spinal cord lesions (Lu et al., 2001). In contrast, NT-3 can induce corticospinal axon growth in the lesioned spinal cord (Schnell et al., 1994;

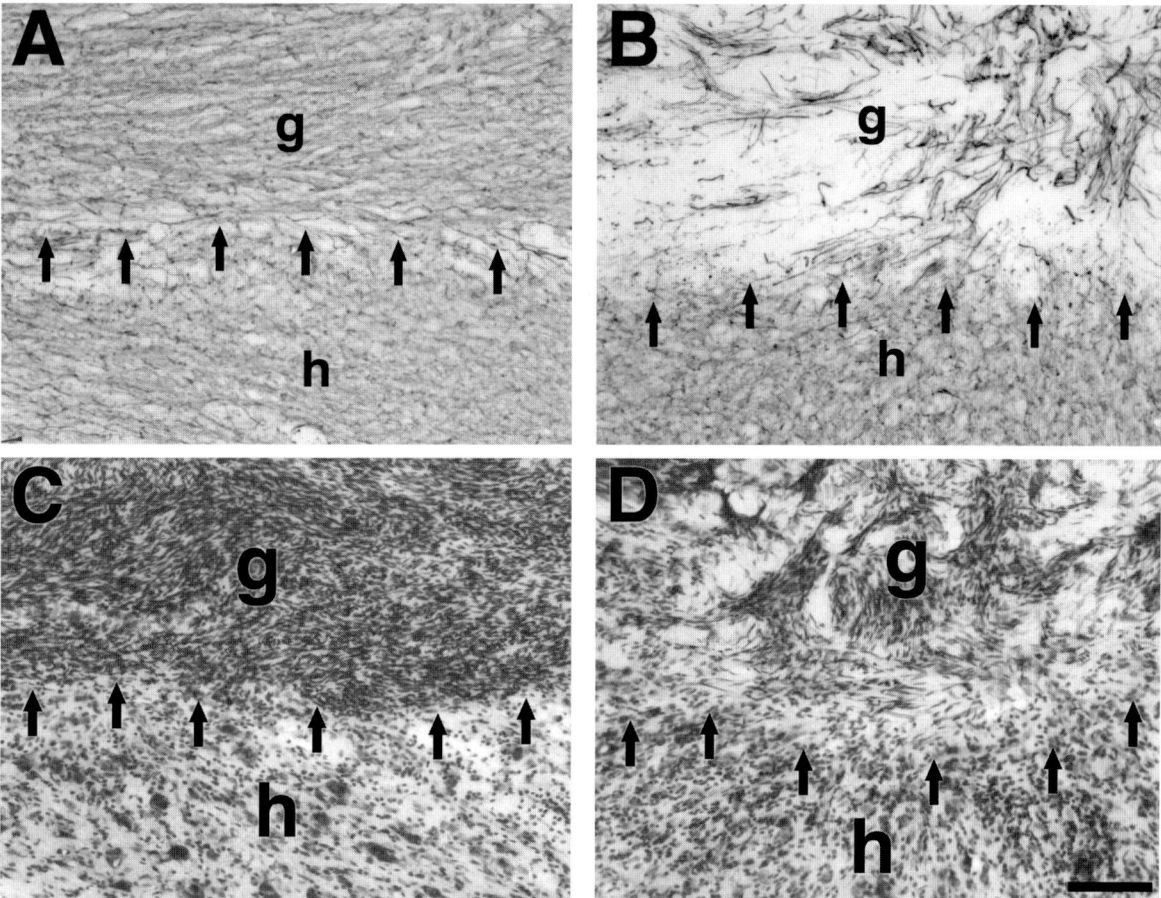

Fig. 1. Axonal penetration of neurotrophin-secreting fibroblast grafts 3 months post-injury and grafting. (A) Grafts of NT-4/5 secreting fibroblasts are densely penetrated by neurofilament labeled axons, whereas few axons are found in (B) control grafts of green fluorescent protein expressing fibroblasts. (C,D) Nissl-stained sections adjacent to the sections in (A,B) show a higher cellular density in (C) NT-4/5 producing grafts compared to (D) control grafts due to an increase in the number of Schwann cells in NT-4/5-secreting cellular grafts. Host (h)/graft (g) interfaces are indicated by arrows. Scale bar: 106 μm.

Grill et al., 1997a; Blits et al., 2000), but its effects on neuronal atrophy are reduced in comparison to BDNF (Giehl and Tetzlaff, 1996). The divergence between neuron survival promoting and axon growth enhancing effects of BDNF might at least partially be due to differential distribution of trkB, the high affinity BDNF receptor. Immunohistochemical analysis shows that trafficking of the trkB protein is restricted to the neuronal soma and dendrites of corticospinal neurons, and trkB is not distributed down corticospinal axons projecting to the spinal cord (Yan et al., 1997; Lu et al., 2001). However, other axonal populations that do grow in response to BDNF-secreting fibroblasts, including motor axons, exhibit

axonal trkB immunoreactivity. Thus, differential receptor distribution might account for the discrepancy between neurotrophism and neurotropism of BDNF for corticospinal motor neurons and their axons.

Behavioral recovery after neurotrophin delivery

Neurotrophin induced behavioral recovery after SCI has been observed in different lesion models and has been attributed to axonal regrowth or influences on the spinal motor pattern generator (Grill et al., 1997a; Jakeman et al., 1998; Liu et al., 1999).

In the first study mentioned above, NT-3 producing genetically modified primary fibroblasts were grafted to a midthoracic dorsal hemisection lesion (Grill et al., 1997a). Functional recovery was observed up to 3 months post-injury and grafting, the longest time point examined. Using a grid task to assess locomotion, animals were trained to cross a horizontal grid and the number of footfalls of the animals' hind limbs was measured (failure to grasp a rung). In this test for sensorimotor integration, animals grafted with NT-3-producing cells made significantly fewer footfalls than control grafted animals, although their function was not fully normalized. This partial functional recovery was accompanied by an increase in corticospinal axon growth up to 8 mm distal to the lesion site. As the increase in corticospinal density over such a relatively short distance is insufficient to reach the lumbar motor neuron pool, the mechanisms responsible for functional improvement are undefined. One mechanism whereby functional recovery might have occurred in this paradigm was the generation of a polysynaptic relay from corticospinal axons to the lumbar motor pattern generators, potentially via propriospinal relays. Alternatively, other axonal systems might have been influenced by cellular NT-3 delivery and contributed to the improvement in function.

In another study reporting functional recovery as a consequence of cellular neurotrophin delivery in the injured adult spinal cord, fibroblasts genetically modified to produce BDNF were grafted to a cervical lateral hemisection lesion (Liu et al., 1999). Animals showed recovery of forelimb function in a glass cylinder test, an exploratory test measuring forelimb use of the unimpaired and impaired side. Behavioral improvement was accompanied by rubrospinal axon growth through the graft and into the distal spinal cord through host gray and white matter.

Thus, in both of the preceding studies, axonal growth was not limited to the graft itself (the neurotrophin delivery site) but continued distal to the lesion site within the host spinal cord. Although the behavioral recovery was morphologically accompanied by axonal growth, no electrophysiological data are available that provide clear evidence that the regenerated axons made functional connections.

Interestingly, infusions of BDNF have also been reported to stimulate hindlimb activity leading to improvements in the rate of recovery and activation of airstepping when the hindlimbs were unloaded (Jakeman et al., 1998). This recovery occurred although no axonal growth bridging through the lesion site was observed. The stepping behavior is likely to be mediated by the spinal pattern generator, intrinsic to the spinal circuitry. Thus, neurotrophins influence not only axonal growth, but may also diminish the threshold for eliciting pattern generator activation in the spinal cord.

Regulated neurotrophin delivery

As summarized in Table I, numerous spinal and supraspinal projections are responsive to neurotrophin delivery. However, in many cases, axonal growth occurs down a concentration gradient, resulting in a dense accumulation of axons within grafts, where growth factor concentrations are maximal, and little extension of axons beyond the graft and into the caudal host spinal cord. The ability to regulate gene expression and to establish spatial and temporal gradients of neurotrophic factors might be a means of allowing axonal growth across a lesion site towards the distal spinal cord. In such a paradigm, neurotrophic factor expression would first be turned *on* at a lesion site to attract the growth of axons. Then, after axons have penetrated the graft, gene expression would be turned *off* at the lesion site and turned *on* at a more distally located site in the caudal host cord, thereby attracting axons from the graft into the distal spinal cord. Such an exogenous regulation of gene expression in grafted cells might be a means of achieving long-distance, highly concentrated axonal growth.

Many studies, including our own, have explored the tetracycline regulatable system for controlled gene expression in the CNS (Gossen and Bujard, 1992; Gossen et al., 1995). Using the 'tet-off' system (i.e., administration of tetracycline turns gene expression off), we have constructed retroviral vectors to express NGF and GFP (green fluorescent protein as control) in primary rat fibroblasts under the control of the tetracycline regulatable promoter (Blesch et al., 2000). In vitro gene expression can be regulated approximately 40–50-fold and levels of doxycycline (a tetracycline analog) as low as 0.1 ng/ml nearly completely turn off gene expression within 24 h.

The regulation of gene expression was also tested in vivo using a model of lesion-induced neuronal degeneration (Blesch et al., 2001). Animals underwent fimbria-fornix lesions leading to degeneration of medial septum cholinergic neurons known to be sensitive to NGF (Hefti, 1986; Williams et al., 1986). Animals received either grafts of cells expressing NGF under the control of the tet-regulatable promoter, or GFP-expressing cells as controls. Two weeks later, there was a significant difference in neuronal rescue in animals that received NGF-secreting grafts in which NGF expression was allowed to remain 'on', compared to animals with NGF-secreting grafts where NGF production was turned 'off' by administering doxycycline in the drinking water. Thus, only animals with NGF-secreting grafts that were not treated with doxycycline (gene expression turned on) showed significant neuronal rescue. In contrast, in animals with regulatable NGF-secreting grafts that were treated with doxycycline, neuronal rescue was reduced to a level that did not differ from control-lesioned animals. Furthermore, significant axonal penetration of grafts was only evident in animals with NGF-secreting grafts that were 'on'; doxycycline-treated animals and control-grafted animals showed very little axonal growth into the grafts. Thus, gene expression could be repressed by doxycycline administration, thereby controlling cell survival and host axonal growth.

Regulation of gene expression for more extended time periods was tested in the injured spinal cord using regulated expression of GFP as a reporter gene. Expression of GFP could be repeatedly turned on and off for at least 3 months in vivo, the longest time point examined (Blesch et al., 2001). Experiments are currently in progress to determine if the regulated expression of neurotrophic factors can enhance axonal growth and re-innervation of the host spinal cord.

In summary, strategies aimed at increasing the intrinsic plasticity of the spinal cord to reorganize and maximize the function of the remaining circuitry and the induction of new axonal growth might enhance functional recovery after spinal cord injury. Neurotrophin delivery in the injured spinal cord is a potential means of achieving this goal. The ability to regulate in vivo gene expression might enhance the safety, practicality and efficiency of neurotrophin gene therapy. The combination of neurotrophic factor therapy with other strategies might optimize functional outcomes after SCI.

Acknowledgements

This study was supported by grants from National Institute of Neurological Disorders and Stroke (NS37083), Veterans Affairs, National Institute for Aging (AG10435), the Hollfelder Foundation, the Brodie Lockart Foundation, the Paralysis Project, and the Stein Institute for Research on Aging.

References

Bamber, N.I., Li, H., Lu, X., Oudega, M., Aebischer, P. and Xu, X.M. (2001) Neurotrophins BDNF and NT-3 promote axonal re-entry into the distal host spinal cord through Schwann cell-seeded mini-channels. *Eur. J. Neurosci.*, 13: 257–268.

Blesch, A. and Tuszynski, M.H. (2001) GDNF gene delivery to injured adult CNS motor neurons promotes axonal growth, expression of the trophic neuropeptide CGRP and cellular protection. *J. Comp. Neurol.*, 436: 399–410.

Blesch, A., Diergardt, N. and Tuszynski, M.H. (1998) Cellularly delivered GDNF induces robust growth of motor and sensory axons in the injured adult spinal cord. *Soc. Neurosci. Abstr.*, 24: 555.

Blesch, A., Diergardt, N., Uy, H.S. and Tuszynski, M.H. (1999a) Cellularly delivered NT-4/5 has axonal growth promoting effects in the injured adult rat spinal cord. *Soc. Neurosci. Abstr.*, 25: 497.

Blesch, A., Uy, H.S., Grill, R.J., Cheng, J.G., Patterson, P.H. and Tuszynski, M.H. (1999b) LIF augments corticospinal axon growth and neurotrophin expression after adult CNS injury. *J. Neurosci.*, 19: 3556–3566.

Blesch, A., Uy, H., Diergardt, N. and Tuszynski, M.H. (2000) Neurite outgrowth can be modulated In vitro using a tetracycline-repressible gene therapy vector expressing human nerve growth factor. *J. Neurosci. Res.*, 59: 402–409.

Blesch, A., Conner, J.M. and Tuszynski, M.H. (2001) Modulation of neuronal survival and axonal growth in vivo by tetracycline-regulated neurotrophin expression. *Gene Ther.*, 8: 954–960.

Blight, A.R. (1983) Cellular morphology of chronic spinal cord injury in the cat: analysis of myelinated axons by line-sampling. *Neuroscience*, 10: 521–543.

Blits, B., Dijkhuizen, P.A., Boer, G.J. and Verhaagen, J. (2000) Intercostal nerve implants transduced with an adenoviral vector encoding neurotrophin-3 promote regrowth of injured rat corticospinal tract fibers and improve hindlimb function. *Exp. Neurol.*, 164: 25–37.

Bradbury, E.J., King, V.R., Simmons, L.J., Priestley, J.V. and McMahon, S.B. (1998) NT-3, but not BDNF, prevents atrophy and death of axotomized spinal cord projection neurons. *Eur. J. Neurosci.*, 10: 3058–3068.

Bregman, B.S. and Goldberger, M.E. (1982) Anatomical plasticity and sparing of function after spinal cord damage in neonatal cats. *Science*, 217: 553–555.

Bregman, B.S. and Goldberger, M.E. (1983) Infant lesion effect:

II. Sparing and recovery of function after spinal cord damage in newborn and adult cats. *Brain Res.*, 285: 119–135.

Bregman, B.S., Kunkel-Bagden, E., Reier, P.J., Dai, H.N., McAtee, M. and Gao, D. (1993) Recovery of function after spinal cord injury: mechanisms underlying transplant-mediated recovery of function differ after spinal cord injury in newborn and adult rats. *Exp. Neurol.*, 123: 3–16.

Brösamle, C. and Schwab, M.E. (1997) Cells of origin, course, and termination patterns of the ventral, uncrossed component of the mature rat corticospinal tract. *J. Comp. Neurol.*, 386: 293–303.

Cotman, C.W., Matthews, D.A., Taylor, D. and Lynch, G. (1973) Synaptic rearrangement in the dentate gyrus: histochemical evidence of adjustments after lesions in immature and adult rats. *Proc. Natl. Acad. Sci. USA*, 70: 3473–3477.

Giehl, K.M. and Tetzlaff, W. (1996) BDNF and NT-3, but not NGF, prevent axotomy-induced death of rat corticospinal neurons in vivo. *Eur. J. Neurosci.*, 8: 1167–1175.

Gossen, M. and Bujard, H. (1992) Tight control of gene expression in mammalian cells by tetracycline-responsive promoters. *Proc. Natl. Acad. Sci. USA*, 89: 5547–5551.

Gossen, M., Freundlieb, S., Bender, G., Muller, G., Hillen, W. and Bujard, H. (1995) Transcriptional activation by tetracyclines in mammalian cells. *Science*, 268: 1766–1769.

Grill, R., Murai, K., Blesch, A., Gage, F.H. and Tuszynski, M.H. (1997a) Cellular delivery of neurotrophin-3 promotes corticospinal axonal growth and partial functional recovery after spinal cord injury. *J. Neurosci.*, 17: 5560–5572.

Grill, R.J., Blesch, A. and Tuszynski, M.H. (1997b) Robust growth of chronically injured spinal cord axons induced by grafts of genetically modified NGF-secreting cells. *Exp. Neurol.*, 148: 444–452.

Hefti, F. (1986) Nerve growth factor promotes survival of septal cholinergic neurons after fimbrial transections. *J. Neurosci.*, 6: 2155–2162.

Jakeman, L.B., Wei, P., Guan, Z. and Stokes, B.T. (1998) Brain-derived neurotrophic factor stimulates hindlimb stepping and sprouting of cholinergic fibers after spinal cord injury. *Exp. Neurol.*, 154: 170–184.

Jones, T.A. (1999) Multiple synapse formation in the motor cortex opposite unilateral sensorimotor cortex lesions in adult rats. *J. Comp. Neurol.*, 414: 57–66.

Jones, T.A. and Schallert, T. (1994) Use-dependent growth of pyramidal neurons after neocortical damage. *J. Neurosci.*, 14: 2140–2152.

Jones, T.A., Kleim, J.A. and Greenough, W.T. (1996) Synaptogenesis and dendritic growth in the cortex opposite unilateral sensorimotor cortex damage in adult rats: a quantitative electron microscopic examination. *Brain Res.*, 733: 142–148.

Jones, T.A., Chu, C.J., Grande, L.A. and Gregory, A.D. (1999) Motor skills training enhances lesion-induced structural plasticity in the motor cortex of adult rats. *J. Neurosci.*, 19: 10153–10163.

Joosten, E.A., Schuitman, R.L., Vermelis, M.E. and Dederen, P.J. (1992) Postnatal development of the ipsilateral corticospinal component in rat spinal cord: a light and electron microscopic anterograde HRP study. *J. Comp. Neurol.*, 326: 133–146.

Kobayashi, N.R., Fan, D.P., Giehl, K.M., Bedard, A.M., Wiegand, S.J. and Tetzlaff, W. (1997) BDNF and NT-4/5 prevent atrophy of rat rubrospinal neurons after cervical axotomy, stimulate GAP-43 and Talpha1-tubulin mRNA expression, and promote axonal regeneration. *J. Neurosci.*, 17: 9583–9595.

Liu, Y., Kim, D., Himes, B.T., Chow, S.Y., Schallert, T., Murray, M., Tessler, A. and Fischer, I. (1999) Transplants of fibroblasts genetically modified to express brain-derived neurotrophic factor promote regeneration of adult rat rubrospinal axons and recovery of forelimb function. *J. Neurosci.*, 19: 4370–4387.

Lu, P., Blesch, A. and Tuszynski, M.H. (2001) Neurotrophism without neurotropism: BDNF promotes survival but not growth of lesioned corticospinal neurons. *J. Comp. Neurol.*, 436: 456–470.

Lynch, G., Gall, C. and Cotman, C. (1977) Temporal parameters of axon 'sprouting' in the brain of the adult rat. *Exp. Neurol.*, 54: 179–183.

McTigue, D.M., Horner, P.J., Stokes, B.T. and Gage, F.H. (1998) Neurotrophin-3 and brain-derived neurotrophic factor induce oligodendrocyte proliferation and myelination of regenerating axons in the contused adult rat spinal cord. *J. Neurosci.*, 18: 5354–5365.

Menei, P., Montero-Menei, C., Whittemore, S.R., Bunge, R.P. and Bunge, M.B. (1998) Schwann cells genetically modified to secrete human BDNF promote enhanced axonal regrowth across transected adult rat spinal cord. *Eur. J. Neurosci.*, 10: 607–621.

Merzenich, M.M., Nelson, R.J., Stryker, M.P., Cynader, M.S., Schoppmann, A. and Zook, J.M. (1984) Somatosensory cortical map changes following digit amputation in adult monkeys. *J. Comp. Neurol.*, 224: 591–605.

Nakamura, M. and Bregman, B. (2001) Differences in neurotrophic factor gene expression profiles between neonate and adult rat spinal cord after injury. *Exp. Neurol.*, 169: 407–415.

Oudega, M. and Hagg, T. (1999) Neurotrophins promote regeneration of sensory axons in the adult rat spinal cord. *Brain Res.*, 818: 431–438.

Raisman, G. (1969) Neuronal plasticity in the septal nuclei of the adult rat. *Brain Res.*, 14: 25–48.

Schnell, L., Schneider, R., Kolbeck, R., Barde, Y.A. and Schwab, M.E. (1994) Neurotrophin-3 enhances sprouting of corticospinal tract during development and after adult spinal cord lesion. *Nature*, 367: 170–173.

Steward, O. (1976) Reinnervation of dentate gyrus by homologous afferents following entorhinal cortical lesions in adult rats. *Science*, 194: 426–428.

Tsukahara, N., Hultborn, H., Murakami, F. and Fujito, Y. (1975) Electrophysiological study of formation of new synapses and collateral sprouting in red nucleus neurons after partial denervation. *J. Neurophysiol.*, 38: 1359–1372.

Tuszynski, M.H., Gabriel, K., Gage, F.H., Suhr, S., Meyer, S. and Rosetti, A. (1996) Nerve growth factor delivery by gene transfer induces differential outgrowth of sensory, motor, and noradrenergic neurites after adult spinal cord injury. *Exp. Neurol.*, 137: 157–173.

Tuszynski, M.H., Murai, K., Blesch, A., Grill, R. and Miller, I. (1997) Functional characterization of NGF-secreting cell grafts to the acutely injured spinal cord. *Cell Transplant.*, 6: 361–368.

Tuszynski, M.H., Peterson, D.A., Ray, J., Baird, A., Nakahara, Y. and Gage, F.H. (1994) Fibroblasts genetically modified to produce nerve growth factor induce robust neuritic ingrowth after grafting to the spinal cord. *Exp. Neurol.*, 126: 1–14.

Tuszynski, M.H., Weidner, N., McCormack, M., Miller, I., Powell, H. and Conner, J. (1998) Grafts of genetically modified Schwann cells to the spinal cord: survival, axon growth, and myelination. *Cell Transplant.*, 7: 187–196.

Vahlsing, H.L. and Feringa, E.R. (1980) A ventral uncrossed corticospinal tract in the rat. *Exp. Neurol.*, 70: 282–287.

Weidner, N., Blesch, A., Grill, R.J. and Tuszynski, M.H. (1999) Nerve growth factor-hypersecreting Schwann cell grafts augment and guide spinal cord axonal growth and remyelinate central nervous system axons in a phenotypically appropriate manner that correlates with expression of L1. *J. Comp. Neurol.*, 413: 495–506.

Weidner, N., Ner, A., Salimi, N. and Tuszynski, M.H. (2001) Spontaneous corticospinal axonal plasticity and functional recovery after adult central nervous system injury. *Proc. Natl. Acad. Sci. USA*, 98: 3513–3518.

Whishaw, I.Q., Pellis, S.M., Gorny, B., Kolb, B. and Tetzlaff, W. (1993) Proximal and distal impairments in rat forelimb use in reaching follow unilateral pyramidal tract lesions. *Behav. Brain Res.*, 56: 59–76.

Widenfalk, J., Lundströmer, K., Jubran, M., Brene, S. and Olson, L. (2001) Neurotrophic factors and receptors in the immature and adult spinal cord after mechanical injury or kainic acid. *J. Neurosci.*, 21: 3457–3475.

Williams, L.R., Varon, S., Peterson, G.M., Wictorin, K., Fischer, W., Bjorklund, A. and Gage, F.H. (1986) Continuous infusion of nerve growth factor prevents basal forebrain neuronal death after fimbria fornix transection. *Proc. Natl. Acad. Sci. USA*, 83: 9231–9235.

Xu, X.M., Guenard, V., Kleitman, N., Aebischer, P. and Bunge, M.B. (1995) A combination of BDNF and NT-3 promotes supraspinal axonal regeneration into Schwann cell grafts in adult rat thoracic spinal cord. *Exp. Neurol.*, 134: 261–272.

Yan, Q., Radeke, M.J., Matheson, C.R., Talvenheimo, J., Welcher, A.A. and Feinstein, S.C. (1997) Immunocytochemical localization of TrkB in the central nervous system of the adult rat. *J. Comp. Neurol.*, 378: 135–157.

Ye, J.H. and Houle, J.D. (1997) Treatment of the chronically injured spinal cord with neurotrophic factors can promote axonal regeneration from supraspinal neurons. *Exp. Neurol.*, 143: 70–81.

L. McKerracher, G. Doucet and S. Rossignol (Eds.)
Progress in Brain Research, Vol. 137

CHAPTER 32

Where the rubber meets the road: netrin expression and function in developing and adult nervous systems

Colleen Manitt and Timothy E. Kennedy [*]

Centre for Neuronal Survival, Montreal Neurological Institute, McGill University, Montreal, QC H3A 2B4, Canada

Abstract: Netrins are a family of secreted proteins that direct the migration of cells and axonal growth cones during neural development. They are bifunctional cues, attracting some cell types and repelling others. Netrins function as either short- or long-range cues, in some circumstances acting close to the surface of the cells that produce them and in other cases at a distance. Two classes of receptors mediate the response to netrin-1, the deleted in colorectal cancer family and the UNC-5 homolog family. Although netrin function has been extensively studied in the embryonic nervous system, netrin-1 is expressed in the adult mammalian spinal cord at a level similar to that in the embryonic CNS. In the adult and embryonic CNS, the majority of netrin-1 protein is not freely soluble but is associated with membranes and extracellular matrix. This distribution is consistent with netrin-1 acting as a short-range cue. Here we present a model whereby netrin-1 in the embryonic neural epithelium could act as a membrane-associated long-range cue. *Netrin-1* is expressed in the adult by multiple types of neurons and by myelinating glia: oligodendrocytes in the CNS and Schwann cells in the PNS. In the white matter of the adult CNS, netrin-1 protein is absent from compact myelin but enriched in periaxonal myelin at the interface between axons and oligodendrocytes. This distribution suggests that in the adult nervous system netrin-1 may function to mediate cell–cell interactions. Furthermore, netrin receptor expression persists in neurons following injury, raising the possibility that netrin-1 may influence axonal regeneration.

Introduction

Extending axons find their way during neural development by following a combination of long- and short-range cues (reviewed by Tessier-Lavigne and Goodman, 1996). Long-range cues interact with neuronal growth cones at a distance from the cell that secreted the cue, while short-range cues influence axon growth on the surface of the cell that produced them.

Netrins are a family of secreted proteins that guide growing axons during embryogenesis. The

* Correspondence to: T.E. Kennedy, Centre for Neuronal Survival, Montreal Neurological Institute, McGill University, 3801 University Street, Montreal, QC H3A 2B4, Canada. Tel.: +1-514-398-7136; Fax: +1-514-398-1319; E-mail: timothy.kennedy@mcgill.ca

first netrins found in vertebrates were purified from embryonic brain on the basis of an in vitro functional assay designed to identify proteins that could promote commissural axon outgrowth (Tessier-Lavigne et al., 1988; Serafini et al., 1994). This assay was based on the proposal and subsequent demonstration that embryonic spinal commissural axons are attracted by a diffusible cue secreted by the floor plate (Fig. 1A; Ramon y Cajal, 1909; Weber, 1938; Tessier-Lavigne et al., 1988; Placzek et al., 1990). *Netrin-1* is expressed by floor plate cells as commissural axons extend toward the ventral midline, and like the floor plate, a source of recombinant netrin-1 protein attracts commissural axons (Kennedy et al., 1994). In mice lacking netrin-1 function, the corpus callosum, hippocampal commissure, and ventral spinal commissure all fail to form, indicating that netrin-1 is required for

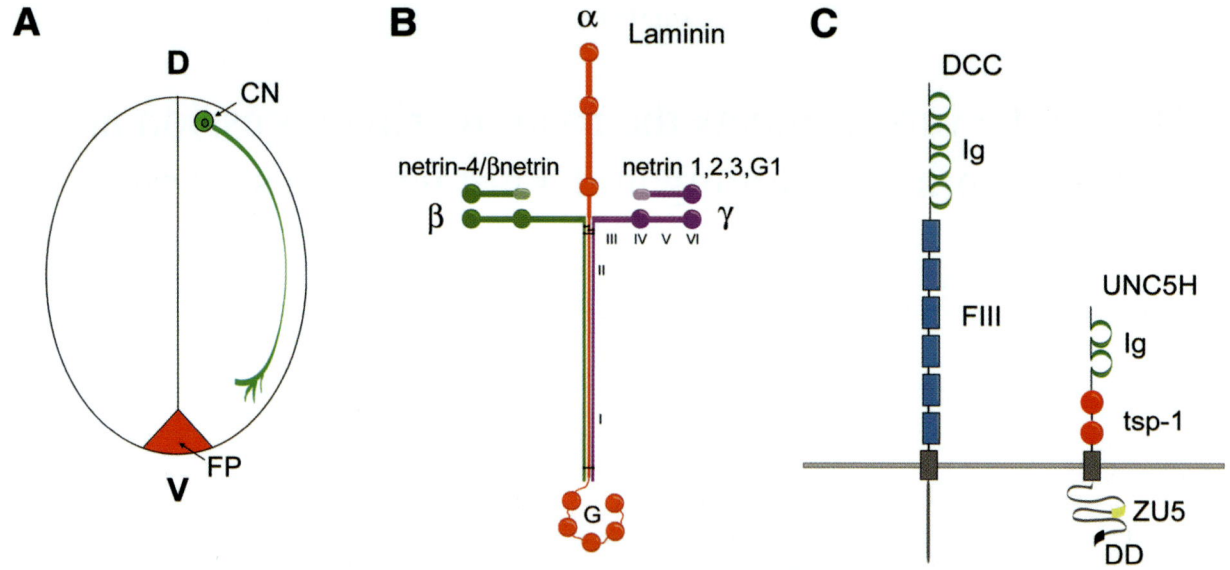

A

D

CN

FP

V

B α   Laminin

netrin-4/βnetrin

β

netrin 1,2,3,G1

γ

III   IV   V   VI

II

I

G

C DCC

Ig

FIII

UNC5H

Ig

tsp-1

ZU5

DD

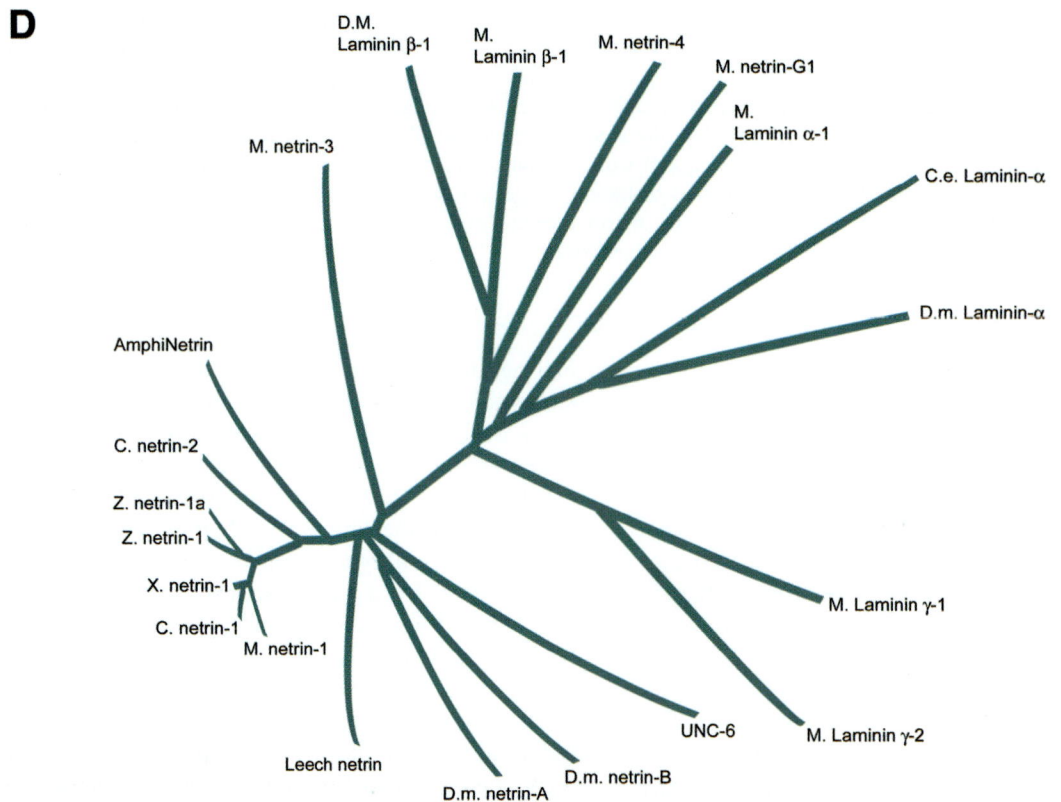

D

D.M. Laminin β-1

M. Laminin β-1

M. netrin-4

M. netrin-G1

M. Laminin α-1

M. netrin-3

C.e. Laminin-α

D.m. Laminin-α

AmphiNetrin

C. netrin-2

Z. netrin-1a

Z. netrin-1

X. netrin-1

C. netrin-1

M. netrin-1

M. Laminin γ-1

Leech netrin

D.m. netrin-A

D.m. netrin-B

UNC-6

M. Laminin γ-2

the development of multiple commissural projections (Serafini et al., 1996). Although initial studies focused on the ability of netrin-1 to attract extending axons, Colamarino and Tessier-Lavigne (1995) demonstrated that netrin-1 also functions as a repellent for other axons. Together, these findings led to the proposal that a gradient of netrin protein emanating from the floor plate orients the growth of multiple populations of axons as they extend circumferentially toward or away from the ventral midline of the embryonic CNS. Netrins not only guide extending axons, but also direct the migration of neuronal cells, glial precursor cells, and mesodermal cells during embryogenesis (Wadsworth et al., 1996; Bloch-Gallego et al., 1999; Kim et al., 1999; Yee et al., 1999; Alcantara et al., 2000; Su et al., 2000; Hamasaki et al., 2001; Sugimoto et al., 2001). Below, we describe additional members of the netrin gene family, netrin receptors, mechanisms of netrin signal transduction, and the recent characterization of netrin and netrin receptor expression in adult nervous systems.

The netrin gene family

Four members of the netrin gene family have been identified in mammals: *netrin-1*, *netrin-3*, *netrin-G1*, and *netrin-4*, also called *β-netrin* (Serafini et al., 1996; Wang et al., 1999; Koch et al., 2000; Nakashiba et al., 2000; Yin et al., 2000). Orthologs of each of these netrin family members have been identified in the human genome (Table I). All encode ∼65 kDa secreted proteins made up of three domains (VI, V, and C) and an amino terminal signal peptide characteristic of secreted proteins. Domains V and VI of netrins are homologous to domains V and VI of laminins (Fig. 1B). No domain homologous to the netrin C domain is present in the laminin family; however the netrin C domain has some similarity to sequences present in the complement and

Fig. 1. Netrins and netrin receptors guide axon extension during vertebrate and invertebrate neural development. (A) *Netrin-1* is highly expressed by floor plate cells (FP) at the ventral (V) midline of the embryonic spinal cord. Netrin-1 functions as an attractant for *dcc* expressing commissural neurons (CN) that extend from the dorsal (D) neural epithelium toward the floor plate. Netrin-1 similarly acts as a chemorepellent for axons extending dorsally away from the ventral midline (not illustrated). (B) Schematic illustrating the relative size of netrins (∼65 kDa) and the heterotrimeric laminin molecule (∼800 kDa). Each laminin polypeptide (α, β, γ) is composed of domains I–VI. The laminin α-chain also contains a globular G domain. Domains III and V are made up of laminin-type epidermal growth factor (EGF) domains (for review see Timpl and Brown, 1994). Domain V and VI of mouse laminin γ-1 and domains V and VI of mouse netrin-1 share ∼45% and ∼52% amino acid identity, respectively. Netrin-4 contains greater sequence identity to the β-chain of laminin than the γ-chain. For the purpose of illustration, netrin-G1 is grouped with the γ-chain of laminin; however, netrin-G1 is the most divergent member of the netrin family isolated thus far and is distantly related to netrin-1 like proteins (see D). (C) Schematic illustrating the structure of DCC and UNC-5 homolog netrin receptors. The extracellular domain of DCC family members is composed of four immunoglobulin-like domains (Ig) and six fibronectin type III domains (FIII), followed by a transmembrane domain and an intracellular domain (Chan et al., 1996). UNC-5 homologs contain two extracellular Ig-like domains, two thrombospondin type 1 (tsp-1) domains, followed by a transmembrane domain and an intracellular domain. The intracellular domain of UNC-5 homologs contains a death domain (DD, Hofmann and Tschopp, 1995) and a ZU5 domain, a region with similarity to sequence present in zona occludens, a protein associated with adherens junctions (Leonardo et al., 1997). (D) A molecular phylogeny illustrating the relationship between members of the netrin and laminin protein families. The branch points linking netrins 1, 2, 3, and UNC-6 cluster together at one end of the tree, while netrins 4, G1 and the laminins cluster at the other. Although composed of the VI, V, C domain structure characteristic of netrins, netrins 4 and G1 contain sequences more closely related to laminins than to other members of the netrin family, as indicated by the position of the branch points leading to netrin-4 and G1 being beyond the branch points separating the α, β and γ laminins. Full-length amino acid sequences of the following proteins were used to generate the tree shown. GenBank accession number are as indicated: mouse netrin-1 (M. netrin-1, AAC52971), mouse netrin-3 (M. netrin-3,AAD40063), mouse netrin-4 (β-NETRIN/M. netrin-4, AAG30823/AAF91404), mouse netrin-G1 (M. netrin-G1, NP_109624), chicken netrin-1 (C. netrin-1, AAA60369), chicken netrin-2 (C. netrin-2, AAA61743), frog netrin-1 (X. netrin-1, AAB87983), zebrafish netrin-1 (Z. netrin-1, AAB70266), zebrafish netrin-1a (Z. netrin-1a, AAC60252), amphioxus netrin (AmphiNetrin, CAB72422), *C. elegans* UNC-6 (C.e. UNC-6, AAA28157), *D. melanogaster* netrin-A (D.m. netrin-A, AAB17547), *D. melanogaster* netrin-B (D.m. netrin-B, AAB17548), *H. medicinalis* netrin (Leech netrin, AAC83376), mouse laminin α-1 (M. laminin α-1, MMMSA), mouse laminin β-1 (M. laminin β-1, MMMSB1), mouse laminin γ-1 (M. laminin γ-1, MMMSB2), mouse laminin γ-2 (M. laminin γ-2, S69000), *C. elegans* laminin α (C.e. laminin α, BAA11828), *D. melanogaster* laminin β-1 (D.m. laminin β-1, P11046), *D. melanogaster* laminin α (D.m. laminin α, AAA28662). Sequences were aligned using CLUSTALW and an unrooted tree generated using DRAWTREE software available at http://bioweb.pasteur.fr/intro-uk.html.

TABLE I

Identified netrins and netrin receptors

Species	Netrin	DCC family	UNC-5 family
Caenorhabditis elegans (nematode)	UNC-6 [1]	UNC-40 [21]	UNC-5 [32]
Drosophila melanogaster (fruit fly)	netrin-A [2,3]	Frazzled [22]	DUnc-5 [33]
	netrin-B [2,3]		
Hirudo medicinalis (medicinal leech)	Leech netrin [4]	N/A	N/A
Ciona intestinalis (sea squirt)	Ci-NET1 [5]	N/A	N/A
Branchiostoma floridae (amphioxus)	AmphiNetrin [6]	N/A	N/A
Perkinsus marinus (sea lamprey)	N/A	N/A	Unc-5 [34]
Xenopus laevis (Clawed frog)	netrin-1 [7]	XDCCa [23]	N/A
		XDCCb [23]	
Danio rerio (zebrafish)	netrin-1 [8]	ZDCC [24]	N/A
	netrin-1a [9]		
Gallus gallus (chicken)	netrin-1 [10]	CDCC [25]	N/A
	netrin-2 [10]	Neogenin [26]	
Mus musculus (house mouse)	netrin-1 [11]	DCC [27]	UNC5H3 [35]
	netrin-3 [12]	Neogenin [28]	
	β-netrin/netrin-4 [13,14]		
	netrin-G1 [15]		
Rattus norvegicus (Norway rat)	netrin-1 [16]	DCC [29,30]	UNC5H1 [36]
	netrin-3 [16]	Neogenin [30]	UNC5H2 [36]
Homo sapiens (human)	NTN1 [11,17]	DCC [29]	UNC5C [37]
	NTN2L [18] (net-3 ortholog)	Neogenin [31]	
	β-netrin/NTN4 [13,19]		
	netrin-G1 [20]		

[1] Ishii et al. (1992). Accession: AAA28157. [2] Harris et al. (1996). Netrin-A, accession: AAB17547. Netrin-B, accession: AAB17548. [3] Mitchell et al. (1996). Netrin-A, accession: AAB17533. Netrin-B, accession: AAB17534. [4] Gan et al. (1999). Accession: AAC83376. [5] Takamura direct submission (06-10-1999). Accession: BAA94302. [6] Shimeld (2000). Accession: CAB72422. [7] de la Torre et al. (1997). Accession: AAB87983. [8] Strahle et al. (1997). Accession: AAB70266. [9] Lauderdale et al. (1997). Accession: AAC60252. [10] Serafini et al. (1994). Netrin-1, accession: AAA60369. Netrin-2, accession: AAA61743. [11] Serafini et al. (1996). Mouse, accession: AAC52971. Human, accession: NP_004813. [12] Wang et al. (1999). Accession: AAD40063. [13] Koch et al. (2000). Mouse β-netrin, accession: AAG30823. Human β-netrin, accession: AAG30822. [14] Yin et al. (2000) Accession: AAF91404. [15] Nakashiba et al. (2000). Accession: NP_109624. [16] Manitt et al. (2001). Netrin-1, accession: AY028417. Netrin-3, accession: AY028418. [17] Meyerhardt et al. direct submission (21-10-1996). Accession: AAD09221. [18] Van Raay et al. (1997). Accession: AAC51246. [19] Strausberg. direct submission (04-09-2001). Accession: AAH13591. [20] Nakashiba et al. (2000). Accession: NP_055732. [21] Chan et al. (1996). Accession: AAB17088. [22] Kolodziej et al. (1996). Accession: AAC47315. [23] Pierceall et al. (1994). XDCCa, accession: AAA70168. XDCCb, accession: AAA70167. [24] Hjorth et al. (2001). [25] Chuong et al. (1994). [26] Vielmetter et al. (1994). Accession: AAC59662. [27] Cooper et al. (1995) Accession: NP_031857. [28] Keeling et al. (1997). Accession: NP_032710. [29] Fearon et al. (1990). Rat, accession: B40098. Human, accession NP_005206. [30] Keino-Masu et al. (1996). DCC, accession: AAB41099. Neogenin, accession: AAB41100. [31] Meyerhardt et al. (1997). Accession: AAB17263. [32] Leung-Hagesteijn et al. (1992). Accession: AAB23867. [33] Keleman and Dickson (2001). Accession: AAF74193. [34] Shifman and Selzer (2000b). Accession: AAF00103. [35] Ackerman et al. (1997). Accession: AAB54103. [36] Leonardo et al. (1997). UNC5H1, accession: NP_071542, UNC5H2, accession: NP_071543. [37] Ackerman and Knowles (1998). Accession: AAC67491.

tissue inhibitors of metalloproteases (TIMPs) protein families (Ishii et al., 1992; Banyai and Patthy, 1999; Sandoval et al., 2000). The functional significance of this homology is unknown. The netrin C domain binds heparin with high affinity (Kappler et al., 2000) and it is likely that components of the cell surface or extracellular matrix (ECM), such as glycosaminoglycans, may bind to the C domain and influence the ability of netrins to diffuse. This type of interaction may function to concentrate netrin locally, present netrin to netrin receptors and determine if netrin functions as a short- or a long-range cue in different contexts. Six alternatively spliced forms of the mRNA encoding netrin-G1 have been reported (Nakashiba et al., 2000), and unlike other netrins, several of these are bound to the plasma membrane via a glycosyl phosphatidyl-inositol lipid anchor linked to the C domain.

Netrin family members identified in non-mammalian vertebrate species include chicken netrin-1 and netrin-2 (Kennedy et al., 1994), zebrafish netrin-1 and netrin-1a (Lauderdale et al., 1997; MacDonald et al., 1997; Strahle et al., 1997), *Xenopus* netrin-1 (de la Torre et al., 1997), and a netrin from *Perkinsus marinus*, the sea lamprey (Shifman and Selzer, 2000a). Netrins have been identified in several invertebrate species including AmphiNetrin from *Branchiostoma floridae*, the cephalochordate amphioxus (Shimeld, 2000), the ascidian *Ciona intestinalis* or sea squirt, also a chordate (Takamura, Genbank BAA94302), *Hirudo medicinalis*, the medicinal leech (Gan et al., 1999), *Drosophila melanogaster* (Harris et al., 1996; Mitchell et al., 1996), and *Caenorhabditis elegans* (Ishii et al., 1992). Fig. 1D presents a molecular phylogeny illustrating the relationship between members of the netrin and laminin families.

UNC-6, the first member of the netrin family identified, was discovered using a genetic assay for defects in neural development by examining *C. elegans* mutants with uncoordinated (unc) phenotypes (Hedgecock et al., 1990; Ishii et al., 1992). Loss of UNC-6 function produces defects in the trajectories of axons that normally extend circumferentially toward or away from the ventral midline of the developing nematode. In a pattern reminiscent of netrin expression by floor plate cells at the ventral midline of the embryonic vertebrate neural tube, *unc-6* is expressed by a row of epidermoblasts at the ventral midline of the developing worm (Wadsworth et al., 1996). Two netrins have been identified in *D. melanogaster*, *netrin-A* and *netrin-B* (Harris et al., 1996; Mitchell et al., 1996). Both are expressed by glial cells at the ventral midline of the embryonic *D. melanogaster* CNS and loss of netrin function causes defects in commissure formation. These findings indicate that netrins perform a highly conserved function, guiding circumferential axon extension in developing vertebrate and invertebrate nervous systems.

Netrin receptors

Candidate netrin receptors were first identified in *C. elegans* based on the similarity of *unc-5*, *unc-40*, and netrin *unc-6* mutant phenotypes. Hedgecock et al. (1990) proposed that the phenotypes of these mutants

revealed the presence of a circumferential guidance mechanism in the developing nematode. Mutation of *unc-5* caused defects in ventral to dorsal migration, away from *unc-6* expressing cells, mutation of *unc-40* produced defects in dorsal to ventral migration, toward *unc-6* expressing cells, and mutation of *unc-6* caused defects in both trajectories. Cloning of *unc-40* and *unc-5* indicated that they encode transmembrane members of the Ig superfamily, and both are expressed by neurons as they extend axons during development in *C. elegans* (Leung-Hagesteijn et al., 1992; Chan et al., 1996). Homologs of *unc-40* and *unc-5* have been identified in many species and make up the deleted in colorectal cancer (DCC) and the UNC-5 homolog families of netrin receptors.

The DCC family of netrin receptors

The DCC family includes DCC and neogenin in vertebrates, frazzled in *D. melanogaster*, and UNC-40 in *C. elegans* (Fearon et al., 1990; Chuong et al., 1994; Pierceall et al., 1994; Vielmetter et al., 1994, 1997; Cooper et al., 1995; Chan et al., 1996; Keino-Masu et al., 1996; Kolodziej et al., 1996; Keeling et al., 1997; Meyerhardt et al., 1997; Hjorth et al., 2001). The extracellular domain of each of these proteins is composed of four immunoglobulin (Ig) domains followed by six fibronectin type III (FNIII) repeats, a transmembrane domain and an intracellular domain (Fig. 1C). Strong evidence indicates that DCC is a receptor mediating the chemoattractant response to netrin-1. In the embryonic vertebrate nervous system, spinal commissural neurons express *dcc* as their axons extend toward the floor plate. DCC binds netrin-1 (Keino-Masu et al., 1996; Stein et al., 2001) and antibodies that block DCC function block the ability of the floor plate to promote commissural axon outgrowth (Keino-Masu et al., 1996). Furthermore, the phenotype of *dcc* knockout mice (Fazeli et al., 1997) is very similar to that generated by loss of netrin-1 (Serafini et al., 1996).

Neogenin, a second member of the DCC family in vertebrates (Vielmetter et al., 1994; Keeling et al., 1997; Meyerhardt et al., 1997) is expressed by neurons and non-neuronal cells in the CNS during embryogenesis (Vielmetter et al., 1994). However, *dcc* expressing embryonic spinal commissural neurons do not express *neogenin* as they extend their axon toward the floor plate (Keino-Masu et al., 1996). Neogenin binds netrin-1 (Keino-Masu et al., 1996) but its function remains unknown. Alternatively spliced mRNA transcripts of both *neogenin* and *dcc* have been identified but their significance is not known (Reale et al., 1994; Vielmetter et al., 1994; Keeling et al., 1997). Two gene products more distantly related to DCC have recently been identified in mammals, Punc and Nope (Salbaum, 1998; Salbaum and Kappen, 2000), but no evidence has been provided to support a functional interaction between either Punc or Nope with any member of the netrin family.

The UNC-5 homolog family of netrin receptors

UNC-5 and its vertebrate homologs are single-pass transmembrane proteins composed of extracellular Ig-like domains, two thrombospondin type I domains, and intracellular sequence that contains a ZU5 domain and a death domain (Fig. 1C). The trajectories of axons extending away from a source of the netrin UNC-6 are disrupted in *C. elegans unc-5* mutants, indicating that the chemorepellent response requires UNC-5 (Hedgecock et al., 1990). In *D. melanogaster*, *unc-5* is expressed by a subset of motoneurons whose axons exit the CNS without crossing the midline and then avoid netrin expressing muscles in the periphery (Keleman and Dickson, 2001). Furthermore, in both *C. elegans* and *D. melanogaster*, ectopic expression of *unc-5* in neurons that either normally do not respond to netrin or are attracted toward a source of netrin, caused their axons to be repelled by netrin in vivo (Hamelin et al., 1993; Keleman and Dickson, 2001). These findings are consistent with UNC-5 mediating a repellent response to netrin.

Three UNC-5 homologs have been identified in mammals, all are transmembrane proteins and all bind netrin-1, suggesting that they function as netrin receptors (Ackerman et al., 1997; Leonardo et al., 1997). Although a role for an UNC-5 homolog directing axon guidance in vivo during mammalian development has not been demonstrated, analysis of the *unc5h3* mouse mutant (rostral cerebellar malformation, rcm, Ackerman et al., 1997; Przyborski et al., 1998) indicates that UNC5H3 is required for the migration of granule cell and Purkinje cell pre-

cursors during cerebellar development. The displacement of the neuronal precursors found in the mutant is consistent with UNC5H3 mediating a repellent migratory response to netrin-1.

Functional interactions between DCC and UNC-5 homolog netrin receptors

Many receptors are activated by multimerization. Interestingly, netrin-1 causes DCC to multimerize and this appears to be required for the axon guidance function of DCC (Stein et al., 2001). This study demonstrated that isolated cytoplasmic domains of DCC interact spontaneously and that this interaction is repressed in the full-length receptors in the absence of netrin-1. The presence of netrin-1 stimulates DCC multimerization both by promoting an association of DCC extracellular domains and via an allosteric effect that allows the intracellular domains to interact.

Members of the DCC and UNC-5 homolog families can respond to netrin independently of the other (Keleman and Dickson, 2001; Merz et al., 2001); however, a straight-forward model accounting for the bifunctional action of netrin, with one receptor family mediating attraction and the other repulsion, is now clearly an oversimplification. Many neurons express members of both the *unc-5* and *dcc* families (Chan et al., 1996; Leonardo et al., 1997). It was noted early on that *C. elegans unc-40* mutants contained subtle defects in ventral to dorsal axon migration, the trajectory more closely associated with *unc-5* function (Hedgecock et al., 1990; McIntire et al., 1992; Colavita and Culotti, 1998). Moreover, biochemical evidence indicates that UNC-5 homologs and DCC can interact directly, forming a netrin receptor complex (Hong et al., 1999). In *D. melanogaster*, ectopic expression of *unc-5* by neurons caused their axons to exhibit a potent repellent response to netrin (Keleman and Dickson, 2001). Interestingly, the short-range repellent function mediated by *unc-5* was independent of frazzled, the *D. melanogaster* homolog of DCC, but the long-range repellent action of netrin required both *unc-5* and *frazzled* expression. Keleman and Dickson (2001) suggest that UNC-5 alone is sufficient to respond to a high concentration of netrin, while UNC-5 and frazzled are required for the long-range repellent response in the presence of lower concentrations of netrin.

Consistent with the results of ectopic expression of *unc-5* in *C. elegans* and *D. melanogaster* (Hamelin et al., 1993; Keleman and Dickson, 2001), neurons isolated from the embryonic *Xenopus* spinal cord engineered to express UNC5H2 switched their response to netrin-1 from attraction to repulsion in vitro (Hong et al., 1999). Significantly, both attraction and repulsion were blocked by an antibody against DCC, indicating that DCC participates in both responses in these cells. Consistent with this functional interaction, the cytoplasmic domains of DCC and UNC5H2 were shown to interact spontaneously (Hong et al., 1999). Like the multimerization of DCC described above, DCC and UNC5H2 cytoplasmic domain interactions are repressed in the full-length receptors, and netrin-1 stimulates multimerization by promoting the association of both extracellular and intracellular domains. These results suggest that the relative number of DCC or UNC-5 homolog receptors present on the surface of a cell may play a key role in determining how an axon responds to netrin-1.

Is the adenosine A2B receptor a netrin-1 receptor?

The adenosine A2B receptor, a G-protein-coupled receptor that triggers an increase in cAMP when bound to adenosine, has recently been proposed to be a receptor for netrin-1 in commissural neurons (Corset et al., 2000). Using a yeast two-hybrid screen, these authors detected an interaction between the intracellular domains of the A2B receptor and DCC. Co-immunoprecipitation experiments using cells over-expressing DCC and A2B suggested that the interaction between these receptors requires netrin-1. However, a careful study by Stein et al. (2001) shows that A2B does not function as a receptor for netrin-1 in rat embryonic commissural neurons. They show that these neurons do not express A2B as they extend axons toward the floor plate. Furthermore, pharmacological manipulation of adenosine receptor activity in these neurons does not affect commissural axon outgrowth in response to netrin-1 protein, a response previously shown to require DCC (Keino-Masu et al., 1996; Fazeli et

al., 1997). Similarly, A2B does not contribute to the netrin-1 induced turning response of the axons of dissociated *Xenopus* embryonic spinal neurons. These findings indicate that A2B is not a netrin-1 receptor in these neurons.

Interaction of netrin family members with identified netrin receptors

Although five netrins have now been identified in vertebrate species, it appears that not all of these interact with known netrin receptors. Evidence has been provided that netrin-1 and netrin-3 bind DCC, neogenin, UNC5H1, UNC5H2, and UNC5H3 (Keino-Masu et al., 1996; Leonardo et al., 1997; Wang et al., 1999). Netrin-1, netrin-2, and netrin-3 promote DCC dependent axon outgrowth from multiple neuronal cell types (Keino-Masu et al., 1996; Deiner et al., 1997; de la Torre et al., 1997; Hong et al., 1999; Wang et al., 1999). Netrin-1 and netrin-3 repel the axons of embryonic trochlear motoneurons (Colamarino and Tessier-Lavigne, 1995; Wang et al., 1999). Recombinant netrin-4/β-netrin evokes the outgrowth of axons from explants of embryonic rat olfactory bulb, but it is not known if this response requires DCC or if these neurons express *dcc* (Koch et al., 2000). Current evidence indicates that none of the known netrin receptors bind netrin-G1. Recombinant netrin-G1 did not promote the outgrowth of cerebellofugal axons from explants of embryonic cerebellar plate (Nakashiba et al., 2000), axons that extend toward a source of netrin-1 (Shirasaki et al., 1995). In summary, these findings indicate that DCC and UNC-5 homologs function as receptors for netrin-1, netrin-2, netrin-3, and possibly netrin-4/β-netrin, and suggest that an unidentified receptor or family of netrin receptors mediates the response to netrin-G1.

Netrin signal transduction and growth cone guidance

As an axon extends, the growth cone encounters cues that may cause it to advance, turn, or retract. Filopodia and lamellipodia are dynamic actin based membrane protrusions found at the edge of neuronal growth cones (reviewed by Bentley and O'Connor, 1994; Tanaka and Sabry, 1995). Contact of the tip of a single filopodium with an appropriate extracellular target is sufficient to change the trajectory of an extending axon (O'Connor et al., 1990; Chien et al., 1993), indicating that the key receptors that interact with guidance cues are present at filopodial tips. Substantial evidence indicates that guidance cues influence motility by remodeling the actin cytoskeleton within the growth cone (reveiwed by Suter and Forscher, 1998). In neuronal and non-neuronal cells, the Rho family of small GPTases are key components of the intracellular signal transduction cascade that regulate the organization of actin. Of particular significance, the Rho family members Cdc42, Rac1, and RhoA regulate the formation of filopodia, lamellipodia, and stress fibers, respectively (reviewed by Hall, 1998; Dickson, 2001).

Although tremendous progress has been made in identifying axon guidance cues and their receptors, the signal transduction mechanisms underlying their mode of action are just beginning to be elucidated. Recently, Shekarabi and Kennedy (2002) reported a striking localization of DCC at the extreme distal tips of filopodia in the growth cones of embryonic rat spinal commissural neurons. This study also demonstrates that expression of DCC causes a netrin-1 dependent increase in the number of filopodia and in cell surface area of rodent neuroblastoma cells (NG108-15) and human embryonic kidney cells (HEK293T). Co-expression of dominant negative Cdc42 or dominant negative Rac1 blocked the netrin-1 induced increase in filopodia number and in cell size, respectively. Furthermore, DCC caused a netrin-1 dependent activation of Cdc42 and Rac1, indicating that these proteins are components of the signal transduction cascade downstream of DCC that is activated by netrin-1. The findings presented in this study suggest that netrin-1 and DCC influence motility by activating the Rho GTPases Cdc42 and Rac1, thereby leading to the reorganization of actin.

Several recent studies indicate that the A kinase plays a key role in determining if a neuronal growth cone is attracted or repelled by netrin-1. Elevating the intracellular concentration of cAMP causes A kinase activation (reviewed by Nairn et al., 1985). Utilizing dissociated neurons from embryonic *Xenopus* spinal cord, Ming et al. (1997) demonstrated that A kinase activation is correlated with chemoattraction to netrin-1, while A kinase inhibition switches the

response to repulsion. RhoA is inhibited by A kinase phosphorylation (Lang et al., 1996) and one way that A kinase activation may influence growth cone guidance is to tip the balance of Rho GTPase activation toward generating a chemoattractant response to netrin-1. A straight forward model suggests that activation of Cdc42 and Rac1 promotes axon growth, while activation of RhoA inhibits growth or induces growth cone collapse (Hall, 1998; Mueller, 1999; Song and Poo, 1999). These findings also suggest that if a growth cone encountered an extracellular cue that altered the intracellular concentration of cAMP, the response of the extending axon to netrin-1 might be reversed. In agreement with this, Hopker et al. (1999) found that retinal ganglion cell axons are attracted to a source of netrin-1 but that this response switches to repulsion if netrin-1 is presented with laminin-1. Importantly, laminin-1 produces this effect by lowering the level of cAMP in the neuron. This study highlights the significance of the extracellular context in which netrin-1 encounters a growth cone.

PI3-kinase activation (Ming et al., 1999) has also been implicated in the turning response made by neurons in response to netrin-1. Rac1 is activated by PI3-kinase in some cells types (reviewed by Hall, 1998), but it remains to be determined if PI-3 kinase is a functional intermediate between DCC and Rac1. Together, these studies have led to the hypothesis that netrin-1 shares signal transduction pathways in the growth cone with other cues that influence axon outgrowth such as myelin-associated glycoprotein (MAG) and the neurotrophins, nerve growth factor (NGF) and brain-derived neurotrophic factor (BDNF) (reviewed by Song and Poo, 1999).

Tong et al. (2001) show that both UNC-40 and UNC-5 homologs are phosphorylated on tyrosine residues. Furthermore, tyrosine phosphorylation of UNC-5 family members is enhanced by netrin in a mammalian cell line and in *C. elegans* in vivo. They also demonstrate netrin-dependent binding of the tyrosine phosphatase Shp2 to phospho-Tyr568 in the intracellular domain of UNC-5. Although it is not yet clear how tyrosine phosphorylation may contribute to netrin-dependent attraction or repulsion, this report provides the first indication that tyrosine phosphorylation may be involved in netrin signal transduction.

Further genetic analysis has implicated eight gene products in UNC-5 function in *C. elegans* (Colavita and Culotti, 1998). Not surprisingly, these included the netrin *unc-6* and the *unc-6* receptor *unc-40* (Hedgecock et al., 1987, 1990). The screen also identified *unc-129*, *unc-34* and *unc-44* (Siddiqui and Culotti, 1991; McIntire et al., 1992; Forrester and Garriga, 1997). *Unc-129* encodes a TGF-β growth factor family member expressed by dorsal muscle cells during *C. elegans* development (Colavita et al., 1998) and loss of UNC-129 function produces a phenotype similar to, but less penetrant than, mutation of *unc-5*. Interestingly, UNC-34 is homologous to the Ena/VASP (enabled/vasodilator-stimulated phosphoprotein) protein family that have also been shown to be required for axon guidance in mouse and *D. melanogaster* (Lanier et al., 1999; Wills et al., 1999). The Ena/VASP family interacts with profilin, a protein that regulates the organization of actin (reviewed by Holt and Koffer, 2001). *Unc-44* encodes ankyrin (Otsuka et al., 1995) a protein that links integral membrane proteins to the actin cytoskeleton (reviewed by Bennet and Chen, 2001). It is not known if UNC-5 interacts directly with ankyrin, but the identification of ankyrin provides one component of what may be a protein complex that links netrin outside the cell to intracellular actin. Three additional genes identified in this screen, *seu-1*, *seu-2* and *seu-3*, remain to be further characterized.

Additional roles for netrin receptors: tumor suppressor and pro-apoptotic effectors?

DCC was first identified as a putative tumor suppressor deleted in some forms of colorectal cancer (Fearon et al., 1990; Hedrick et al., 1994). An increase in tumor frequency was not found in *dcc* knockout mice; however the full significance of this finding is difficult to interpret because the mice die shortly after birth and tumors may not have had time to develop (Fazeli et al., 1997). Re-expression of *dcc* in tumor cells has been shown to suppress tumorigenicity (Tanaka et al., 1991; Klingelhutz et al., 1995) and analysis of chromosomal deletions continue to correlate loss of *dcc* expression with tumorigenesis in many types of cancer (Thiagalingam et al., 1996; Hilgers et al., 2000). Correlations made

between *dcc* expression and the phenotypes of primary tumor cells suggest that DCC does not influence tumor formation but inhibits a later step in tumor development, such as tumor cell migration and metastasis (Reale et al., 1996; Kong et al., 1997a,b; Reyes-Mugica et al., 1998). These findings suggest that DCC may function as a tumor suppressor by restraining cell motility. If DCC inhibits cell migration in this context, it may use a mechanism similar to that underlying the repellent action of netrin-1. Although an attractive hypothesis, this remains to be demonstrated. Because of its relationship to DCC, a role for neogenin in tumorigenesis has been investigated, but no changes in its expression have been found (Meyerhardt et al., 1997).

Recent studies of *dcc* over-expression in HEK293T cells suggest that DCC functions as a tumor suppressor by acting as a pro-apoptotic dependence receptor (Mehlen et al., 1998). These authors provide evidence that, in the absence of netrin-1, DCC promotes apoptosis through activation of a novel pro-apoptotic caspase-dependent pathway (Forcet et al., 2001). Chen et al. (1999) confirmed that overexpression of *dcc* induces apoptosis in several carcinoma cell lines; but that netrin-1 did not rescue DCC induced cell death. Furthermore, these authors reported that in some cell lines, overexpression of *dcc* produced cell cycle arrest but not apoptosis.

Mehlen and his colleagues have recently provided evidence that UNC-5 homologs also function as dependence receptors that promote apoptosis in the absence of netrin-1 (Llambi et al., 2001). However, all of the results supporting a pro-apoptotic role for netrin receptors have been obtained using cell lines overexpressing *dcc* or an *unc-5* homolog. Convincing evidence has not been provided that cells expressing physiologically relevant levels of netrin receptors die, either in vitro or in vivo, in the absence of netrin. Furthermore, the proposal that UNC-5 homologs act as pro-apoptotic dependence receptors generates an immediate paradox. The model suggests that when an axon becomes lost and wanders away from a netrin-secreting target, it will be eliminated by an apoptotic mechanism induced by the absence of ligand (Llambi et al., 2001). However, if an UNC-5 homolog functions to appropriately lead a growth cone away from a source of netrin, the model proposed by Llambi et al. (2001) suggests that the neuron extending this correctly migrating axon will by killed due to the absence of ligand. It seems unlikely that UNC-5 homologs function simultaneously as pro-apoptotic dependence receptors and as mediators of the repellent response to netrin.

Long- and short-range actions of netrin-1

Analysis of netrin-1 function during embryogenesis suggests that it can act as a long-range cue or a short-range cue in different circumstances (reviewed by Kennedy, 2000). Several lines of evidence indicate that netrin-1 can function as a long-range cue. First, netrin-1 protein can diffuse away from its source through a collagen matrix in vitro to attract or repel growing axons (Kennedy et al., 1994; Colamarino and Tessier-Lavigne, 1995; Shirasaki et al., 1996; Deiner et al., 1997; Metin et al., 1997; Varela-Echavarria et al., 1997; Wang et al., 1999). Second, axons extending through explants of embryonic neuroepithelium reorient their growth and turn toward an ectopic source of netrin-1 (Kennedy et al., 1994). Growth cones turn up to 250 μm away from the source of netrin-1, suggesting that netrin-1 protein can diffuse through the neuroepithelium for at least this distance. Third, the growth cones of neurons dissociated from the embryonic *Xenopus laevis*

CNS turn when challenged in vitro with a gradient of netrin-1 puffed from a micropipette (de la Torre et al., 1997; Ming et al., 1997). Together, these results support the hypothesis that following secretion, netrin-1 can diffuse several hundred microns and act as a long-range cue to direct axon extension.

Netrins have also been suggested to function as a short-range cue. A target derived short-range function for netrin has been proposed to contribute to the development of nerve–muscle synapses in *D. melanogaster* (Mitchell et al., 1996; Winberg et al., 1998). Netrin-1 expressed by cells at the optic disc also appears to function as a short-range cue for retinal ganglion cell axons as they exit the retina during mouse embryogenesis (Deiner et al., 1997).

Analysis of the subcellular distribution of netrin-1 protein in the adult rat spinal cord demonstrated that the majority of netrin-1 protein is not freely soluble but is associated with ECM or cell membranes (Fig. 2B; Manitt et al., 2001). When netrin-1 was initially purified from embryonic day 10 (E10) chick brains, the axon outgrowth promoting activity corresponding to netrin-1 fractionated as a membrane-associated protein (Serafini et al., 1994), while only very limited activity was present in the fraction containing soluble proteins. Western blot analysis following subcellular fractionation of homogenates

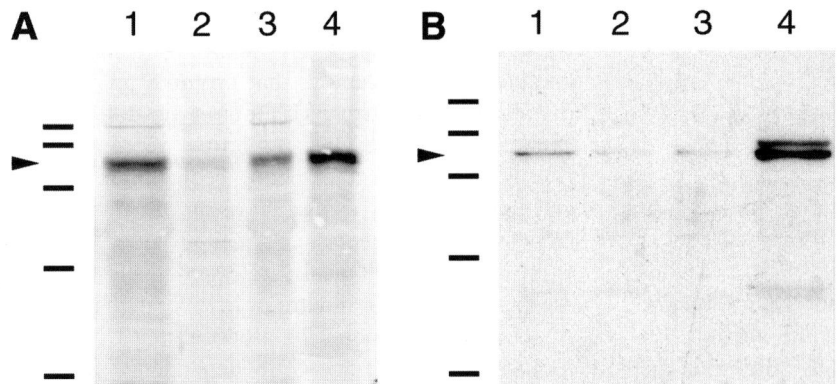

Fig. 2. The majority of netrin-1 protein is not freely soluble in the embryonic or adult CNS. Western blot analysis illustrating the relative enrichment of netrin-1 protein in subcellular fractions of embryonic day 10 chick brain (A) and adult rat spinal cord (B). Fractionation was carried out as described (Manitt et al., 2001). Lane 1 corresponds to a high speed pellet made up of microsomes, cargo proteins inside membrane vesicles, integral membrane proteins, and membrane-associated proteins. Lane 2 corresponds to the high speed supernatant that contains soluble proteins, but relatively little netrin-1. Lanes 3 and 4 are the product of high salt extraction of the high speed pellet, followed by high speed centrifugation to separate membranes from solubilized membrane-associated proteins. Lane 3 contains the high salt extract pellet composed of salt stripped membranes and lane 4 the high salt extract supernatant, containing membrane-associated proteins and the majority of netrin-1 (10% PAGE; ∼20 μg of total protein loaded per lane; Molecular weight markers correspond to 116, 97.4, 66.2, 45, and 31 kDa).

of E10 chick brains confirmed this distribution. The vast majority of netrin-1 protein was found to be membrane-associated with only a small amount of netrin-1 detected in the fraction containing soluble protein (Fig. 2A). These findings suggest that following secretion netrin-1 may not diffuse a great distance, if at all, from the surface of the cells producing it, and that a major function of netrin-1 in the embryonic and adult CNS may be short-range, mediating cell–cell interactions.

If the majority of netrin-1 is not freely soluble following secretion, how might a gradient of netrin-1 in the embryonic neural epithelium be produced? Fig. 3 presents two models illustrating extreme examples of how a graded distribution could be generated around a source of netrin-1. Fig. 3A shows a gradient formed by protein freely diffusing away from the cells that secrete it. However, if netrin-1 binds to cell surfaces and the ECM, this would dramatically limit diffusion. Fig. 3B illustrates an alternative model that incorporates secretion, limited diffusion, cell surface binding, cell division and cell migration in the embryonic neuroepithelium. Here, netrin-1 is secreted and diffuses a short distance from its source, but is rapidly captured on cell surfaces. As these cells divide and migrate they dilute the concentration of netrin-1 on their surface, generating a graded distribution of netrin-1 protein that extends many cell diameters away from the source. Via this mechanism, a protein can function as a long-range cue in the absence of long distance diffusion in an environment like the developing CNS. It is important to note that these models are caricatures of extremes. The distribution of netrin protein in the embryonic CNS in vivo is likely to result from a combination of secretion, limited diffusion, and redistribution on the surface of migrating cells. Due to very limited cell migration in the adult CNS, this model predicts that netrin-1 would predominantly function as a short-range cell and ECM-associated cue (Manitt et al., 2001).

Expression of netrins and netrin receptors in the adult CNS

Netrins and netrin receptors are expressed in the adult CNS and PNS (Kennedy et al., 1994; Livesey and Hunt, 1997; Volenec et al., 1997, 1998; Madison et al., 2000; Petrausch et al., 2000; Ellezam et al., 2001; Manitt et al., 2001). Netrin-1 expression has been well documented in motoneurons, spinal sensory interneurons (Manitt et al., 2001), and in retinal ganglion cells in the eye (Ellezam et al., 2001). In addition, *netrin-1* is expressed by myelinating glia: Schwann cells in the PNS (Madison et al., 2000; Ellezam et al., 2001) and oligodendro-

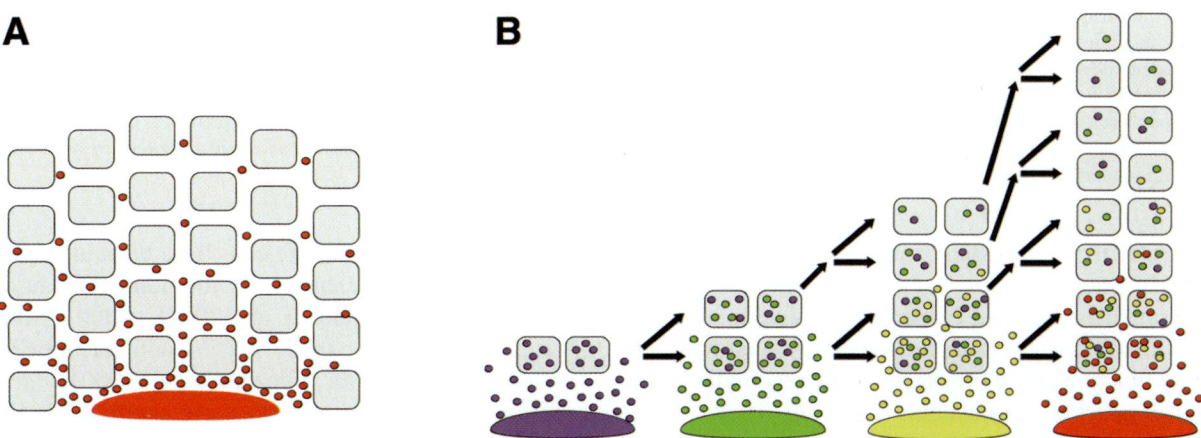

Fig. 3. Several mechanisms could contribute to generating a graded distribution of netrin-1 in the embryonic neural tube. (A) Netrin protein (red) freely diffusing away from a source of netrin secreting cells. Unlike this model, most netrin protein is not freely soluble in vivo (see Fig. 2). In B, netrin protein diffuses away from its source but is rapidly captured on the surface of proliferating cells. As these cells divide and migrate, they both dilute the concentration of netrin on their surface and carry the protein away from its source, generating a graded distribution of protein bound to cell surfaces. The different colors in B represent netrin protein secreted from the source at different time points.

436

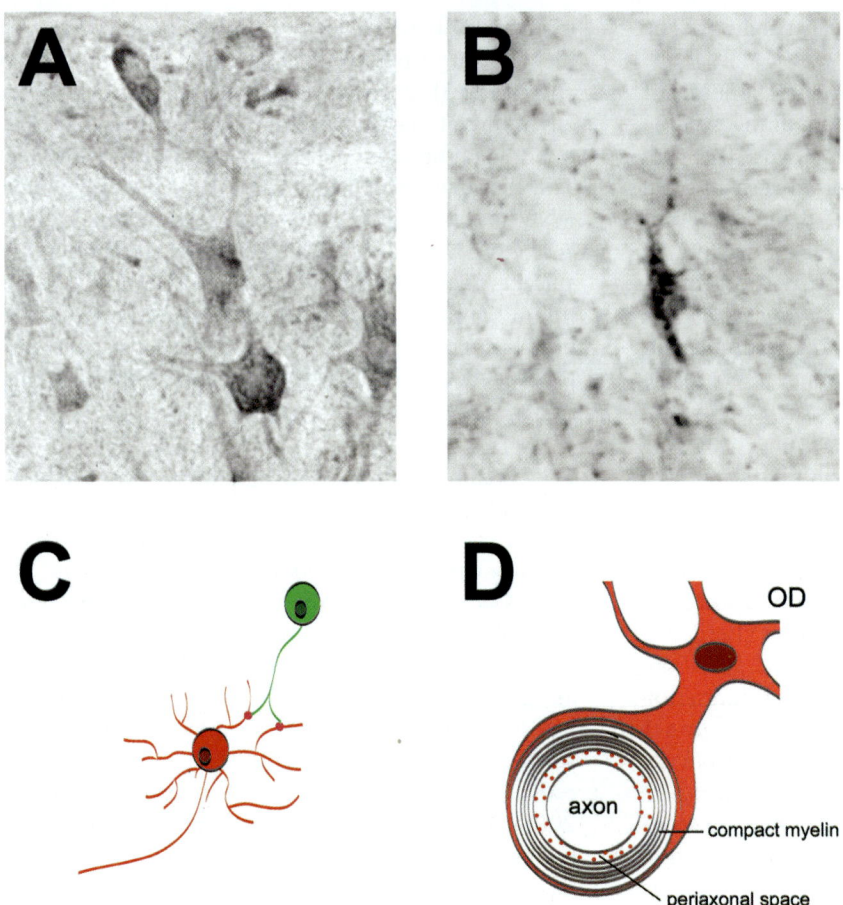

Fig. 4. Distribution of netrin-1 associated with neurons and oligodendroglia in the adult spinal cord. (A) Neuronal netrin-1 immunoreactivity in adult rat spinal cord, showing staining of the cell body, neurites, and neuropil. (B) Netrin-1 immunoreactivity associated with an oligodendrocyte in adult rat spinal cord white matter. The cell body and processes are netrin-1 immunoreactive. Subcellular fractionation suggests that netrin-1 is enriched in periaxonal myelin (Manitt et al., 2001) the interface between axons and oligodendrocytes (OD). Cartoons in C and D illustrate how netrin (red) presented on cell membranes may contribute to mediating cell–cell contacts such as synaptic connections (C) or axon oligodendroglial interactions (D). In D, illustrating the presence of netrin-1 protein in periaxonal myelin, the cell body, axon, and compact myelin are not drawn to scale.

cytes in the CNS (Manitt et al., 2001). Subcellular fractionation of white matter indicates that netrin-1 protein is enriched in periaxonal myelin (Manitt et al., 2001), supporting the hypothesis that netrin-1 may function as a short-range cue that mediates cell–cell interactions in the adult CNS (Fig. 4). *Netrin-3*, *netrin-4/βnetrin*, and *netrin-G1* are all expressed in the adult brain, but the cell types involved have not been identified (Wang et al., 1999; Koch et al., 2000; Nakashiba et al., 2000).

Dopaminergic neurons of the substantia nigra compacta (Volenec et al., 1998), retinal ganglion

cells, and retinal amacrine cells have been identified as *dcc* expressing neurons in the adult (Petrausch et al., 2000; Ellezam et al., 2001). Adult retinal ganglion cells also express *unc5h1* and *unc5h2* (Petrausch et al., 2000; Ellezam et al., 2001). *dcc*, *neogenin*, and *unc-5* homologs are expressed in the adult rat spinal cord (Manitt and Kennedy, unpublished observations). Interestingly, the relative level of expression of *unc-5* homologs compared to *dcc* in the adult is greater than in the embryo.

A limited number of studies have addressed the functional role of netrin protein produced by neurons. Netrin-1 immunoreactivity is associated with neurites in the adult CNS (Fig. 4), but it is not clear if netrin-1 is secreted from neurons via dendrites, axons, or both, or if the protein is secreted by neighboring cells and then captured on the neuronal surface. Netrin-1 produced by a neuron might signal neighboring cells or, alternatively, function as an autocrine cue. During neural development in *C. elegans*, some pioneer neurons that extend an axon in response to a source of netrin/UNC-6 later express *unc-6* themselves and this neuronal source of UNC-6 influences the growth of other axons (Wadsworth et al., 1996). Furthermore, analysis of the distribution of netrin protein in *D. melanogaster* revealed that the fly homolog of DCC, frazzled, can capture netrin protein and present it on axonal surfaces where it acts as a guidance cue for other axons (Hiramoto et al., 2000). These findings indicate that netrin presented on the surface of a neuron can influence a neighboring cell and that the distribution of netrin receptors may localize and present netrin protein to nearby cells. Interestingly, in *D. melanogaster*, netrin has been shown to function as a target derived cue regulating synapse formation (Mitchell et al., 1996; Winberg et al., 1998). Although the distribution of netrin protein in the mammalian CNS suggests that it is associated with neurites (Fig. 4), a role for netrin at the synapse has not been demonstrated. Additional studies will be required to reveal the function of netrin produced by neurons in the adult mammalian CNS.

Netrin and netrin receptor expression following CNS injury

Although many CNS neurons have the capacity to regenerate a severed axon (David and Aguayo, 1981) the onset of myelination in the mammalian CNS coincides with a dramatic drop in the ability of injured axons to regenerate. Substantial evidence indicates that CNS white matter contains factors that inhibit axon outgrowth (reviewed by Schwab et al., 1993) and multiple inhibitory components of myelin have been identified (McKerracher et al., 1994; Mukhopadhyay et al., 1994; Chen et al., 2000; GrandPre et al., 2000; Prinjha et al., 2000). The expression of netrin-1 by oligodendrocytes in the adult CNS raises the possibility that netrin-1 may be a

myelin-associated inhibitor of axonal regeneration. If this is the case, neurons attempting to regenerate following injury would be predicted to express members of the *unc-5* homolog family of netrin receptors. Ellezam et al. (2001) report that both *dcc* and *unc5h2* expression persists, albeit downregulated, in axotomized retinal ganglion cell neurons as they attempt to regenerate into the optic nerve or into a peripheral nerve graft, both of which contain netrin-1 expressing cells (Madison et al., 2000; Petrausch et al., 2000; Ellezam et al., 2001). Interestingly, a study carried out in lamprey, a primitive vertebrate with the capacity to recover significant function following transection of its spinal cord (Cohen et al., 1988), reports a correlation between the expression of *unc-5* by neurons and poor axonal regeneration following injury (Shifman and Selzer, 2000b). It may be the case that the relative level of *dcc* and *unc-5* homolog receptors expressed by a neuron influences how the axon responds to netrin-1. It is intriguing that the relative level of UNC-5 homolog expression increases in the adult spinal cord and the level of DCC expression decreases when compared to the embryonic CNS (Manitt and Kennedy, unpublished observations) suggesting that a repellent function may be the dominant action of netrin-1 in the adult CNS.

An additional series of observations supports the suggestion that netrin-1 functions as a repellent in the adult CNS. As described above, the intracellular level of cAMP in a neuron can modulate the response to netrin-1: high levels of cAMP associated with attraction and low levels with repulsion (Ming et al., 1997). During late embryonic and early postnatal development, the intracellular concentration of cAMP is downregulated in neurons (Cai et al., 2001). This correlates with the loss of the capacity of these neurons to regenerate an axon in the presence of myelin or myelin-associated proteins, such as MAG. Furthermore, lowering the concentration of cAMP in neurons in the early postnatal rat spinal cord blocked their ability to regenerate in vivo (Cai et al., 2001). Consistent with this, increasing the level of intracellular cAMP can overcome the inhibition of axon outgrowth exerted by MAG and myelin in vitro (Ming et al., 2001). Extracellular cues, such as laminin-1, can lower the level of cAMP and shift the response to netrin-1 from attraction to repulsion. An attractive hypothesis is that a component of myelin lowers the axonal concentration of cAMP during maturation, changing the response of growth cones to myelin-associated proteins. As such, netrin-1 may be one of several components of the extracellular milieu associated with myelin that inhibits axon extension.

Although we have focused on the possibility that netrin-1 may inhibit axon regeneration, it may equally be the case that netrin-1 promotes axonal regeneration following injury. Perhaps the most likely scenario is that netrin-1 will continue to act as it does during embryogenesis, inhibiting the regeneration of some classes of axons and promoting the regeneration of others. This may depend on the intracellular state of second-messenger systems in the neurons involved, the presence of components of the ECM that modulate the response to netrin-1, and the type and relative number of netrin-1 receptors present on the surface of the axons attempting to regenerate. Future studies will determine how netrin-1, a potent axon guidance cue in the embryonic nervous system, influences axon regeneration in the adult mammalian CNS following injury.

Acknowledgements

We thank Cecilia Flores, Adriana Di Polo, Katherine M. Thompson, Jean-Francois Bouchard, Andrew Jarjour and Masoud Shekarabi for comments on the manuscript, Phil H. Crossley for helpful discussions about gradients, and Phil A. Barker for assistance with analysis of molecular phylogeny. This research was supported by the Canadian Institutes of Health Research (CIHR), The Paralyzed Veterans of America Spinal Cord Research Foundation, and the Multiple Sclerosis Society of Canada. T.E.K. is a scholar of the CIHR.

References

Ackerman, S.L. and Knowles, B.B. (1998) Cloning and mapping of the UNC5C gene to human chromosome 4q21–q23. *Genomics*, 52: 205–208.

Ackerman, S.L., Kozak, L.P., Przyborski, S.A., Rund, L.A., Boyer, B.B. and Knowles, B.B. (1997) The mouse rostral cerebellar malformation gene encodes an UNC-5-like protein. *Nature*, 386: 838–842.

Alcantara, S., Ruiz, M., De Castro, F., Soriano, E. and Sotelo, C. (2000) Netrin 1 acts as an attractive or as a repulsive cue for distinct migrating neurons during the development of the cerebellar system. *Development*, 127: 1359–1372.

Altman, J. and Bayer, S.A. (1984) The development of the rat spinal cord. *Adv. Anat. Embryol. Cell Biol.*, 85: 1–164.

Banyai, L. and Patthy, L. (1999) The NTR module: domains of netrins, secreted frizzled related proteins, and type I procollagen C-proteinase enhancer protein are homologous with tissue inhibitors of metalloproteases. *Protein Sci.*, 8: 1636–1642.

Bennet, V. and Chen, L. (2001) Ankyrins and cellular targeting of diverse membrane proteins to physiological sites. *Curr. Opin. Cell Biol.*, 13: 61–67.

Bentley, D. and O'Connor, T.P. (1994) Cytoskeletal events in growth cone steering. *Curr. Opin. Neurobiol.*, 4: 43–48.

Bloch-Gallego, E., Ezan, F., Tessier-Lavigne, M. and Sotelo, C. (1999) Floor plate and netrin-1 are involved in the migration and survival of inferior olivary neurons. *J. Neurosci.*, 19: 4407–4420.

Cai, D., Qiu, J., Cao, Z., McAtee, M., Bregman, B.S. and Filbin, M.T. (2001) Neuronal cyclic AMP controls the developmental loss in ability of axons to regenerate. *J. Neurosci.*, 21: 4731–4739.

Chan, S.S., Zheng, H., Su, M.W., Wilk, R., Killeen, M.T., Hedgecock, E.M. and Culotti, J.G. (1996) UNC-40, a *C. elegans* homolog of DCC (Deleted in Colorectal Cancer), is required in motile cells responding to UNC-6 netrin cues. *Cell*, 87: 187–195.

Chen, M.S., Huber, A.B., van der Haar, M.E., Frank, M., Schnell, L., Spillmann, A.A., Christ, F. and Schwab, M.E. (2000) Nogo-A is a myelin-associated neurite outgrowth inhibitor and an antigen for monoclonal antibody IN-1. *Nature*, 403: 434–439.

Chen, Y.Q., Hsieh, J.T., Yao, F., Fang, B., Pong, R.C., Cipriano, S.C. and Krepulat, F. (1999) Induction of apoptosis and G2/M cell cycle arrest by DCC. *Oncogene*, 18: 2747–2754.

Chien, C.B., Rosenthal, D.E., Harris, W.A. and Holt, C.E. (1993) Navigational errors made by growth cones without filopodia in the embryonic *Xenopus* brain. *Neuron*, 11: 237–251.

Chuong, C.M., Jiang, T.X., Yin, E. and Widelitz, R.B. (1994) cDCC (chicken homologue to a gene deleted in colorectal carcinoma) is an epithelial adhesion molecule expressed in the basal cells and involved in epithelial–mesenchymal interaction. *Dev. Biol.*, 164: 383–397.

Cohen, A.H., Mackler, S.A. and Selzer, M.E. (1988) Behavioral recovery following spinal transection: functional regeneration in the lamprey CNS. *Trends Neurosci.*, 11: 227–231.

Colamarino, S.A. and Tessier-Lavigne, M. (1995) The axonal chemoattractant netrin-1 is also a chemorepellent for trochlear motor axons. *Cell*, 81: 621–629.

Colavita, A. and Culotti, J.G. (1998) Suppressors of ectopic UNC-5 growth cone steering identify eight genes involved in axon guidance in *Caenorhabditis elegans*. *Dev. Biol.*, 194: 72–85.

Colavita, A., Krishna, S., Zheng, H., Padgett, R.W. and Culotti, J.G. (1998) Pioneer axon guidance by UNC-129, a *C. elegans* TGF-beta. *Science*, 281: 706–709.

Cooper, H.M., Armes, P., Britto, J., Gad, J. and Wilks, A.F. (1995) Cloning of the mouse homologue of the deleted in colorectal cancer gene (mDCC) and its expression in the developing mouse embryo. *Oncogene*, 11: 2243–2254.

Corset, V., Nguyen-Ba-Charvet, K.T., Forcet, C., Moyse, E., Chedotal, A. and Mehlen, P. (2000) Netrin-1-mediated axon outgrowth and cAMP production requires interaction with adenosine A2b receptor. *Nature*, 407: 747–750.

David, S. and Aguayo, A.J. (1981) Axonal elongation into peripheral nervous system 'bridges' after central nervous system injury in adult rats. *Science*, 214: 931–933.

de la Torre, J.R., Hopker, V.H., Ming, G.L., Poo, M.M., Tessier-Lavigne, M., Hemmati-Brivanlou, A. and Holt, C.E. (1997) Turning of retinal growth cones in a netrin-1 gradient mediated by the netrin receptor DCC. *Neuron*, 19: 1211-1224.

Deiner, M.S., Kennedy, T.E., Fazeli, A., Serafini, T., Tessier-Lavigne, M. and Sretavan, D.W. (1997) Netrin-1 and DCC mediate axon guidance locally at the optic disc: loss of function leads to optic nerve hypoplasia. *Neuron*, 19: 575–589.

Dickson, B.J. (2001) Rho GTPases in growth cone guidance. *Curr. Opin. Neurobiol.*, 11: 103–110.

Ellezam, B., Selles-Navarro, I., Manitt, C., Kennedy, T.E. and McKerracher, L. (2001) Expression of netrin-1 and its receptors DCC and UNC5H2 after axotomy and during regeneration of adult rat retinal ganglion cells. *Exp. Neurol.*, 168: 105–115.

Fazeli, A., Dickinson, S.L., Hermiston, M.L., Tighe, R.V., Steen, R.G., Small, C.G., Stoeckli, E.T., Keino-Masu, K., Masu, M., Rayburn, H., Simons, J., Bronson, R.T., Gordon, J.I., Tessier-Lavigne, M. and Weinberg, R.A. (1997) Phenotype of mice lacking functional Deleted in colorectal cancer (dcc) gene. *Nature*, 386: 796–804.

Fearon, E.R., Cho, K.R., Nigro, J.M., Kern, S.E., Simons, J.W., Ruppert, J.M., Hamilton, S.R., Preisinger, A.C., Thomas, G. and Kinzler, K.W. (1990) Identification of a chromosome 18q gene that is altered in colorectal cancers. *Science*, 247: 49–56.

Forcet, C., Ye, X., Granger, L., Corset, V., Shin, H., Bredesen, D.E. and Mehlen, P. (2001) The dependence receptor DCC (deleted in colorectal cancer) defines an alternative mechanism for caspase activation. *Proc. Natl. Acad. Sci. USA*, 98: 3416–3421.

Forrester, W.C. and Garriga, G. (1997) Genes necessary for *C. elegans* cell and growth cone migrations. *Development*, 124: 1831–1843.

Gan, W.B., Wong, V.Y., Phillips, A., Ma, C., Gershon, T.R. and Macagno, E.R. (1999) Cellular expression of a leech netrin suggests roles in the formation of longitudinal nerve tracts and in regional innervation of peripheral targets. *J. Neurobiol.*, 40: 103–115.

GrandPre, T., Nakamura, F., Vartanian, T. and Strittmatter, S.M. (2000) Identification of the Nogo inhibitor of axon regeneration as a Reticulon protein. *Nature*, 403: 439–444.

Hall, A. (1998) Rho GTPases and the actin cytoskeleton. *Science*, 279: 509–514.

Hamasaki, T., Goto, S., Nishikawa, S. and Ushio, Y. (2001) A role of netrin-1 in the formation of the subcortical structure striatum: repulsive action on the migration of late-born striatal neurons. *J. Neurosci.*, 21: 4272–4280.

Hamelin, M., Zhou, Y., Su, M.W., Scott, I.M. and Culotti, J.G. (1993) Expression of the UNC-5 guidance receptor in the touch neurons of *C. elegans* steers their axons dorsally. *Nature*, 364: 327–330.

Harris, R., Sabatelli, L.M. and Seeger, M.A. (1996) Guidance cues at the *Drosophila* CNS midline: identification and characterization of two *Drosophila* Netrin/UNC-6 homologs. *Neuron*, 17: 217–228.

Hedgecock, E.M., Culotti, J.G., Hall, D.H. and Stern, B.D. (1987) Genetics of cell and axon migrations in *Caenorhabditis elegans*. *Development*, 100: 365–382.

Hedgecock, E.M., Culotti, J.G. and Hall, D.H. (1990) The unc-5, unc-6, and unc-40 genes guide circumferential migrations of pioneer axons and mesodermal cells on the epidermis in *C. elegans*. *Neuron*, 4: 61–85.

Hedrick, L., Cho, K.R., Fearon, E.R., Wu, T.C., Kinzler, K.W. and Vogelstein, B. (1994) The DCC gene product in cellular differentiation and colorectal tumorigenesis. *Genes Dev.*, 8: 1174–1183.

Hilgers, W., Song, J.J., Haye, M., Hruban, R.R., Kern, S.E. and Fearon, E.R. (2000) Homozygous deletions inactivate DCC, but not MADH4/DPC4/SMAD4, in a subset of pancreatic and biliary cancers. *Genes Chrom. Cancer*, 27: 353–357.

Hiramoto, M., Hiromi, Y., Giniger, E. and Hotta, Y. (2000) The *Drosophila* Netrin receptor Frazzled guides axons by controlling Netrin distribution. *Nature*, 406: 886–889.

Hjorth, J.T., Gad, J., Cooper, H. and Key, B. (2001) A zebrafish homologue of deleted in colorectal cancer (zdcc) is expressed in the first neuronal clusters of the developing brain. *Mech. Dev.*, 109: 105–109.

Hofmann, K. and Tschopp, J. (1995) The death domain motif found in Fas (Apo-1) and TNF receptor is present in proteins involved in apoptosis and axonal guidance. *FEBS Lett.*, 371: 321–323.

Holt, M.R. and Koffer, A. (2001) Cell motility: proline-rich proteins promote protrusions. *Trends Cell Biol.*, 11: 38–46.

Hong, K., Hinck, L., Nishiyama, M., Poo, M.M., Tessier-Lavigne, M. and Stein, E. (1999) A ligand-gated association between cytoplasmic domains of UNC5 and DCC family receptors converts netrin-induced growth cone attraction to repulsion. *Cell*, 97: 927–941.

Hong, K., Nishiyama, M., Henley, J., Tessier-Lavigne, M. and Poo, M. (2000) Calcium signalling in the guidance of nerve growth by netrin-1. *Nature*, 403: 93–98.

Hopker, V.H., Shewan, D., Tessier-Lavigne, M., Poo, M. and Holt, C. (1999) Growth-cone attraction to netrin-1 is converted to repulsion by laminin-1. *Nature*, 401: 69–73.

Ishii, N., Wadsworth, W.G., Stern, B.D., Culotti, J.G. and Hedgecock, E.M. (1992) UNC-6, a laminin-related protein, guides cell and pioneer axon migrations in *C. elegans*. *Neuron*, 9: 873–881.

Kappler, J., Franken, S., Junghans, U., Hoffmann, R., Linke, T., Muller, H.W. and Koch, K.W. (2000) Glycosaminoglycan-binding properties and secondary structure of the C-terminus of netrin-1. *Biochem. Biophys. Res. Commun.*, 271: 287–291.

Keeling, S.L., Gad, J.M. and Cooper, H.M. (1997) Mouse Neogenin, a DCC-like molecule, has four splice variants and is expressed widely in the adult mouse and during embryogenesis. *Oncogene*, 15: 691–700.

Keino-Masu, K., Masu, M., Hinck, L., Leonardo, E.D., Chan, S.S., Culotti, J.G. and Tessier-Lavigne, M. (1996) Deleted in Colorectal Cancer (DCC) encodes a netrin receptor. *Cell*, 87: 175–185.

Keleman, K. and Dickson, B.J. (2001) Short- and long-range repulsion by the *Drosophila* unc5 netrin receptor. *Neuron*, 32: 605–617.

Kennedy, T.E. (2000) Cellular mechanisms of netrin function: long-range and short-range actions. *Biochem. Cell Biol.*, 78: 569–575.

Kennedy, T.E., Serafini, T., de la Torre, J.R. and Tessier-Lavigne, M. (1994) Netrins are diffusible chemotropic factors for commissural axons in the embryonic spinal cord. *Cell*, 78: 425–435.

Kim, S., Ren, X.C., Fox, E. and Wadsworth, W.G. (1999) SDQR migrations in *Caenorhabditis elegans* are controlled by multiple guidance cues and changing responses to netrin UNC-6. *Development*, 126: 3881–3890.

Klingelhutz, A.J., Hedrick, L., Cho, K.R. and McDougall, J.K. (1995) The DCC gene suppresses the malignant phenotype of transformed human epithelial cells. *Oncogene*, 10: 1581–1586.

Koch, M., Murrell, J.R., Hunter, D.D., Olson, P.F., Jin, W., Keene, D.R., Brunken, W.J. and Burgeson, R.E. (2000) A novel member of the netrin family, beta-netrin, shares homology with the beta chain of laminin: identification, expression, and functional characterization. *J. Cell Biol.*, 151: 221–234.

Kolodziej, P.A., Timpe, L.C., Mitchell, K.J., Fried, S.R., Goodman, C.S., Jan, L.Y. and Jan, Y.N. (1996) frazzled encodes a *Drosophila* member of the DCC immunoglobulin subfamily and is required for CNS and motor axon guidance. *Cell*, 87: 197–204.

Kong, X.T., Choi, S.H., Inoue, A., Takita, J., Yokota, J., Hanada, R., Yamamoto, K., Bessho, F., Yanagisawa, M. and Hayashi, Y. (1997a) Alterations of the tumour suppressor gene DCC in neuroblastoma. *Eur. J. Cancer*, 33: 1962–1965.

Kong, X.T., Choi, S.H., Inoue, A., Xu, F., Chen, T., Takita, J., Yokota, J., Bessho, F., Yanagisawa, M., Hanada, R., Yamamoto, K. and Hayashi, Y. (1997b) Expression and mutational analysis of the DCC, DPC4, and MADR2/JV18-1 genes in neuroblastoma. *Cancer Res.*, 57: 3772–3778.

Lang, P., Gesbert, F., Delespine-Carmagnat, M., Stancou, R., Pouchelet, M. and Bertoglio, J. (1996) Protein kinase A phosphorylation of RhoA mediates the morphological and functional effects of cyclic AMP in cytotoxic lymphocytes. *EMBO J.*, 15: 510–519.

Lanier, L.M., Gates, M.A., Witke, W., Menzies, A.S., Wehman, A.M., Macklis, J.D., Kwiatkowski, D., Soriano, P. and Gertler, F.B. (1999) Mena is required for neurulation and commissure formation. *Neuron*, 22: 313–325.

Lauderdale, J.D., Davis, N.M. and Kuwada, J.Y. (1997) Axon tracts correlate with netrin-1a expression in the zebrafish embryo. *Mol. Cell. Neurosci.*, 9: 293–313.

Leonardo, E.D., Hinck, L., Masu, M., Keino-Masu, K., Ackerman, S.L. and Tessier-Lavigne, M. (1997) Vertebrate homologues of *C. elegans* UNC-5 are candidate netrin receptors. *Nature*, 386: 833–838.

Leung-Hagesteijn, C., Spence, A.M., Stern, B.D., Zhou, Y., Su,

M.W., Hedgecock, E.M. and Culotti, J.G. (1992) UNC-5, a transmembrane protein with immunoglobulin and thrombospondin type 1 domains, guides cell and pioneer axon migrations in *C. elegans*. *Cell*, 71: 289–299.

Livesey, F.J. and Hunt, S.P. (1997) Netrin and netrin receptor expression in the embryonic mammalian nervous system suggests roles in retinal, striatal, nigral, and cerebellar development. *Mol. Cell. Neurosci.*, 8: 417–429.

Llambi, F., Causeret, F., Bloch-Gallego, E. and Mehlen, P. (2001) Netrin-1 acts as a survival factor via its receptors UNC5H and DCC. *EMBO J.*, 20: 2715–2722.

MacDonald, R., Scholes, J., Strahle, U., Brennan, C., Holder, N., Brand, M. and Wilson, S.W. (1997) The Pax protein Noi is required for commissural axon pathway formation in the rostral forebrain. *Development*, 124: 2397–2408.

Madison, R.D., Zomorodi, A. and Robinson, G.A. (2000) Netrin-1 and peripheral nerve regeneration in the adult rat. *Exp. Neurol.*, 161: 563–570.

Manitt, C., Colicos, M.A., Thompson, K.M., Rousselle, E., Peterson, A.C. and Kennedy, T.E. (2001) Widespread expression of netrin-1 by neurons and oligodendrocytes in the adult mammalian spinal cord. *J. Neurosci.*, 21: 3911–3922.

McIntire, S.L., Garriga, G., White, J., Jacobson, D. and Horvitz, H.R. (1992) Genes necessary for directed axonal elongation or fasciculation in *C. elegans*. *Neuron*, 8: 307–322.

McKerracher, L., David, S., Jackson, D.L., Kottis, V., Dunn, R.J. and Braun, P.E. (1994) Identification of myelin-associated glycoprotein as a major myelin-derived inhibitor of neurite growth. *Neuron*, 13: 805–811.

Mehlen, P., Rabizadeh, S., Snipas, S.J., Assa-Munt, N., Salvesen, G.S. and Bredesen, D.E. (1998) The DCC gene product induces apoptosis by a mechanism requiring receptor proteolysis. *Nature*, 395: 801–804.

Merz, D.C., Zheng, H., Killeen, M.T., Krizus, A. and Culotti, J.G. (2001) Multiple signaling mechanisms of the UNC-6/netrin receptors UNC-5 and UNC-40/DCC in vivo. *Genetics*, 158: 1071–1080.

Metin, C., Deleglise, D., Serafini, T., Kennedy, T.E. and Tessier-Lavigne, M. (1997) A role for netrin-1 in the guidance of cortical efferents. *Development*, 124: 5063–5074.

Meyerhardt, J.A., Look, A.T., Bigner, S.H. and Fearon, E.R. (1997) Identification and characterization of neogenin, a DCC-related gene. *Oncogene*, 14: 1129–1136.

Ming, G., Song, H., Berninger, B., Inagaki, N., Tessier-Lavigne, M. and Poo, M. (1999) Phospholipase C-gamma and phosphoinositide 3-kinase mediate cytoplasmic signaling in nerve growth cone guidance. *Neuron*, 23: 139–148.

Ming, G., Henley, J., Tessier-Lavigne, M., Song, H. and Poo, M. (2001) Electrical activity modulates growth cone guidance by diffusible factors. *Neuron*, 29: 441–452.

Ming, G.L., Song, H.J., Berninger, B., Holt, C.E., Tessier-Lavigne, M. and Poo, M.M. (1997) cAMP-dependent growth cone guidance by netrin-1. *Neuron*, 19: 1225–1235.

Mitchell, K.J., Doyle, J.L., Serafini, T., Kennedy, T.E., Tessier-Lavigne, M., Goodman, C.S. and Dickson, B.J. (1996) Genetic analysis of Netrin genes in *Drosophila*: netrins guide CNS commissural axons and peripheral motor axons. *Neuron*, 17: 203–215.

Mitchison, T.J. and Cramer, L.P. (1996) Actin-based cell motility and cell locomotion. *Cell*, 84: 371–379.

Mueller, B.K. (1999) Growth cone guidance: first steps towards a deeper understanding. *Annu. Rev. Neurosci.*, 22: 351–388.

Mukhopadhyay, G., Doherty, P., Walsh, F.S., Crocker, P.R. and Filbin, M.T. (1994) A novel role for myelin-associated glycoprotein as an inhibitor of axonal regeneration. *Neuron*, 13: 757–767.

Nairn, A.C., Hemmings Jr., H.C. and Greengard, P. (1985) Protein kinases in the brain. *Annu. Rev. Biochem.*, 54: 931–976.

Nakashiba, T., Ikeda, T., Nishimura, S., Tashiro, K., Honjo, T., Culotti, J.G. and Itohara, S. (2000) Netrin-G1: a novel glycosyl phosphatidylinositol-linked mammalian netrin that is functionally divergent from classical netrins. *J. Neurosci.*, 20: 6540–6550.

O'Connor, T.P., Duerr, J.S. and Bentley, D. (1990) Pioneer growth cone steering decisions mediated by single filopodial contacts in situ. *J. Neurosci.*, 10: 3935–3946.

Otsuka, A.J., Franco, R., Yang, B., Shim, K.H., Tang, L.Z., Zhang, Y.Y., Boontrakulpoontawee, P., Jeyaprakash, A., Hedgecock, E. and Wheaton, V.I. (1995) An ankyrin-related gene (unc-44) is necessary for proper axonal guidance in *Caenorhabditis elegans*. *J. Cell Biol.*, 129: 1081–1092.

Petrausch, B., Jung, M., Leppert, C.A. and Stuermer, C.A. (2000) Lesion-induced regulation of netrin receptors and modification of netrin-1 expression in the retina of fish and grafted rats. *Mol. Cell. Neurosci.*, 16: 350–364.

Pierceall, W.E., Reale, M.A., Candia, A.F., Wright, C.V., Cho, K.R. and Fearon, E.R. (1994) Expression of a homologue of the deleted in colorectal cancer (DCC) gene in the nervous system of developing *Xenopus* embryos. *Dev. Biol.*, 166: 654–665.

Placzek, M., Tessier-Lavigne, M., Jessell, T. and Dodd, J. (1990) Orientation of commissural axons in vitro in response to a floor plate-derived chemoattractant. *Development*, 110: 19–30.

Prinjha, R., Moore, S.E., Vinson, M., Blake, S., Morrow, R., Christie, G., Michalovich, D., Simmons, D.L. and Walsh, F.S. (2000) Inhibitor of neurite outgrowth in humans. *Nature*, 403: 383–384.

Przyborski, S.A., Knowles, B.B. and Ackerman, S.L. (1998) Embryonic phenotype of Unc5h3 mutant mice suggests chemorepulsion during the formation of the rostral cerebellar boundary. *Development*, 125: 41–50.

Ramon y Cajal, S. (1909) *Histologie du System Nerveux de l'Homme et des Vertebres*. Consejo Superior de investigaciones Cientificas, Madrid.

Reale, M.A., Hu, G., Zafar, A.I., Getzenberg, R.H., Levine, S.M. and Fearon E.R. (1994) Expression and alternative splicing of the deleted in colorectal cancer (DCC) gene in normal and malignant tissues. *Cancer Res.*, 54: 4493–4501.

Reale, M.A., Reyes-Mugica, M., Pierceall, W.E., Rubinstein, M.C., Hedrick, L., Cohn, S.L., Nakagawara, A., Brodeur, G.M. and Fearon, E.R. (1996) Loss of DCC expression in neuroblastoma is associated with disease dissemination. *Clin. Cancer Res.*, 2: 1097–1102.

Reyes-Mugica, M., Lin, P., Yokota, J. and Reale, M.A. (1998) Status of deleted in colorectal cancer gene expression correlates with neuroblastoma metastasis. *Lab. Invest.*, 78: 669–675.

Salbaum, J.M. (1998) Punc, a novel mouse gene of the immunoglobulin superfamily, is expressed predominantly in the developing nervous system. *Mech. Dev.*, 71: 201–204.

Salbaum, J.M. and Kappen, C. (2000) Cloning and expression of nope, a new mouse gene of the immunoglobulin superfamily related to guidance receptors. *Genomics*, 64: 15–23.

Sandoval, A., Ai, R., Ostresh, J.M. and Ogata, R.T. (2000) Distal recognition site for classical pathway convertase located in the C345C/netrin module of complement component C5. *J. Immunol.*, 165: 1066–1073.

Schwab, M.E., Kapfhammer, J.P. and Bandtlow, C.E. (1993) Inhibitors of neurite growth. *Annu. Rev. Neurosci.*, 16: 565–595.

Serafini, T., Kennedy, T.E., Galko, M.J., Mirzayan, C., Jessell, T.M. and Tessier-Lavigne, M. (1994) The netrins define a family of axon outgrowth-promoting proteins homologous to *C. elegans* UNC-6. *Cell*, 78: 409–424.

Serafini, T., Colamarino, S.A., Leonardo, E.D., Wang, H., Beddington, R., Skarnes, W.C. and Tessier-Lavigne, M. (1996) Netrin-1 is required for commissural axon guidance in the developing vertebrate nervous system. *Cell*, 87: 1001–1014.

Shekarabi, M. and Kennedy, T.E. (2002) The netrin-1 receptor DCC promotes filopodia formation and cell spreading by activating Cdc42 and Rac1. *Mol. Cell. Neurosci.*, 19: 1–17.

Shifman, M.I. and Selzer, M.E. (2000a) In situ hybridization in wholemounted lamprey spinal cord: localization of netrin mRNA expression. *J. Neurosci. Methods*, 104: 19–25.

Shifman, M.I. and Selzer, M.E. (2000b) Expression of the netrin receptor UNC-5 in lamprey brain: modulation by spinal cord transection. *Neurorehabil. Neural Repair*, 14: 49–58.

Shimeld, S. (2000) An amphioxus netrin gene is expressed in midline structures during embryonic and larval development. *Dev. Genes Evol.*, 210: 337–344.

Shirasaki, R., Tamada, A., Katsumata, R. and Murakami, F. (1995) Guidance of cerebellofugal axons in the rat embryo: directed growth toward the floor plate and subsequent elongation along the longitudinal axis. *Neuron*, 14: 961–972.

Shirasaki, R., Mirzayan, C., Tessier-Lavigne, M. and Murakami, F. (1996) Guidance of circumferentially growing axons by netrin-dependent and – independent floor plate chemotropism in the vertebrate brain. *Neuron*, 17: 1079–1088.

Siddiqui, S.S. and Culotti, J.G. (1991) Examination of neurons in wild type and mutants of Caenorhabditis elegans using antibodies to horseradish peroxidase. *J. Neurogenet.*, 7: 193–211.

Song, H.J. and Poo, M.M. (1999) Signal transduction underlying growth cone guidance by diffusible factors. *Curr. Opin. Neurobiol.*, 9: 355–363.

Stein, E., Zou, Y., Poo, M. and Tessier-Lavigne, M. (2001) Binding of DCC by netrin-1 to mediate axon guidance independent of adenosine A2B receptor activation. *Science*, 291: 1976–1982.

Strahle, U., Fischer, N. and Blader, P. (1997) Expression and regulation of a netrin homologue in the zebrafish embryo. *Mech. Dev.*, 62: 147–160.

442

Su, M., Merz, D.C., Killeen, M.T., Zhou, Y., Zheng, H., Kramer, J.M., Hedgecock, E.M. and Culotti, J.G. (2000) Regulation of the UNC-5 netrin receptor initiates the first reorientation of migrating distal tip cells in *Caenorhabditis elegans*. *Development*, 127: 585–594.

Sugimoto, Y., Taniguchi, M., Yagi, T., Akagi, Y., Nojyo, Y. and Tamamaki, N. (2001) Guidance of glial precursor cell migration by secreted cues in the developing optic nerve. *Development*, 128: 3321–3330.

Suter, D.M. and Forscher, P. (1998) An emerging link between cytoskeletal dynamics and cell adhesion molecules in growth cone guidance. *Curr. Opin. Neurobiol.*, 8: 106–116.

Tanaka, E. and Sabry, J. (1995) Making the connection: cytoskeletal rearrangements during growth cone guidance. *Cell*, 83: 171–176.

Tanaka, K., Oshimura, M., Kikuchi, R., Seki, M., Hayashi, T. and Miyaki, M. (1991) Suppression of tumorigenicity in human colon carcinoma cells by introduction of normal chromosome 5 or 18. *Nature*, 349: 340–342.

Tessier-Lavigne, M. and Goodman, C.S. (1996) The molecular biology of axon guidance. *Science*, 274: 1123–1133.

Tessier-Lavigne, M., Placzek, M., Lumsden, A.G., Dodd, J. and Jessell, T.M. (1988) Chemotropic guidance of developing axons in the mammalian central nervous system. *Nature*, 336: 775–778.

Thiagalingam, S., Lengauer, C., Leach, F.S., Schutte, M., Hahn, S.A., Overhauser, J., Willson, J.K., Markowitz, S., Hamilton, S.R., Kern, S.E., Kinzler, K.W. and Vogelstein, B. (1996) Evaluation of candidate tumour suppressor genes on chromosome 18 in colorectal cancers. *Nat. Genet.*, 13: 343–346.

Timpl, R. and Brown, J.C. (1994) The laminins. *Matrix Biol.*, 14: 275–281.

Tong, J., Killeen, M., Steven, R., Binns, K.L., Culotti, J. and Pawson, T. (2001) Netrin stimulates tyrosine phosphorylation of the UNC-5 family of netrin receptors and induces Shp2 binding to the RCM cytodomain. *J. Biol. Chem.*, 276: 40917–40925.

Van Raay, T.J., Foskett, S.M., Connors, T.D., Klinger, K.W., Landes, G.M. and Burn, T.C. (1997) The NTN2L gene encoding a novel human netrin maps to the autosomal dominant polycystic kidney disease region on chromosome 16p13.3. *Genomics*, 41: 279–282.

Varela-Echavarria, A., Tucker, A., Puschel, A.W. and Guthrie, S. (1997) Motor axon subpopulations respond differentially to the chemorepellents netrin-1 and semaphorin D. *Neuron*, 18: 193–207.

Vielmetter, J., Kayyem, J.F., Roman, J.M. and Dreyer, W.J. (1994) Neogenin, an avian cell surface protein expressed during terminal neuronal differentiation, is closely related to the human tumor suppressor molecule deleted in colorectal cancer. *J. Cell Biol.*, 127: 2009–2020.

Vielmetter, J., Chen, X.N., Miskevich, F., Lane, R.P., Yamakawa, K., Korenberg, J.R. and Dreyer, W.J. (1997) Molecular characterization of human neogenin, a DCC-related protein, and the mapping of its gene (NEO1) to chromosomal position 15q22.3–q23. *Genomics*, 41: 414–421.

Volenec, A., Bhogal, R.K., Moorman, J.M., Leslie, R.A. and Flanigan, T.P. (1997) Differential expression of DCC mRNA in adult rat forebrain. *NeuroReport*, 8: 2913–2917.

Volenec, A., Zetterstrom, T.S. and Flanigan, T.P. (1998) 6-OHDA denervation substantially decreases DCC mRNA levels in rat substantia nigra compacta. *NeuroReport*, 9: 3553–3556.

Wadsworth, W.G., Bhatt, H. and Hedgecock, E.M. (1996) Neuroglia and pioneer neurons express UNC-6 to provide global and local netrin cues for guiding migrations in *C. elegans*. *Neuron*, 16: 35–46.

Wang, H., Copeland, N.G., Gilbert, D.J., Jenkins, N.A. and Tessier-Lavigne, M. (1999) Netrin-3, a mouse homolog of human NTN2L, is highly expressed in sensory ganglia and shows differential binding to netrin receptors. *J. Neurosci.*, 19: 4938–4947.

Weber, A. (1938) Croissance des fibres nerveuses commissurales lors de lesions de la moelle epiniere chez de jeunes embryons de Poulet. *Biomorphosis*, 1: 30–35.

Wills, Z., Bateman, J., Korey, C.A., Comer, A. and Van Vactor, D. (1999) The tyrosine kinase Abl and its substrate enabled collaborate with the receptor phosphatase Dlar to control motor axon guidance. *Neuron*, 22: 301–312.

Winberg, M.L., Mitchell, K.J. and Goodman, C.S. (1998) Genetic analysis of the mechanisms controlling target selection: complementary and combinatorial functions of netrins, semaphorins, and IgCAMs. *Cell*, 93: 581–591.

Yee, K.T., Simon, H.H., Tessier-Lavigne, M. and O'Leary, D.M. (1999) Extension of long leading processes and neuronal migration in the mammalian brain directed by the chemoattractant netrin-1. *Neuron*, 24: 607–622.

Yin, Y., Sanes, J.R. and Miner, J.H. (2000) Identification and expression of mouse netrin-4. *Mech. Dev.*, 96: 115–119.

L. McKerracher, G. Doucet and S. Rossignol (Eds.)
Progress in Brain Research, Vol. 137

CHAPTER 33

Reinnervation of the pretectum in adult rats by regenerated retinal ganglion cell axons: anatomical and functional studies

Manuel Vidal-Sanz [1,*], Marcelino Avilés-Trigueros [2], Simon J.O. Whiteley [3], Yves Sauvé [4] and Raymond D. Lund [4]

[1] *Laboratorio de Oftalmología Experimental, Universidad de Murcia, 30100 Murcia, Spain*
[2] *Instituto de Bioingeniería, Universidad Miguel Hernández, 03550 San Juan (Alicante), Spain*
[3] *Department of Psychology, University of Sheffield, Sheffield S10 2TP, UK*
[4] *Moran Eye Center, Health Science Center, University of Utah, 50 North Medical Drive, Salt Lake City, UT 84132, USA*

Abstract: We have investigated the specificity of reinnervation and terminal arborization of injured retinal ganglion cell (RGC) axons in the brainstem with the object of studying in a simple situation the degree to which regenerating axons are able to replicate the characteristic patterns of terminal arborization and restore normal function. We have focussed here on the pathway that is responsible for the pupillary light reflex, which is mediated through the olivary pretectal nucleus (OPN). In adult rats, the left optic nerve was transected and a segment of peripheral nerve (PN) graft was used to bridge between the retina and different regions of the ipsilateral brainstem, including the superior colliculus. After 4–13 months, regenerated RGC axons were examined in coronal sections stained for cholera toxin B subunit. RGC axons were found extending into the ipsilateral brainstem for distances of up to 6 mm. Within the pretectum, axons innervated the OPN and the nucleus of the optic tract preferentially, and formed distinctive terminal arbors within each. Within the SC axons extended laterally into the visual layers and formed a different type of arborization. On testing the pupillary light reflex, it was found in best cases to show response amplitudes which were comparable to those recorded from control intact animals. However, unlike normals, the response amplitude tended to diminish with repeated stimulation and also appeared to deteriorate with age, although responses could still be detected in some cases as long as 15 months after grafting. These results indicate that regenerating axons can selectively reinnervate denervated nuclei, where they form typical terminal arborizations, and provide the substrates for restoring functional circuitry.

Introduction

In the adult mammalian central nervous system (CNS) severed axons do not regenerate and re-establish their original connections to restitute func-

tion. This failure for spontaneous axonal regeneration has been explained by changes in the neurons and their environment, which are associated with the normal development and maturation of the CNS (Chen et al., 1995; Cai et al., 2001). However, experiments aimed at modifying the axonal environment have proven the capacity of severed CNS axons to regenerate. Within the adult mammalian spinal cord, for example, several studies have shown axonal regeneration under experimental conditions, such as: at the site of the lesion placing a segment of periph-

* Correspondence to: M. Vidal-Sanz, Laboratorio de Oftalmología Experimental, Universidad de Murcia, 30100 Murcia, Spain. Tel: +34-96-836-3961; Fax: +34-96-836-3962; E-mail: ofmmv01@fcu.um.es

eral nerve graft (David and Aguayo, 1981), Schwann cells (Xu et al., 1999), olfactory ensheathing cells (Li et al., 1997; Ramón-Cueto et al., 1998), fetal cells (Diener and Bregman, 1998; Giménez y Ribotta et al., 2000), activated macrophages (Lazarov-Spiegler et al., 1996, 1998), trophic factors (Cheng et al., 1996; Menei et al., 1998) or antibodies against growth-inhibitory molecules present in the CNS (Schnell and Schwab, 1990; Z'Graggen et al., 1998), producing a conditioning lesion (Richardson and Issa, 1984; Neumann and Woolf, 1999), using microtransplants of sensory neurons (Davies et al., 1997), accelerating the immune cell response to clear myelin debris (Ousman and David, 2000) or modifying the animal's immune response against some of the adult myelin components (Huang et al., 1999; Hauben et al., 2000).

While it is obviously important to find ways of promoting the regeneration of damaged axons across an injury site, it is equally important to know how well such axons can restore normal connectivity in the target region and the degree to which such circuitry can mediate restitution of lost relay functions. It is difficult to examine this problem in the spinal cord, however, because of the complex interactions of converging systems. The primary optic pathway provides several advantages for such studies, however (Vidal-Sanz et al., 1993). It is a single relay pathway, isolated from terminal neuropil; it has clearly circumscribed central distributions to regions which subserve a range of individual visual functions; the visual input signals which it relays to the CNS can be clearly defined; and it regenerates after injury in response to extrinsic treatments. Thus, if the optic nerve (ON) is transected in the orbit and a segment of peripheral nerve (PN) is grafted to the ocular stump of the ON, a small proportion of the retinal ganglion cell (RGC) population will consistently innervate these PN grafts (Vidal-Sanz et al., 1987). Furthermore, if regenerated retinal axons are placed in the vicinity of retino-recipient regions, such as the superior colliculus (SC), these axons will extend for short distances (Vidal-Sanz et al., 1987, 1991; Carter et al., 1989, 1994; Thanos and Mey, 1995; Carter and Jhaveri, 1997; Thanos et al., 1997), form synapses within host primary visual centers (Vidal-Sanz et al., 1987; Carter et al., 1989) that persist for long periods of time (Vidal-Sanz et al.,

1991; Carter et al., 1994), which are capable of driving postsynaptic cells in response to light (Keirstead et al., 1989; Sauvé et al., 1995, 2001), and mediating visually driven behaviors such as light-induced EEG desynchronization (Sasaki et al., 1996) and the pupillary light reflex (PLR) (Thanos, 1992; Whiteley et al., 1998). There is evidence too that while the regenerated axons may not form a normal topological map they do distribute in a non-random fashion, with a degree of topological specificity (Sauvé et al., 2001).

Here we review recent studies on the adult rat visual system with PN grafts linking the retina with several retinorecipient regions in the midbrain to provide insights into mechanisms of axonal reinnervation (Avilés-Trigueros et al., 2000) and functional restoration (Whiteley et al., 1998) in the CNS of adult mammals.

Methods

Experiments were performed on adult female pigmented (Piebald Virol Glaxo, PVG) and albino (Sprague–Dawley) rats. Animal care and experimental procedures were performed according to Home Office (UK) and European Union regulations.

Peripheral nerve grafting

Adult rats (150–200 g) received autologous peripheral nerve grafts linking the retina with the brainstem according to previously described methods (Vidal-Sanz et al., 1987). In short, under chloral hydrate anesthesia (0.42 mg/g, i.p.), the left optic nerve was exposed intraorbitally, and sectioned close to the sclera without affecting the retinal blood supply. One end of an autologous common peroneal nerve segment was apposed to the ocular stump with three 10/0 monofilament sutures, while the distal end was inserted superficially into the ipsilateral midbrain, using a fine glass probe, in one of two different sites: laterally into the diencephalon or adjacent to the olivary pretectal nucleus (OPN). These two respective sites were chosen to allow comparisons of the pattern of axonal growth within the brainstem and the capacity of regenerating axons to innervate different retinorecipient pretectal nuclei. Finally, in order to examine the pattern of RGC axons growth as well as the capacity of axons to reinnervate their main target region, an additional group of animals had the distal end of the PN grafts inserted superficially in the lateral aspect of the superior colliculus (SC). For all experiments, immediately following PN-graft insertion, the contralateral eye was removed to deprive the pretectum of its normal visual input. The rationale was to ensure that the normal optic input would not diminish the efficacy of the regenerated pathway (Radel et al., 1991).

Histological assessment

To investigate the course of regenerated retinal axons we have used a method that demonstrates retinofugal projections with great sensitivity (Angelucci et al., 1996; Avilés-Trigueros et al., 2000). This consists of intraocular administration of the orthograde neuroanatomical tracer cholera toxin subunit B (CTb) and its immunolocalization. In brief, at different time periods (4–13 months) post-grafting, 5 μl of 1% CTb (List Biologic, Campbell, CA) were injected into the vitreous chamber of the PN-grafted eye and 5 days later the rats were sacrificed. Orthogradely transported CTb was immunolocalized on frozen coronal sections (40 μm thick) using the protocol of Angelucci et al. (1996). Sections were examined under bright field or stereoscopic microscopy for CTb-labeled fibers. Drawings of CTb-labeled axons and terminal arborizations were made from printed photographs and with the aid of a camera lucida attached to the microscope.

Pupillary light reflex

The pupil constricts in response to light. This reflex starts with light stimulus on the retina being conducted to the OPN, which projects to the Edinger–Westphal nucleus (Sillito and Zbrozyna, 1970; Young and Lund, 1994) and this in turn innervates the sphincter muscles of the iris (Klooster et al., 1993). Two parameters of the pupillary light reflex (PLR), amplitude and latency, may be measured to provide a quantified assessment of this visual behavior in normal conditions and after experimental restoration (Klassen and Lund, 1987, 1988, 1990).

To investigate the capacity of regenerated retinal axons to restore a visual behavior, a group of adult albino Sprague–Dawley rats with PN segments linking the retina with the pretectum was examined for PLR, following already described methods (Whiteley et al., 1996, 1998). In brief, 5, 7 and 11 months after surgery animals were dark-adapted and anesthetized. The rats were placed in the view of a CCD camera. A white light source measuring 30,000 cd/m^2 intensity provided a light stimulus, which was focussed on the eye for 5 s followed by a recovery period of 60 s. An infrared light source provided illumination for a CCD camera that recorded the pupil image via a VCR. The camera image was observed on a video monitor allowing direct observation of the pupil while testing. Responses were registered using a video tape recorder and analysis of pupil diameter and latency was done over stop-frame images on the 25 frames/s recorded.

Results

Anatomical studies

Anatomical investigation of the regenerated projection showed considerable variation among animals. In approximately two-thirds of the experiments, there was no axonal ingrowth into the brainstem or very few fibers were seen to extend for very short distances within the surrounding brainstem. In the remaining one-third of the animals analyzed, there was profuse reinnervation of several retinorecipient nuclei within the brainstem.

Within the group of animals in which the distal end of the PN graft had been inserted laterally into the ipsilateral SC 10 or 12 months before, axons extended for up to approximately 4 mm through the neuropil of the stratum griseum superficiale (SGS) and formed elaborated arborizations exhibiting numerous bouton-like endings (Fig. 1), that were similar to those observed in control animals, but differed from those observed within the pretectal area.

Within the group of animals in which the distal end of the PN graft was inserted in the ipsilateral pretectum 4–13 months before, there were two different preparations; one had the distal end of the PN graft inserted adjacent to the OPN and the other had an insertion more lateral in the diencephalon, in a region corresponding to the junction of the lateral geniculate and the lateral posterior nuclei. Retinal

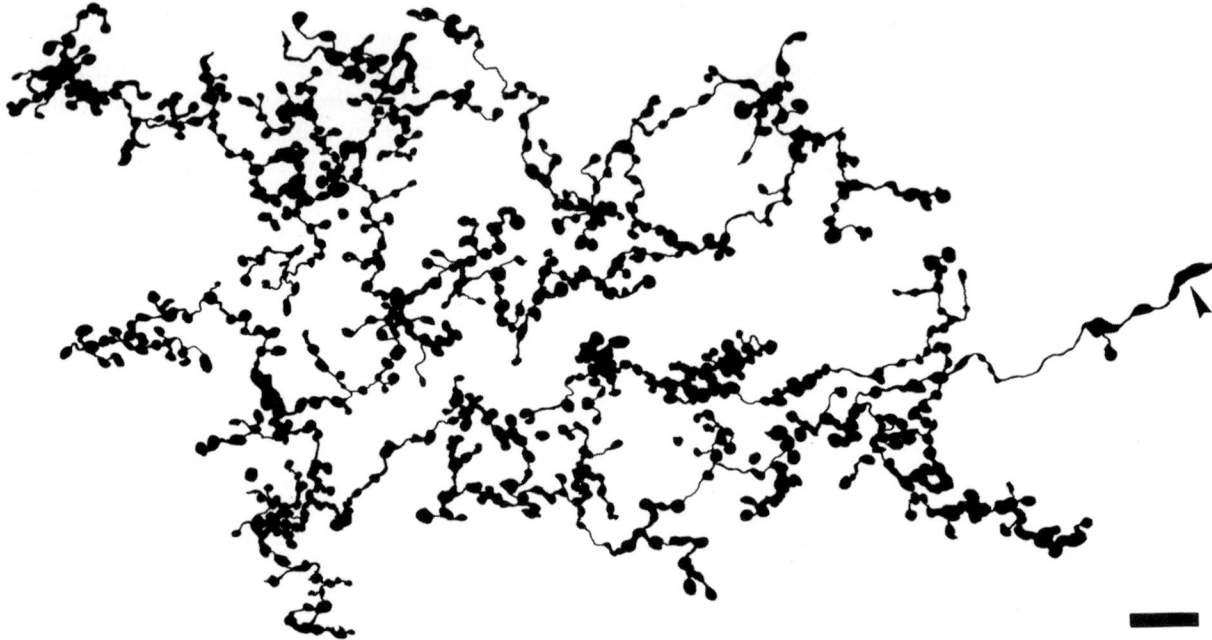

Fig. 1. Camera lucida drawing illustrating regenerated retinal fiber in the stratum griseum superficiale (SGS) of a 40-μm-thick cryostat section of the midbrain 48 weeks after grafting an autologous segment of peripheral nerve between the left eye and the lateral side of the ipsilateral superior colliculus (SC) and 5 days after intraocular injection of cholera toxin subunit B. A single regenerated retinal ganglion cell axon in the SGS of the SC forming many branches that bear multiple varicosities of similar appearance and uniform size. The stem axon is illustrated by an arrowhead. Scale bar: 9 μm. (Reproduced from Fig. 9b of Avilés-Trigueros et al., 2000, with permission.)

axons in PN grafts inserted close to the OPN invaded the surrounding neuropil and innervated the OPN and nucleus of the optic tract (NOT), with some axons extending towards the midline to innervate the contralateral side. In the group of animals with PN grafts inserted more laterally in the diencephalon, retinal axons also extended for up to 6 mm through the brainstem and profusely innervated the NOT and OPN (Fig. 2). Thus, in general, animals with PN grafts inserted in the pretectum showed retinal axons following the course of the OPN and NOT and formed terminal arborizations and bouton-like structures within these nuclei.

The morphology of the regenerated retinal arbors compared with the respective types in NOT and OPN described in intact hamsters (Ling et al., 1998). Within the NOT area, regenerated CTB-labeled retinal axons divided into small branches which were decorated with numerous medium and small size varicosities and terminal swellings. In contrast, axons within the OPN exhibited little branching and

were decorated with large elliptical varicosities along the axons and with terminal swellings of different sizes (Avilés-Trigueros et al., 2000).

Functional studies

To study in more detail the efficacy of the regenerated optic pathway, animals with PN segments connecting the left eye and the ipsilateral pretectal region were tested for pupillary light responses. In approximately two-thirds of the animals prepared for this functional test, the PLR was recorded at some stage between 5 and 11 months. The proportion of responders was similar for the group of animals with the PN graft inserted adjacent to the OPN (62%, 10 out of 16) and for the group with the graft inserted more laterally in the diencephalons (60%, 12 out of 20).

Amplitude and latency of the PLR responses varied greatly between PN-grafted animals, and in general these were smaller than those recorded from in-

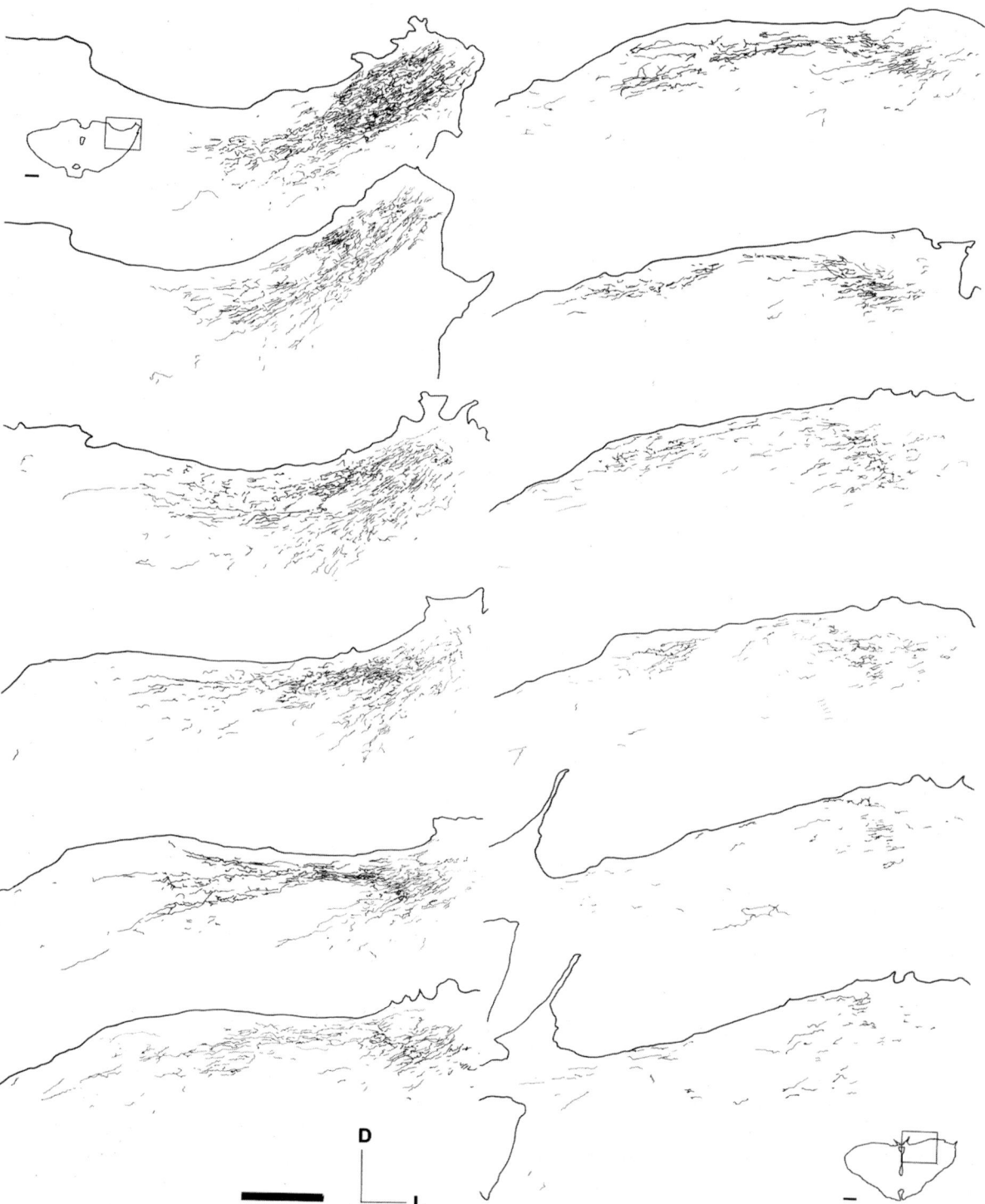

Fig. 2. Drawings of alternate 40-µm-thick cryostat coronal sections through the brainstem, from caudal (top left) to rostral (bottom right), of a rat 16 weeks after grafting a peripheral nerve segment between the left retina and the lateral aspect of the left diencephalon. The drawings illustrate the distribution of regenerated retinal fibers orthogradely labeled with CTB injected 5 days earlier into the PN-grafted retina. Note the extensive reinnervation through the pretectum. Scale bar: 0.5 mm. The inserts are drawings of the most caudal and rostral sections, respectively. Scale bar: 1 mm. (Reproduced from Fig. 2 of Avilés-Trigueros et al., 2000, with permission.)

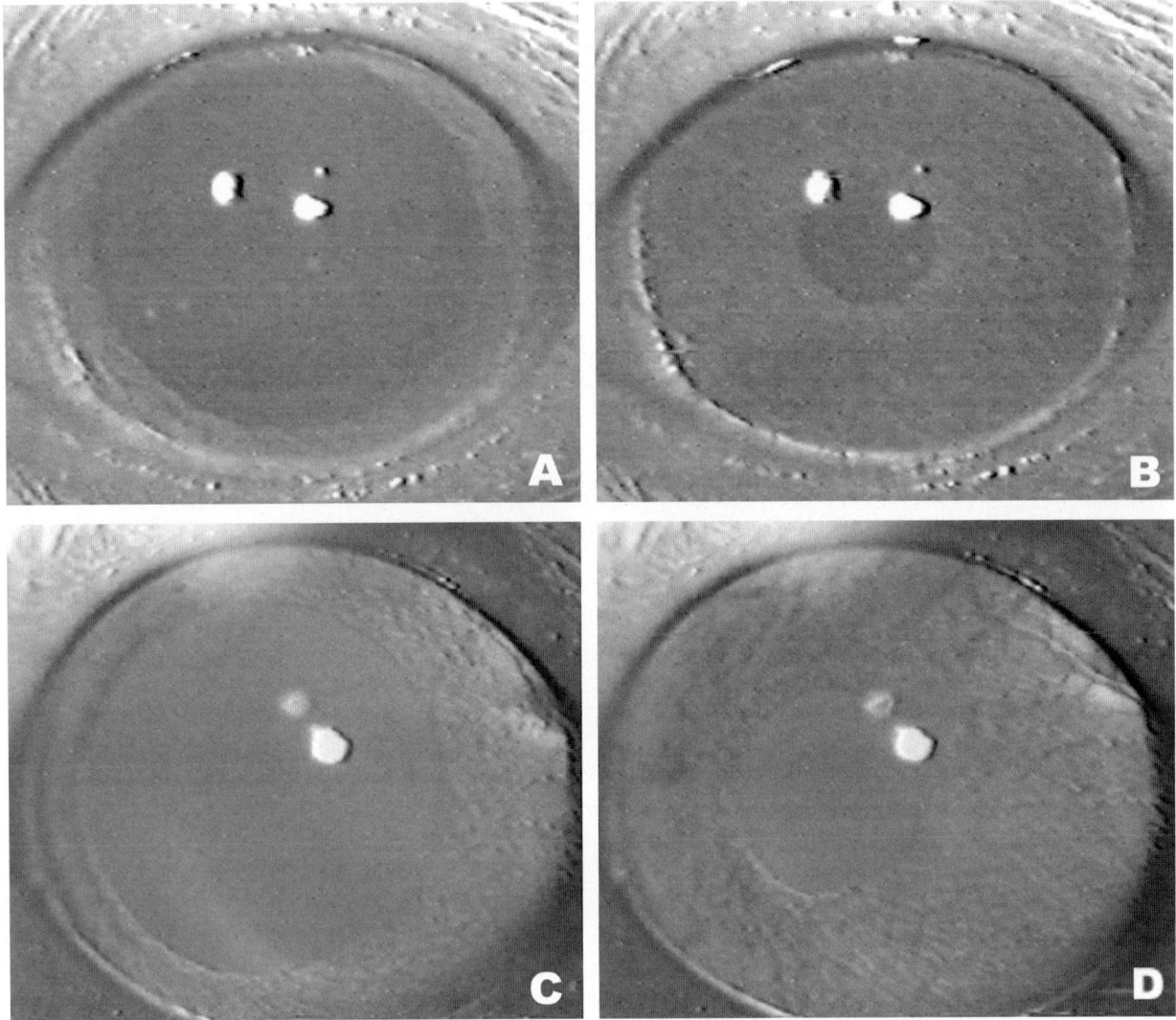

Fig. 3. Video images of pupils recorded from albino rats at the start (A,C) and end (B,D) of the stimulus presentation. There are two white reflections apparent in the pictures: one is the infrared illumination and the other is the light stimulus, which has the appearance of being slightly dimmer due to the infrared sensitivity of the camera. (A,B) Pupil recorded from an unoperated control rat. (C,D) Pupil changes to the same light intensity, recorded from a PN grafted rat. As can be seen, the change in diameter is substantial for both animals. (Reproduced with permission from Fig. 2 of Whiteley et al., 1998.)

tact animals. The amplitude of the pupillary constriction in intact animals was approximately 64% of its baseline diameter. In the PN-grafted rats, mean amplitudes varied between 10 and 40% of the baseline value. The time elapsed between the light stimulus presentation and the beginning of pupil constriction, that is the latency, was around 330 ms in intact animals. For the PN-grafted rats, latencies varied from 500 to over 1500 ms. Some individual trials

delivered amplitudes of 62% and latencies of 500 ms, values which resembled closely those found in control rats (Fig. 3).

In the PN-grafted animals, the responses progressively worsened when elicited repeatedly in three consecutive trials; that is, the amplitude was smaller and the latency increased. There was also a tendency for the responses to deteriorate with time. Overall, the amplitude and latency of the responses at 11 months showed a clear sign of deterioration when compared to those elicited at 7 months.

Discussion

These studies were designed to investigate the potential of severed adult retinal ganglion cell axons to extend, arborize and establish functional connections within the brainstem, a regions that contains several small (i.e., NOT and OPN) and large (i.e. the superficial layers of the SC) retinorecipient nuclei. We have used sensitive neuroanatomical tracing methods to examine the course and termination of regenerated retinal axons within the brainstem and have investigated the efficacy of newly established synaptic connections by recording pupillary responses to light stimulus presentation on the retina.

Our results document the potential of adult injured RGCs for extensive axonal regrowth within the brainstem. In approximately one-third of the animals analyzed with anatomical techniques axons extended for distances that were in the range of 4 (in the SC) to 6 (in the pretectum) millimeters. This extensive axonal regeneration in the CNS was obtained without the additional use of growth-promoting factors (Cheng et al., 1996; Menei et al., 1998; Z'Graggen et al., 1998), or cells (Lazarov-Spiegler et al., 1996; Li et al., 1997; Ramón-Cueto et al., 1998; Xu et al., 1999). Most of the axons, however, were observed coursing through the dorsal brainstem, or the superficial layers of the SC, regions that are relatively poor in myelin, which is known to inhibit axonal growth (Caroni and Schwab, 1988; McKerracher et al., 1994). Not all animals showed evidence of such robust regenerative ingrowth, however. Possible explanations for this failure include the formation of a glial scar and the expression of growth inhibitory molecules at the PN–CNS interface (Davies et al., 1997, 1999; Dusart et al., 1999; Shearer and Fawcett, 2001), or secondary degenerative events occurring over time.

Along their course within the SC or the pretectum, retinal axons targeted the main retinorecipient regions including the SGS, the OPN and NOT, suggesting that reinnervation was selective for optic target regions. These results are in accordance with previous studies showing certain degree of specificity in the reinnervation of SC; regenerated axons preferred to extend on the superficial layers versus the deep nonvisual layers of the SC (Vidal-Sanz et al., 1991; Carter et al., 1994) and showed a tendency for acquiring a degree of appropriate topological distribution within the rostrocaudal axis of the SC (Sauvé et al., 2001). Our present results also show that the morphology of regenerated retinal arbors is different for the OPN, the NOT and the visual layers of the SC. Furthermore, these different types of terminal arborizations were reminiscent of those found in control animals (Ling et al., 1998). This indicates that retinal axons adopt different patterns of arborizations depending on the nuclei they innervate (Carter and Jhaveri, 1997), and further suggests specificity for axonal distribution (Sauvé et al., 2001) and terminal arborization in the retinorecipient reinnervated nuclei. Because in our anatomical studies, most animals were analyzed after long periods of time, that is between 4 and 12 months after PN grafting, we have not explored whether there may have been projections to non-retinorecipient targets at earlier time points, which subsequently disappeared. Such transient projections have been previously described during development (Frost, 1986).

Our studies also indicate that a large proportion of the animals tested showed at some stage a pupil constriction in response to light. The wide range of PLR recorded, including some responses that had amplitude and latency values that reached nearly normal parameters, may well correlate with the varying degree of successful OPN reinnervation, as observed with neuroanatomical methods. We were not able to estimate the number of axons successfully reinnervating the OPN, but previous studies have shown that the number of RGCs regenerating their axons along PN grafts varies between approximately 1 and 10% of the RGC population (Vidal-Sanz et al., 1987; Villegas-Pérez et al., 1988). Thus, it is possible that varying degrees of success in the growth of RGC axons into the PN graft and out of the graft into the surrounding brainstem might have contributed to different levels of OPN reinnervation, and this might reflect in turn the variability in the strength of the PLR responses. The absence of anatomical evidence for retinal fibers reinnervating the OPN in similar proportions of animals analyzed with neuroanatomical methods would explain the limited number of responders observed in the functional studies.

The functional tests also indicated that most animals showed a deterioration of the PLR over a series of consecutive tests, an event that may be explained by changes in the inner circuitry of the retina secondary to massive loss of RGCs (Villegas-Pérez et al., 1993) as well as by changes in the local circuits within the lesioned and denervated host OPN (Whiteley et al., 1998). In many of the functionally tested animals, the response efficacy deteriorated when elicited serially at increasing survival intervals; suggesting that while functional circuitry has clearly been restored, it is not as robust as the normal input in driving postsynaptic cells. Most important in this respect may be the reorganization of local circuitry after primary deafferentation that has been reported in visual centers such as the superior colliculus (Lund and Lund, 1971) and pretectum (Campbell and Lieberman, 1985). There was also a clear deterioration of the response parameters between 7 and 11 months after PN grafting. It is possible that this time-related deterioration of the PLR might be explained by degeneration of the regenerated retinal projection to the OPN or their parent cells in the retina (Keirstead et al., 1985; Villegas-Pérez et al., 1993). Nevertheless, the presence of PLR in some animals that were analyzed 15 months after PN grafting (Whiteley et al., 1998) demonstrated that reformed retinal connections can remain functional for long periods of time in these laboratory animals (Whiteley et al., 1998). Indeed, the anatomical studies corroborated OPN reinnervation by RGC axons in animals that were analyzed as late as 12 months after PN grafting, suggesting that in some experiments regenerated axons maintain their connections for long periods of time. The reason why some axons would remain while others might degenerate with time is presently unknown.

In summary, these results show that adult injured optic nerve axons conveyed through PN grafts to the proximity of their main targets may re-extend for considerable distances into the host neuropil and show a high level of selectively in reaching their target nuclei to form specific types of arborizations. The potential of the primary optic pathway for repair studies is highlighted by the fact that it may also subserve a simple visual function, such as the pupillary light reflex. The results do suggest that the responses are not as robust as the normal optic projection and offer caution that while it may be possible to promote axon growth across an area of injury within the CNS, and while regenerated axons can distribute in appropriate target regions, functional efficacy may still be compromised. What the factors involved are and how they may be manipulated or overridden are issues that clearly deserve further investigation.

Abbreviations

CNS	central nervous system
CTb	subunit B of cholera toxin
NOT	nucleus of the optic tract
ON	optic nerve
OPN	olivary pretectal nucleus
PLR	pupillary light reflex
PN	peripheral nerve
RGC	retinal ganglion cell
SC	superior colliculus
SGS	stratum griseum superficiale

Acknowledgements

This study was supported by Spanish (FIS 98/0341) and European Union (Biomed-2 CT-96-09076) research grants.

References

Angelucci, A., Clasca, F. and Sur, M. (1996) Anterograde axonal tracing with the subunit B of the cholera toxin: a highly sensitive immunohistochemical protocol for revealing fine axonal morphology in adult and neonatal brains. *J. Neurosci. Methods*, 65: 101–112.

Avilés-Trigueros, M., Sauvé, Y., Lund, R.D. and Vidal-Sanz, M. (2000) Selective innervation of retinorecipient brainstem nuclei by retinal ganglion cell axons regenerating through peripheral nerve grafts in adult rats. *J. Neurosci.*, 20: 361–374.

Cai, D., Qiu, J., Cao, Z., McAtee, M., Bregman, B.S. and Filbin, T. (2001) Neuronal cyclic AMP controls the developmental loss in ability of axons to regenerate. *J. Neurosci.*, 21: 4731–4739.

Campbell, G. and Lieberman, A.R. (1985) The olivary pretectal nucleus: experimental anatomical studies in the rat. *Philos. Trans. R. Soc. Lond. B. Biol. Sci.*, 310: 573–609.

Caroni, P. and Schwab, M.E. (1988) Antibody against myelin-associated inhibitor of neurite growth neutralises nonpermissive substrate properties of CNS white matter. *Neuron*, 1: 85–96.

Carter, D.A. and Jhaveri, S. (1997) Retino-geniculate axons regenerating in adult hamsters are able to form morphologically distinct terminals. *Exp. Neurol.*, 146: 315–322.

Carter, D.A., Bray, G.M. and Aguayo, A.J. (1989) Regenerated retinal ganglion cell axons can form well-differentiated synapses in the superior colliculus of adult hamsters. *J. Neurosci.*, 9: 4042–4050.

Carter, D.A., Bray, G.M. and Aguayo, A.J. (1994) Long-term growth and remodeling of regenerated retino-collicular connections in adult hamsters. *J. Neurosci.*, 14: 590–598.

Chen, D.F., Jhaveri, S. and Schneider, G.E. (1995) Intrinsic changes in developing retinal neurons result in regenerative failure of their axons. *Proc. Natl. Acad. Sci. USA*, 92: 7287–7291.

Cheng, H., Cao, Y. and Olson, L. (1996) Spinal cord repair in adult paraplegic rats: partial restoration of hind limb function. *Science*, 273: 510–513.

David, S. and Aguayo, A.J. (1981) Axonal elongation into peripheral nervous system 'bridges' after central nervous system injury in adult rats. *Science*, 214: 931–933.

Davies, S.J.A., Fitch, M.T., Memberg, S.P., Hall, A.K., Raisman, G. and Silver, J. (1997) Regeneration of adult axons in white matter tracts of the central nervous system. *Nature*, 390: 680–684.

Davies, S.J.A., Goucher, D.R., Doller, C. and Silver, J. (1999) Robust regeneration of adult sensory axons in degenerating white matter of the adult rat spinal cord. *J. Neurosci.*, 19: 5810–5822.

Diener, P.S. and Bregman, B.S. (1998) Fetal spinal cord transplants support growth of supraspinal and segmental projections after cervical spinal cord hemisection in the neonatal rat. *J. Neurosci.*, 18: 779–793.

Dusart, I., Morel, M.P., Wehrle, R. and Sotelo, C. (1999) Late axonal sprouting of injured Purkinje cells and its temporal correlation with permissive changes in the glial scar. *J. Comp. Neurol.*, 408: 399–418.

Frost, D.O. (1986) Development of anomalous retinal projections to non-visual thalamic nuclei in Syrian hamsters: a quantitative study. *J. Comp. Neurol.*, 252: 95–105.

Giménez y Ribotta, M., Provencher, J., Feraboli-Lohnherr, D., Rossignol, S., Privat, A. and Orsal, D. (2000) Activation of locomotion in adult chronic spinal rats is achieved by transplantation of embryonic raphe cells reinnervating a precise lumbar level. *J. Neurosci.*, 20: 5144–5152.

Hauben, E., Butovsky, O., Nevo, U., Yoles, E., Moalem, G., Agranov, E., Mor, F., Leibowitz-Amit, R., Pevsner, E., Akselrod, S., Neeman, M., Cohen, I.R. and Schwartz, M. (2000) Passive or active immunization with myelin basic protein promotes recovery from spinal cord contusion. *J. Neurosci.*, 20: 6421–6430.

Huang, D.W., McKerracker, L., Braun, P.E. and David, S. (1999) A therapeutic vaccine approach to stimulate axon regeneration in the adult mammalian spinal cord. *Neuron*, 24: 639–647.

Keirstead, S.A., Vidal-Sanz, M., Rasminsky, M., Aguayo, A.J., Levesque, M. and So, K.F. (1985) Responses to light of retinal neurons regenerating axons into peripheral nerve grafts in the rat. *Brain Res.*, 359: 402–406.

Keirstead, S.A., Rasminsky, M., Fukuda, Y., Carter, D.A., Aguayo, A.J. and Vidal-Sanz, M. (1989) Electrophysiologic responses in hamster superior colliculus evoked by regenerating retinal axons. *Science*, 246: 255–257.

Klassen, H. and Lund, R.D. (1987) Retinal transplants can drive a pupillary light reflex in host brains. *Proc. Natl. Acad. Sci. USA*, 84: 6958–6960.

Klassen, H. and Lund, R.D. (1988) Anatomical and behavioural correlates of a xenograft-mediated pupillary reflex. *Exp. Neurol.*, 102: 102–108.

Klassen, H. and Lund, R.D. (1990) Parameters of retinal graft-mediated responses are related to underlying target innervation. *Brain Res.*, 533: 181–191.

Klooster, J., Beckers, H.J.M., Vrensen, G.F.J.M. and van der Want, J.J.L. (1993) The peripheral and central projections of the Edinger–Westphal nucleus in the rat. A light and electron microscopic tracing study. *Brain Res.*, 632: 260–273.

Lazarov-Spiegler, O., Solomon, A.S., Zeev-Brann, A.B., Hirschberg, D.L., Lavie, V. and Schwartz, M. (1996) Transplantation of activated macrophages overcomes central nervous system regrowth failure. *FASEB J.*, 10: 1296–1302.

Lazarov-Spiegler, O., Solomon, A.S. and Schwartz, M. (1998) Peripheral nerve-stimulated macrophages simulate a peripheral nerve-like regenerative response in rat transected optic nerve. *Glia*, 24: 329–337.

Li, Y., Field, P.M. and Raisman, G. (1997) Repair of adult corticospinal tract by transplants of olfactory ensheathing cells. *Science*, 277: 2000–2002.

Ling, C., Schneider, G.E. and Jhaveri, S. (1998) Target-specific morphology of retinal axon arbors in the adult hamster. *Vis. Neurosci.*, 15: 559–579.

Lund, R.D. and Lund, J.S. (1971) Synaptic adjustment after deafferentation of the superior colliculus of the rat. *Science*, 171: 804–807.

McKerracher, L., David, S., Jackson, D.L., Kottis, V., Dunn, R.J. and Braun, P.E. (1994) Identification of myelin-associated glycoprotein as a major myelin-derived inhibitor of neurite growth. *Neuron*, 13: 805–811.

Menei, P., Montero-Menei, C., Whittemore, S.R., Bunge, R.P. and Bunge, M.B. (1998) Schwann cells genetically modified to secrete human BDNF promote enhanced axonal regrowth across transected adult rat spinal cord. *Eur. J. Neurosci.*, 10: 607–621.

Neumann, S. and Woolf, C.J. (1999) Regeneration of dorsal column fibers into and beyond the lesions site following adult spinal cord injury. *Neuron*, 23: 83–91.

Ousman, S.S. and David, S. (2000) Lysophosphatidylcholine induces rapid recruitment and activation of macrophages in the adult mouse spinal cord. *Glia*, 30: 92–104.

Radel, J.D., Kustra, D.J. and Lund, R.D. (1991) Rapid enhancement of transplant-mediated pupilloconstriction after elimination of competing host optic input. *Dev. Brain Res.*, 60: 275–278.

Ramón-Cueto, A., Plant, G.W., Avila, J. and Bunge, M.B. (1998) Long-distance axonal regeneration in the transected adult rat spinal cord is promoted by olfactory ensheathing glia transplants. *J. Neurosci.*, 18: 3803–3815.

Richardson, P. and Issa, V.M. (1984) Peripheral injury enhances regeneration of primary sensory neurones. *Nature*, 309: 791–793.

Sasaki, H., Coffey, P., Villegas-Pérez, M.P., Vidal-Sanz, M., Young, M.J., Lund, R.D. and Fukuda, Y. (1996) Light induced EEG desynchronization and behavioural arousal in rats with re-stored retinocollicular projection by peripheral nerve graft. *Neurosci. Lett.*, 218: 45–48.

Sauvé, Y., Sawai, H. and Rasminsky, M. (1995) Functional synaptic connections made by regenerated retinal ganglion cell axons in the superior colliculus of adult hamsters. *J. Neurosci.*, 15: 665–675.

Sauvé, Y., Sawai, H. and Rasmisky, M. (2001) Topological specificity in reinnervation of the superior colliculus by regenerated retinal ganglion cell axons in adult hamsters. *J. Neurosci.*, 21: 951–960.

Schnell, L. and Schwab, M.E. (1990) Axonal regeneration in the rat spinal cord produced by an antibody against myelin-associated neurite growth inhibitors. *Nature*, 343: 269–272.

Shearer, M.C. and Fawcett, J.W. (2001) The astrocyte/meningeal interface — a barrier to successful regeneration? *Cell Tissue Res.*, 305: 267–273.

Sillito, A.M. and Zbrozyna, A.W. (1970) The localization of pupilloconstrictor function within the midbrain of the cat. *J. Physiol.*, 211: 461–477.

Thanos, S. (1992) Adult retinofugal axons regenerating through peripheral nerve grafts can restore the light-induced pupilloconstriction reflex. *Eur. J. Neurosci.*, 4: 691–699.

Thanos, S. and Mey, J. (1995) Type-specific stabilization and target-dependent survival of regenerating ganglion cells in the retina of adult rats. *J. Neurosci.*, 15: 1057–1079.

Thanos, S., Naskar, R. and Heiduschka, P. (1997) Regenerating ganglion cell axons in the adult rat establish retinofugal topography and restore visual function. *Exp. Brain Res.*, 114: 483–491.

Vidal-Sanz, M., Bray, G.M., Villegas-Pérez, M.P., Thanos, S. and Aguayo, A.J. (1987) Axonal regeneration and synapse formation in the superior colliculus by retinal ganglion cells in the adult rat. *J. Neurosci.*, 7: 2894–2909.

Vidal-Sanz, M., Bray, G.M. and Aguayo, A.J. (1991) Regenerated synapses persist in the superior colliculus after the regrowth of retinal ganglion cell axons. *J. Neurocytol.*, 20: 940–952.

Vidal-Sanz, M., Villegas-Pérez, M.P., Bray, G.M. and Aguayo, A.J. (1993) Use of peripheral nerve grafts to study regeneration after CNS injury. *Neuroprotocols*, 3: 29–33.

Villegas-Pérez, M.P., Vidal-Sanz, M., Bray, G.M. and Aguayo, A.J. (1988) Influences of peripheral nerve grafts on the survival and regrowth of axotomized retinal ganglion cells in adult rats. *J. Neurosci.*, 8: 265–280.

Villegas-Pérez, M.P., Vidal-Sanz, M., Rasminsky, M., Bray, G.M. and Aguayo, A.J. (1993) Rapid and protracted phases of retinal ganglion cell loss follow axotomy in the optic nerve of adult rats. *J. Neurobiol.*, 24: 23–36.

Whiteley, S.J.O., Litchfield, T.M., Coffey, P.J. and Lund, R.D. (1996) Improvement of the pupillary light reflex of Royal College of Surgeons rats following RPE cell grafts. *Exp. Neurol.*, 140: 100–104.

Whiteley, S.J.O., Avilés-Trigueros, M., Sauvé, Y., Vidal-Sanz, M. and Lund, R.D. (1998) Extent and duration of recovered pupillary light reflex following retinal ganglion cell axon regeneration through peripheral nerve grafts directed to the pretectum in adult rats. *Exp. Neurol.*, 154: 560–572.

Xu, X.M., Zhang, S.X., Li, H., Aebisher, P. and Bunge, M.B. (1999) Regrowth of axons into the distal spinal cord through a Schwann-cell-seeded mini-channel implanted into hemisected adult rat spinal cord. *Eur. J. Neurosci.*, 11: 1723–1740.

Young, M.J. and Lund, R.D. (1994) The anatomical substrates subserving the pupillary light reflex in rats: Origin of the consensual pupillary response. *Neuroscience*, 62: 481–496.

Z'Graggen, W.J., Metz, G.A., Kartje, G.L., Thallmair, M. and Schwab, M.E. (1998) Functional recovery and enhanced corticofugal plasticity after unilateral pyramidal tract lesion and blockade of myelin-associated neurite growth inhibitors in adult rats. *J. Neurosci.*, 18: 4744–4757.

L. McKerracher, G. Doucet and S. Rossignol (Eds.)
Progress in Brain Research, Vol. 137
© 2002 Elsevier Science B.V. All rights reserved

CHAPTER 34

Seeking axon guidance molecules in the adult rat CNS

Guy Doucet * and Audrey Petit

*Département de Pathologie et Biologie Cellulaire and Centre de Recherche en Sciences Neurologiques, Université de Montréal,
C.P. 6128, succursale Centre-ville, Montreal, QC H3C 3J7, Canada*

Introduction

The last decade has been particularly rich in developments in the field of neural regeneration, as discussed in several chapters of this volume. Most of the efforts — and the most fruitful, up to now — were devoted to the identification of inhibitory factors responsible for growth limitations, and possible means to overcome them (McKeon et al., 1991; Fawcett, 1994; McKerracher et al., 1994; Mukhopadhyay et al., 1994; Smith-Thomas et al., 1994; Fitch and Silver, 1997; Chen et al., 2000; GrandPre et al., 2000). This craze for inhibitory factors left in the lurch the search for cellular and molecular factors, other than the neurotrophins, that might stimulate and direct axonal growth in a context of regeneration. Now, in spite of the progress in the identification of inhibitory molecules, blocking the action of these molecules has yielded only partial regeneration of lesioned axonal pathways and incomplete functional recovery. However, axonal regeneration is probably not limited solely by inhibitory molecules in the environment of the mature CNS. Oriented axonal growth, during development, results from several factors that attract, repulse or impede the movement of neuronal processes and thereby determine the

adopted direction. Regenerative growth would likely depend on similar vectorial combination of forces. Neurons being living elements, the driving forces are intrinsic to the growing cells, not in their environment. It is the neurons themselves which express the whole motor machinery, constituted by their cytoskeleton (microtubules microfilaments, neurofilaments and their associated molecules) and their energy metabolism. The elaboration of the axonal cytoskeleton in any given direction is influenced by signals present in the external environment — extracellular matrix molecules, cell adhesion molecules, attractant and repellant, short- or long-range molecules (see Tessier-Lavigne and Goodman, 1996) — but recognition of all these signals depends on the expression of receptors at the surface of the growing cell (the response to netrins, for example, see Manitt and Kennedy, 2002, this volume). It is then the state of the intracellular signaling pathways and their action on the cytoskeleton that determines whether any given signal will have attractant, repellant or stabilizing effects (see Qiu et al., 2002, this volume; Manitt and Kennedy, 2002, this volume; Ellezam et al., 2002, this volume). It is therefore essential to identify the molecules that are susceptible to guide axon growth in the adult CNS, as well as the involved receptors and intracellular signaling pathways, in order to better understand, and eventually manipulate the potential for regeneration in the adult CNS. The search and study of guidance molecules is naturally hindered by the preponderance of axon growth inhibition in the adult CNS. However, substantial experimentation over the last

---

* Correspondence to: G. Doucet, Département de Pathologie et Biologie Cellulaire, Université de Montréal, C.P. 6128, succursale Centre-ville, Montréal, QC H3C 3J7, Canada. Tel.: +1-514-343-6255; Fax: +1-514-343-5755; E-mail: guy.doucet@umontreal.ca

four decades, using neural lesions and transplantation, has demonstrated that axon guidance cues still exist in the adult CNS. The task consists henceforth of identifying these molecular cues, which might be molecules that serve the same ends during development.

In this paper, we will first review succinctly lesion and transplantation experiments showing the existence of axon guidance cues in the adult CNS, as well as the capacity of mature neurons to recognize and respond to such cues in the mature CNS, or in grafted peripheral or fetal neural tissues. We will then describe our own experimental model, which will hopefully lead to the identification of axon guidance molecules for mature 5-HT neurons.

Axon guidance in the adult CNS

Most of the lesion experiments demonstrating anatomical plasticity in the adult CNS were conducted before the 1980s (reviewed by Björklund and Stenevi, 1979; Kiernan, 1979; Björklund et al., 1981; Cotman et al., 1981). The anatomical plasticity thus disclosed consisted generally in a local sprouting of the lesioned axons or of unlesioned homo- or heterotypic pathways. These studies demonstrated that the mature CNS was not immutable and that its axons could still respond appropriately, but sometimes also aberrantly, to local guidance cues. Nevertheless, some lesion experiments, using specific cytotoxic drugs (5,6- or 5,7-dihydroxytryptamine) and producing less structural damage, demonstrated that serotoninergic (5-HT) neurons were capable of long-distance regeneration — down to the lumbar spinal cord or up to the forebrain (reviewed in Björklund and Stenevi, 1979; Björklund et al., 1981).

In the 1970s–1980s, neural transplantation was used extensively to study anatomical plasticity in the CNS (reviewed in Björklund and Stenevi, 1979, 1984). Since adult CNS neurons do not survive transplantation, these studies used transplants of fetal nervous tissue in adult animals, either to test for the presence, in the mature CNS, of guidance cues that could be recognized by fetal neurons or, inversely, to examine the response of adult host neurons to tropic molecules present in neural grafts.

Most of these studies demonstrated that grafted fetal neurons could establish specific projections in the adult host brain, but usually with only short-distance projections (see Björklund and Stenevi, 1984). More recently, however, long-distance projections were observed in xenograft experiments — human or porcine fetal neural tissue in adult rat CNS (Wictorin et al., 1990; Wictorin and Björklund, 1992; Wictorin et al., 1992; Isacson and Deacon, 1996, 1997). These projections were specific for their usual targets, even after ectopic placement. For example, fetal human dopamine neurons implanted in the adult rat substantia nigra, following a 6-hydroxydopamine lesion of the host dopamine neurons, extended axons exclusively in the rostral direction, towards the striatum (Wictorin et al., 1992); confirming the existence of long-range guidance in the adult CNS. Moreover, some of these results could best be interpreted as axonal responses to long-range attractant, since ectopic nigral graft-derived axons could reach their normal target, the thalamus, by taking unusual pathways (Isacson and Deacon, 1996). It remains to be seen whether intact or severed adult neurons could also respond to such cues.

Recent experiments with endogenous adult neural stem cells, have also demonstrated the persistence of axon guidance signals in the adult hippocampus, allowing for the integration of newly generated neurons into its circuitry (Markakis and Gage, 1999).

Although mature axons rarely grow for long distances in the adult CNS environment, their responses to neural grafts indicate that they can recognize some guidance molecules. Indeed, work by Björklund and colleagues (see Björklund and Stenevi, 1979) showed that noradrenaline neurons of the locus coeruleus could reproduce the sympathetic innervation pattern of the iris implanted into the mature brain. The brain-derived cholinergic innervation of the implanted iris being different, these observations suggested the existence of guidance signals in the grafted iris, to which monoamine or cholinergic axons were able to react. Moreover, 5-HT neurons could also innervate the implanted iris with the sympathetic pattern, if there had been a prior destruction of the host noradrenaline neurons of the locus coeruleus; suggesting that CNS neurons of different types were able to respond to the same guidance molecules expressed in the iris, although with different affinities. Several other studies with fetal neural tissues implanted into the adult CNS have demonstrated that monoamine and cholinergic neurons could respond more readily to graft-derived signals than other types of CNS neurons (Björklund et al., 1981; Björklund and Stenevi, 1984; Nothias et al., 1988; Wictorin et al., 1988, 1989b; Nothias et al., 1990; Labandeira-Garcia et al., 1991; Triarhou et al., 1992). Other lightly myelinated axons, such as the primary dorsal root ganglion afferents expressing CGRP, also grow readily into neural grafts; suggesting that myelination may be an important factor in this phenomenon (Tessler et al., 1988; Itoh and Tessler, 1990; Nothias and Peschanski, 1990; Itoh et al., 1992). Other types of point-to-point CNS projection neurons could also innervate neural grafts, but only when there had been a prior lesion of their endogenous target (Björklund and Stenevi, 1984; Armengol et al., 1989; Tønder et al., 1989; Wictorin and Björklund, 1989; Field et al., 1991; Labandeira-Garcia et al., 1991; Girman, 1993; Schulz et al., 1993; Girman, 1994), of parallel projections (Sørensen et al., 1986), or of peripheral branches (Erzurumlu and Ebner, 1988; Ebner et al., 1989). In such cases, either the development of the grafts was modified by lesions of the host brain, so as to make them produce more attractant molecules, or the lesions changed the response of the host target-deprived neurons, which then became more responsive to signals from the grafts (by inducing the expression of receptors or changing the state of intracellular signaling pathways). In any case, these experiments show that mature neurons can respond, or can be induced to respond, to guidance cues.

At present the identity of these signals of the adult CNS, or of the neural grafts, that are acting on adult neurons is unknown. Adult and fetal neurons can have divergent responses to the same signals (e.g., Debellard et al., 1996; Fawcett, 1997; Borisoff et al., 2000). Even during neural development, the neuronal response to axon guidance signals changes along the way to the final destination of the axon tip (e.g., Stein and Tessier-Lavigne, 2001). It will therefore be important to define in space and time the specific guidance cues that may be acting on selective groups of axons, in order to promote their functional regeneration. Indeed, many of the above-mentioned lesion or grafting experiments have disclosed the formation of aberrant connections, particularly after ectopic placement of neural grafts (Wiklund and Møllgård,

1979; Hallas et al., 1980; Oblinger and Das, 1982; Itoh and Tessler, 1990; Bosler et al., 1992; Zwimpfer et al., 1992); a situation that may have some similarity with that of lesioned axons, following trauma. Indeed, lesioned axons growing in the adult CNS must find their targets along pathways that greatly differ from those they had followed during development. Extensive knowledge of the molecules expressed in the intact or lesioned adult CNS that could be used by growing axons as guidance cues would help to manipulate their expression in order to minimize aberrant connections and to optimize those appropriate for recovery of function.

There has been immense progress lately in the identification of axon guidance molecules acting during neural development (e.g., Tessier-Lavigne, 1994; Tessier-Lavigne and Goodman, 1996; Brose and Tessier-Lavigne, 2000; Stein and Tessier-Lavigne, 2001). What is still missing is the knowledge of their expression, distribution and roles in the adult CNS. We need to know if these molecules can serve to guide the axon growth of adult neurons, i.e., if they might promote or, inversely, hinder regeneration; and also how they might be affected by CNS injury. Considering the number of genes that are still unknown (Bork and Copley, 2001; Hogenesch et al., 2001), it is also likely that a fair number of such molecules remain to be identified.

Most of the currently known guidance molecules have been discovered by studying experimental models in which axon growth from defined populations of neurons could be manipulated in vivo or in vitro. Many of the above transplantation experiments showing axon guidance activities might contribute to the discovery of new guidance molecules, if analyzed further. Combined with the recent advances in genomic (DNA chips) and proteomic (2D gel electrophoresis and mass spectrometry) approaches, such models could contribute to the progress in the field of CNS injury and regeneration. The experiments described below represent an attempt in this direction.

Use of neural transplants into the striatum as a model to study axon guidance in adult rat brain

To determine whether adult host neurons could innervate ectopic grafts, we have first studied the innervation by host brain neurons of ventral mesencephalic (VM) grafts implanted into the neostriatum of adult rats — in collaboration with Anders Björklund and Patrick Brundin (Doucet et al., 1989). We examined the projections from the frontal cortex (anterograde transport of PHA-L), the neostriatum (DARPP-32 immunohistochemistry and PHA-L anterograde transport) and the mesencephalic raphe (5-HT immunohistochemistry), i.e., the major afferent projections common to both transplanted (VM) and recipient (neostriatum) target regions. It was expected that 5-HT axons would be the most profuse inside the grafts, since they project densely to the substantia nigra, and since most of the dorsal raphe 5-HT neurons projecting to the nigra have collaterals into the neostriatum.

However, the densest host projections into the core of VM grafts were those from the frontal cortex. Neostriatal projections were also profuse, but remained confined within 100–300 μm of the inner graft border; whereas 5-HT axons showed very little growth into the grafts: only few axons were detected inside the graft, essentially near the graft–host border (Fig. 1). This contrasted with the observation of profuse 5-HT innervations into grafts of fetal striatal tissue implanted into the ibotenic acid-lesioned neostriatum (Wictorin et al., 1988). Thus, in spite of their so-called 'diffuse' mode of projection, adult 5-HT axons appear to display anatomical selectivity in their reaction to a new innervation target. It was therefore of particular interest to define the conditions in which they would or would not grow.

Serotonin innervation of VM and striatal transplants into the neostriatum

These experiments also demonstrated that the grafted VM tissue was not inhibitory to 5-HT axon growth, at least for immature 5-HT axons. Indeed, when VM grafts included even very few co-grafted 5-HT perikarya (4–5 per 50-μm-thick section), they were filled with a very dense 5-HT axonal network (Doucet et al., 1989; Mounir et al., 1994). This dense 5-HT innervation was present even when the host 5-HT neurons had been destroyed by 5,7-DHT (Mounir et al., 1994), confirming that it took origin in the grafted 5-HT neurons. We therefore examined the hypothesis that immature 5-HT axons

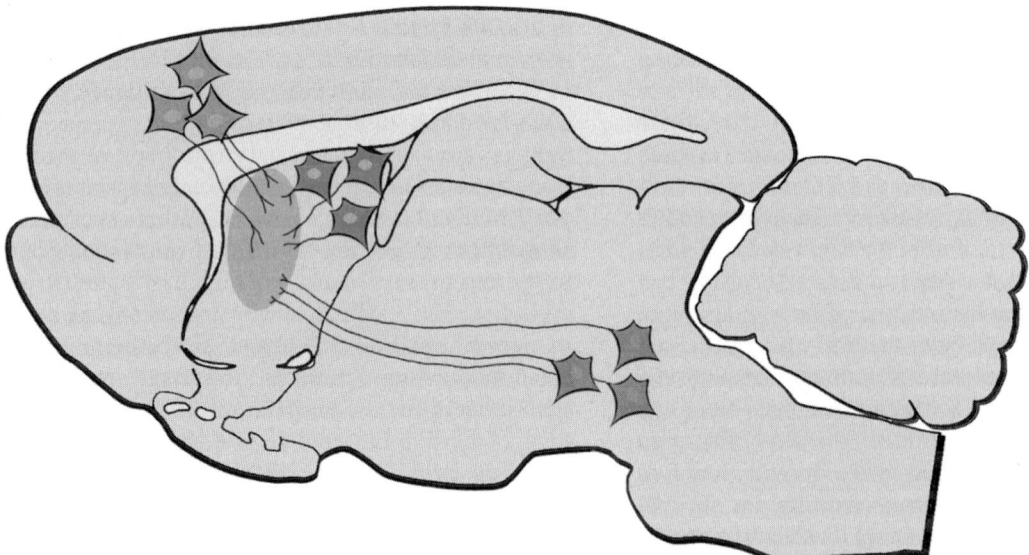

Fig. 1. Diagram summarizing the results of axonal tracing from the host cerebral cortex, striatum and dorsal raphe (serotonin) into intrastriatal ventral mesencephalic grafts. The most profuse projections from the host brain came from the frontal cortex, with axons innervating all areas of the grafts. Host striatal axons remained essentially confined within a 100–300-μm-large band in the peripheral zones of the grafts, whereas serotonin axons were virtually absent from the core of the grafts and only occasional in the periphery (see Doucet et al., 1989).

would have a higher affinity than adult ones for VM tissue, by quantifying host-derived 5-HT axons in VM grafts following implantation into immature and adult recipients. Transplants were done in newborn (postnatal days 5–7 or P5–P7), juvenile (P15) and adult (body weight 200–250 g) rats and examined 2 months later by 5-HT immunohistochemistry. We then found a much denser innervation of the grafts in newborn recipients than in juvenile or adult ones. Indeed, with recipient ages P15 and above at the time of implantation, there were practically no 5-HT axons in the core of VM grafts (Mounir et al., 1994), in keeping with our earlier observations (Doucet et al., 1989).

The 5-HT innervation of fetal striatal — but not VM — grafts had been reported to be less dense after implantation in intact rather than ibotenic acid-lesioned striatum (Labandeira-Garcia et al., 1991; Lu et al., 1991). To rule out the possibility that the differences in 5-HT innervation we had observed between striatal and VM grafts be due to the prior excitotoxic lesion, we compared the 5-HT innervation of VM and striatal grafts following implantation into intact neostriatum. Since no data were available on the 5-HT innervation of striatal grafts implanted in newborns, the study included VM or striatal grafts implanted in neonatal, juvenile and adult rat striatum. To quantify the innervation, we used a method based on the uptake of tritiated 5-HT, in vitro, followed by autoradiography and image analysis, 6 months after transplantation (Doucet and Descarries, 1993). Brain slices were incubated with 10^{-6} M $[^3H]5$-HT, in the presence of a monoamine oxidase inhibitor and of an inhibitor of monoamine uptake by dopaminergic neurons. These slices were then fixed with glutaraldehyde, embedded in epoxy resin and sectioned at a thickness of 4 μm for autoradiography. Serotonin axon varicosities were then counted within the grafts (see Fig. 2B,D). Adjacent semi-thin sections from the same brain slices were processed by post-embedding immunohistochemistry for tryptophan hydroxylase (TPH), tyrosine hydroxylase (TH, Fig. 2A) or dopamine- and adenosine-regulated phosphoprotein-32 (DARPP-32, Fig. 2C) (Ouimet et al., 1984). Sections immunostained for TPH confirmed the absence of 5-HT neurons inside the grafts, whereas TH or DARPP-32 staining was used to assess the distribution of 5-HT fibers in relation to that

of dopamine or striatal neurons, in VM or striatal grafts (Wictorin et al., 1989a), respectively.

The quantitative analyses demonstrated that the DARPP-32-positive patches, representing the true striatal compartments of 'striatal' grafts, were three to four times more densely innervated by host 5-HT axons than VM grafts, or DARPP-32-immunonegative (non-striatal) regions of 'striatal' grafts. In all types of grafts (VM as well as DARPP-32-positive and DARPP-32-negative regions of striatal grafts), the amount of 5-HT innervation decreased by 75–80% between grafts implanted in neonatal versus adult rats (and examined 6 months later) (Pierret et al., 1998). Therefore, the proportion of 5-HT innervation in VM and striatal grafts remained unchanged between newborn and adult recipients. These results demonstrated that the relative affinity of the 5-HT axons present in the host striatum for VM or striatal grafts remained constant between newborns and adults. The differences between adult and neonatal 5-HT innervations of the grafts was likely the result of an intrinsic developmental decrease in the growth capacity of the mature host 5-HT neurons (Goldberg et al., 2001).

Nevertheless, the 5-HT innervation of striatal grafts decreased gradually in juvenile and adult recipients, whereas the amount of 5-HT innervation of VM grafts in juvenile recipients was as low as that in adult recipients, as in our previous study (Mounir et al., 1994). Therefore, the intrinsic developmental decrease in growth capacity for a given type of neuron may not follow the same time course for different targets, i.e., in their response to different guidance molecules. It follows from this idea that different signaling pathways involved in axon growth and guidance might mature at different rates in a given neuron. It would then be imaginable to selectively reactivate one signaling pathway, in order to promote the regeneration of specific projections.

Influence of the glial scar or chondroitin sulfate proteoglycans

A difference in the glial scar, or in the expression of axon growth inhibitory molecules, such as chondroitin sulfate proteoglycans (CSPG), might have explained the difference in 5-HT innervation between VM and striatal grafts. We therefore ex-

458

amined the glial scar and expression of CSPG by immunohistochemistry at different time points after transplantation of VM tissue in newborn, juvenile or adult rats, as well as of striatal tissue in adults (Petit et al., 2002). Ten days after transplantation, immunohistochemistry for GFAP showed the presence of astrocytes inside and around the grafts, forming a glial scar, in all cases. This glial scar appeared only slightly less dense around VM grafts implanted in newborns. Also, the distribution of GFAP-immunostained elements was more heterogeneous in striatal grafts, as previously reported by others (Gates et al., 1996). The expression of CSPG was very similar in all types of grafts and in recipients of any age, at 10 days. Serotonin immunoreactive axons were already profuse in VM grafts implanted in newborns, but rare in VM and striatal grafts implanted in adults. Therefore, the presence of a glial scar or CSPG had no negative impact on the ingrowth of immature 5-HT axons.

At longer time points, GFAP and CSPG immunoreactivities subsided gradually in striatal grafts implanted in adults, but remained highly heterogeneous, such that patches of intense staining remained present between 10 days and 2 months. Serotonin axons gradually invaded these striatal grafts and were clearly more profuse in DARPP-32-positive patches, although many were also present in DARPP-32-negative zones. Interestingly, the DARPP-32-positive patches corresponded to GFAP- and CSPG-negative zones of these grafts (the latter two being then largely overlapping), 2 months after transplantation. Thus, for striatal grafts, the time course of appearance and distribution of 5-HT axons was in inverse correlation with those of GFAP and CSPG. Nevertheless, a similarly heterogeneous 5-HT innervation of striatal grafts, inversely correlated with GFAP, had also been demonstrated following implantation in newborn rats (Pierret et al., 1998). Therefore,

since neonatal 5-HT axons were not inhibited by the glial scar or CSPG around or in the VM grafts, as stated above, this heterogeneity in 5-HT innervation of striatal grafts could not be explained by the complementary distribution of GFAP or CSPG. Other elements — attractant or repellant — in the different compartments of striatal grafts must be responsible of the differential affinity of host 5-HT axons.

The situation was different for VM grafts. Serotonin axons remained rare in these grafts, even after 2 months, as observed in our previous studies; even though GFAP immunoreactive elements were greatly reduced and the expression of CSPG was totally abolished. It was then concluded that the absence of 5-HT innervation inside VM grafts could not be attributed to the astrocyte scar or the expression of CSPG in the graft.

Our interpretation was that either VM grafts contained molecules that were inhibitory to the ingrowth of 5-HT axons or, else, that striatal grafts (and particularly their DARPP-32-positive zones) contained molecules that were attractant for these axons. To settle this issue, it was crucial to determine the type of cells that expressed the molecules responsible for the repellent or attractant activity.

Role of astrocytes in the graft

In view of the complexity of the grafted tissue, it is not easy to identify molecules that may attract 5-HT axons into striatal grafts, or repel them from VM grafts. A more simple model was needed for that purpose. Because astrocytes had been shown in several instances to have different regional phenotypes that could affect the growth of dopamine or 5-HT neurons (Denis-Donini et al., 1983, 1984; Chamak et al., 1987; Liu and Lauder, 1992a), it was proposed that they might be the cells that influenced 5-HT axon ingrowth into the grafts.

Fig. 2. Ventral mesencephalic (A,B) and striatal (C,D) grafts in juvenile (P15) rats. The animals were sacrificed 6 months after transplantation. (A) Semi-thin section from a brain slice incubated with tritiated 5-HT. The section was treated for post-embedding TH-immunohistochemistry, showing grafted dopamine neurons and processes. (B) An adjacent section of the same brain slice, but exposed to a nuclear emulsion, for autoradiography of 5-HT nerve terminals, showing that serotonin axon terminals were very sparse in the graft. (C) A section treated in post-embedding DARPP-32-immunohistochemistry, showing the striatal neurons. Part of the graft contains true striatal tissue, and part of it contains non-striatal tissue (DARPP-32-negative). (D) Adjacent section showing that the DARPP-32-positive area is more densely innervated by host 5-HT axons. From Pierret et al. (1998). Reproduced with permission.

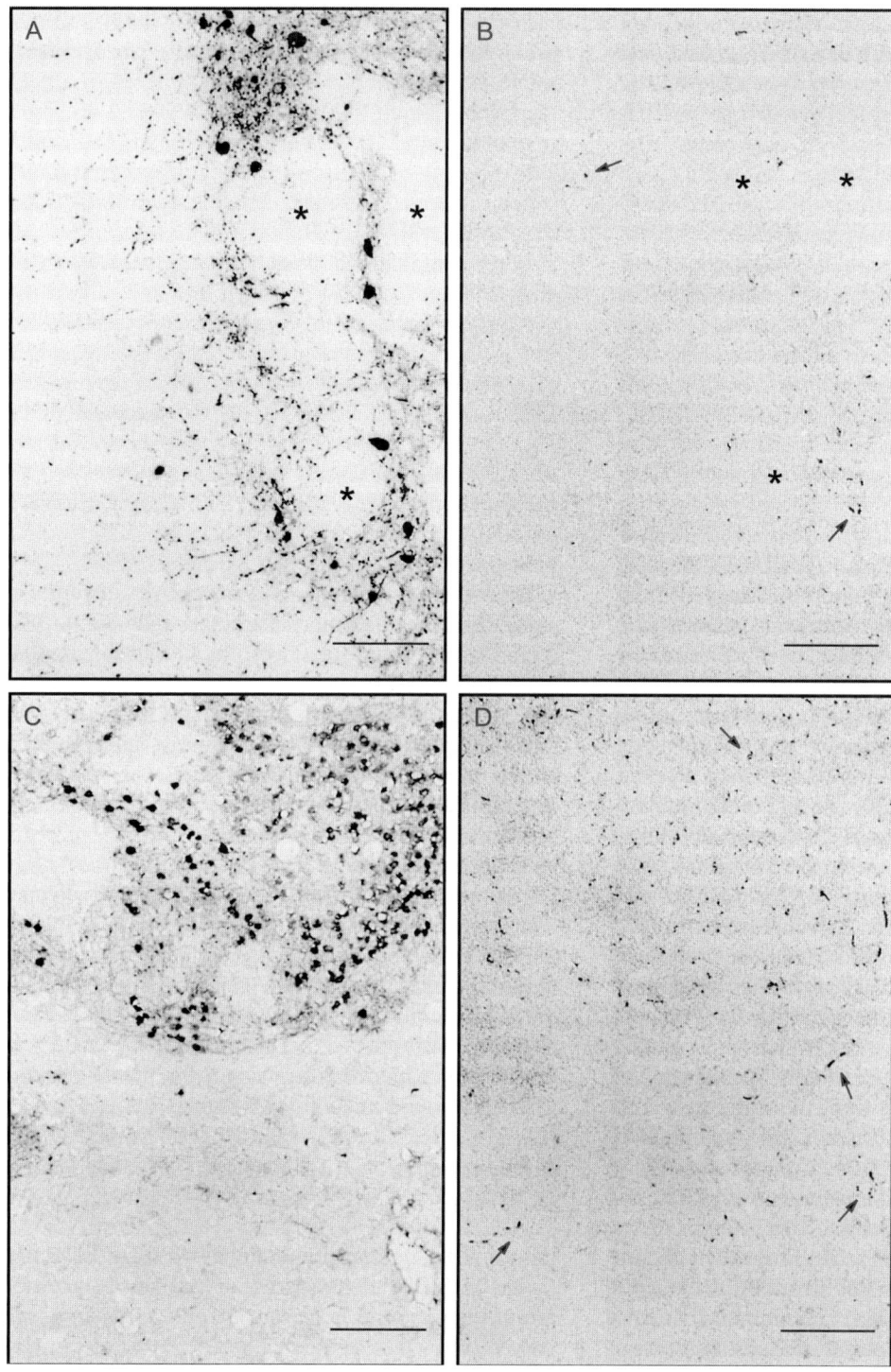

460

Dissection and culture of neonatal astrocytes

Co-implantation of cultured astrocytes with ventral mesencephalic (or striatal) tissue

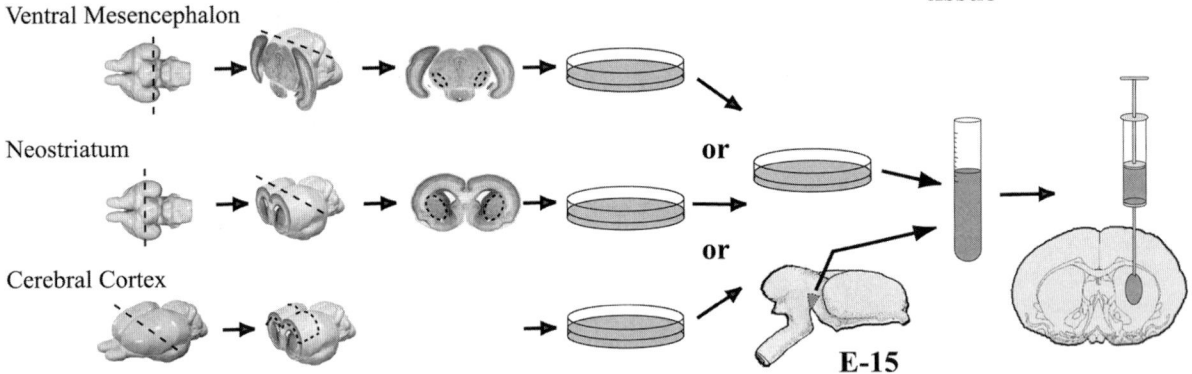

Ventral Mesencephalon

Neostriatum

or

or

Cerebral Cortex

E-15

Fig. 3. Technique used for co-transplantation of astrocytes cultured from the neonatal ventral mesencephalon, neostriatum or cerebral cortex, and then mixed with dissociated fetal (E14–E15) ventral mesencephalic or striatal tissue, before implantation into the striatum of adult rats. From Petit et al. (2001). Reprinted with permission

To test this hypothesis, cultured astrocytes from three different brain regions were co-implanted with fetal VM or striatal tissue into the intact striatum of adult rats (Petit et al., 2001) (see Fig. 3). The same autoradiographic technique, described above, was used to determine the density of 5-HT innervation in each type of graft. This quantitative analysis clearly showed that co-grafts of VM containing striatal or neocortical astrocytes were three to four times more densely innervated by host 5-HT axons than control VM grafts or co-grafts of VM enriched with cultured VM astrocytes (Fig. 4). Moreover, co-grafts of striatal tissue with VM astrocytes were innervated as profusely as single striatal grafts, demonstrating that VM astrocytes were not inhibitory to 5-HT axon ingrowth.

To ensure that this difference in the density of 5-HT innervation resulting from the addition of cortical or striatal astrocytes was not due to some indirect effect on the glial scar or on the expression of CSPG in the graft, we also examined the different types of grafts by GFAP and CSPG immunohistochemistry (Petit et al., 2001). No difference between graft types were found in the distribution of these molecules. The density of CSPG immunostaining, as well as the surface area of GFAP immunoreactive processes in the core of the grafts, at the graft–host border, and in the adjacent host striatal tissue were also quantified. The results showed no difference in

CSPG immunoreactivity. As for GFAP, all types of co-grafts contained more astrocytes than single VM grafts, as expected for grafts that had been enriched with astrocytes; but there was no difference between the groups of co-grafts, including VM grafts with VM astrocytes which were as poorly innervated by 5-HT axons as single VM grafts. It was concluded that the differences in 5-HT innervation between co-grafts were not due to a reduction in the glial reaction or in the expression of CSPG.

Altogether, the latter observations rather indicated that cortical and striatal astrocytes attracted adjacent host 5-HT axons normally fated to innervate the striatum. Interestingly, some of these axons might have been collaterals of axons innervating the ventral midbrain (van der Kooy and Hattori, 1980; Imai et al., 1986), which might account for the few axons that were found in control VM grafts.

Influence of co-grafted astrocytes on other graft afferents

To test the possibility that these effects of astrocytes on 5-HT axons represented a general growth-promoting action on all surrounding host axons, we also examined the influence of the different populations of astrocytes on the other types of host afferents that had previously been demonstrated into the VM grafts, i.e., cortical and striatal afferents (see above).

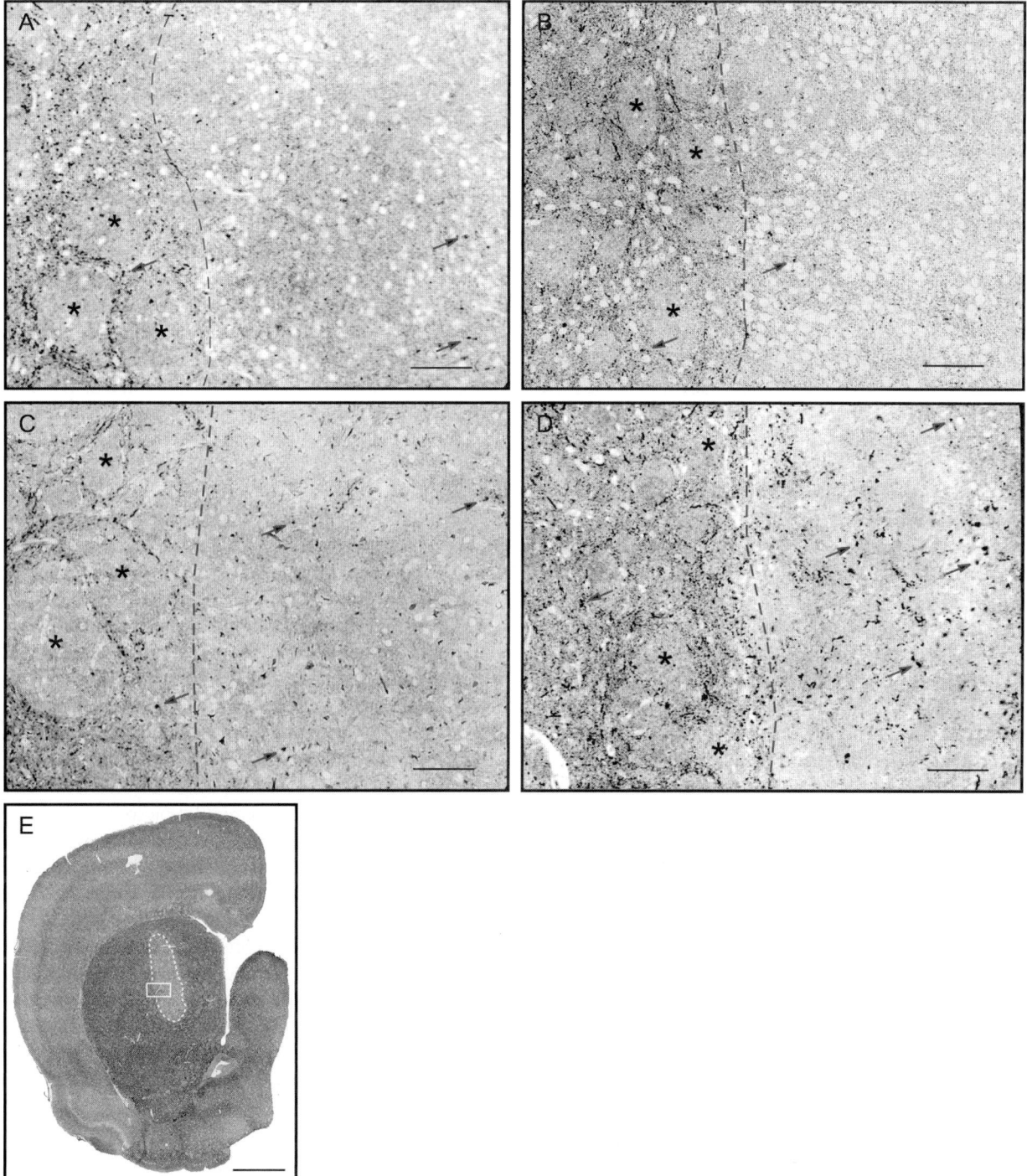

Fig. 4. Grafts of ventral mesencephalic tissue, with or without co-grafted astrocytes, into the striatum of adult rats. Pictures are from 4-μm-thick sections from 200-μm-thick brain slices processed in vitro for tritiated serotonin uptake and autoradiography, 2 months after transplantation. (A) Single ventral mesencephalic graft. (B) Co-graft containing ventral mesencephalic astrocytes. (C) Co-graft with striatal astrocytes. (D) Co-graft with cortical astrocytes. (E) The complete section of the graft in A, to show the size of the pictures in A–D (white rectangle). In all cases the left part displays host striatum and the right part the graft. Arrows point to silver grain aggregates representing labeled serotonin varicosities. From Petit et al. (2001). Reprinted with permission.

We found no increases or decreases in the number of labeled axons following multiple injections of biotinylated dextran in the frontoparietal cortex or after DARPP-32 immunohistochemistry. Therefore, it appears that the growth-promoting effects of striatal or cortical astrocytes were specific for 5-HT axons.

Advantages of the model for the search of axon guidance molecules

Now, since we have three highly purified populations of astrocytes in culture, with different effects on 5-HT axons, it becomes possible to use a comparison of gene and protein expression between them, in the hope of finding candidate molecules with the same biological activity on 5-HT axons as in cografts. Some molecules with known action on 5-HT axons are among such candidates, such as brain-derived neurotrophic factor (BDNF), glial cell line-derived neurotrophic factor (GDNF) or S100β (Liu and Lauder, 1992b; Beck et al., 1996; Mamounas et al., 2000; Nishi et al., 2000), but the probability is high that the observed effects were due to unknown molecules. Indeed, recent estimates of the total human genome are in the order of 30,000–60,000 genes (Bork and Copley, 2001; Hogenesch et al., 2001), and the total number of genes in the rat or mouse genomes are probably near the same order of magnitude. Among these genes, the number of those with a known protein product is about 15,000, which represents 25–50% of the total estimate. Therefore, a newly detected activity has approximately a 50–75% chance of being due to an unidentified molecule.

We are currently running experiments with gene chips and 2D gel electrophoresis, comparing gene and protein expression in different astrocyte populations in culture. Preliminary results already ruled out BDNF, GDNF and S100β as candidates for the effects. They also indicate that the number of gene products expressed differently among astrocyte populations from the cortex or VM is relatively low, in the order of a few hundred. Taking into account the numbers of proteins involved in structural or metabolic functions, and the structure expected from presumed intercellular signaling molecules, such numbers should be reducible to a manageable number of candidates to be tested with appropriate tests in vitro.

We are also developing tests in vitro that will reproduce the features of the transplantation model described above; based on the collagen gel explant technique of Tessier-Lavigne (Tessier-Lavigne et al., 1988; Kennedy et al., 1994). Serotoninergic axons innervating neostriatal explants will thus be challenged with VM tissue, with or without added cortical or striatal astrocytes. Such in vitro models should help to further characterize the nature of the molecules involved (membrane or matrix-bound, diffusible, etc.), allowing the number of criteria that candidate molecules will need to fulfil to account for the observed activity to be increased. These in vitro characterizations will thus be useful to reduce the number of molecules to be tested and the same techniques will then serve to test the candidate molecules generated from genomic and proteomic data.

Conclusion

Several inhibitory molecules have been identified as being responsible for the poor regenerative capacities of CNS neurons. However, a reduction in the level of growth-promoting or axon guidance molecules might also contribute in turning the balance towards inhibition. Lesion and transplantation experiments suggested that guidance molecules are still present in the adult CNS, but adult neurons might require some priming to respond to these signals. A better knowledge of growth-promoting or guidance molecules might allow their manipulation to turn back the balance towards appropriately directed axon growth. Several models suggesting tropic activities in the adult CNS exist, but need to be developed further in vitro to allow identification of the molecules that underlie the observed effects. A better knowledge of 5-HT axon guidance molecules would certainly be relevant for spinal cord injury, in view of the role of 5-HT in the control of locomotion in brain and the spinal cord (Jacobs and Fornal, 1995; Schmidt and Jordan, 2000; see also Rossignol et al., 2002, this volume).

Acknowledgements

We thank Dr. Laurent Descarries for his critical revision of this manuscript. This work was supported by the Canadian Institutes for Health Research (CIHR), the Fonds de la recherche en santé du Québec (FRSQ), the Fonds pour la formation des chercheurs et l'aide à la recherche (FCAR) and Groupe de recherche sur le système nerveux central (FCAR Center).

References

Armengol, J.A., Sotelo, C., Angaut, P. and Alvarado-Mallart, R.-M. (1989) Organization of host afferents to cerebellar grafts implanted into kainate lesioned cerebellum in adult rats. *Eur. J. Neurosci.*, 1: 75–93.

Beck, K.D., Irwin, I., Valverde, J., Brennan, T.J., Langston, J.W. and Hefti, F. (1996) GDNF induces a dystonia-like state in neonatal rats and stimulates dopamine and serotonin synthesis. *Neuron*, 16: 665–673.

Björklund, A. and Stenevi, U. (1979) Regeneration of monoaminergic and cholinergic neurons in the mammalian central nervous system. *Physiol. Rev.*, 59: 62–100.

Björklund, A. and Stenevi, U. (1984) Intracerebral neural implants: neuronal replacement and reconstruction of damaged circuitries. *Annu. Rev. Neurosci.*, 7: 279–308.

Björklund, A., Wiklund, L. and Descarries, L. (1981) Regeneration and plasticity of central serotoninergic neurons: a review. *J. Physiol. (Paris)*, 77: 247–255.

Borisoff, J.F., Pataky, D.M., McBride, C.B. and Steeves, J.D. (2000) Raphe-spinal neurons display an age-dependent differential capacity for neurite outgrowth compared to other brainstem–spinal neuron populations. *Exp. Neurol.*, 166: 16–28.

Bork, P. and Copley, R. (2001) The draft sequences. Filling in the gaps. *Nature*, 409: 818–820.

Bosler, O., Vuillon-Cacciuttolo, G. and Saidi, H. (1992) Long-term serotonin reinnervation of the suprachiasmatic nucleus after 5,7-dihydroxytryptamine axotomy in the adult rat. *Neurosci. Lett.*, 143: 159–163.

Brose, K. and Tessier-Lavigne, M. (2000) Slit proteins: key regulators of axon guidance, axonal branching, and cell migration. *Curr. Opin. Neurobiol.*, 10: 95–102.

Chamak, B., Fellous, A., Glowinski, J. and Prochiantz, A. (1987) MAP2 expression and neuritic outgrowth and branching are coregulated through region-specific neuro-astroglial interactions. *J. Neurosci.*, 7: 3163–3170.

Chen, M.S., Huber, A.B., van der Haar, M.E., Frank, M., Schnell, L., Spillmann, A.A., Christ, F. and Schwab, M.E. (2000) Nogo-a is a myelin-associated neurite outgrowth inhibitor and an antigen for monoclonal antibody IN-1. *Nature*, 403: 434–439.

Cotman, C.W., Nieto-Sampedro, M. and Harris, E.W. (1981) Synapse replacement in the nervous system of adult vertebrates. *Physiol. Rev.*, 61: 684–784.

Debellard, M.E., Tang, S., Mukhopadhyay, G., Shen, Y.J. and Filbin, M.T. (1996) Myelin-associated glycoprotein inhibits axonal regeneration from a variety of neurons via interaction with a sialoglycoprotein. *Mol. Cell. Neurosci.*, 7: 89–101.

Denis-Donini, S., Glowinski, J. and Prochiantz, A. (1983) Specific influence of striatal target neurons on the in vitro outgrowth of mesencephalic dopaminergic neurites: a morphological quantitative study. *J. Neurosci.*, 3: 2292–2299.

Denis-Donini, S., Glowinski, J. and Prochiantz, A. (1984) Glial heterogeneity may define the three dimensional shape of mouse mesencephalic dopaminergic neurones. *Nature*, 307: 641–643.

Doucet, G. and Descarries, L. (1993) Quantification of monoamine innervations by light microscopic autoradiography following tritiated monoamine uptake in brain slices. *Neurosci. Protocols*: 93-050-09-01-15.

Doucet, G., Murata, Y., Brundin, P., Bosler, O., Mons, N., Geffard, M., Ouimet, C.C. and Björklund, A. (1989) Host afferents into intrastriatal transplants of fetal ventral mesencephalon. *Exp. Neurol.*, 106: 1–19.

Ebner, F.F., Erzurumlu, R.S. and Lee, S.M. (1989) Peripheral nerve damage facilitates functional innervation of brain grafts in adult sensory cortex. *Proc. Natl. Acad. Sci. USA*, 86: 730–734.

Ellezam, B., Dubreuil, C., Winton, M., Loy, L., Dergham, P., Sellés-Navarro, I. and McKerracher, L. (2002) Inactivation of intracellular Rho to stimulate axon growth and regeneration. In: L. McKerracher, G. Douchet and S. Rossignol (Eds.), *Spinal Cord Trauma: Neural Repair and Functional Recovery. Progress in Brain Research*, Vol. 137. Elsevier Science, Amsterdam, pp. 371–380.

Erzurumlu, R.S. and Ebner, F.F. (1988) Peripheral nerve transection induces innervation of embryonic neocortical transplants by specific thalamic fibers in adult mice. *J. Comp. Neurol.*, 272: 536–544.

Fawcett, J.W. (1994) Astrocytes and axon regeneration in the central nervous system. *J. Neurol.*, 241: S25–S28.

Fawcett, J.W. (1997) Astrocytic and neuronal factors affecting axon regeneration in the damaged central nervous system. *Cell Tissue Res.*, 290: 371–377.

Field, P.M., Seeley, P.J., Frotscher, M. and Raisman, G. (1991) Selective innervation of embryonic hippocampal transplants by adult host dentate granule cell axons. *Neuroscience*, 41: 713–727.

Fitch, M.T. and Silver, J. (1997) Glial cell extracellular matrix: boundaries for axon growth in development and regeneration. *Cell Tissue Res.*, 290: 379–384.

Gates, M.A., Laywell, E.D., Fillmore, H. and Steindler, D.A. (1996) Astrocytes and extracellular matrix following intracerebral transplantation of embryonic ventral mesencephalon or lateral ganglionic eminence. *Neuroscience*, 74: 579–597.

Girman, S.V. (1993) Retinal afferents innervate functionally tectal but not neocortical grafts placed in lesioned superior colliculus of adult rats. *Brain Res.*, 607: 167–176.

Girman, S.V. (1994) Neocortical grafts receive functional afferents from the same neurons of the thalamus which have innervated the visual cortex replaced by the graft in adult rats. *Neuroscience*, 60: 989–997.

Goldberg, J.L., Cameron, M.E. and Barres, B.A. (2001) What is the molecular basis for the developmental loss of intrinsic regenerative ability by retinal ganglion cells? *Soc. Neurosci. Abstr.*, 27: Program No: 257.8.

GrandPre, T., Nakamura, F., Vartanian, T. and Strittmatter, S.M.

(2000) Identification of the nogo inhibitor of axon regeneration as a reticulon protein. *Nature*, 403: 439–444.

Hallas, B.H., Oblinger, M.M. and Das, G.D. (1980) Heterotopic neural transplants in the cerebellum of the rat: their afferents. *Brain Res.*, 196: 242–246.

Hogenesch, J.B., Ching, K.A., Batalov, S., Su, A.I., Walker, J.R., Zhou, Y., Kay, S.E., Schultz, P.G. and Cooke, M.P. (2001) A comparison of the celera and ensembl predicted gene sets reveals little overlap in novel genes. *Cell*, 106: 413–415.

Imai, H., Steindler, D.A. and Kitai, S.T. (1986) The organization of divergent axonal projections from the midbrain raphe nuclei in the rat. *J. Comp. Neurol.*, 243: 363–380.

Isacson, O. and Deacon, T.W. (1996) Specific axon guidance factors persist in the adult brain as demonstrated by pig neuroblasts transplanted to the rat. *Neuroscience*, 75: 827–837.

Isacson, O. and Deacon, T. (1997) Neural transplantation studies reveal the brain's capacity for continuous reconstruction. *Trends Neurosci.*, 20: 477–482.

Itoh, Y. and Tessler, A. (1990) Regeneration of adult dorsal root axons into transplants of fetal spinal cord and brain — a comparison of growth and synapse formation in appropriate and inappropriate targets. *J. Comp. Neurol.*, 302: 272–293.

Itoh, Y., Sugawara, T., Kowada, M. and Tessler, A. (1992) Time course of dorsal root axon regeneration into transplants of fetal spinal cord. 1. A light microscopic study. *J. Comp. Neurol.*, 323: 198–208.

Jacobs, B.L. and Fornal, C.A. (1995) Activation of 5-HT neuronal activity during motor behavior. *Semin. Neurosci.*, 7: 401–408.

Kennedy, T.E., Serafini, T., de la Torre, J.R. and Tessier-Lavigne, M. (1994) Netrins are diffusible chemotropic factors for commissural axons in the embryonic spinal cord. *Cell*, 78: 425–435.

Kiernan, J.A. (1979) Hypotheses concerned with axonal regeneration in the mammalian nervous system. *Biol. Rev.*, 54: 155–197.

Labandeira-Garcia, J.L., Wictorin, K., Cunningham, E.T. and Björklund, A. (1991) Development of intrastriatal striatal grafts and their afferent innervation from the host. *Neuroscience*, 42: 407–426.

Liu, J.P. and Lauder, J.M. (1992a) Serotonin promotes region-specific glial influences on cultured serotonin and dopamine neurons. *Glia*, 5: 306–317.

Liu, J.P. and Lauder, J.M. (1992b) S-100beta and insulin-like growth factor-II differentially regulate growth of developing serotonin and dopamine neurons in vitro. *J. Neurosci. Res.*, 33: 248–256.

Lu, S.Y., Shipley, M.T., Norman, A.B. and Sanberg, P.R. (1991) Striatal, ventral mesencephalic and cortical transplants into the intact rat striatum — a neuroanatomical study. *Exp. Neurol.*, 113: 109–130.

Manitt, C. and Kennedy, T.E. (2002) Where the rubber meets the road: netrin expression and function in developing and adult nervous systems. In: L. McKerracher, G. Douchet and S. Rossignol (Eds.), *Spinal Cord Trauma: Neural Repair and Functional Recovery. Progress in Brain Research*, Vol. 137. Elsevier Science, Amsterdam, pp. 425–442.

Mamounas, L.A., Altar, C.A., Blue, M.E., Kaplan, D.R., Tessarollo, L. and Lyons, W.E. (2000) BDNF promotes the regenerative sprouting, but not survival, of injured serotonergic axons in the adult rat brain. *J. Neurosci.*, 20: 771–782.

Markakis, E.A. and Gage, F.G. (1999) Adult-generated neurons in the dentate gyrus send axonal projections to field CA3 and are surrounded by synaptic vesicles. *J. Comp. Neurol.*, 406: 449–460.

McKeon, R.J., Schreiber, R.C., Rudge, J.S. and Silver, J. (1991) Reduction of neurite outgrowth in a model of glial scarring following CNS injury is correlated with the expression of inhibitory molecules on reactive astrocytes. *J. Neurosci.*, 11: 3398–3411.

McKerracher, L.J., David, S., Jackson, D.L., Kottis, V., Dunn, R.J. and Braun, P.E. (1994) Identification of myelin-associated glycoprotein as a major myelin-derived inhibitor of neurite growth. *Neuron*, 13: 805–811.

Mounir, A., Chkirate, M., Vallée, A., Pierret, P., Geffard, M. and Doucet, G. (1994) Host serotonin axons innervate intrastriatal ventral mesencephalic grafts after implantation in newborn rat. *Eur. J. Neurosci.*, 6: 1307–1315.

Mukhopadhyay, G., Doherty, P., Walsh, F.S., Crocker, P.R. and Filbin, M.T. (1994) A novel role for myelin-associated glycoprotein as an inhibitor of axonal regeneration. *Neuron*, 13: 757–767.

Nishi, M., Kawata, M. and Azmitia, E.C. (2000) Trophic interactions between brain-derived neurotrophic factor and S100beta on cultured serotonergic neurons. *Brain Res.*, 868: 113–118.

Nothias, F., Onteniente, B., Geffard, M. and Peschanski, M. (1988) Rapid growth of host afferents into fetal thalamic transplants. *Brain Res.*, 463: 341–345.

Nothias, F., Onténiente, B., Geffard, M. and Peschanski, M. (1990) Dissimilar responses of adult thalamic monoaminergic and somatosensory afferent fibers to implantation of thalamic fetal cells. *Neuroscience*, 37: 353–366.

Nothias, F. and Peschanski, M. (1990) Homotypic fetal transplants into an experimental model of spinal cord neurodegeneration. *J. Comp. Neurol.*, 301: 520–534.

Oblinger, M.M. and Das, G.D. (1982) Connectivity of neural transplants in adult rats: analysis of afferents and efferents of neocortical transplants in the cerebellar hemisphere. *Brain Res.*, 249: 31–49.

Ouimet, C.C., Miller, P.E., Hemmings, H.C.J., Walaas, S.I. and Greengard, P. (1984) Darpp-32, a dopamine- and adenosine 3′:5′-monophosphate-regulated phosphoprotein enriched in dopamine-innervated brain regions. III. Immunocytochemical localization. *J. Neurosci.*, 4: 111–124.

Petit, A., Pierret, P., Vallée, A. and Doucet, G. (2001) Astrocytes from cerebral cortex or striatum attract adult host serotoninergic axons into intrastriatal ventral mesencephalic co-grafts. *J. Neurosci.*, 21: 7182–7193.

Petit, A., Quenneville, N., Vallée, A., Pierret, P. and Doucet, G. (2002) Differences in host serotonin innervation of intrastriatal grafts are not related to a glial scar or chondroitin sulfate proteoglycans. *Exp. Neurol.*, in press.

Pierret, P., Vallée, A., Bosler, O., Dorais, M., Moukhles, H., Abbaszadeh, R., Lepage, Y. and Doucet, G. (1998) Serotonin axons of the neostriatum show a higher affinity for striatal than for ventral mesencephalic transplants: a quantitative study in adult and immature recipient rats. *Exp. Neurol.*, 152: 101–115.

Qiu, J., Cai, D. and Filbin, M.T. (2002) A role for cAMP in regeneration during development and after injury. In: L. McKerracher, G. Douchet and S. Rossignol (Eds.), *Spinal Cord Trauma: Neural Repair and Functional Recovery. Progress in Brain Research*, Vol. 137. Elsevier Science, Amsterdam, pp. 381–387.

Rossignol, S., Chau, C., Giroux, N., Brustein, E., Bouyer, L., Marcoux, J., Langlet, C., Barthélemy, D., Provencher, J., Leblond, H., Barbeau, H. and Reader, T.A. (2002) The cat model of spinal injury. In: L. McKerracher, G. Douchet and S. Rossignol (Eds.), *Spinal Cord Trauma: Neural Repair and Functional Recovery. Progress in Brain Research*, Vol. 137. Elsevier Science, Amsterdam, pp. 151–168.

Schmidt, B.J. and Jordan, L.M. (2000) The role of serotonin in reflex modulation and locomotor rhythm production in the mammalian spinal cord. *Brain Res. Bull.*, 53: 689–710.

Schulz, M.K., Hogan, T.P. and Castro, A.J. (1993) Connectivity of fetal neocortical block transplants in the excitotoxically ablated cortex of adult rats. *Exp. Brain Res.*, 96: 480–486.

Smith-Thomas, L.C., Fokseang, J., Stevens, J., Du, J.S., Muir, E., Faissner, A., Geller, H.M., Rogers, J.H. and Fawcett, J.W. (1994) An inhibitor of neurite outgrowth produced by astrocytes. *J. Cell Sci.*, 107: 1687–1695.

Sørensen, T., Jensen, S., Møller, A. and Zimmer, J. (1986) Intracephalic transplants of freeze-stored rat hippocampal tissue. *J. Comp. Neurol.*, 252: 468–482.

Stein, E. and Tessier-Lavigne, M. (2001) Hierarchical organization of guidance receptors: Silencing of netrin attraction by slit through a robo/DCC receptor complex. *Science*, 291: 1928–1938.

Tessier-Lavigne, M. (1994) Axon guidance by diffusible repellants and attractants. *Curr. Opin. Genet. Dev.*, 4: 596–601.

Tessier-Lavigne, M. and Goodman, C.S. (1996) The molecular biology of axon guidance. *Science*, 274: 1123–1133.

Tessier-Lavigne, M., Placzek, M., Lumsden, A.G.S., Dodd, J. and Jessell, T.M. (1988) Chemotropic guidance of developing axons in the mammalian central nervous system. *Nature*, 336: 775–778.

Tessler, A., Himes, B.T., Houle, J. and Reier, P.J. (1988) Regeneration of adult dorsal root axons into transplants of embryonic spinal cord. *J. Comp. Neurol.*, 270: 537–548.

Tønder, N., Sørensen, T. and Zimmer, J. (1989) Enhanced host perforant path innervation of neonatal dentate tissue after grafting to axon sparing, ibotenic acid lesions in adult rats. *Exp. Brain Res.*, 75: 483–496.

Triarhou, L.C., Low, W.C. and Ghetti, B. (1992) Serotonin fiber innervation of cerebellar cell suspensions intraparenchymally grafted to the cerebellum of pcd mutant mice. *Neurochem. Res.*, 17: 475–482.

van der Kooy, D. and Hattori, T. (1980) Dorsal raphe cells with collateral projections to the caudate-putamen and substantia nigra: a fluorescent retrograde double study in the rat. *Brain Res.*, 186: 1–7.

Wictorin, K. and Björklund, A. (1989) Connectivity of striatal grafts implanted into the ibotenic acid-lesioned striatum — II. Cortical afferents. *Neuroscience*, 30: 297–311.

Wictorin, K. and Björklund, A. (1992) Axon outgrowth from grafts of human embryonic spinal cord in the lesioned adult rat spinal cord. *NeuroReport*, 3: 1045–1048.

Wictorin, K., Isacson, O., Fischer, W., Nothias, F., Peschanski, M. and Björklund, A. (1988) Connectivity of striatal grafts implanted into the ibotenic acid-lesioned striatum — 1. Subcortical afferents. *Neuroscience*, 27: 547–562.

Wictorin, K., Ouimet, C.C. and Björklund, A. (1989a) Intrinsic organization and connectivity of intrastriatal striatal transplants in rats as revealed by DARPP-32 immunohistochemistry: specificity of connections with the lesioned host brain. *Eur. J. Neurosci.*, 1: 690–701.

Wictorin, K., Simerly, R.B., Isacson, O., Swanson, L.W. and Björklund, A. (1989b) Connectivity of striatal grafts implanted into the ibotenic acid-lesioned striatum — III. Efferent projecting graft neurons and their relation to host afferents within the grafts. *Neuroscience*, 30: 313–330.

Wictorin, K., Brundin, P., Gustavii, B., Lindvall, O. and Björklund, A. (1990) Reformation of long axon pathways in adult rat central nervous system by human forebrain neuroblasts. *Nature*, 347: 556–558.

Wictorin, K., Brundin, P., Sauer, H., Lindvall, O. and Björklund, A. (1992) Long distance directed axonal growth from human dopaminergic mesencephalic neuroblasts implanted along the nigrostriatal pathway in 6-hydroxydopamine lesioned adult rats. *J. Comp. Neurol.*, 323: 475–494.

Wiklund, L. and Møllgård, K. (1979) Neurotoxic destruction of the serotoninergic innervation of the rat subcommissural organ is followed by reinnervation through collateral sprouting of non-monoaminergic neurons. *J. Neurocytol.*, 8: 469–480.

Zwimpfer, T.J., Aguayo, A.J. and Bray, G.M. (1992) Synapse formation and preferential distribution in the granule cell layer by regenerating retinal ganglion cell axons guided to the cerebellum of adult hamsters. *J. Neurosci.*, 12: 1144–1159.

Subject Index